Congenital Heart Disease in Adults

Congenital Heart Disease in Adults

THIRD EDITION

JOSEPH K. PERLOFF, MD
Streisand/American Heart Association Professor of Medicine and Pediatrics, Emeritus
Ahmanson/UCLA Adult Congenital Heart Disease Center
David Geffen School of Medicine at UCLA
Los Angeles, California

JOHN S. CHILD, MD
Professor of Medicine
David Geffen School of Medicine at UCLA
Director
Ahmanson/UCLA Adult Congenital Heart Disease Center
UCLA Center for the Health Sciences
Los Angeles, California

JAMIL ABOULHOSN, MD
Assistant Clinical Professor of Medicine
Division of Cardiology
Ahmanson/UCLA Adult Congenital Heart Disease Center
David Geffen School of Medicine at UCLA
Los Angeles, California

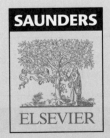

SAUNDERS

ELSEVIER

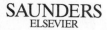

1600 John F. Kennedy Blvd.
Ste 1800
Philadelphia, PA 19103-2899

CONGENITAL HEART DISEASE IN ADULTS, THIRD EDITION   ISBN: 978-1-4160-5894-6

Library of Congress Cataloging-in-Publication Data
Perloff, Joseph K., 1924-
  Congenital heart disease in adults / Joseph K. Perloff, John S. Child, Jamil Aboulhosn.—3rd ed.
    p. ; cm.
  Includes bibliographical references and index.
  ISBN 978-1-4160-5894-6
1. Congenital heart disease. I. Child, John S. II. Aboulhosn, Jamil.
III. Title
  [DNLM: 1. Heart Defects, Congenital. 2. Adult. WG 220 P451ca 2008]
  RC687.P39 2008
  616.1'2043—dc22.

                                                    2008003109

Acquisitions Editor: Natasha Andjelkovic
Developmental Editor: Isabel Trudeau
Project Manager: Bryan Hayward
Design Direction: Gene Harris

Printed in United States of America
Last digit is the print number: 9   8   7   6   5   4   3   2   1

CONTRIBUTORS

JAMIL ABOULHOSN, MD
Assistant Clinical Professor of Medicine
Division of Cardiology
Ahmanson/UCLA Adult Congenital Heart Disease
  Center
David Geffen School of Medicine at UCLA
Los Angeles, California

FABIAN CHEN, MD
Physician, Cardiology
Assistant Professor, Medicine
Assistant Professor-In-Residence, Pediatric
  Cardiology
Member, ACCESS Department—MCIP
David Geffen School of Medicine at UCLA
Los Angeles, California

JOHN S. CHILD, MD
Professor of Medicine
David Geffen School of Medicine at UCLA
Director
Ahmanson/UCLA Adult Congenital Heart Disease
  Center
UCLA Center for the Health Sciences
Los Angeles, California

EMMANUÈLE DÉLOT, PhD
Department of Pediatrics
Pediatric Cardiology
David Geffen School of Medicine at UCLA
Los Angeles, California

HOWARD DINH, MD
Chief Cardiology Fellow
Cardiology/Medicine
David Geffen School of Medicine at UCLA
Los Angeles, California

JOHN PAUL FINN, MD
Department of Radiological Sciences
David Geffen School of Medicine at UCLA
Los Angeles, California

BARRY H. GUZE, MD
Department of Psychiatry and Biobehavioural Sciences
David Geffen School of Medicine at UCLA
Resnick Neuropsychiatric Hospital at UCLA
Los Angeles, California

LINDA HOUSER
Assistant Dean for Evaluation and Program
  Improvement
Indiana University
Bloomington, Indiana

JON A. KOBASHIGAWA, MD
Clinical Professor of Medicine
Cardiology
David Geffen School of Medicine at UCLA
UCLA Medical Center
Medical Director
UCLA Heart Transplant Program
Los Angeles, California

BRIAN KOOS, MD, DPHIL
Department of Obstetrics and Gynecology
UCLA Medical Center
Los Angeles, California

HILLEL LAKS, MD
Director, Heart and Heart-Lung Transplant Program
UCLA Medical Center
Division of Cardiac Surgery
David Geffen School of Medicine at UCLA
Los Angeles, California

DANIEL LEVI, MD
Assistant Professor
Division of Pediatric Cardiology
Mattel Children's Hospital at UCLA
Los Angeles, California

DANIEL MARELLI, MD
David Geffen School of Medicine at UCLA
Los Angeles, California

PAMELA D. MINER, NP
Nurse Practitioner
Ahmanson/UCLA Adult Congenital Heart Disease
  Center
UCLA Medical Center
Los Angeles, California

JOHN W. MOORE, MD
Director, Diagnostic and Interventional Catheterization
  Program
UCLA Medical Center
Los Angeles, California

ELISA A. MORENO
Department of Psychiatry and Biobehavioural Sciences
David Geffen School of Medicine at UCLA
Resnick Neuropsychiatric Hospital at UCLA
Los Angeles, California

DAVID A. PEGUES, MD
Professor of Clinical Medicine
Division of Infectious Disease, Department of Medicine
Hospital Epidemiologist
David Geffen School of Medicine at UCLA
Los Angeles, California

JOSEPH K. PERLOFF, MD
Streisand/American Heart Association Professor of
  Medicine and Pediatrics, Emeritus
Ahmanson/UCLA Adult Congenital Heart Disease
  Center
David Geffen School of Medicine at UCLA
Los Angeles, California

MARK D. PLUNKETT, MD
Associate Professor
Division of Cardiothoracic Surgery
David Geffen School of Medicine at UCLA
Los Angeles, California

JEFFREY L. SAVER, MD
Director, Stroke and Vascular Neurology
Stroke Center and Department of Neurology
UCLA Medical Center
Los Angeles, California

KALYANAM SHIVKUMAR, MD, PhD
Director, Cardiac Arrhythmia Center
Director, Interventional Cardiac Electrophysiology
Associate Professor of Medicine and Radiological
  Sciences
Los Angeles, California

MICHAEL SOPHER, MD
Clinical Professor
Department of Anesthesiology
David Geffen School of Medicine at UCLA
Los Angeles, California

AMY VERSTAPPEN, MED
President and Chief Executive Officer
Adult Congenital Heart Association
Philadelphia, Pennsylvania

PREFACE

Since publication of the second edition of *Congenital Heart Disease in Adults* a decade ago, progress has been rapid and impressive. The third edition is designed to keep the reader abreast of the current status of this evolving field. Worldwide recognition is reflected in the *International Society for Adult Congenital Cardiac Disease (ISACCD)* that is represented in more than 30 countries (Chapter 2), and American recognition is reflected in the *Adult Congenital Heart Association (ACHA)*, the first national patient advocacy organization (Chapter 2).

Survival has changed dramatically, literally reversing traditional norms. In developed countries, approximately 85% of infants born with congenital heart disease are expected to reach adulthood. In the United States today, there are more adults than infants and children with what was once considered a disorder of the young. Congenital heart disease is no longer defined by the age of onset but more appropriately by the age range that survival permits. Interest has broadened to include the quality of extended life spans.

The third edition consists of 23 chapters grouped in five sections—Background and Facilities, Survival Patterns, Medical Considerations, Surgical Considerations, and Residua and Sequelae After Surgery or Interventional Catheterization. Three chapters are entirely new—Chapter 2: "National and International Scope," Chapter 7: "Cardiac Magnetic Resonance Imaging and Computed Tomography in the Assessment of Adult Congenital Heart Disease," and Chapter 17: "Cardiac Transplantation in Patients with Congenital Heart Disease." Thirteen of the remaining chapters were virtually rewritten—"Echocardiography in Anatomic Imaging and Hemodynamic Evaluation of Adults with Congenital Heart Disease," "Infective Endocarditis and Congenital Heart Disease," "Management of Pregnancy and Contraception in Congenital Heart Disease," "Genetics, Epidemiology, and Counseling," "Exercise and Athletics in Adults with Congenital Heart Disease," "Cyanotic Congenital Heart Disease: A Multisystem Disorder," "Psychiatric and Psychosocial Disorders in Congenital Heart Disease," "Neurologic Disorders," "Cardiac Surgery in Adults with Congenital Heart Disease: Operation and Reoperation," "Prosthetic Materials: Selection, Use, and Long-Term Effects," "Transcatheter Interventions in Adult Congenital Heart Disease," "Electrophysiologic Abnormalities: Unoperated Occurrence and Postoperative Residua and Sequelae," and "Myocardial Growth and the Development and Regression of Increased Ventricular Mass."

As was the case in the first two editions, the final version of each chapter was drafted by one author (Joseph K. Perloff) to ensure that the book reads stylistically as a single-authored text while retaining the advantages of expert collaborators, all of whom were affiliated with the Ahmanson/University of California, Los Angeles (UCLA) Adult Congenital Heart Disease Center.

Although the third edition, like its predecessors, is designed to chart advances in the field, it also recognizes that progress has not been without a price—indeed, it has created problems of its own. There are too few pediatric cardiologists to care for the large and growing adult population and too few adult congenital heart disease facilities to handle the influx, concerns that are the subject of Chapter 3,

"Specialized Facilities for Adults with Congenital Heart Disease." A generation ago, survival was the chief objective—to make it possible for infants and children with congenital heart disease to reach adulthood. However, prolongation of life is often eclipsed by problems inherent in increased longevity, the very goal that we have labored to achieve. Psychosocial and neurologic problems (Chapters 13 and 14), only some of which were anticipated, accompany survival into adulthood. Cures in the literal sense are few and far between. Postoperative residua and sequelae vary from minor to serious and, with few exceptions, require long-term medical attention (Chapter 3). Congenital heart disease is now recognized by the National Heart, Lung, and Blood Institute as a chronic illness. Although life span has increased considerably, longevity is not normal. Hence patients are confronted with the prospect of premature mortality and with the emotional, social, educational, and occupational problems associated with chronic illness (Chapter 13). Neurologic complications have revealed themselves and are the subject of Chapter 14. The cardiovascular and the central nervous systems form almost simultaneously in early gestation, so structural abnormalities of the heart may coincide with structural abnormalities of the brain. Disorders of intellectual development, cognition, and higher cortical function are major postoperative concerns.

Pediatric cardiology evolved as a specialized field when advances in diagnostic techniques and surgical management created an air of optimism for infants and children. Congenital heart disease in adults evolved as a specialized field because the success of pediatric cardiologists and cardiac surgeons profoundly affected survival patterns. The third edition of this book brings up to date the gratifying progress that has characterized this field during the past decade.

In 1936, Maude Abbott published her landmark *Atlas of Congenital Heart Disease,* and in 1944, Alfred Blalock sutured the end of a subclavian artery to the side of a pulmonary artery in an infant with tetralogy of Fallot, establishing the now legendary Blalock-Taussig anastomosis. A century has now passed, and a new patient population has emerged—adults with congenital heart disease. The hopeless futilities to whom Helen Taussig devoted herself to in the Harriet Lane Children's Clinic have come of age. Worldwide adult congenital heart disease facilities are gratifying achievements and testimonies to progress.

ACKNOWLEDGMENTS

Our largest debt is to the Ahmanson Foundation, whose generous endowment to the UCLA Adult Congenital Heart Disease Center made possible the experience that set the stage for the third edition.

Our thanks to Yelba Castellon, to whom we turned to resolve many problems and who was responsible for the endnote arrangements of virtually all 23 chapters.

Pamela Miner and Linda Houser, nurse practitioners, were dedicated partners.

CONTENTS

SECTION **IV**

SURGICAL CONSIDERATIONS

SECTION **V**

RESIDUA AND SEQUELAE AFTER SURGERY OR INTERVENTIONAL CATHETERIZATION

BACKGROUND
AND FACILITIES

CHAPTER 1

Historical Perspective

JOSEPH K. PERLOFF

> We have seen from our observations that cyanosis, especially in the adult, is the result of a small number of cardiac malformations well determined.
>
> —*Etienne-Louis Arthur Fallot, 1888*[1]

The Hospital for Sick Children, established in London in 1852 with the aid of Charles Dickens, was the first major medical facility in the English-speaking world dedicated to treatment of the young. The second major pediatric hospital, Children's Hospital of Philadelphia, was founded in 1855, and Children's Hospital of Boston followed in 1869. However, these institutions were little more than dim lights of hope in the darkness of pediatric medicine. Congenital heart disease, the bedrock of pediatric cardiology, had not yet surfaced. L. Emmett Holt's *The Diseases of Infancy and Childhood* (1897), a book of more than 1100 pages, included a 35-page section devoted to Diseases of the Circulatory System.[2] Chapter II of that section (all of seven pages) was titled "Congenital Anomalies of the Heart" and dealt with eight malformations. William Osler's *The Principles and Practice of Medicine* (1892), a book of just under 1100 pages, included a 102-page section devoted to Diseases of the Circulatory System.[3] Chapter VI (five pages in all), "Congenital Affections of the Heart," began by stating, "These have only a limited clinical interest, as in a large proportion of the cases the anomaly is not compatible with life, and in others nothing can be done to remedy the defect or even to relieve the symptoms."[3] Congenital heart disease in adults was an oxymoron—not even a theoretical consideration.

The first major step forward was the untiring work of Maude Elizabeth Seymour Abbot (Fig. 1–1) who was born in March 1869 in St. Andrews, a small village on the north shore of the Ottawa River.[4] As class Valedictorian and winner of the Lord Stanley Gold Medal, she set her mind on the McGill Medical School and petitioned for admission. The Registrar replied, "I'm sorry to inform you that the Faculty of Medicine can hold out no hope of being able to comply with your request." The prevailing view was voiced by G. E. Fenwick, professor of surgery, "I will resign if women are allowed to take the medical course."[4]

Maude Abbott's interest in congenital heart disease began in 1900 when she came across at McGill Museum a specimen that she described as "a remarkable cardiac anomaly, an adult heart with no ventricular septum, but a small supplementary cavity at its right upper angle, giving off the pulmonary trunk."[5] She wrote to William Osler, who informed her that the specimen had been reported by Andrew F. Holmes, McGill's first dean, and came to be known as the "Holmes heart."[6] Osler advised Maude Abbott to take advantage of holdings in the McGill Museum, advice that culminated in her remarkable *Atlas of Congenital Cardiac Disease* (1936), which was based on 1000 pathology specimens personally studied while she was the museum curator.[7] The *Atlas* was a landmark in the orderly classification of congenital cardiac anomalies and remains an invaluable source of information on the clinical course of patients before the advent of cardiac surgery. In the frontispiece (Fig. 1–2), Abbott recognized five distinguished predecessors: (1) Jean Baptiste de Senac, who wrote the two-volume book *Diseases of the Heart* (1749), the precision of its observations making it a classic; (2) Giovanni Battista Morgagni, whose *De Sedibus et Causis Morborum per Anatomen Indagatis* (1761) was a high-water mark of

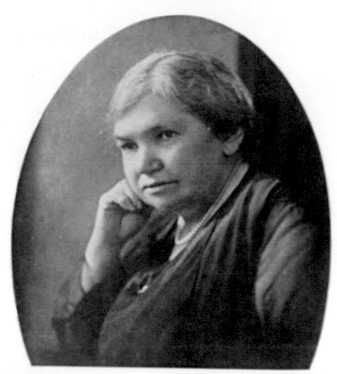

FIGURE 1-1   Maude E. Abbott (1869–1940), McGill University, Montreal. *(Courtesy of Dr. H. E. MacDermott, Montreal.)*

clinical-pathological achievement; (3) Karl Rokitansky, one of the greatest gross descriptive pathologists, who by 1866 had performed no fewer than 30,000 necropsies; (4) Thomas B. Peacock, whose great work, *Malformations of the Heart*, appeared in 1858; and (5) Sir Arthur Keith, who, with Martin Flack in 1907, discovered the sinus node—a remarkable structure that governs the heartbeat. The seminal contributions of Gross (Fig. 1–3), Crafoord (Fig. 1–4), and Blalock and Taussig (Fig. 1–5) soon followed, and the sense of despair that had surrounded congenital malformations of the heart—those "hopeless futilities"—began to dissipate.

In 1888, John C. Munro of Boston established the technical feasibility of ligating a patent ductus arteriosus in an infant cadaver, and in 1907, Munro proposed the operation to the Philadelphia Academy of Surgery.[8] However, he did not act on his proposal because of the difficulty in arriving at an accurate clinical diagnosis.[9] In 1938, Graybiel, Strieder, and Boyer ligated a patent ductus in an unsuccessful attempt to save the life of a 22-year-old woman with infective endocarditis.[10] The conventional history of successful ductal ligation dates from August 1938 (publication date 1939) when Robert E. Gross, a pediatric surgeon at Boston Children's Hospital (see Fig. 1–3), ligated the patent ductus of a 7-year-old girl "in the hope of preventing subsequent bacterial endocarditis and with the immediate purpose of reducing the work of the heart caused by the shunt between the

aorta and the pulmonary artery." [11,12] Also in 1938, Emil Karl Frey (Fig. 1–6), a surgeon at the Medizinische Akademie in Dusseldorf, successfully ligated the patent ductus of a 14-year-old boy.[13] Frey did not report his experience because he hoped to operate on additional patients with patent ductus and because he was told that Gross in the United States had already published an account of ductal ligation.[12] During the bombing of Dusseldorf in World War II, Frey's hospital records were destroyed.

Robert Gross (see Fig. 1–3) and Charles Hufnagel, in 1938, undertook the first experimental studies that anticipated surgical resection of coarctation of the aorta. A "direct attack could be made on the lesion by cutting out the constricted segment, freeing the aortic arch and thoracic aorta, and bringing the remaining ends together by primary end-to-end suture.[14] Clarence Crafoord of Stockholm (see Fig. 1–4) was aware of this experimental work on coarctation and, while operating on a patient with patent ductus arteriosus, "took the risk of placing clamp forceps on the aorta above and below the point of entry of the duct into this artery and of keeping them attached during the time necessary to divide the duct and suture the aorta."[15] Crafoord "began to wonder whether it might not also be possible to treat congenital coarctation of the aortic isthmus by surgical means," and in 1944, he resected a coarctation and sutured the ends of the aorta together in two patients, both of whom recovered and improved.[15] In the United States, Gross continued his work on coarctation, planning to combine cooling the lower part of the body during aortic cross-clamping to prevent paralysis. The operations by Gross and Crafoord had a major impact on the progress of cardiac surgery.

In 1939, James W. Brown underscored the feasibility—and desirability—of clinical recognition of congenital malformations of the heart in his seminal book, *Congenital Heart Disease*.[16] Brown noted that "The main purpose of this volume is to present a brief account of congenital heart disease with special emphasis on those lesions capable of clinical recognition when modern methods are employed. My friends have sometimes suggested that congenital heart disease is largely a matter for the postmortem room, but my own experience has been the reverse. Eight years of work in five clinics devoted to the study of heart disease in children has made it possible to observe more than 350 cases of congenital heart disease, and these observations form the basis of this work."[16] Brown's book received scant attention because it was published during the Second World War, but it was a forerunner of Paul Wood's book, *Diseases of the Heart and Circulation* (1950),[17] and my subsequent book, *Clinical Recognition of Congenital Heart Disease* (1972).[18]

Helen Brooke Taussig (see Fig. 1–5, *B*), a younger contemporary of Maude Abbott, was born in May 1898 in Cambridge, Massachusetts.[19] Her father was a professor of economics at Harvard University, the medical school of which did not then admit women.[20] The aspiring

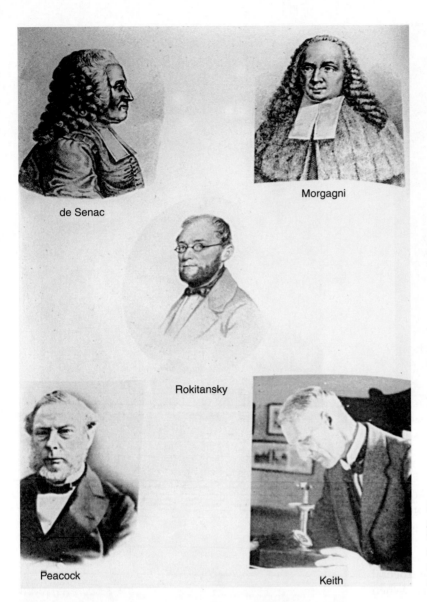

de Senac

Morgagni

Rokitansky

Peacock

Keith

FIGURE 1-2 Frontispiece from Abbott ME: *Atlas of Congenital Cardiac Disease.* New York, American Heart Association, 1936. *(Photographed by J. K. Perloff in the Bibliotheca Osleriana, McGill University, Montreal. Reproduced with permission. © Atlas of Congenital Cardiac Disease, 1936. Copyright American Heart Association.)*

young Helen was permitted to attend certain lectures but was not allowed to speak to the male students.[20] She subsequently studied gross morphology at Boston University, where Alexander Begg, professor of anatomy and dean of the Medical School, gave her a beef heart to examine ("that was how I got into cardiology") and urged her to enroll at Johns Hopkins, the first American medical school to admit women. Taussig later observed that cyanotic neonates often died when their ductus arteriosus closed spontaneously after birth, and many acyanotic neonates became cyanotic following ductal closure. Her thoughts turned to the possibility of constructing an artificial ductus for the cyanotic child with deficient pulmonary blood flow.[21] After trying unsuccessfully to interest Robert Gross in creating a ductus in cyanotic children, Taussig turned to Alfred Blalock (see Fig. 1–5, *A*), a vascular surgeon at Hopkins who, in animal studies on coarctation, had developed a technique of anastomosing a brachiocephalic artery to the aorta.[22] "If that is possible,"

thought Taussig, "why not put the subclavian artery into the pulmonary artery?"[21] This idea was greeted with the highest skepticism by some of the most eminent cardiac surgeons, but Alfred Blalock accepted the challenge. With Vivian Thomas—his exceptionally skilled technical assistant who a half century later was duly recognized by the American Heart Association's Vivian Thomas Young Investigator's Award—tested the idea on dogs.[19] In 1944, the end of a subclavian artery was sutured to the side of a pulmonary artery in a patient with tetralogy of Fallot, establishing the now-legendary Blalock-Taussig anastomosis and proving that a deeply cyanosed child could tolerate operation and improve substantially.[23] The anesthesiologist for that seminal operation was Dr. Merel Harmel, a junior anesthesiologist at Hopkins (Fig. 1–7) who used open-drip ether. Blalock had asked Austin Lamont, the chief of anesthesiology, to administer the anesthesia, but Lamont refused, commenting, "I will not put that child to death."[24]

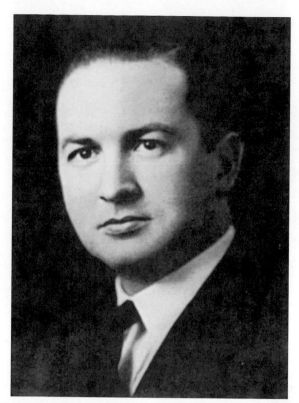

FIGURE 1–3 Robert E. Gross (1905–1988), Children's Hospital, Boston. *(With permission from Nissen, R.: Erlebtes Aus Der Thoraxchirurgie. Stuttgart, Georg Thieme, 1955.)*

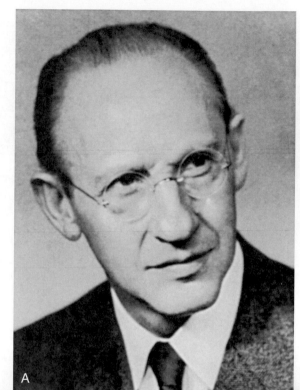

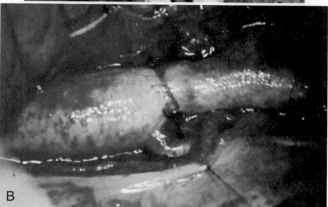

FIGURE 1–4 **(A)** Clarence Crafoord (1899–1984), Karolinska Institute, Stockholm. **(B)** Coarctation resection with end-to-end anastomosis. *(A, with permission from Nissen, R.: Erlebtes Aus Der Thoraxchirurgie. Stuttgart, Georg Thieme, 1955.)*

Helen Taussig recalled the glacial pace of her academic promotions. "Dr Blalock was Professor of Surgery and he was elected to the Academy of Science. I was not even promoted from being an Assistant to an Associate Professor.[20] Taussig devoted 10 years to the preparation of *Congenital Malformations of the Heart*,[25] the monumental clinical counterpart to Maude Abbott's *Atlas*. When Taussig began work on her book, the surgical treatment of congenital heart disease was not even a dream, but when the book was published in 1947, it included ligation of patent ductus arteriosus, resection of coarctation of the aorta, and the Blalock-Taussig operation.[19]

In 1711, Steven Hales, an English scientist, inserted brass pipes into the ventricles of a horse via the jugular vein and carotid artery. The pressure in the tube's water column rose to over 9 feet. In 1844, Claude Bernard catheterized the right and left ventricles of a horse, and in 1861, Aime Cheveau and Etienne Jules Marey measured intracardiac pressures by the method of Bernard. In 1831, F. J. Dieffenbach, professor at the University of Berlin, employed a retrograde arterial catheter to access the central circulation in a misguided attempt to perform a therapeutic phlebotomy in a patient with cholera who was dying of dehydration.[26] It is unclear whether the catheter tip reached the left ventricle.

Werner Forssmann (Fig. 1–8A), then a medical student, saw an etching that depicted the cardiac catheterization of Cheveau and Marey.[27] The picture made an indelible impression on the young Forssmann, who became convinced that "these experimental studies could be performed in man without any danger."[28] In 1929, just a year after finishing his medical studies and while working in the surgical department of the Augusta-Viktoria Hospital in Eberswalde near Berlin, Forssmann performed the first cardiac catheterization on a living human being—himself. As he later recalled,

The anatomy of the venous system is such that starting from any site, except of course from the portal region, one arrives in the vessels of the heart. ... Thus, I catheterized

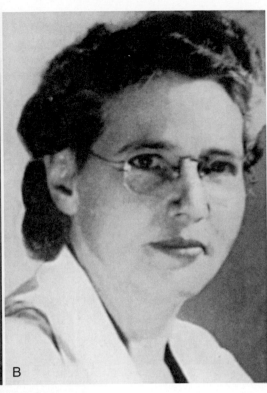

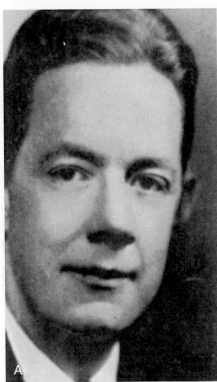

FIGURE 1-5 **(A)** Alfred Blalock (1899–1964) and **(B)** Helen B. Taussig (1898–1986), the Johns Hopkins Hospital, Baltimore. *(Reprinted with permission from cover of Science Vol. 107, Copyright American Association for the Advancement of Science, April 16, 1948.)*

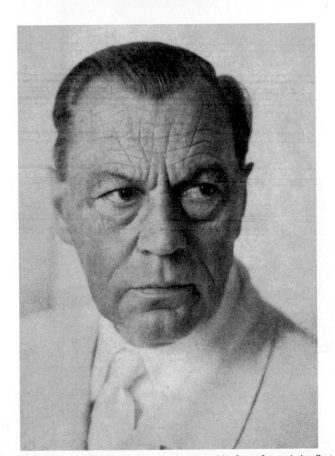

FIGURE 1-6   E. K. Frey, a surgeon in Dusseldorf, performed the first successful ligation of a patent ductus in 1938 on a 14-year-old boy. Hospital documents were destroyed during the Second World War. The case was not reported.

(cadavers) from an elbow vein toward the heart and reached the right atrium without encountering resistance and with feather-like gliding. ... The location of the catheter was later checked by autopsy. ... After experiments in cadavers had been successful, I undertook the first experiments in living man by experimenting upon myself. I carried out under local anesthesia a venesection in my left elbow and introduced the catheter without resistance in its whole length of 65 cm. This distance appeared to me, according to the measurement on the body surface, to correspond to the route from the left elbow to the heart. ... I checked the position of the catheter in a roentgen picture [see Fig. 1-8, *B*], and I observed the forward advance of the catheter in a mirror held in front of the fluoroscope screen by a nurse. ... The catheter, coming straight up my left arm, lies on the thoracic wall. It disappears behind the clavicle and, at the site of the discharge from the jugular vein, makes a downward curve, joins the right margin of the vessel shadow, and there—partially covered by the shadow margin of the vertebral column—can be followed into the right atrium [see Fig. 1-8, *B*]. The length of the catheter was not sufficient for a further catheterization.[27]

Measurement of cardiac output—an illusive objective of physiologists—involved the principle described by Fick and Grollman in 1870.[28-30] Catheterization in dogs had been employed in New York since 1937 by Andre F. Cournand and Dickenson W. Richards, but Forssmann's cardiac catheter provided a practical means of directly applying the Fick principle. Cournand and Richards

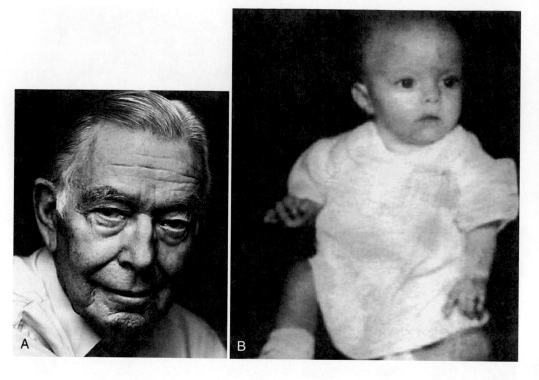

FIGURE 1-7   (A) Merel Harmel. **(B)** Eileen Saxon, the "blue baby." The anesthesiologist for the seminal operation was Merel Harmel, a junior anesthesiologist at Johns Hopkins, who used open-drip ether.

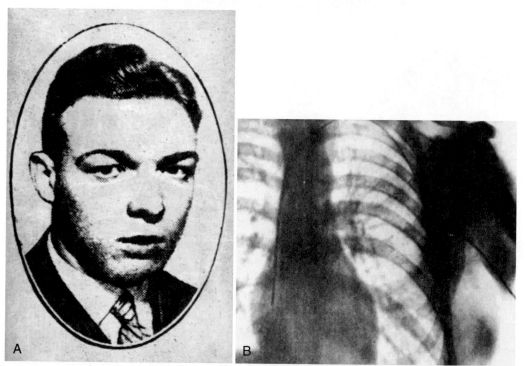

FIGURE 1-8   (A) Werner Forssman. **(B)** "The catheter extends from the left cephalic vein down into the right atrium."

proposed the use of a cardiac catheter and an arterial needle to measure cardiac output by a direct Fick method.[31] In 1956, Cournand, Richards, and Forssmann shared the Nobel Prize in medicine or physiology "for their discoveries concerning heart catheterization and pathological changes in the circulatory system."[32,33]

Soon after Wilhelm Konrad Roentgen's discovery of "a new kind of rays" in 1896[34] (Fig. 1–9), angiography had its inception with injections of contrast material into blood vessels of cadavers and animals. Angiocardiography was first performed in 1937 when Castellanos, Pereiras, and Garcia, in Havana, visualized the right cardiac chambers in

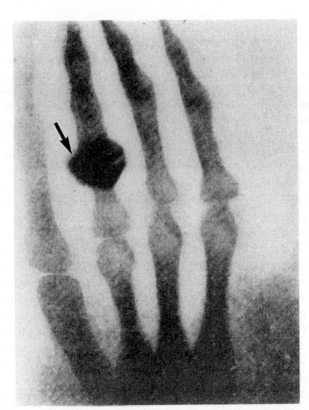

FIGURE 1–9 Photograph of the bones in the fingers of a living human hand. The third finger has a ring upon it *(arrow). (From Roentgen, W. K.:* Nature *1896;53:274. Reprinted with permission from* Nature. *Copyright 1896, Macmillan Magazines Limited.)*

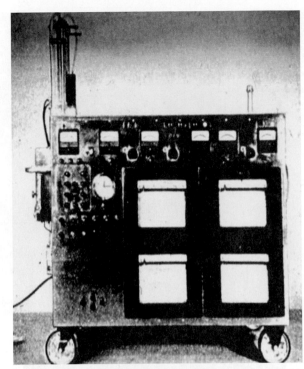

FIGURE 1–10 The first successful intracardiac operation (1953) employed the Gibbon heart/lung bypass system for closure of an atrial septal defect in an 18-year-old woman.

infants and children using the agent Diadrast.[35] Independently, George Potts Robb and Israel Steinberg in New York employed angiography in adults and stated, with poetic eloquence, "The internal structure of the living heart had been revealed for the first time."[36] In the late 1940s, selective angiocardiography was introduced by Ignacio Chavez in Mexico.[36]

As early as the 19th century, physiologists had been interested in techniques that permitted the maintenance of organs or tissues by artificial circulation of the blood. John H. Gibbon, of Philadelphia, conceived of a heart/lung bypass machine in 1931 when, as a surgical fellow in Boston, he witnessed the death of a young woman following a pulmonary embolus. "[T]he patient's life might have been saved if some of the blue blood in her veins could be continuously withdrawn into an extracorporeal blood circuit, exposed to an atmosphere of oxygen, and then returned to the patient by way of a systemic artery. ... Cardiorespiratory function might be temporarily performed by the blood circuit while the massive pulmonary embolus was surgically removed." By the early 1950s, Gibbon was ready to undertake heart/lung bypass in patients. In 1953, the first successful intracardiac operation employing Gibbon's heart/lung bypass system (Fig. 1–10) was done for closure of an atrial septal defect in an 18-year-old woman.[37] Success was confirmed several

months later by cardiac catheterization. However, the next two patients on whom Gibbon used his heart/lung machine died, and he did not use it again. In 1955, C. Walton Lillihei employed controlled cross-circulation for "direct-vision intracardiac correction of congenital anomalies,"[38] with a parent acting as the "oxygenator." In the same year, the Mayo Clinic reported intracardiac surgery in eight patients with the aid of a modified Gibbon-type mechanical pump oxygenator.[39,40] John W. Kirklin[41] (Fig. 1–11) wrote that "accurate visualization of structures within the heart for a period sufficient to permit precise corrective measures" had been achieved.[40] Decades then elapsed before Aldo Casteneda at the Boston Children's Hospital established the feasibility of intracardiac surgery in neonates and infants.

Legend ascribed to Pien Ch'iao, who practiced in China in the second century BC such skillful use of anesthesia that he was able to operate painlessly and to exchange the hearts of two patients. In 1960, Lower and Shumway (Fig. 1–12) performed the first orthotopic cardiac transplantation, and in 1966, the Pien Ch'iao legend was followed by reality when Christiaan Barnard, a charismatic, controversial South African surgeon, performed the first human-to-human cardiac transplantation.[41,42] The succeeding decades witnessed major advances in surgical techniques and immunosuppression that permitted cardiac transplantation to be applied successfully in patients with congenital heart disease (see Chapter 17).

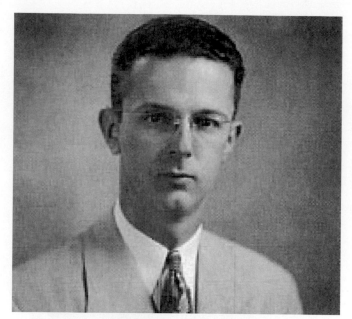

FIGURE 1-11   John Kirklin.

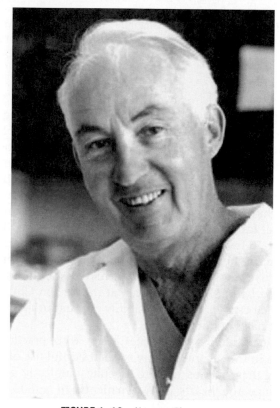

FIGURE 1-12   Norman Shumway.

The pivotal role of anesthesia must now be underscored. Within a span of four years—1842 to 1846—anesthesia was born in the United States, a feat that ranks among the nation's greatest contributions to medicine. Without anesthesia, cardiac surgery would not exist. Without cardiac surgery, congenital heart disease in adults would not exist.

In 1818, Michael Faraday discovered that sulfuric ether had anesthetic properties. In March 1842, Crawford W. Long, a modest country practitioner in Jefferson County, Georgia, first used ether in surgery. Seven years elapsed before Long published his observations, which received little attention, although no greater boon has ever come to mankind than the power thus granted to induce temporary but complete insensibility to pain. In October 1846, at the Massachusetts General Hospital, William Thomas Green Morton used ether anesthesia, and within a month, the event was published in the *Boston Medical and Surgical Journal.* Within another month, ether was used in London, and in the succeeding year, ether anesthesia became widespread throughout Europe.

These historical events heralded one of the most successful rehabilitation programs that medicine has witnessed. Formidable technical resources at our disposal permit remarkably accurate anatomic and physiologic cardiac diagnoses and astonishing feats of reparative surgery.[43,44] Survival patterns have dramatically improved, and thus congenital heart disease is no longer considered simply in terms of age at onset but also in terms of the age range that survival now permits—a continuum from fetal life to the neonate, the child, the adolescent, the young adult, and on to advanced age.[18,45]

Worldwide prevalence of congenital heart disease has long been a topic of interest,[46-52] but certain qualifications and definitions are necessary to interpret epidemiologic information.[45] Congenital heart disease (*con,* "together"; *genitus,* "born") is generally taken to connote the presence at birth of a gross structural abnormality of the heart, great arteries, or great veins that is actually or potentially of functional significance.[48,52] Included in this definition, however, are congenital complete heart block, which is not a gross structural abnormality, and small ventricular defects that close spontaneously within 6 months of life. Excluded is an isolated patent ductus arteriosus in an infant with a gestational age younger than 38 weeks, without heart failure, and with ductal closure by 2 weeks.[47,48]

Forssmann's innovation—the cardiac catheter—was soon employed for the diagnosis of congenital heart disease.[32] A major step forward is current use of the catheter for therapeutic interventions,[26] which is the subject of Chapter 18.

Incidence of congenital heart disease varies significantly if a sibling or parent is so afflicted (see Chapter 10). When one sibling is affected, subsequent incidence is 2.3%; when two siblings are affected, the subsequent incidence rises to 7.3%. If a mother has congenital heart disease, the incidence of transmission is as high at 6.7%, with expression coupled considerably to the maternal malformation (concordance). If the father has congenital heart disease, the incidence is 2.1%, much lower than maternal transmission. This is so because a distinguishing feature of cytoplasmic material such as mitochondria is a tendency for inheritance through the female line, in addition to which non-Mendelian behavior of certain autosomal genes results in expression that depends on the sex of the parent from which the gene is inherited.[53] The pattern of transgene expression correlates with the state of parentally imprinted methylation.[53] The prevalence of functionally trivial or clinically subtle anomalies, such as tiny ventricular septal defects, reflects the advent of high-technology diagnostic methods. Moderate malformations occur in approximately 3 per 1000 live births (0.3%) and complex malformations in approximately 2.5 to 3 per 1000 live births with significant lesion-specific variation.[49] Collective incidence is estimated at 0.6% of live births,[45] excluding the bicuspid aortic valve, which occurs in approximately 2.0% of live births.[45,54–57]

In the United States, there are currently more adults with congenital heart disease than there are infants and children, and approximately 20,000 open operations are performed annually in this patient population. Approximately 85% of infants born with congenital heart disease in developed countries can expect to reach adulthood.[58,59] Because the prevalence of congenital heart disease in the offspring of parents with congenital heart disease exceeds the 0.6% in the general population, the number of patients is increasing at a rate of about 5% per year,[58] with an adult population in the United States approaching 1 million.[59,60] There are about 32,000 new cases per year in the United States[56, 61] and about 1.5 million new cases worldwide.[54]

Long-term care necessarily remains concerned with unoperated patients who reach adulthood but is increasingly concerned with the growing number of patients who reach adulthood because of operation and who need continuing medical surveillance.[59,61,62] The traditional quality of care provided by pediatric cardiologists from birth to maturity must be matched with care of equal quality for adults, and herein lies a problem. In the United States, there are about 1200 board-certified pediatric cardiologists and about 20,000 board certifications in cardiovascular medicine. This number of pediatric cardiologists is far too small to cope with the current number of adults with congenital heart disease, in addition to which the relative geographic mobility of the population makes it unlikely that patients with congenital heart disease will remain under the long-term care of their pediatric cardiologists. The need for care cannot be met from the relatively large pool of adult cardiovascular specialists because only a small percentage have an interest in or knowledge of congenital heart disease. Who, then, will assume responsibility for the growing number of adults? This question is the subject of Chapter 3—"Specialized Centers for the Comprehensive Care of Adults with Congenital Heart Disease."

"The natural history of any disease is a description of what happens to people with that disease who do not receive treatment for it."[55] Unoperated adults enjoy the

Table 1-1   Survival Patterns of Adults with Congenital Heart Disease

Survival without Operation
Malformations that do not require operation
Malformations that remain amenable to operation in adulthood
Malformations that are inoperable except for organ transplantation

Postoperative Survival
Expected adult survival enhanced by operation
Adult survival related chiefly or solely to operation

Table 1-2   Types of Surgery for Congenital Heart Disease

SURGERY TYPE	CHARACTERISTICS
Curative	No postoperative residua, sequelae, or complications
Reparative	Anatomic repair or reconstruction with obligatory
	Postoperative of residua or sequela
Palliative	Basic morphologic anomaly is neither repaired nor reconstructive
Reoperative	Late reoperation after reparative or palliative surgery
Organ transplantation	Heart, lung, heart/lung

benefits of a host of advances in medical treatment—pharmacologic and electrophysiologic, to name but two—none of which is "natural." The term *natural history* is therefore a misnomer and is not used in this text. Instead, reference is made to survival patterns and clinical course without cardiac surgery or interventional catheterization, and to postoperative or postinterventional survival patterns (Table 1–1). Proper care of patients after operation requires knowledge of the preoperative congenital heart disease; the type and effects of the surgical or catheter intervention; and the presence, type, and degree of postoperative or postinterventional residua and sequelae (Table 1–2). Cure in the literal sense is rarely achieved. Accordingly, a wide range of residua and sequelae remain and require prolonged, if not indefinite, medical attention. These residua and sequelae are the subjects of Chapter 20.

Congenital heart disease in adults has emerged as a major area of cardiovascular medicine[61]—a recognized subspecialty.[60,62] Long-term care is essential if the concerns inherent in this increasing patient population are to be addressed. Importance worldwide is reflected in the International Society for Adult Congenital Cardiac Disease; importance in the United States is reflected in the Adult Congenital Heart Association, which are the subjects of Chapter 2.

References

1. Fallot A. Contribution a l'anatomie pathologique de la maladie bleue (cyanose cardiaque). *Marseilles Med.* 1888;25:418–420.
2. Holt LE. *The Disease of Infancy and Childhood.* New York: D. Appleton; 1894.
3. Olser W. *The Principles and Practice of Medicine.* New York: D. Appleton; 1892.
4. Waugh D. *Maudie of Mcgill. Dr. Maude Abbott and the Foundations of Heart Surgery.* Toronto and Oxford: Hannah Institute & Dundurn Press; 1990.
5. Holmes AF. Case of malformation of the heart. *Edinburgh Trans Medico-Chir Soc.* 1824;252–254.
6. Dobell AR, Van Praagh R. The Holmes heart: historic associations and pathologic anatomy. *Am Heart J.* 1996;132:437–445.
7. Abbott ME. *Atlas of Congenital Cardiac Disease.* New York: American Heart Association; 1936.
8. Munro JC. Ligation of the ductus arteriosus. *Ann Surg.* 1907; 46:335–338.
9. Acierno LJ. *The History of Cardiology.* London: Parthenon; 1994.
10. Graybiel A, Strieder JW, Boyer NH. An attempt to obliterate the patent ductus arteriosus in a patient with subacute bacterial endarteritis. *Am Heart J.* 1938;15:621.
11. Castaneda AR. Classics in thoracic surgery. Patent ductus arteriosus: a commentary (Robert E. Gross). *The Ann Thorac Surg.* 1981;31:92–96.
12. Gross RE, Hubbard JP. Surgical ligation of a patent ductus arteriosus: report of first successful case. *JAMA.* 1939;112:729–731.
13. Kaemmerer H, Meisner H, Hess J, Perloff JK. Surgical treatment of patent ductus arteriosus: a new historical perspective. *Am J Cardiol.* 2004;94:1153–1154.
14. Gross RE, Hufnagel CA. Coarctation of the aorta: experimental studies regarding its surgical correction. *N Engl J Med.* 1945; 233:287.
15. Crafoord C, Nylin G. Congenital coarctation of the aorta and its surgical treatment. *J Thorac Surg.* 1945;14:347.
16. Brown JW. *Congenital Heart Disease.* London: John Bale Medical.; 1939.
17. Wood PH. *Diseases of the Heart and Circulation.* London: Eyre & Spottiswoode; 1950.
18. Perloff JK. *Clinical Recognition of Congenital Heart Disease.* 5th ed. Philadelphia: WB Saunders; 2003.
19. McNamara DG, Manning JA, Engle MA, et al. Helen Brooke Taussig: 1898 to 1986. *J Am Coll Cardiol.* 1987;10:662–671.
20. Taussig HB. *Letter dated October 3, 1966 to Dr. Robert J. Glasser, Dean, Stanford University of Medicine, signed by Helen B. Taussig, Professor Emeritus of Pediatrics, The Johns Hopkins Hospital.* 1966.
21. Taussig HB. On the evolution of our knowledge of congenital malformations of the heart; the T. Duckett Jones Memorial Lecture. *Circulation.* 1965;31:768–777.
22. Blalock A, Park EA The surgical treatment of experimental coarctation (atresia) of the aorta. *Ann Surg.* 1944;119:445–456.
23. Blalock A, Taussig HB. Surgical treatment of malformations of the heart in which there is pulmonary stenosis or pulmonary atresia. *JAMA.* 1945;128:189–202.
24. Neill CA, Clark EB. Tetralogy of Fallot. The first 300 years. *Texas Heart Inst J.* 1994;21:272–279.
25. Taussig HB. *Congenital Malformations of the Heart* New York: Commonwealth Fund; 1947.
26. Mueller RL, Sanborn TA. The history of interventional cardiology: cardiac catheterization, angioplasty, and related interventions. *Am Heart J.* 1995;129:146–172.
27. Forssmann W. Die Sondierung des rechten Herzens (catheterization of the right heart). *Klin Wochenschr.* 1929;8:2085.
28. Grollman A. *The Cardiac Output of Man in Health and Disease.* Baltimore: Williams & Wilkins; 1932.
29. Fick A. Ueber die Messung des Blutquantums in den Herzventrikeln. *Sitzungsb Phys-Med Ges Wu-rzb.* 1870.
30. Richards DW, Riley CB, Hiscock M. Congenital heart disease, measurements of the circulation. *Arch Int Med.* 1931;47:484–499.
31. Cournand A, Ranges HA, Riley RL. Comparison of results of the normal ballistocardiogram and a direct Fick method in measuring the cardiac output in man. *J Clin Invest.* 1942;21:287–294.
32. Cournand A, Baldwin JS, Himmelstein A. *Catheterization in Congenital Heart Disease.* New York: The Commonwealth Fund; 1949.
33. Sourkes TL. *Nobel Prize Winners in Medicine and Physiology, 1901–1965.* Revised ed. New York: Abelard-Schuman; 1966.
34. Roentgen WK. On a new kind of rays. *Nature.* 1896;53:274–276.
35. Castellanos A, Pereiras R, Garcia A. La angiocardiografia radio-opaqua. *Arch Soc Estud Habana.* 1937;31:523.
36. Chavez I, Dorbecker N, Celis A. Direct intracardiac angiography: its diagnostic value. *Am Heart J.* 1947;33:560–566.
37. Miller BJ, Gibbon JH, Fineberg C. An improved mechanical heart and lung apparatus; its use during open cardiotomy in experimental animals. *Med Clin North Am.* 1953;1:1603–1624.
38. Lillehei CW, Cohen M, Warden HE, Varco RL. The direct-vision intracardiac correction of congenital anomalies by controlled cross circulation; results in thirty-two patients with ventricular septal defects, tetralogy of Fallot, and atrioventricularis communis defects. *Surgery.* 1955;38:11–29.
39. Cooley DA, Kirklin JWM. 1917–2004. *Circulation.* 2004;109: 2928–2929.
40. Kirklin JW, Dushane JW, Patrick RT, et al. Intracardiac surgery with the aid of a mechanical pump-oxygenator system (Gibbon type): report of eight cases. *Mayo Clin Proc.* 1955;30:201–206.
41. Cooper KC, Cooley DA. Christiaan Neethling Barnard 1922–2001. *Circulation.* 2001;104:2756–2757.
42. Barnard CN. The operation. A human cardiac transplant: an interim report of a successful operation performed at Groote Schuur Hospital, Cape Town. *S Afr Med J.* 1967;41:1271–1274.
43. Engle MA, Perloff JK. Postoperative congenital heart disease in adults. *Am J Cardiol.* 1982;50:541–543.
44. Rashkind WJ. Pediatric cardiology: a brief historical perspective. *Pediatr Cardiol.* 1979;1:63–73.
45. Marelli AJ, Mackie AS, Ionescu-Ittu R, et al. Congenital heart disease in the general population: changing prevalence and age distribution. *Circulation.* 2007;115:163–172.
46. Akang EE, Osinusi KO, Pindiga HU, et al. Congenital malformations: a review of 672 autopsies in Ibadan, Nigeria. *Pediatr Path.* 1993;13:659–670.
47. Fixler DE, Pastor P, Chamberlin M, et al. Trends in congenital heart disease in Dallas County births. 1971–1984. *Circulation.* 1990;81: 137–142.
48. Hoffman JI, Christianson R. Congenital heart disease in a cohort of 19,502 births with long-term follow-up. *Am J Cardiol.* 1978;42: 641–647.
49. Hoffman JI, Kaplan S, Liberthson RR. Prevalence of congenital heart disease. *Am Heart J.* 2004;147:425–439.
50. Khalil A, Aggarwal R, Thirupuram S, Arora R. Incidence of congenital heart disease among hospital live births in India. *Indian Pediatr.* 1994;31:519–527.
51. Kidd SA, Lancaster PA, McCredie RM. The incidence of congenital heart defects in the first year of life. *J Paediatr Child Health.* 1993;29:344–349.
52. Mitchell SC, Korones SB, Berendes HW. Congenital heart disease in 56,109 births. Incidence and natural history. *Circulation.* 1971;43: 323–332.
53. Barlow DP. Gametic imprinting in mammals. *Science.* 1995;270: 1610–1613.
54. Hoffman JI. Congenital heart disease: incidence and inheritance. *Pediatr Clin North Am.* 1990;37:25–43.
55. Hoffman JI. Reflections on the past, present and future of pediatric cardiology. *Cardiol Young.* 1994;4:208–223.
56. Moller JH, Taubert KA, Allen HD, et al. Cardiovascular health and disease in children: current status. A Special Writing Group from

the Task Force on Children and Youth, American Heart Association. *Circulation.* 1994;89:923–930.

57. Roberts WC. The congenitally bicuspid aortic valve. A study of 85 autopsy cases. *Am J Cardiol.* 1970;26:72–83.

58. Moodie DS. Adult congenital heart disease. *Curr Opin Cardiol.* 1994;9:137–142.

59. Reid GJ, Webb GD, Barzel M, et al. Estimates of life expectancy by adolescents and young adults with congenital heart disease. *J Am Coll Cardiol.* 2006;48:349–355.

60. Ritchie JL, Cheitlin MD, Hlatky MA, et al. Task Force 5: Profile of the cardiovascular specialist: trends in needs and supply and implications for the future. *J Am Coll Cardiol.* 1994;24:313–321.

61. Perloff JK. Pediatric congenital cardiac becomes a postoperative adult. The changing population of congenital heart disease. *Circulation.* 1973;47:606–619.

62. Perloff JK. Congenital heart disease in adults. A new cardiovascular subspecialty. *Circulation.* 1991;84:1881–1890.

CHAPTER 2

National and International Scope

JOSEPH K. PERLOFF ▪ AMY VERSTAPPEN

Congenital heart disease in adults was formally recognized as a new cardiovascular subspecialty in 1990 at the 22nd Bethesda Conference, Congenital Heart Disease After Childhood: An Expanding Patient Population.[1,2] The 32nd Bethesda Conference a decade later,[3] Care of the Adult with Congenital Heart Disease, marked the first time two Bethesda Conferences had been devoted to the same topic. Gary Webb from the Toronto General Hospital was invited to participate in the 22nd Conference, at which the International Society of Adult Congenital Cardiac Disease (ISACCD) had its inception during a casual but extended conversation that focused on patient care, training, education, and research. With our mutual interests aroused, it was agreed to continue the discussion at the forthcoming American Heart Association meeting. Thereafter, biannual meetings were planned at the American Heart Association and the American College of Cardiology Scientific Sessions.

A few selected colleagues were invited to join us. Small sums were taken from meager fiscal resources to pay for a hotel room modestly equipped with a table and a dozen or so chairs that were seldom filled, at least initially. The first meeting in Dallas, held in April 1992, included Daniel Murphy, Timothy Garson, Richard Liberthson, David Skorton, and Carole Warnes, in addition to Gary Webb and Joseph Perloff. In the meantime, Webb had been energized by the 22nd Bethesda Conference and mounted an impressive initiative, mobilizing the abundant resources of the renamed Toronto Hospital and the Hospital for Sick Children. In response to joint efforts in the United States and Canada, attendance at the biannual meetings grew appreciably, and before long, a sizeable formal organization evolved. I nominated Gary Webb as the organization's first president. He was elected by acclamation and served two successful terms. The organization's name, the Society for Adult Congenital Cardiac Disease, was changed to the International Society of Adult Congenital Cardiac Disease to underscore its worldwide scope (Fig. 2–1). "Cardiac" disease rather than "heart" disease was Webb's preference.

Carole Warnes (Mayo Clinic) and Richard Liberthson (Massachusetts General Hospital) respectively succeeded Webb as President. Michael Gatzoulis was ISACCD's first president from outside North America. Successive presidents outdid themselves to make the biannual meetings more and more attractive, with programs that included guest speakers, collaborative research initiatives, and development of an international database. David Skorton, now president of Cornell University, was the first treasurer of ISACCD; his witty reports on tenuous fiscal solvency provided comic relief.

A dedicated nonprofessional staff was soon in place, and the ISACCD Newsletter appeared, together with a Web site (http://www.isaccd.org) that defined the missions, goals, and objectives of the society. The International Journal of Cardiology became the official affiliated publication, the initial issue of which featured an editorial by Michael Gatzoulis and Thomas Graham, "International Society for Adult Congenital Cardiac Disease: An Introduction to the Readership and an Invitation to Join."[4] In 1995, more than half of the 94 registered members attended the semiannual ISACCD meeting during the American College of Cardiology Scientific Sessions. By 2006, membership had increased to nearly 300, with representatives from 30 countries. The founding group from the United States, Canada, and the United Kingdom was followed by a worldwide array that included, alphabetically, Argentina, Australia, Austria, Belgium, China, Colombia, France, Germany, Greece, Hong Kong, India, Ireland, Israel, Italy, Japan, the Republic of Korea, Kuwait, the Netherlands, the Netherlands Antilles, New Zealand, Pakistan, the Philippines, Saudi Arabia, Singapore, Slovenia, Spain, Sweden, Switzerland, Trinidad and Tobago, the United Arab Emirates, and Venezuela. The American College of

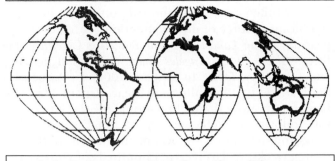

FIGURE 2-1   International Society for Adult Congenital Cardiac Disease.

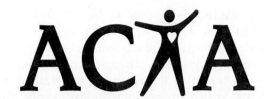

Adult Congenital Heart Association

FIGURE 2-2   Adult Congenital Heart Association.

Cardiology soon included adult congenital heart disease (ACHD) in its Accredited Cardiac Training Program, as recommended by ISACCD. The *Canadian Adult Congenital Heart Council Newsletter* was launched, together with the Canadian Adult Congenital Heart (CACH) Network.

In her "President's Message," Carole Warnes proposed that a support and advocacy group be established in the United States for patients with congenital heart disease, analogous to patient advocacy groups for Marfan syndrome and Down syndrome.[5] The Adult Congenital Heart Association (ACHA), which was conceived by patients and their families, evolved to meet this need[6] (Fig. 2-2). Incorporated in 1998, the first "board" consisted of the five patient founders, with a makeshift "office" in one of their homes. ACHA took advantage of the Internet and began to serve as an authentic advocate for patients with ACHD. The Worldwide Web provided national and international reach.

The first ACHA mission statement defined its purpose: "support and education of patients and their families." Initial focus was on the ACHA Web site (http://www .achaheart.org) and its newsletter. In 1999, an online discussion board was created as a lifeline for patients and families. Most ACHD patients had never known anyone else who had struggled with congenital heart disease, and many patients mistakenly believed that their experience was unique. When asked why ACHA matters, the commonest response was, "It was the first time I realized I wasn't alone." The wide variety of congenital heart diseases, the diversity of outcomes, and the differences in impact on quality of life made it difficult for patients to find others with comparable experiences, hence the potential for isolation and the struggle for self-identity. The online message board attracts English-speaking ACHD patients from around the world, enabling even those with rare disorders to find a "heart buddy."

The Web site also permits 24-hour participation from the privacy and security of one's own home or other venue with Internet access and is readily accessed even by severely limited patients. The ACHA Discussion Board has a strict "no medical advice" policy, emphasizing that assumptions about care should not be extrapolated from the experiences of others. Adults with congenital heart defects are often poorly informed about their illness and its potential risks and are ill-prepared to deal with practical issues, of which health insurance is a prime example. Posted messages are reviewed, and when concerns arise, action is taken to ensure that misinformation is not promulgated. *ACHA Newsletter* articles by ACHD specialists are available on the Web site, and access to additional information is provided through extensive links.

The ACHA Tool Kit provides online information and resources as an innovative educational tool containing a Personal Health Passport that can be readily updated and easily accessed and that is available in both print and electronic formats. The Passport contains key information such as prior and current cardiac and noncardiac issues, diagnoses, previous surgeries, birth control and reproductive recommendations, and exercise limitations. "Red flags" include information on anticoagulants, oxygen saturation, endocarditis risk, and the need for intravenous filtration devices. The Passport also contains drawings and descriptions of individual malformations and operations, is designed to be carried when traveling or when consulting new physicians, and functions as an educational device when filled out by the patient under the supervision of the patient's cardiologist. An electronic version, which is similar to the Electronic Medical Passport of the International Society for Adult Congenital Cardiac Disease, is a password-protected device on which patients and families can store and update information and print copies. With support from the American College of Cardiology Foundation, in excess of 15,000 copies of the Passport have been distributed in more than 50 pediatric and ACHD facilities nationwide. The importance of long-term specialized care is emphasized. The ISACCD/ACHA Clinic Directory is fully searchable by clinic name.

The ACHA Conferences, Web site, online discussion board, and health passport emphasize the founding mission of support and education. A large number of congenital heart disease survivors surveyed throughout the United States provided a startling revelation—that most postoperative patients with complex congenital heart disease perceived themselves as "fixed" and had often received little or no cardiac care for decades at a time. When care was provided, it was usually by nonspecialized community cardiologists. These concerns were subsequently addressed in the report of the 32nd Bethesda Conference, which stressed that survivors with complex congenital heart defects faced high rates of ongoing health problems, a striking unawareness of special health care needs, and a lack of access to appropriate health care resources. In early 2002, the *32nd Bethesda Conference Guidelines* became available in a variety of patient-friendly formats. The need for long-term specialized care was emphasized yet again, making it clear that congenital heart disease, with few exceptions, is analogous to other forms of chronic illnesses that require a lifetime of specialized medical surveillance. In 2004, a new Mission Statement more fully reflected the ACHA's commitment to advocacy and acknowledged an increasing commitment to promoting lifelong care:

> The Adult Congenital Heart Association is a nonprofit organization that seeks to improve the quality of life and extend the lives of adults with congenital heart defects. Through education, outreach, advocacy, and promotion of research, ACHA serves and supports the million or more adults with congenital heart defects, their families, and the medical community.

Regional ACHA Conferences have been held in Washington, DC; Chicago; San Francisco; New York; Los Angeles; and Kissimmee, Florida. The first National Conference in 2000 was cosponsored by the Boston Adult Congenital Heart Clinic, and subsequent National Conferences were hosted by the Loyola Medical Center and the Mayo Clinic. In 2006, the ACHA's Fourth National Conference was cosponsored by Stanford University and the University of California San Francisco and brought together more than 300 patients, families, and health care professionals for a 3-day program that included experts from 13 states and 4 countries. More than $25,000 in registration scholarships and travel assistance permitted income-limited and handicapped patients and their families to attend.

A major unresolved problem is the large number of patients who are unaware that they need long-term cardiac care and who thus have been lost to follow-up.[7] The ACHA/ISACCD Clinic Survey confirmed that a relatively small portion of adults with complex congenital heart disease were receiving recommended levels of care. According to the survey, the aggregate number of patients seen annually in the United States at all self-described ACHD centers is under 40,000. The discrepancy between 40,000 and the estimated 500,000 patients with complex ACHD is unsettling, especially because patients who have been seen at more than one center are likely to be double-counted and because the 40,000 includes both complex and simple malformations.

In 2004, the Medical Advisory Board targeted "lost patients" as a primary strategic goal. In 2005, efforts by board members, staff, and supporters resulted in a significant upsurge of media attention, with articles appearing in the *Lancet, the San Francisco Chronicle, the Boston Globe, the Los Angeles Times, the Washington Post,* and *Cardiology Today.* In January 2006, an Associated Press article titled "Childhood Heart Repairs May Not Last" ran in more than 700 national media outlets and was followed by televised reports on CNN and Fox News and in a variety of local media outlets. In the following weeks, ACHA received hundreds of e-mails and phone calls from concerned patients and families. Availability of the Clinic Survey enabled ACHA to connect with cardiologists throughout the country.

In the fall of 2004, ACHA served on the first National Heart, Lung, and Blood Institute working group dedicated to research in ACHD. The recommendations were published in the February 2006 *Journal of the American College of Cardiology* and included the establishment of a national adult congenital heart disease research network and federal efforts to identify the "lost" patients with ACHD. In response to these recommendations and to the need for federal awareness and funding, ACHA held its first Congenital Heart Lobby Day in February 2006 in collaboration with the Congenital Heart Information Network and the Children's Heart Foundation. Seventy-eight patients, family members, and health professionals converged from 27 states and made more than 75 congressional visits to solicit funds for a National Adult Congenital Heart Disease Registry and for research in ACHD.

ACHA's mission, programs, impact, and resources have increased substantially since 1998. Membership has risen from a handful in 1992 to about 200 in 2000 to more than 1600 in 2006. A fledgling organization run by volunteers has evolved into an organization with a dedicated professional staff available to execute its primary functions. Funding from the Schooler Family Foundation has made it possible for the ACHA to create a development position with the primary goal of core funding. In 2002, the ACHA Medical Advisory Board authorized funding for the first paid chief executive—a president and CEO. With the objectives outlined in its 2006 Strategic Plan having been achieved, the Board is developing objectives for 2009, including membership growth, increased services, expansion of media outlets, and rededication to the unmet needs of congenital heart disease survivors. With the ACHD population in the United States growing at a rate of 5% per year and with patients who have survived because of 20th-century breakthroughs now approaching middle age, action is needed to prevent avoidable disabilities and premature mortality. A concerted effort is planned to achieve a 21st-century health system that ensures lifelong care for patients with congenital heart disease—from the neonate to whatever age survival permits.

References

1. Perloff JK. Congenital heart disease in adults. A new cardiovascular subspecialty. *Circulation*. 1991;84:1881–1890.
2. Perloff JK. 22nd Bethesda Conference. Congenital heart disease after childhood: an expanding patient population. *J Am Coll Cardiol*. 1991;18:311–342.
3. Webb GD, Williams RG. Care of the adult with congenital heart disease: introduction. *J Am Coll Cardiol*. 2001;37:1166.
4. Gatzoulis MA, Graham TP Jr. International Society for Adult Congenital Cardiac Disease: an introduction to the readership and an invitation to join. *Int J Cardiol*. 2003;88:127–128.
5. Warnes CA, Liberthson R, Danielson GK, et al. Task force 1: the changing profile of congenital heart disease in adult life. *J Am Coll Cardiol*. 2001;37:1170–1175.
6. Verstappen A, Pearson D, Kovacs AH. Adult congenital heart disease: the patient's perspective. *Cardiol Clin*. 2006;24:515–529.
7. Perloff JK, Warnes CA. Challenges posed by adults with repaired congenital heart disease. *Circulation*. 2001;103:2637–2643.

Specialized Facilities for Adults with Congenital Heart Disease

JOSEPH K. PERLOFF ▪ PAMELA D. MINER ▪ LINDA HOUSER

Specialized facilities for adults with congenital heart disease include tertiary care, training, education, and research—a combination difficult, if not impossible, to duplicate in hospitals not so designed.[1] This chapter focuses on the faculty, patient population, cardiac and noncardiac consultants, outpatient and inpatient services, noninvasive and imaging laboratories, diagnostic and interventional catheterization laboratories, and the opportunities for training, education, and research.

FACULTY AND PATIENT POPULATION

The faculty includes medical (adult) and pediatric cardiologists, cardiac surgeons, nurse practitioners, and physician assistants. The faculty functions most effectively when engaged in collaborative efforts in a university hospital in which intellectual interchange, teaching, and research are as paramount as optimal patient care.

Close association with pediatric cardiologists is essential despite the evolution of a generation of cardiologists with specialized training and expertise in adult congenital heart disease (ACHD).[2,3] This evolution is altogether appropriate because existing resources are insufficient to cope with the current and projected numbers of adults with congenital heart disease.[4,5] A glance at the figures shows why this is so.

Eighty-five percent of infants born with congenital heart disease in developed countries are expected to reach adulthood. In the United States today, there are already more adults with congenital heart disease then there are infants and children. With current and projected advances in surgical techniques and in catheter-based interventions, the numbers are expected to increase at a rate of 5% per year.[6] It is conservatively estimated that there are 800,000 adults with congenital heart disease in the United States, with a top estimate in excess of a million. More than half of these patients have moderate to complex disease that requires long-term care in specialized tertiary facilities.[4,6-9] Because of relative geographic mobility, it is unlikely that these patients will remain under the care of their pediatric cardiologists, whose numbers in any event are insufficient to cope with the current and projected adult patient population.[4,5,8,9] There are more than 10 times more board-certified medical cardiologists in the United States than board-certified pediatric cardiologists, but despite the abundant supply, medical cardiologists for the most part have little interest in or knowledge of congenital heart disease, and pediatric cardiologists are generally not trained in acquired heart diseases of adults.[9,10]

The professional personnel in ACHD facilities must be well versed in the arcane language of congenital heart disease and must understand the diverse manifestations of the disorders; the reparative and palliative surgical procedures; the postoperative residua and sequalae; the cardiovascular and general medical illnesses that adults with congenital heart disease acquire during the course of aging; the related echocardiographic, hemodynamic, electrophysiologic, and angiographic information; and the current imaging techniques.

Infants and children with congenital heart disease have, as a rule, one illness—their congenital malformation—but this singularity is replaced in adults by a complex interplay between the preoperative or postoperative congenital cardiac disease and acquired cardiac and noncardiac diseases. Surgeons trained largely, if not exclusively, in acquired heart disease of adults are seldom equipped to deal with congenital malformations of the heart, especially complex ones. However, surgeons with the knowledge and skills necessary to deal with congenital heart disease can generally adapt those advantages to coexisting acquired heart disease so that two cardiac surgeons are not required to perform one operation.[10]

Nurse practitioners (NPs) and physician assistants (PAs) are recognized by the American College of Cardiology and the 2001 Bethesda Conference as key members of ACHD faculties.[10] NPs with master's degrees often have training in pediatric and medical cardiology and further specialize in ACHD. Qualified NPs take comprehensive histories, perform physical examinations, order and interpret diagnostic information, implement or modify treatment regimens, and are authorized to write prescriptions in many states.[11] They also counsel and educate patients, collaborate in research, and assume administrative responsibilities.[12-15] PAs are certified to assume responsibilities similar to those of NPs.[16]

ACHD cardiologists use their time more effectively when an NP or PA assists in the coordination of outpatient and inpatient care. NPs or PAs (also known as "mid-level" providers), oversee inpatient management including treatment plans under the supervision of an attending cardiologist, facilitate communication with community physicians, provide discharge planning and education, and maintain a seamless link between patients and their cardiac providers in an outpatient setting. NPs and PAs monitor exercise tests and pacemaker/implantable cardioverter defibrillator interrogations, understand echocardiographic interpretations, and assist in the cardiac catheterization laboratory.[10]

One of the most demanding aspects of care for adults with congenital heart disease is the unending need to deal with the sum of physical, psychological, and emotional burdens[17] (see Chapter 13). Although cardiologists are sensitive to these issues, they often require help from a consulting psychiatrist. Alternatively, psychosocial problems can fall within the expertise of the NP or PA, who can provide counseling or referral.[19]

Adults with congenital heart disease all too often have major gaps in knowledge and understanding of their disorder.[18] NPs or PAs counsel patients regarding lifestyle, exercise, diet, smoking cessation, endocarditis prophylaxis, contraception, pregnancy, and insurability and play a major role in the transition of patients from a pediatric to an adult congenital cardiac facility.[20]

Appropriate use of NPs or PAs is a key factor in reducing the frequency of hospital admissions and emergency department visits, improving patient compliance and satisfaction, and minimizing morbidity caused by patients' inadequate understanding of their medical management.

Supervising patients for data collection, knowledge of research protocols, and oversight of databases provide the necessary backdrops for successful investigations. Collaboration in multicenter research is an important responsibility of the NP or PA.

CARDIAC AND NONCARDIAC CONSULTANTS

Consultants formally affiliated with an ACHD facility rapidly gain experience with the special problems about which they will be called on to consult. Ad hoc advice is often misleading, even when given by otherwise qualified consultants. Quality of care suffers when access to specialists is restricted and when general physicians unrealistically broaden the scope of their care.[21]

The list of cardiac and noncardiac consultants is long but worth stating (in alphabetical order): advanced cardiac imaging, anesthesiology, cardiac pathology, cardiovascular surgery, developmental biology, electrophysiology, general surgery, genetics, hematology, infectious disease, interventional catheterization, nephrology, obstetrics, gynecology, pathology, psychiatry, pulmonary medicine, and rheumatology.[22,23] A cardiac pathologist with expertise in congenital heart disease underscores the important role still played by the postmortem examination despite the current array of impressive imaging modalities.

Children are not small adults, and adults are not large children. Patients with congenital heart disease can qualify as adults at age 18 years or when judged to have reached appropriate psychological and physical maturity. However, the transition is not necessarily clear. Some postadolescents are too immature to warrant transfer, whereas occasional mature preadolescents look on themselves as young adults. Every effort must be taken to avoid reinforcing a sense of immature dependency by unnecessarily delaying the transition to adult care (see Chapter 13).

Adolescents are sui generis— a special category requiring special expertise. The American Board of Pediatrics considers adolescent medicine as a certified subspecialty, and there is subcertification for house officers who complete training in general medicine and pediatrics. The *Archives of Pediatrics and Adolescent Medicine* reflects this interest.

Referrals to an ACHD facility in a university hospital often originate from pediatric cardiology in the same institution. It is reassuring for patients know that their pediatric cardiologists will be kept abreast of their progress and will periodically see them as outpatients or inpatients, albeit in an adult setting. Referrals from outside the parent institution are from general physicians, general pediatricians, family practitioners, and general cardiologists. Patients referred directly to a cardiac surgeon should be seen by a cardiologist in the ACHD facility in anticipation of or during admission for operation.

OUTPATIENT SERVICES

Adults with congenital heart disease are best managed in an adult setting whether outpatient or inpatient. Pediatric cardiology clinics reinforce a sense of dependency that must be overcome if patients are to function as mature adults (see earlier in this chapter and Chapter 13).

The location of the outpatient clinic and its nursing staff should be the same for each visit insofar as possible to provide patients with a sense of familiarity, continuity, and security. Outpatient laboratories, especially echocardiography, should be readily accessible to the clinic area. Clinical laboratories should be nearby and staffed with personnel who are acquainted with the special techniques that apply to specimens from adults with congenital heart disease (see Chapter 12). Transcutaneous fingertip pulse oximetry for systemic arterial oxygen saturation should be readily available and routinely obtained. The nursing staff should be responsive to the occasional need for phlebotomy and with the techniques employed (see Chapter 12).

Follow-up and consultation reports should be dictated by staff cardiologists, NPs, or PAs to ensure high-quality documents that serve as reliable components of a computerized database and that provide educational, as well as practical, information for referring physicians (discussed subsequently). Patients should be given Personal Health Passports, as recommended in Chapter 2, to ensure ready access to accurate up-to-date information if they relocate or present in an emergency department.

INPATIENT SERVICES

Inpatient policy depends in large part on whether medicine and pediatrics share the same hospital. When that is the case, adults with congenital heart disease are admitted to adult inpatient facilities under the care of an ACHD cardiologist.

Inpatients include elective and emergency admissions for cardiac or noncardiac surgery, for cardiac intensive care which is usually electrophysiologic, less often heart failure, for coexisting general medical illnesses, and for labor and delivery. When inpatients are referred directly to a cardiac surgeon, an ACHD staff cardiologist should serve as the attending cardiologist before and after operation. Upon discharge, the NP or PA arranges follow-up appointments. The referring physician receives an immediate telephone call followed by a discharge summary. The cardiac surgeon sends operative reports separately.

NONINVASIVE AND IMAGING LABORATORIES

Echocardiography laboratories are staffed by cardiologists and technologists equally adept at transthoracic and transesophageal techniques (see Chapter 6). Technologists must have training and expertise in preoperative and postoperative ACHD. Laboratories employing current and evolving magnetic resonance and computerized tomography imaging are the topics of Chapter 7.

DIAGNOSTIC AND INTERVENTIONAL CATHETERIZATION LABORATORIES

Diagnostic catheterization, electrophysiologic, and angiographic laboratories for adults with congenital heart disease must maintain standards set by pediatric cardiology laboratories. Assignment of patients to a pediatric or adult interventional catheterization laboratory should be individualized according to specific therapeutic needs and according to the skill and experience of the interventional cardiologist, who is more important than the laboratory in which the procedure is performed.

TRAINING, EDUCATION, AND RESEARCH

A major responsibility of an ACHD facility is the training and education of fellows, residents, NPs, and PAs. Medical cardiology fellows should have block assignments devoted to inpatient and outpatient pediatric and ACHD. Similarly, pediatric cardiology fellows should have assignments in ACHD to familiarize them with the long-term consequences of decisions made during infancy and childhood. If pediatric cardiologists fail to take advantage of this opportunity, important insights into the decision-making process are lost. The ultimate justification for therapeutic decisions in infants and children is long-term survival and quality of life in the adult with congenital heart disease.[3]

Education extends to community physicians, visiting cardiologists, and the patients themselves. The ACHD facility should be responsive to cardiologists who wish to continue their medical education by attending outpatient clinics and inpatient activities. Practicing physicians must be made aware that the care of adults with congenital heart disease requires special expertise seldom available in community hospitals. Their patients can then be channeled to appropriate tertiary care facilities.

A major step forward is the Adult Congenital Heart Association, the first national advocacy resource for this patient population (see Chapter 2). Adults with congenital heart disease now have access to a wealth of reliable information via the Internet.

Visits to an ACHD facility should be an educational opportunity for the patient and his or her family. The extra time taken to clarify terminology and answer questions is a requisite in the care of adults with congenital heart disease.

The UCLA Adult Congenital Heart Disease Center has long maintained a dual record system, with one set of records readily available to the staff of the center and a second set available in hospital files. Electronic storage and computer retrieval are modifying but not replacing this policy. When patients move to another geographic area, the Personal Health Passport ensures that their records move with them. Patients are responsible emissaries.

FUNCTIONAL CLASSIFICATIONS

The New York Heart Association Functional Classification, introduced in 1964, was based on the absence, presence, and degree of symptoms according to the norm of "ordinary physical activity."[24] Subsequent revisions of the classification, for all practical purposes, dealt with ischemic heart disease and with the heart failure of acquired heart disease.[25,26] The more detailed Canadian Cardiovascular Society Functional Classification (1972) was analogous.[27] Modifications of these two classifications have been proposed because of the need to include variables in addition to symptoms, the need to resolve whether symptoms should be "generalized" or "particularized," and to decide whether functional status should be supplemented by prognosis.[28] If the term *functional* is to be retained, the classification must necessarily deal with *function*. New terms should be avoided when established terms suffice. Simplicity encourages acceptance. Emphasis on symptoms in the New York Heart Association and Canadian Cardiovascular Society Classifications was highly successful. That emphasis should be retained. The Functional Classification in Table 3–1 is recommended.

Physical activity best refers to ordinary activities that sustain a satisfactory quality of everyday life as perceived by the patient. Symptoms should be considered in general rather than in specific terms to encompass the many and often unusual causes unique to congenital heart disease, as well as causes due to the acquired heart diseases that accrue with age. A functional classification appropriate for adults with congenital heart disease must take into account a diverse population that includes cyanotic and acyanotic patients who have not undergone cardiac surgery or interventional catheterization, patients who have undergone cardiac surgery or interventional catheterization and require no further intervention, those who have had palliative procedures in anticipation of reparative surgery, and those who are inoperable apart from organ transplantation.

Adult congenital heart disease facilities, especially in university hospitals, must be committed to research prompted by a desire to address unresolved questions inherent in this patient population. Research experience must be provided for fellows with career interests in ACHD. Investigations typically require collaboration with colleagues in other disciplines, thus stimulating valuable interdisciplinary interchange. A rich harvest is in store when advantage is taken of these opportunities.[29]

References

1. Perloff JK. Congenital heart disease after childhood: an expanding patient population. 22nd Bethesda Conference. *J Am Coll Cardiol.* 1991;18:311.
2. Ritchie JL, Cheitlin MD, Hlatky MA, et al. Task Force 5: profile of the cardiovascular specialist: trends in needs and supply and implications for the future. *J Am Coll Cardiol.* 1994;24:275.
3. Skorton DJ, Cheitlin MD, Freed MD, et al. Training in the care of adult patients with congenital heart disease. *J Am Coll Cardiol.* 1995;25:31–33.
4. Hoffman J, Kaplan S, Liberthson RR. Prevalence of congenital heart disease. *Am Heart J.* 2004;147:425–439.
5. Gurvitz MZ, Chang RK, Ramos FJ, et al. Variations in adult congenital heart disease training in adult and pediatric cardiology fellowship programs. *J Am Coll Cardiol.* 2005;46:893–898.
6. Warnes, CA, Liberthson, R., Danielson GK. Task Force 1: the changing profile of congenital heart disease in adult life. *J Am Coll Cardiol.* 2001;37:1170–1175.
7. Niwa K, Perloff JK, Webb GD. Survey of specialized tertiary care facilities for adults with congenital heart disease. *Int J Cardiol.* 2004;96:211–216.
8. Moller JH, Gaubert KA, Allan HD, et al. Cardiovascular health and disease in children: current status. *Circulation.* 1994;89:923.
9. 1993 Heart and Stroke Facts Statistics. Dallas: American Heart Association, 1992.
10. Child JS, Collins-Nakai RL, Alpert JS, et al. Task Force 3: workforce description and educational requirements for the care of adults with congenital heart disease. *J Am Coll Cardiol.* 2001;5:1183–1187.
11. Pearson LJ. Annual update of how each state stands on legislative issues affecting advanced nursing practice. *Nurs Pract.* 1995;20:13.
12. Moodie DS. Adult congenital heart disease. *Curr Opin Cardiol.* 1994;9:137.
13. Canobbio MM, Day MJ. The role of the clinical specialist in an adult congenital heart disease program. *Nurs Clin North Am.* 1994;29:357.
14. Cronin C, Maklebust J. Case-managed care: capitalizing on the CNS. *Nurs Manage.* 1989;20:38.
15. Davies B. Clarification of advanced nursing practice: characteristics and competencies. *Clin Nurs Spec.* 1995;9:156.
16. Dracup K, DeBusk RF, DeMots H, et al. Task Force 3: partnerships in delivery of cardiovascular care. *J Am Coll Cardiol.* 1994;24:296.
17. Foster E, Graham TP, Driscoll DJ, et al. Task Force 2: special health care needs of adults with congenital heart disease. *J Am Coll Cardiol.* 2001;5:1176–1183.
18. Moons P, De Volder E, Budts W, et al. What do adult patients know about their disease, treatment, and prevention of complications? A call for structured patient education. *Heart.* 2001;86:74–80.
19. Moons P, De Geest S, Budts W. Comprehensive care for adults with congenital heart disease: expanding roles for nurses. *Eur J Cardiovasc. Nurs* 2002;1:23–28.
20. Van Deyk K, Moons P, Gewilling M, Budts W. Educational and behavioral issues in transitioning from pediatric cardiology to adult centered health care. *Nurs Clin North Am.* 2004;39:755–768.
21. Kassirer JP. Access to specialty care. *N Engl J Med.* 1994;331:1151.
22. Landzberg MJ, Murphy DJ, Davidson WR, et al. Task Force 4: organization of delivery systems for adults with congenital heart disease. *J Am Coll Cardiol.* 2001;5:1187–1193.

Table 3–1 UCLA Congenital Heart Disease Functional Classification (Presence and Degree of Symptoms)

Class 1	Asymptomatic at all levels of activity
Class 2	Symptoms are present but do not curtail average, everyday activity
Class 3	Symptoms significantly curtail most but not all average, everyday activity
Class 4	Symptoms significantly curtail virtually all average, everyday activity and may be present at rest

23. Webb CL, Jenkins KJ, Karpawich PP. Collaborative care for adults with congenital heart disease. *Circulation.* 2002;105:2318–2323.

24. The Criteria Committee of the New York Heart Association. *Diseases of the Heart and Blood Vessels: Nomenclature and Criteria for Diagnosis.* 6 ed. Boston, Little, Brown, 1964.

25. Harvey RM, Doyle EF, Ellis K., et al. Major changes made by the Criteria Committee of the New York Heart Association. *Circulation.* 1974;49:390.

26. The Criteria Committee of the New York Heart Association. *Nomenclature and Criteria for Diagnosis of the Diseases of Heart and Great Vessels.* 8 ed. New York, New York Heart Association/Little, Brown, 1979.

27. Campeau L. Grading of angina pectoris. *Circulation.* 1976;54:522.

28. Goldman L, Hashimoto B, Cook EF, Loscalzo A. Comparative reproducibility and validity of systems for assessing cardiovascular functional class: advantages of a new specific activity scale. *Circulation.* 1981;64:1227.

29. Mackie, AS, Pilote L, Ionescu-Ittu R, et al. Health care resource utilization in adults with congenital heart disease. *Am J Cardiol.* 2007;99:839–843.

SURVIVAL PATTERNS

Survival Patterns Without Cardiac Surgery or Interventional Catheterization: A Narrowing Base

JOSEPH K. PERLOFF

This chapter deals with common and uncommon defects in which unoperated adult survival is either expected or exceptional. It must be made clear at the outset that *unoperated* is not synonymous with *natural history,* and *unnatural* should not be applied to postoperative survival patterns. Surgeons should not be cast in the role of perpetrators of the unnatural.

The *Oxford Dictionary of Natural History* defines the term *natural* as "a community that would develop if human influences were removed completely and permanently."[1] More focused and more relevant to the topic of this chapter is Julien Hoffman's definition: "The natural history of any disease is a description of what happens to people with the disease who do not receive treatment for it." Yet publications carry titles with wordings such as "natural history: results of treatment."[2] Pharmacologic therapeutics are not natural. Anticoagulants are not natural. Pacemakers are not natural. Electrical cardioversion and defibrillation are not natural. Radiofrequency ablation is not natural. The term *natural history* is therefore a misnomer and is inappropriate in contemporary medicine.

Maude Abbott's *Atlas of Congenital Cardiac Diseases* (1936) was a landmark in the orderly classification of the malformations and was also an invaluable source of longevity before the advent of cardiac surgery.[3] Survival patterns for unoperated adults with congenital heart disease are shown in Table 4–1 and include malformations that do not require operation (Table 4–2), malformations that are amenable to operation in adulthood, and mal-

formations that are inoperable apart from organ transplantation. Medical management of unoperated adults with congenital heart disease deals not only with the congenital cardiac malformations per se but also with acquired disorders of the heart and circulation and with noncardiovascular illnesses that coexist and modify the physiologic and clinical expressions of the basic congenital anomaly.

BICUSPID AORTIC VALVE

Congenitally malformed aortic valves can be unicuspid, bicuspid, tricuspid, or quadricuspid.[4-6] A bicuspid aortic valve (Fig. 4–1) is the most common congenital anomaly to which that structure is subject and one of the most common gross morphologic congenital anomalies of the heart or great arteries.[4,5,7-11] Incidence of congenital bicuspid aortic valves in the general population is approximately 1% to 2% with a 2:1 male:female ratio.[9,11] Prevalence in the United States is approximately 4 million. In patients 15 years or older, a bicuspid aortic valve accounts for 98% of congenital aortic valve malformations.[4,5] Three percent of congenitally malformed aortic valves are unicuspid, and less than 1% are tricuspid or quadricuspid (discussed later).[6]

Congenital bicuspid aortic valves do not result simply from nonseparation of cusps but are a complex developmental process. Normal aortic valves are composed of a

Table 4-1   Congenital Heart Disease in Adults—Unoperated Survival

Common Defects
1. Expected adult survival
2. Exceptional adult survival
Uncommon Defects
1. Expected adult survival
2. Exceptional adult survival

Table 4-2   Congenital Heart Diseases That Do Not Require Operation

Situs inversus or situs solitus with dextrocardia (uncomplicated)
Functionally normal bicuspid aortic valve
Mild pulmonary valve stenosis
Idiopathic dilatation of the pulmonary trunk
Congenital pulmonary valve regurgitation (mild to moderate)
Isolated left superior vena cava
Isolated inferior vena caval interruption with azygous continuation
Isolated right aortic arch
Isolated anomalous connection of a single pulmonary vein
Small interatrial communication (usually sinus venosus)
Ventricular septal defect, spontaneously closed or nearly closed
Mild Ebstein's anomaly without Wolff-Parkinson-White bypass tracts
Uncomplicated congenitally corrected transposition of the great
   arteries

connective tissue framework of interstitial cells and a matrix covered by endothelial cells. During valvulogenesis, extracellular matrix proteins govern cell differentiation and cusp formation. Differentiation of mesenchymal cells into mature aortic valve cells correlates with the expression of the matrix protein fibrillin-1, which is deficient in bicuspid aortic valve tissue.[12] Inadequate fibrillin-1 expression during valvulogenesis disrupts normal formation of aortic cusps and can result in a bicuspid aortic valve. How does a bicuspid aortic valve function? Why does it fail? Distensibility of the aortic root permits a normal closed trileaflet aortic valve to open as a triangle and then as a circle without causing flexion deformity of cuspal tissue. Endothelial cells on the ventricular surface of the valve are, however, subjected to high mechanical stress. For a bicuspid aortic valve, in contrast to a normal trileaflet aortic valve, opening and closing stress are modified by inherently abnormal histology and ultrastructure whether the bicuspid valve is functionally normal, stenotic, or incompetent. Cuspal inequality inherent in a bicuspid aortic valve exaggerates the mechanical stress during opening and closing, predisposing the valve to fibrocalcific transformation (Fig. 4–1, B), which is an active process that is also influenced by atherosclerotic risk factors amenable to the salutatory effects of statins.

The bicuspid aortic cusps are oriented in either an anteroposterior or a right-to-left arrangement[7,11] (Fig. 4–2). When the two cusps are anteroposterior, both coronary arteries arise on the side of the anterior sinus. When the

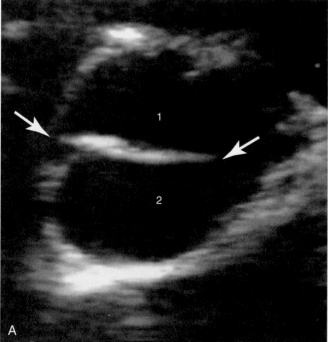

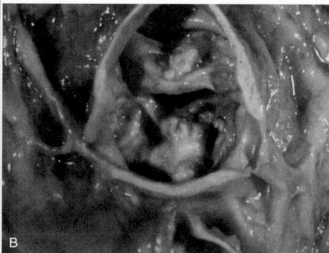

FIGURE 4-1   **(A)** Short-axis echocardiographic image of a functionally normal bicuspid aortic valve in a 13-year-old boy. A single diastolic closure line *(arrows)* separates two cusps (1, 2) that are in an anteroposterior relationship. **(B)** Necropsy specimen from a patient with severe bicuspid aortic stenosis. The two cusps are thickened and calcified. There is a calcified false raphe (FR) at the lower rim. *(Courtesy of William C. Roberts, MD, National Heart, Lung and Blood Institute, Bethesda, MD.)*

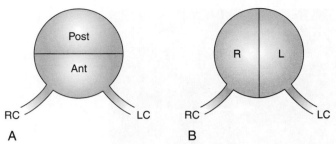

FIGURE 4-2 Origin of the coronary ostia with a bicuspid aortic valve. **(A)** When the two cusps are posteroanterior, both the right (RC) and the left (LCA) coronary arteries originate in the sinus of the anterior cusp. **(B)** When the two cusps are oriented right-left, the RC and the LCA each arise concordantly from the right coronary sinus (R) and the left coronary sinus (L).

bicuspid arrangement is right-to-left, the two coronary arteries arise concordantly from the right and left sinuses.[7,13] A distinctive fibrous tissue ridge, the false raphe, resides at the peripheral margin of one cusp (see Fig. 4-1, *B*), but occasionally the raphe extends to the free edge and sometimes consists of a fenestrated strand that runs from the aortic wall to the free edge.[9,11] Bicuspid aortic valves can be functionally normal, that is, nonstenotic with minimal or no regurgitation. Functionally normal bicuspid aortic valves may remain so throughout a normal life span, but as a rule, the cusps undergo fibrocalcific thickening with progressive obstruction, which accounts for approximately half of surgical cases of isolated calcific aortic stenosis in adults.[4,5,7,9,10,14,15] Fibrocalcific transformation of a bicuspid aortic valve tends to be more prevalent when the right and noncoronary cusps are fused, whereas coarctation of the aorta is more prevalent when fusion is in the right and left coronary cusps.[7] Exceptionally, one of the cusps can be aneurysmal.[16]

Functionally normal bicuspid aortic valves are usually mildly incompetent because the free edge of one or both cusps must be sufficiently longer than the diameter of the aortic ring to permit unobstructed antegrade flow. Not surprisingly, bicuspid aortic valves with marked cuspal inequality and little or no fibrocalcific derangement are more likely to develop pure regurgitation,[4] which is the most prevalent form of chronic severe aortic regurgitation in adults.[5,17] Survival depends on the degree and chronicity of regurgitant flow and on the adaptive response of the left ventricle to volume overload[4] (see Chapter 21). Progression is usually insidious, but a functionally normal bicuspid aortic valve can be rendered suddenly and severely incompetent by infective endocarditis to which the structure is highly susceptible,[15] a point emphasized by William Osler over a century ago and reaffirmed by Maude Abbott[3] (see Chapter 8).

Maude Abbott wrote in 1928, "The presence of a bicuspid aortic valve appears to indicate, at least in a portion of the cases in which it occurs, a tendency for spontaneous rupture." In the same year, Gsell coined the term

"medionecrosis," and in 1930, Erdheim referred to "medionecrosis aortae idiopathica cystica."[18] Cystic medionecrosis soon became part of the medical vocabulary, but the term is open to question because the so-called cysts are in fact noncystic medial structural faults, and necrosis is rare. The ascending aortic media above a congenitally bicuspid aortic valve is abnormal whether the valve is functionally normal, stenotic, or incompetent, that is, irrespective of the functional state of the valve, because the medial structural fault is inherently associated with the bicuspid condition of the valve.[18-21] The fibrillin-1 deficiency found in bicuspid aortic leaflets is also expressed in the ascending aortic media.[12] These associations imply that the bicuspid aortic valve is one component of a genetically determined disease of the thoracic aorta. "Poststenotic" dilatation is therefore a misnomer. The turbulence of bicuspid aortic stenosis and the increased pulsatile flow of bicuspid aortic regurgitation promote further dilatation but are not primarily causative.

The clinical course of patients with a bicuspid aortic valve is sometimes dramatically punctuated by a dissecting aortic aneurysm[18] (Fig. 4-3, *A*), which abruptly and significantly affects morbidity and longevity. In XO Turner's syndrome, aortic dilatation with rupture is dramatic and fatal and occurs with or without a bicuspid aortic valve (see Fig. 4-3, *B*). Noonan's syndrome, sometimes called Turner phenotype (see Fig. 4-3, *C*), is rarely complicated by ascending aortic dilatation and dissection.[22]

UNICUSPID AORTIC VALVE

These valves are acommissural or unicommissural[10] and have an even greater male prevalence than bicuspid aortic valves.[11] The *acommissural* type is characterized by a single leaflet with a stenotic central orifice and three rudimentary commissures that do not divide the valve.[10] The *unicommissural* type is characterized by a single leaflet with a single commissural attachment to the aortic wall.[10,23,24] Acommissural unicuspid aortic valves are rare at any age, whereas unicommissural unicuspid aortic valves are uncommon if not rare after infancy. The typical unicommissural valve is intrinsically stenotic at birth, but if the free edge is sufficiently redundant and the single commissure is not fused, obstruction may initially be mild or absent, developing later in life when valve mobility is reduced by fibrosis and calcification[23] (Fig. 4-4). Of 21 adults with calcific unicuspid aortic valve stenosis, the average age was 25 years, with nine patients older than 50 years.[23]

QUADRICUSPID AORTIC VALVE

Isolated quadricuspid aortic valves are rare and usually function normally in early life despite cuspal inequality.[6,25-28] When a quadricuspid aortic valve functions

FIGURE 4-3 **(A)** Transesophageal echocardiogram from a 37-year-old male with a bicuspid aortic valve (BAV) and a dissecting aneurysm of the ascending aorta (Ao). The flap of the dissection moved freely within the dilated aortic root. LVOT, left ventricular outflow tract. **(B)** Aortogram (digital vascular image) from a 28-year-old woman with 45 XO Turner syndrome. The ascending aortic aneurysm (Asc Ao) ruptured 8 weeks later. DA, descending aorta; LV, left ventricle. **(C)** 24-year-old man with Noonan's syndrome (46 XY), who experienced a dissecting aneurysm of the ascending aorta. *(From Shachter, N., Perloff, J.K., and Mulder, D.G.: Aortic dissection in Noonan's syndrome (46XY Turner). Am J Cardiol 1984;54:465.)*

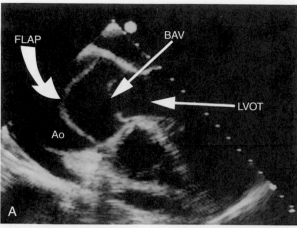

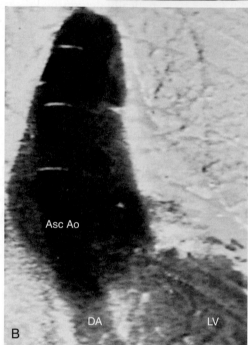

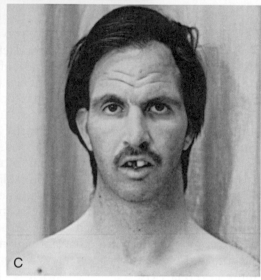

abnormally, the derangement is almost always regurgitation, which is seldom significant until adulthood.[25,27,29] Occasionally, a functionally normal isolated quadricuspid aortic valve is found incidentally at necropsy or on echocardiography (Fig. 4–5).

COARCTATION OF THE AORTA

Coarctation of the aorta tends to cause symptoms either in early infancy or after the beginning of the third or fourth decade.[13,30]

The majority of patients who survive infancy reach adulthood, but appreciable attrition begins by age 20 years, and more than three fourths of unoperated patients die by age 50 years.[30-33] Sporadic examples of exceptional longevity should not obscure the inherent risks that significantly limit life span.[32,34-37] Figure 4–6 is from two patients with

coarctation of the aorta, one aged 47 years and the other aged 70 years, who had virtually complete obstruction at the coarctation site. The longest recorded survivor was a 92-year-old man reported by Reynaud in 1828.[35] A variation on the theme—isolated *atresia* of the aortic arch—was reported in a 65-year-old man.[37]

Morbidity and mortality in adults with aortic coarctation are influenced by certain predictable coexisting congenital or acquired cardiac and vascular disorders.[30,32-34,38-42] The most common associated congenital malformation is a bicuspid aortic valve that superimposes its own inherent risks (see earlier discussion). A potentially lethal but uncommon coexisting anomaly is a congenital aneurysm of the circle of Willis that characteristically announces itself by rupture (see Chapter 14).[39,42] The majority of patients who die from cerebral hemorrhage do so in the second or third decade.[32,36,39,42] Systemic hypertension does not necessarily predispose

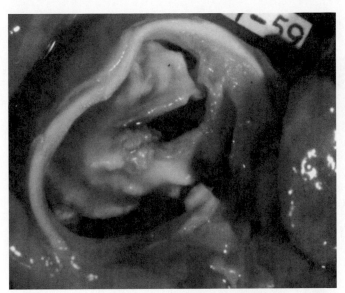

FIGURE 4-4   Calcified unicommissural unicuspid aortic valve in a 47-year-old man.

to rupture of a cerebral aneurysm because hemorrhage may occur in normotensive patients long after successful repair of coarctation (see Chapter 14).[13,43] Rupture of the aorta or dissecting aneurysm is a dramatic complication of aortic coarctation, with peak incidence in the third and fourth decades.[32,36,38]

The paracoarctation aorta harbors medial abnormalities qualitatively similar to those of Marfan's syndrome and those of great arterial wall in congenital heart disease.[18,44-46] The abnormalities are inherent because they are present in neonates and are identical in the high-pressure, low-velocity proximal paracoarctation segment and in the low-pressure, high-velocity distal segment.[18] Pregnancy increases the risk of aortic rupture by superimposing the medial changes that characterize gestation upon the medial abnormalities of the paracoarctation aorta (see Chapter 9). Ascending aortic dissection coincides with the presence of a bicuspid aortic valve (see earlier discussion). Left ventricular failure in patients with unoperated coarctation follows a bimodal probability curve, with two thirds of patients either younger than age 1 year or older than age 40 years.[36]

FIXED SUBAORTIC STENOSIS

Fixed or discrete subaortic stenosis accounts for 15% to 20% of all types of congenital obstruction to left ventricular outflow and occurs in two principal varieties.[13,47,48] The first variety is characterized by a thin, fibrous, crescent-shaped membrane located immediately below the aortic valve[10,47-51] (Fig. 4-7). The less common variety is called *tunnel* or *tubular* subaortic stenosis because it is represented by a long, narrow fibromuscular channel occupying several centimeters within the left ventricular outflow tract.[49,52-54] In both varieties of subaortic stenosis, aortic cusp abnormalities result from proximity of the subaortic obstruction to the aortic leaflets and from injury to the leaflets caused by the eccentric jet.

Fixed subaortic stenosis as just defined can evolve from little or no gradient to appreciable obstruction, but once present, the obstruction tends to be progressive.[52,53,55,56] The change with age is one of both degree

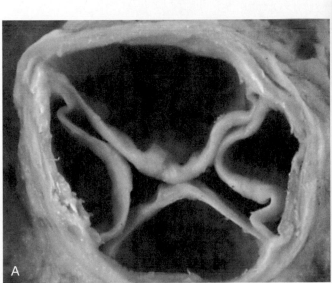
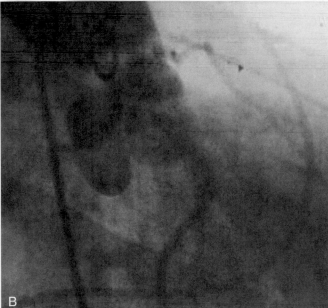

FIGURE 4-5   **(A)** Isolated quadricuspid aortic valve that was an incidental finding at necropsy in a 56-year-old man. **(B)** Isolated quadricuspid aortic valve found incidentally during thoracic aortography in a 62-year-old man.

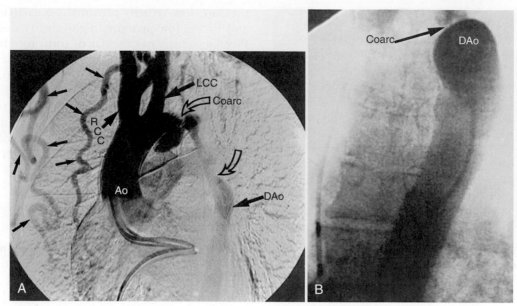

FIGURE 4-6 **(A)** Angiogram with contrast medium injected into the ascending aorta (Ao) of a 47-year-old man with coarctation of the aorta (Coarc). The right common carotid (RCC) and left common carotid (LCC) arteries are visualized, but the left subclavian artery does not opacify because the coarctation compromised its orifice. Accordingly, the collateral arterial circulation was unilateral on the right *(unlabeled small black arrows)*. A long hypoplastic segment of aorta is shown distal to the coarctation *(unlabeled open arrows)*. DAo, descending aorta. **(B)** Contrast injection into the descending aorta (DAo) of a 70-year-old woman with virtually complete obstruction of the site of coarctation of the aorta (Coarc).

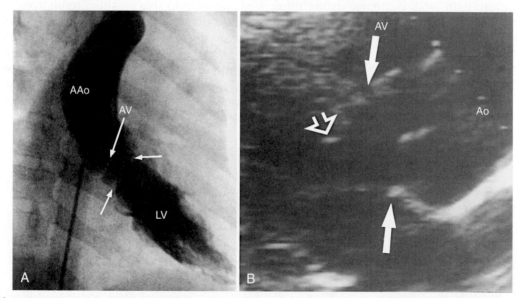

FIGURE 4-7 **(A)** Angiocardiogram from a 13-year-old boy with discrete subaortic stenosis, a systolic gradient of 40 mm Hg, and mild aortic regurgitation. The unmarked paired arrows identify a localized zone of stenosis just beneath the aortic valve (AV). The ascending aorta (AAo) is only moderately dilatated. LV, left ventricle. **(B)** Two-dimensional echocardiogram (parasternal long axis) from a 27-year-old man with a nonobstructive subaortic membrane *(open arrow)* that was relatively remote from the AV *(paired arrows)*. There was no aortic regurgitation. Ao, aortic root.

(severity) and morphology.[48,50] The magnitude of obstruction sometimes progresses rapidly.[55] The fibromembranous variety accounts for 11% to 15% of patients younger than age 40 years, whereas tunnel subaortic stenosis seldom occurs in adults.[47,48] Average longevity of fixed discrete subaortic stenosis was 35 years in one necropsy study.[51] Our oldest patient was a 54-year-old man.[57] The cumulative risk of progressive aortic regurgitation provides a substrate for infective endocarditis (see Chapter 8). In contrast to rapid progression in infants and children, both of these varieties of fixed subaortic stenosis progress slowly in adults.

SUPRAVALVE AORTIC STENOSIS

This form of aortic stenosis, the least common variety of congenital obstruction to left ventricle outflow, is characterized by a localized hourglass narrowing immediately above the aortic sinuses associated with thickening of the aortic media and fibrous intimal proliferation.[7,10] Supravalvular aortic stenosis can be *familial* or *nonfamilial* and sporadic.[13] In addition to the degree of stenosis, three features influence longevity: (1) the condition of the extramural coronary arteries, (2) the condition of the aortic leaflets, and (3) the association with Williams syndrome.

Obstruction, even obliteration, of a coronary ostium can result from adherence of a distorted aorta leaflet or by extension of aortic medial proliferation[10,58] (Fig. 4–8). Because the coronary ostia are proximal to the zone of supravalvular obstruction, the extramural coronary arteries are exposed to high left ventricle systolic pressure, which makes them prone to premature atherosclerosis.[10,59] In approximately one third of patients, the aortic leaflets are thickened, and occasionally a cusp is fused to the site of obstruction or to a coronary orifice.[10,59] Williams syndrome is characterized by supravalvular aortic stenosis, pulmonary artery stenosis, characteristic facial dysmorphism, mental retardation, infantile hypercalcemia, small stature, and a number of vascular anomalies that include renal or renovascular disorders and systemic hypertension.[60-68] The striking conceptual deficits in Williams syndrome are counterbalanced by exceptional auditory and musical skills that include a high incidence of absolute pitch.[69] Unoperated adult survival in Williams syndrome is uncommon if not rare, even when supravalvular aortic stenosis exists as an isolated cardiac malformation.[63,64,66]

EBSTEIN'S ANOMALY OF THE TRICUSPID VALVE

Longevity in unoperated Ebstein's anomaly ranges from intrauterine or neonatal death to asymptomatic survival into adulthood (Fig. 4–9) or advanced age.[70-91] The main factors governing survival beyond infancy are the degree of tricuspid regurgitation reflected in cardiac size, cyanosis (right-to-left interatrial shunt), and recurrent paroxysmal rapid heart action, especially when associated with bypass tracts.[73,75,77,81,86,90] Only 5% of patients live beyond the fifth decade, a figure that includes the 50% mortality in neonates, infants, and young children.[74,77,81,86,90,92,93] Intermittent or persistent cyanosis occurs in 50% to 80% of patients, but the presence and degree do not necessarily correlate with the symptomatic state.[76,81] However, after symptoms develop, disability tends to be progressive even in patients who had few or no symptoms until adolescence or adulthood. With advancing age, the enlarged right atrium predisposes to atrial fibrillation or atrial flutter, which with reentrant supraventricular tachycardia occur in approximately one third of patients (see Chapter 20).[74] The advent of chronic atrial fibrillation, even in patients without bypass tracts, generally predicts death within 5 years,[75] but accelerated conduction sets the stage for potential ventricular rates of

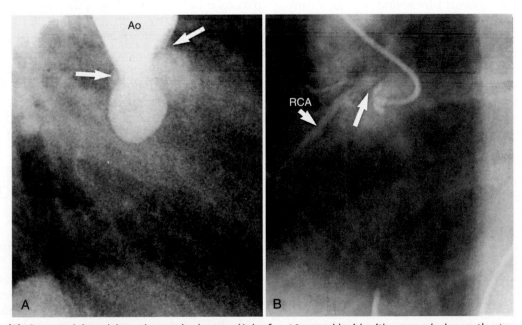

FIGURE 4-8   **(A)** Contrast injected into the proximal aorta (Ao) of a 16-year-old girl with supravalvular aortic stenosis *(paired arrows)*. **(B)** Obstruction *(unmarked arrow)* of the ostium of the right coronary artery (RCA) was caused by aortic medial proliferation. The right coronary artery was perfused by collaterals from the left coronary artery (not shown).

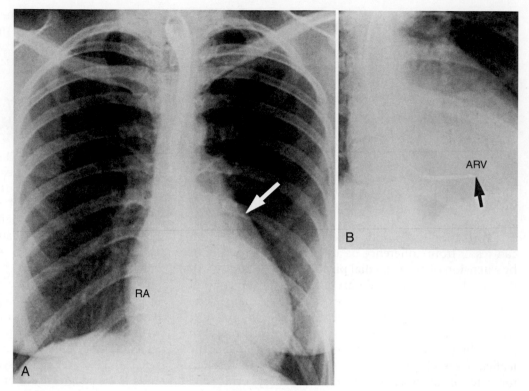

FIGURE 4–9 Radiographs from a 33-year-old woman with mild Ebstein's anomaly. **(A)** The film illustrates how close to normal the cardiac silhouette can appear. The left border is straightened by the infundibulum *(arrow)*. The right atrial (RA) contour is only slightly more prominent than normal. **(B)** The catheter tip *(arrow)* is in the atrialized right ventricle (ARV) far to the left of the sternal edge.

300 beats per minute, which are not long tolerated and can result in syncope or sudden death, a consequence believed to account for the drop-off in survival in the fifth decade.[74,75,94]

Bradyarrhythmias are uncommon despite PR interval prolongation and have little impact on morbidity and mortality.[74] One of our patients, a 56-year-old woman, had complete heart block, and only two similar cases have been reported.[80] In our case, pacemaker leads were attached to the left ventricular epicardium because of the risk of inducing ventricular tachycardia by stimulating the endocardium of the arrhythmogenic atrialized right ventricle (see Chapter 22).[95] Infective endocarditis is rare in patients with Ebstein's anomaly, presumably because of the low velocity of tricuspid regurgitant flow and the lack of a jet impact site (see Chapter 8).[74,80]

Despite qualifications, there are legendary accounts of astonishing longevity in patients with Ebstein's malformation. Survivals into the ninth decade have been reported.[70,72,73,81,84,88,90,96] Ebstein's anomaly was discovered at necropsy in a 75-year-old man who, as a youth, had been a lumberjack working on log booms.[70] He was asymptomatic until his 50s, when he was obliged to outrun an irate female bear. Twenty-five years later at necropsy, his tricuspid valve was found to be significantly malformed, and the right atrium was thin-walled and greatly dilatated. The oldest patient on record with Ebstein's anomaly had no cardiac symptoms until age 79 years and survived until age 85 years.[88]

UHL'S ANOMALY

Sometimes mistaken for Ebstein's malformation, Uhl's anomaly is characterized by a structurally normal and functionally competent tricuspid valve but with hypoplasia or aplasia of most, if not all, of the myocardium of the trabecular or inflow portion of the right ventricle.[97–100] In contrast to the electrically unstable atrialized right ventricle of Ebstein's anomaly, the parchment right ventricle of Uhl's anomaly is characteristically "inexcitable."[101] The Uhl right ventricle functions chiefly as a passive conduit from right atrium to pulmonary artery, with forward flow in response to brisk paradoxical movement of the ventricular septum.[97] Despite the functionally inadequate right ventricle, adult survival is the rule (Fig. 4–10).

CONGENITALLY CORRECTED TRANSPOSITION OF THE GREAT ARTERIES (VENTRICULAR INVERSION)

Longevity depends largely on the presence and degree of coexisting congenital cardiac malformations.[102–107] In isolated congenitally corrected transposition, longevity patterns are good (Fig. 4–11) but not normal because of the functional vulnerability of a subaortic morphologic right ventricle.[103] Incompetence of the inverted tricuspid valve caused by an Ebstein-like anomaly may be misdiagnosed as acquired mitral regurgitation[71,79] and serves to volume

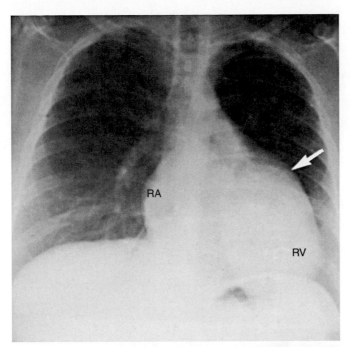

FIGURE 4-10 Radiograph from a 25-year-old woman with Uhl's anomaly. The thin-walled right ventricle (RV) is dilatated. The uninvolved infundibular portion *(arrow)* imparts a hump-shaped appearance to the left upper cardiac border. The right atrium (RA) is moderately enlarged.

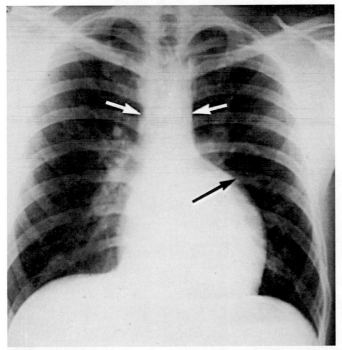

FIGURE 4-11 Radiograph from a 34-year-old man with congenitally corrected transposition of the great arteries and mild left atrioventricular valve regurgitation. The vascular pedicle is narrow *(paired white arrows)* because the ascending aorta rises vertically and anterior, and the pulmonary trunk is medial and posterior. The hump-shaped appearance of the left upper cardiac silhouette is caused by the inverted infundibulum *(black arrow)*.

overload the vulnerable systemic right ventricle. An important longevity variable is abnormal atrioventricular conduction that varies from PR interval prolongation to complete heart block (see Chapter 20). When all ages are included, more than 75% of patients with congenitally corrected transposition exhibit varying degrees of atrioventricular block, and approximately 30% develop complete heart block.[104,106,108-112] The accrued risk of complete atrioventricular block occurs at a rate as high as 2% per year.[102,103,110]

Survival into the sixth or seventh decade is uncommon but not unknown, with two patients reaching their eighth decade,[105,106,110,113-118] and two reaching age 80 years.[119,120] Clinically stable adults with uncomplicated congenitally corrected transposition and no acquired heart disease may develop failure of the morphologic right ventricle, an eventuality that may first become manifest during pregnancy in previously asymptomatic women.[13,121]

CONGENITAL MITRAL REGURGITATION

Regurgitation of an inverted right atrioventricular valve in congenitally corrected transposition of the great arteries is tricuspid, not mitral (see earlier discussion). Congenital mitral regurgitation is caused by accessory commissures with anomalous chordal insertions, congenital perforations, congenitally short or absent chordae, a cleft posterior mitral leaflet, or an isolated component of an atrioventricular septal defect.[13] Survival patterns depend on the degree of regurgitation, the adaptive response of the volume-loaded left ventricle, and the size of the left atrium, enlargement of which predisposes to atrial fibrillation.

PULMONARY VALVE STENOSIS

In its typical form, pulmonary valve stenosis is characterized as a pliant, mobile dome-shaped structure with a narrow outlet at its apex. The anomaly is usually isolated and uncomplicated and is the most common variety of congenital obstruction to right ventricular outflow.[13,122-138] With the exception of pinpoint pulmonary valve stenosis in neonates, survival into adolescence and adulthood is the rule. In a review of 69 anatomically proved cases, 7 patients lived to age 50 years and 3 survived to ages 70 to 75 years.[138] Survival into the sixth, seventh, and eighth decades has been recorded, with one patient living for 78 years.[123,126,128-131,134,136,138-140]

Longevity depends chiefly on four variables: (1) the initial severity, (2) whether a given degree of stenosis remains constant or progresses, (3) the functional adequacy (adaptive response) of the pressure-overloaded right ventricle, and (4) the degree of tricuspid regurgitation that adds volume to the pressure-overloaded right ventricle.[132-135,137] Dilatation of the pulmonary trunk is inherently related to the mobile dome congenital valve, just as dilatation of the ascending aorta is inherently related to the bicuspid aortic valve.[18] In neither condition is dilatation related to the functional derangement of the malformed valve—that is, to the degree of pulmonary or aortic stenosis—but is related instead to the inherent medial abnormality of the pulmonary trunk or ascending aorta. However, dilatation of the pulmonary trunk, even when aneurysmal, rarely influences longevity because unlike the systemic pressure ascending aorta above a bicuspid aortic valve, the dilated low-pressure pulmonary trunk above a mobile dome pulmonary valve is not prone to rupture.[135]

The orifice size of typical mobile pulmonary valve stenosis usually increases appropriately with age, although the development of secondary hypertrophic subpulmonary stenosis (Fig. 4–12) or rarely fibrocalcific thickening (Fig. 4–13) augments the degree of obstruction. Subinfundibular stenosis or double-chambered right ventricle occurs with a normal pulmonary valve and is characterized by muscle bundles that cause varying degrees of fixed obstruction[13] (see Fig. 4–12, B and C).

Symptoms associated with pulmonary valve stenosis become more prevalent with time; however, equivalent degrees of stenosis may limit one patient in childhood but leave another relatively unaffected as an adult. An appreciable number of adults with moderate to severe pulmonary valve stenosis remain virtually free of symptoms.[124,141] One group of patients with right ventricular systolic pressures between 50 and 100 mm Hg included a long-distance swimmer, a long-distance runner, and a hockey captain.[124,141] One of our patients, a 17-year-old

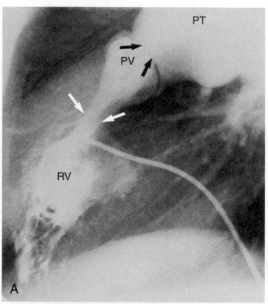

FIGURE 4–12 **(A)** Right ventriculogram (lateral projection) from a 37-year-old man with severe pulmonary valve stenosis, secondary hypertrophic subpulmonary stenosis *(paired white arrows)*, and a right ventricular (RV) systolic pressure of 145 mm Hg. The mobile pulmonary valve (PV) exhibits typical systolic doming. The pulmonary trunk (PT) is conspicuously dilated. **(B)** Chest radiograph from a 40-year-old woman with double-chambered right ventricle caused by obstructing subinfundibular muscle bundles. The infundibulum (INF) is slightly convex, but the pulmonary trunk (PT) is not dilatated. The right atrium (RA) is somewhat convex. The right ventricle (RV) occupies the apex. Ao, transverse aorta. **(C)** Right ventriculogram identifies the obstructing muscle bundles *(three white arrows)* that extend to the ostium of a slightly dilated infundibulum.

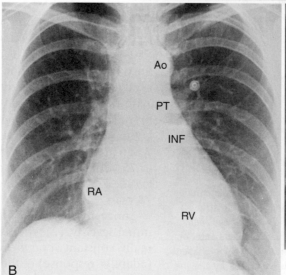

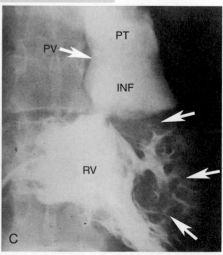

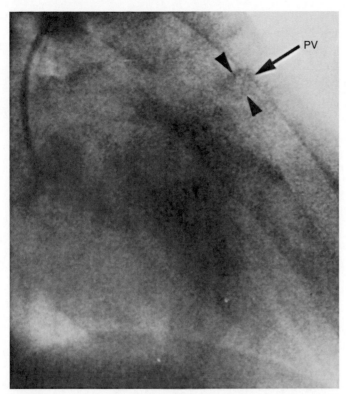

FIGURE 4-13   Cineframe (right anterior oblique) from a 64-year-old man with a calcified, stenotic pulmonary valve stenosis (PV) and a nonrestrictive perimembranous ventricular septal defect that extended into the inlet septum.

boy, played baseball despite a right ventricular systolic pressure of nearly 200 mm Hg; a 32-year-old man with a right ventricular systolic pressure of 75 mm Hg had run the quarter mile in high school; and an asymptomatic patient who had been a star high school track sprinter underwent percutaneous balloon valvuloplasty at age 37 years for severe pulmonary valve stenosis with hypertrophic subpulmonary stenosis[57] (see Fig. 4-12, A). Nevertheless, the most common cause of death is right ventricular failure, usually after the fourth decade.[138,142] Infective endocarditis carries a risk of 2% to 7%, except in very mild pulmonary valve stenosis (see Chapter 8).[128,142] The impact on longevity depends on the degree and chronicity of pulmonary regurgitation.

PULMONARY VALVE REGURGITATION

One, two, or three cusps may undergo faulty development, all three cusps may be rudimentary, one cusp may be absent and the other two rudimentary, or cusps may fail to develop altogether—congenital absence of the pulmonary valve, which usually coexists with tetralogy of Fallot[143,144] (discussed later). Longevity depends on the degree of regurgitation and on the adaptive response of the right ventricle. Children, adolescents, and young adults are typically asymptomatic when congenital pul-

monary regurgitation is discovered.[145-148] Because regurgitant flow is usually moderate or less and because an otherwise normal right ventricle readily adapts to low-pressure volume overload, the majority of patients survive through middle age and occasionally into the eighth decade.[146-155] Two exceptional examples of isolated congenital absence of the pulmonary valve were reported at age 69 years[156] and 73 years.[144]

Although most patients tolerate the anomaly well into adulthood, acquired cardiopulmonary disorders that accrue with advancing age become potential hazards because the accompanying rise in pulmonary arterial pressure increases regurgitant flow across the congenitally incompetent valve. The risk of infective endocarditis is relatively low (see Chapter 8) but potentially augments the degree of regurgitation and modifies the clinical course.

PULMONARY ARTERY STENOSIS

Stenosis (or stenoses) of the pulmonary artery and its branches is usually an isolated malformation that can be unilateral or bilateral, single or multiple, and located in the pulmonary trunk, at its bifurcation, or in its primary or peripheral branches.[157-160] Obstruction may involve a localized site with segmental narrowing or varying lengths of a pulmonary artery segment culminating in diffuse tubular hypoplasia. Isolated pulmonary artery stenosis is uncommon, but the unoperated malformation is likely to be seen in adulthood because surgical repair and balloon dilatation are seldom efficacious.

OSTIUM SECUNDUM ATRIAL SEPTAL DEFECT

These defects are common congenital cardiac malformations in adults, accounting for up to 40% of acyanotic shunt lesions in unoperated patients older than age 40 years.[161-177] The malformation may go unrecognized for decades because symptoms are absent and physical signs are subtle. Detection often awaits a routine chest radiograph in an otherwise healthy adult. Survival into adulthood is the rule, with many patients living to an advanced age.[161-164,166,168-173,175,176,178] Paul Wood remarked, "In any series of geriatric necropsies, atrial septal defect is always represented."[178] Ostium secundum atrial is twice as common in females. Unoperated longevity extends into adulthood, so it can be anticipated that women will frequently reach childbearing age (see Chapter 9).

Unoperated survival beyond the fifth or sixth decade seldom exceeds 50%, with subsequent attrition of about 6% per year.[164,168,169] Sporadic examples of isolated ostium secundum atrial septal defects have been reported in patients beyond 70 years of age[177] and occasionally in patients in their 80s or 90s.[161,162,166,169,170,172,173,175,176,178,179] One of our patients lived relatively comfortably until

3 months before his 95th birthday, and another died at age 87 years following the onset of atrial fibrillation and right ventricular failure[171] (Fig. 4–14).

With few exceptions, patients who survive beyond the sixth decade are symptomatic. Older patients deteriorate chiefly on three counts: first, because an age-related decrease in left ventricular distensibility augments the left-to-right shunt[13,173,175,180–183] (the left ventricle during diastole at a greater modulus of elastic stiffness[184]). Second, supraventricular tachyarrhythmias (atrial fibrillation, atrial flutter, and, less commonly, reentrant atrial tachycardia) increase in frequency after the fourth decade, augmenting the left-to-right shunt and precipitating right ventricular failure. Third, symptomatic adults older than 40 years commonly have mild to moderate elevations of pulmonary arterial pressure in the presence of a persistent large left-to-right shunt, so the aging volume-overloaded right ventricle is also beset by pressure overload.[13,175,178]

A left-to-right shunt in a neonate with an ostium secundum atrial septal defect depends on the relative compliances of the right and left ventricles, which are similar *in utero* and at birth but then diverge as left ventricular mass exceeds right ventricular mass during the process of normal extrauterine growth.[185] The left-to-right shunt awaits this decrease in right ventricular mass and increase in compliance, a time course during which the pulmonary arterioles involute (normalize), permitting the pulmonary bed to evolve into a low-resistance, low-pressure circulation. The pulmonary arterial pressure remains normal because the left-to-right shunt, after it is established, is into a compliant low-resistance vascular bed, and thus an appreciable increment in pulmonary arterial blood flow is tolerated without a rise in pulmonary arterial pressure. Pulmonary vascular disease with reversed shunt occurs in less than 10% of patients with an ostium secundum atrial septal defect, with a preponderance in young females.[164,176,186–189] The high pulmonary vascular resistance in these young female patients is believed to represent the coincidence of primary pulmonary hypertension rather than a sequel of the atrial septal defect shunt (discussed later).[13] At high altitude, otherwise uncomplicated ostium secundum atrial septal defects are likely to be accompanied by substantial elevations in pulmonary arterial pressure, even in the young.[164,186,190–192]

An interatrial communication improves longevity in patients with primary pulmonary hypertension because the right-to-left shunt decompresses the right atrium and maintains left ventricular stroke volume and cardiac output,[13] hence the rationale for atrial septostomy as bridge to lung transplantation.[193] Thrombus in the dilatated hypertensive proximal pulmonary arteries is not uncommon in cyanotic patients with atrial septal defect[194] (see Chapter 12).

Age-related abnormalities of the mitral valve sufficient to cause significant regurgitation occur in about 15% of adults with an ostium secundum atrial septal defect.[13,195–200] The lesions are acquired and have been attributed to disturbed leaflet movement associated with deformity of the underfilled left ventricular cavity and abnormal position and motion of the ventricular septum in response to right ventricular volume overload.[13,196,201] Superior systolic displacement is increased because leaflets with normal area and chordal length are housed in a left ventricular cavity that is reduced in size. In Lutembacher's syndrome, the mitral valve lesion is acquired rheumatic (discussed later).[202]

Infective endocarditis in uncomplicated ostium secundum atrial septal defect is exceedingly rare (see Chapter 8). Occurrence depends on incompetence of a structurally abnormal mitral valve, as just described. The normal pulmonary valve is not susceptible to infective endocarditis despite an increased velocity of flow across the orifice; only one case has been reported.[203]

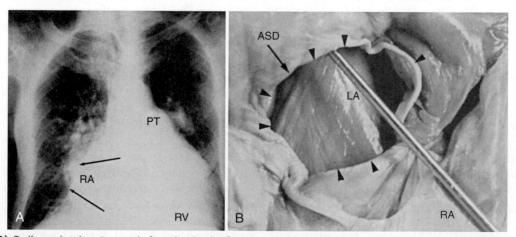

FIGURE 4–14 **(A)** Radiograph taken 2 years before the death of a 96-year-old male with an ostium secundum atrial septal defect. Pulmonary vascularity is increased. The pulmonary trunk (PT) and its branches are dilatated, the right atrium (RA) is enlarged, and a dilatated right ventricle (RV) occupies the apex. **(B)** Necropsy specimen from an 87-year-old woman with an ostium secundum atrial septal defect (ASD), outlined by the arrowheads. The probe is through the defect. LA, left atrium.

IDIOPATHIC PULMONARY HYPERTENSION

Defined as an intrinsic, obstructive disease residing in the small pulmonary arteries and arterioles, idiopathic (primary) pulmonary hypertension has been ascribed to abnormalities of vasoconstrictor endothelin-1 homeostasis together with defects in voltage-gated potassium channels and abnormalities in metalloproteinase and elastase activity, in transforming growth factor ß, and in bone morphogenetic protein.[13,204-206] The disease usually becomes clinically manifest in female young adults and only occasionally in childhood.[205,207] Early in the course, vasoreactivity can be demonstrated in response to pulmonary vasodilators, but, with few exceptions, the pulmonary vascular disease is progressive, and the resistance becomes fixed[208,209] because of morphologic alterations elegantly described by Heath and Edwards.[208,210,211] The combination of ostium secundum atrial septal defects and pulmonary vascular resistance at or above systemic is usually found in young women who are believed to represent the concurrence of primary pulmonary hypertension and atrial septal defect (see earlier discussion).

Longevity is determined chiefly by the response of right ventricle to afterload imposed by increased pulmonary vascular resistance.[212] Right ventricular failure is the commonest cause of death. In three large studies, mean patient age was 21 to 30 years.[13] Syncope is ominous and can herald sudden death, which can be precipitated by seemingly innocuous stress. Longevity is significantly influenced by lifestyle. Patients should be counseled to avoid abrupt, strenuous, or isometric exercise; to desist from any form of exercise at the onset of symptoms; and to avoid exposure to circumstances that provoke systemic vasodilatation such as heat and humidity, hot baths, or hot showers. The majority of patients with primary pulmonary hypertension are young women who should be warned that the risk of pregnancy is prohibitive with maternal mortality as high as 50% (see Chapter 9).[212] High altitude is an avoidable risk, and air travel is a corollary (see Chapter 12). A commercial jetliner flying at 33,000 to 36,000 feet has cabin atmospheric conditions that are altitude equivalents of approximately 6,000 to 8,000 feet, which is comparable to breathing 15% oxygen at sea level.[13] Also to be reckoned with are the risks of nonflight–related stress and travel fatigue. Myocardial ischemia can be caused by compression of the left main coronary artery by the dilatated pulmonary trunk. Hemoptysis is not a feature of primary pulmonary hypertension as it is in Eisenmenger syndrome (see Chapter 12). Cigarette smoking is proscribed.

Oral anticoagulants have been advocated on the basis of data that *in situ* thrombosis is an important component of the progressive rise in pulmonary vascular resistance.[213] However, anticoagulants should be used cautiously if at

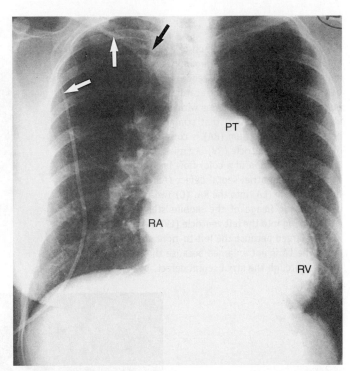

FIGURE 4-15   Chest radiograph from a 34-year-old woman with primary pulmonary hypertension. The catheter *(white arrows)* with tip *(black arrow)* in the right subclavian vein was inserted for continuous infusion of prostacyclin. The pulmonary trunk (PT) is dilatated, and the right atrium (RA) is moderately prominent. The right ventricle (RV) occupies the apex.

all in cyanotic patients because of the risk of reinforcing intrinsic hemostatic defects (see Chapter 12).

Continuous prostacyclin infusion has been employed to reduce pulmonary vascular resistance even in patients in whom vasoreactivity cannot be demonstrated and who are presumed to have irreversible morphologic changes in the pulmonary vascular bed (see earlier)[214,215] (Fig. 4–15). The long-term salutary responses have been attributed to effects on pulmonary vascular endothelium, vascular growth, remodeling of the pulmonary resistance vessels, and platelet function.[214,216-218] Prostanoids[216] have largely been superseded by endothelial receptor antagonists (bosentan)[219] and phosphodiesterase inhibitors (sildenafil)[220-222] (see earlier discussion).

LUTEMBACHER SYNDROME

In 1750, Johann Friedrich Meckel described a case of atrial septal defect with mitral stenosis,[97] a combination that carries the eponym referring to Rene Lutembacher who reported the disorder in 1916.[97] Lutembacher's syndrome consists of a congenital defect in the atrial septum that coexists with rheumatic mitral stenosis[12,319] (Fig. 4–16). When an atrial septal defect and mitral stenosis coexist, each modifies the hemodynamics and clinical expressions of the other.[319] The idea that an interatrial communication

FIGURE 4–16 **(A)** Radiograph of a 45-year-old man with Lutembacher's syndrome. Pulmonary arterial vascularity is moderately increased. The ascending aorta is inconspicuous because the shunt was intracardiac. The border-forming pulmonary trunk (PT) merges with the shadow of the left atrial appendage (LAAp) that straightens the left cardiac border. The right atrium (RA) is conspicuously enlarged. A dilatated right ventricle (RV) occupies the apex. **(B)** Black-and-white rendition of a color flow image showing the ostium secundum atrial septal defect (ASD) with shunt from the left atrium (LA) into the RA. **(C)** Two-dimensional echocardiographic image of the mobile stenotic mitral valve (MS) doming into the left ventricle (LV) during diastole. The RV is enlarged because the left-to-right shunt was at atrial level. The LA is not enlarged because the chamber decompresses through the atrial septal defect.

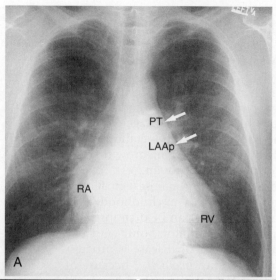

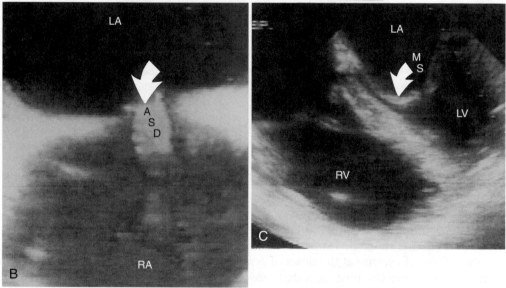

might exert a favorable effect on mitral stenosis was proposed by Firkett in 1880.[12] Mitral stenosis increases resistance to blood flow from left atrium into left ventricle and, in so doing, augments the left-to-right shunt. The coexisting nonrestrictive atrial septal defect decompresses the left atrium so that the mitral gradient diminishes or may disappear altogether except during exercise. Cardiac output necessarily declines.

Lutembacher's original patient was a 61-year-old woman who endured seven pregnancies, and Firkett's patient was a 77-year-old woman who been pregnant 11 times.[13] Survival to advanced age was reconfirmed,[13] and in one instance an 81-year-old woman experienced no cardiac symptoms until her 75th year.[223] These reports should not obscure the fact that the long-term outlook of an unoperated ostium secundum atrial septal defect is unfavorably influenced by mitral stenosis, which predisposes to atrial fibrillation and right ventricular failure by augmenting the left-to-right shunt.[13,224]

SINUS VENOSUS ATRIAL SEPTAL DEFECTS

Sinus venosus atrial septal defects constitute 2% to 3% of interatrial communications.[225] Defects of the *superior vena caval* type are situated immediately beneath the orifice of the superior vena cava as it enters the right atrium, vary from small to nonrestrictive, and are generally associated with anomalous connection of the right superior pulmonary vein to the superior vena cava. Sinus venosus defects of the *inferior caval* type are located below the foramen ovale, merge with the orifice of the inferior vena cava, and vary from restrictive to nonrestrictive (Fig. 4–17). Longevity is analogous to that of other atrial septal defects of equivalent size and equivalent left-to-right shunts (see earlier discussion). Because a superior vena caval sinus venosus defect is located at the site normally occupied by the sinoatrial node, the normal right sinoatrial pacemaker is often absent.[13] An

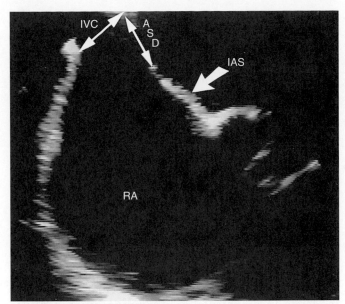

FIGURE 4-17 Transesophageal echocardiogram from a 32-year-old man with a nonrestrictive inferior vena caval (IVC) sinus venous atrial septal defect (ASD). IAS, intact interatrial septum; RA, right atrium.

ectopic atrial pacemaker generally serves the purpose, with little or no negative effect on longevity. The oldest recorded patient with a superior vena caval sinus venosus atrial septal defect died of right ventricular failure at age 88 years.[226] In contrast to ostium secundum defects, superior vena caval sinus venosus defects do not lend themselves to paradoxical emboli, which usually enter the systemic circulation in the midportion of the atrial septum (fossa ovalis region).[13]

PARTIAL ANOMALOUS PULMONARY VENOUS CONNECTION

The term *partial anomalous pulmonary venous connection* applies when one or more—but not all—pulmonary veins connect to the right atrium.[227-230] *Isolated* partial anomalous pulmonary venous connection applies when the atrial septum is intact and represents an uncommon malformation with expected adult survival. The volume of blood entering the right atrium in the presence of isolated partial anomalous pulmonary venous connection tends to be greater than anticipated because right atrial pressure is lower than left atrial pressure owing to an intact atrial septum. Accordingly, the pressure gradient across the lung that drains anomalously is greater than the gradient across the normally draining lung.[231]

The term *scimitar* refers to a radiographic shadow that resembles a scimitar, or Turkish sword. Scimitar syndrome is a rare disorder characterized by anomalous connection to the inferior vena cava of most, if not all, pulmonary venous drainage pathways of the right lung.[232-234] The left

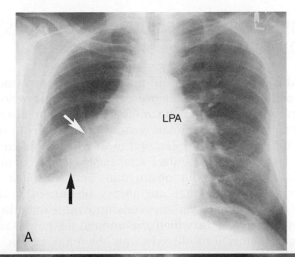

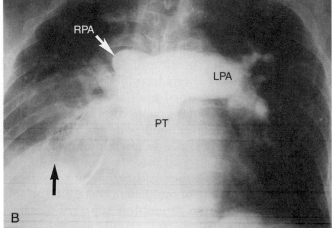

FIGURE 4-18 **(A)** Chest radiograph from a 67-year-old man with scimitar syndrome (anomalous pulmonary venous drainage of the entire right lung with infradiaphragmatic connection to the inferior vena cava), an ostium secundum atrial septal defect, and moderate pulmonary hypertension with a left-to-right shunt of 1.7 to 1. The white arrow identifies the confluence of the right pulmonary veins. Elevation of the right hemidiaphragm *(black arrow)* and rightward shift of the cardiac silhouette are due to hypoplasia of the right lung. A dilatated left pulmonary artery (LPA) is just visible. **(B)** Angiogram with contrast injected into the pulmonary trunk (PT). The right pulmonary artery (RPA) is atretic, and the left pulmonary artery (LPA) is dilatated. The black arrow tip is at the level of the elevated right hemidiaphragm.

lung is rarely involved.[158] Adult survival is expected, but longevity depends on a number of variables in addition to and apart from the volume of blood channeled through the anomalous right pulmonary veins. The right lung and right pulmonary artery are hypoplastic, the mediastinum is shifted to the right, the lower portion of the right lung is perfused by systemic arteries that arise from the abdominal aorta, and the left lung is hyperflated.[233,234] One of our patients, an asymptomatic 26-year-old woman, experienced an uncomplicated full-term pregnancy. Our oldest patient with scimitar syndrome died at age 67 years with chronic atrial fibrillation and right ventricular failure (Fig. 4-18).

TOTAL ANOMALOUS PULMONARY VENOUS CONNECTION

In this malformation, all pulmonary veins connect anomalously to a confluence or to a systemic venous tributary of the right atrium or to the right atrium proper, with no pulmonary venous connections to the left atrium.[235] The simplest and most widely used clinical classification recognizes *supradiaphragmatic* connections with or without obstruction, and *infradiaphragmatic* connections that are always obstructed.[13] The supradiaphragmatic varieties constitute more than three fourths of cases, in which the anomalous pulmonary venous connections directly join the right atrium or coronary sinus, or join a confluence that gives rise to a left vertical vein that attaches to an innominate bridge and a right superior vena cava. An interatrial communication is the only access to the left side of the heart and systemic circulation. The 10% of patients who survive their first year almost always have low pulmonary vascular resistance, a nonrestrictive atrial septal defect, and supradiaphragmatic venous connections. Exceptionally, such patients reach adulthood with surprisingly little disability and a clinical course resembling isolated ostium secundum atrial septal defect except for mild cyanosis.[236] Survival sometimes reaches the third, fourth, or fifth decade.[237-242] One of our patients with total anomalous pulmonary venous connection, suprasystemic pulmonary vascular resistance, and a confluence that joined a left vertical vein died at age 54 years (Fig. 4–19). Another died at age 62 years,[239] and one underwent surgical repair at age 66 years.[243]

COMMON ATRIUM

This rare variety of interatrial communication is characterized by absence or virtual absence of the atrial septum, vestigial remnants of which occasionally remain.[244] Complete absence of the atrial septum necessarily includes the atrioventricular septum, so a "cleft" anterior mitral leaflet almost always coexists. Physiologic consequences resemble those of nonrestrictive atrial septal defects, although venoarterial mixing and cyanosis are obligatory, incompetence of the malformed mitral valve is frequent, and symptoms occur earlier and are more pronounced. Occasional patients are relatively well into adolescence,[244,245] and one adult had a common atrium, mitral regurgitation, and the Ellis-van Creveld syndrome.[246] Our oldest patient was a 57-year-old woman with common atrium, pulmonary vascular disease, and moderate incompetence of a common atrioventricular valve (Fig. 4–20).

ATRIOVENTRICULAR SEPTAL DEFECT

Down syndrome exerts an important independent influence on longevity. The proclivity for pulmonary vascular disease is coupled with Down syndrome per se rather than with the presence and type of coexisting malformation.[13]

The physiologic consequences and longevity patterns of an isolated ostium primum atrial septal defect are the same as for other interatrial communications of equivalent size, provided the malformed left atrioventricular valve remains competent and pulmonary vascular disease

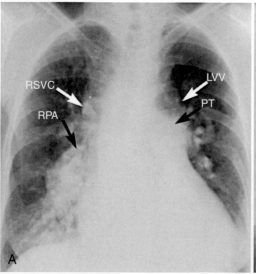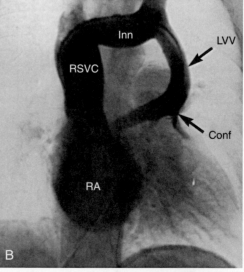

FIGURE 4–19 **(A)** Chest radiograph from a 54-year-old cyanotic woman with total anomalous pulmonary venous connection and pulmonary vascular disease. The pulmonary trunk (PT) and its right branch (RPA) are considerably enlarged. **(B)** Angiogram (levophase after contrast injection into the pulmonary artery) shows all four pulmonary veins joining a confluence (Conf) that gives rise to a left vertical vein (LVV). An innominate bridge (Inn) crosses to a large right superior vena cava (RSVC). RA, right atrium.

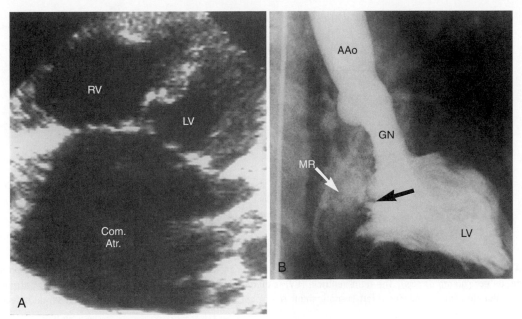

FIGURE 4-20   **(A)** Two-dimensional echocardiogram from a 57-year-old cyanotic female patient with a common atrium (Com. Atr.) and pulmonary vascular disease. The right and left atrioventricular valves are at the same level because of absence of the atrioventricular septum. The right ventricle (RV) is dilatated. LV, left ventricle. **(B)** Left ventriculogram delineates the "cleft" in the anterior mitral leaflet *(black arrow)*. There is mitral regurgitation (MR) and the typical goose neck (GN) deformity of the left ventricular outflow tract. AAo, ascending aorta.

is not present.[247-249] However, coexisting mitral regurgitation reinforces the left-to-right interatrial shunt, and a large ostium primum defect decompresses the left atrium as it receives the regurgitant flow. When mitral regurgitation is absent, mild, or moderate, adult survival can be anticipated. In a report of 52 adult patients, 12% were aged 60 years or older, although all of those older than age 45 years were symptomatic.[250] The oldest reported survivors were aged 69, 75, and 79 years.[250-252] The patient whose echocardiogram is shown in Figure 4-21 underwent successful cardiac surgery at age 71 years. The cumulative risk of infective endocarditis, which may alter the clinical course, is related to mitral regurgitation, not to the ostium primum atrial septal defect (see Chapter 8). An isolated nonrestrictive inlet ventricular septal defect is functionally equivalent to other ventricular septal defects of comparable size, including Eisenmenger syndrome (discussed earlier). Complete, common atrioventricular canals are typically symptomatic in early life. Prolonged survival is exceptional; one patient lived to age 46 years,[252] and another lived to age 73 years.[253]

PATENT DUCTUS ARTERIOSUS

After the first year of life, the majority of patients with patent ductus arteriosus are asymptomatic, and by the beginning of the second decade, the risk of infective endarteritis exceeds the risk of congestive heart failure.[254-256] In the third decade (occasionally earlier), more and more patients with sizable left-to-right shunts develop cardiac

failure, whereas those with small shunts across a restrictive ductus remain asymptomatic.[254-258] A number of reports have called attention to survival beyond the sixth decade,[259] with one death at age 85 and another at age 92 years.[254-256,258,260-265] One of our patients was an 84-year-old woman with a restrictive patent ductus, and another was an 84-year-old woman with a moderately restrictive ductus, atrial fibrillation, and congestive heart failure. The risk of infective endocarditis is cumulative, especially if the ductus is restrictive (see Chapter 8), but susceptibility has not been established in patients with a tiny, clinically silent ductus detected only by echocardiographic color flow imaging.[266] A sizeable vegetation at the narrower pulmonary arterial end of the ductus may result in ductal closure, albeit rarely.[267]

In 1947, Taussig confirmed the presence of a valve at the pulmonary arterial end of a ductus arteriosus.[268] This veil-like structure has been held responsible for intermittent appearance and disappearance of the continuous murmur,[269] and rupture of the ductal valve was held responsible for the abrupt appearance of a loud continuous murmur in a 55-year-old man.[270] The ductal valve sometimes results in spontaneous closure in young adults. Rarely, the lumen of a sealed ductus is reestablished by spontaneous intramural dissection of a ductal aneurysm.[271] Also rarely, a ductal aneurysm is complicated by systemic embolism, laryngeal nerve paralysis, compression of the pulmonary trunk, and rupture or erosion with hemorrhage into the esophagus or tracheobronchial tree.[272-274] There are reports of spontaneous postpartum rupture of a patent ductus[275] and of a case of

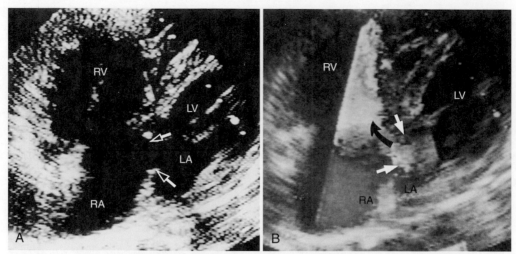

FIGURE 4-21 **(A)** Two-dimensional echocardiogram from a 71-year-old woman with a large left-to-right shunt through a nonrestrictive ostium primum atrial septal defect *(paired arrows)*. The right ventricle (RV) is dilated. LA, left atrium; LV, left ventricle; RA, right atrium. **(B)** Black-and-white rendition of a color flow image showing a left-to-right shunt *(black arrow)* through the ostium primum atrial septal defect *(white arrows)*.

unoperated patent ductus with dissecting aneurysm of the pulmonary artery.[276]

Patients with a nonrestrictive patent ductus arteriosus seldom reach adulthood unless a rise in pulmonary vascular resistance relieves the left ventricle of excessive volume overload.[192,254,277] Birth at a high altitude has been implicated in both persistent patency of ductus arteriosus and the development of pulmonary vascular disease.[13] A rare example of benefit from pulmonary vascular disease with reversed shunt through a nonrestrictive patent ductus arteriosus is the ductal-dependent circulation in an adult with complete interruption of the aortic arch.[278]

VENTRICULAR SEPTAL DEFECT

In his remarks on adult survival in congenital heart disease, Paul Wood asked, "Where's the maladie de Roger? Assuming it does not provide immortality, it must either close spontaneously in middle life or have long since run its mortal course."[178] Spontaneous closure was recognized in 1919 when French described the case of a boy whose murmur and thrill disappeared at age 5 years.[279] The incidence of spontaneous closure depends on the population under study and the method of diagnosis.[280,281] With few exceptions, spontaneous closure is a feature of perimembranous or muscular (trabecular septal) ventricular septal defects, with an incidence that is almost equally divided between these two sites.[13] It has been estimated that 25% of ventricular septal defects in these locations close spontaneously, but when observed from birth, the incidence of spontaneous closure increases to 50% to 75% of asymptomatic patients with restrictive defects.[280,282-285] Five to ten percent of moderately large to nonrestrictive ventricular septal defects also close spontaneously.[284,286] Many, if not most, defects that

close spontaneously do so within the first year of life,[280,281,287] with approximately 60% closing before age 3 years and 90% closing before age 8 years.[282-285] However, late spontaneous closure has been reported in older children and young adults[284,288,289] and has been sporadically documented after age 23 years,[290] between ages 26 and 33 years,[283,291] and after age 46 years.[292]

The physiologic consequences of an isolated ventricular septal defect depend chiefly on two variables—namely, the size of the communication and the behavior of the pulmonary vascular bed, that is, pulmonary vascular resistance. Patients who survive into adulthood comprise two main groups: (1) those whose defects have closed spontaneously (see earlier) or have decreased in size and are clinically occult (Fig. 4–22) and (2) those with nonrestrictive defects accompanied by elevated pulmonary vascular resistance that relieves the left ventricle of excessive volume overload while imposing no additional afterload on the already systemic right ventricle (Eisenmenger's physiology)[202,283,290-302] (see Fig. 4–22, *B*). Exceptionally, patients with a moderately restrictive or nonrestrictive ventricular septal defect and a significant left-to-right shunt survive to adulthood,[303] with one reaching 79 years of age.[51] When aortic regurgitation coexists with a moderately restrictive or nonrestrictive ventricular septal defect, the left ventricle confronts the sum of volume overload imposed by aortic regurgitant flow together with the left-to-right shunt.[13] When aortic regurgitation coexists with a restrictive ventricular septal defect, the left ventricle essentially confronts the aortic regurgitation per se, the presence of which increases susceptibility to infective endocarditis (see Chapter 8).

Sporadic adult survivors with a restrictive perimembranous ventricular septal defect (see Fig. 4–22) are exposed to the cumulative risk of infective endocarditis (see Chapter 8). Longevity is otherwise normal, with the

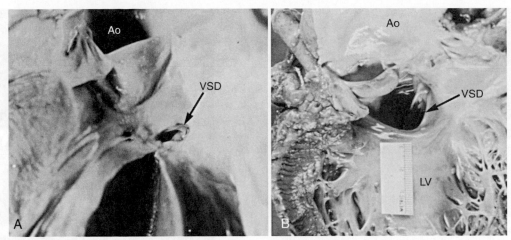

FIGURE 4-22   (A) Tiny membranous ventricular septal defect (VSD) that was an incidental necropsy finding in a 60-year-old man. Ao, aorta. **(B)** Nonrestrictive perimembranous ventricular septal defect (VSD) at necropsy in a 44-year-old man with Eisenmenger syndrome. LV, left ventricle.

disconcerting exception of occasionally serious distur-bances in cardiac rhythm, including ventricular tachycar-dia.[2] Patients with defects that have closed spontane-ously but with septal aneurysm formation can develop abnormal atrioventricular conduction, even complete heart block (see Chapter 20). Although aneurysmal transformation tends to decrease the size or even close the ventricular septal defect,[304] there is a relatively high incidence of development of left ventricular to right atrial shunts with a concomitant increase in the risk of infective endocarditis.[304]

In the normal fetus, pulmonary arterial and systemic arterial pressures are the same because of the presence of a nonrestrictive ductus arteriosus. In infants with a nonre-strictive ventricular septal defect, equalization of these pres-sures persists, so the direction of shunt flow depends on the relative resistances in the pulmonary and systemic vascular beds.[185] At birth, pulmonary vascular resistance falls pre-cipitously, then continues to fall during the next few months. Survival depends on an inverse interplay between flow and resistance because increased resistance curtails flow and prevents death from congestive heart failure. In approximately 10% of patients with nonrestrictive ventricu-lar septal defects, pulmonary vascular resistance rises to suprasystemic levels with reversed shunt—Eisenmenger syndrome—as defined by Paul Wood in 1958).[2,192,298] Be-cause right ventricular afterload is determined by systemic vascular resistance, and because the right ventricle has been adapted to systemic afterload from birth, right ventricular failure is uncommon.[192,305-308] Eisenmenger syndrome, like all forms of cyanotic congenital heart disease in adults, is a multisystem systemic disorder[301] that includes hematologic disorders in red blood cell mass and platelets, the systemic and coronary vascular beds,[309-311] bilirubin kinetics, the kidneys,[312] the digits and long bones, the lungs,[185,194] the central nervous system (see Chapter 14), and gynecologic endocrinology (see Chapter 9). Meticulous medical man-agement has had a significant impact on morbidity and

longevity.[302] Mean age at death has been reported at 37 ± 8.1 years[301] and 45.3 ± 15.8 years,[302] which is approxi-mately 1 to 2 decades longer than in earlier reports. How-ever, longer life spans expose patients to proximal pulmo-nary arterial aneurysms and thrombi[194] and to a substantial increase in the risk of massive fatal intrapulmonary hemor-rhage[301] (Fig. 4-23) as in Eisenmenger's original patient[192] (see Chapter 12). Advancing age, however, does not incur the risk of atherosclerotic coronary artery disease in cya-notic patients because of the antiatherogenic effects of hy-pocholesterolemia, upregulated nitric oxide, hyperbilirubi-nemia, hypoxemia, and low platelet counts.[310] A patient with Eisenmenger syndrome experienced a noncardiac death 3 months before her 70th birthday. The outlook promises to improve still further as prostanoids[216] are su-perseded by phosphodiesterase inhibitors (sildenafil)[220,221] and endothelial receptor antagonists (bosentan).[219]

DEFECTS IN THE INFUNDIBULAR SEPTUM

These are located in the cephalic portion of the infun-dibular or outlet septum immediately beneath the valves of both great arterial trunks (doubly committed subarterial).[297,313] Interventricular communications in the infundibular septum account for 5% to 7% of ven-tricular septal defects in North America and Western Europe but for approximately 30% of defects in Asian patients.[314,315] Because the defects are subarterial, an inherently normal aortic valve lacks adequate sup-port. The right and noncoronary sinuses tend to move into the right ventricular outflow tract, causing aortic regurgitation and sometimes subpulmonary obstruc-tion.[316,317] Long-term survival is influenced by the size of the ventricular septal defect, which tends to remain constant, and by coexisting aortic regurgitation, which imposes volume load on both ventricles and is suscep-tible to infective endocarditis (see Chapter 8).

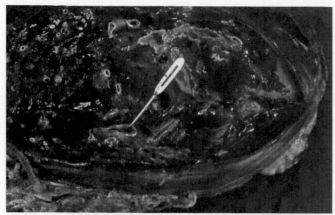

FIGURE 4-23 Massive intrapulmonary hemorrhage causing sudden death in a 54-year-old woman with a nonrestrictive ventricular septal defect and Eisenmenger syndrome. The cross-sections of the small hypertensive intrapulmonary arteries are prominent.

SINUS OF VALSALVA ANEURYSM

The typical congenital sinus of Valsalva aneurysm is a fingerlike or nipplelike projection that originates from a localized fault in an aortic sinus that is otherwise normal.[318] Ninety to ninety-five percent of these congenital aortic sinus aneurysms originate in the right or noncoronary sinus.[319,320] Aneurysms arising in the noncoronary sinus almost always rupture into the right atrium, and those arising in the right coronary sinus generally rupture into the right ventricle, occasionally into the right atrium.[318] Aortic sinus aneurysms that rupture into the right ventricle or right atrium may be associated with a ventricular septal defect, especially subpulmonary, that is clinically overt years before the ruptured sinus announces itself. The association is not fortuitous.[13] Ruptured aortic sinus aneurysms typically occur in males and usually express themselves after puberty but before age 30 years, with a range of 11 to 67 years.[318,321-324] Longevity depends chiefly on four variables: (1) the rapidity with which the rupture develops, (2) the amount of blood flowing through the rupture, (3) the chamber that receives the rupture, and (4) a coexisting ventricular septal defect (discussed earlier). The clinical picture usually reflects a sudden large perforation, less commonly the gradual development of a small perforation, and still less commonly an unruptured aneurysm.[318,321] An unoperated acute large perforation culminates in death after a relatively short time course. Sudden death results from rupture into the pericardium or rupture into the base of the ventricular septum, which can also cause complete heart block and syncope.[13] A small perforation may initially go unnoticed, as was the case in one of our patients, an asymptomatic 35-year-old man who came to attention because of a soft, high-frequency continuous murmur; a small perforation of a noncoronary sinus of Valsalva aneurysm into the right atrium was identified on

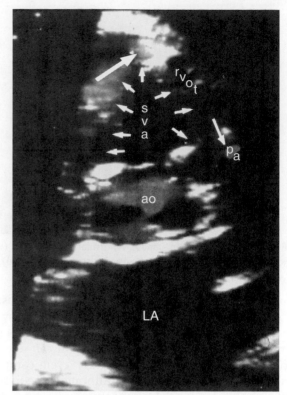

FIGURE 4-24 Unruptured sinus of Valsalva aneurysm (sva) in an 85-year-old man. ao, aorta; LA, left atrium; pa, pulmonary artery; rvot, right ventricular outflow tract.

transesophageal echocardiography (see Chapter 6). Small, chronic perforations are susceptible to infective endocarditis[318,325,326] (see Chapter 8).

Approximately 20% of congenital sinus of Valsalva aneurysms are unperforated and are chance findings at necropsy or cardiac surgery.[327,328] With the advent of echocardiography, however, unruptured congenital aortic sinus aneurysms are being diagnosed with increasing frequency (see Chapter 6).[329-331] An 85-year-old asymptomatic man was found to have an unruptured aortic sinus aneurysm when he was referred for an echocardiogram because of a prominent murmur that was thought to be continuous (Fig. 4-24). In an 82-year-old man, an unruptured clinically occult aneurysm of the right coronary sinus was an incidental necropsy finding.[329] Rarely, an unruptured aneurysm projects into the right ventricular outflow tract, causing obstruction[332,333]; compresses a coronary artery, causing angina pectoris; or myocardial infarction[334-336]; or compresses the base of the ventricular septum, causing atrioventricular conduction defects.[337,338]

TRUNCUS ARTERIOSUS

Truncus arteriosus is characterized by a single great artery that leaves the base of the heart and gives rise to coronary, pulmonary, and systemic arteries.[339-343] The single arterial trunk receives the output of both ventricles. The truncal semilunar valve is quadricuspid in 40% to 50% of cases and in most of the rest is equipped with three leaflets that tend to be focally or diffusely thickened or dysplastic.[13]An obligatory ventricular septal defect, which is almost always nonrestrictive, results from absence or deficiency of the infundibular septum and is roofed by the truncal valve, setting the stage for inadequate support and truncal regurgitation.

By far the most common type of truncus arteriosus is characterized by a short main pulmonary artery that originates from the side of the truncus and gives rise to right and left pulmonary arterial branches.[343] A second type is characterized by right and left pulmonary arterial branches that originate directly from the truncus by two separate orifices.[339,341,343] The physiologic consequences and longevity patterns depend chiefly on the presence of stenoses of the pulmonary arteries and on the resistance to flow through the peripheral pulmonary vascular bed. Right ventricular pressure is identical with systemic pressure because both ventricles communicate directly with the biventricular truncus through a nonrestrictive ventricular septal defect. When resistance is low, pulmonary blood flow is increased and cyanosis is mild, advantages gained at the price of volume overload of the left ventricle and congestive heart failure. Truncal valve regurgitation, less commonly stenosis, adds to the burden of the volume-overloaded left ventricle, and these hemodynamic derangements are necessarily imposed on the right ventricle because the truncus is biventricular. A rise in pulmonary vascular resistance relieves the left ventricle of volume overload and improves longevity, albeit at the price of increasing cyanosis.[344-347] Less commonly, narrowing of pulmonary artery branches as they arise from the truncus curtails pulmonary blood flow and improves longevity. Although the majority of patients die of congestive heart failure before their first birthday, occasional survivors with elevated pulmonary vascular resistance reach the fifth decade, with an exceptional survival to age 52 years.[339,345,347]

One of our patients was a 41-year-old man with a calcified stenotic and incompetent truncal valve (Fig. 4–25), and 14 of our truncus patients are aged 25 to 47 years.

COMPLETE TRANSPOSITION OF THE GREAT ARTERIES

This malformation is characterized by atrioventricular concordance and ventricular/great artery *discordance* in hearts with two noninverted ventricles.[348-352] The systemic and pulmonary circulations are in parallel and do not cross, so there is no interchange between the two unless a communication exists at atrial, ventricular, or great arterial levels. Survival is tightly coupled to the delicate interplay between these intercirculatory connections and pulmonary blood flow. Survival is poorest when the foramen ovale is restrictive, the ventricular septum is intact, and the ductus is closed.[353] The salutary effect of an adequate-sized interatrial communication is underscored by the immediate response to balloon atrial septostomy.[354] The majority of patients who reach their teens have a large ventricular septal defect with either pulmonary vascular disease or, less commonly, pulmonary stenosis.[355,356] Isolated examples of unusual longevity have been recorded in the fourth and fifth decades.[245,356-359] A 56-year-old patient had complete transposition documented at necropsy.[360] Our oldest survivor was a 42-year-old woman with pulmonary vascular disease, a nonrestrictive ventricular septal defect, a moderately restrictive interarterial communication, and a restrictive patent ductus arteriosus (Fig. 4–26).

DOUBLE-OUTLET VENTRICLE

Double-outlet ventricle as considered here refers to hearts with concordant atrioventricular connections to each of two ventricles (biventricular-atrioventricular connection)

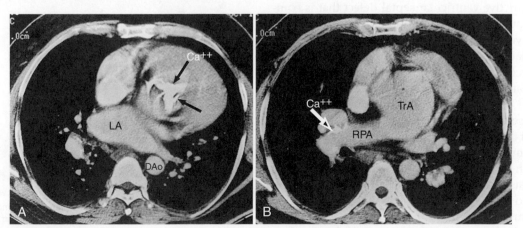

FIGURE 4-25 Computed tomographic scans from a 41-year-old man with truncus arteriosus Type I. **(A)** The calcified truncal valve (CA++) was quadricuspid. DAo=descending aorta; LA, left atrium. **(B)** Calcium (CA++) in the right pulmonary artery (RPA), which originated from a common pulmonary trunk that arose from the truncus arteriosus (TrA).

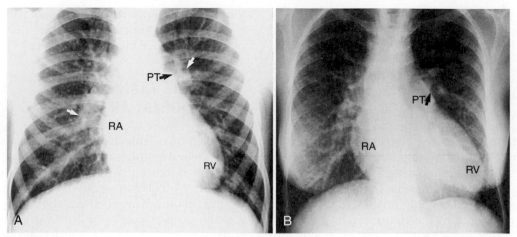

FIGURE 4-26 Chest radiographs from a cyanotic patient with complete transposition of the great arteries, a nonrestrictive ventricular septal defect, a moderately restrictive atrial septal defect, and pulmonary vascular disease. **(A)** At age 11 years the hypertensive dilatated posterior pulmonary trunk (PT) is barely border-forming *(black arrow)*. The right and left pulmonary arteries *(white arrows)* are dilatated. The right atrium (RA) is moderately prominent. A convex right ventricle (RV) occupies the apex. The lacy appearance in the lungs represents neovascularity. **(B)** At age 34 years, the dilatated hypertensive posterior pulmonary trunk is border-forming, right atrium is prominent, and a dilatated right ventricle occupies the apex. The lower lobe neovascularity appears more prominent because of soft tissue attenuation (breasts).

but with both great arteries originating from only one ventricular chamber.[13] In double-outlet right ventricle, two great arterial trunks separated by the outlet septum are housed exclusively in the right ventricle.[361] A subaortic or subpulmonary ventricular septal defect provides the left ventricle with its only exit.[362-364] When the ventricular septal defect is committed to the aorta and when the pulmonary vascular resistance is low, cyanosis is absent because oxygenated left ventricular blood preferentially streams into the aortic root, and unoxygenated right ventricular blood preferentially streams into the pulmonary trunk. Longevity is analogous to isolated perimembranous ventricular septal defects of similar size and similar pulmonary vascular resistance (see earlier discussion). One of our patients underwent intracardiac repair at age 53 years (Fig. 4–27). Less than 10% of double-outlet right ventricles have a nonrestrictive ventricular septal defect that is committed to the pulmonary trunk (subpulmonary), and thus saturated left ventricular blood selectively enters the pulmonary circulation, whereas unsaturated right ventricular blood selectively enters the aorta (see subsequent discussion on the Taussig-Bing anomaly).[365-367] Cyanosis exists with increased pulmonary blood flow. When pulmonary vascular disease occurs with nonrestrictive ventricular septal defects and double-outlet ventricles, longevity is similar to isolated nonrestrictive perimembranous ventricular septal defects with Eisenmenger syndrome. When pulmonary stenosis coexists with double-outlet right ventricle, longevity is similar to tetralogy of Fallot (discussed later), which it closely resembles.

Double-outlet left ventricle—the rarest of the ventricular/great artery malalignments—is characterized by a nonrestrictive ventricular septal defect and a clinical

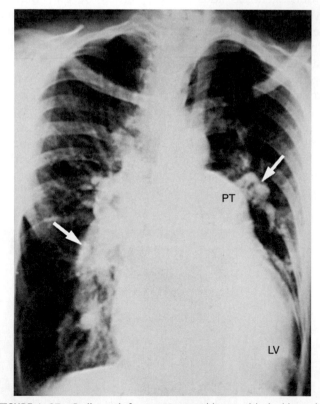

FIGURE 4-27 Radiograph from a 53-year-old man with double-outlet right ventricle, a subaortic ventricular septal defect, and a pulmonary-to-systemic flow ratio of 1.7 to 1. The pulmonary trunk (PT) and its branches *(arrows)* are conspicuously dilatated, pulmonary vascularity is increased, and an enlarged left ventricle (LV) occupies the apex. Thoracic distortion is due to scoliosis.

course resembling that of an isolated nonrestrictive ventricular septal defect with comparable pulmonary vascular resistence.[368] Pulmonary stenosis occasionally exerts a favorable effect on longevity by regulating pulmonary blood flow so that it is adequate for oxygenation but not hemodynamically excessive.[369]

TAUSSIG-BING ANOMALY

Double-outlet right ventricle with a nonrestrictive ventricular septal defect committed to the pulmonary trunk—the Taussig-Bing anomaly—comprises less than 10% of cases of right ventricular origin of both great arteries.[268,367] Right ventricular blood enters the aorta, whereas left ventricular blood selectively enters the pulmonary trunk.[365,367] Cyanosis is initially mild, but if survival permits, hypoxemia increases as pulmonary vascular resistance rises and diverts right ventricular blood into the aorta. The rise in pulmonary resistance occasionally regulates pulmonary blood flow and ameliorates congestive heart failure without seriously compromising systemic arterial oxygenation. Longevity improves, and an occasional patient lives into the second, third, or fourth decade.[370] Our oldest patient was a 42-year-old woman with suprasystemic pulmonary vascular resistance and a reversed ductal shunt (reversed differential cyanosis, acyanotic feet, cyanotic hands) (Fig. 4–28). Longevity is curtailed in the 50% of Taussig-Bing patients with coexisting

aortic arch malformations that include coarctation and isthmic hypoplasia or interruption.[13]

TETRALOGY OF FALLOT

In 1888, Arthur Fallot wrote, "We have seen from our observations that cyanosis, especially in the adult, is the result of a small number of cardiac malformations well determined."[371] Survival in unoperated patients with tetralogy of Fallot is linked to the degree of right ventricular outflow obstruction. Attrition is highest in deeply cyanotic infants with severe pulmonary stenosis and lowest when the degree of pulmonary stenosis is sufficiently modest to permit adequate but not excessive pulmonary blood flow and mild or absent cyanosis.

An analysis of unoperated survival based on 566 necropsy cases disclosed 66% attrition at age 1 year; 50% reached age 3 years, approximately 25% completed the first decade, and thereafter the attrition rate was 6% to 7% per year.[283,372–374] Put differently, for unoperated patients with tetralogy of Fallot of all degrees of severity, 11% are alive at age 20 years, 6% at age 30 years, and 3% at age 40 years. There are a number of reports of survival between the fifth and seventh decades.[372,373,375–385] Arthur Fallot's oldest patient was 36 years of age.[371] A 64-year-old woman with the tetralogy was examined in 1895 by G. A. Gibson (best known for his description of the continuous murmur of patent ductus arteriosus).[383] In 1929,

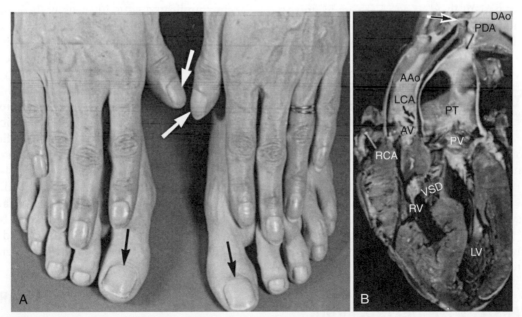

FIGURE 4–28 **(A)** The hands and feet of a 40-year-old woman with reversed differential cyanosis. The thumbs *(white arrows)* and fingers are clubbed and more cyanotic than the toes, which are not clubbed *(black arrows)*. **(B)** Necropsy specimen at age 42 years shows the mechanism of reversed differential cyanosis. Unoxygenated blood entered an ascending aorta (AAo) that arose from the right ventricle (RV), so the hands were cyanosed. Oxygenated blood from the left ventricle (LV) entered a biventricular pulmonary trunk (PT) and flowed through a nonrestrictive patent ductus arteriosus (PDA) to the feet (suprasystemic pulmonary resistance). The ventricular septal defect (VSD) was subpulmonary. AV, PV, aortic and pulmonary valves; DAo, descending aorta; LCA, RCA, left and right coronary arteries. *(From Perloff, J.K., Urschell C.W., Roberts, W.C., and Caulfield, W.H.: Aneurysmal dilatation of the coronary arteries in cyanotic congenital heart disease. Am. J. Med. 1968;45:802.)*

White and Sprague published an account of the American composer Henry F. Gilbert, who lived to age 60 years.[385] Another patient played cricket and football as a schoolboy and survived to age 62 years.[373]

Systemic arterial hypertension or acquired fibrocalcific aortic stenosis in adults with tetralogy of Fallot poses a special problem because the increase in afterload is imposed on both the left and right ventricles (biventricular aorta).[375] Augmented resistance to right ventricular discharge serves to improve pulmonary blood flow and reduce cyanosis but at the price of right ventricular or biventricular failure.

The greater the degree of anterior and rightward deviation of the malaligned infundibular septum, the more severe the obstruction to right ventricular outflow, the larger the aorta, and the higher the incidence of aortic regurgitation that accrues decade by decade.[386] However, the size of the ascending aorta is determined not only by the degree of right ventricular outflow obstruction but also by a coexisting abnormality of the media.[18] Although aortic regurgitation imposes volume load on both ventricles, the right ventricle is more adversely affected because it is already confronted with systemic afterload.[387] Infective endocarditis on the susceptible, incompetent biventricular aortic valve can result in catastrophic acute severe regurgitation into both right and left ventricles (see Chapter 8).

In tetralogy of Fallot with pulmonary atresia, unoperated life expectancy is approximately 50% in 1 year and 8% in the first decade.[372] Adequate but not excessive aortic-to-pulmonary arterial collateral blood flood occasionally permits survival into adolescence and adulthood.[166-171] One patient lived to age 54 years,[388] and another of our patients survived until 6 months before her 55th birthday despite acquired calcific aortic stenosis and regurgitation[389] (Fig. 4-29).

TETRALOGY OF FALLOT WITH ABSENT PULMONARY VALVE

In 2% to 6% of patients with tetralogy of Fallot, pulmonary valve tissue is either absent or consists of rudimentary remnants of cellular, vascular, myxomatous, or primitive connective tissue.[390-392] Occasionally patients go through infancy with relatively few symptoms, but respiratory distress (tracheobronchial obstruction) and right ventricular failure conspire to limit longevity. One patient survived to age 22 years.[393]

SITUS INVERSUS WITH DEXTROCARDIA

When situs inversus with dextrocardia occurs with a structurally normal heart, which is usually the case, longevity is normal, but when congenital heart disease coexists, longevity is determined by the coexisting cardiac anomalies.[13] The uncomplicated malposition is usually discovered by

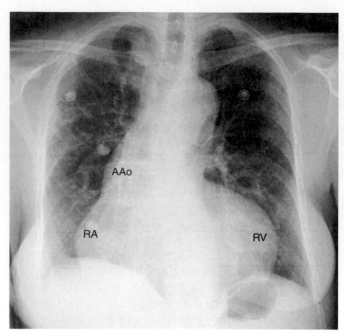

FIGURE 4-29   Chest radiograph taken 6 months before the death of a 55-year-old cyanotic woman with tetralogy of Fallot and pulmonary atresia. The aortic valve was calcified, stenotic, and moderately regurgitant. AAo, dilatated ascending aorta; RA, dilatated right atrium; RV, right ventricle that occupies the apex.

chance on a routine chest x-ray, but when the film is inadvertently reversed before reading, it is misinterpreted as normal, so the positional anomaly escapes detection.

Uncomplicated situs inversus with dextrocardia is accompanied by age-related acquired cardiac and noncardiac diseases because longevity is not curtailed. Symptoms so related may lead to discovery of the previously unsuspected cardiac malposition. Angina pectoris or myocardial infarction is accompanied by pain in the right anterior chest with radiation to the right shoulder and right arm.[394,395] Because of mirror image locations of the abdominal viscera, the pain of acute appendicitis is located in the left lower quadrant,[396] and the pain of biliary colic is located in the left upper quadrant (Fig. 4-30). In 1933, Kartagener called attention to the association of situs inversus with sinusitis and bronchiectasis (Kartagener's syndrome), which was subsequently found to be an inherited ciliary disorder that included the upper and lower respiratory tracts and immobile sperm (male infertility).[13]

SITUS SOLITUS WITH DEXTROCARDIA

This malposition occasionally occurs with a structurally normal heart that delays clinical recognition and permits normal longevity.[13] A routine chest radiograph may provide the first evidence (abdominal situs solitus with a right thoracic heart, Fig. 4-31). Coexisting congenital cardiac malformations are usually present and determine longevity.[13]

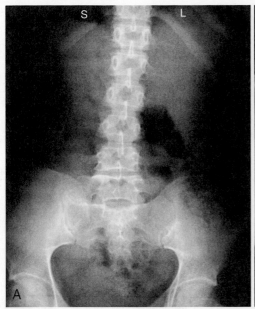
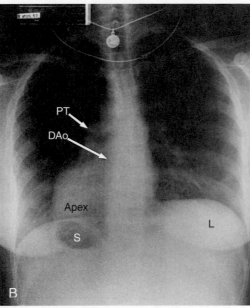

FIGURE 4–30   Radiographs from a 34-year-old woman who presented with acute left upper quadrant colic. **(A)** Abdominal radiograph disclosed the stomach bubble (S) on the right and the liver (L) on the left, establishing the diagnosis of abdominal situs inversus, appropriate for left upper quadrant biliary colic. **(B)** Chest radiograph identified the heart and stomach (S) on the right and the liver (L) on the left. The aorta descended along the right edge of the vertebral column (DAo, descending aorta), and the pulmonary trunk (PT) was convex in its mirror image location.

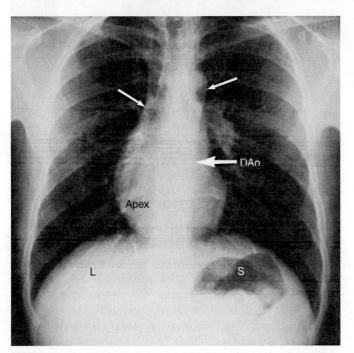

FIGURE 4–31   Radiograph from a 20-year-old man in situs solitus with dextrocardia. There were no associated congenital anomalies. The stomach (S) and liver (L) are in their normal positions. The base-to-apex axis of the heart points downward and to the right. The ascending aorta, aortic knuckle *(unmarked arrows)*, and descending aorta (DAo) are in their normal positions.

VISCERAL HETEROTAXY WITH LEFT ISOMERISM (BILATERAL LEFT-SIDEDNESS)

A distinctive and diagnostically important feature of this malposition is inferior vena caval interruption with azygos vein continuation, which occurs in 70% to 80% of cases

and rarely in otherwise normal individuals[13] (Fig. 4–32). Because of bilateral left-sidedness, a right superior vena cava joins a morphologic left atrium, and thus the sinus node is usually absent or hypoplastic. A 22-year-old man with visceral heterotaxy, left isomerism, and inferior vena caval interruption with azygos continuation came to attention because of syncope caused by ectopic atrial bradycardia (Fig. 4–33). Complete atrioventricular block occurs in approximately 20% of patients with left isomerism and can present in the fetus and neonate with a significant impact on mortality.[13] Conduction is interrupted at the level of the penetrating bundle, resulting in nodo-ventricular discontinuity and an escape rhythm with a narrow QRS complex.

ISOLATED CONGENITAL COMPLETE HEART BLOCK

Complete heart block *in utero* is strongly associated with maternal antibodies to ribonucleoproteins and is also strongly associated with the neonatal lupus syndrome (see Chapter 20).[13,397] Long-term morbidity therefore involves both mother and offspring. The conduction injury is believed to be in response to active transport of maternal IgG autoantibodies into the fetal circulation.[13] As many as 70% of pregnant women with lupus are asymptomatic at the time of delivery and are diagnosed as such because of the birth of an infant with heart block.[398,399] Maternal lupus erythematosus may not be recognized until many years after the birth of an affected child.[400,401] Long-term follow-up of these mothers, however, is more reassuring than previously assumed.[398,399] Less clear is the long-term immunologic prognosis for infants with congenital complete heart block who survive the neonatal period. A small number develop connective tissue disorders as adults, but the

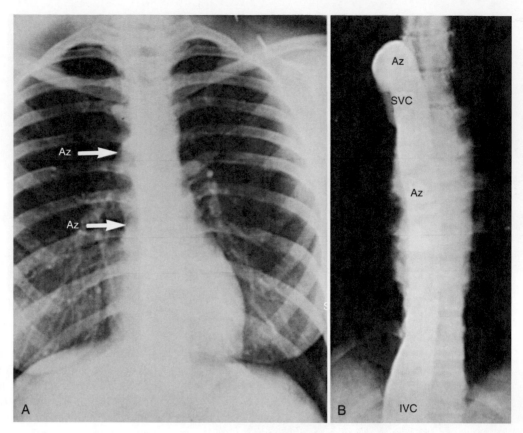

FIGURE 4-32 (A) Radiograph from a 28-year-old woman with isolated uncomplicated inferior vena caval interruption and azygos (Az) continuation. The spleen was present and single. The azygos vein ascends along the right margin of the vertebral column. **(B)** Inferior vena cavogram (IVC) shows the course of the azygos vein (Az) to the right superior vena cava (SVC).

likelihood of doing so is unknown.[398,399] Familial heart block is well recognized.[13]

The key determinants of clinical stability and longevity in isolated congenital complete heart block are the ventricular rate, hemodynamic adjustments to exercise, and the presence of intrinsically normal ventricular myocardium.[402-406] However, dilatated cardiomyopathy may become manifest, and a strong relationship has been reported between the earlier-described antibodies and subsequent development of cardiomyopathy.[13]

The clinical course of children with uncomplicated congenital complete heart block is good, but the ultimate fate of large numbers of adolescents and adults dampens optimism.[13,407-412] Although a substantial majority of young patients are asymptomatic, serious or even fatal sequelae sometimes occur.[407,409,411,412] Syncope and sudden death are usually due to excessive bradycardia, but the cause is occasionally ventricular tachycardia or fibrillation.[13]

Normal tolerance to endurance exercise is uncommon but not rare with congenital complete heart block.[406] Adults have included ice hockey and cricket players and Air Force pilots, one of whom was a 48-year-old man. At age 23 years, he experienced a normal response to a Royal Canadian Air Force decompression chamber, engaged in competitive sports, and subsequently flew jet aircraft.[403,405,406,413,414]

VENA CAVAL TO LEFT ATRIAL COMMUNICATIONS

Congenital communications between a vena cava or both vena cavae and the left atrium are rare anomalies that seldom occur in isolation[415-420] (Fig. 4-34). Isolated communications between vena cavae and the left atrium permit survival into adulthood, with cases recorded in the sixth decade.[415-420] Most rarely, both the superior and inferior vena cavae communicate with the left atrium–total anomalous caval connection (see Fig. 4-34, *B* and *C*).

Patients with caval to left atrial communications are necessarily cyanotic with normal or reduced pulmonary arterial blood flow. An important variation is cyanosis with increased pulmonary blood flow that occurs when an ostium secundum atrial septal defect exists with a large eustachian valve that extends from the orifice of the inferior vena cava to the margin of the secundum defect selectively channeling inferior caval blood into the left atrium in amounts sufficient to cause clinical cyanosis.[421-423] Survival patterns are believed to be the same as for uncomplicated ostium secundum atrial septal defect, as described earlier, but the risk of paradoxical embolism is increased.

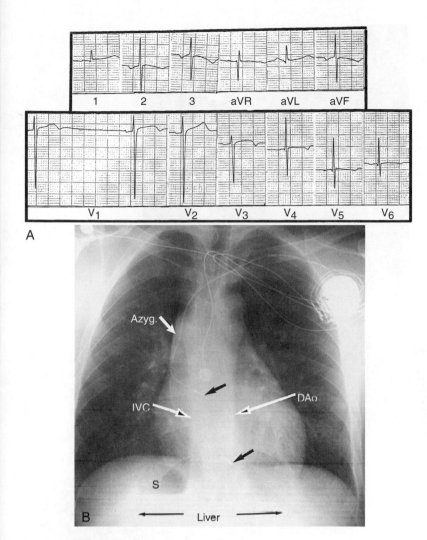

FIGURE 4-33   **(A)** Electrocardiogram from a 22-year-old man with left isomerism. He presented with syncope caused by ectopic atrial bradycardia. The normal sinus node pacemaker was absent because there was no right superior vena caval/right atrial junction. The inverted P waves in leads 2, 3, and aVF indicate an ectopic atrial focus. **(B)** Radiograph shows the stomach (S) on the right, a transverse liver, inferior vena caval (IVC) interruption with azygos (Azyg.) continuation, a left descending aorta (DAo), and a dual-chamber pacemaker *(black arrows)*.

CORONARY ARTERIAL FISTULA

Coronary arterial fistulae are the most frequent clinically overt congenital malformations of the coronary circulation.[424-430] Both coronary arteries arise from their assigned aortic sinus, but a fistulous branch of one or more of these arteries communicates directly with a cardiac chamber or with the pulmonary trunk, coronary sinus, vena cava, or a pulmonary vein.[13] The general terms *coronary artery* or *coronary arterial* fistula apply to all of these, but when the fistula drains into a right cardiac chamber or into the pulmonary trunk, it is *arteriovenous*. Adult survival is expected, although life span is not normal. Longevity depends on the magnitude of flow through the fistulous communication, the chamber or vascular bed that receives the fistula, myocardial ischemia from a coronary steal caused by the low resistance vascular channels, and complications that include infective endocarditis, rupture and sudden death.[13] Survivals have been recorded from ages 63 through 75 years [425,428,431,432] (Fig. 4-35, *A*) and up to age 85 years.[433-436] A 68-year-old professional athlete was undiagnosed until acquired atherosclerotic coronary artery disease prompted angiography that identified bilateral coronary arterial fistulae.[437] In a 63-year-old woman, a coronary arterial fistula was incidentally diagnosed during routine coronary angiography (see Fig. 4-35, *B*). Spontaneous closure of a coronary arterial fistula is uncommon but not rare,[438-444] exerting a favorable effect on longevity.

ANOMALOUS ORIGIN OF THE LEFT CORONARY ARTERY FROM THE PULMONARY TRUNK

This is the most important high-risk congenital malformation of the coronary circulation. Immediately after birth, high pulmonary arterial pressure provides an antegrade perfusion gradient that promotes flow into the anomalous left coronary artery. The fall in neonatal pulmonary vascular resistance is accompanied by a parallel fall in antegrade flow through the anomalous coronary artery. As flow falls, myocardial ischemia ensues unless adequate circulation is established through right-to-left intercoronary

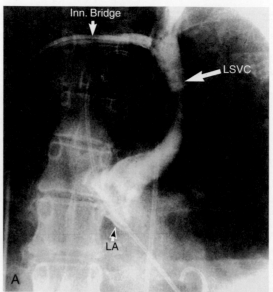

FIGURE 4–34 **(A)** Angiogram from a 53-year-old woman with Ebstein's anomaly of the tricuspid valve. A left superior vena cava (LSVC) connected to the left atrium (LA) was an incidental angiographic finding. The innominate bridge (Inn Bridge) was restrictive. **(B** and **C)** Radiographs from a 28-year-old woman with drainage of both superior and inferior vena cavas into the left atrium (total anomalous systemic venous connection). An ostium secundum atrial septal defect coexisted. The size and shape of the heart and great arteries are virtually normal. Increased markings in the lower lung fields are due to soft tissue attenuation (breasts). In the lateral film, the inferior vena caval shadow is conspicuous by its absence *(arrow)*.

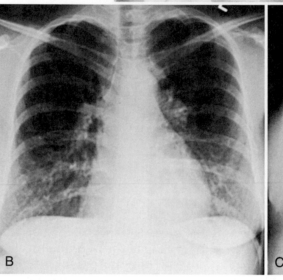

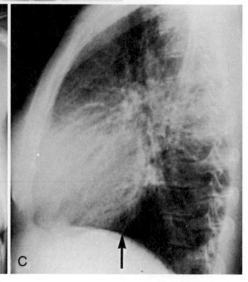

anastomoses on which survival largely depends.[445-447] Flow into the anomalous left coronary artery through large intercoronary anastomoses has opposing effects: (1) the desirable effect of reestablishing left coronary arterial perfusion; (2) the undesirable effect of acting as a low-resistance coronary steal that bypasses the capillary bed, thus reducing myocardium oxygen delivery; (3) mitral regurgitation caused by ischemic papillary muscle dysfunction; and (4) the undesirable effect of establishing a left-to-right shunt that is occasionally large enough to volume overload the left venticle.[445,446] Two quite different cellular, pathologic, and clinical derangements result from hypoxemia imposed on *immature* ventricular cardiomyocytes (see Chapter 21): (1) ischemic myocardium is injured and replaced with connective tissue resulting in depressed left ventricular contractility, and conversely, (2) the segment of hypoperfused but viable immature left ventricular myocardium responds with myocyte replication and a regional increase in mass (see Chapter 21).

The clinical course of patients with unoperated anomalous origin of the left coronary artery from the pulmonary trunk is a continuum ranging from death in infancy to asymptomatic adult survival, with all gradations in between.[446,448-452] One of the first known patients with the anomaly was a 60-year-old woman described by Maude Abbott in 1908.[453] Our oldest patient was a 68-year-old woman whose electrocardiogram and chest radiograph are shown in Fig. 4–36. An occasional infant with cardiac failure subsequently improves, only to die suddenly during a relatively asymptomatic childhood or adolescence.[454] The anomalous left coronary artery is sometimes discovered in adults during diagnostic studies of the mitral regurgitation[455]; less commonly, adults present with a continuous murmur via intercoronary anastomoses initially mistaken for patent ductus arteriosus, or a previously asymptomatic adult experiences angina pectoris, cardiac failure, syncope, or sudden death.[449-452,456-458] The

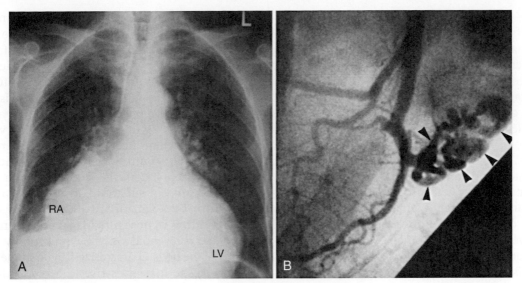

FIGURE 4-35   (A) Radiograph from a 75-year-old man with a congenital right coronary arterial-to-right atrial fistula. The pulmonary-to-systemic flow ratio was 1.7 to 1. The right atrium (RA) is considerably enlarged, and a dilated left ventricle (LV) occupies the apex. There is a small right pleural effusion. **(B)** Coronary arteriogram from a 63-year-old woman with a small congenital coronary arteriovenous fistula *(arrowheads)* arising from the left anterior descending artery and communicating with the pulmonary trunk.

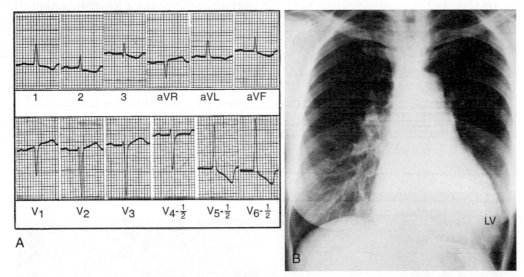

FIGURE 4-36   (A) Electrocardiogram from a 68-year-old woman with anomalous origin of the left coronary artery from the pulmonary trunk. The PR interval is prolonged. There is poor r wave progression in the precordial leads with left ventricular hypertrophy in leads V_{5-6} (half standardized). Limb leads show nonspecific repolarization abnormalities. **(B)** Chest radiograph shows an enlarged left ventricle (LV). Soft tissue densities in right lower lung field are due to the overlying breast tissue.

frequency of sudden death—even in patients with little or no clinically evident heart disease—warrants emphasis.[454,459,460]

PULMONARY ARTERIOVENOUS FISTULAE

Pulmonary arteriovenous fistulae consist of one or more vascular trunks, a thin vascular sac, or a tangle of distended tortuous vascular channels and are either solitary or multiple, minute or large, unilateral or bilateral, or diffuse in both lungs.[461-464] Approximately 75% of congenital pulmonary arteriovenous fistulae involve the lower lobes or right middle lobe and tend to increase in size with age.[465] The intrapulmonary right-to-left shunt is sufficient to cause cyanosis but not sufficient to cause hemodynamic overload with the rare exception of massive pulmonary arteriovenous fistulae in the neonate.[466]

A substantial majority of these fistulae go undiagnosed until adult life, with the distinct minority of clinically recognized patients aged younger than 20 years.[461] Longevity and morbidity are determined by complications of the fistulae per se—rupture into a bronchus causing hemoptysis that varies from mild and intermittent to recurrent and massive[13,461]—and by the coexisting Rendu-Osler-Weber syndrome—hemorrhagic telangiectasia—characterized by tiny localized arteriovenous fistulae that readily rupture because of fragile, dilatated vascular membranes [461,463] (Fig. 4–37). A constellation of peculiar cerebral symptoms occurs in the Rendu-Osler-Weber syndrome, including dizziness, vertigo, paresthesias, tinnitus, visual disturbances, speech defects, headaches, weakness of limbs, hemiplegia, mental confusion, and convulsions.[13]

Appropriately placed lesions cause melena, hematuria, intraocular hemorrhage, vaginal bleeding, and cerebrovascular accidents.[13] Insidious gastrointestinal blood loss is a major cause of symptomatic iron deficient anemia, which can be profound.[467] Epistaxis, which is frequently the first overt manifestation of telangiectasia, ultimately affects 90% of patients and can be copious and recurrent.

Patients without the coexisting Rendu-Osler-Weber association fare better. Two of our patients with pulmonary arteriovenous fistulae without telangiectasia were siblings aged 71 and 73 years (Fig. 4–37).

UNIVENTRICULAR HEART

In this malformation, two atria and their atrioventricular junctions are exclusively or primarily related to a single ventricular compartment that qualifies on morphologic grounds as a left or right ventricle.[468-473] When the single ventricular compartment is a morphologic left ventricle, it incorporates at its base an outlet chamber that, with few exceptions, gives rise to the aorta, whereas the pulmonary trunk originates from the single ventricle.[468,471,474] When the single ventricular compartment is a morphologic right ventricle—10% to 24% of cases—a rudimentary trabecular pouch is incorporated into its posterior, lateral, or inferior wall, and both great arteries arise from the single right ventricle.[469-471] In univentricular hearts of the left ventricular type, obstruction to outflow can involve either great artery (subpulmonary stenosis or stenosis of a bicuspid pulmonary valve, or subaortic obstruction in the outlet foramen or by a subaortic conus), but in univentricular hearts of the right ventricular type, obstruction to outflow is represented only by pulmonary stenosis. The Holmes heart is characterized by a single morphologic left ventricle that gives rise to a concordant aorta and pulmonary stenosis that usually results from obstruction of the outlet foramen of the concordant subpulmonary outlet chamber.[13] The types of atrioventricular connections that guard the inlet of a univentricular heart consist of two separate valves, a common valve, or atresia of the right or left component.[468,474-476]

Longevity depends on the morphology of the single ventricle; the absence, presence, and degree of pulmonary stenosis or subaortic stenosis; the pulmonary vascular resistance in patients without pulmonary stenosis; and the morphology and function of the valve or valves that guard the atrioventricular junction. All else being equal, univentricular hearts of the left ventricle type have a better outlook than univentricular hearts of the right ventricle type, reflecting the inherent deficits of morphologic

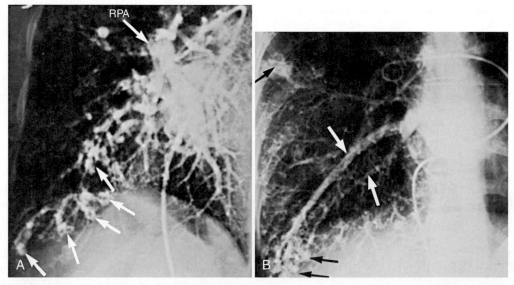

FIGURE 4–37 **(A)** Selective right pulmonary arteriogram (RPA) from a 73-year-old woman. Both she and her 71-year-old brother had congenital bilateral pulmonary arteriovenous fistulae (*arrows,* right lower lobe) *without* telangiectasia. **(B)** Selective right pulmonary arteriogram from a 57-year-old woman with bilateral pulmonary arteriovenous fistulae (*black arrows,* right middle and lower lobes) and Rendu-Osler-Weber syndrome. The afferent and efferent vascular channels that join and leave the lower lobe fistulae are identified by *white arrows.* *(A from Wong, L. B., and Perloff, J. K.: Am. J. Cardiol. 1988;62:149.)*

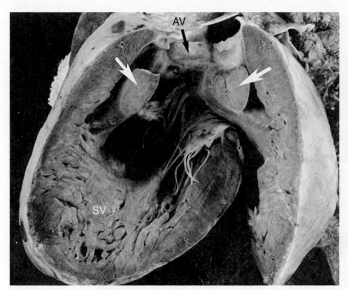

FIGURE 4-38   Necropsy specimen from a 21-year-old cyanotic man with pulmonary vascular disease and a single ventricle (SV) of the indeterminate type. White arrows identify an obstructing subaortic conus. AV, aortic valve.

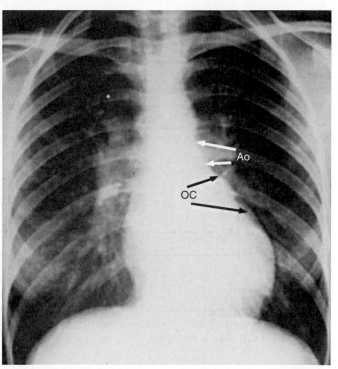

FIGURE 4-39   Radiograph from a 30-year-old woman with a univentricular heart of the left ventricular type and pulmonary stenosis (gradient 85 mm Hg). The heart size is normal. An inverted outlet chamber (OC) gives rise to the aorta (Ao).

right ventricles.[477,478] Subaortic stenosis augments already excessive pulmonary blood flow or, in the presence of pulmonary stenosis or pulmonary vascular disease, imposes additional afterload on the single ventricle (Fig. 4–38). Pulmonary stenosis is more effective than pulmonary vascular resistance in achieving favorable regulation of pulmonary arterial blood flow. Survival benefits from two-competent atrioventricular valves or a competent common atrioventricular valve.

Longevity is best when univentricular hearts of the left ventricular type benefit from moderate pulmonary stenosis and a functionally adequate atrioventricular valve mechanism (Fig. 4–39) Survival into early adulthood is not rare, and longevity occasionally extends into the fifth decade, with one patient reaching age 56 years.[473,479,480] Women have occasionally experienced successful pregnancies.[481,482] Our adults with single ventricle and pulmonary vascular disease include 16 patients aged 25 to 45 years. The oldest reported survivor was a 59-year-old man.[483]

TRICUSPID ATRESIA

The consistent anatomic features of this anomaly are as follows: (1) absence of an anatomic connection between the morphologic right atrium and morphologic right ventricle, (2) hypoplasia of the morphologic right ventricle, (3) an interatrial communication, and (4) a left ventricle and mitral valve that are morphologically normal. In the presence of an adequate-sized interatrial communication, longevity depends chiefly on the absence, presence, and degree of obstruction to pulmonary blood flow and on whether the great arteries are normally related or transposed. In the more common variety of tricuspid atresia, the great arteries are normally related, and a restrictive ventricular septal defect constitutes a zone of subpulmonary stenosis.[484,485] When pulmonary blood flow is adequate but not excessive—a balance seldom achieved—survivals have been recorded from the second through the fifth decades (Fig. 4–40), with two patients living to age 57 years.[51,486–491] Life span is shortest when tricuspid atresia exists with *pulmonary atresia* that takes the form of either spontaneous closure of a restrictive ventricular septal defect or an inherently intact ventricular septum.[488,492,493] Unusual survivals include an 18-year-old[488] and a 27-year-old with tricuspid atresia and late spontaneous closure of a ventricular septal defect,[494] a patient who lived for 21 years with tricuspid atresia and an intact ventricular septum,[495] a 21-year-old woman with tricuspid atresia and pulmonary atresia who survived because pulmonary blood flow was derived from an anomalous artery connecting the ascending aorta to the pulmonary trunk,[496] and a 22-year-old woman with a patent ductus arteriosus.[497] The most extraordinary survival was a 65-year-old man with tricuspid atresia, pulmonary atresia, an ostium secundum atrial septal defect, and large aortic-to-pulmonary arterial collaterals.[498]

Tricuspid atresia with a nonrestrictive ventricular septal defect and no pulmonary stenosis typically occurs with complete transposition of the great arteries.[488,499,500]

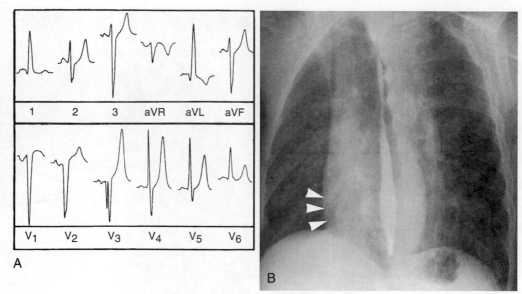

FIGURE 4-40 **(A)** Electrocardiogram from a 28-year-old man with tricuspid atresia, a restrictive ventricular septal defect, and normally related great arteries. There are biatrial P wave abnormalities, left axis deviation with left ventricular hypertrophy (lead aVL), and unexplained Q waves in leads V_{2-3}. **(B)** Left oblique radiograph shows flattening at the site of the underdeveloped right ventricle *(arrowheads)*.

Whether or not the great arteries are transposed, pulmonary blood flow in the absence of pulmonary stenosis is determined by pulmonary vascular resistance, which seldom achieves a balance between adequate and excessive flow.[488,499] However, occasional survivals have been reported between 32 and 45 years of age,[491] with one exceptional survival to age 57 years.[490] Rarely, tricuspid atresia with a nonrestrictive ventricular septal defect, complete transposition, and pulmonary stenosis permits a desirable regulation of pulmonary blood flow with longevity into the second, third, and fourth decades.[51,489,491] One patient survived to age 56 years.[51]

CONGENITAL OBSTRUCTION TO LEFT ATRIAL FLOW

Of the three major types of congenital obstruction to left atrial flow—pulmonary vein stenosis, mitral stenosis, and cor triatriatum—it is the latter that occasionally permits adult survival.[501-504] The clinical manifestations and longevity patterns of uncomplicated cor triatriatum depend on the degree of obstruction, which ranges from functionally insignificant ridges of tissue to complete absence of a direct communication between upper and lower atrial compartments.[503,505] Cor triatriatum usually comes to light in infants or young children, but symptoms may await adolescence or adulthood.[13] Mild cor triatriatum in asymptomatic adults can be an incidental finding at necropsy or an incidental echocardiographic finding, as was the case in a 70-year-old man.[506] One of our patients, a 24-year-old woman, was undiagnosed until she presented with dyspnea initially mistaken for asthma (Fig. 4–41).

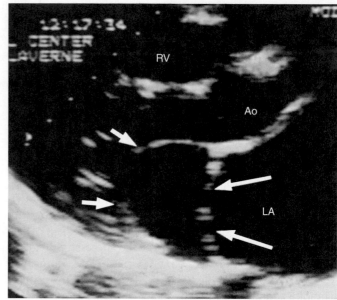

FIGURE 4-41 Two-dimensional echocardiogram (parasternal long-axis) from a 24-year-old woman with cor triatriatum. Longer arrows on the right identify the obstructing membrane well above the normal mitral leaflets *(shorter arrows on the left)*. Symptoms began at age 24 years. Ao, aorta; LA, left atrium; RV, right ventricle.

VASCULAR RINGS

Eighty percent of these aortic arch anomalies occur without coexisting congenital cardiac or vascular malformations.[507] Symptoms vary with the degree of tracheoesophageal compression. Some vascular rings cause no symptoms and are discovered incidentally at

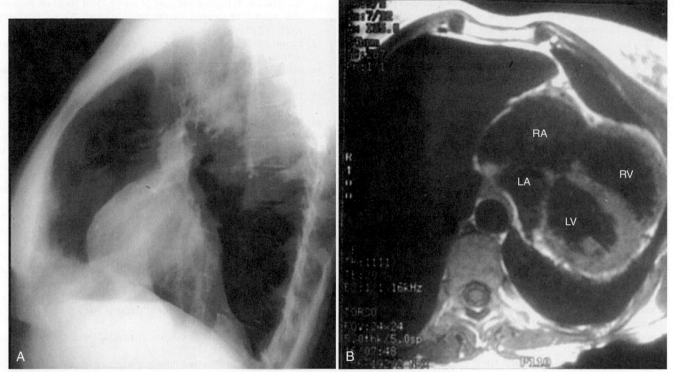

FIGURE 4-42   **(A)** Lateral chest x-ray from a 38-year-old woman with congenital complete absence of the pericardium showing striking retrodisplacement of the heart. **(B)** Magnetic resonance image axial view showing a strikingly mobile heart displaced into the left thoracic cavity. Ao, aorta; LA/RA, left and right atrium; LV/RV, left and right ventricle.

necropsy. More commonly, stridor, wheezing, and cough during the first few months of life result from tracheal compression, although dysphagia (esophageal compression) is relatively uncommon. Symptoms in a 17-year-old boy were misdiagnosed for years as bronchial asthma (Fig. 4-42).

CONGENITAL COMPLETE ABSENCE OF THE PERICARDIUM

This rare anomaly is accompanied by an increase in right ventricular size because the parietal pericardium normally exerts myocardial contact stress that limits dilatation.[508] Pain is believed to originate from torsion of the thoracic inlet caused by striking mobility of the heart (Fig. 4-42). Longevity has not been established in congenital complete absence of the pericardium, but our patient was 38 years old,[508] and another survived to the eighth decade.[13]

References

1. Allaby M. *The Oxford Dictionary of Natural History*. Oxford: Oxford University; 1985.
2. Hoffman JDE. Reflections on the past, present and future of pediatric cardiology. *Cardiol Young*. 1994;4:208–212.
3. Abbott ME. *Atlas of Congenital Cardiac Diseases*. New York: American Heart Association; 1936.
4. Waller BF, Howard J, Fess S. Pathology of mitral valve stenosis and pure mitral regurgitation—Part II. *Clin Cardiol*. 1994;17:395–402.
5. Waller BF, Howard J, Fess S. Pathology of mitral valve stenosis and pure mitral regurgitation—Part I. *Clin Cardiol*. 1994;17:330–336.
6. Waller BF, Taliercio CP, Dickos DK, et al. Rare or unusual causes of chronic, isolated, pure aortic regurgitation. *Clin Cardiol*. 1990;13: 577–581.
7. Beppu S, Suzuki S, Matsuda H, et al. Rapidity of progression of aortic stenosis in patients with congenital bicuspid aortic valves. *Am J Cardiol*. 1993;71:322–327.
8. Fenoglio JJ Jr, McAllister HA Jr, DeCastro CM, et al. Congenital bicuspid aortic valve after age 20. *Am J Cardiol*. 1977;39:164–169.
9. Roberts WC. The congenitally bicuspid aortic valve. A study of 85 autopsy cases. *Am J Cardiol*. 1970;26:72–83.
10. Roberts WC. Valvular, subvalvular and supravalvular aortic stenosis: morphologic features. *Cardiovasc Clin*. 1973;5:97–126.
11. Walley VM AD, Kyrollos AG, Chan KL. Congenitally bicuspid aortic valve: study of a variant with fenestrated raphe. *Can J Cardiol*. 1994;10:535–542.
12. Fedak PW, Verma S, David TE, et al. Clinical and pathophysiological implications of a bicuspid aortic valve. *Circulation*. 2002;106: 900–904.
13. Perloff J. *The Clinical Recognition of Congenital Heart Disease*. 5th ed. Philadelphia: WB Saunders; 2003.
14. Carter JB, Sethi S, Lee GB, Edwards JE. Prolapse of semilunar cusps as causes of aortic insufficiency. *Circulation*. 1971;43:922–932.
15. Morganroth J, Perloff JK, Zeldis SM, Dunkman WB. Acute severe aortic regurgitation. Pathophysiology, clinical recognition, and management. *Ann Intern Med*. 1977;87:223–232.
16. Ratib O, Perloff JK, Child JS. Images in cardiovascular medicine. Bicuspid aortic valve aneurysm. *Circulation*. 2004;109:671.

17. Roberts WC, Ko JM, Moore TR, Jones WH 3rd. Causes of pure aortic regurgitation in patients having isolated aortic valve replacement at a single US tertiary hospital (1993 to 2005). *Circulation.* 2006;114: 422–429.
18. Niwa K, Perloff JK, Bhuta SM, et al. Structural abnormalities of great arterial walls in congenital heart disease: light and electron microscopic analyses. *Circulation.* 2001;103:393–400.
19. Hahn RT, Roman MJ, Mogtader AH, Devereux RB. Association of aortic dilation with regurgitant, stenotic and functionally normal bicuspid aortic valves. *J Am Coll Cardiol.* 1992;19:283–288.
20. Larson EW, Edwards WD. Risk factors for aortic dissection: a necropsy study of 161 cases. *Am J Cardiol.* 1984;53:849–855.
21. Roberts CS, Roberts WC. Dissection of the aorta associated with congenital malformation of the aortic valve. *J Am Coll Cardiol.* 1991;17:712–716.
22. Shachter N, Perloff JK, Mulder DG. Aortic dissection in Noonan's syndrome (46 XY turner). *Am J Cardiol.* 1984;54:464–465.
23. Falcone MW, Roberts WC, Morrow AG, Perloff JK. Congenital aortic stenosis resulting from a unicommissural valve. Clinical and anatomic features in twenty-one adult patients. *Circulation.* 1971;44:272–280.
24. Simon AL, Reis RL. The angiographic features of bicuspid and unicommissural aortic stenosis. *Am J Cardiol.* 1971;28:353–358.
25. Brouwer MH, de Graaf JJ, Ebels T. Congenital quadricuspid aortic valve. *Int J Cardiol.* 1993;38:196–198.
26. Fernicola DJ, Mann JM, Roberts WC. Congenitally quadricuspid aortic valve: analysis of six necropsy patients. *Am J Cardiol.* 1989;63:136–138.
27. Fischler D, Fitzmaurice M, Ratliff NB Jr. Quadricuspid aortic valve. *Am J Cardiovasc Pathol.* 1990;3:91–94.
28. Hurwitz LE, Roberts WC. Quadricuspid semilunar valve. *Am J Cardiol.* 1973;31:623–626.
29. Feldman BJ, Khandheria BK, Warnes CA, et al. Incidence, description and functional assessment of isolated quadricuspid aortic valves. *Am J Cardiol.* 1990;65:937–938.
30. Mitchell SC, Korones SB, Berendes HW. Congenital heart disease in 56,109 births. Incidence and natural history. *Circulation.* 1971;43: 323–332.
31. Abbott M. Coarctation of the aorta of adult type: II. Statistical study and historical retrospect of 200 recorded cases, with autopsy, of stenosis or obliteration of descending arch in subjects above the age of two years. *Am Heart J.* 1928;3:392.
32. Campbell M. Natural history of coarctation of the aorta. *Br Heart J.* 1970;32:633–640.
33. Reifenstein GH, Levine SA, Gross RE. Coarctation of the aorta: a review of 104 autopsied cases of the "adult type," 2 years of age or older. *Am Heart J.* 1947;33:146–168.
34. Haldane JH. Coarctation of the aorta in an elderly man. *Can Med Assoc J.* 1983;128:1298–1299.
35. Jarcho S. Coarctation of the aorta (Reynaud, 1828). *Am J Cardiol.* 1962;9:591–597.
36. Liberthson RR, Pennington DG, Jacobs ML, Daggett WM. Coarctation of the aorta: review of 234 patients and clarification of management problems. *Am J Cardiol.* 1979;43:835–840.
37. Milo S, Massini C, Goor DA. Isolated atresia of the aortic arch in a 65-year-old man. Surgical treatment and review of published reports. *Br Heart J.* 1982;47:294–297.
38. Edwards JE. Aneurysms of the thoracic aorta complicating coarctation. *Circulation.* 1973;48:195–201.
39. Hodes HL, Steinfeld L, Blumenthal S. Congenital cerebral aneurysms and coarctation of the aorta. *Arch Pediatr.* 1959;76:28–43.
40. Schneeweiss A, Sherf L, Lehrer E, et al. Segmental study of the terminal coronary vessels in coarctation of the aorta: a natural model for study of the effect of coronary hypertension on human coronary circulation. *Am J Cardiol.* 1982;49:1996–2002.
41. Vlodaver Z, Neufeld HN. The coronary arteries in coarctation of the aorta. *Circulation.* 1968;37:449–454.
42. Woltman HW, Shelden WD. Neurologic complications associated with congenital stenosis of the isthmus of the aorta; case of cerebral aneurysm with rupture and case of intermittent lameness presumably related to stenosis of the isthmus. *Arch Neurol Psychiatry.* 1927;17:303.
43. Simon AL, Reis RL. The angiographic features of bicuspid and unicommissural aortic stenosis. *Am J Cardiol.* 1971;28:353–358.
44. Balis JU, Chan AS, Conen PE. Morphogenesis of human aortic coarctation. *Exp Mol Pathol.* 1967;6:25–38.
45. Dunnill MS. Histology of the aorta in coarctation. *J Pathol Bacteriol.* 1959;78:203–207.
46. Isner JM, Donaldson RF, Fulton D, et al. Cystic medial necrosis in coarctation of the aorta: a potential factor contributing to adverse consequences observed after percutaneous balloon angioplasty of coarctation sites. *Circulation.* 1987;75:689–695.
47. Greenspan AM, Morganroth J, Perloff JK. Discrete fibromembranous aortic stenosis in middle age. Natural history and case report. *Cardiology.* 1979;64:306–316.
48. Katz NM, Buckley MJ, Liberthson RR. Discrete membranous subaortic stenosis. Report of 31 patients, review of the literature, and delineation of management. *Circulation.* 1977;56:1034–1038.
49. Freedom RM, Pelech A, Brand A, et al. The progressive nature of subaortic stenosis in congenital heart disease. *Int J Cardiol.* 1985;8: 137–148.
50. Newfeld EA, Muster AJ, Paul MH, et al. Discrete subvalvular aortic stenosis in childhood. Study of 51 patients. *Am J Cardiol.* 1976;38: 53–61.
51. Fontana RS, Edwards JE. *Congenital Cardiac Disease.* Philadelphia: WB Saunders; 1962.
52. Choi JY, Sullivan ID. Fixed subaortic stenosis: anatomical spectrum and nature of progression. *Br Heart J.* 1991;65:280–286.
53. Firpo C, Maitre Azcarate MJ, et al. Discrete subaortic stenosis (DSS) in childhood: a congenital or acquired disease? Follow-up in 65 patients. *Eur Heart J.* 1990;11:1033–1040.
54. Maron BJ, Redwood DR, Roberts WC, et al. Tunnel subaortic stenosis: left ventricular outflow tract obstruction produced by fibromuscular tubular narrowing. *Circulation.* 1976;54:404–416.
55. Freedom RM, Fowler RS, Duncan WJ. Rapid evolution from "normal" left ventricular outflow tract to fatal subaortic stenosis in infancy. *Br Heart J.* 1981;45:605–609.
56. Leichter DA, Sullivan I, Gersony WM. "Acquired" discrete subvalvular aortic stenosis: natural history and hemodynamics. *J Am Coll Cardiol.* 1989;14:1539–1544.
57. Child JS. Echo-Doppler and color-flow imaging in congenital heart disease. *Cardiol Clin.* May 1990;8:289–313.
58. Martin MM, Lemmer JH Jr, Shaffer E, et al. Obstruction to left coronary artery blood flow secondary to obliteration of the coronary ostium in supravalvular aortic stenosis. *Ann Thorac Surg.* 1988;45: 16–20.
59. Pansegrau DG, Kioshos JM, Durnin RE, Kroetz FW. Supravalvular aortic stenosis in adults. *Am J Cardiol.* 1973;31:635–641.
60. Daniels SR, Loggie JM, Schwartz DC, et al. Systemic hypertension secondary to peripheral vascular anomalies in patients with Williams syndrome. *J Pediatr.* 1985;106:249–251.
61. Ino T, Nishimoto K, Iwahara M, et al. Progressive vascular lesions in Williams-Beuren syndrome. *Pediatr Cardiol.* 1988;9:55–58.
62. Lopez-Rangel E, Maurice M, et al. Williams syndrome in adults. *Am J Med Genet.* 1992;44:720–729.
63. Morris CA, Carey JC. Three diagnostic signs in Williams syndrome. *Am J Med Genet Suppl.* 1990;6:100–101.
64. Morris CA, Demsey SA, Leonard CO, et al. Natural history of Williams syndrome: physical characteristics. *J Pediatr.* 1988;113: 318–326.
65. Williams JC, Barratt-Boyes BG, Lowe JB. Supravalvular aortic stenosis. *Circulation.* 1961;24:1311–1318.
66. Williams RL, Azouz EM. Aortic anomalies in an adolescent with the Williams' elfin facies syndrome. *Pediatr Radiol.* 1984;14:122–124.
67. Beuren AJ, Apitz J, Harmjanz D. Supravalvular aortic stenosis in association with mental retardation and a certain facial appearance. *Circulation.* 1962;26:1235–1240.

68. Ingelfinger JR, Newburger JW. Spectrum of renal anomalies in patients with Williams syndrome. *J Pediatr.* Nov 1991;119:771–773.

69. Sacks O. Musical ability. *Science.* 1995;268:621–622.

70. Adams JC, Hudson R. A case of Ebstein's anomaly surviving to the age of 79. *Br Heart J.* 1956;18:129–132.

71. Anderson KR, Zuberbuhler JR, Anderson RH, et al. Morphologic spectrum of Ebstein's anomaly of the heart: a review. *Mayo Clin Proc.* 1979;54:174–180.

72. Bialostozky D, Horwitz S, Espino-Vela J. Ebstein's malformation of the tricuspid valve. A review of 65 cases. *Am J Cardiol.* 1972;29: 826–836.

73. Cabin HS, Roberts WC. Ebstein's anomaly of the tricuspid valve and prolapse of the mitral valve. *Am Heart J.* 1981;101:177–180.

74. Celermajer DS, Bull C, Till JA, et al. Ebstein's anomaly: presentation and outcome from fetus to adult. *J Am Coll Cardiol.* 1994;23: 170–176.

75. Gentles TL, Calder AL, Clarkson PM, Neutze JM. Predictors of long-term survival with Ebstein's anomaly of the tricuspid valve. *Am J Cardiol.* 1992;69:377–381.

76. Genton E, Blount SG Jr. The spectrum of Ebstein's anomaly. *Am Heart J.* 1967;73:395–425.

77. Giuliani ER, Fuster V, Brandenburg RO, Mair DD. Ebstein's anomaly: the clinical features and natural history of Ebstein's anomaly of the tricuspid valve. *Mayo Clin Proc.* 1979;54:163–173.

78. Harris RH. Ebstein's anomaly: discovered in a 75-year-old subject in the dissecting laboratory. *Can Med Assoc J.* 1960;83:653–655.

79. Hong YM, Moller JH. Ebstein's anomaly: a long-term study of survival. *Am Heart J.* 1993;125:1419–1424.

80. Jaiswal PK, Balakrishnan KG, Saha A, et al. Clinical profile and natural history of Ebstein's anomaly of tricuspid valve. *Int J Cardiol.* 1994;46:113–119.

81. Kumar AE, Fyler DC, Miettinen OS, Nadas AS. Ebstein's anomaly. Clinical profile and natural history. *Am J Cardiol.* 1971;28: 84–95.

82. Leung MP, Baker EJ, Anderson RH, Zuberbuhler JR. Cineangiographic spectrum of Ebstein's malformation: its relevance to clinical presentation and outcome. *J Am Coll Cardiol.* 1988;11:154–161.

83. Mair DD. Ebstein's anomaly: natural history and management. *J Am Coll Cardiol.* 1992;19:1047–1048.

84. Makous N, Vander Veer JB. Ebstein's anomaly and life expectancy. Report of a survival to over age 79. *Am J Cardiol.* 1966;18: 100–104.

85. Nihoyannopoulos P, McKenna WJ, Smith G, Foale R. Echocardiographic assessment of the right ventricle in Ebstein's anomaly: relation to clinical outcome. *J Am Coll Cardiol.* 1986;8:627–635.

86. Radford DJ, Graff RF, Neilson GH. Diagnosis and natural history of Ebstein's anomaly. *Br Heart J.* 1985;54:517–522.

87. Saxena A, Fong LV, Tristam M, et al. Late noninvasive evaluation of cardiac performance in mildly symptomatic older patients with Ebstein's anomaly of tricuspid valve: role of radionuclide imaging. *J Am Coll Cardiol.* 1991;17:182–186.

88. Seward JB, Tajik AJ, Feist DJ, Smith HC. Ebstein's anomaly in an 85-year-old man. *Mayo Clin Proc.* 1979;54:193–196.

89. Shiina A, Seward JB, Edwards WD, et al. Two-dimensional echocardiographic spectrum of Ebstein's anomaly: detailed anatomic assessment. *J Am Coll Cardiol.* 1984;3:356–370.

90. Watson H. Natural history of Ebstein's anomaly of tricuspid valve in childhood and adolescence. An international co-operative study of 505 cases. *Br Heart J.* 1974;36:417–427.

91. Attenhofer Jost CH, Connolly HM, Dearani JA, et al. Ebstein's anomaly. *Circulation.* 2007;115:277–285.

92. Celermajer DS, Cullen S, Sullivan ID, et al. Outcome in neonates with Ebstein's anomaly. *J Am Coll Cardiol.* 1992;19:1041–1046.

93. Celermajer DS, Dodd SM, Greenwald SE, et al. Morbid anatomy in neonates with Ebstein's anomaly of the tricuspid valve: pathophysiologic and clinical implications. *J Am Coll Cardiol.* 1992;19:1049–1053.

94. Rossi L, Thiene G. Mild Ebstein's anomaly associated with supraventricular tachycardia and sudden death: clinicomorphologic features in 3 patients. *Am J Cardiol.* 1984;53:332–334.

95. Tede NH, Shivkumar K, Perloff JK, et al. Signal-averaged electrocardiogram in Ebstein's anomaly. *Am J Cardiol.* 2004;93:432–436.

96. Vacca JB, Bussmann DW, Mudd JG. Ebstein's anomaly; complete review of 108 cases. *Am J Cardiol.* 1958;2:210–226.

97. Child JS, Perloff JK, Francoz R, et al. Uhl's anomaly (parchment right ventricle): clinical, echocardiographic, radionuclear, hemodynamic and angiocardiographic features in 2 patients. *Am J Cardiol.* 1984;53:635–637.

98. Cote M, Davignon A, Fouron JC. Congenital hypoplasia of right ventricular myocardium (Uhl's anomaly) associated with pulmonary atresia in a newborn. *Am J Cardiol.* 1973;31:658–661.

99. French JW, Baum D, Popp RL. Echocardiographic findings in Uhl's anomaly. Demonstration of diastolic pulmonary valve opening. *Am J Cardiol.* 1975;36:349–353.

100. Perez Diaz L, Quero Jimenez M, Moreno Granados F, et al. Congenital absence of myocardium of right ventricle: Uhl's anomaly. *Br Heart J.* 1973;35:570–572.

101. Bharati S, Ciraulo DA, Bilitch M, et al. Inexcitable right ventricle and bilateral bundle branch block in Uhl's disease. *Circulation.* 1978;57:636–644.

102. Bjarke BB, Kidd BS. Congenitally corrected transposition of the great arteries. A clinical study of 101 cases. *Acta Paediatr Scand.* 1976;65:153–160.

103. Connelly MS, Liu PP, Williams WG, et al. Congenitally corrected transposition of the great arteries in the adult: functional status and complications. *J Am Coll Cardiol.* 1996;27:1238–1243.

104. Friedberg DZ, Nadas AS. Clinical profile of patients with congenital corrected transposition of the great arteries. A study of 60 cases. *N Engl J Med.* 1970;282:1053–1059.

105. Presbitero P, Somerville J, Rabajoli F, et al. Corrected transposition of the great arteries without associated defects in adult patients: clinical profile and follow-up. *Br Heart J.* 1995;74:57–59.

106. Schiebler GL, Edwards JE, Burchell HB, et al. Congenital corrected transposition of the great vessels: a study of 33 cases. *Pediatrics.* 1961;27:849–888.

107. Graham TP Jr, Bernard YD, Mellen BG, et al. Long-term outcome in congenitally corrected transposition of the great arteries: a multi-institutional study. *J Am Coll Cardiol.* 2000;36:255–261.

108. Anderson RH, Becker AE, Arnold R, Wilkinson JL. The conducting tissues in congenitally corrected transposition. *Circulation.* 1974;50:911–923.

109. Daliento L, Corrado D, Buja G, et al. Rhythm and conduction disturbances in isolated, congenitally corrected transposition of the great arteries. *Am J Cardiol.* 1986;58:314–318.

110. Huhta JC, Danielson GK, Ritter DG, Ilstrup DM. Survival in atrioventricular discordance. *Pediatr Cardiol.* 1985;6:57–60.

111. Kupersmith J, Krongrad E, Gersony WM, Bowman FO Jr. Electrophysiologic identification of the specialized conduction system in corrected transposition of the great arteries. *Circulation.* 1974;50: 795–800.

112. Lundstrom U, Bull C, Wyse RK, Somerville J. The natural and "unnatural" history of congenitally corrected transposition. *Am J Cardiol.* 1990;65:1222–1229.

113. Benchimol A, Sundararajan V. Congenital corrected transposition of the great vessels in a 58-year-old man. *Chest.* 1971;59: 634–638.

114. Lieberson AD, Schumacher RR, Childress RH, Genovese PD. Corrected transposition of the great vessels in a 73-year-old man. *Circulation.* 1969;39:96–100.

115. Nagle JP, Cheitlin MD, McCarty RJ. Corrected transposition of the great vessels without associated anomalies: report of a case with congestive failure at age 45. *Chest.* 1971;60:367–370.

116. Rotem CE, Hultgren HN. Corrected transposition of the great vessels without associated defects. *Am Heart J.* 1965;70:305–318.

117. Schwartz HA, Wagner PI. Corrected transposition of the great vessels in a 55-year-old woman; diagnosis by coronary angiography. *Chest.* 1974;66:190–192.

118. Cummings GR. Congenital corrected transposition of the great vessels without associated intracardiac anomalies. *Am J Cardiol.* 1962;10:605–614.

119. Attie F, Rijlaarsdam M, Zabal C, et al. [Corrected transposition of the great arteries in patients over 65]. *Arch Inst Cardiol Mex.* 1995;65:57–64.

120. Melero-Pita A, Alonso-Pardo F, Bardaji-Mayor JL, Higueras J. Corrected transposition of the great arteries. *N Engl J Med.* 1996;334:866–867.

121. Lam D, Cheitlin MD, Popper RW, Szarnicki RJ. Rapid development of biventricular heart failure in corrected transposition of the great arteries during pregnancy. *Am Heart J.* 1988;116:1111–1115.

122. Abrahams DG, Wood P. Pulmonary stenosis with normal aortic root. *Br Heart J.* 1951;13:419–448.

123. Barritt DW. Simple pulmonary stenosis. *Br Heart J.* 1954;16:381–386.

124. Blount SG Jr, Komesu S, McCord MC. Asymptomatic isolated valvular pulmonary stenosis; diagnosis by clinical methods. *N Engl J Med.* 1953;248:5–11.

125. Campbell M. Simple pulmonary stenosis; pulmonary valvular stenosis with a closed ventricular septum. *Br Heart J.* 1954;16:273–300.

126. Campbell M. Natural history of congenital pulmonary stenosis. *Br Heart J.* 1969;31:394.

127. Danilowicz D, Hoffman JI, Rudolph AM. Serial studies of pulmonary stenosis in infancy and childhood. *Br Heart J.* 1975;37:808–818.

128. Engle MA, Ito T, Goldberg HP. The fate of the patient with pulmonic stenosis. *Circulation.* 1964;30:554–561.

129. Genovese PD, Rosenbaum D. Pulmonary stenosis with survival to the age of 78 years. *Am Heart J.* 1951;41:755–761.

130. Geraci JE, Burchell HB, Edwards JE. Cardiac clinics. 140. Congenital pulmonary stenosis with intact ventricular septum in persons more than 50 years of age: report of 2 cases. *Mayo Clin Proc.* 1953;28:346–352.

131. Johnson LW, Grossman W, Dalen JE, Dexter L. Pulmonic stenosis in the adult. Long-term follow-up results. *N Engl J Med.* 1972;287:1159–1163.

132. Lueker RD, Vogel JH, Blount SG Jr. Regression of valvular pulmonary stenosis. *Br Heart J.* 1970;32779–32782.

133. Moller JH, Adams P Jr. The natural history of pulmonary valvular stenosis. Serial cardiac catheterizations in 21 children. *Am J Cardiol.* 1965;16:654–664.

134. Nugent EW, Freedom RM, Nora JJ, et al. Clinical course in pulmonary stenosis. *Circulation.* 1977;56:I38–I47.

135. Tami LF, McElderry MW. Pulmonary artery aneurysm due to severe congenital pulmonic stenosis. Case report and literature review. *Angiology.* 1994;45:383–390.

136. White PD, Hurst JW, Fennell RH. Survival to the age of seventy-five years with congenital pulmonary stenosis and patent foramen ovale. *Circulation.* 1950;2:558–564.

137. Stone FM, Bessinger FB Jr, Lucas RV Jr, Moller JH. Pre- and postoperative rest and exercise hemodynamics in children with pulmonary stenosis. *Circulation.* 1974;49:1102–1106.

138. Greene DG, Baldwin ED, Baldwin JS, et al. Pure congenital pulmonary stenosis and idiopathic congenital dilatation of the pulmonary artery. *Am J Med.* 1949;6:24–40.

139. Campbell M, Missen GA. Survival in good health until 65 years with pulmonary valvar stenosis. *Guys Hosp Rep.* 1959;108:390–402.

140. Wild JB, Eckstein JW, Van Epps EF, Culbertson JW. Three patients with congenital pulmonic valvular stenosis surviving for more than fifty-seven years; medical histories and physiologic data. *Am Heart J.* 1957;53:393–403.

141. Wood P. *Diseases of the Heart and Circulation.* 2nd ed. Philadelphia: JB Lippincott; 1956.

142. Levine OR, Blumenthal S. Pulmonic stenosis. *Circulation.* 1965;32:III33–III41.

143. Berman W Jr, Fripp RR, Rowe SA, Yabek SM. Congenital isolated pulmonary valve incompetence: neonatal presentation and early natural history. *Am Heart J.* 1992;124:248–251.

144. Pouget JM, Kelly CE, Pilz CG. Congenital absence of the pulmonic valve. Report of a case in a seventy-three-year-old man. *Am J Cardiol.* 1967;19:732–740.

145. Ansari A. Isolated pulmonary valvular regurgitation: current perspectives. *Prog Cardiovasc Dis.* 1991;33:329–344.

146. Cortes FM, Jacoby WJ. Isolated congenital pulmonary valvular insufficiency. *Am J Cardiol.* 1962;10:287–290.

147. Lendrum BL, Shaffer AB. Isolated congenital pulmonic valvular regurgitation. *Am Heart J.* 1959;57:298–308.

148. Price BO. Isolated incompetence of the pulmonic valve. *Circulation.* 1961;23:596–602.

149. Brayshaw JR, Perloff JK. Congenital pulmonary insufficiency complicating idiopathic dilatation of the pulmonary artery. *Am J Cardiol.* 1962;10:282–286.

150. Collins NP, Braunwald E, Morrow AG. Isolated congenital pulmonic valvular regurgitation. Diagnosis by cardiac catheterization and angiocardiography. *Am J Med.* 1960;28:159–164.

151. Fish RG, Takaro T, Crymes T. Prognostic considerations in primary isolated insufficiency of the pulmonic valve. *N Engl J Med.* 1959;261:739–742.

152. Goldberg E, Katz I. Isolated pulmonic regurgitation with intermittent pulmonary artery dilatation. *Am J Cardiol.* 1962;9:619–625.

153. Hamby RI, Gulotta SJ. Pulmonic valvular insufficiency: etiology, recognition, and management. *Am Heart J.* 1967;74:110–125.

154. Kelly DT. Isolated congenital pulmonary incompetence. *Br Heart J.* 1965;27:777–780.

155. Laneve SA, Uesu CT, Taguchi JT. Isolated pulmonic valvular regurgitation. *Am J Med Sci.* 1962;244:446–458.

156. Tanabe Y, Takahashi M, Kuwano H, et al. Long-term fate of isolated congenital absent pulmonary valve. *Am Heart J.* 1992;124:526–529.

157. Arvidsson H, Carlsson E, Hartmann A Jr, et al. Supravalvular stenoses of the pulmonary arteries. Report of eleven cases. *Acta Radiol.* 1961;56:466–480.

158. D CL, Arcilla RA. Anomalous venous drainage of the left lung into the inferior vena cava. a case report. *Am Heart J.* 1964;67:539–544.

159. Delaney TB, Nadas AS. Peripheral pulmonic stenosis. *Am J Cardiol.* 1964;13:451–461.

160. Franch RH, Gay BB Jr. Congenital stenosis of the pulmonary artery branches. A classification, with postmortem findings in two cases. *Am J Med.* 1963;35:512–529.

161. Adams CW. A reappraisal of life expectancy with atrial shunts of the secundum type. *Dis Chest.* 1965;48:357–375.

162. Campbell M. Natural history of atrial septal defect. *Br Heart J.* 1970;32:820–826.

163. Colmers RA. Atrial septal defects in elderly patients; report of three patients aged 68, 72 and 78. *Am J Cardiol.* 1958;1:768–773.

164. Craig RJ, Selzer A. Natural history and prognosis of atrial septal defect. *Circulation.* 1968;37:805–815.

165. Dexter L. Atrial septal defect. *Br Heart J.* 1956;18:209–225.

166. Forfang K, Simonsen S, Andersen A, Efskind L. Atrial septal defect of secundum type in the middle-aged. Clinical results of surgery and correlations between symptoms and hemodynamics. *Am Heart J.* 1977;94:44–54.

167. Kelly JJ Jr, Lyons HA. Atrial septal defect in the aged. *Ann Intern Med.* 1958;48:267–283.

168. Markman P, Howitt G, Wade EG. Atrial septal defect in the middle-aged and elderly. *Quart J Med.* 1965;34:409–426.

169. Mattila S, Merikallio E, Tala P. ASD in patients over 40 years of age. *Scand J Thorac Cardiovasc Surg.* 1979;13:21–24.

170. Paolillo V, Dawkins KD, Miller GA. Atrial septal defect in patients over the age of 50. *Int J Cardiol.* 1985;9:139–147.

171. Perloff JK. Ostium secundum atrial septal defect—survival for 87 and 94 years. *Am J Cardiol.* 1984;53:388–389.

172. Rodstein M, Zeman FD, Gerber IE. Atrial septal defect in the aged. *Circulation.* 1961;23:665–674.

173. Sanders C, Bittner V, Nath PH, et al. Atrial septal defect in older adults: atypical radiographic appearances. *Radiology.* 1988;167:123–127.

174. Shub C, Tajik AJ, Seward JB. Clinically "silent" atrial septal defect: diagnosis by two-dimensional and Doppler echocardiography. *Am Heart J.* 1985;110:665–667.

175. St John Sutton MG, Tajik AJ, et al. Assessment of left ventricular function in secundum atrial septal defect by computer analysis of the M-mode echocardiogram. *Circulation.* 1979;60:1082–1090.

176. Gault JH, Morrow AG, Gay WA, Ross J. Atrial septal defect in patients over the age of forty years: clinical and hemodynamic studies and the effects of operation. *Circulation.* 1968;37:261–272.

177. Landi F, Cipriani L, Cocchi A, et al. Ostium secundum atrial septal defect in the elderly. *J Am Geriatric Soc.* 1991;39:60–63.

178. Wood P. Forward. In: Bedford ED, Caird FL, ed. *Valvular Disease of the Heart in Old Age.* Boston: Little, Brown; 1960.

179. Zaver AG, Nadas AS. Atrial septal defect—secundum type. *Circulation.* 1965;32:III24–III32.

180. Bonow RO, Borer JS, Rosing DR, et al. Left ventricular functional reserve in adult patients with atrial septal defect: pre- and postoperative studies. *Circulation.* 1981;63:1315–1322.

181. Carabello BA, Gash A, Mayers D, Spann JF. Normal left ventricular systolic function in adults with atrial septal defect and left heart failure. *Am J Cardiol.* 1982;49:1868–1873.

182. Popio KA, Gorlin R, Teichholz LE, et al. Abnormalities of left ventricular function and geometry in adults with an atrial septal defect. Ventriculographic, hemodynamic and echocardiographic studies. *Am J Cardiol.* 1975;36:302–308.

183. Wanderman KL, Ovsyshcher I, Gueron M. Left ventricular performance in patients with atrial septal defect: evaluation with noninvasive methods. *Am J Cardiol.* 1978;41:487–493.

184. Booth DC, Wisenbaugh T, Smith M, DeMaria AN. Left ventricular distensibility and passive elastic stiffness in atrial septal defect. *J Am Coll Cardiol.* 1988;12:1231–1236.

185. Sheehan R, Perloff JK, Fishbein MC, et al. Pulmonary neovascularity: a distinctive radiographic finding in Eisenmenger syndrome. *Circulation.* 2005;112:2778–2785.

186. Cherian G, Uthaman CB, Durairaj M, et al. Pulmonary hypertension in isolated secundum atrial septal defect: high frequency in young patients. *Am Heart J.* 1983;105:952–957.

187. Dave KS, Pakrashi BC, Wooler GH, Ionescu MI. Atrial septal defect in adults. Clinical and hemodynamic results of surgery. *Am J Cardiol.* 1973;31:7–13.

188. Saksena FB, Aldridge HE. Atrial septal defect in the older patient. A clinical and hemodynamic study in patients operated on after age 35. *Circulation.* 1970;42:1009–1020.

189. Steele PM, Fuster V, Cohen M, et al. Isolated atrial septal defect with pulmonary vascular obstructive disease—long-term follow-up and prediction of outcome after surgical correction. *Circulation.* 1987;76:1037–1042.

190. Dalen JE, Bruce RA, Cobb LA. Interaction of chronic hypoxia of moderate altitude on pulmonary hypertension complicating defect of the atrial septum. *N Engl J Med.* 1962;266:272–277.

191. Khoury GH, Hawes CR. Atrial septal defect associated with pulmonary hypertension in children living at high altitude. *J Pediatr.* 1967;70:432–435.

192. Wood P. The Eisenmenger syndrome or pulmonary hypertension with reversed central shunt. *Br Med J.* 1958;2:755–762.

193. Rothman A, Sklansky MS, Lucas VW, et al. Atrial septostomy as a bridge to lung transplantation in patients with severe pulmonary hypertension. *Am J Cardiol.* 1999;84:682–686.

194. Perloff JK, Hart EM, Greaves SM, et al. Proximal pulmonary arterial and intrapulmonary radiologic features of Eisenmenger syndrome and primary pulmonary hypertension. *Am J Cardiol.* 2003;92:182–187.

195. Boucher CA, Liberthson RR, Buckley MJ. Secundum atrial septal defect and significant mitral regurgitation: incidence, management and morphologic basis. *Chest.* 1979;75:697–702.

196. Davies MJ. Mitral valve in secundum atrial septal defects. *Br Heart J.* 1981;46:126–128.

197. Furuta S, Wanibuchi Y, Ino T, Aoki K. Etiology of mitral regurgitation in secundum atrial septal defect. *Jpn Circ J.* 1982;46:346–351.

198. Hynes KM, Frye RL, Brandenburg RO, et al. Atrial septal defect (secundum) associated with mitral regurgitation. *Am J Cardiol.* 1974;34:333–338.

199. Liberthson RR, Boucher CA, Fallon JT, Buckley MJ. Severe mitral regurgitation: a common occurrence in the aging patient with secundum atrial septal defect. *Clin Cardiol.* 1981;4:229–232.

200. Nagata S, Nimura Y, Sakakibara H, et al. Mitral valve lesion associated with secundum atrial septal defect. Analysis by real time two dimensional echocardiography. *Br Heart J.* 1983;49:51–58.

201. Schreiber TL, Feigenbaum H, Weyman AE. Effect of atrial septal defect repair on left ventricular geometry and degree of mitral valve prolapse. *Circulation.* 1980;61:888–896.

202. Weidman WH, DuShane JW, Ellison RC. Clinical course in adults with ventricular septal defect. *Circulation.* 1977;56:I78–I79.

203. Garcia R, Taber RE. Bacterial endocarditis of the pulmonic valve. Association with atrial septal defect of the ostium secundum type. *Am J Cardiol.* 1966;18:275–280.

204. Abman SH, Chatfield BA, Hall SL, McMurtry IF. Role of endothelium-derived relaxing factor during transition of pulmonary circulation at birth. *Am J Physiol.* 1990;259:H1921–H1927.

205. Rich S, Brundage BH. Pulmonary hypertension: a cellular basis for understanding the pathophysiology and treatment. *J Am Coll Cardiol.* 1989;14:545–550.

206. McLaughlin VV, McGoon MD. Pulmonary arterial hypertension. *Circulation.* 2006;114:1417–1431.

207. Rich S, Dantzker DR, Ayres SM, et al. Primary pulmonary hypertension. A national prospective study. *Ann Intern Med.* 1987;107:216–223.

208. Heath D, Edwards JE. The pathology of hypertensive pulmonary vascular disease; a description of six grades of structural changes in the pulmonary arteries with special reference to congenital cardiac septal defects. *Circulation.* 1958;18:533–547.

209. Palevsky HI, Schloo BL, Pietra GG, et al. Primary pulmonary hypertension. Vascular structure, morphometry, and responsiveness to vasodilator agents. *Circulation.* 1989;80:1207–1221.

210. Heath D, Smith P, Gosney J, et al. The pathology of the early and late stages of primary pulmonary hypertension. *Br Heart J.* 1987;58:204–213.

211. Wagenvoort CA, Wagenvoort N. *Pathology of Pulmonary Hypertension.* 2nd ed. New York: John Wiley; 1977.

212. D'Alonzo GE, Barst RJ, Ayres SM, et al. Survival in patients with primary pulmonary hypertension. Results from a national prospective registry. *Ann Intern Med.* 1991;115:343–349.

213. Fuster V, Steele PM, Edwards WD, et al. Primary pulmonary hypertension: natural history and the importance of thrombosis. *Circulation.* 1984;70:580–587.

214. Barst RJ, Rubin LJ, Long WA, et al. A comparison of continuous intravenous epoprostenol (prostacyclin) with conventional therapy for primary pulmonary hypertension. The Primary Pulmonary Hypertension Study Group. *N Engl J Med.* 1996;334:296–302.

215. Barst RJ, Maislin G, Fishman AP. Vasodilator therapy for primary pulmonary hypertension in children. *Circulation.* 1999;99:1197–1208.

216. Badesch DB, McLaughlin VV, Delcroix M, et al. Prostanoid therapy for pulmonary arterial hypertension. *J Am Coll Cardiol.* 2004;43:56S–61S.

217. Nagaya N, Uematsu M, Okano Y, et al. Effect of orally active prostacyclin analogue on survival of outpatients with primary pulmonary hypertension. *J Am Coll Cardiol.* 1999;34:1188–1192.

218. Rich S, McLaughlin VV. The effects of chronic prostacyclin therapy on cardiac output and symptoms in primary pulmonary hypertension. *J Am Coll Cardiol.* 1999;34:1184–1187.

219. Gatzoulis MA, Rogers P, Li W, et al. Safety and tolerability of bosentan in adults with Eisenmenger physiology. *Int J Cardiol.* 2005;98:147–151.

220. Ghofrani HA, Pepke-Zaba J, Barbera JA, et al. Nitric oxide pathway and phosphodiesterase inhibitors in pulmonary arterial hypertension. *J Am Coll Cardiol.* 2004;43:68S–72S.

221. Humpl T, Reyes JT, Holtby H, et al. Beneficial effect of oral sildenafil therapy on childhood pulmonary arterial hypertension: twelve-month clinical trial of a single-drug, open-label, pilot study. *Circulation.* 2005;111:3274–3280.

222. Channick RN, Sitbon O, Barst RJ, et al. Endothelin receptor antagonists in pulmonary arterial hypertension. *J Am Coll Cardiol.* 2004;43:62S–67S.

223. Rosenthal L. Atrial septal defect with mitral stenosis (Lutembacher's syndrome) in a woman of 81. *Br Med J.* 1956;2:1351.

224. Bashi VV, Ravikumar E, Jairaj PS, et al. Coexistent mitral valve disease with left-to-right shunt at the atrial level: clinical profile, hemodynamics, and surgical considerations in 67 consecutive patients. *Am Heart J.* 1987;114:1406–1414.

225. Davia JE, Cheitlin MD, Bedynek JL. Sinus venosus atrial septal defect: analysis of fifty cases. *Am Heart J.* 1973;85:177–185.

226. Bates ER. Survival for 88 years with sinus venosus atrial septal defect. *Am Geriatr Soc.* 1986;33:151.

227. Alpert JS, Dexter L, Vieweg WV, et al. Anomalous pulmonary venous return with intact atrial septum: diagnosis and pathophysiology. *Circulation.* 1977;56:870–875.

228. Frye RL, Krebs M, Rahimtoola SH, et al. Partial anomalous pulmonary venous connection without atrial septal defect. *Am J Cardiol.* 1968;22:242–250.

229. Snellen HA, van Ingen HC, Hoefsmit EC. Patterns of anomalous pulmonary venous drainage. *Circulation.* 1968;38:45–63.

230. Stewart JR, Schaff HV, Fortuin NJ, Brawley RK. Partial anomalous pulmonary venous return with intact atrial septum: report of four cases. *Thorax.* 1983;38:859–862.

231. McGaughey MD, Traill TA, Brinker JA. Partial left anomalous pulmonary venous return: a diagnostic dilemma. *Cathet Cardiovasc Diagn.* 1986;12:110–115.

232. Dupuis C, Charaf LA, Breviere GM, et al. The "adult" form of the scimitar syndrome. *Am J Cardiol.* 1992;70:502–507.

233. Honey M. Anomalous pulmonary venous drainage of right lung to inferior vena cava ("scimitar syndrome"): clinical spectrum in older patients and role of surgery. *Q J Med.* 1977;46:463–483.

234. Oakley D, Naik D, Verel D, Rajan S. Scimitar vein syndrome: report of nine new cases. *Am Heart J.* 1984;107:596–598.

235. Edwards JE, Helmholz HF Jr. A classification of total anomalous pulmonary venous connection based on developmental considerations. *Mayo Clin Proc.* 1956;31:151–160.

236. Rodriguez-Collado J, Attie F, Zabal C, et al. Total anomalous pulmonary venous connection in adults. Long-term follow-up. *J Thorac Cardiovasc Surg.* 1992;103:877–880.

237. Arbona GL, Kilman JW, Van Aman ME. Type IV total anomalous pulmonary venous connection. Unusual survival and review of the literature. *J Cardiovasc Surg.* 1982;23:49–53.

238. Gardner F, Oram S. Persistent left superior vena cava draining the pulmonary veins. *Br Heart J.* 1953;15:305–318.

239. McManus BM, Luetzeler J, Roberts WC. Total anomalous pulmonary venous connection: survival for 62 years without surgical intervention. *Am Heart J.* 1982;103:298–301.

240. Miller G, Pollock BE. Total anomalous pulmonary venous drainage. *Am Heart J.* 1955;49:127–134.

241. Pastore JO, Akins CW, Zir LM, et al. Total anomalous pulmonary venous connection and severe pulmonic stenosis in a 52-year-old man. *Circulation.* 1977;55:206–209.

242. Jensen JB, Blount SG Jr. Total anomalous pulmonary venous return. A review and report of the oldest surviving patient. *Am Heart J.* 1971;82:387–407.

243. McMullan MH, Fyke FE 3rd. Total anomalous pulmonary venous connection: surgical correction in a 66-year-old man. *Ann Thorac Surg.* 1992;53:520–521.

244. Munoz-Armas S, Gorrin JR, Anselmi G, et al. Single atrium. Embryologic, anatomic, electrocardiographic and other diagnostic features. *Am J Cardiol.* 1968;21:639–652.

245. Shaher RM. Prognosis of transposition of the great vessels with and without atrial septal defect. *Br Heart J.* 1963;25:211–218.

246. Hurst JW. The examination of the heart: the importance of initial screening. *Dis Mon.* 1990;36:245–313.

247. Brandenburg RO, Dushane JW. Clinical features of persistent common atrioventricular canal. *Mayo Clin Proc.* 1956;31:509–513.

248. Brockenbrough EC, Braunwald E, Roberts WC, Morrow AG. Partial persistent atrioventricular canal simulating pure mitral regurgitation. *Am Heart J.* 1962;63:9–17.

249. MacLeod CA. Endocardial cushion defects with severe mitral insufficiency and small atrial septal defect. *Circulation.* 1962;26:755.

250. Hynes JK, Tajik AJ, Seward JB, et al. Partial atrioventricular canal defect in adults. *Circulation.* 1982;66:284–287.

251. Heath D. Long survival in partial persistent common atrioventricular canal. *Br J Dis Chest.* 1968;62:207–210.

252. Tandon R, Moller JH, Edwards JE. Unusual longevity in persistent common atrioventricular canal. *Circulation.* 1974;50:619–626.

253. Zion MM, Rosenman D, Balkin J, Glaser J. Complete atrioventricular canal with survival to the eighth decade. *Chest.* 1984;85:437–438.

254. Campbell M. Natural history of persistent ductus arteriosus. *Br Heart J.* 1968;30:4–13.

255. Fisher RG, Moodie DS, Sterba R, Gill CC. Patent ductus arteriosus in adults—long-term follow-up: nonsurgical versus surgical treatment. *J Am Coll Cardiol.* 1986;8:280–284.

256. Marquis RM, Miller HC, McCormack RJ, et al. Persistence of ductus arteriosus with left to right shunt in the older patient. *Br Heart J.* 1982;48:469–484.

257. Morgan JM, Gray HH, Miller GA, Oldershaw PJ. The clinical features, management and outcome of persistence of the arterial duct presenting in adult life. *Int J Cardiol.* 1990;27:193–199.

258. Ng AS, Vlietstra RE, Danielson GK, et al. Patent ductus arteriosus in patients more than 50 years old. *Int J Cardiol.* 1986;11:277–285.

259. Hang CL, Sullebarger JT. Patent ductus arteriosus presenting in old age. *Cathet Cardiovasc Diagn.* 1993;28:228–230.

260. Aiken JE, Bifulco E, Sullivan JJ Jr. Patent ductus arteriosus in the aged. Report of this disease in a 74-year-old female. *JAMA.* 1961;177:330–331.

261. Bain CW. Longevity in patients ductus arteriosus. *Br Heart J.* 1957;19:574–576.

262. Boe J, Humerfelt S. Patent ductus arteriosus Botalli in an octogenarian followed for fifty years. *Acta Med Scand.* 1960;167:73–75.

263. Fishman L. Patent ductus arteriosus in a patient surviving to seventy-four years. *Am J Cardiol.* 1960;6:685–688.

264. Hornsten TR, Hellerstein HK, Ankeney JL. Patent ductus arteriosus in a 72-year-old woman. Successful corrective surgery. *JAMA.* 1967;199:580–582.

265. White PD, Mazurkie SJ, Boschetti AE. Patency of the ductus rteriosus at 90. *N Engl J Med.* 1969;280:146–147.

266. Houston AB, Gnanapragasam JP, Lim MK, et al. Doppler ultrasound and the silent ductus arteriosus. *Br Heart J.* 1991;65:97–99.

267. Chiles NH, Smith HL, Christensen NA, Geraci JE. Spontaneous healing of subacute bacterial endarteritis with closure of patent ductus arteriosus. *Mayo Clin Proc.* 1953;28:520–525.

268. Taussig HB. *Congenital Malformations of the Heart.* New York: Commonwealth Fund; 1947.

269. Keith TR, Sagarminaga J. Spontaneously disappearing murmur of patent ductus arteriosus. A case report. *Circulation*. 1961;24: 1235-1238.

270. Umebayashi Y, Taira A, Morishita Y, Arikawa K. Abrupt onset of patient ductus arteriosus in a 55-year-old man. *Am Heart J*. 1989;118:1067-1069.

271. Borow KM, Hessel SJ, Sloss LJ. Fistulous aneurysm of ductus arteriosus. *Br Heart J*. 1981;45:467-470.

272. Cruickshank B, Marquis RM. Spontaneous aneurysm of the ductus arteriosus; a review and report of the tenth adult case. *Am J Med*. 1958;25:140-149.

273. Lund JT, Jensen MB, Hjelms E. Aneurysm of the ductus arteriosus. A review of the literature and the surgical implications. *Eur J Cardiothorac Surg*. 1991;5:566-570.

274. Ohtsuka S, Kakihana M, Ishikawa T, et al. Aneurysm of patent ductus arteriosus in an adult case: findings of cardiac catheterization, angiography, and pathology. *Clin Cardiol*. 1987;10: 537-540.

275. Jayakrishnan AG, Loftus B, Kelly P, Luke DA. Spontaneous postpartum rupture of a patent ductus arteriosus. *Histopathology*. 1992;21:383-384.

276. Sardesai SH, Marshall RJ, Farrow R, Mourant AJ. Dissecting aneurysm of the pulmonary artery in a case of unoperated patent ductus arteriosus. *Eur Heart J*. 1990;11:670-673.

277. Espino-Vela J, Cardenas N, Cruz R. Patent ductus arteriosus. With special reference to patients with pulmonary hypertension. *Circulation*. 1968;38:45-60.

278. Kerkar P, Dalvi B, Kale P. Interruption of the aortic arch with associated cardiac anomalies. Survival to adulthood. *Chest*. 1993;103:279-280.

279. French H. The possibility of a loud congenital murmur disappearing when a child grows up. *Guy Hosp Gaz*. 1919;32:87.

280. Moe DG, Guntheroth WG. Spontaneous closure of uncomplicated ventricular septal defect. *Am J Cardiol*. 1987;60:674-678.

281. Krovetz LJ. Spontaneous closure of ventricular septal defect. *Am J Cardiol*. 1998;81:100-101.

282. Alpert BS, Mellits ED, Rowe RD. Spontaneous closure of small ventricular septal defects. probability rates in the first five years of life. *Am J Dis Child*. 1973;125:194-196.

283. Bloomfield DK. The natural history of ventricular septal defect in patients surviving infancy. *Circulation*. 1964;29:914-955.

284. Hoffman JI. Natural history of congenital heart disease. Problems in its assessment with special reference to ventricular septal defects. *Circulation*. 1968;37:97-125.

285. Hoffman JI, Rudolph AM. The natural history of ventricular septal defects in infancy. *Am J Cardiol*. 1965;16:634-653.

286. Glancy DL, Roberts WC. Complete spontaneous closure of ventricular septal defect: necropsy study of five subjects. *Am J Med*. 1967;43:846-853.

287. Trowitzsch E, Braun W, Stute M, Pielemeier W. Diagnosis, therapy, and outcome of ventricular septal defects in the 1st year of life: a two-dimensional colour-Doppler echocardiography study. *Eur J Pediatr*. 1990;149:758-761.

288. Freedom RM, White RD, Pieroni DR, et al. The natural history of the so-called aneurysm of the membranous ventricular septum in childhood. *Circulation*. 1974;49:375-384.

289. Suzuki H, Lucas RV Jr. Spontaneous closure of ventricular septal defects. Anatomic evidence in three patients. *Arch Pathol*. 1967;84:31-36.

290. Schott GD. Documentation of spontaneous functional closure of a ventricular septal defect during adult life. *Br Heart J*. 1973;35: 1214-1216.

291. Wise JR Jr, Wilson WS. Angiographic documentation of spontaneous closure of ventricular septal defect in an adult. *Chest*. 1979;75:90-93.

292. Campbell M. Natural history of ventricular septal defect. *Br Heart J*. 1971;33:246-257.

293. Corone P, Doyon F, Gaudeau S, et al. Natural history of ventricular septal defect. A study involving 790 cases. *Circulation*. 1977;55: 908-915.

294. Hu DC, Giuliani ER, Downing TP, Danielson GK. Spontaneous closure of congenital ventricular septal defect in an adult. *Clin Cardiol*. 1986;9:587-588.

295. Keith JD, Rose V, Collins G, Kidd BS. Ventricular septal defect. Incidence, morbidity, and mortality in various age groups. *Br Heart J*. 1971;33(Suppl):81-87.

296. Kusumoto M, Amemiya K. Congenital heart disease in patients over 40 years old who have not undergone cardiac surgery. *Jpn Circ J*. 1981;45:243-248.

297. Momma K, Toyama K, Takao A, et al. Natural history of subarterial infundibular ventricular septal defect. *Am Heart J*. 1984;108: 1312-1317.

298. Otterstad JE, Nitter-Hauge S, Myhre E. Isolated ventricular septal defect in adults. Clinical and haemodynamic findings. *Br Heart J*. 1983;50:343-348.

299. Ramaciotti C, Keren A, Silverman NH. Importance of (perimembranous) ventricular septal aneurysm in the natural history of isolated perimembranous ventricular septal defect. *Am J Cardiol*. 1986;57:268-272.

300. Suzuki H. Spontaneous closure of ventricular septal defects. Anatomic evidence in six adult patients. *Am J Clin Pathol*. 1969;52: 391-402.

301. Niwa K, Perloff JK, Kaplan S, et al. Eisenmenger syndrome in adults: ventricular septal defect, truncus arteriosus, univentricular heart. *J Am Coll Cardiol*. 1999;34:223-232.

302. Cantor WJ, Harrison DA, Moussadji JS, et al. Determinants of survival and length of survival in adults with Eisenmenger syndrome. *Am J Cardiol*. 1999;84:677-681.

303. Sadamatsu K, Harasawa Y, Ozono K, et al. A rare case of large ventricular septal defect with minimal pulmonary vascular obstructive changes in a 41-year-old woman. *Heart Vessels*. 1995;10:218-220.

304. Wu MH, Wu JM, Chang CI, et al. Implication of aneurysmal transformation in isolated perimembranous ventricular septal defect. *Am J Cardiol*. 1993;72:596-601.

305. Brammell HL, Vogel JH, Pryor R, Blount SG Jr. The Eisenmenger syndrome. A clinical and physiologic reappraisal. *Am J Cardiol*. 1971;28:679-692.

306. Clarkson PM, Frye RL, DuShane JW, et al. Prognosis for patients with ventricular septal defect and severe pulmonary vascular obstructive disease. *Circulation*. 1968;38:129-135.

307. Hopkins WE, Waggoner AD. Right and left ventricular area and function determined by two-dimensional echocardiography in adults with the Eisenmenger syndrome from a variety of congenital anomalies. *Am J Cardiol*. 1993;72:90-94.

308. Young D, Mark H. Faith of the patient with Eisenmenger syndrome. *Am J Cardiol*. 1972;28:658.

309. Brunken RC, Perloff JK, Czernin J, et al. Myocardial perfusion reserve in adults with cyanotic congenital heart disease. *Am J Physiol*. 2005;289:H1798-H1806.

310. Fyfe A, Perloff JK, Niwa K, et al. Cyanotic congenital heart disease and coronary artery atherogenesis. *Am J Cardiol*. 2005;96:283-290.

311. Dedkov EI, Perloff JK, Tomanek RJ, et al. The coronary microcirculation in cyanotic congenital heart disease. *Circulation*. 2006;114: 196-200.

312. Perloff JK, Latta H, Barsotti P. Pathogenesis of the glomerular abnormality in cyanotic congenital heart disease. *Am J Cardiol*. 2000;86:1198-1204.

313. Van Praagh R, Geva T, Kreutzer J. Ventricular septal defects: how shall we describe, name and classify them? *J Am Coll Cardiol*. 1989;14:1298-1299.

314. Anzai T, Iijima T, Yoshida I, et al. The natural history and timing of the radical operation for subpulmonic ventricular septal defects. *Jpn J Surg*. 1991;21:487-493.

315. Griffin ML, Sullivan ID, Anderson RH, Macartney FJ. Doubly committed subarterial ventricular septal defect: new morphological criteria with echocardiographic and angiocardiographic correlation. *Br Heart J.* 1988;59:474–479.

316. Nadas AS, Thilenius OG, Lafarge CG, Hauck AJ. Ventricular septal defect with aortic regurgitation: medical and pathologic aspects. *Circulation.* 1964;29:862–873.

317. Van Praagh R, McNamara JJ. Anatomic types of ventricular septal defect with aortic insufficiency. Diagnostic and surgical considerations. *Am Heart J.* 1968;75:604–619.

318. Sakakibara S, Konno S. Congenital aneurysm of the sinus of Valsalva. Anatomy and classification. *Am Heart J.* 1962;63:405–424.

319. Tahir MZ, Rustom M, al Ebrahim K. Left coronary sinus of Valsalva aneurysm: an extremely rare malformation. A case report. *Angiology.* 1995;46:753–758.

320. D'Silva SA, Dalvi BV, Lokhandwala YY, et al. Unruptured congenital aneurysm of the left sinus of Valsalva presenting as acute right ventricular failure. *Chest.* 1992;101:578–579.

321. Winfield ME. Rupture of an aneurysm of the posterior sinus of Valsalva into the right atrium. *Am J Cardiol.* 1959;3:688–691.

322. Lukacs L, Bartek I, Haan A, et al. Ruptured aneurysms of the sinus of Valsalva. *Eur J Cardiothorac Surg.* 1992;6:15–17.

323. Boutefeu JM, Moret PR, Hahn C, Hauf E. Aneurysms of the sinus of Valsalva. Report of seven cases and review of the literature. *Am J Med.* 1978;65:18–24.

324. Mayer ED, Ruffmann K, Saggau W, et al. Ruptured aneurysms of the sinus of Valsalva. *Ann Thorac Surg.* 1986;42:81–85.

325. Conde CA, Meller J, Donoso E, Dack S. Bacterial endocarditis with ruptured sinus of Valsalva and aorticocardiac fistula. *Am J Cardiol.* 1975;35:912–917.

326. Jick H, Kasarjian PJ, Barsky M. Rupture of aneurysm of aortic sinus of Valsalva associated with acute bacterial endocarditis. *Circulation.* 1959;19:745–749.

327. Fishbein MC, Obma R, Roberts WC. Unruptured sinus of Valsalva aneurysm. *Am J Cardiol.* 1975;35:918–922.

328. Lewis BS, Agathangelou NE. Echocardiographic diagnosis of unruptured sinus of Valsalva aneurysm. *Am Heart J.* 1984;107:1025–1027.

329. Desai AG, Sharma S, Kumar A, et al. Echocardiographic diagnosis of unruptured aneurysm of right sinus of Valsalva: an unusual cause of right ventricular outflow obstruction. *Am Heart J.* 1985;109:363–364.

330. Dev V, Shrivastava S. Echocardiographic diagnosis of unruptured aneurysm of the sinus of Valsalva dissecting into the ventricular septum. *Am J Cardiol.* 1990;66:502–503.

331. Kiefaber RW, Tabakin BS, Coffin LH, Gibson TC. Unruptured sinus of Valsalva aneurysm with right ventricular outflow obstruction diagnosed by two-dimensional and Doppler echocardiography. *J Am Coll Cardiol.* 1986;7:438–442.

332. Bulkley BH, Hutchins GM, Ross RS. Aortic sinus of Valsalva aneurysms simulating primary right-sided valvular heart disease. *Circulation.* 1975;52:696–699.

333. Kerber RE, Ridges JD, Kriss JP, et al. Unruptured aneurysm of the sinus of Valsalva producing right ventricular outflow obstruction. *Am J Med.* 1972;53:775–783.

334. Gallet B, Combe E, Saudemont JP, et al. Aneurysm of the left aortic sinus causing coronary compression and unstable angina: successful repair by isolated closure of the aneurysm. *Am Heart J.* 1988;115:1308–1310.

335. Eliot RS, Wolbrink A, Edwards JE. Congenital aneurysm of the left aortic sinus. A rare lesion and a rare cause of coronary insufficiency. *Circulation.* 1963;28:951–956.

336. Hiyamuta K, Ohtsuki T, Shimamatsu M, et al. Aneurysm of the left aortic sinus causing acute myocardial infarction. *Circulation.* 1983;67:1151–1154.

337. Metras D, Coulibaly AO, Ouattara K. Calcified unruptured aneurysm of sinus of Valsalva with complete heart block and aortic regurgitation. Successful repair in one case. *Br Heart J.* 1982;48:507–509.

338. Sebag C, Davy JM, Scheuble C, et al. [Atrioventricular block disclosing an isolated congenital aneurysm of the sinus of Valsalva, extending into the septum and not ruptured]. *Arch Mal Coeur Vaiss.* 1981;74:1233–1239.

339. Calder L, Van Praagh R, Van Praagh S, et al. Truncus arteriosus communis. Clinical, angiocardiographic, and pathologic findings in 100 patients. *Am Heart J.* 1976;92:23–38.

340. Ceballos R, Soto B, Kirklin JW, Bargeron LM Jr. Truncus arteriosus. An anatomical-angiographic study. *Br Heart J.* 1983;49:589–599.

341. Collett RW, Edwards JE. Persistent truncus arteriosus: classification according to anatomic types. *Surg Clin North Am.* 1949;29:1245.

342. Van Praagh R. Editorial: Classification of truncus arteriosus communis (TAC). *Am Heart J.* 1976;92:129–132.

343. Van Praagh R, Van Praagh S. The anatomy of common aorticopulmonary trunk (truncus arteriosus communis) and its embryologic implications. A study of 57 necropsy cases. *Am J Cardiol.* 1965;16:406–425.

344. Carr FB, Goodale RH, Rockwell AEP. Persistent truncus arteriosus in a man aged 36 years *Br Heart J.* 1966;28:284.

345. Carter JB, Blieden LC, Edwards JE. Persistent truncus arteriosus. Report of survival to age of 52 years. *Minn Med.* 1973;56:280–282.

346. Hicken P, Evans D, Heath D. Persistent truncus arteriosus with survival to the age of 38 years. *Br Heart J.* 1966;28:284–286.

347. Marcelletti C, McGoon DC, Mair DD. The natural history of truncus arteriosus. *Circulation.* 1976;54:108–111.

348. de la Cruz MV, Arteaga M, Espino-Vela J, et al. Complete transposition of the great arteries: types and morphogenesis of ventriculoarterial discordance. *Am Heart J.* 1981;102:271–281.

349. Elliott LP, Neufeld HN, Anderson RC, et al. Complete transposition of the great vessels: I. An anatomic study of sixty cases. *Circulation.* 1963;27:1105–1117.

350. Lev M, Rimoldi HJ, Paiva R, Arcilla RA. The quantitative anatomy of simple complete transposition. *Am J Cardiol.* 1969;23:409–416.

351. Van Praagh R. Transposition of the great arteries. II. Transposition clarified. *Am J Cardiol.* 1971;28:739–741.

352. Warnes CA. Transposition of the great arteries. *Circulation.* 2006;114:2699–2709.

353. Bonnet D, Coltri A, Butera G, et al. Detection of transposition of the great arteries in fetuses reduces neonatal morbidity and mortality. *Circulation.* 1999;99:916–918.

354. Rashkind WJ, Miller WW. Creation of an atrial septal defect without thoracotomy. A palliative approach to complete transposition of the great arteries. *JAMA.* 1966;196:991–992.

355. Kidd L, Humphries JO. Transposition of the great arteries in the adult. *Cardiovasc Clin.* 1979;10:365–381.

356. Shaher RM. *Complete Transposition of the Great Arteries.* New York: Academic Press; 1973.

357. Johnson CD. Longevity in transposition of the great arteries. *Bol Asoc Med P R.* 1981;73:344–350.

358. Messeloff CR, Weaver JC. A case of transposition of the large vessels in an adult who lived to the age of 38 years. *Am Heart J.* 1951;42:467–471.

359. Nichol AD, Segal AJ. Complete transposition of the main arterial stems; report of a case. *J Am Med Assoc.* 1951;147:645–648.

360. Kato K. Congenital transposition of the vessels: clinical and pathologic study. *Am J Dis Child.* 1930;39:363.

361. Roberson DA, Silverman NH. Malaligned outlet septum with subpulmonary ventricular septal defect and abnormal ventriculoarterial connection: a morphologic spectrum defined echocardiographically. *J Am Coll Cardiol.* 1990;16:459–468.

362. Anderson RH, Becker AE, Lucchese FA, et al. Double outlet right ventricle. *Morphology of Congenital Heart Disease.* Baltimore: University Park Press; 1983.

363. Neufeld HN, Dushane JW, Edwards JE. Origin of both great vessels from the right ventricle. II. With pulmonary stenosis. *Circulation.*1961;23:603–612.

364. Van Praagh S, Davidoff A, Chin A, et al. Double outlet right ventricle: anatomic types and developmental implications based on a study of 101 autopsied cases. *Coeur.* 1982;8:389.

365. Sondheimer HM, Freedom RM, Olley PM. Double outlet right ventricle: clinical spectrum and prognosis. *Am J Cardiol.* 1977;39:709–714.

366. Taussig HB, Bing RJ. Complete transposition of aorta and levoposition of pulmonary artery: clinical, physiological, and pathological findings. *Am Heart J.* 1949;37:551.

367. Van Praagh R. What is the Taussig-Bing malformation? *Circulation.* 1968;38:445–449.

368. Coto EO, Jimenez MQ, Anderson RH, et al. Double outlet ventricle. In: Anderson RH, McCartney FJ, Shinebourne EA, Tynan M, ed. *Paediatric Cardiology* Edinburgh: Churchill Livingstone; 1983.

369. Dadourian BJ, Perloff JK, Drinkwater DC, et al. Double outlet left ventricle—long survival after surgical correction. *Ann Thorac Surg.* 1991;51:159–160.

370. Campbell M, Hudson RE. A case of Taussig-Bing transposition with survival for 34 years. *Guys Hosp Rep.* 1958;107:14–22.

371. Fallot A. Contribution à l'anatomie pathologique de la maladie bleue (cyanose cardiaque). *Marseille Med.* 1888;25:418.

372. Bertranou EG, Blackstone EH, Hazelrig JB, et al. Life expectancy without surgery in tetralogy of Fallot. *Am J Cardiol.* 1978;42:458–466.

373. Meindok H. Longevity in the tetralogy of Fallot. *Thorax.* 1964;19:12–15.

374. Rygg IH, Olesen K, Boesen I. The life history of tetralogy of Fallot. *Dan Med Bull.* 1971;18(Suppl 2):25–30.

375. Abraham KA, Cherian G, Rao VD, et al. Tetralogy of Fallot in adults. A report on 147 patients. *Am J Med.* 1979;66:811–816.

376. Bain GO. Tetralogy of Fallot: survival to seventieth year; report of a case. *AMA Arch Pathol.* 1954;58:176–179.

377. Bedford DE. Two cases of Fallot's tetralogy, shown at the section in 1929, exhibiting unusual longevity. *Proc R Soc Med.* 1956;49:314–316.

378. Bowie EA. Longevity in tetralogy and trilogy of Fallot: discussion of cases in patients surviving 40 years and presentation of two further cases. *Am Heart J.* 1961;62:125.

379. Chin J, Bashour T, Kabbani S. Tetralogy of Fallot in the elderly. *Clin Cardiol.* 1984;7:453–456.

380. Friesinger GC, Bahnson HT. Tetralogy of Fallot. Report of case with total correction at 54 years of age. *Am Heart J.* 1966;71:107–111.

381. Higgins CB, Mulder DG. Tetralogy of Fallot in the adult. *Am J Cardiol.* 1972;29:837–846.

382. Holladay WE Jr, Witham AC. The tetralogy of Fallot; the variability of its clinical manifestations. *AMA Arch Intern Med.* 1957;100:400–414.

383. Marquis RM. Longevity and the early history of the tetralogy of Fallot. *Br Med J.* 1956;1:819–822.

384. Phadke AR, Phadke SA, Handy, Iunnarkar RV. Acyanotic Fallot's tetralogy with survival to the age of 70 years: case report. *Indian Heart J.* 1977;29:46–49.

385. White PD, Sprague HB. Tetralogy of Fallot: report of a case in a noted musician who lived to his 60th year. *JAMA.* 1929;92:787.

386. Marelli AJ, Perloff JK, Child JS, Laks H. Pulmonary atresia with ventricular septal defect in adults. *Circulation.* 1994;89:243–251.

387. Capelli H, Ross D, Somerville J. Aortic regurgitation in tetrad of Fallot and pulmonary atresia. *Am J Cardiol.* 1982;49:1979–1983.

388. Smitherman TC, Nimetz AA, Friedlich AL. Pulmonary atresia with ventricular septal defect: report of the oldest known surviving case. *Chest.* 1975;67:603–606.

389. Fallon MD, Schwartz DJ, Perez BM. Pseudotruncus arteriosus: Its occurrence with acquired aortic stenosis in an adult. *Arch Pathol Lab Med.* 1981;105:250–252.

390. Lev M, Eckner FA. The pathologic anatomy of tetralogy of Fallot and its variations. *Dis Chest.* 1964;45:251–261.

391. Rao BN, Anderson RC, Edwards JE. Anatomic variations in the tetralogy of Fallot. *Am Heart J.* 1971;81:361–371.

392. Rao PS, Lawrie GM. Absent pulmonary valve syndrome. Surgical correction with pulmonary arterioplasty. *Br Heart J.* 1983;50:586–589.

393. Harris BC, Shaver JA, Kroetz FW, Leonard JJ. Congenital pulmonary valvular insufficiency complicating tetralogy of Fallot. Intracardiac sound and pressure correlates. *Am J Cardiol.* 1969;23:864–871.

394. Hynes KM, Gau GT, Titus JL. Coronary heart disease in situs inversus totalis. *Am J Cardiol.* 1973;31:666–669.

395. Jacoby WJ Jr, Jacobson WA. Dextrocardia complicated by myocardial infarction. *Am J Cardiol.* 1963;11:119–122.

396. Nagaratnam N, Kotagama LS. Dextrocardia, situs inversus totalis and appendicular abscess. *Postgrad Med J.* 1957;33:287–288.

397. Frohn-Mulder IM, Meilof JF, Szatmari A, et al. Clinical significance of maternal anti-Ro/SS-A antibodies in children with isolated heart block. *J Am Coll Cardiol.* 1994;23:1677–1681.

398. Brucato A, Franceschini F, Gasparini M, et al. Isolated congenital complete heart block: long-term outcome of mothers, maternal antibody specificity and immunogenetic background. *J Rheumatol.* 1995;22:533–540.

399. Brucato A, Gasparini M, Vignati G, et al. Isolated congenital complete heart block: longterm outcome of children and immunogenetic study. *J Rheumatol.* 1995;22:541–543.

400. Kasinath BS, Katz AI. Delayed maternal lupus after delivery of offspring with congenital heart block. *Arch Intern Med.* 1982;142:2317.

401. Lockshin MD, Bonfa E, Elkon K, Druzin ML. Neonatal lupus risk to newborns of mothers with systemic lupus erythematosus. *Arthritis Rheum.* 1988;31:697–701.

402. Campbell M, Thorne MG. Congenital heart block. *Br Heart J.* 1956;18:90–101.

403. Corne RA, Mathewson FA. Congenital complete atrioventricular heart block. A 25 year follow-up study. *Am J Cardiol.* 1972;29:412–415.

404. Dewey RC, Capeless MA, Levy AM. Use of ambulatory electrocardiographic monitoring to identify high-risk patients with congenital complete heart block. *N Engl J Med.* 1987;316:835–839.

405. McHenry MM. Factors influencing longevity in adults with congenital complete heart block. *Am J Cardiol.* 1972;29:416–421.

406. Reybrouck T, Vanden Eynde B, Dumoulin M, Van der Hauwaert LG. Cardiorespiratory response to exercise in congenital complete atrioventricular block. *Am J Cardiol.* 1989;64:896–899.

407. Camm AJ, Bexton RS. Congenital complete heart block. *Eur Heart J.* 1984;5(Suppl A):115–117.

408. Campbell M, Emanuel R. Six cases of congenital complete heart block followed for 34–40 years. *Br Heart J.* 1967;29:577–587.

409. Esscher E. Review article. Congenital complete heart block. *Acta Paediatr Scand.* 1981;70:131–136.

410. Esscher EB. Congenital complete heart block in adolescence and adult life. A follow-up study. *Eur Heart J.* 1981;2:281–288.

411. Michaelsson M, Engle MA. Congenital complete heart block: an international study of the natural history. *Cardiovasc Clin.* 1972;4:85–101.

412. Pinsky WW, Gillette PC, Garson A Jr, McNamara DG. Diagnosis, management, and long-term results of patients with congenital complete atrioventricular block. *Pediatrics.* 1982;69:728–733.

413. Mathewson FA, Harvie FH. Complete heart block in an experienced pilot. *Br Heart J.* 1957;19:253–258.

414. Turner LB. Asymptomatic congenital heart block in an Army Air Force pilot. *Am Heart J.* 1947;34:426.

415. Ezekowitz MD, Alderson PO, Bulkley BH, et al. Isolated drainage of the superior vena cava into the left atrium in a 52-year-old man: a rare congenital malformation in the adult presenting with cyanosis, polycythemia, and an unsuccessful lung scan. *Circulation.* 1978;58:751–756.

416. Konstam MA, Levine BW, Strauss HW, McKusick KA. Left superior vena cava to left atrial communication diagnosed with radionuclide angiocardiography and with differential right to left shunting. *Am J Cardiol.* 1979;43:149–153.

417. Meadows WR, Bergstrand I, Sharp JT. Isolated anomalous connection of a great vein to the left atrium. The syndrome of cyanosis and clubbing, "normal" heart, and left ventricular hypertrophy on electrocardiogram. *Circulation.* 1961;24:669–676.

418. Meadows WR, Sharp JT. Persistent left superior vena cava draining into the left atrium without arterial oxygen unsaturation. *Am J Cardiol.* 1965;16:273–279.

419. Shapiro EP, Al-Sadir J, Campbell NP, et al. Drainage of right superior vena cava into both atria. Review of the literature and description of a case presenting with polycythemia and paradoxical embolization. *Circulation.* 1981;63:712–717.

420. Bourdillon PD, Foale RA, Sommerville J. Persistent left superior vena cava with coronary sinus and left atrial connection *Eur J Cardiol.* 1979;11:227–234.

421. Bashour T, Kabbani S, Saalouke M, Cheng TO. Persistent Eustachian valve causing severe cyanosis in atrial septal defect with normal right heart pressures. *Angiology.* 1983;34:79–83.

422. Morrison JG, Merrill WH, Friesinger GC, Bender HW Jr. Cyanosis, interatrial communication, and normal pulmonary vascular resistance in adults. *Am J Cardiol.* 1986;58:1128–1129.

423. Seward JB, Hayes DL, Smith HC, et al. Platypnea-orthodeoxia: clinical profile, diagnostic workup, management, and report of seven cases. *Mayo Clin Proc.* 1984;59:221–231.

424. Levin DC, Fellows KE, Abrams HL. Hemodynamically significant primary anomalies of the coronary arteries. Angiographic aspects. *Circulation.* 1978;58:25–34.

425. Liberthson RR, Sagar K, Berkoben JP, et al. Congenital coronary arteriovenous fistula. Report of 13 patients, review of the literature and delineation of management. *Circulation.* 1979;59:849–854.

426. McLellan BA, Pelikan PC. Myocardial infarction due to multiple coronary-ventricular fistulas. *Cathet Cardiovasc Diagn.* 1989;16:247–249.

427. Rose AG. Multiple coronary arterioventricular fistulae. *Circulation.* 1978;58:178–180.

428. Sakakibara S, Yokoyama M, Takao A, et al. Coronary arteriovenous fistula. Nine operated cases. *Am Heart J.* 1966;72:307–314.

429. Shakudo M, Yoshikawa J, Yoshida K, Yamaura Y. Noninvasive diagnosis of coronary artery fistula by Doppler color flow mapping. *J Am Coll Cardiol.* 1989;13:1572–1577.

430. Slater J, Lighty GW Jr, Winer HE, et al. Doppler echocardiography and computed tomography in diagnosis of left coronary arteriovenous fistula. *J Am Coll Cardiol.* 1984;4:1290–1293.

431. Brooks CH, Bates PD. Coronary artery-left ventricular fistula with angina pectoris. *Am Heart J.* 1983;106:404–406.

432. Harris A, Jefferson K, Chatterjee K. Coronary arteriovenous fistula with aneurysm of coronary sinus. *Br Heart J.* 1969;31:400–403.

433. Brack MJ, Hubner PJ, Firmin RK. Successful operation on a coronary arteriovenous fistula in a 74 year old woman. *Br Heart J.* 1991;65:107–108.

434. Colbeck JC, Shaw JM. Coronary aneurysm with arteriovenous fistula. *Am Heart J.* 1954;48:270–274.

435. Yenel F. Coronary arteriovenous communication. Report of a case and review of the literature. *N Engl J Med.* 1961;265:577–580.

436. Paul O, Sweet RH, White PD. Coronary arteriovenous fistula: case report. *Am Heart J.* 1949;37:441.

437. Baim DS, Kline H, Silverman JF. Bilateral coronary artery—pulmonary artery fistulas. Report of five cases and review of the literature. *Circulation.* 1982;65:810–815.

438. Glynn TP Jr, Fleming RG, Haist JL, Hunteman RK. Coronary arteriovenous fistula as a cause for reversible thallium-201 perfusion defect. *J Nucl Med.* 1994;35:1808–1810.

439. Griffiths SP, Ellis K, Hordof AJ, et al. Spontaneous complete closure of a congenital coronary artery fistula. *J Am Coll Cardiol.* 1983;2:1169–1173.

440. Hackett D, Hallidie-Smith KA. Spontaneous closure of coronary artery fistula. *Br Heart J.* 1984;52:477–479.

441. Mahoney LT, Schieken RM, Lauer RM. Spontaneous closure of a coronary artery fistula in childhood. *Pediatr Cardiol.* 1982;2:311–312.

442. Muthusamy R, Gupta G, Ahmed RA, et al. Fistula between a branch of left anterior descending coronary artery and pulmonary artery with spontaneous closure. *Eur Heart J.* 1990;11:954–956.

443. Rein AJ, Yatsiv I, Simcha A. An unusual presentation of right coronary artery fistula. *Br Heart J.* 1988;59:598–600.

444. Said SA, Austermann-Kaper T, Bucx JJ. Congenital coronary arteriovenous fistula associated with atrioventricular valvular regurgitation in an octogenarian. *Int J Cardiol.* 1993;38:96–97.

445. Case RB, Morrow AG, Stainsby W, Nestor JO. Anomalous origin of the left coronary artery; the physiologic defect and suggested surgical treatment. *Circulation.* 1958;17:1062–1068.

446. Nadas AS, Gamboa R, Hugenholtz PG. Anomalous left coronary artery originating from the pulmonary artery. Report of two surgically treated cases with a proposal of hemodynamic and therapeutic classification. *Circulation.* 1964;29:167–175.

447. Sabiston DC Jr, Neill CA, Taussig HB. The direction of blood flow in anomalous left coronary artery arising from the pulmonary artery. *Circulation.* 1960;22:591–597.

448. Hurwitz RA, Caldwell RL, Girod DA, et al. Clinical and hemodynamic course of infants and children with anomalous left coronary artery. *Am Heart J.* 1989;118:1176–1181.

449. Letcher JR, McCormick D, Tendler S, et al. Left main coronary artery arising from the pulmonary trunk in a 56-year-old patient presenting with acute myocardial infarction. *Am J Cardiol.* 1991;68:1257–1258.

450. Purut CM, Sabiston DC Jr. Origin of the left coronary artery from the pulmonary artery in older adults. *J Thorac Cardiovasc Surg.* 1991;102:566–570.

451. Suzuki Y, Murakami T, Kawai C. Detection of anomalous origin of left coronary artery from pulmonary artery by real-time Doppler color flow mapping in a 53-year-old asymptomatic female. *Int J Cardiol.* 1992;34:339–342.

452. Vesterlund T, Thomsen PE, Hansen OK. Anomalous origin of the left coronary artery from the pulmonary artery in an adult. *Br Heart J.* 1985;54:110–112.

453. Abbott M. Congenital cardiac disease In: Osler W, ed. *Modern Medicine, Its Theories and Practice.* Philadelphia: Lee & Febiger; 1908.

454. Wesselhoeft H, Fawcett JS, Johnson AL. Anomalous origin of the left coronary artery from the pulmonary trunk. Its clinical spectrum, pathology, and pathophysiology, based on a review of 140 cases with seven further cases. *Circulation.* 1968;38:403–425.

455. Usman A, Fernandez B, Uricchio JF, Nichols HT. Aberrant origin of left coronary artery combined with mitral regurgitation in an adult. *Am J Cardiol.* 1961;8:130–134.

456. Gasior RM, Winters WL, Glick H, et al. Anomalous origin of left coronary artery from pulmonary artery. Treatment by aorto-left coronary saphenous vein bypass. *Am J Cardiol.* 1971;27:215–220.

457. Harthorne JW, Scannell JG, Dinsmore RE. Anomalous origin of the left coronary artery. Remediable cause of sudden death in adults. *N Engl J Med.* 1966;275:660–663.

458. Roche AH. Anomalous origin of the left coronary artery from the pulmonary artery in the adult. Report of uneventful ligation in two cases. *Am J Cardiol.* 1967;20:561–565.

459. George JM, Knowlan DM. Anomalous origin of the left coronary artery from the pulmonary artery in an adult. *N Engl J Med.* 1959;261:993–998.

460. Roberts WC. Major anomalies of coronary arterial origin seen in adulthood. *Am Heart J.* 1986;111:941–963.

461. Dines DE, Seward JB, Bernatz PE. Pulmonary arteriovenous fistulas. *Mayo Clin Proc.* 1983;58:176–181.

462. Foley RE, Boyd DP. Pulmonary arteriovenous aneurysm. *Surg Clin North Am.* 1961;41:801–806.

463. Moyer JH, Glantz G, Brest AN. Pulmonary arteriovenous fistulas; physiologic and clinical considerations. *Am J Med*. 1962;32: 417–435.

464. Terry PB, Barth KH, Kaufman SL, White RI Jr. Balloon embolization for treatment of pulmonary arteriovenous fistulas. *N Engl J Med*. 1980;302:1189–1190.

465. Teragaki M, Akioka K, Yasuda M, et al. Hereditary hemorrhagic telangiectasia with growing pulmonary arteriovenous fistulas followed for 24 years. *Am J Med Sci*. 1988;295:545–547.

466. Hall RJ, Nelson WP, Blake HA, Geiger JP. Massive pulmonary arteriovenous fistula in the newborn; a correctable form of "cyanotic heart disease;" an additional cause of cyanosis with left axis deviation. *Circulation*. 1965;31:762–767.

467. Phillips MD. Stopping bleeding in hereditary telangiectasia. *N Engl J Med*. 1994;330:1822–1823.

468. Goldberg HL, Sniderman K, Devereux RB, Levin A. Prolonged survival (62 years) with single ventricle. *Am J Cardiol*. 1983;52: 214–215.

469. Shinebourne EA, Lau KC, Calcaterra G, Anderson RH. Univentricular heart of right ventricular type: clinical, angiographic and electrocardiographic features. *Am J Cardiol*. 1980;46:439–445.

470. Soto B, Bertranou EG, Bream PR, et al. Angiographic study of univentricular heart of right ventricular type. *Circulation*. 1979;60: 1325–1334.

471. Soto B, Pacifico AD, Di Sciascio G. Univentricular heart: an angiographic study. *Am J Cardiol*. 1982;49:787–794.

472. Vanpraagh R, Ongley PA, Swan HJ. Anatomic types of single or common ventricle in man. Morphologic and geometric aspects of 60 necropsied cases. *Am J Cardiol*. 1964;13:367–386.

473. Vanpraagh R, Vanpraagh S, Vlad P, Keith JD. Diagnosis of the anatomic types of single or common ventricle. *Am J Cardiol*. 1965;15: 345–366.

474. Freedom RM, Rowe RD. Morphological and topographical variations of the outlet chamber in complex congenital heart disease: an angiocardiographic study. *Cathet Cardiovasc Diagn*. 1978;4: 345–371.

475. Shiraishi H, Silverman NH. Echocardiographic spectrum of double inlet ventricle: evaluation of the interventricular communication. *J Am Coll Cardiol*. 1990;15:1401–1408.

476. Stein JI, Smallhorn JF, Coles JG, et al. Common atrioventricular valve guarding double inlet atrioventricular connexion: natural history and surgical results in 76 cases. *Int J Cardiol*. 1990;28: 7–17.

477. Moodie DS, Ritter DG, Tajik AJ, O'Fallon WM. Long-term follow-up in the unoperated univentricular heart. *Am J Cardiol*. 1984;53:1124–1128.

478. Sano T, Ogawa M, Yabuuchi H, et al. Quantitative cineangiographic analysis of ventricular volume and mass in patients with single ventricle: relation to ventricular morphologies. *Circulation*. 1988;77:62–69.

479. Klaus AP, Smith RM, Schneider AB, Parker BM. Single ventricle with normal relationship of the great vessels and pulmonic stenosis. A case report of an adult with the "Holmes heart." *Am Heart J*. 1969;78:530–536.

480. Sagar KB, Mauck HP. Univentricular heart in adults: report of nine cases with review of the literature. *Am Heart J*. 1985;110: 1059–1062.

481. Leibbrandt G, Munch U, Gander M. Two successful pregnancies in a patient with single ventricle and transposition of the great arteries. *Int J Cardiol*. 1982;1:257–262.

482. Stiller RJ, Vintzileos AM, Nochimson DJ, et al. Single ventricle in pregnancy: case report and review of the literature. *Obstet Gynecol*. 1984;64:18S–20S.

483. Habeck JO, Reinhardt G, Findeisen V. A case of double inlet left ventricle in a 59-year-old man. *Int J Cardiol*. 1991;30:119–120.

484. Edwards JE, Burchell HB. Congenital tricuspid atresia: classification. *Med Clin North Am*. 1949;33:1177.

485. Sade RM, Fyfe DA. Tricuspid atresia: current concepts in diagnosis and treatment. *Pediatr Clin North Am*. 1990;37:151–169.

486. Brown JW, Heath D, Morris TL, Whitaker W. Tricuspid atresia. *Br Heart J*. 1956;18:499–518.

487. Cooley RN, Sloan RD, Hanlon CR, Bahnson HT. Angiocardiography in congenital heart disease of cyanotic type. II. Observations on tricuspid stenosis or atresia with hypoplasia of the right ventricle. *Radiology*. 1950;54:848–868.

488. Dick M, Fyler DC, Nadas AS. Tricuspid atresia: clinical course in 101 patients. *Am J Cardiol*. 1975;36:327–337.

489. Jordan JC, Sanders CA. Tricuspid atresia with prolonged survival. A report of two cases with a review of the world literature. *Am J Cardiol*. 1966;18:112–119.

490. Patel MM, Overy DC, Kozonis MC, Hadley-Fowlkes LL. Long-term survival in tricuspid atresia. *J Am Coll Cardiol*. 1987;9:338–340.

491. Patterson W, Baxley WA, Karp RB, Soto B, Bargeron LL. Tricuspid atresia in adults. *Am J Cardiol*. 1982;49:141–152.

492. Franklin RC, Spiegelhalter DJ, Sullivan ID, et al. Tricuspid atresia presenting in infancy. Survival and suitability for the Fontan operation. *Circulation*. 1993;87:427–439.

493. Rao PS, Sissman NJ. Spontaneous closure of physiologically advantageous ventricular septal defects. *Circulation*. 1971;43:83–90.

494. Roberts WC, Morrow AG, Mason DT, Braunwald E. Spontaneous closure of ventricular septal defect, anatomic proof in an adult with tricuspid atresia. *Circulation*. 1963;27:90–94.

495. Breisch EA, Wilson DB, Laurenson RD, et al. Tricuspid atresia (type Ia):survival to 21 years of age. *Am Heart J*. 1983;106:149–151.

496. Anderson RH, Rigby ML. The morphologic heterogeneity of tricuspid atresia. *Int J Cardiol*. 1987;16:67.

497. Voci G, Diego JN, Shafia H, et al. Type Ia tricuspid atresia with extensive coronary artery abnormalities in a living 22 year old woman. *J Am Coll Cardiol*. 1987;10:1100–1104.

498. Beaver TR, Shroyer KR, Muro-Cacho CA, et al. Survival to age 65 years with tricuspid and pulmonic valve atresia. *Am J Cardiol*. 1988;62:165–166.

499. Marcano BA, Riemenschneider TA, Ruttenberg HD, et al. Tricuspid atresia with increased pulmonary blood flow. An analysis of 13 cases. *Circulation*. 1969;40:399–410.

500. Tandon R, Edwards JE. Tricuspid atresia. A re-evaluation and classification. *J Thorac Cardiovasc Surg*. 1974;67:530–542.

501. Ehrich DA, Vieweg WV, Alpert JS, et al. Cor triatriatum: report of a case in a young adult with special reference to the echocardiographic features and etiology of the systolic murmur. *Am Heart J*. 1977;94:217–221.

502. Fuster-Siebert M, Llorens R, Arcas-Meca R, et al. Cor triatriatum with mitral valve disease in adults. *Tex Heart Inst J*. 1982;9:363–366.

503. McGuire LB, Nolan TB, Reeve R, Dammann JF Jr. Cor Triatriatum as a problem of adult heart disease. *Circulation*. 1965;31:263–272.

504. Ostman-Smith I, Silverman NH, Oldershaw P, et al. Cor triatriatum sinistrum. Diagnostic features on cross sectional echocardiography. *Br Heart J*. 1984;51:211–219.

505. Feld H, Shani J, Rudansky HW, et al. Initial presentation of cor triatriatum in a 55-year-old woman. *Am Heart J*. 1992;124:788–791.

506. Loeffler E. Unusual malformation of left atrium: pulmonary sinus. *Arch Pathol*. 1949;48:371.

507. van Son JA, Julsrud PR, Hagler DJ, et al. Surgical treatment of vascular rings: the Mayo Clinic experience. *Mayo Clin Proc*. 1993;68:1056–1063.

508. Ratib O, Perloff JK, Williams WG. Congenital complete absence of the pericardium. *Circulation*. 2001;103:3154–3155.

CHAPTER 5

Survival Patterns After Cardiac Surgery or Interventional Catheterization: A Broadening Base

JOSEPH K. PERLOFF ▪ MARK D. PLUNKETT

Long-term outcomes of cardiac surgery or interventional catheterization in congenital heart disease are best understood in light of knowledge of the basic malformation, the nature and effects of the therapeutic procedure(s), and the subsequent residua and sequelae (see Chapter 20). Success is measured by the quality of life as well as the length of survival (see Chapter 13). It is axiomatic that surgical techniques continue to evolve and affect long-term outcome, often significantly. Myocardial protection has materially improved, and prosthetic materials—valves, patches, and conduits—that were once state of the art have been superseded by new generations of improved materials and improved techniques of insertion (see Chapter 16).

CONGENITALLY MALFORMED CARDIAC VALVES

Interventional catheterization employs balloon valvuloplasty and most recently, transcatheter valve replacement.[1] Surgery employs valve reconstruction or replacement with repair of coexisting defects.

Isolated Mobile Pulmonary Valve Stenosis

Late results of *surgical valvotomy* for typical mobile dome-shaped pulmonary valve stenosis are excellent, regardless of whether the valve has discernible commissures.[2,3] Balloon dilatation has superseded surgical valvulotomy with similar salutary results and similar minor residua and sequelae[4-7] (see Chapter 18). Relief of obstruction incurs relatively minor degrees of regurgitation that are usually of little or no physiologic consequence.[8] Dilatation of the pulmonary trunk persists[9] but is of no clinical importance, even when marked. The relatively low risk of infective endocarditis after successful balloon dilatation or surgical valvotomy is dealt with in Chapter 8.

Prognosis is excellent if pulmonary valve stenosis—even severe—is relieved during childhood. When gradients are reduced to less than 20 mm Hg and when right ventricular mass and function normalize, survival patterns are similar to age- and sex-matched control subjects, with patients generally achieving asymptomatic adulthood and normal lifestyles.[2,3] Repair after 21 years of age continues to yield good results, but not surprisingly, the more severe the stenosis and the longer the right ventricle confronts increased afterload, the more qualified the long-term outcome, including the prospect of late death from right ventricular failure.[2,3,10,11] These conclusions support the practice of early intervention and underscore the desirability of long-term surveillance.

Dysplastic Pulmonary Valve Stenosis

The dysplastic stenotic pulmonary valve represents a different therapeutic problem.[12] Dysplastic pulmonary valves are occasionally found in otherwise normal children but are especially likely to occur with Noonan's syndrome. Because obstruction is caused by thick, poorly mobile leaflets without commissural fusion, surgical relief requires excision of one or more leaflets, so postoperative pulmonary regurgitation is inevitable and usually appreciable (see Chapter 15). Pulmonary valve replacement is ultimately necessary because of dilatation and failure of the volume-overloaded right ventricle. Balloon dilatation is of no therapeutic value.

Isolated Pulmonary Valve Regurgitation

Isolated congenital pulmonary valve regurgitation is a rare disorder that is usually well tolerated because regurgitation is seldom more than moderate, which is a volume overload to which the right ventricle readily adapts.[12] A rare exception is isolated congenital *absence* of the pulmonary valve in which severe regurgitation warrants valve replacement. There is little or no information regarding long-term results, but it can be plausibly assumed that the longer the duration of severe regurgitation, the less likely that the postoperative right ventricle will achieve normal function. Congenital absence of the pulmonary valve is more likely to occur with tetralogy of Fallot (albeit rarely; see later), is necessarily accompanied by severe regurgitation, and is typically associated with aneurysmal dilatation of the branch pulmonary arteries.

Congenital Abnormalities of the Aortic Valve Causing Stenosis

These abnormalities include unicuspid, bicuspid, or tricuspid aortic valves.[12] Unicuspid aortic valves are either acommissural or unicommissural and are usually inherently stenotic. Bicuspid valves occur with or without commissural fusion and can be inherently stenotic, incompetent (see later), or functionally normal. Tricuspid aortic valves are inherently stenotic when there is a small aortic ring with a miniature or dysplastic valve.

The bicuspid valve is far and away the most common cause of congenital aortic stenosis; hence information on long-term postoperative or postinterventional results is greatest. Surgical or balloon valvotomy or valvuloplasty presupposes that the structure is a pliant noncalcified bicuspid valve in which obstruction is caused by congenital fusion (nonseparation) of commissures. Given this substrate, the best that valvotomy or valvuloplasty can achieve is the creation of a functionally normal bicuspid aortic valve, that is, little or no obstruction and no more than mild regurgitation. These postoperative valves have at least the same if not a greater tendency to thicken, calcify, and become stenotic with the passage of time, and the risk of infective endocarditis remains unchanged[13-17] (see Chapter 8). Many patients who underwent aortic valvotomy before 1970 subsequently required reoperation; still others have died.[16] The probability of remaining free

of serious complications—reoperation, endocarditis, or death—is 92% at 5 years, 87% at 10 and 15 years, 82% at 20 years, and 77% at 22 years.[14] Unfavorable indicators include restenosis or progressive aortic regurgitation, which usually develops gradually, but infective endocarditis can cause sudden, severe incompetence that requires urgent valve replacement. Among 516 patients, there were 54 late deaths (10.5%), the majority of which were related to the residual aortic valve disease.[13-17] Of the 54 deaths, 20 (37%) were sudden, 14 (26%) were related to reoperation, 10 (18%) were related to infective endocarditis, and two (4%) were ascribed to heart failure and aortic regurgitation. The longer the interval after initial operation, the greater the incidence of reoperation. By actuarial analysis, the probability of reoperation was 2% at 5 years, 8% at 10 years, 19% at 15 years, 35% at 20 years, and 44% at 22 years.[14] The risk of sudden death was calculated at 0.4% per year.[14,16,18] More than half the patients who died suddenly had significant aortic stenosis, regurgitation, or both; the majority were asymptomatic at the time of sudden death.

The incidence of infective endocarditis is not reduced by valvotomy or valvuloplasty, even if stenosis is successfully relieved[19,20] (see earlier and see Chapter 8). Morbidity and mortality are significant, with a death rate of 31% and a 23% incidence of aortic valve replacement.[14] The clinical course of bicuspid aortic stenosis can be dramatically altered by a dissecting ascending aortic aneurysm,[9] which can occur years after valvotomy or valve replacement[21] (Fig. 5–1).

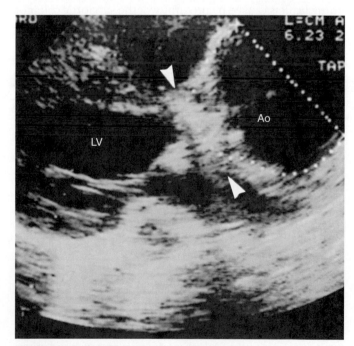

FIGURE 5–1 Two-dimensional echocardiogram from a 26-year-old man who experienced an acute dissection of the proximal ascending aorta (Ao) several years after replacement *(arrowheads)* of a stenotic bicuspid aortic valve. LV, left ventricle.

Balloon aortic valvuloplasty is the initial procedure for the treatment of typical pliant, dome-shaped congenital bicuspid aortic stenosis in young adults[16] (see Chapter 18). Balloon dilatation does not lend itself to the controlled meticulous technical relief of commissural fusion that is possible at open operation, hence the greater the likelihood of inducing aortic regurgitation. Monitoring the interventional procedure by transesophageal echocardiography reduces that risk. When a stenotic unicommissural unicuspid aortic valve is mistaken for a stenotic bicuspid aortic valve, balloon dilatation can induce significant if not severe regurgitation[22,23] (see Chapter 18).

Isolated Fixed Subaortic Stenosis

There are two varieties of isolated fixed (discrete) subaortic stenosis. The first variety is characterized by a crescent-shaped membrane immediately beneath the aortic valve usually forming a collar that extends across an otherwise normal left ventricular outflow tract and inserts onto the anterior leaflet of the mitral valve. Long-term results after surgical resection are good, provided the obstruction does not recur and the aortic leaflets function normally.[18,24] The mechanism responsible for recurrence of obstruction is unclear but has been attributed to regrowth of tissue or to impaired growth of the outflow tract from fibrosis. Current surgical techniques provide excellent relief with low risk of injury to aortic or mitral leaflets, and low risk of perforation of the ventricular septum or of injury to the bundle of His (see Chapter 15). Long-term survival is qualified by coexisting aortic regurgitation that results from damage to aortic leaflets caused by proximity of the subaortic collar or by impact of the systolic stenotic jet. An important objective of resection, even when obstruction is comparatively mild, is to prevent the development or progression of aortic regurgitation. The incompetent aortic valve is susceptible to infective endocarditis (see Chapter 8), and progressive regurgitation may require repair or replacement many years after subaortic resection.

The second and less common variety of fixed subaortic stenosis is represented by a fibromuscular channel that can occupy several centimeters of the outflow tract and is therefore referred to as *tubular* or *tunnel obstruction*. The malformation is not present at birth but becomes manifest after the first year of life and then changes in morphology and severity. Aortic regurgitation is common but usually mild and nonprogressive. The narrow tunnel-like obstruction is often associated with marked left ventricular hypertrophy and diminished left ventricular chamber size. Surgical resection of the fibromuscular obstruction together with septal myomectomy through the aortic valve is the initial approach to this form of stenosis. Care must be taken to avoid creating a ventricular septal defect and to avoid injury to the adjacent mitral and aortic valves or the conduction system. Surgical intervention may relieve obstruction but is associated with a high incidence of late recurrence of steno-

sis and progressive aortic regurgitation.[25] To achieve adequate relief of obstruction, enlargement of the outflow tract may be necessary. The septum is exposed and incised through a right ventriculotomy and augmented with patch material to enlarge the left ventricular outflow tract and aortic annulus (Kono procedure). The aortic valve is then replaced with an adequate-sized prosthetic valve, homograft, or pulmonary autograft (Ross-Konno procedure). Low operative mortality (0%–6%) and excellent outcomes have been reported, with freedom from recurrent subaortic stenosis as high as 86% at 5 years.[26-28]

Supravalvular Aortic Stenosis

This is the least common variety of congenital obstruction to left ventricular outflow. The localized type usually takes the form of a segmental hourglass deformity immediately above the aortic sinuses with medial thickening and fibrous intimal proliferation (Fig. 5–2). Less commonly, there is a localized fibrous membrane with a central opening. Late results of operation are good, with little need for reoperation.[29,30] Postoperative survival has been reported as 94% in 10 years and 91% in 20 years.[31] Long-term outcome is affected by three variables: (1) aortic valve abnormalities, (2) coronary arterial abnormalities, and (3) the coexistence of Williams syndrome.[12]

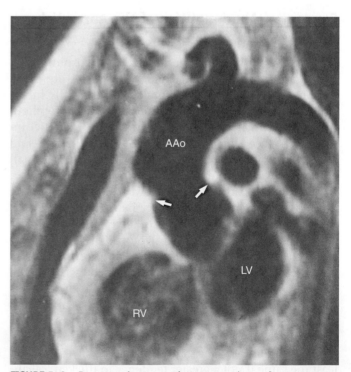

FIGURE 5–2 Postoperative magnetic resonance image from a 24-year-old man with Williams syndrome. He underwent repair of supravalvular aortic stenosis at age 16 years. Arrows identify the site of repair across which there was no gradient. AAo, ascending aorta; LV and RV, left and right ventricles. The patient had postoperative systemic hypertension with no discernible vascular cause.

In about one third of patients, the aortic cusps are thickened and distorted. An adherent aortic cusp may obstruct a coronary ostium. Premature coronary atherosclerosis results from systolic hypertension in the segment of aorta proximal to the supravalvular obstruction. Williams syndrome with characteristic facies and mental retardation is complicated by renal or renovascular abnormalities and systemic hypertension that affect longevity in nearly half of afflicted patients[12,32] (see Chapters 10 and 20).

An uncommon variety of supravalvular aortic stenosis is represented by diffuse tubular hypoplasia of the ascending aorta beginning above the sinuses of Valsalva, with narrowing of the aortic arch and the orifices of the brachiocephalic arteries.[14] The aortic leaflets are usually thickened and occasionally dysplastic, but regurgitation is mild. Surgical treatment involves the placement of a patch, starting from the sinuses of Valsalva and extending to include the entire aortic arch, with augmentation of the proximal innominate and left common carotid arteries. Endarterectomy of the ascending aorta and aortic arch is occasionally employed with relief of obstruction and improved long-term survival.[33] Occasionally encountered are patients with apical-to-descending aorta valved conduits implanted to relieve diffuse supravalvar aortic stenosis.

Congenital Aortic Regurgitation

A bicuspid aortic valve is the most common cause of isolated congenital aortic regurgitation of sufficient severity to warrant surgical intervention.[12] Longevity after operation is determined by the chronicity and degree of regurgitation, the functional state of the volume overloaded left ventricle, and the type of operation—reconstruction, a Ross procedure or valve replacement with a rigid prosthesis, or a tissue valve[34] (see Chapter 15). Isolated quadricuspid aortic valve regurgitation is rare (Fig. 5–3). Replacement is the only surgical option.

The prime objectives of operation for congenital aortic valve regurgitation are relief of left ventricular volume overload and preservation or restoration of left ventricular function and functional reserve. Long-term postoperative survival is good and relates chiefly to patients who have undergone valve replacement as young adults. The long-term fate of reparative (valve-sparing) operations remains to be established. The Ross operation is dealt with in Chapter 15. The inherent medial abnormality that attenuates the ascending aorta above an incompetent congenitally bicuspid valve poses the risk of dissection[9] (see Fig. 5–1).

Congenital Mitral Valve Disease

Congenital stenosis of the mitral valve takes one of several forms:[12] (1) the "typical" form with short chordae tendineae, fibrous reduction or obliteration of interchordal spaces, and a decrease in interpapillary muscle distance; (2) the parachute mitral valve characterized by insertion into a single eccentric papillary muscle of fused chordae tendineae from both leaflets; (3) a "mitral arcade" characterized by little or no chordal interposition between mitral leaflet tissue or by multiple papillary muscles in close proximity; and (4) accessory mitral valve tissue or anomalous papillary muscle bundles. Congenital obstruction *immediately above* the mitral leaflets consists of a supravalvular stenosing ring, which is a curtain or diaphragm originating at the base of the atrial surfaces of the leaflets. An isolated supravalvular stenosing ring is amenable to surgical resection with good long-term results, but the malformation seldom occurs in isolation.

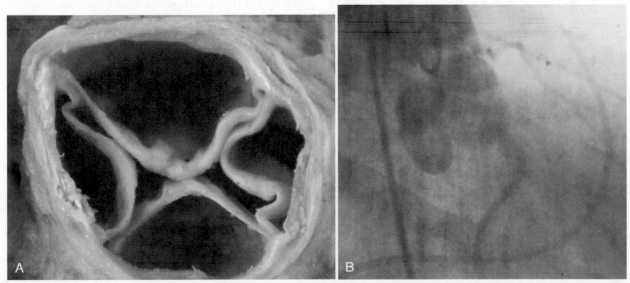

FIGURE 5–3   **(A)** Isolated quadricuspid aortic valve, an incidental necropsy finding in a 56-year-old male. **(B)** Isolated quadricuspid aortic valve, an incidental angiographic finding in a 62-year-old male.

Congenital stenosis of the mitral valve itself usually requires early valve replacement. Perioperative mortality is high, with survival beyond 5 to 10 years of approximately 30% to 60%.[29] Long-term survival is adversely affected by recurrence of obstruction as the child outgrows the size of the prosthesis, the need for anticoagulants, the risk of infective endocarditis, the almost invariable presence of other congenital malformations, and the need for reoperation.

Isolated congenital *mitral regurgitation* is rare. Immediate postoperative results are good after repair of posterior leaflet clefts, but the long-term outcome is unknown.

Congenital Tricuspid Valve Disease

Isolated congenital tricuspid valve malformations requiring surgical intervention almost always take the form of regurgitation rather than stenosis. *Ebstein's anomaly* is by far the most common of these abnormalities. The objectives of operation are to relieve volume overload of the functionally inadequate right ventricle, to exclude the arrhythmogenic atrialized right ventricle, to reduce recurrences of atrial tachyarrhythmias by a Maze procedure, to eliminate bypass tracts that were not ablated preoperatively (see Chapter 22), and to close a foramen ovale or atrial septal defect. Every attempt should be made to reconstruct rather than replace the tricuspid valve[29,35-37] (Fig. 5-4). Whether Ebstein's malformation lends itself to tricuspid reconstruction can almost always be determined by transesophageal echocardiography (see Chapter 6) that identifies a large mobile anterior leaflet suitable for creation of a unicuspid right atrioventricular valve. If most (or all) of these objectives can be achieved, there is significant improvement in functional class and in longevity.[35,38,39] Closure of the interatrial communication removes the hazard of paradoxic emboli.[32] Supraventricular tachyarrhythmias occur postoperative in 10% to 20% of patients, but if accessory pathways have been eliminated,

the risk of a rapid ventricular response to atrial flutter or fibrillation is obviated[40,41] (see Chapter 20).

Residual abnormalities of a reconstructed tricuspid valve necessarily persist, but tricuspid valve replacement carries a late mortality of 10% to 15%.[35,37,39] Tissue valves are preferred (see Chapter 16). Mechanical valves incur thromboembolic complications even with anticoagulation. Potential long-term effects of operation on abnormal left ventricular geometry and function in adults with Ebstein's anomaly are unknown.[38,40,41]

In congenitally corrected transposition of the great arteries (see later), incompetence of the inverted tricuspid valve is caused by an Ebstein-like malformation. When surgical relief is indicated, the malformed valve requires replacement with few or no exceptions (see Chapter 15). Long-term outcome is determined largely by the duration of preoperative regurgitation and by the functional state of a morphologic right ventricle in the systemic location.

INTRAATRIAL SURGERY

Ostium Secundum Atrial Septal Defect

When surgical repair is performed in childhood, right atrial and right ventricular dimensions decrease, often strikingly, and usually normalize.[42,43] When repair awaits adulthood, dimensions remain abnormal in about 80% of patients.[42,43] Dilatation of the pulmonary trunk decreases but seldom normalizes because the enlargement is caused by an intrinsic medial fault[9,44] (Fig. 5-5), but the dilatation is of little or no prognostic significance. Preoperative abnormalities of left ventricular geometry tend to normalize within 6 months after operation.[45-47] However, in adults with preoperative tricuspid regurgitation and right ventricular failure, late postoperative right atrial and right ventricular dilatation persist, and right ventricular ejection fraction seldom normalizes.

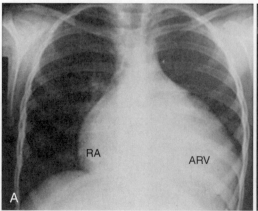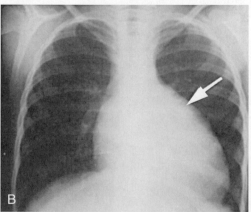

FIGURE 5-4 Chest radiographs from a 32-year-old cyanotic patient with Ebstein's anomaly of the tricuspid valve. **(A)** The cardiac silhouette is typical of the malformation, with a large right atrium (RA) and an atrialized right ventricle (ARV). **(B)** Chest radiograph 2 years after tricuspid valve reconstruction. There is a significant decrease in cardiac size. The hump-shaped infundibulum persists *(arrow).*

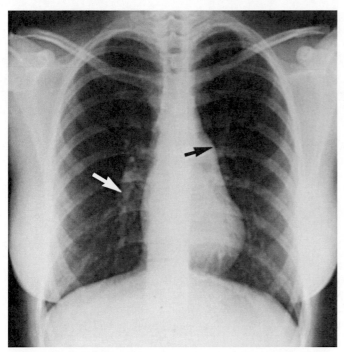

FIGURE 5–5   Chest radiograph from a 17-year-old girl who had repair of an ostium secundum atrial septal defect at age 6 years. The radiograph is normal except for mild residual dilatation of the pulmonary trunk *(black arrow)* and of the right pulmonary artery *(white arrow)*.

There is a relatively uniform consensus that closure of an ostium secundum atrial septal defect before the early 20s is followed by long-term survival not significantly different from an age- and sex-matched control population.[48] Repair between 25 and 41 years of ages is followed by long-term survival that is good but shorter than normal, and closure after 41 years of age is associated with a substantial increase in late mortality and morbidity.[48] Despite 4 decades of surgical intervention, there is no consensus on whether closure is preferable to medical management for middle-aged and elderly patients with an ostium secundum atrial septal defect. However, data from 179 consecutive patients older than 40 years of age have been assembled from two hospitals in which all patients were treated surgically or medically by the same professional staff.[49] The mean (± SD) age of the surgically treated patients was 54 ± 7 years; for medically managed patients, it was 57 ± 10 years ($p = .01$). There were no statistically significant differences between the two groups with regard to other clinical characteristics. Surgical closure was performed in 84 patients (47%), and medical management was employed for 95 patients (53%). On the basis of Cox proportional-hazards analysis and after adjustments for a number of covariates, the estimated probability of survival among the surgically treated patients was 98% after 5 years and 95% at 10 years, compared with 93% and 84%, respectively, among the medically managed patients. The New York Heart Association

(NYHA) functional class improved in 32% of the surgically treated patients and deteriorated in only 11%. The favorable effect of surgical intervention was especially evident in the subgroup of patients with severe heart failure (NYHA functional class III or IV). Conversely, only 3% of the medically treated patients had long-term improvement in the severity of heart failure, and 34% deteriorated. These data argue persuasively that surgical or interventional closure of atrial septal defects in middle-aged and elderly patients is superior to medical management, improving longevity and reducing functional limitations. Nevertheless, the risk of atrial tachyarrhythmias, especially fibrillation and flutter, and the attendant risk of thromboembolic events are not reduced by closure of the defect. It has often been assumed, but without a firm basis, that these atrial tachyarrhythmias are more amenable to anti-arrhythmic therapy if operation eliminates the stimulus of the left-to-right interatrial shunt and if right atrial size decreases. In addition, radiofrequency ablation is now an option[50] (see Chapter 22). A minority of patients who undergo atrial septal defect closure during childhood experience late-onset atrial flutter or fibrillation, which has been attributed to patchy fibrosis of the shunt-induced right atrial dilatation.[51] Sinus node injury has become a rarity with current techniques of surgical repair or interventional closure.[52–54]

Increased pulmonary vascular resistance in adults with isolated uncomplicated ostium secundum atrial septal defects occurs in two chronologically disparate age groups. An elevation in pulmonary vascular resistance in patients in their late teens or 20s is believed to represent primary pulmonary hypertension in young females in whom the ostium secundum atrial septal defect is coincidental.[12,55] These patients should not undergo atrial septal defect closure because pulmonary vascular disease was not initiated by the shunt and progresses whether or not the defect is closed. Indeed, longevity benefits from the presence of the atrial septal defect (see Chapter 4). The second age group with elevated pulmonary arterial pressure consists chiefly, if not exclusively, of adults beyond 40 years of age, so the aging right ventricle is beset by both pressure and volume overload.[12,56] These patients respond favorably to closure of the atrial septal defect (see earlier discussion).

Sinus Venosus Atrial Septal Defect

Superior vena caval sinus venosus defects, which represent the principal type, vary from small to nonrestrictive and are located immediately inferior to the junction of the superior vena cava and right atrium. *Inferior vena caval sinus venosus defects* are located below the foramen ovale and merge with the floor of the inferior vena cava. The long-term outcome after surgical closure of sinus venosus atrial septal defects, either superior or inferior vena caval, is similar to outcome in ostium secundum atrial septal

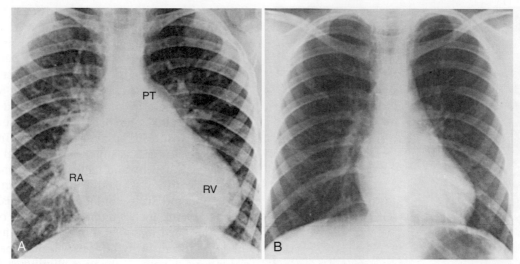

FIGURE 5-6 Chest radiographs from a patient with a clinically isolated nonrestrictive ostium primum atrial septal defect. **(A)** The preoperative radiograph at age 7 years shows increased pulmonary arterial vascularity, a prominent pulmonary trunk (PT), and enlargement of the right atrium (RA) and right ventricle (RV). The ascending aorta is inconspicuous because the shunt was intracardiac. **(B)** Six years after operation, the cardiac size and shape are virtually normal, the pulmonary vascularity is normal, and the pulmonary trunk is no longer dilatated.

defects of equivalent size, with the following exceptions.[57] Because the location of a superior vena caval defect is at the superior vena caval–right atrium junction, the sinus node is often defective or absent before operation or injured during repair.[57-59] An ectopic atrial pacemaker usually provides satisfactory coordinated atrial depolarization (see Chapter 22). Rarely, a pressure gradient at the superior vena caval–right atrium site of repair persists late postoperatively, generally without ill effect.[58,59]

Atrioventricular Septal Defects—Partial and Complete

The *partial form* of these malformations consists of an ostium primum defect with a "cleft" anterior mitral leaflet that may or may not render the mitral valve incompetent. Long-term results after closure of the defect are similar to results after closure of an ostium secundum atrial septal defect of equivalent size and shunt magnitude (Fig. 5–6). Patients between ages 40 and 71 years have undergone repair of ostium primum atrial septal defects (Fig. 5–7) with an early mortality of 6%.[60] Postoperative electrophysiologic residua that have an impact on late survival are dealt with in Chapter 22. A cleft but functionally normal mitral valve is an important postoperative residuum (see Chapter 20). How long such a valve will function normally after the advent of age-related changes in left ventricular geometry, ischemic heart disease, or systemic hypertension is open to question,[11] but it is unlikely that the competent mitral valve of a partial atrioventricular septal defect will, in the long run, prove as durable as its normal counterpart[61,62] (see Chapter 20).

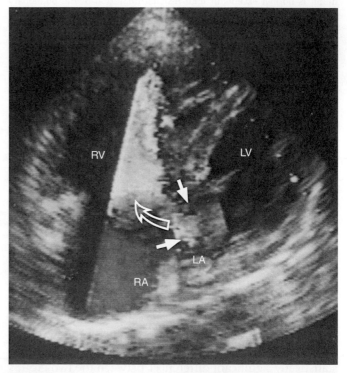

FIGURE 5-7 Black-and-white photograph of a color flow image from a 71-year-old woman with a nonrestrictive ostium primum atrial septal defect *(paired white arrows)* and a cleft anterior mitral leaflet without significant mitral regurgitation. An inlet ventricular septal defect had closed spontaneously by intrusion of atrioventricular valve tissue. The curved arrow identifies the left-to-right shunt through the ostium primum atrial septal defect with flow from left atrium (LA) into right atrium (RA) and then into right ventricle (RV). LV, left ventricle. The patient underwent intracardiac repair just before her 72nd year.

The physiologic consequences of a *complete common atrioventricular canal* are the sum of the interatrial and interventricular communications and the degree of incompetence of the left and right components of the common atrioventricular canal. Down syndrome often coexists and necessarily persists as an important noncardiac postoperative residuum that significantly affects survival patterns because of an inherently shorter life span (see Chapter 20). In addition, there is a proclivity for patients with Down syndrome to develop premature pulmonary vascular disease that tends to persist and progress after operation.

Successful closure of the ostium primum atrial septal defect and the inlet ventricular septal defect can be achieved in infancy. Postoperative pulmonary vascular resistance remains normal or normalizes, and chamber sizes may virtually normalize (Fig. 5-8). Long-term outlook is good but qualified by the adequacy and durability of repair of the abnormal atrioventricular valve.[63] Postoperative electrophysiologic residua are described in Chapter 22 and are similar to those in partial atrioventricular septal defects (discussed earlier).

Total Anomalous Pulmonary Venous Connection

Three features must be taken into account:[14] (1) the pathway by which pulmonary venous blood reaches the right atrium, (2) the presence or absence of obstruction along the course of the pathway, and (3) the nature of the interatrial communication. *Supradiaphragmatic* connections constitute more than three quarters of cases and occur with or without obstruction. The *unobstructed* types are functionally analogous to large left-to-right shunts through a nonrestrictive ostium secundum atrial septal defect except for obligatory venoarterial mixing.[12] *Infradiaphragmatic* connections are almost always obstructed.

In the *unobstructed supradiaphragmatic* types, surgical repair in infancy, childhood, or adolescence is generally followed by a late postoperative course similar to that described earlier for ostium secundum atrial septal defect (Fig. 5-9). In the *obstructed* types of total anomalous pulmonary venous connection, surgical repair in infancy is obligatory.[12] After operation, the majority of patients are asymptomatic and remain so. Long-term outlook is good to excellent.[64] Late recurrence of obstruction is uncommon and originates at the site of anastomosis of the confluence to the left atrium or from stenoses of the pulmonary veins remote from the confluence. Recurrent stenosis is more likely to be associated with repair in neonates with venous obstruction. The results of reoperation have been disappointing but more recently have improved.

Cor Triatriatum

Anatomic varieties of cor triatriatum are referred to as *diaphragmatic*, which is the most common; *hourglass*, which is a developmentally intermediate form; and *tubular*, which is the most primitive and least common. The diaphragmatic type is characterized by a fibrous or fibromuscular membrane that partitions the left atrium into a proximal accessory chamber that receives the pulmonary veins and a distal left atrial chamber that contains the atrial appendage and fossa ovalis. The diaphragmatic type of cor triatriatum lends itself to complete resection of the obstruction, which can be curative, especially if the diagnosis and operation are accomplished in early life.[65] The hourglass and tubular varieties are less amenable to complete repair.

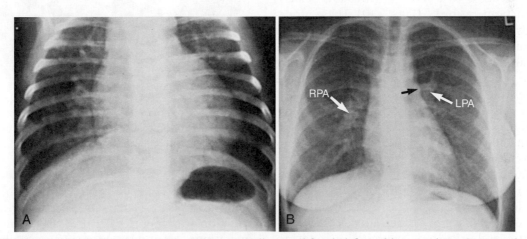

FIGURE 5-8   (A) Chest radiograph from a 24-month-old phenotypically normal female infant with a complete common atrioventricular canal. Pulmonary vascularity is increased, and the heart is enlarged. **(B)** Radiograph from the same patient 18 years after intracardiac repair. Pulmonary vascularity and heart size are normal, and the patient was clinically well. The pulmonary trunk *(black arrow)* is not dilatated, but the right pulmonary artery (RPA) and left pulmonary artery (LPA) remain moderately prominent.

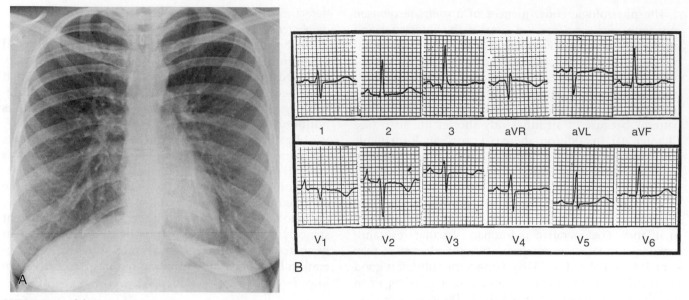

FIGURE 5–9   **(A)** Chest radiograph from a 24-year-old woman who at age 4 months underwent repair of total anomalous pulmonary venous connection. The four pulmonary veins joined a confluence from which a left vertical vein arose to join an innominate bridge and a right superior vena cava. The confluence was anastomosed to the posterior wall of the left atrium. The cardiac silhouette shown here is normal. The right and left pulmonary arteries are somewhat prominent, but the pulmonary trunk is not dilated. **(B)** Electrocardiogram recorded from the same patient at age 24 years. There are peaked right atrial P waves in leads V_1 and V_2, and the QRS frontal plane axis is +100 degrees, but the electrocardiogram is otherwise normal.

INTRAATRIAL SURGERY FOR COMPLEX CYANOTIC CONGENITAL HEART DISEASE

Complete Transposition of the Great Arteries

In the 1960s and 1970s, the standard management of simple transposition of the great arteries was a Rashkind balloon atrial septostomy performed in the neonate and followed by an intraatrial redirection of venous return at age 3 to 6 months (Mustard or Senning atrial switch operation)[66] (Fig. 5–10). These procedures have given way to the *arterial switch* operation (see later), but the large numbers of patients who underwent atrial switch repairs in infancy or early childhood are presenting as adults, often encumbered with major residua and sequelae[67] (see Chapter 20). Ten-year survival after the Mustard operation has been reported at 83% and 20-year survival at 80%[66,67] (Fig. 5–11). The 10-year survival after a Senning operation has been reported at 92%.[68] A fundamental determinant of long-term survival is the performance of a subaortic morphologic right ventricle, which is designed as a low-pressure, low-resistance pulmonary pump.[8,66–72] As patients grow older, an accrued incidence of aortic and tricuspid regurgitation adds to the functional inadequacy of the systemic right ventricle. The intraatrial baffle is responsible for a number of important late postoperative residua, sequelae, or

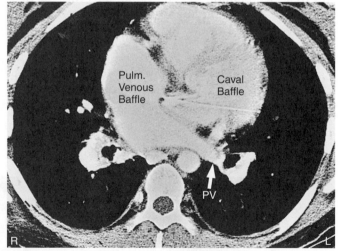

FIGURE 5–10   Magnetic resonance image from a 26-year-old woman with complete transposition of the great arteries and a Mustard repair at age 18 months. The pulmonary venous baffle and the caval baffle are clearly delineated. PV, pulmonary vein.

complications (see Chapter 20). Inferior vena caval obstruction was reported in the early series of Mustard operations,[73,74] and superior vena caval obstruction has been reported late postoperatively in 5% to 10% of patients.[29] Protein-losing enteropathy occasionally develops years after operation because of obstruction of

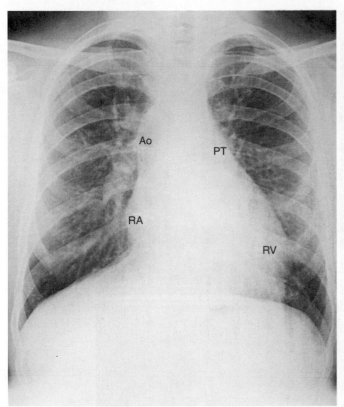

FIGURE 5-11 Chest radiograph from a 27-year-old man with complete transposition of the great arteries and a Mustard atrial switch operation at age 5 months. The long-term result was unusually salutary. The subaortic systemic right ventricle (RV) is not dilatated, and the right atrium (RA) is only slightly convex. The ascending aorta (Ao) is border forming at the right thoracic inlet, and the pulmonary trunk (PT) is border forming at the left thoracic inlet.

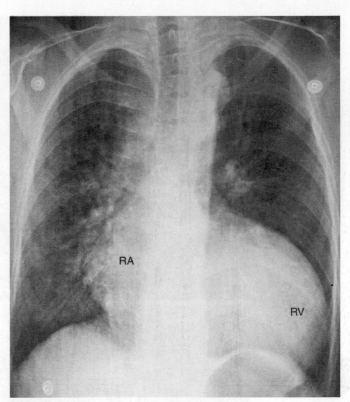

FIGURE 5-12 Chest radiograph from a 22-year-old man with complete transposition of the great arteries and a Mustard atrial switch operation at age 10 months. The increased vascularity in the right lung is the result of baffle obstruction of the right pulmonary veins. The right atrium (RA) and right ventricle (RV) are enlarged. The pulmonary trunk is not border forming.

both superior and inferior venae cavae.[75] Obstruction of the pulmonary venous baffle usually becomes manifest in the first few weeks or months after surgery, less commonly in late survivors (Fig. 5-12). Trivial baffle leaks with bidirectional shunts (dominant left-to-right) occur in about 15% of patients.[29] Large baffle leaks are unusual and require reoperation. Postoperative electrophysiologic sequelae (see Chapter 22) are almost invariable and have a major impact on long-term morbidity and mortality.

Pulmonary vascular disease seldom develops when an atrial switch operation is performed in the first 3 months of life[76] but develops postoperatively in 5% to 10% of older infants.[77-79] A postoperative fall in pulmonary resistance without normalization is generally followed by a subsequent fatal rise in resistance.

"Palliative" Mustard or Senning Operations

Mustard or Senning operations can be performed in patients with complete transposition of the great arteries and a nonrestrictive ventricular septal defect that cannot be closed because of pulmonary vascular disease—hence the term *palliative*[78,80] (Fig. 5-13). Hypoxemia improves because oxygenated systemic flow increases significantly. Failure of the systemic right ventricle is predictably high.

Complete Transposition of the Great Arteries with Ventricular Septal Defect and Pulmonary Stenosis

Surgical experience with this combination of malformations has employed the Rastelli procedure in which left ventricular flow is baffled into the aorta, and right ventricular flow is channeled into the pulmonary artery through an external valved conduit.[29] Varying degrees of right and left ventricular dysfunction persist for years after operation, in addition to long-term concerns related to the durability of the intraventricular tunnel and the external valved conduit[29] (see Chapter 16) and to postoperative electrophysiologic residua and sequelae[81] (see Chapter 22). One of our patients survived to age 46 years with a Blalock-Taussig shunt (Fig. 5-14), then underwent a successful Rastelli procedure.

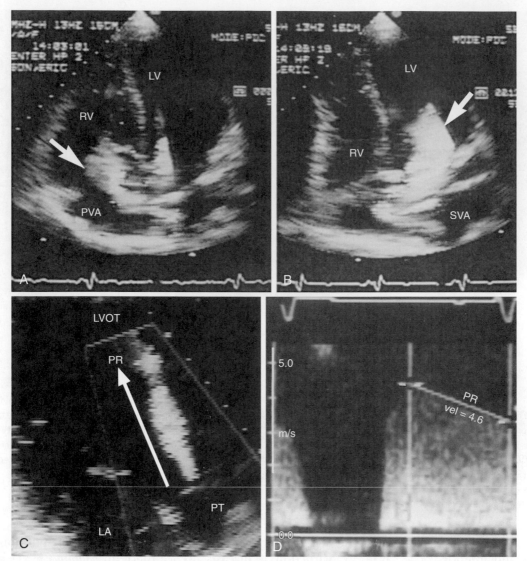

FIGURE 5–13 Two-dimensional echocardiogram (black-and-white photographs of apical four-chamber color flow image) from a 31-year-old man with complete transposition of the great arteries, nonrestrictive ventricular septal defect, pulmonary vascular disease, and a palliative Mustard repair. **(A)** The intraatrial baffle directs blood *(arrow)* from the pulmonary venous atrium (PVA) into the right ventricle (RV) for delivery into the aorta. LV, left ventricle. **(B)** The intraatrial baffle directs blood flow *(arrow)* from the systemic venous atrium (SVA) into the left ventricle (LV) for delivery into the pulmonary circulation. **(C** and **D)** Echocardiographic images from a 28-year-old man with complete transposition of the great arteries, nonrestrictive ventricular septal defect, pulmonary vascular disease, and a palliative Mustard repair. **(C)** Black-and-white photograph of color flow image showing the high-velocity pulmonary regurgitation (PR) prompted by suprasystemic pulmonary vascular resistance. The regurgitation is from the pulmonary trunk (PT) into the left ventricular outflow tract (LVOT) of the morphologic left ventricle. LA, left atrium. **(D)** Continuous-wave Doppler recording aligned parallel to the color flow pulmonary regurgitation shown in part C of this figure. The velocity of 4.6 m/s reflects the increase in diastolic pulmonary arterial pressure in response to the high pulmonary vascular resistance.

Complete Transposition of the Great Arteries with Intact Ventricular Septum and No Pulmonary Stenosis

The procedure of choice is the arterial switch (Jatene) operation within the first 2 weeks of life.[82] Because the operation had its inception in 1976, some patients are now adolescents and young adults. Operative mortality was initially high, but the risk has steadily declined. In a series of 208 consecutive patients who underwent the arterial

switch operation between 1989 and 1992, hospital mortality with or without a ventricular septal defect was less than 5%.[83] In a multi-institutional report of 513 neonates, the 1-month, 1-year, and 5-year survival rates were 84%, 82%, and 82%, respectively.[84] In 475 patients from the Boston Children's Hospital, there were 10 late deaths (2.1%) caused by coronary artery obstruction incurred during implantation, less commonly by intimal proliferation.[85] Long-term outlook depends chiefly on coronary implantations that grow without kinking. Morbidity from

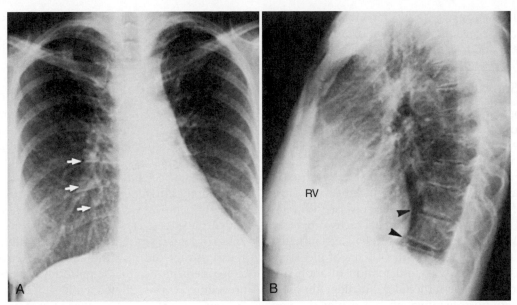

FIGURE 5-14   Chest radiograph from a 46-year-old woman with complete transposition of the great arteries, nonrestrictive ventricular septal defect, and severe pulmonary stenosis. She had undergone a right Blalock-Taussig shunt at age 5 years and a Rastelli repair shortly after these radiographs were taken. **(A)** The right pulmonary artery and its intrapulmonary branches *(arrows)* are relatively prominent. The heart is not enlarged. **(B)** Lateral chest radiograph shows the right ventricle (RV) in contact with the sternum. The left ventricle *(arrowheads)* is not enlarged.

compromised coronary flow (Fig. 5-15) varies from asymptomatic occlusion with exuberant coronary arterial collaterals to sudden death.[85-87] Gradients exceeding 40 mm Hg at the pulmonary arterial anastomotic site occur with an incidence of less than 10%[85] and are generally managed with balloon angioplasty (see Chapter 18). Dilatation of the neoaortic root is another concern.

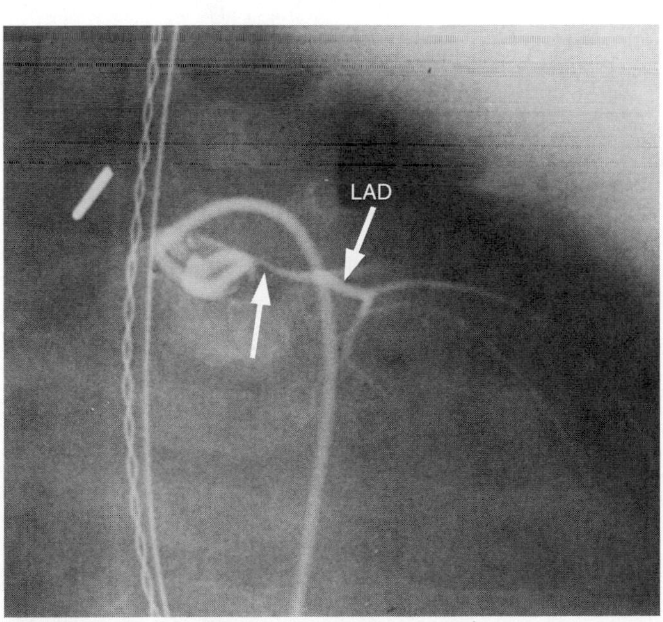

FIGURE 5-15   Semiselective coronary arteriogram after an arterial switch repair in an infant with complete transposition of the great arteries. The left anterior descending (LAD) artery is obstructed in its proximal course *(unmarked arrow)*.

After technically successful arterial switch operations with unimpaired coronary flow, left ventricular mechanics are similar to those of age-matched control subjects.[85,88] Recall that before atrial septostomy, mortality in unoperated patients with complete transposition of the great arteries was 90% in the first year of life. How remarkable it is that adult survival is now expected in most patients after atrial and arterial switch operations.

Congenitally Corrected Transposition of the Great Arteries

This malformation is characterized by discordant ventriculoarterial alignments (transposition of the great arteries) with discordant atrioventricular alignments that physiologically "correct" the transposition. Blood from a morphologic right atrium reaches the pulmonary artery after traversing a morphologic mitral valve and a morphologic left ventricle, and blood from a morphologic left atrium reaches the aorta after traversing a morphologic tricuspid valve and a morphologic right ventricle. When this malformation occurs in children or adults with a large ventricular septal defect and pulmonary stenosis, intracardiac repair is feasible.[29,89] Functional results are good, but qualifications abound. Apart from relatively high operative mortality, four major concerns influence long-term postoperative survival: (1) left atrioventricular valve regurgitation (see earlier), (2) a high incidence of heart block incurred at operation or by a 2% per year accrued incidence of acquired high-degree infranodal heart block[12] (see Chapter 22), (3) the durability of a long external valved conduit extending from left ventricle to pulmonary artery (see Chapter 16), and (4) a progressive decrease in function of a morphologic right ventricle in the systemic location (see Chapter 4).

Ventricular Septal Defects

Perimembranous and inlet ventricular defects are generally repaired from the right atrium (see Chapter 15). Right ventriculotomy is usually reserved for subarterial defects, and left ventriculotomy is reserved for trabecular or muscular defects that cannot otherwise be effectively closed.[90] Transatrial repair reduces the risk of right ventriculotomy-induced sites of slowed conduction that serve as substrates for reentry and monomorphic ventricular tachycardia (see Chapter 22). When transatrial closure of a ventricular septal defect is performed in the first 2 years of life, long-term outlook is excellent with anticipation of adult survival.[91-93] When surgery is undertaken in older children, an increase in late postoperative left ventricular size and mass may persist together with reduced left ventricular systolic function.[94,95] Moderately restrictive or nonrestrictive ventricular septal defects seldom present for operation in adults because a reduction in size or spontaneous closure obviates the need, because large left-to-right shunts induce congestive heart failure that seldom permits adult survival, or because pulmonary vascular disease results in inoperable Eisenmenger syndrome[92,96-101] (Fig. 5–16) (see Chapter 4). When preoperative pulmonary vascular resistance exceeds 10 units/m^2 and the postoperative decline in resistance is relatively small, the attrition rate is about 25% within 5 years.[29,102-104]

Mild preoperative aortic regurgitation usually remains mild.[105] Moderate to marked regurgitation is generally amenable to aortic valve reconstruction[105] (see Chapter 15).

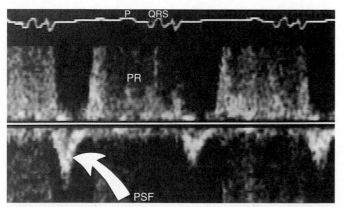

FIGURE 5–16 Pulsed Doppler recording from a 45-year-old man with a moderately restrictive perimembranous ventricular septal defect that was associated with elevated pulmonary vascular resistance before the defect was surgically closed at age 9 years. A progressive postoperative increase in pulmonary vascular resistance resulted in depressed right ventricular systolic function reflected in the low velocity pulmonary systolic flow (PSF, *arrow*). The elevated diastolic pressure generated pulmonary regurgitation (PR).

Postoperative risk of infective endocarditis is determined by aortic regurgitation or by an aortic valve prosthesis (see Chapter 8).

Tetralogy of Fallot

Long-term survival after intracardiac repair is good to excellent.[106] Even when surgery was performed as long ago as 1955 to 1960, the 32-year actuarial survival rate for 163 patients was 86%, compared with a survival rate of 96% in an age- and sex-matched control population.[106] Survival rates in patients 11 years of age or younger at the time of operation were 90% to 93%, whereas survival in patients aged 12 years or older at the time of surgery was 76% compared with an expected rate of 93%. A Blalock-Taussig shunt did not influence long-term survival after subsequent intracardiac repair, but a Potts or Waterston procedure was associated with significant reduction in 30-year survival (73%) because of progressive pulmonary vascular disease or depressed function of the volume overload left ventricle, complications that rarely occur after a Blalock-Taussig anastomosis (Fig. 5–17).

Repair of tetralogy of Fallot is now undertaken in infants. Early operation improves cumulative longevity, with an actuarial survival rate of 93% at 15 years.[83] The incidence of complications is reduced, and quality of life is improved.[107] Patients who undergo repair before 2 years of age are usually symptom free and, for all practical purposes, lead normal lives.[108] The reoperation rate has been reported as less than 5%.[108-112] Symptoms within 2 years of operation occur because of inadequate relief of right ventricular outflow obstruction, severe pulmonary regurgitation, or residual defects in the ventricular septum.[109]

Patients who reach adulthood after palliative shunts in early life fall into two general categories: first, those who have undergone Potts anastomoses and are likely to present with inoperable pulmonary vascular disease (Fig. 5–18) and second, those who have undergone early Blalock-Taussig shunts and live to undergo intracardiac repair as adults[113,114] (Fig. 5–19).

The majority of adults who have undergone early intracardiac repair of tetralogy of Fallot are clinically well,[115,116] but continued surveillance is mandatory because of postoperative residua that involve the right ventricle, its outflow tract (Fig. 5–20), the pulmonary valve, the left ventricle, the aortic valve, electrophysiologic residua and sequelae (see later in this chapter and see Chapter 22), and sequelae associated with prosthetic valves, patches (Fig. 5–21), and conduits (see Fig. 5–20). When intracardiac repair is performed within the first 5 years of life, right ventricular end-diastolic volume and ejection fraction are normal provided obstruction to right ventricular outflow is absent or insignificant, and pulmonary regurgitation is no more than moderate.[117,118] A transannular patch (Fig. 5–22) incurs immediate severe pulmonary

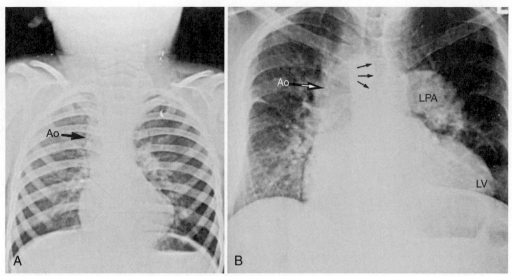

FIGURE 5–17   (A) Chest radiograph before a left Blalock-Taussig shunt in a 4.5-year-old cyanotic boy with the typical boot-shaped heart and right aortic arch (Ao) of tetralogy of Fallot. **(B)** Chest radiograph from the same patient at age 50 years. The left pulmonary arch (LPA) is strikingly dilated, pulmonary vascularity is increased, the right aortic arch (Ao) indents the trachea toward the left *(small arrows),* and an enlarged left ventricle (LV) occupies the apex. The patient underwent intracardiac repair with revision of the shunt.

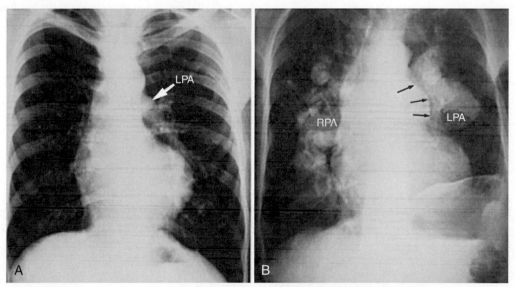

FIGURE 5–18   (A) Chest radiograph from a 32-year-old man with tetralogy of Fallot. A Potts anastomosis in early childhood was followed by progressive pulmonary vascular disease. The patient died 2 years after this radiograph was taken. The cardiac silhouette retains its boot-shaped appearance, reflecting the rapidity with which pulmonary blood flow was curtailed by postoperative pulmonary vascular disease. The left pulmonary artery (LPA) is conspicuously dilatated. **(B)** Chest radiograph from a 39-year-old man with tetralogy of Fallot. After a Potts anastomosis in infancy, the patient developed progressive pulmonary vascular disease. The pulmonary trunk *(arrows)* is markedly dilatated, and the right pulmonary artery (RPA) and left pulmonary artery (LPA) are aneurysmal. The left hemidiaphragm is elevated because of gas in the stomach and splenic flexure.

regurgitation that imposes an appreciable volume load on the incised right ventricle. A subannular incision compromises infundibular support for the pulmonary valve, resulting in slowly developing but potentially severe pulmonary regurgitation. In either case, severe regurgitation serves as a trigger that activates slow conduction reentrant substrates for monomorphic ventricular tachycardia[119] (discussed later).

Postoperative elevation of right ventricular systolic pressure defined as a resting peak-to-peak gradient greater than 40 mm Hg results from a persistently small pulmonary valve annulus, a small pulmonary arterial trunk, or obstruction at the pulmonary arterial bifurcation or within the proximal branches.

Postoperative aneurysms of the right ventricular outflow tract were frequent when earlier surgical techniques

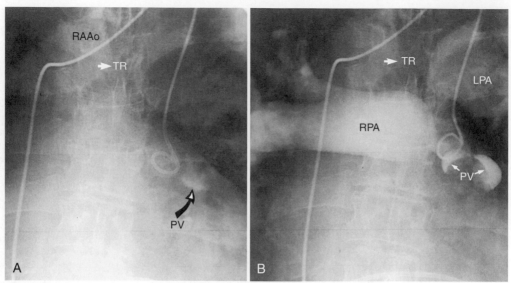

FIGURE 5-19 **(A)** Overpenetrated selected portion of a chest radiograph from a 54-year-old man with tetralogy of Fallot and a left Blalock-Taussig shunt at age 9 years. The pulmonary valve (PV) is calcified, and a dilatated right aortic arch (RAAo) indents the trachea (TR, *arrow*) toward the left. **(B)** Pulmonary arteriogram via the left Blalock-Taussig shunt. The bicuspid pulmonary valve (PV) is still mobile (doming) despite radiologic calcification shown in part A of this figure. The left pulmonary artery (LPA) is disproportionately enlarged because it received the shunt. RPA, right pulmonary artery. The trachea (TR) is indented on its right margin *(arrow)* because of the right aortic arch. The patient underwent revision of the shunt together with closure of the ventricular septal defect and replacement of the calcified pulmonary valve with a tissue prosthesis.

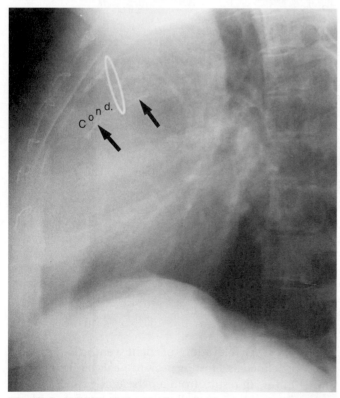

FIGURE 5-20 Lateral chest radiograph from a 19-year-old woman with tetralogy of Fallot and an external valved conduit (Cond.) that is calcified *(arrows)* and obstructed above and below a porcine valve identified by the metallic sewing ring.

were employed but are uncommon with current techniques. Small aneurysms generally do not progress (see Fig. 5–21) and do not require repair,[120] but reoperation is required in patients with large incisional aneurysms and depressed right ventricular function (see Fig. 5–22).

A small but not insignificant group of patients with tetralogy of Fallot die suddenly years after intracardiac repair via a right ventriculotomy.[81] These patients tend to have prolonged QRS durations and positive signal-averaged electrocardiograms that indicate substrates of slowed conduction capable of sustained reentrant monomorphic ventricular tachycardia. Older age has been implicated as a risk factor in postventriculotomy reentrant monomorphic ventricular tachycardia because of an age-related increase in scarring at the incision site.[113] Ventricular tachyarrhythmias are rare when intracardiac repair is performed before age 5 years.[81] Severe pulmonary regurgitation serves as a trigger that activates the arrhythmogenic substrate[81] (see Chapter 22). Reoperation with pulmonary valve replacement, excision and revision of the ventriculotomy scar, and radiofrequency ablation of residual sites of slowed conduction obviate the risk of monomorphic ventricular tachycardia, improve right ventricular function, and substantially increase the prospects of long-term survival.

Depressed left ventricular function in tetralogy of Fallot is due to excess volume overload from a previous shunt[121] (discussed earlier; see Fig. 5–19). However,

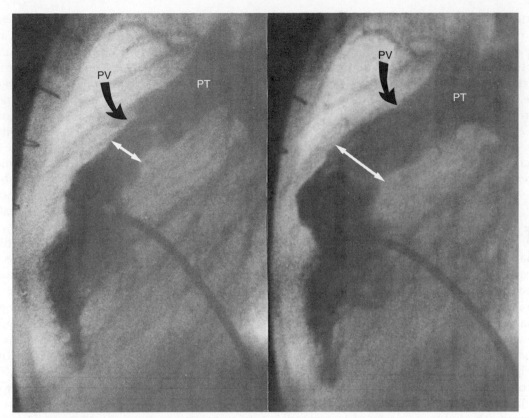

FIGURE 5-21   Lateral right ventriculogram from a 27-year-old woman who had undergone intracardiac repair of tetralogy of Fallot by means of a vertical right ventriculotomy 3 years earlier. Mild to moderate dyskinesis of the right ventricular outflow tract is illustrated by its increasing width from diastole on the left to systole on the right *(paired white arrows)*. PV, pulmonary valve; PT, pulmonary trunk.

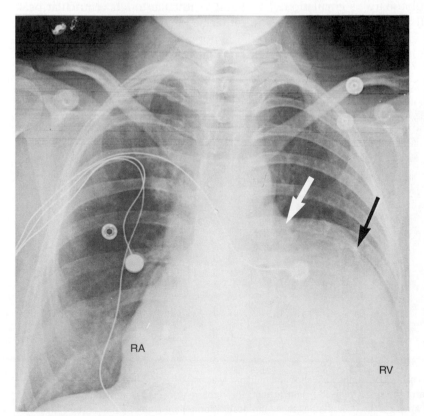

FIGURE 5-22   Chest radiograph from a 21-year-old woman with tetralogy of Fallot and a dramatic postoperative aneurysm at the site of a transannular patch (non-valved conduit). The black and white arrows identify calcium in the wall of the aneurysm. The right ventricle (RV) and right atrium (RA) are dilatated because of severe pulmonary and tricuspid regurgitation.

severe cyanotic tetralogy of Fallot is accompanied by a substantial decrease in pulmonary blood flow with a comparable decrease in left ventricular volume and ejection fraction—left ventricular volume "underload."[122] When intracardiac repair is performed after 2 years of age, left ventricular volume normalizes, but left ventricular function often remains subnormal[122,123] (see Chapter 20). When repair is performed in the first 2 years of life, normalization of left ventricular volume is usually accompanied by a normal or near normal physiologic response to loading conditions[122,123] (see Chapter 11).

Tetralogy of Fallot with Pulmonary Atresia

This malformation is characterized by a right ventricle that terminates blindly against an atretic pulmonary valve or against imperforate muscle—the ultimate expression of severity in tetralogy of Fallot. The pulmonary trunk is either a vestigial chord or a hypoplastic funnel-shaped channel that widens slightly as it approaches hypoplastic proximal branches that may be discontinuous. The entire output of the right ventricle necessarily enters the systemic circulation through a malaligned ventricular septal defect. The biventricular aorta is dilatated and often continues as a right aortic arch. The lungs are perfused by systemic-to-pulmonary arterial collaterals that serve both nutritive and respiratory functions and on which survival depends. Systemic arterial collaterals are classified according to their origins as *bronchial* that anastomose to pulmonary arteries within the lungs, *direct systemic arterials* that originate from the descending aorta, enter the hilum, and then assume the structure and distribution of intrapulmonary

arteries, and *indirect systemic arterial collaterals* that originate from major branches of the aorta and anastomose to proximal pulmonary arteries outside the lungs.

About 65% of patients are symptomatic in infancy because pulmonary blood flow is inadequate, and about 25% have symptomatic congestive heart failure because pulmonary blood flow is excessive.[124] Approximately 60% of symptomatic infants survive their first birthday with or without operation, and about 65% of those alive at 1 year survive to age 10 years.[124] Without operation, mortality thereafter is high, with only 16% surviving to adulthood[124] (see Chapter 4). At the other end of the spectrum are occasional patients with adequate but not excessive aortic-to-pulmonary collateral arterial blood flow that permits survival into adolescence or adulthood.[12] This uncommon survival pattern includes 62% of unoperated patients and 39% who were palliated before age 18 years.[125] Twenty-three percent died during follow-up at a mean age of 31 years, with only two patients surviving beyond age 40 years.[125] Our adult survivors were all symptomatic, of whom half were NYHA class II and half class III (see Chapter 4). Moderate to severe aortic regurgitation was present in 77%, and 38% experienced heart failure.[125] Ten patients older than 18 years underwent staged unifocalization repairs (see Chapters 15 and 16; Fig. 5–23) with significant improvement in exercise tolerance and near-normal lifestyles. Long-term outcome depends on the degree of residual obstruction to right ventricular outflow and on the adequacy of flow into the reconstructed pulmonary circulation.[126,127] Right ventricular-to-left ventricular peak systolic pressure ratios between 0.8 and 1.0 are due to pulmonary arterial hypoplasia or residual pulmonary artery branch stenoses that were not accessible to surgical

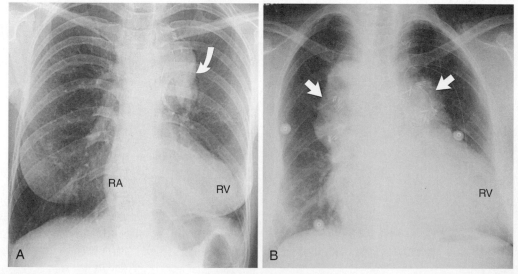

FIGURE 5–23 (**A**) Chest radiograph from a 26-year-old woman with tetralogy of Fallot and pulmonary atresia after the first stage of a unifocalization repair. Arrow points to the unilateral pericardial tube of the first stage. RA, right atrium; RV, right ventricle. (**B**) Chest radiograph from a 28-year-old woman with tetralogy of Fallot and pulmonary atresia after a completed staged unifocalization repair. Arrows point to the silhouettes of the bilateral pericardial tubes employed in the completed repair (see Chapter 15).

repair and were not responsive to balloon angioplasty (see Chapter 18). The right ventricular-to-pulmonary artery conduits require replacement, and unrepaired aortic regurgitation may progress and require valve repair or replacement (see Chapter 16). Large aortic-to-pulmonary arterial collaterals left unattended risk volume overload of the left ventricle, so transcatheter occlusion should be attempted before unifocalization[128] (see Chapter 18). One of our patients with incomplete unifocalization developed segmental pulmonary vascular disease and died suddenly at age 25 years of a ruptured central shunt (Fig. 5–24).

Surgically Created Shunts Between Aorta and Pulmonary Artery

Three major shunts between the aorta and pulmonary artery have been employed—the Blalock-Taussig (1945), the Potts (descending aorta-to-left pulmonary artery, 1946), and the Waterston (ascending aorta-to right pulmonary artery, 1962). The latter two have fallen into disuse, but modified Blalock-Taussig shunts are used for short-term palliation in infants with deficient pulmonary blood flow as Taussig originally proposed, as a bridge to subsequent repair, or as palliation in adults with unrepaired cyanotic congenital heart disease.

Patients with tetralogy of Fallot occasionally undergo intracardiac repair 40 years or more after Blalock-Taussig shunts that were inserted in infancy or early childhood (see Figs. 5–19 and 5–20). Shunts inserted decades earlier have served admirably as a bridge to subsequent intracardiac repair in adults with malformations other than the tetralogy (Fig. 5–25).

A subclavian-to-pulmonary arterial shunt rarely provokes an increase in pulmonary vascular resistance, but one of our patients operated on by Dr. Alfred Blalock at 3 years of age died 40 years later from rupture of an aneurysmal hypertensive pulmonary trunk[129] (see Fig. 5–17).

The ipsilateral arm may be a little smaller than normal after a classic Blalock-Taussig shunt, but blood flow is generally sufficient so that the arm functions normally.[130] Occasionally, a *subclavian steal* becomes manifest years after placement of the shunt.

Potts anastomoses, because of their size, were frequently complicated by pulmonary vascular disease, but patients often reached adulthood (see Fig. 5–18). Less commonly, ideal Potts anastomoses permitted adult survival without the development of cardiac failure or pulmonary vascular disease (Fig. 5–26, *B*).

Waterston anastomoses established shunts that were more readily controlled than Potts anastomoses, but the Waterston often caused kinking of the right pulmonary artery (see Chapter 15). The takedown of Potts and Waterston shunts can be technically difficult and hazardous especially in older patients (see Chapter 15).

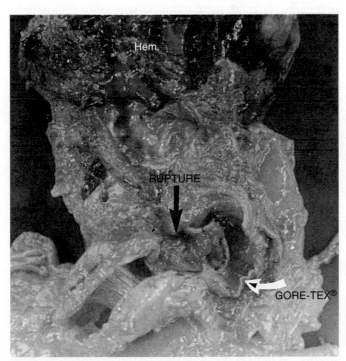

FIGURE 5–24   Necropsy specimen from a 25-year-old man with tetralogy of Fallot and pulmonary atresia. An incomplete unifocalization operation was followed by segmental pulmonary vascular disease that resulted in sudden death caused by rupture of a central shunt (GORE-TEX®; see Chapter 16) with intrapulmonary and intrapleural hemorrhage (Hem.).

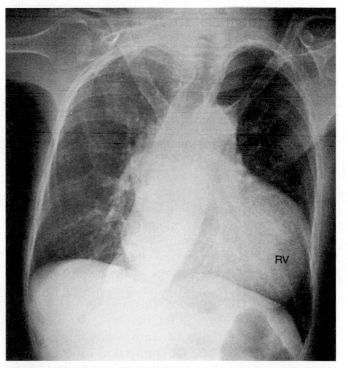

FIGURE 5–25   Chest radiograph from a 66-year-old man with double-outlet right ventricle (RV) and pulmonary stenosis. The clinical diagnosis was tetralogy of Fallot, for which the patient underwent a Blalock-Taussig shunt procedure performed by Dr. Alfred Blalock.

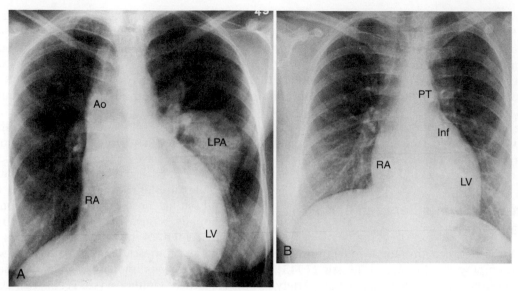

FIGURE 5–26 **(A)** Chest radiograph from a 23-year-old woman with tricuspid atresia, normally related great arteries, and spontaneous closure of a restrictive perimembranous ventricular septal defect after a Potts anastomosis. A continuous murmur through the anastomosis remained audible. The left pulmonary artery (LPA) is strikingly dilatated, but pulmonary arterial blood flow is not visibly increased. The ascending aorta (Ao) is conspicuous because of the persistent shunt. A convex left ventricle (LV) occupies the apex, and a moderately enlarged right atrium (RA) occupies the right lower cardiac silhouette. The patient did not meet the criteria for a Fontan repair. **(B)** Chest radiograph from a 20-year-old woman with tricuspid atresia, normally related great arteries, a restrictive ventricular septal defect (subpulmonary stenosis), and an ideal Potts anastomosis at age 13 months. The right atrium (RA) is moderately enlarged, the left ventricle (LV) is not significantly dilatated, and the pulmonary trunk (PT) is normal. The patient underwent a successful Fontan repair. Inf, infundibulum.

Glenn Operation

The original Glenn operation consisted of end-to-side anastomosis of the superior vena cava to the distal end of a divided right pulmonary artery, with closure of the junction of the superior vena cava and right atrium. A modified Glenn operation (superior vena caval flow to both pulmonary arteries, or the bidirectional Glenn) is used for patients in whom total caval to pulmonary arterial flow is not acceptable because of elevated pulmonary arterial pressure or an increase in left ventricular filling pressure. The bidirectional Glenn sometimes achieves symptomatic improvement that is maintained for years.[131,132]

A 30-year follow-up after the classic Glenn procedure for a variety of cyanotic congenital malformations disclosed an actuarial survival rate of 84% and 66% at 10 and 20 years, with 22% late deaths.[133] Follow-up after the bidirectional Glenn procedure has necessarily been shorter, with a survival rate of 87% in 129 patients followed for an average of just over 2 years.[134] Results were not as good when a morphologic right ventricle was in the subaortic position.[134] If ventricular function improves and pulmonary vascular resistance falls after a bidirectional Glenn operation, an inferior caval-to-pulmonary arterial connection can be undertaken, resulting in the physiology of a completed Fontan repair (total caval-to-pulmonary artery).

Right lower lobe pulmonary arteriovenous fistulae develop late postoperatively in 19% to 25% of patients

with classic Glenn shunts[133,135,136] (Fig. 5–27). The pathogenesis of these fistulae is speculative, but proposed mechanisms include nonpulsatile pulmonary blood flow with maldistribution reflected in a relative increase in lower lobe flow,[135] lack of an hepatic substance,[137] or response to the relatively low volume of superior vena caval return that is delivered to the larger volume right lung. These arteriovenous fistulae are amenable to occlusion by interventional catheterization (see Chapter 18) and may regress after Fontan completion.

Fontan Operation

The Fontan operation evolved from a model proposed in 1955 and was first employed in 1968 to tricuspid atresia with pulmonary stenosis.[138] The procedure has undergone many significant modifications[139] and is now applied to lesions in addition to tricuspid atresia or single ventricle with pulmonary stenosis (see Fig. 5–26). Few cardiac operations demand stricter adherence to preoperative criteria, which are discussed in Chapter 15, together with surgical techniques.[83,140–148] Hospital mortality after a Fontan procedure has steadily declined and is now less than 10%.[142,143,148] One to five years after operation, most patients are active and NYHA functional class I or II. Ten years after operation, functional class decreases in 44% of patients,[29,149] with 15-year survival predicted to be 73%.[29,150]

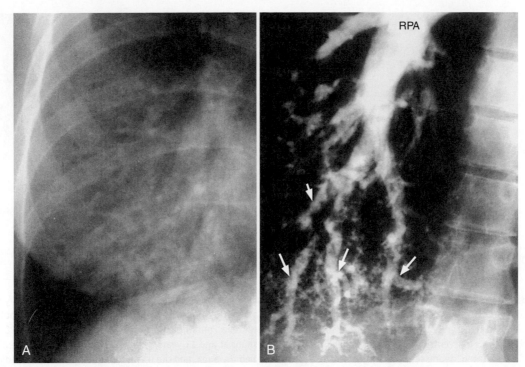

FIGURE 5–27   **(A)** Close-up of the right lower lobe (posteroanterior chest radiograph) from a 20-year-old woman with tricuspid atresia, pulmonary stenosis, and a classic Glenn operation 12 years earlier. The radiodensities are typical of right lower lobe pulmonary arteriovenous fistulae. **(B)** Selective right pulmonary arteriogram (RPA) identifying the fistulae *(arrows)*, which were subsequently closed by coil embolization (see Chapter 15).

Late postoperative results depend heavily on ventricular function and on the maintenance of sinus rhythm (see Chapter 22). Long-term functional adequacy is best realized when there is a morphologic left ventricle, as in tricuspid atresia or univentricular heart of the left ventricular type (Fig. 5–28). Successful operation is accompanied by a reduction in ventricular size, a normal mass-to-volume ratio, and improved contractility[151] (Fig. 5–29). The largest and longest follow-ups include patients who underwent Fontan procedures for tricuspid atresia or for univentricular hearts of the left ventricular type.[141,152-155] When the procedure is performed in patients with univentricular hearts of the right ventricular type, long-term function is not as good because a single morphologic right ventricle serves the systemic circulation.[154] Operation in patients 18 years or older sometimes achieves remarkable rehabilitation (Fig. 5–30), with 93% of these adults functional NYHA class II or I.[156]

Right atrial pressure after a classic right atrial-to-pulmonary artery Fontan procedure rises to the mean pulmonary arterial pressure and increases further with exercise.[149,157-159] Atrial fibrillation or flutter elevates right atrial mean pressure still more because of the effect of the tachyarrhythmia on left ventricular filling pressure, which is transmitted to the pulmonary artery (discussed later). Pleural effusions, ascites, and peripheral edema can be severe for months after a Fontan operation,[153,156] but total caval to pulmonary arterial connections with an intraatrial tunnel or extracardiac conduit preclude right atrial distention and tend to reduce postoperative fluid retention.[141]

After a Fontan operation, as many as 12% of patients have late-onset protein-losing enteropathy expressed as edema, pleural effusions, ascites, diarrhea, excessive loss of serum protein into the gastrointestinal lumen, low serum albumin, increased mesenteric vascular resistance, prominent lymphatic vessels in the jejunal mucosa,[160] high α_1-antitrypsin clearance, and low serum calcium levels.[29] Percutaneous atrial fenestration has resulted in clinical improvement and occasional resolution.[161]

Disturbances in atrial rhythm are among the most serious late sequelae of a Fontan repair (see Chapter 22). Atrial fibrillation, flutter, and ectopic atrial tachycardia deprive the subaortic ventricle of an atrial contribution to filling, adversely affecting ventricular function, impairing forward flow through the Fontan connection, and increasing the risk of thrombosis and obstruction (Fig. 5–31). Late conduit obstruction from any cause is a serious complication that requires prompt recognition and reoperation. Sinus node dysfunction or impaired atrioventricular node conduction may require a pacemaker.

Pulmonary Atresia with Intact Ventricular Septum

This malformation is represented by an imperforate pulmonary valve, a well-formed main pulmonary artery and proximal branches, a ventricular septum that by

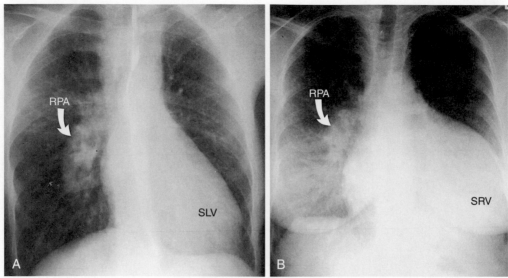

FIGURE 5–28 **(A)** Chest radiograph from a 24-year-old man with single ventricle of the left ventricular type, pulmonary stenosis, and a right Blalock-Taussig shunt in childhood. Dilatation of the right pulmonary artery (RPA) reflects previous shunt flow. The mean pulmonary arterial pressure and the size and function of the single left ventricle (SLV) were ideal for a Fontan repair. **(B)** Chest radiograph from a 28-year-old woman with single ventricle of the right ventricular type and right Blalock-Taussig shunt at age 11 years, reflected in the increased size of the right pulmonary artery (RPA). The dilatated, depressed single right ventricle (SRV) occupied the apex, and the increase in filling pressure is indicated by radiographic pulmonary edema shown better in the right hemithorax. A Fontan repair was not feasible. The radiographs shown here underscore the difference in functional adequacy of a single morphologic left ventricle compared with a single morphologic right ventricle.

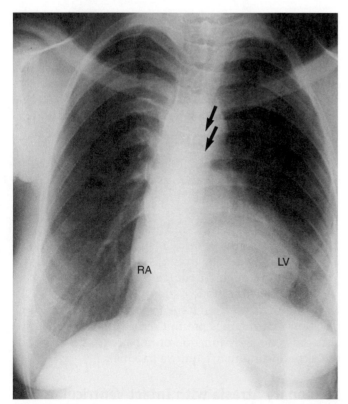

FIGURE 5–29 Chest radiograph from a 20-year-old woman with tricuspid atresia and pulmonary stenosis 14 years after a right atrial-to-pulmonary artery Fontan operation. Except for the telltale metal sutures *(arrows)*, the radiograph could be read as normal. RA, right atrium; LV, left ventricle.

definition is intact, and an obligatory interatrial communication.[12] Right ventricular size varies from diminutive with a correspondingly small tricuspid annulus and valve, to dilatated with an incompetent Ebstein-like tricuspid valve.[12] Important variables are adequacy of the right ventricular size and tricuspid valve mechanism and the state of the coronary circulation. Surgery performed in infants is designed to increase pulmonary blood flow, decompress the right ventricle, minimize tricuspid regurgitation, and promote right ventricular growth (see Chapter 15). Pulmonary valvotomy or valvectomy combined with a systemic-to-pulmonary arterial shunt permits an occasional patient to reach young adulthood and reoperation (Fig. 5–32).

Double-Chambered Right Ventricle

The right ventricle is divided by muscle bundles that consist of a hypertrophied moderator band or trabecular septomarginalis (Fig. 5–33) or a fibromuscular diaphragm. An accompanying ventricular septal defect in the proximal high-pressure compartment results in a right-to-left shunt.[12,162] The results 20 years after intracardiac repair have been good.[163] Postoperative residua include right ventricular outflow obstruction and aortic regurgitation, not necessarily present before repair. Reoperation has been reported in 10% of patients[163] but has been much less frequent with current surgical techniques.

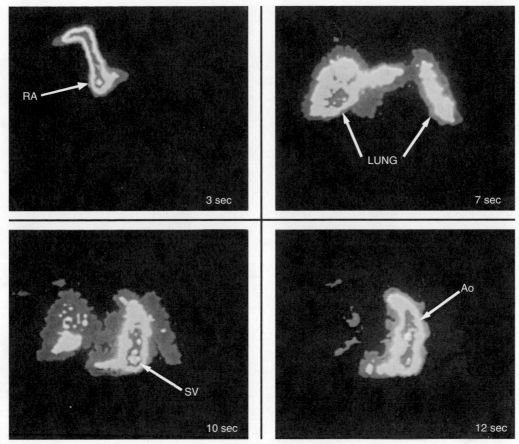

FIGURE 5–30   Nuclear angiogram after a Fontan repair (right atrial to pulmonary artery anastomosis) in a 38-year-old man with a univentricular heart of the left ventricular type and pulmonary stenosis. The radionuclide injection was made into the right antecubital vein and shows the bolus (*arrows*) traversing in sequence the right atrium (RA), lungs, single ventricle (SV), and ascending aorta (Ao). Postoperative improvement was remarkable despite age at operation.

Double-Outlet Right Ventricle

Three essential morphologic features characterize this malformation: the ventricular–great artery connections; the relationship of the ventricular septal defect to the great arteries; and the absence, presence, and degree of pulmonary stenosis. By definition, both great arteries arise from the morphologic right ventricle. The common types of double-outlet right ventricle occur without pulmonary stenosis and with either a subaortic or subpulmonic ventricular septal defect. Less commonly, the ventricular septal defect is doubly committed or uncommitted, or, rarely, the ventricular septum is intact. Double-outlet right ventricle with a *subaortic* ventricular septal defect and *pulmonary stenosis* resembles tetralogy of Fallot, and double-outlet right ventricle with a *subpulmonary* ventricular septal defect and *no pulmonary stenosis* resembles complete transposition of the great arteries. One of our patients, a 67-year-old man with double-outlet right ventricle, a subaortic ventricular septal defect, and pulmonary stenosis, had a shunt placed by Dr. Blalock for an understandably mistaken diagnosis of tetralogy of Fallot (see Fig. 5–25).

Although postoperative survival is good when the ventricular septal defect is subaortic or doubly committed and when flow from the left ventricle is successfully baffled into the aorta,[164] there is a relatively high incidence of sudden death many years after repair. Of 89 patients, 22 died, 16 of whom (73%) died suddenly.[165]

Double-Outlet Left Ventricle

Data on long-term survival after surgery are scanty because double-outlet left ventricle is the rarest of the ventricular–great arterial malalignments.[12] Two of our patients underwent re-repairs in their mid-20s after initial shunt operations (Figs. 5–34 and 5–35).

CENTRAL ARTERIAL SURGERY

Patent Ductus Arteriosus

Division of an isolated, restrictive patent ductus arteriosus in childhood represents one of the few cures of congenital malformations of the heart and circulation. Transcatheter ductal closure (see Chapter 18) promises to compete with this record. After surgical or interventional closure of the ductus, patients are normal in the literal sense.

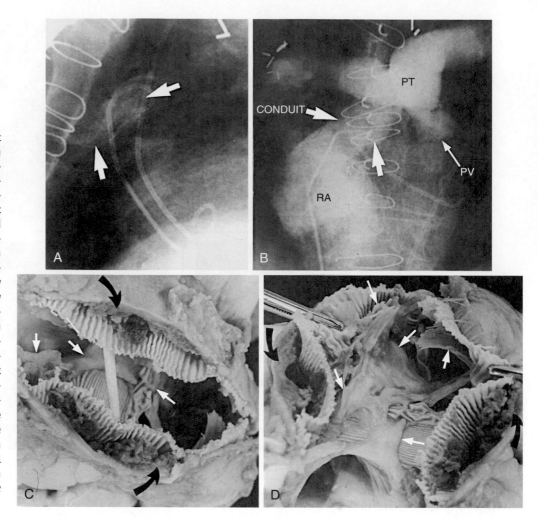

FIGURE 5–31 **(A)** Lateral chest radiograph from a 47-year-old man with tricuspid atresia, two Blalock-Taussig shunts, and a right atrial-to-pulmonary arterial Fontan conduit at age 34 years. Arrows point to calcification in the obstructed conduit. **(B)** Contrast medium injection into the right atrium (RA) shows the obstructed conduit connected to a well-formed pulmonary trunk (PT). The sealed pulmonary valve (PV) is identified by the arrow. **(C and D)** Necropsy specimen from a 42-year-old man with tricuspid atresia and a right atrial-to-pulmonary arterial Fontan conduit at age 20 years. He presented moribund. Transesophageal echocardiography identified a large mobile thrombus in the conduit. These necropsy specimens show the open conduit with obstructing internal peel *(white arrows)* and separation of the wall by fresh thrombus *(black arrows)*.

When the ductus is moderately restrictive or nonrestrictive, division in childhood is typically followed by regression of left atrial and left ventricular enlargement and in normalization of pulmonary arterial and right ventricular systolic pressures. If a relatively large or nonrestrictive ductus remains patent after childhood, the long-term outcome after closure is guarded and depends on the preoperative pulmonary vascular resistance and the chronic effects of left ventricular volume overload.[166] Premature infants who undergo ductal closure because of heart failure and respiratory distress experience long-term complications that are usually related to prematurity, including bronchopulmonary dysplasia, retrolental fibroplasia, and cerebral palsy.[167]

Aortopulmonary Window

This malformation is physiologically but not morphogenetically akin to a nonrestrictive patent ductus arteriosus and is characterized by a communication, usually nonrestrictive, between adjacent walls of the ascending aorta and pulmonary trunk. Early repair permits good long-term survival provided that (1) preoperative pulmonary vascular resistance is less than 8 units/m² of body surface area, (2) the pulmonary-to-systemic resistance ratio is less than 0.4, and (3) there are no major coexisting cardiac anomalies.[168]

Truncus Arteriosus

A single great artery with a single semilunar valve leaves the base of the heart and gives rise to the pulmonary, systemic, and coronary circulations. The single arterial trunk receives the output from both ventricles through an obligatory ventricular septal defect. Long-term survival is compromised if patients are older than 3 months at the time of surgical ventricular septal effect closure and conduit placement, if there is significant truncal valve regurgitation, and if only a single pulmonary artery branch emerges from the truncus.[169] Right ventricular-to-pulmonary artery conduit replacement is always required[170] (see Chapter 16). Mild preoperative truncal valve regurgitation may become hemodynamically significant years later. When patients are operated on in

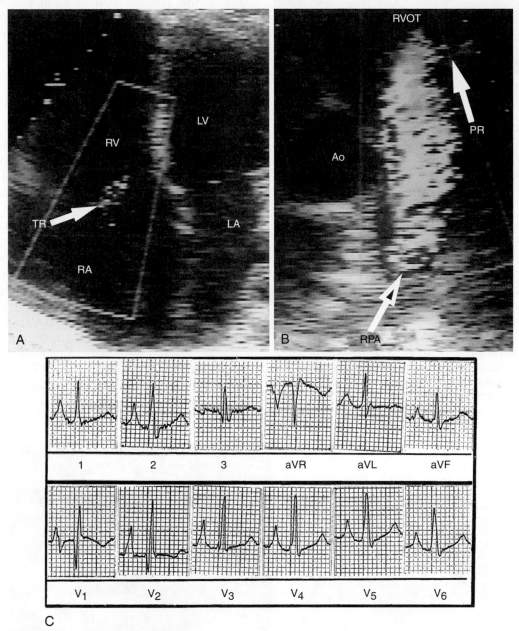

FIGURE 5-32   Images from a 19-year-old man with pulmonary atresia, intact ventricular septum, a well-formed right ventricle, and severe neonatal tricuspid regurgitation. At age 3 months, the patient underwent pulmonary valvectomy. **(A)** The right ventricle (RV) was dilatated and akinetic, but tricuspid regurgitation (TR) was mild. The right atrium (RA) was nevertheless enlarged. LA, left atrium; LV, left ventricle. **(B)** Black-and-white photograph of a color flow image shows severe low-pressure pulmonary regurgitation (PR) into a dilatated right ventricular outflow tract (RVOT). The right pulmonary artery (RPA) together with the pulmonary trunk and left branch were enlarged. Ao, aorta. **(C)** Scalar electrocardiogram shows strikingly tall peaked right atrial P waves in leads 1, 2, and V_{2-6}. The Q wave in lead V_1 indicates that an enlarged right atrium was topographically beneath the V_1 electrode position.

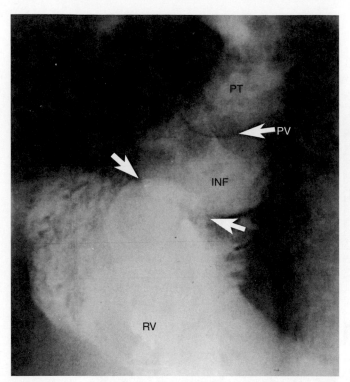

FIGURE 5-33 Right ventriculogram (RV) from a 40-year-old woman with double-chambered right ventricle caused by obstructing subinfundibular muscle bundles that extended up to the ostium of the infundibulum (INF) *(paired arrows)*. The INF per se is moderately dilatated. A tiny perimembranous ventricular septal defect was identified with intraoperative transesophageal echocardiography. PV, pulmonary valve that functioned normally; PT, pulmonary trunk.

infancy, pulmonary vascular resistance usually decreases and remains normal or nearly so. When operation is performed in older children, pulmonary vascular disease is progressive with 13-year survival reportedly 68%.[171] One of our patients had bilateral pulmonary arterial banding in early infancy, an intracardiac repair at age 5 years using a Hancock conduit that was replaced at age 12 years (Fig. 5-36). She is now gainfully employed at age 42 years.

Anomalous Origin of the Left Coronary Artery from the Pulmonary Trunk

Long-term postoperative outcome depends on patient age at operation, on the type of surgical procedure employed, on the presence and degree of preoperative myocardial ischemic injury, on the presence and degree of mitral regurgitation (papillary muscle dysfunction), and less on the increase in ventricular mass (hyperplasia) of hypoperfused but viable myocardium (see Chapter 23). The first operation for this malformation was ligation of the anomalous left coronary artery at its origin from the pulmonary trunk, creating a functional single coronary artery. Early deaths were frequent,[83] but a few postligation patients reached asymptomatic adulthood.[172] The current surgical procedure creates a two-coronary arterial system by attaching the anomalous left coronary artery to an aortic sinus[83,173] (see Chapter 15). Operative mortality has steadily declined, and long-term survival has steadily increased, with significant

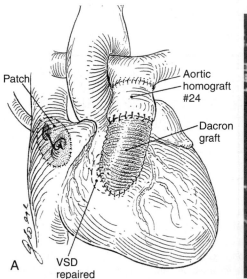

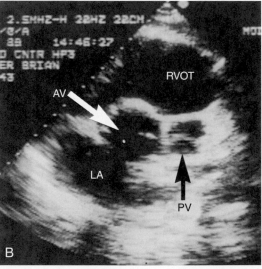

FIGURE 5-34 **(A)** Illustration from the third operation of a 26-year-old man with double-outlet left ventricle and pulmonary stenosis. The initial operation at age 7 years was a Waterston shunt for a mistaken diagnosis of tetralogy of Fallot. The second operation was an intracardiac repair that consisted of oversewing the pulmonary valve, closure of the ventricular septal defect (VSD), and insertion of a nonvalved Dacron conduit between right ventricle and pulmonary trunk. The illustration shown here is from the third operation 14 years later. A large right ventricular aneurysm was resected, a small ventricular septal patch leak was repaired, and the conduit was replaced with an aortic homograft with right ventricular extension of albumen-treated Dacron. An anomalous right superior pulmonary vein was incorporated into the left atrium during repair of an atrial septal defect (Patch). **(B)** Postoperative short-axis two-dimensional echocardiogram showing residual enlargement of the right ventricular outflow tract (RVOT). The aortic valve (AV) and pulmonary valve (PV) are side by side. LA, left atrium.

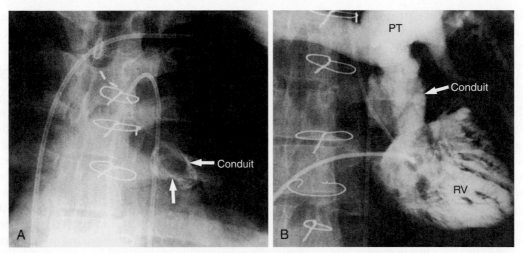

FIGURE 5-35 **(A)** Close-up of a chest radiograph from a 28-year-old man with double-outlet left ventricle and a right ventricular to pulmonary arterial external valved conduit that was calcified *(arrows)* and obstructed. **(B)** Selective angiography shows, in sequence, the dilatated heavily trabeculated right ventricle (RV), the obstructed, calcified conduit, and a well-formed pulmonary trunk (PT) with disproportionate dilatation of the left branch. The patient underwent replacement of the conduit with an aortic homograft.

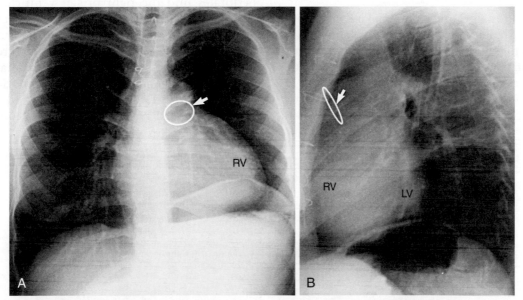

FIGURE 5-36 **(A)** Chest radiograph from a 25-year-old woman with type 1 truncus arteriosus. Banding of both pulmonary artery branches was accomplished as a neonate, followed by the initial intracardiac repair at age 5 years, and re-repair at age 12 years for conduit replacement. Arrow identifies the ring of the valve within the conduit. A moderately enlarged, convex right ventricle (RV) occupies the apex. **(B)** In the lateral film, the enlarged right ventricle is shown together with the ring *(arrow)* of the valve within the conduit. The left ventricle is of normal size.

reductions in heart size and improvement if not normalization in left ventricular function and wall motion.[174] However, survival is compromised by mitral regurgitation and the residual effects of left ventricular ischemic injury.[175] Determination of myocardial blood flow and metabolism by position emission tomography serves to identify the presence and degree of postoperative ischemic injury.[176]

In the 10% to 15% of unoperated patients who reach adulthood, a two-coronary arterial system is readily established surgically, with good results[177] (see Chapter 15). Angina pectoris disappears, left ventricular size decreases, and function improves. Late outcome depends chiefly on the extent of residual myocardial injury and on the presence and degree of mitral regurgitation (discussed earlier).

Congenital Coronary Arteriovenous Fistulae

Both coronary arteries arise from their normal aortic sinuses, but a fistulous branch of one or both of these arteries communicates directly with the right ventricle (approximately 40%), right atrium (approximately 25%), pulmonary trunk (approximately 15%), coronary sinus (approximately 7%), or, most rarely, the superior vena cava.[12] Long-term results of surgical repair are related to the volume of blood traversing the fistulous communication, the chamber or vessel into which the fistula drains, and the potential for myocardial ischemia (coronary steal) that is believed to result from the fistulous bypass.[12] Survival into adulthood is expected, but life span is not normal.[12,178] Because symptoms and complications increase appreciably with age, and because of the safety and efficacy of operation, surgery is undertaken unless the fistula is single and small and the shunt is trivial[29] (see Chapter 15). Late results of repair are excellent. The dilatated, elongated, tortuous coronary artery that forms the fistula involutes after early repair.[29]

Congenital Atresia of the Left Main Coronary Artery

In this malformation, the atretic proximal left main coronary artery and the left anterior descending and circumflex arteries are filled by collaterals from a normally arising right coronary artery.[12] Survival depends on the adequacy of the collateral circulation. If symptoms of myocardial ischemia are deferred beyond adolescence, satisfactory coronary artery bypass can be achieved with

good results, provided postoperative myocardial perfusion is normal at rest and after exercise (Fig. 5–37).

Congenital Sinus of Valsalva Aneurysm

The aneurysm, which is usually single, begins as a blind pouch or diverticulum that originates from a localized developmental fault at the junction of the aortic sinus media and the annulus fibrosis and protrudes as a finger-like or nipple-like projection that perforates at its tip. The anatomic relationship to adjacent structures determines the site into which the congenital aneurysm ruptures. As many as 90% to 95% originate in the right or noncoronary sinus and project into the right atrium or right ventricle. Those arising in the noncoronary sinus almost always rupture into the right atrium.[12] Those arising in the right coronary sinus rupture into the right ventricle, or less frequently into the right atrium.[12] Rarely, a sinus aneurysm dissects into the ventricular septum and either remains unruptured or perforates into the right or left ventricle. Perforation typically occurs well after puberty but before age 30 years. Sudden large ruptures announce themselves dramatically with acute severe aortic regurgitation, whereas the gradual development of a small rupture or an unruptured aneurysm may go unnoticed, at least initially. Surgical mortality is low, and the 20-year survival rate is 95%.[29,179] One qualification is gradually

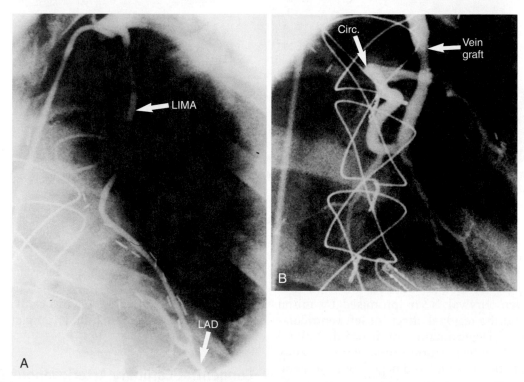

FIGURE 5–37 Selective arteriograms after coronary bypass surgery in an 18-year-old woman with congenital atresia of the left main coronary artery. **(A)** A left internal mammary artery (LIMA) was inserted into the left anterior descending (LAD) coronary artery. **(B)** A vein graft was used to bypass the circumflex (Circ.) artery. Postoperative exercise radionuclide myocardial perfusion scans were normal, and the electrocardiogram was normal at rest and after exercise.

progressive aortic regurgitation, especially when a right sinus of Valsalva aneurysm perforates into the right ventricle.[179] Postoperative survival patterns are influenced by a significant correlation with perimembranous ventricular septal defects.[179]

Coarctation of the Aorta

The postoperative residua, sequelae, and complications make long-term follow-up obligatory[180,181] (see Chapter 20). There are five major concerns: (1) recoarctation, (2) residual systolic hypertension despite absence of recoarctation, (3) a paracoarctation aneurysm, (4) a coexisting bicuspid aortic valve, and (5) a potentially coexisting cerebral berry aneurysm. Exercise stress testing determines the response of the systolic blood pressure (see Chapter 11) and identifies an exercise-induced difference in arm-to-leg systolic pressure and a stress-induced gradient across the coarctation site using color flow imaging and continuous-wave Doppler (see Chapter 6). Morphologic evaluation of the site of coarctation repair (reobstruction, aneurysm formation) is now accomplished with transesophageal echocardiography (see Chapter 6), computed tomography, or magnetic resonance imaging[182] (Fig. 5–38). A coexisting bicuspid aortic valve is identified by echocardiography (see Chapter 6). The dilatated aortic root above a bicuspid aortic valve typically harbors medial abnormalities (see Chapter 4). Late postoperative survival is also affected by premature atherosclerotic coronary artery disease, cerebrovascular accidents (see Chapter 14), and congenital anomalies of the mitral apparatus (discussed later).

In addition to these variables, longevity is influenced by age at operation.[183] When isolated coarctation is repaired in infancy, late survival is approximately 92%.[29] Repair of isolated coarctation during childhood results in 89% survival at 15 years and 83% at 25 years.[29] When coarctation repair is performed between ages 20 and 40 years, the 25-year survival is 75%. However, when surgery is performed on patients older than 40 years of age, only 50% are alive 15 years after operation.[29] Balloon angioplasty of unoperated coarctation or recoarctation[184–193] is discussed in Chapter 18. In anticipation of childbearing, females with unoperated coarctation or recoarctation should undergo resection with end-to-end anastomosis to remove the abnormal paracoarctation aortic medial abnormality and thus reduce the risk of gestational rupture (see Chapter 9).

The major risk factor for postoperative systemic hypertension is the duration of preoperative coarctation hypertension.[183,194] In patients older than 5 years of age at operation, 90% are normotensive 5 years later, 50% are normotensive 20 years later, and 25% are normotensive 25 years later.[29] In patients operated on at age 20 years or more, especially those older than 40 years, 67% are alive 25 years after operation, but only 20% are

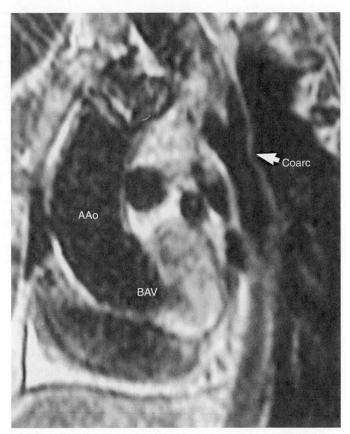

FIGURE 5–38   Magnetic resonance image from a 40-year-old man after resection of coarctation of the aorta (Coarc) with end-to-end anastomosis and mild residual narrowing at the coarctation site *(arrow)*. The ascending aorta (AAo) is dilatated above a functionally normal bicuspid aortic valve (BAV).

normotensive.[194–198] Strategies considered for the management of postoperative hypertension are shown in Fig. 5–39. Children with postoperative systolic hypertension but with no obstruction at the site of coarctation repair have abnormal increases in blood pressure during exercise[199] (see Chapter 11). An additional concern is the postoperative normotensive patient without recoarctation but with a hypertensive response to exercise. These responses are not due to sympathetic overdrive or to disorders of the angiotensin-aldosterone system[200] but instead are believed to reflect baroreceptor abnormalities and structural (compliance) changes in the great arterial walls.

A coexisting bicuspid aortic valve materially influences long-term morbidity and survival patterns after coarctation repair. The clinical course of a bicuspid aortic valve with coarctation of the aorta is the same as that of an isolated congenitally bicuspid aortic valve, including the risks of infective endocarditis (see Chapter 8) and dissecting aneurysm because of the medial abnormalities of the ascending aorta (see Chapter 4). Seven percent of patients who underwent coarctectomy in infancy required surgery for bicuspid aortic stenosis between the ages of 3 and

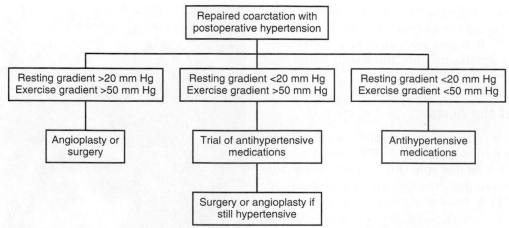

FIGURE 5–39 Management strategies in patients with hypertension after coarctation repair. *(Adapted from Rocchini, A. P.: Exercise evaluation after repair of coarctation of the aorta. Prog. Pediatr. Cardiol. 1993;2:14, with kind permission from Elsevier Science Ireland Ltd., Bay 15K, Shannon Industrial Estate, Co. Clare, Ireland.)*

7 years.[29] When coarctectomy was performed in children older than 1 year, 21% had bicuspid aortic stenosis, regurgitation, or both, but only a few required aortic surgery at that time.[29] Forty-eight percent of patients from Craaford's original series (observed by Bjork and associates[201] for more than 26 years) developed aortic valve disease, and most required aortic valve surgery.[200]

Recurrence of coarctation is diagnosed when the resting arm-to-leg systolic gradient exceeds 20 mm Hg and the postexercise gradient exceeds 50 mm Hg. The frequency of recurrence is related to the technique employed for the initial repair. After infancy, end-to-end anastomosis has the lowest incidence of recoarctation[29] (Fig. 5–40). End-to-end anastomosis in neonates is followed by recurrent obstruction in 50% of patients, an incidence materially reduced when the subclavian flap repair is used.[202] Recurrence rates are also lower in neonates after the "extended" end-to-end technique.[203]

Patch aortoplasty leaves behind the abnormal paracoarctation media, so aneurysm formation is relatively frequent[204–207] and prone to rupture, especially during pregnancy[208] (see Chapter 9).

Left ventricular mass may not regress entirely after successful coarctation repair, presumably because of postoperative systolic hypertension, especially with exercise.[209] Diastolic function may not normalize because of a residual increase in left ventricular mass.[210] Preoperative supranormal left ventricular ejection fraction may persist after successful repair (see Chapter 23).

Preoperative systemic hypertension causes intimal proliferation and medial thickening of extramural coronary arteries and is a risk factor for premature atherosclerotic coronary artery disease.[12] Myocardial infarction, congestive heart failure, and complications of coronary atherosclerosis were major causes of death in 12% of patients 11 to 25 years after coarctation repair.[211]

Cerebral hemorrhage is usually due to rupture of an aneurysm of the circle of Willis (see Chapter 14). Hypertension is not a necessary precondition for rupture because hemorrhage occurs in normotensive patients long after successful coarctation repair.[212] Rarely, coexisting fibromuscular dysplasia of intracranial arteries announces itself by cerebral infarction.[213]

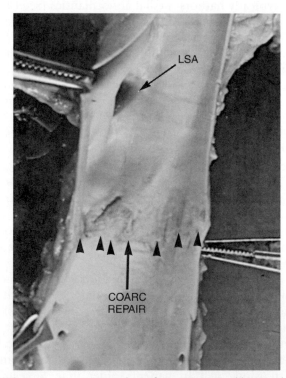

FIGURE 5–40 Necropsy specimen from a 35-year-old man who, at age 4 years, underwent resection of coarctation of the aorta with an ideal end-to-end anastomosis *(arrowheads)*. He was left with a nonrestrictive ventricular septal defect and pulmonary vascular disease that culminated in death 31 years after the coarctation repair. LSA, left subclavian artery.

There is a close association between coarctation of the aorta and congenital anomalies of the mitral apparatus, with an incidence of 26% to 58%.[12] Malformations vary from clinically occult to grossly overt and produce stenosis or incompetence of the mitral valve. With the advent of echocardiographic interrogation, major abnormalities of the mitral valve have been demonstrated echocardiographically in 20% of patients with coarctation.[214]

Degenerative disease of hip joints has been reported in about 20% of postoperative patients who were followed for more than 26 years.[201] The relationship to coarctation remains uncertain.

Vascular Rings and Slings

Developmental anomalies of the aortic arch that encircles and compresses the esophagus and trachea—vascular rings and slings—include (1) double aortic arch, (2) right aortic arch with a retroesophageal segment and an aberrant left subclavian artery, (3) right aortic arch with mirror-image branching and a left ductus arteriosus, (4) aberrant retroesophageal right subclavian artery, and (5) left aortic arch with a retroesophageal segment and an aberrant right subclavian artery. These vascular rings and slings are usually isolated, hence successful early operation yields excellent long-term results. Patients are generally asymptomatic after operation and are believed to have normal longevity. Occasionally, a significantly obstructing vascular ring remains undiagnosed until the teens or young adulthood (Fig. 5-41). Late postoperative results in these older patients are necessarily qualified by their preoperative course and clinical presentation.

Heart and Heart-Lung Transplantation

Transplantation of a heart, a single lung, both lungs, or a heart and lung is the subject of Chapter 17.

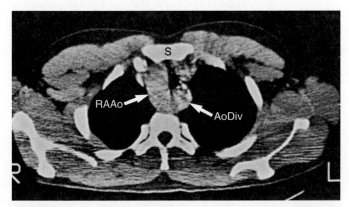

FIGURE 5-41   Magnetic resonance image from a 15-year-old boy with an obstructing vascular ring caused by a right ascending aorta (RAAo), a retroesophageal aortic diverticulum (AoDiv), and a left ligamentum arteriosum (not shown). Five years after repair, he remained clinically well. S, sternum; V, vertebral column.

References

1. Bonhoeffer P, Boudjemline Y, Saliba Z, et al. Percutaneous replacement of pulmonary valve in a right-ventricle to pulmonary-artery prosthetic conduit with valve dysfunction. *Lancet.* 2000;356: 1403-1405.
2. Hayes CJ, Gersony WM, Driscoll DJ, et al. Second natural history study of congenital heart defects. Results of treatment of patients with pulmonary valvar stenosis. *Circulation.* 1993;87(2 Suppl): I28-37.
3. Kopecky SL, Gersh BJ, McGoon MD, et al. Long-term outcome of patients undergoing surgical repair of isolated pulmonary valve stenosis. Follow-up at 20-30 years. *Circulation.* 1988;78(5 Pt 1):1150-1156.
4. Kan JS, White RI Jr, Mitchell SE, Gardner TJ. Percutaneous balloon valvuloplasty: a new method for treating congenital pulmonary-valve stenosis. *N Engl J Med.* 1982;307:540-542.
5. Masura J, Burch M, Deanfield JE, Sullivan ID. Five-year follow-up after balloon pulmonary valvuloplasty. *J Am Coll Cardiol.* 1993;21: 132-136.
6. McCrindle BW, Kan JS. Long-term results after balloon pulmonary valvuloplasty. *Circulation.* 1991;83:1915-1922.
7. Mullins CE. Pediatric and congenital therapeutic cardiac catheterization. *Circulation.* 1989;79:1153-1159.
8. Kaplan S, Adolph RJ, Murphy DJ. Pulmonary valve stenosis. In: Roberts WC, ed. *Adult Congenital Heart Disease.* Philadelphia: F.A. Davis; 1987.
9. Niwa K, Perloff JK, Bhuta SM, et al. Structural abnormalities of great arterial walls in congenital heart disease: light and electron microscopic analyses. *Circulation.* 2001;103:393-400.
10. Jones M, Ferrans VJ. Myocardial ultrastructure in children and adults with congenital heart disease. *Cardiovasc Clin.* 1979;10:501-530.
11. Perloff JK. Late postoperative concerns in adults with congenital heart disease. *Cardiovasc Clin.* 1981;11:431-447.
12. Perloff JK. The Clinical Recognition of Congenital Heart Disease. 5th ed. Philadelphia, W.B. Saunders; 2003.
13. Ankeney JL, Tzeng TS, Liebman J. Surgical therapy for congenital aortic valvular stenosis. A 23 year experience. *J Thorac Cardiovasc Surg.* 1983;85:41-48.
14. Hsieh KS, Keane JF, Nadas AS, et al. Long-term follow-up of valvotomy before 1968 for congenital aortic stenosis. *Am J Cardiol.* 1986;58:338-341.
15. Presbitero P, Somerville J, Revel-Chion R, Ross D. Open aortic valvotomy for congenital aortic stenosis. Late results. *Br Heart J.* 1982;47:26-34.
16. Sandor GG, Olley PM, Trusler GA, et al. Long-term follow-up of patients after valvotomy for congenital valvular aortic stenosis in children: a clinical and actuarial follow-up. *J Thorac Cardiovasc Surg.* 1980;80:171-176.
17. Stewart JR, Paton BC, Blount SG Jr, Swan H. Congenital aortic stenosis: ten to 22 years after valvulotomy. *Arch Surg.* 1978;113:1248-1252.
18. Whitmer JT, James FW, Kaplan S, et al. Exercise testing in children before and after surgical treatment of aortic stenosis. *Circulation.* 1981;63:254-263.
19. Gersony WM, Hayes CJ. Bacterial endocarditis in patients with pulmonary stenosis, aortic stenosis, or ventricular septal defect. *Circulation.* 1977;56(1 Suppl):I84-I87.
20. Jones M, Barnhart GR, Morrow AG. Late results after operations for left ventricular outflow tract obstruction. *Am J Cardiol.* 1982;50:569-579.
21. Larson EW, Edwards WD. Risk factors for aortic dissection: a necropsy study of 161 cases. *Am J Cardiol.* 1984;53:849-855.
22. Choy M, Beekman RH, Rocchini AP, et al. Percutaneous balloon valvuloplasty for valvar aortic stenosis in infants and children. *Am J Cardiol.* 1987;59:1010-1013.
23. Helgason H, Keane JF, Fellows KE, et al. Balloon dilation of the aortic valve: studies in normal lambs and in children with aortic stenosis. *J Am Coll Cardiol.* 1987;9:816-822.

24. Somerville J, Stone S, Ross D. Fate of patients with fixed subaortic stenosis after surgical removal. *Br Heart J.* 1980;43:629–647.

25. de Vries AG, Hess J, Witsenburg M, et al. Management of fixed subaortic stenosis: a retrospective study of 57 cases. *J Am Coll Cardiol.* 1992;19:1013–1017.

26. Jahangiri M, Nicholson IA, del Nido PJ, et al. Surgical management of complex and tunnel-like subaortic stenosis. *Eur J Cardiothorac Surg.* 2000;17:637–642.

27. Reddy VM, Rajasinghe HA, Teitel DF, et al. Aortoventriculoplasty with the pulmonary autograft: the "Ross-Konno" procedure. *J Thorac Cardiovasc Surg.* 1996;111:158–165.

28. Roughneen PT, DeLeon SY, Cetta F, et al. Modified Konno-Rastan procedure for subaortic stenosis: indications, operative techniques, and results. *Ann Thorac Surg.* 1998;65:1368–1375.

29. Kirklin JW, Barratt-Boyes BG. *Cardiac Surgery.* 2nd ed. New York, Churchill Livingstone; 1993.

30. Myers JL, Waldhausen JA, Cyran SE, et al. Results of surgical repair of congenital supravalvular aortic stenosis. *J Thorac Cardiovasc Surg.* 1993;105:281–287.

31. van Son JA, Danielson GK, Puga FJ, et al. Supravalvular aortic stenosis. Long-term results of surgical treatment. *J Thorac Cardiovasc Surg.* 1994;107:103–114.

32. Daniels SR, Loggie JM, Schwartz DC, et al. Systemic hypertension secondary to peripheral vascular anomalies in patients with Williams syndrome. *J Pediatr.* 1985;106:249–251.

33. Sharma BK, Fujiwara H, Hallman GL, et al. Supravalvar aortic stenosis: a 29-year review of surgical experience. *Ann Thorac Surg.* 1991;51:1031–1039.

34. Trusler GA, Williams WG, Smallhorn JF, Freedom RM. Late results after repair of aortic insufficiency associated with ventricular septal defect. *J Thorac Cardiovasc Surg.* 1992;103:276–281.

35. Barbero-Marcial M, Verginelli G, Awad M, et al. Surgical treatment of Ebstein's anomaly. Early and late results in twenty patients subjected to valve replacement. *J Thorac Cardiovasc Surg.* 1979;78:416–422.

36. Danielson GK, Fuster V. Surgical repair of Ebstein's anomaly. *Ann Surg.* 1982;196:499–504.

37. Westaby S, Karp RB, Kirklin JW, et al. Surgical treatment in Ebstein's malformation. *Ann Thorac Surg.* 1982;34:388–395.

38. Benson LN, Child JS, Schwaiger M, et al. Left ventricular geometry and function in adults with Ebstein's anomaly of the tricuspid valve. *Circulation.* 1987;75:353–359.

39. Driscoll DJ, Mottram CD, Danielson GK. Spectrum of exercise intolerance in 45 patients with Ebstein's anomaly and observations on exercise tolerance in 11 patients after surgical repair. *J Am Coll Cardiol.* 1988;11:831–836.

40. Ng R, Somerville J, Ross D. Ebstein's anomaly: late results of surgical correction. *Eur J Cardiol.* 1979;9:39–52.

41. Raj Behl P, Blesovsky A. Ebstein's anomaly: sixteen years' experience with valve replacement without plication of the right ventricle. *Thorax.* 1984;39:8–13.

42. Liberthson RR, Boucher CA, Strauss HW, et al. Right ventricular function in adult atrial septal defect. Preoperative and postoperative assessment and clinical implications. *Am J Cardiol.* 1981;47:56–60.

43. Pearlman AS, Borer JS, Clark CE, et al. Abnormal right ventricular size and ventricular septal motion after atrial septal defect closure: etiology and functional significance. *Am J Cardiol.* 1978;41:295–301.

44. Meyer RA, Korfhagen JC, Covitz W, Kaplan S. Long-term follow-up study after closure of secundum atrial septal defect in children: an echocardiographic study. *Am J Cardiol.* 1982;50:143–148.

45. Bonow RO, Borer JS, Rosing DR, et al. Left ventricular functional reserve in adult patients with atrial septal defect: pre- and postoperative studies. *Circulation.* 1981;63:1315–1322.

46. Schreiber TL, Feigenbaum H, Weyman AE. Effect of atrial septal defect repair on left ventricular geometry and degree of mitral valve prolapse. *Circulation.* 1980;61:888–896.

47. Wanderman KL, Ovsyshcher I, Gueron M. Left ventricular performance in patients with atrial septal defect: evaluation with noninvasive methods. *Am J Cardiol.* 1978;41:487–493.

48. Murphy JG, Gersh BJ, McGoon MD, et al. Long-term outcome after surgical repair of isolated atrial septal defect. Follow-up at 27 to 32 years. *N Engl J Med.* 1990;323:1645–1650.

49. Konstantinides S, Geibel A, Olschewski M, et al. A comparison of surgical and medical therapy for atrial septal defect in adults. *N Engl J Med.* 1995;333:469–473.

50. Perloff JK. Surgical closure of atrial septal defect in adults. *N Engl J Med.* 1995;333:513–514.

51. Bink-Boelkens MT, Velvis H, van der Heide JJ, et al. Dysrhythmias after atrial surgery in children. *Am Heart J.* 1983;106:125–130.

52. Bolens M, Friedli B. Sinus node function and conduction system before and after surgery for secundum atrial septal defect: an electrophysiologic study. *Am J Cardiol.* 1984;53:1415–1420.

53. Esscher E, Michaelsson M. Long-term results following closure of isolated ostium secundum atrial septal defect in children and adults. *Eur J Cardiol.* 1977;6:109–116.

54. Magilligan DJ Jr, Lam CR, Lewis JW Jr, Davila JC. Late results of atrial septal defect repair in adults. *Arch Surg.* 1978;113:1245–1247.

55. Sheehan R, Perloff JK, Fishbein MC, et al. Pulmonary neovascularity: a distinctive radiographic finding in Eisenmenger syndrome. *Circulation.* 2005;112:2778–2785.

56. Steele PM, Fuster V, Cohen M, et al. Isolated atrial septal defect with pulmonary vascular obstructive disease—long-term follow-up and prediction of outcome after surgical correction. *Circulation.* 1987;76:1037–1042.

57. Kyger ER 3rd, Frazier OH, Cooley DA, et al. Sinus venosus atrial septal defect: early and late results following closure in 109 patients. *Ann Thorac Surg.* 1978;25:44–50.

58. Friedli B, Guerin R, Davignon A, et al. Surgical treatment of partial anomalous pulmonary venous drainage. A long-term follow-up study. *Circulation.* 1972;45:159–170.

59. Trusler GA, Kazenelson G, Freedom RM, et al. Late results following repair of partial anomalous pulmonary venous connection with sinus venosus atrial septal defect. *J Thorac Cardiovasc Surg.* 1980;79:776–781.

60. Bergin ML, Warnes CA, Tajik AJ, Danielson GK. Partial atrioventricular canal defect: long-term follow-up after initial repair in patients > or = 40 years old. *J Am Coll Cardiol.* 1995;25:1189–1194.

61. McGrath LB, Gonzalez-Lavin L. Actuarial survival, freedom from reoperation, and other events after repair of atrioventricular septal defects. *J Thorac Cardiovasc Surg.* 1987;94:582–590.

62. Portman MA, Beder SD, Ankeney JL, et al. A 20-year review of ostium primum defect repair in children. *Am Heart J.* 1985;110:1054–1058.

63. Berger TJ, Blackstone EH, Kirklin JW, et al. Survival and probability of cure without and with operation in complete atrioventricular canal. *Ann Thorac Surg.* 1979;27:104–111.

64. Karamlou T, Gurofsky R, Sukhni EA, et al. Factors associated with mortality and reoperation in 377 children with total anomalous pulmonary venous connection. *Circulation.* 2007;115:1591–1598.

65. Bisset GS 3rd, Kirks DR, Strife JL, Schwartz DC. Cor triatriatum: diagnosis by MR imaging. *AJR Am J Roentgenol.* 1987;149:567–568.

66. Williams WG, Trusler GA, Kirklin JW, et al. Early and late results of a protocol for simple transposition leading to an atrial switch (Mustard) repair. *J Thorac Cardiovasc Surg.* 1988;95:717–726.

67. Lange R, Horer J, Kostolny M, et al. Presence of a ventricular defect and the mustard operation are risk factors for late mortality after the atrial switch operation. *Circulation.* 2006;114:1905–1913

68. Turina M, Siebenmann R, Nussbaumer P, Senning A. Long-term outlook after atrial correction of transposition of great arteries. *J Thorac Cardiovasc Surg.* 1988;95:828–835.

69. Mathews RA, Fricker FJ, Beerman LB, et al. Exercise studies after the Mustard operation in transposition of the great arteries. *Am J Cardiol.* 1983;51:1526–1529.

70. Musewe NN, Reisman J, Benson LN, et al. Cardiopulmonary adaptation at rest and during exercise 10 years after Mustard atrial repair for transposition of the great arteries. *Circulation.* 1988;77:1055–1061.

71. Parrish MD, Graham TP Jr, Bender HW, et al. Radionuclide angiographic evaluation of right and left ventricular function during exercise after repair of transposition of the great arteries. Comparison with normal subjects and patients with congenitally corrected transposition. *Circulation.* 1983;67:178–183.

72. Ramsay JM, Venables AW, Kelly MJ, Kalff V. Right and left ventricular function at rest and with exercise after the Mustard operation for transposition of the great arteries. *Br Heart J.* 1984;51:364–370.

73. Stark J, Silove ED, Taylor JF, Graham GR. Obstruction to systemic venous return following the Mustard operation for transposition of the great arteries. *J Thorac Cardiovasc Surg.* 1974;68:742–749.

74. Venables AW, Edis B, Clarke CP. Vena caval obstruction complicating the Mustard operation for complete transposition of the great arteries. *Eur J Cardiol.* 1974;1:401–410.

75. Kirk CR, Gibbs JL, Wilkinson JL, et al. Protein-losing enteropathy caused by baffle obstruction after Mustard's operation. *Br Heart J.* 1988;59:69–72.

76. Mahony L, Turley K, Ebert P, Heymann MA. Long-term results after atrial repair of transposition of the great arteries in early infancy. *Circulation.* 1982;66:253–258.

77. Newfeld EA, Paul MH, Muster AJ, Idriss FS. Pulmonary vascular disease in transposition of the great vessels and intact ventricular septum. *Circulation.* 1979;59:525–530.

78. Lindesmith GG, Stiles QR, Tucker BL, et al. The Mustard operation as a palliative procedure. *J Thorac Cardiovasc Surg.* 1972;63:75–80.

79. Rosengart R, Fisbein M, Emmanouilides GC. Progressive pulmonary vascular disease after surgical correction (Mustard procedure) of transposition of great arteries with intact ventricular septum. *Am J Cardiol.* 1975;35:107–111.

80. Mair DD, Ritter DG, Danielson GK, et al. The palliative Mustard operation: rationale and results. *Am J Cardiol.* 1976;37:762–768.

81. Perloff JK, Middlekauf HR, Child JS, et al. Usefulness of postventriculotomy signal averaged electrocardiograms in congenital heart disease. *Am J Cardiol.* 2006;98:1646–1651.

82. Jatene AD, Fontes VF, Paulista PP, et al. Anatomic correction of transposition of the great vessels. *J Thorac Cardiovasc Surg.* 1976;72:364–370.

83. Castaneda AR, Jonas RA, Mayer JE, Hanley FL. *Cardiac Surgery in the Neonate and Infant.* Philadelphia, W.B. Saunders, 1994.

84. Kirklin JW, Blackstone EH, Tchervenkov CI, Castaneda AR. Clinical outcomes after the arterial switch operation for transposition. Patient, support, procedural, and institutional risk factors. Congenital Heart Surgeons Society. *Circulation.* 1992;86:1501–1515.

85. Wernovsky G, Hougen TJ, Walsh EP, et al. Midterm results after the arterial switch operation for transposition of the great arteries with intact ventricular septum: clinical, hemodynamic, echocardiographic, and electrophysiologic data. *Circulation.* 1988;77:1333–1344.

86. Arensman FW, Sievers HH, Lange P, et al. Assessment of coronary and aortic anastomoses after anatomic correction of transposition of the great arteries. *J Thorac Cardiovasc Surg.* 1985;90:597–604.

87. Kaplan S, Allada V. Evolution of therapy for D-transposition of the great arteries. *Circulation.* 1992;86:1654–1656.

88. Colan SD, Trowitzsch E, Wernovsky G, et al. Myocardial performance after arterial switch operation for transposition of the great arteries with intact ventricular septum. *Circulation.* 1988;78:132–141.

89. Hwang B, Bowman F, Malm J, Krongrad E. Surgical repair of congenitally corrected transposition of the great arteries: results and follow-up. *Am J Cardiol.* 1982;50:781–785.

90. Griffiths SP, Turi GK, Ellis K, et al. Muscular ventricular septal defects repaired with left ventriculotomy. *Am J Cardiol.* 1981;48:877–886.

91. Feldt RH, Brandhagen DJ, Schwenk WF 2nd. Height and weight of adults with ventricular septal defect detected in infancy or childhood. *Am J Cardiol.* 1994;73:715–716.

92. Meijboom F, Szatmari A, Utens E, et al. Long-term follow-up after surgical closure of ventricular septal defect in infancy and childhood. *J Am Coll Cardiol.* 1994;24:1358–1364.

93. Moller JH, Patton C, Varco RL, Lillehei CW. Late results (30 to 35 years) after operative closure of isolated ventricular septal defect from 1954 to 1960. *Am J Cardiol.* 1991;68:1491–1497.

94. Jarmakani JM, Graham TP Jr, Canent RV Jr. Left ventricular contractile state in children with successfully corrected ventricular septal defect. *Circulation.* 1972;45(1 Suppl):I102–I110.

95. Jarmakani JM, Graham TP Jr, Canent RV Jr, Capp MP. The effect of corrective surgery on left heart volume and mass in children with ventricular septal defect. *Am J Cardiol.* 1971;27:254–258.

96. Ellis JH 4th, Moodie DS, Sterba R, Gill CC. Ventricular septal defect in the adult: natural and unnatural history. *Am Heart J.* 1987;114:115–120.

97. Lillehei CW AR, Eliot RE, Wang Y, Ferlic RM. Pre and postoperative cardiac catheterization in 200 patients undergoing closure through right atrium. *Ann Thorac Surg.* 1971;12:29.

98. Maron BJ, Redwood DR, Hirshfeld JW Jr, et al. Postoperative assessment of patients with ventricular septal defect and pulmonary hypertension. Response to intense upright exercise. *Circulation.* 1973;48:864–874.

99. Mattila S, Kostiainen S, Kyllonen KE, Tala P. Repair of ventricular septal defect in adults. *Scand J Thorac Cardiovasc Surg.* 1985;19:29–31.

100. Otterstad JE, Froysaker T, Erikssen J, Simonsen S. Long-term results in isolated ventricular septal defect surgically repaired after age 10. Comparison with the natural course in similarly-aged patients. *Scand J Thorac Cardiovasc Surg.* 1985;19:221–229.

101. Sigmann JM, Perry BL, Gehrendt DM, et al. Ventricular septal defect: results after repair in infancy. *Am J Cardiol.* 1977;39:66–71.

102. Blackstone EH, Kirklin JW, Bradley EL, et al. Optimal age and results in repair of large ventricular septal defects. *J Thorac Cardiovasc Surg.* 1976;72:661–679.

103. Friedli B, Kidd BS, Mustard WT, Keith JD. Ventricular septal defect with increased pulmonary vascular resistance. Late results of surgical closure. *Am J Cardiol.* 1974;33:403–409.

104. Hallidie-Smith KA, Hollman A, Cleland WP, et al. Effects of surgical closure of ventricular septal defects upon pulmonary vascular disease. *Br Heart J.* 1969;31:246–260.

105. Tatsuno K, Konno S, Ando M, Sakakibara S. Pathogenetic mechanisms of prolapsing aortic valve and aortic regurgitation associated with ventricular septal defect. Anatomical, angiographic, and surgical considerations. *Circulation.* 1973;48:1028–1037.

106. Murphy JG, Gersh BJ, Mair DD, et al. Long-term outcome in patients undergoing surgical repair of tetralogy of Fallot. *N Engl J Med.* 1993;329:593–599.

107. Walsh EP, Rockenmacher S, Keane JF, et al. Late results in patients with tetralogy of Fallot repaired during infancy. *Circulation.* 1988;77:1062–1067.

108. Wennevold A, Rygg I, Lauridsen P, et al. Fourteen- to nineteen-year follow-up after corrective repair for tetralogy of Fallot. *Scand J Thorac Cardiovasc Surg.* 1982;16:41–45.

109. Fuster V, McGoon DC, Kennedy MA, et al. Long-term evaluation (12 to 22 years) of open heart surgery for tetralogy of Fallot. *Am J Cardiol.* 1980;46:635–642.

110. Abe T, Asai Y, Sugiki K, Komatsu S. Reoperation after initial correction of tetralogy of Fallot. *J Cardiovasc Surg (Torino).* 1985;26:568–572.

111. Katz NM, Blackstone EH, Kirklin JW, et al. Late survival and symptoms after repair of tetralogy of Fallot. *Circulation.* 1982;65:403–410.

112. Zhao HX, Miller DC, Reitz BA, Shumway NE. Surgical repair of tetralogy of Fallot. Long-term follow-up with particular emphasis on late death and reoperation. *J Thorac Cardiovasc Surg.* 1985;89:204–220.

113. Hu DC, Seward JB, Puga FJ, et al. Total correction of tetralogy of Fallot at age 40 years and older: long-term follow-up. *J Am Coll Cardiol.* 1985;5:40–44.

114. Hughes CF, Lim YC, Cartmill TB, et al. Total intracardiac repair for tetralogy of Fallot in adults. *Ann Thorac Surg.* 1987;43:634–638.

115. Rosenthal A. Adults with tetralogy of Fallot—repaired, yes; cured, no. *N Engl J Med.* 1993;329:655–656.

116. Shampaine EL, Nadelman L, Rosenthal A, et al. Longitudinal psychological assessment in tetralogy of Fallot. *Pediatr Cardiol.* 1989;10:135–140.

117. Finnegan P, Haider R, Patel RG, et al. Results of total correction of the tetralogy of Fallot. Long-term haemodynamic evaluation at rest and during exercise. *Br Heart J.* 1976;38:934–942.

118. Murphy JD, Freed MD, Keane JF, et al. Hemodynamic results after intracardiac repair of tetralogy of Fallot by deep hypothermia and cardiopulmonary bypass. *Circulation.* 1980;62:I168.

119. Bove EL, Byrum CJ, Thomas FD, et al. The influence of pulmonary insufficiency on ventricular function following repair of tetralogy of Fallot. Evaluation using radionuclide ventriculography. *J Thorac Cardiovasc Surg.* 1983;85:691–696.

120. Rosenthal A, Gross RE, Pasternac A. Aneurysms of right ventricular outflow patches. *J Thorac Cardiovasc Surg.* 1972;63:735–740.

121. Lange PE, Onnasch DG, Bernhard A, Heintzen PH. Left and right ventricular adaptation to right ventricular overload before and after surgical repair of tetralogy of Fallot. *Am J Cardiol.* 1982;50:786–794.

122. Jarmakani JM, Graham TP Jr, Canent RV Jr, Jewett PH. Left heart function in children with tetralogy of Fallot before and after palliative or corrective surgery. *Circulation.* 1972;46:478–490.

123. Borow KM, Green LH, Castaneda AR, Keane JF. Left ventricular function after repair of tetralogy of Fallot and its relationship to age at surgery. *Circulation.* 1980;61:1150–1158.

124. Bull K, Somerville J, Ty E, Spiegelhalter D. Presentation and attrition in complex pulmonary atresia. *J Am Coll Cardiol.* 1995;25: 491–499.

125. Marelli AJ, Perloff JK, Child JS, Laks H. Pulmonary atresia with ventricular septal defect in adults. *Circulation.* 1994;89:243–251.

126. Kirklin JW, Blackstone EH, Shimazaki Y, et al. Survival, functional status, and reoperations after repair of tetralogy of Fallot with pulmonary atresia. *J Thorac Cardiovasc Surg.* 1988;96:102–116.

127. Millikan JS, Puga FJ, Danielson GK, et al. Staged surgical repair of pulmonary atresia, ventricular septal defect, and hypoplastic, confluent pulmonary arteries. *J Thorac Cardiovasc Surg.* 1986;91: 818–825.

128. Benson LN, Laks H, Lois J, et al. Surgical correction of pulmonary atresia and ventricular septal defect with large systemic-pulmonary collaterals. *Ann Thorac Surg.* 1984;38:522–525.

129. Donohue BC, Binder SW, Perloff JK, Child JS. Rupture of an aneurysmal pulmonary trunk 40 years after Blalock-Taussig anastomosis. *Am J Cardiol.* 1988;61:477–478.

130. Joyner MJ, Chase PB, Allen HD, Seals DR. Response of upper limb blood flow to handgrip exercise after Blalock-Taussig operation (for tetralogy of Fallot) or subclavian flap operation (for aortic isthmic coarctation). *Am J Cardiol.* 1989;63:1379–1384.

131. di Carlo D, Williams WG, Freedom RM, et al. The role of cavapulmonary (Glenn) anastomosis in the palliative treatment of congenital heart disease. *J Thorac Cardiovasc Surg.* 1982;83:437–442.

132. Laks H, Mudd JG, Standeven JW, et al. Long-term effect of the superior vena cava-pulmonary artery anastomosis on pulmonary blood flow. *J Thorac Cardiovasc Surg.* 1977;74:253–260.

133. Kopf GS, Laks H, Stansel HC, et al. Thirty-year follow-up of superior vena cava-pulmonary artery (Glenn) shunts. *J Thorac Cardiovasc Surg.* 1990;100:662–670.

134. Alejos JC, Williams RG, Jarmakani JM, et al. Factors influencing survival in patients undergoing the bidirectional Glenn anastomosis. *Am J Cardiol.* 1995;75:1048–1050.

135. Bernstein HS, Brook MM, Silverman NH, Bristow J. Development of pulmonary arteriovenous fistulae in children after cavopulmonary shunt. *Circulation.* 1995;92(9 Suppl):II309–314.

136. Cloutier A, Ash JM, Smallhorn JF, et al. Abnormal distribution of pulmonary blood flow after the Glenn shunt or Fontan procedure: risk of development of arteriovenous fistulae. *Circulation.* 1985;72:471–479.

137. Srivastava D, Preminger T, Lock JE, et al. Hepatic venous blood and the development of pulmonary arteriovenous malformations in congenital heart disease. *Circulation.* 1995;92:1217–1222.

138. Fontan F, Baudet E. Surgical repair of tricuspid atresia. *Thorax.* 1971;26:240–248.

139. Cowgill LD. The Fontan procedure: a historical review. *Ann Thorac Surg.* 1991;51:1026–1030.

140. Bridges ND, Lock JE, Castaneda AR. Baffle fenestration with subsequent transcatheter closure. Modification of the Fontan operation for patients at increased risk. *Circulation.* 1990;82:1681–1689.

141. de Leval MR, Kilner P, Gewillig M, Bull C. Total cavopulmonary connection: a logical alternative to atriopulmonary connection for complex Fontan operations. Experimental studies and early clinical experience. *J Thorac Cardiovasc Surg.* 1988;96:682–695.

142. Fontan F, Fernandez G, Costa F, et al. The size of the pulmonary arteries and the results of the Fontan operation. *J Thorac Cardiovasc Surg.* 1989;98:711–719.

143. Fontan F, Kirklin JW, Fernandez G, et al. Outcome after a "perfect" Fontan operation. *Circulation.* 1990;81:1520–1536.

144. Kuhn MA, Jarmakani JM, Laks H, et al. Effect of late postoperative atrial septal defect closure on hemodynamic function in patients with a Lateral tunnel Fontan procedure. *J Am Coll Cardiol.* 1995;26:259–265.

145. Laks H. The partial Fontan procedure. A new concept and its clinical application. *Circulation.* 1990;82:1866–1867.

146. Laks H, Pearl JM, Haas GS, et al. Partial Fontan: advantages of an adjustable interatrial communication. *Ann Thorac Surg.* 1991;52: 1084–1094.

147. Mavroudis C, Zales VR, Backer CL, et al. Fenestrated Fontan with delayed catheter closure. Effects of volume loading and baffle fenestration on cardiac index and oxygen delivery. *Circulation.* 1992;86(5 Suppl):II85–II92.

148. Mayer JE Jr, Bridges ND, Lock JE, et al. Factors associated with marked reduction in mortality for Fontan operations in patients with single ventricle. *J Thorac Cardiovasc Surg.* 1992;103:444–451.

149. Shachar GB, Fuhrman BP, Wang Y, et al. Rest and exercise hemodynamics after the Fontan procedure. *Circulation.* 1982;65:1043–1048.

150. Driscoll DJ, Offord KP, Feldt RH, et al. Five- to fifteen-year follow-up after Fontan operation. *Circulation.* 1992;85:469–496.

151. Gewillig MH, Lundstrom UR, Deanfield JE, et al. Impact of Fontan operation on left ventricular size and contractility in tricuspid atresia. *Circulation.* 1990;81:118–127.

152. Fontan F, Deville C, Quaegebeur J, et al. Repair of tricuspid atresia in 100 patients. *J Thorac Cardiovasc Surg.* 1983;85:647–660.

153. Humes RA, Porter CJ, Mair DD. Intermediate follow-up and predicted survival after the modified Fontan procedure for tricuspid atresia and double-inlet ventricle. *Circulation.* 1987;76:III67–71.

154. Matsuda H, Kawashima Y, Kishimoto H, et al. Problems in the modified Fontan operation for univentricular heart of the right ventricular type. *Circulation.* 1987;76:III45–III52.

155. Stefanelli G, Kirklin JW, Naftel DC, et al. Early and intermediate-term (10-year) results of surgery for univentricular atrioventricular connection ("single ventricle"). *Am J Cardiol.* 1984;54:811–821.

156. Humes RA, Mair DD, Porter CB, et al. Results of the modified Fontan operation in adults. *Am J Cardiol.* 1988;61:602–604.

157. Coles JG, Kielmanowicz S, Freedom RM, et al. Surgical experience with the modified Fontan procedure. *Circulation.* 1987;76: III61–III66.

158. de Vivie ER, Rupprath G. Long-term results after Fontan procedure and its modifications. *J Thorac Cardiovasc Surg.* 1986;91:690–697.

159. Laks H, Milliken JC, Perloff JK, et al. Experience with the Fontan procedure. *J Thorac Cardiovasc Surg.* 1984;88:939–951.

160. Davis CA, Driscoll DJ, Perrault J, et al. Enteric protein loss after the Fontan operation. *Mayo Clin Proc.* 1994;69:112–114.

161. Jacobs ML, Rychik J, Byrum CJ, Norwood WI Jr. Protein-losing enteropathy after Fontan operation: resolution after baffle fenestration. *Ann Thorac Surg.* 1996;61:206–208.

162. Rowland TW, Rosenthal A, Castaneda AR. Double-chamber right ventricle: experience with 17 cases. *Am Heart J.* 1975;89:455–462.

163. Kveselis D, Rosenthal A, Ferguson P, et al. Long-term prognosis after repair of double-chamber right ventricle with ventricular septal defect. *Am J Cardiol.* 1984;54:1292–1295.

164. Stewart RW, Kirklin JW, Pacifico AD, et al. Repair of double-outlet right ventricle. An analysis of 62 cases. *J Thorac Cardiovasc Surg.* 1979;78:502–514.

165. Shen WK, Holmes DR Jr, Porter CJ, et al. Sudden death after repair of double-outlet right ventricle. *Circulation.* 1990;81:128–136.

166. Fisher RG, Moodie DS, Sterba R, Gill CC. Patent ductus arteriosus in adults—long-term follow-up: nonsurgical versus surgical treatment. *J Am Coll Cardiol.* 1986;8:280–284.

167. Brandt B, Marvin WJ, Ehrenhaft JL, et al. Ligation of patent ductus arteriosus in premature infants. *Ann Thorac Surg.* 1981;32:166–172.

168. van Son JA, Puga FJ, Danielson GK, et al. Aortopulmonary window: factors associated with early and late success after surgical treatment. *Mayo Clin Proc.* 1993;68:128–133.

169. Hanley FL, Heinemann MK, Jonas RA, et al. Repair of truncus arteriosus in the neonate. *J Thorac Cardiovasc Surg.* 1993;105:1047–1056.

170. Ebert PA, Turley K, Stanger P, et al. Surgical treatment of truncus arteriosus in the first 6 months of life. *Ann Surg.* 1984;200:451–456.

171. Di Donato RM, Fyfe DA, Puga FJ, et al. Fifteen-year experience with surgical repair of truncus arteriosus. *J Thorac Cardiovasc Surg.* 1985;89:414–422.

172. Shrivastava S, Casteneda AR, Moller JH. Anomalous left coronary artery from pulmonary trunk. Long-term follow-up after ligation. *J Thorac Cardiovasc Surg.* 1978;76:130–134.

173. Takeuchi S, Imamura H, Katsumoto K, et al. New surgical method for repair of anomalous left coronary artery from pulmonary artery. *J Thorac Cardiovasc Surg.* 1979;78:7–11.

174. Laborde F, Marchand M, Leca F, et al. Surgical treatment of anomalous origin of the left coronary artery in infancy and childhood. Early and late results in 20 consecutive cases. *J Thorac Cardiovasc Surg.* 1981;82:423–428.

175. Vouhe PR, Baillot-Vernant F, Trinquet F, et al. Anomalous left coronary artery from the pulmonary artery in infants. Which operation? When? *J Thorac Cardiovasc Surg.* 1987;94:192–199.

176. Allada V, Schelbert HR. Position emission tomography. In: Emmanouilides GC, Riemenschneider TA, Allen HD, Gutgesell HP, eds. *Heart Disease in Infants, Children and Adolescents.* Baltimore, Williams & Wilkins; 1995.

177. Moodie DS, Fyfe D, Gill CC, et al. Anomalous origin of the left coronary artery from the pulmonary artery (Bland-White-Garland syndrome) in adult patients: long-term follow-up after surgery. *Am Heart J.* 1983;106:381–388.

178. Liberthson RR, Sagar K, Berkoben JP, et al. Congenital coronary arteriovenous fistula. Report of 13 patients, review of the literature and delineation of management. *Circulation.* 1979;59:849–854.

179. van Son JA, Danielson GK, Schaff HV, et al. Long-term outcome of surgical repair of ruptured sinus of Valsalva aneurysm. *Circulation.* 1994;90:II20–II29.

180. Kappetein AP, Zwinderman AH, Bogers AJ, et al. More than thirty-five years of coarctation repair. An unexpected high relapse rate. *J Thorac Cardiovasc Surg.* 1994;107:87–95.

181. Koller M, Rothlin M, Senning A. Coarctation of the aorta: review of 362 operated patients. Long-term follow-up and assessment of prognostic variables. *Eur Heart J.* 1987;8:670–679.

182. Kaemmerer H, Theissen P, Konig U, et al. Follow-up using magnetic resonance imaging in adult patients after surgery for aortic coarctation. *Thorac Cardiovasc Surg.* 1993;41:107–111.

183. Daniels SR, James FW, Loggie JM, Kaplan S. Correlates of resting and maximal exercise systolic blood pressure after repair of coarctation of the aorta: a multivariable analysis. *Am Heart J.* 1987;113:349–353.

184. Beekman RH, Rocchini AP, Dick M 2nd, et al. Percutaneous balloon angioplasty for native coarctation of the aorta. *J Am Coll Cardiol.* 1987;10:1078–1084.

185. Cooper SG, Sullivan ID, Wren C. Treatment of recoarctation: balloon dilation angioplasty. *J Am Coll Cardiol.* 1989;14:413–419.

186. Harrison JK, Sheikh KH, Davidson CJ, et al. Balloon angioplasty of coarctation of the aorta evaluated with intravascular ultrasound imaging. *J Am Coll Cardiol.* 1990;15:906–909.

187. Hellenbrand WE, Allen HD, Golinko RJ, et al. Balloon angioplasty for aortic recoarctation: results of Valvuloplasty and Angioplasty of Congenital Anomalies Registry. *Am J Cardiol.* 1990;65:793–797.

188. Mendelsohn AM, Lloyd TR, Crowley DC, et al. Late follow-up of balloon angioplasty in children with a native coarctation of the aorta. *Am J Cardiol.* 1994;74:696–700.

189. Morrow WR, Vick GW 3rd, Nihill MR, et al. Balloon dilation of unoperated coarctation of the aorta: short- and intermediate-term results. *J Am Coll Cardiol.* 1988;11:133–138.

190. Rao PS, Najjar HN, Mardini MK, et al. Balloon angioplasty for coarctation of the aorta: immediate and long-term results. *Am Heart J.* 1988;115:657–665.

191. Saul JP, Keane JF, Fellows KE, Lock JE. Balloon dilation angioplasty of postoperative aortic obstructions. *Am J Cardiol.* 1987;59:943–948.

192. Sohn S, Rothman A, Shiota T, et al. Acute and follow-up intravascular ultrasound findings after balloon dilation of coarctation of the aorta. *Circulation.* 1994;90:340–347.

193. Tynan M, Finley JP, Fontes V, et al. Balloon angioplasty for the treatment of native coarctation: results of Valvuloplasty and Angioplasty of Congenital Anomalies Registry. *Am J Cardiol.* 15 1990;65:790–792.

194. Presbitero P, Demarie D, Villani M, et al. Long term results (15–30 years) of surgical repair of aortic coarctation. *Br Heart J.* 1987;57:462–467.

195. Behl PR, Sante P, Blesovsky A. Surgical treatment of isolated coarctation of the aorta: 18 years' experience. *Thorax.* 1987;42:309–314.

196. Clarkson PM, Nicholson MR, Barratt-Boyes BG, et al. Results after repair of coarctation of the aorta beyond infancy: a 10 to 28 year follow-up with particular reference to late systemic hypertension. *Am J Cardiol.* 1983;51:1481–1488.

197. Cohen M, Fuster V, Steele PM, et al. Coarctation of the aorta. Long-term follow-up and prediction of outcome after surgical correction. *Circulation.* 1989;80:840–845.

198. Liberthson RR, Pennington DG, Jacobs ML, Daggett WM. Coarctation of the aorta: review of 234 patients and clarification of management problems. *Am J Cardiol.* 1979;43:835–840.

199. James FW, Kaplan S. Systolic hypertension during submaximal exercise after correction of coarctation of aorta. *Circulation.* 1974;50(2 Suppl):II27–II34.

200. Simsolo R, Grunfeld B, Gimenez M, et al. Long-term systemic hypertension in children after successful repair of coarctation of the aorta. *Am Heart J.* 1988;115:1268–1273.

201. Bjork VO, Bergdahl L, Jonasson R. Coarctation of the aorta. The world's longest follow-up. *Adv Cardiol.* 1978:205–215.

202. Penkoske PA, Williams WG, Olley PM, et al. Subclavian arterioplasty. Repair of coarctation of the aorta in the first year of life. *J Thorac Cardiovasc Surg.* 1984;87:894–900.

203. Backer CL, Mavroudis C, Zias EA, et al. Repair of coarctation with resection and extended end-to-end anastomosis. *Ann Thorac Surg.* 1998;66:1365–1370.

204. Hesslein PS, McNamara DG, Morriss MJ, et al. Comparison of resection versus patch aortoplasty for repair of coarctation in infants and children. *Circulation.* 1981;64:164–168.

205. Ala-Kulju K, Jarvinen A, Maamies T, et al. Late aneurysms after patch aortoplasty for coarctation of the aorta in adults. *Thorac Cardiovasc Surg.* 1983;31:301–306.

206. Bromberg BI, Beekman RH, Rocchini AP, et al. Aortic aneurysm after patch aortoplasty repair of coarctation: a prospective analysis

of prevalence, screening tests and risks. *J Am Coll Cardiol.* 1989;14:734–741.

207. Kreitmann P, Schmitt R, Jourdan J, et al. Aneurysms complicating coarctation of the aorta: anatomic aspects and evolution. Report of six successful surgical cases. *Thorac Cardiovasc Surg.* 1982;30:315–318.

208. Parks WJ, Ngo TD, Plauth WH Jr, et al. Incidence of aneurysm formation after Dacron patch aortoplasty repair for coarctation of the aorta: long-term results and assessment utilizing magnetic resonance angiography with three-dimensional surface rendering. *J Am Coll Cardiol.* 1995;26:266–271.

209. Krogmann ON, Kramer HH, Rammos S, et al. Non-invasive evaluation of left ventricular systolic function late after coarctation repair: influence of early vs late surgery. *Eur Heart J.* 1993;14:764–769.

210. Krogmann ON, Rammos S, Jakob M, et al. Left ventricular diastolic dysfunction late after coarctation repair in childhood: influence of left ventricular hypertrophy. *J Am Coll Cardiol.* 1993;21:1454–1460.

211. Maron BJ, Humphries JO, Rowe RD, Mellits ED. Prognosis of surgically corrected coarctation of the aorta. A 20-year postoperative appraisal. *Circulation.* 1973;47:119–126.

212. Simon AB, Zloto AE. Coarctation of the aorta. Longitudinal assessment of operated patients. *Circulation.* 1974;50:456–464.

213. Malloy DS, Sangalang VE, Fraser GM. Cerebral infarction secondary to unsuspected intracranial fibromuscular dysplasia following bypass of aortic coarctation. *Stroke.* 1984;15:908–911.

214. Celano V, Pieroni DR, Morera JA, et al. Two-dimensional echocardiographic examination of mitral valve abnormalities associated with coarctation of the aorta. *Circulation.* 1984;69:924–932.

MEDICAL CONSIDERATIONS

SECTION III

MEDICAL
CONSIDERATIONS

Echocardiography in Anatomic Imaging and Hemodynamic Evaluation of Adults with Congenital Heart Disease

JOHN S. CHILD

Transthoracic, transesophageal, and intracardiac echocardiography and Doppler techniques are central to the diagnosis and management of congenital heart disease from the fetus to senescence.[1-13] This chapter describes the use of echocardiography with color flow imaging and spectral Doppler for the comprehensive anatomic and functional characterization of the major unoperated and operated malformations in adults with congenital heart disease.

In the second half of the 20th century, surgical and medical advances in developed countries resulted in adult survival of more than 85% of patients with congenital cardiovascular malformations[14,15] (see Chapters 4 and 5). It is currently estimated that in the United States alone, there are more adults with congenital heart disease than infants and children, in addition to the increasing complexity of malformations in adult survivors.[16] Similar results have been reported from Canada.[17] Specialized centers have evolved for the care of these patients[18] (see Chapter 3). The 32nd Bethesda Conference addressed the needs, and special programs were proposed to train cardiologists in the unique and demanding management of congenital heart disease in adults[19] (see Chapter 3).

Patients in this growing population are often first identified in an adult echocardiography laboratory. A bicuspid aortic valve, an isolated ostium secundum atrial septal defect, and uncomplicated congenitally corrected transposition of the great arteries[20] are examples.

COMPREHENSIVE ANATOMIC AND HEMODYNAMIC ECHOCARDIOGRAPHY

Despite impressive advances in surgery for congenital heart disease, cures in the literal sense are few and far between. Postoperative residua and sequelae are the rule[21] (see Chapters 20-22). Transthoracic echocardiography (TTE) plays an essential role in the periodic evaluation of these patients. Successful use of TTE requires proper selection, application, and interpretation of the modalities necessary for anatomic imaging and hemodynamic assessment, in addition to detailed knowledge of the anatomy and physiology of unoperated malformations, the changes that occur over time, the reparative and palliative surgical and interventional catheterization techniques, postoperative or postinterventional residua and sequelae, and the effects of acquired cardiac and vascular diseases of adulthood[1-3,5,7,9,10,12,13,22] (Table 6-1).

Acquisition of this knowledge is an ongoing process accomplished by visits to the necropsy laboratory; by comparing tomographic echocardiographic anatomy with classic angiography, magnetic resonance imaging, and multidetector computed tomography (CT; see Chapter 7); and by visits to the operating room to observe the living cardiac surgical anatomy. Familiarity with terminology and controversies among experts regarding the most appropriate terminology permit

Table 6-1 Knowledge Required
for Echocardiographic Imaging in Adults
with Congenital Heart Disease

Spectrum of congenital cardiac lesions including usual and unusual
  associated anomalies
Dynamic nature of the malformations
Various surgical techniques—remote and current
Effects of acquired heart disease on the congenital malformation
  before and after operation
The segmental anatomic approach to echocardiographic imaging
Echocardiographic imaging and Doppler hemodynamics in congenital
  cardiac malformations
Transesophageal echocardiography, including intraoperative, in
  simple and complex congenital heart disease

optimal conveyance of information to those who will use the clinical data.[23]

It should be emphasized at the outset that highly qualified echocardiographic laboratories where the volume is largely, if not exclusively, confined to standard acquired cardiac and vascular diseases are not equipped to study congenital malformations of the heart.[1,10,24-27] The resulting information is often incomplete, incorrect, or misinterpreted, requiring that the imaging be performed properly in a laboratory proficient in the study of unoperated and postoperative congenital heart disease in adults. Guidelines have been published.[24-29]

A comprehensive echocardiographic evaluation includes thorough anatomic delineation of intracardiac and extracardiac structures using two-dimensional imaging and color flow.[1,5-13,24-26] Anatomic information must be obtained from all available windows, including unusual ones. Subcostal views and anatomically correct views (apical and subcostal windows with apex down) often result in clearer understanding and interpretation of complex lesions.[1,5-7,12] Echo contrast using intravenous agitated saline refines the interpretation of directions and locations of shunts.

Color flow based on a mean of pulsed-wave (PW) Doppler velocities for each pixel, with color encoding for that mean velocity and direction of flow, provides blood flow images in real time with an angiographic quality and is of great value in following the course of arteries and veins, detecting small septal defects or small aortic-to-pulmonary connections, and delineating stenotic and regurgitant lesions. PW and continuous-wave (CW) spectral Doppler, particularly in conjunction with color flow imaging, permit identification and quantification of valvular, subvalvular, or supravalvular stenosis, valvular regurgitation, extracardiac and intracardiac conduit stenoses, pulmonary and systemic venous obstructions, septal defects, surgical shunts, and intracardiac anatomy and hemodynamics. Details regarding quantification of valvular stenosis or regurgitation or the intricacies of assessment of intracardiac and

pulmonary pressures are beyond the scope of this chapter. The reader is referred to excellent reviews.[30-33]

Transesophageal echocardiography (TEE) has been a major step forward in the evaluation of regions of the heart and circulation not readily accessible to surface imaging, for securing refined details of complex anatomy, for monitoring therapeutic interventions in the cardiac catheterization laboratory, and for intraoperative online assistance to the cardiac surgeon[1-4,10,13,34] (Table 6-2). For best results, TEE imaging with a multiplane probe is preferable. In pediatric patients, size limitations require a smaller biplane or monoplane probe. In adults, TEE studies are especially useful when acoustic windows are poor or when the distances of certain structures from the transducer render the power of the ultrasound beam inadequate. When employing TEE, the data must be acquired promptly and efficiently in real time. Accordingly, the operator must have immediate knowledge of both simple and complex congenital malformations and of the many surgical inventions that modify the basic anomalies. TEE anatomic and hemodynamic imaging must be thorough and complete to avoid overlooking unsuspected lesions that might be missed and therefore go unrepaired. TEE permits good visualization of the origins of the coronary arteries, of the main pulmonary artery and its branches, and of the entire aorta, and it lends itself to interrogation of conduit course and obstruction, to pulmonary artery branches, and to aortopulmonary collaterals.[1-4,10,13,34]

When optimal delineation requires angiography or magnetic resonance imaging (MRI), those techniques can then be applied selectively. Origins and proximal courses of coronary arteries are often well seen in children with transthoracic echocardiograms and color flow imaging, but in adults, coronary artery imaging requires TEE, MRI angiography, multidetector CT angiography, or standard selective radiographic angiography.

Transthoracic and transesophageal echocardiography and MRI have largely relegated diagnostic cardiac catheterization in congenital heart disease to preoperative selective coronary angiography in adults, to quantification

Table 6-2 Advantages of Transesophageal
Echocardiography over Transthoracic
Echocardiography in Adults with Congenital Heart
Disease

Superior vena caval anatomy and Glenn shunts
Pulmonary veins
Atrial septum, especially sinus venosus defects
Atrial baffles and Fontan connections
Back side of prosthetic valves and patches
Ventricular outflow tracts, including ventricular-to-pulmonary
  arterial conduits
Pulmonary trunk and main branches
Aorta and aortopulmonary shunts
Origins and proximal courses of coronary arteries

of ventricular filling pressures, or to answer specific unresolved diagnostic questions such as the patterns of collateral blood flow. Echocardiography plays a role in the cardiac catheterization laboratory by using injections of saline echo contrast to reduce the amount of angiographic dye required to identify valvular incompetence and to establish the size and location of shunts, catheter position or course, and device position. When TEE is used to monitor interventional catheterization, efficacy and safety improve and radiation exposure is reduced.

Intraoperative TEE is in standard use during surgery for complex congenital heart disease.[2-4,9,10,13,35,36] TEE refines anatomic diagnoses and detects unsuspected lesions before the patient is put on cardiopulmonary bypass. TEE before chest closure determines the adequacy of repair,[2-4,9,10,13] and TEE immediately after cardiopulmonary bypass defines the residua and sequelae.

TEE plays a major role in the postoperative intensive care unit by determining the etiology of complications such as hypotension (tamponade, ventricular dysfunction, hypovolemia) or complications associated with a specific operation (Fontan lateral tunnel thrombus). A high level of skill, proficiency, and experience is required.[37]

DIGITAL ECHOCARDIOGRAPHY

Transition from the analog videotape of the 1970s and 1980s to digital echo equipment of the 1990s has fully evolved into sophisticated imaging equipment permitting storage and review of all recorded data and the capability of accurate online and offline quantification. Current digitally acquired and displayed images are better than previous analog videotape systems and are not hampered during the review process by the need to speed back and forth on the tape to re-review or compare data. Remeasurement of digital data offline when questions arise regarding accuracy of the initial online measurements improves the interpretation process. Stored digital data from previous studies can be retrieved and placed side by side for direct comparison. Ready retrieval of all studies with a given diagnostic label allows clinical review for trainee education, assessment for quality control, and research. For the science and setup of such a digital laboratory, the reader is referred to the equipment manufacturers and to the relevant literature.[38-48]

VENTRICULAR FUNCTION

Evaluation of left and right ventricular morphology, size, mass, volume, and function are essential uses of echocardiography in both acquired and congenital heart disease. For comprehensive reviews, the reader is referred to the American Society of Echocardiography standards.[49-51]

In a two-ventricle heart with normally related chambers, the ventricles are believed to consist of a single continuous myofiber band that originates in the right ventricle just below the pulmonary valve and forms a double helix that terminates in the left ventricle just below the aortic valve.[52,53] The helical shape results in twisting that generates ejection, followed by untwisting that generates suction and rapid filling in preparation for the next beat. Standard two-dimensional echocardiographic linear measurements provide an assessment of chamber size, mass, and shape. Digital online or offline biplane quantification of left ventricular (LV) volumes using the modified Simpson's rule is useful when greater precision is required. The most common functional determination is calculation of the ejection fraction (EF), which is load dependent.[50,54,55]

A potential error in any imaging technique is the degree to which left ventricular regional contraction is not simultaneous, symmetric, or in a straight line from base to apex (see *torsion*, discussed later). Accordingly, the endocardial targets in any one echo view may move out of the imaging plane, an effect that is decreased by relatively orthogonal views of biplane volumes.[53,56]

Right ventricular form and shape are more complicated and technically more challenging to image than the form and shape of the left ventricle, even in the normal heart, and often substantially more so in congenitally malformed hearts or in the case of a systemic subaortic right ventricle.[57-62] In contrast to acquired heart disease, the right ventricle in congenital heart disease is just as or more important than the left. The free wall of each ventricle affects the contralateral ventricle—ventricular-ventricular interaction—because of the single myofiber band that originates at the right ventricular (RV) outflow tract and extends to the LV outflow tract (discussed earlier). RV function affects LV function, and LV function affects RV function.

The noninverted right ventricle is a complex crescent-shaped structure that wraps around the left ventricle from which it is separated by a shared ventricular septum.[49,58,59,62,63] In assessing the function of either ventricle, ventricular-ventricular interaction, as well as the interplay of intrinsic myocardial performance versus loading conditions within an individual ventricle, must be taken into account.[62-66] Asymmetry or heterogeneity is a feature of the timing and degree of contraction of segments of the right and left ventricles.[67] A simple measure of RV systolic function is a two-dimensional echo targeted M-mode recording of the basal lateral wall excursion toward the apex.[59,68,69] However, this measurement is qualified by failure to account for displacement of the RV inflow tract from the imaging plane, and failure to account for the RV outflow tract. For detailed reviews of various approaches to evaluation of the right ventricle, the reader is referred to recent reviews.[49,57-59,62]

The myocardial performance index (or *Tei Index*) is a measure of global ventricular function based on measurements of the isovolumic periods (technically not accurate in the presence of significant atrioventricular valve regurgitation). Ventricular ejection time suffers no geometric constraints but is relatively load dependent.[70-78] The basic formula divides the combined isovolumic times (isovolumic contraction and relaxation times) by the ejection time to give a dimensionless "index." The isovolumic periods are best obtained by measuring the atrioventricular regurgitant signal duration and subtracting the ejection time, items that have been validated by MRI and brain natriuretic peptide levels in tetralogy of Fallot and transposition of the great arteries.[73,74,78]

A valuable adjunct in the evaluation of ventricular function is spectral CW Doppler sampling of a jet of atrioventricular valve regurgitation. This regurgitation signal, when technically performed well at high-speed display, allows measurement of the positive and negative dP/dt, relatively load-independent measures of ventricular contractility and early relaxation rates.[30,79,80] Evaluation of ventricular filling parameters—diastolic function—is elucidated by measurements of atrioventricular valve velocity inflow signals and venous inflow profiles into the atria.[72,81-84] These measurements are more accurate and predictive of diastolic function and atrial pressures when supplemented by tissue Doppler imaging[72,81,85-98] (discussed later).

Atria enlargement in the absence of significant atrioventricular valve regurgitation or chronic atrial fibrillation reflects ventricular distensability.[49,99,100] Measuring the systemic and pulmonary venous flow dynamics into the atria with PW Doppler profiles significantly assists in estimating atrial pressures, the severity of valvular regurgitation, and ventricular filling characteristics.[1,30,33,72,81,87,94,101-103]

NEW AND EVOLVING ECHO-DOPPLER TECHNIQUES

Tissue harmonic imaging is a commonly used and valuable transducer technology that enhances the edge detection of images. When ultrasound propagates through tissue, higher frequencies are created that are multiples of the original fundamental frequency. These higher frequencies are due to compressibility and density changes of the tissue impacted by the sound waves; sound travels faster through denser tissue. The energy of the harmonic frequency is greater at deeper depths, and the scattering and reverberation artifacts are fewer, thus improving differentiation of tissue from blood pool. Accordingly, display of these harmonic frequencies improves edge detection and improves endocardial imaging.

Tissue Doppler imaging (TDI) uses PW Doppler technology to focus selectively on myocardial regions and to assess myocardial velocities. Myocardial velocity gradients provide insight into systolic, diastolic, and isovolumetric indices.[72,81,85-98,104-107] For diastolic function and prediction of atrial pressures, these measurements are best combined with the atrioventricular inflow velocities. Dividing the standard spectral PW Doppler peak mitral E velocity by the TDI basal lateral LV velocity (E') provides a ratio (E/E') that is relatively load independent and reasonably predictive of significantly elevated atrial pressure. A ratio of ≤ 8 is normal, whereas E/E' ≥ 15 indicates a mean left atrial pressure ≥ 20 mm Hg.[72,95,96,98,106] These parameters are effective even in the presence of atrial fibrillation.[94]

TDI of the systolic amplitude of basal ventricular contraction at the level of the tricuspid annulus reflects systolic function (normal values generally 16.4 ± 1.2).[108] In a study of the right ventricle in operated tetralogy of Fallot, TDI systolic and diastolic parameters compared favorably with brain natriuretic peptide levels and RV size.[108]

In unoperated tetralogy of Fallot, a ratio of early tricuspid inflow PW Doppler spectral velocity to the annular tissue Doppler velocity ≥ 4 provides a noninvasive estimate of RV filling pressure, with right atrial pressure ≥ 10 mm Hg. In postoperative adults, the relationship is less predictive.[109] Systolic and early diastolic RV basal wall TDI velocities are frequently abnormal in asymptomatic operated tetralogy of Fallot and transposition of the great arteries, even though RV function otherwise appears normal, suggesting subclinical abnormalities of RV performance.[110]

Myocardial acceleration during isovolumic contraction, which measures the regional peak myocardial acceleration during isovolumic contraction by TDI, is also believed to be useful in predicting ventricular function, including a systemic right ventricle and the univentricular heart.[111-116]

Because of the load dependence of many of the standard parameters of ventricular function, *strain rate imaging* is emerging as a useful method for quantification of regional and global tissue deformation in systole and diastole.[97,117,118] The myocardial velocities obtained by TDI may be overestimated because of myocardial translational motion or underestimated because of the effects of myocardial tethering.[97] Measurement of strain and strain rate imaging helps overcome these limitations. Strain represents tissue deformation during the cardiac cycle and is calculated as change of length divided by original length; it is thus dimensionless and represents a percentage change in the given dimension. Simply put, strain occurs when muscle shortens and thickens (systole) in the longitudinal and circumferential dimensions (a negative strain) or lengthens in the radial direction in diastole (positive strain).[118]

Strain rate imaging measures the time course of tissue deformation and is the primary parameter of tissue deformation obtained from TDI. *Strain rate* correlates with the rate of change of pressure (dP/dt)—a reflection of contractility—whereas *strain* is related more to E.F.[97,118] In animal models, longitudinal strain has been used to quantify RV contractile function.[119] In operated tetralogy of Fallot, the degree of RV deformation using Doppler strain and strain rate imaging has been more abnormal in patients with a transannular patch or with electrical depolarization abnormalities.[120] These findings are consistent with observations suggesting adverse mechanical-electrical interaction and risk for ventricular arrhythmias or sudden death in operated tetralogy of Fallot.[121,122]

Speckle tracking is a new, noninvasive echo technique applied for assessment of ventricular *rotation, twist,* and *torsion* (see section on LV helical coil motion). Because of scattering, reflection, and interference of the ultrasound beams in myocardial tissue, speckle formations in gray-scale echo images represent "tissue markers" that can be tracked frame by frame throughout the cardiac cycle.[123] The speckle tracking imaging technique enhances the accuracy of displacement estimation by filtering out random speckles and then performing autocorrelation, which allows estimation of motion of stable structures.[123-126] Quantification of ventricular rotation has previously been possible only with MRI and tissue tagging;[127] recent studies show that the echo speckle tracking technique provides results comparable to MRI.[123,126]

Further investigation in ventricular mechanics, including "twist" and "untwist" that represent systolic and diastolic function, promises to further our understanding not only of the disease process but potentially of treatment.[128-131] In normal hearts, the technique has disclosed enhanced LV untwisting during exercise, linked temporally to early base-to-apex pressure gradients, a mechanistic manifestation of the elastic recoil described by TDI.[124] Left ventricular torsion and subsequent untwisting are therefore manifestations of elastic recoil that links systolic contraction to diastolic suction and ventricular filling.[124] The techniques have not been adequately studied in congenital heart disease, but TDI observations from infancy to adulthood provide insight into the maturational and adaptive modulation of normal LV torsion mechanics.[125] These findings are beginning to offer insight into changes in contractility and myocardial function after birth, perhaps in part due to changing isoforms of myocardial sarcomeric proteins, such as titin, the "giant sarcomeric spring" that resists passive stretch and helps in myocyte recoil after contraction.[132-135] Net torsion increases gradually from infancy through adulthood but with different determinants between the age groups, perhaps related in part to the initially thicker-walled right ventricle in the neonate.[125] A torsion decline in adulthood has been ascribed to aging changes in the myocardium, as well as to the development of abnormal arterial compliance and potentially adverse ventriculoarterial coupling that affects systolic and diastolic function.[136-140] In light of the value of MRI in defining three-dimensional anatomy and ventricular tagging mechanics[64,65,141-145] and because echo speckle tracking provides similar information, the technique of speckle tracking holds great promise for elucidating myocardial mechanics in complex congenital heart disease.

Intracardiac echocardiography (ICE) is now well established and available for specialized applications.[146] ICE is an invasive technique that requires insertion of the ultrasound catheter and probe into the vascular bed but has the advantage over TEE of being better tolerated and requiring only one operator. Potential applications of ICE include use during device closure of atrial and ventricular septal defects (ASDs and VSDs) or during electrophysiologic mapping and ablation.[146] A detailed description of the technique can be found in *The Echo Manual* of the Mayo Clinic.[146]

Three-dimensional echocardiography (3DE) has been evolving for more than 3 decades. Images were initially created freehand as a composite of multiple two-dimensional (2D) images from a linear, fanlike, or rotational format, then digitally reformatted into rectangular pixels creating data sets in the shape of a cone, pyramid, or rectangle.[68,147] Missing data were reconstructed using interpolation techniques. Three-dimensional echocardiography (3DE) has advanced considerably because of more powerful computers and improved transducer technologies, such as real-time 3DE and 3D-TEE.[147-174] 3DE can be performed from the same transducer positions used for 2DE, and multiple 2DE images can be displayed simultaneously with real-time 3DE images. Software allows shading or coloring to display depth within the images. After the data sets are obtained, the 3DE images can be rotated for additional viewing planes. 3DE in motion is actually *four-dimensional echocardiography (4DE)* with time as the fourth dimension. 3DE is time consuming and computer intensive and less useful for experienced echocardiographers with a well-developed ability to form rapid 3D mental images simultaneously with 2DE imaging.

The major advantage of 3DE is improved accuracy in evaluating cardiac chamber volumes, an advantage achieved by eliminating assumed geometric modeling and by eliminating errors caused by foreshortened or off-axis views.[148,150-155] 4DE measurements of RV volumes, including stroke volume and EF, use newly developed software that has been validated against 3-Tesla MRI.[154] All patients studied had congenital heart disease ranging in age from 4 months to 16 years.[154]

Measurement of volumetric flow using 3DE is feasible for the mitral, aortic, and pulmonic valves but is less accurate for flow through the tricuspid valve.[170] Valve anatomy, even for complex atrioventricular septal defects, quantification of stenoses and regurgitation, various septal defects,[148,149,156-169] and cor triatriatum are well shown by 3DE.[171] Anomalous connection of the left coronary artery to the pulmonary artery has been delineated, and the morphology of the coronary arteries in Kawasaki disease has been reported.[172,173]

3DE has the advantage of conveying complex anatomy in a more recognizable form[174] (Figs. 6–1 through 6–4).

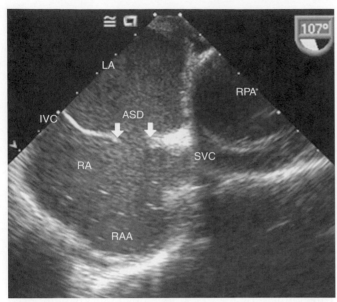

FIGURE 6-1 Transesophageal echocardiogram (standard two-dimensional display) of a small 10-mm secundum atrial septal defect (ASD) in a vertical plane or bicaval view. IVC, inferior vena cava; LA, left atrium; RA, right atrium; RAA, RA appendage; RPA; right pulmonary artery; SVC, superior vena cava.

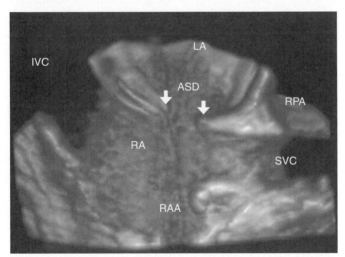

FIGURE 6-2 Three-dimensional transesophageal echocardiogram in the patient referred to in Figure 6-1. Same viewing plane but a more topographic visualization of the 10-mm atrial septal defect and adjacent anatomy. In real time, the image was rotated around the vertical axis through a 90-degree angle for better anatomic appreciation (see Fig. 6-3). IVC, inferior vena cava; LA, left atrium; RA, right atrium; RAA, RA appendage; RPA; right pulmonary artery; SVC, superior vena cava.

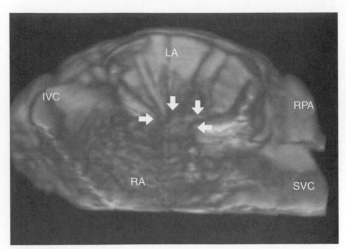

FIGURE 6-3 Three-dimensional transesophageal echocardiogram and viewing plane in the patient referred to in Figures 6-1 and 6-2 with a topographic visualization of the 10-mm atrial septal defect (ASD). The figure is now rotated 60 degrees around the vertical axis from that of Figure 6-2, allowing visualization of the enface ASD from above. IVC, inferior vena cava; LA, left atrium; RA, right atrium; RAA, RA appendage; RPA; right pulmonary artery; SVC, superior vena cava.

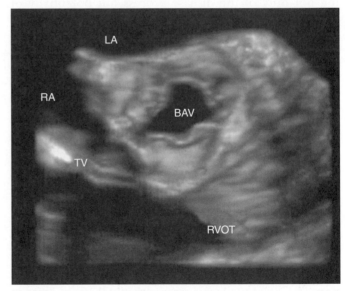

FIGURE 6-4 Three-dimensional image of a bicuspid aortic valve (BAV) providing a topographic appreciation of the adjacent anatomy. LA, left atrium; RA, right atrium; RVOT, right ventricular outflow tract; TV, tricuspid valve.

Real-time 3DE may also be valuable to surgeons during intraoperative echo assessment of complex anatomy that requires 3D interpretation before and after repair.[148,156,158–162,168,175] 3DE during interventional catheterization and in the electrophysiology laboratory are additional applications.[148,149,167]

SEGMENTAL APPROACH TO THE DIAGNOSIS OF CONGENITAL HEART DISEASE

Image interpretation is best achieved by sequential interrogation of the atrial, ventricular, and great arterial segments with determination of (1) atrial and ventricular situs, (2) connections of the atria to the ventricles and of the ventricles to the great arteries, and (3) the

Table 6–3   Sequence of Echocardiographic Analysis

The atria and their venous connections
The atrioventricular junction
The atrioventricular valves
The ventricles
The semilunar valves
The great arteries and veins

Table 6–4   Segmental Anatomic Approach

Identification of *segments*: atrial and ventricular situs
Connections: atrioventricular, ventriculoarterial
Relationships of ventricles and great arteries

Table 6–5   Atria and Their Venous Connections

Intraatrial switch procedures (Mustard, Senning)
Preoperative evaluation
Atrial situs
Atrial septal defects, size and location
Anomalous pulmonary venous connections
Cor triatriatum
Left superior vena cava
Postoperative evaluation
Glenn shunts
Fontan connections

Table 6–6   Atrioventricular Anatomy

Atrioventricular relationships: identification of ventricular anatomy
Atrioventricular septal defects
Straddling atrioventricular valves
Criss-cross relationships
Ebstein's anomaly
Cleft leaflets, accessory valve tissue, parachute deformities, supra-
   valvular rings
Tricuspid/mitral atresia/hypoplasia
Postoperative evaluation of valve repairs

Table 6–7   Ventricles

Ventricular morphology
Ventricular size and function
Ventricular septal defects
Ventricular outflow tracts and semilunar valve anatomy
Intraventricular (ventricular septal defect to aortic conduit)
Extracardiac (ventricular to pulmonary arterial conduit)
Ventricular relationships (inverted, superior-inferior)
Ventricular/great arterial connections (double-outlet ventricle,
   concordant or discordant connections)

Table 6–8   Great Arteries

Size, position, and relationships (transposition, malpositions,
   right aortic arch)
Pulmonary trunk and branches
Coronary arterial origins and proximal courses
Truncus arteriosus
Patent ductus arteriosus, aortopulmonary window
Systemic to pulmonary arterial collaterals
Surgical aortopulmonary connections (Blalock-Taussig, Potts,
   Waterston)
Aortic coarctation

relationships of the ventricles and great arteries.[1-10,12,13] (Tables 6–3 through 6–8).

It is useful to interpret and reconstruct the anatomic data according to the direction of blood flow, even if the initial images were not obtained in that order.[1-4,10] Begin with the abdominal vessels. Determine whether the inferior vena cava lies on the right side of the vertebral column and whether the abdominal aorta lies on the left side of the vertebral column (normal). Determine whether the inferior vena cava connects to the right-sided atrium, then focus on the superior vena cava(s), both left and right, and their connections. Does the right-sided atrium have a

morphologic right atrial appendage (blunt, triangular), and does that atrium connect to a morphologic right ventricle via a tricuspid valve (atrioventricular concordance)?

The tricuspid valve is not only trileaflet but also has chordal attachments from the septal leaflet to the ventricular septum. The right-sided ventricle exhibits the anatomic features of a morphologic right ventricle—heavily trabeculated inflow to apical portion, broad angle between inflow and outflow portions, smooth outflow portion, and a moderator band. Does this ventricle give rise to the pulmonary artery (identified by right and left branches), indicating ventriculo-arterial concordance?

A similar analysis can then be applied to left-sided structures—pulmonary veins, left atrium, mitral valve (bileaflet without chordal attachments to the ventricular septum), morphologic left ventricle (smooth trabeculae, two papillary muscles, acute inflow/outflow angle), and aorta. On what side does the ascending and descending aorta lie? Is there coarctation? During this segmental evaluation, search should be made for septal defects, valvular abnormalities, aortic-to-pulmonary connections, and abnormal relationships and positions of the cardiac chambers and great arteries.

After completion of the segmental anatomic analysis, attention is turned to cardiac situs and malpositions that depend chiefly on the location of the atria and cardiac apex. After establishing the atrioventricular and ventriculoarterial connections as concordant or discordant, the ventricular/ great arterial relationships must be established.[2-4,9,10,13]

Despite a meticulous TTE, additional information may be required to complete the segmental analysis. TEE provides most of that information. MRI angiography, CT angiography with 3-dimensional reconstructions (see Chapter 7), and standard catheterization-based angiography play important roles in the segmental evaluation. Situs and malpositions are established by identifying bronchial anatomy on chest x-ray; by the positions of the stomach, liver, abdominal aorta and inferior vena cava; and by the presence of a transverse liver on x-ray or abdominal echocardiography. The presence or absence of a spleen (or spleens) can be determined by abdominal echocardiography or a splenic scan. These data provide most if not all of the information required for the diagnosis of left or right isomerism.

SIMPLE SHUNT LESIONS

Shunt Identification

The location of a shunt is readily identified by 2D transthoracic echocardiographic imaging, provided that the shunt is sufficiently large and the acoustic window is acceptable. Shunts are best characterized with 2DE in combination with color flow imaging or echo contrast.[2-4,9,10,13] Flow accelerates as blood arrives at the relatively narrow entrance to the shunt. Acceleration is a clue to the location of the defect, which is further defined with a combination of 2DE and color flow imaging that focuses on the defect and the curvilinear shunt. In the catheterization laboratory, contrast echocardiography using either peripheral venous injection or injection into specific chambers assists in determining the site of right-to-left and left-to-right shunts. PW Doppler techniques are indispensable in identifying the location and direction of shunts, particularly when the anatomic site cannot otherwise be imaged. Limitations of TTE windows in adults often make TEE necessary.

Shunt Quantification

The physiologic consequences of a shunt can be inferred from the effects of chronic volume overload on the receiving chamber or chambers.[1,12] In an uncomplicated ASD, the larger the right ventricle, the larger the left-to-right shunt. Shunt quantification can also be estimated by direct measurement of the orifice of the shunt in conjunction with color flow imaging. Limitations include artifactual dropout, too much or too little gain of the color flow image, and failure to intersect the maximal width of the defect and the color flow stream owing to inadequate transducer angulation. Shunt quantification is best achieved by TEE with color flow imaging.

Doppler estimation of shunt size is possible by employing a combination of 2D TTE and PW Doppler velocity to estimate flow volume across the pulmonary and

Table 6–9 Sites to Measure Echo-Doppler Stroke Volume for Determination of QP and QS
Atrial Septal Defects
Tricuspid inflow or pulmonary outflow = QP Mitral inflow or aortic outflow = QS
Ventricular Septal Defects
Mitral inflow or pulmonary outflow = QP Tricuspid inflow or aortic outflow = QS
Patent Ductus Arteriosus
Mitral inflow or aortic outflow = QP Tricuspid inflow or pulmonary outflow = QS

systemic circulations expressed as QP:QS (Table 6–9). The flow volume is the product of the time velocity integral of blood flow through a given cross-sectional area (stroke volume = mean velocity × time × cross-sectional area). Measurements of the dimension of an outflow or inflow tract by 2DE target the site of the PW Doppler velocity profile. Measurements are most accurate if the echocardiographic beam is perpendicular to the site of interest. Conversely, the Doppler recording must be parallel to flow to obtain the maximum waveform deflection. For an outflow tract area, a circular orifice is assumed. It is also assumed that the tricuspid annulus is circular and that the mitral annulus is oval shaped. Measurements generally use mean velocity with online or offline planimetry. For the outflow tracts, peak velocities alone allow adequate estimation of the QP:QS ratios and are recommended for simplicity. Use of the *outflow tract* or *great artery* method is simpler and more reproducible than use of the *inflow* or *atrioventricular valve* method, although both methods allow separation of shunts with QP:QS ≥ 2:1 from ratios < 2:1. Drawbacks include difficulties in measuring the pulmonary annulus in adults, the inherent inaccuracy of the inflow method due in part to an elliptical orifice, and inaccurate Doppler velocities in the presence of turbulence due to obstruction or to disturbed blood flow jets that extend from a VSD into the RV outflow tract.

Clinical decisions are not based on Doppler QP:QS alone. Instead, shunt estimates should be considered in conjunction with the size of the volume-loaded chamber or chambers and in the context of the physical examination, electrocardiogram, and chest radiograph.[1,12] Additional inferences regarding shunt size are derived from spectral CW Doppler hemodynamics. Isolated uncomplicated VSDs are classified as small, moderately restrictive, and nonrestrictive on the basis of the estimated RV systolic pressure obtained from the peak left-to-right ventricular systolic velocity and from the calculated left-to-right ventricle pressure gradient across the VSD, together with corroborative data from the tricuspid regurgitant velocity (right ventricular-to-right atrial systolic gradient + estimated mean right atrial pressure).[1,12]

SPECIFIC SIMPLE SHUNT LESIONS

Atrial Septal Defects

These malformations are among the most common congenital heart defects seen in adults—unoperated and postoperative—and are often first discovered in an echocardiography laboratory.[1,176] Previously unrecognized ASDs are encountered with regularity.[20] An ASD is defined by its location in the atrial septum.[1–4,11,20,176,177] Knowledge of the anatomic-echocardiographic correlations assists in imaging and assessment of ASDs and associated lesions such as anomalous pulmonary venous connections.[2–4,9,10,13,177] An *ostium secundum* ASD is most prevalent and consists of tissue deficiency in the midportion of the atrial septum. A *sinus venosus* ASD of the superior vena caval type is located, as the name implies, at the junction of the superior vena cava and right atrium[12,20,176,178] (Figs. 6–5 through 6–7). Anomalous connection of the right superior pulmonary vein usually coexists.[1,12,20,176,178] The relatively rare *sinus venosus ASD of the inferior vena caval* type resides at the junction of the inferior cava and right atrium. An *ostium*

primum ASD is one component of an atrioventricular septal defect (AVSD).[1,12] A *coronary sinus* ASD, rarest of the interatrial communications, is represented by a sinoseptal defect in the roof of the coronary sinus resulting in a shunt between left and right atria. More than one type of ASD may coexist, a circumstance for which the examiner must be prepared.[12]

The magnitude of the left-to-right shunt depends on the size of the ASD, the relative diastolic distensibilities of the right and left ventricles, and the relative vascular resistances in the systemic and pulmonary arterial circulations. 2DE imaging establishes the consequences of the shunt, that is, right atrial and RV dilatation and abnormal ventricular septal motion.[12] An ASD is usually visualized with TTE subcostal, right parasternal, and left parasternal modified views, but TEE is occasionally required for identification and localization. In adults, a sinus venosus ASD of the superior vena caval type tends to be difficult to image by TTE. Subcostal views are required with angulation of the transducer toward the superior atrial septum adjacent to the aortic root and superior vena cava. TEE is the diagnostic method of choice for a sinus venosus ASD of the superior vena caval type, and for the commonly associated anomalous pulmonary venous connection or connections[12] (see Figs. 6–5 through 6–7). An *inferior* vena caval sinus venous ASD is seldom identified by TTE in an adult and may be misinterpreted on TEE. The most easily imaged ASD is in the ostium primum location, with the two

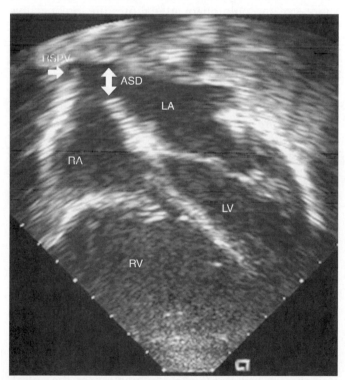

FIGURE 6–5   Transthoracic echo in a teenage girl with a sinus venosus atrial septal defect (ASD) and partial anomalous pulmonary venous connection. End-diastolic frame of a four-chamber, apex-down, anatomically correct view. The superior sinus venosus ASD extends high in the atrial septum. The superior vena cava portion is not well seen. The right superior pulmonary vein (RSPV) is directed to the right atrium (RA). LA, left atrium; LV, left ventricle; RV, right ventricle.

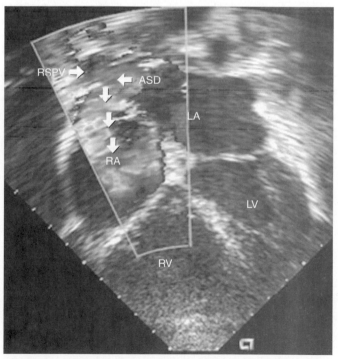

FIGURE 6–6   Sinus venosus atrial septal defect (ASD) in the patient referred to in Figure 6–5. Color flow imaging at end-systole shows the left to right shunt from LA to RA and from the RSPV to the RA. LA, left atrium; LV, left ventricle; RV, right ventricle.

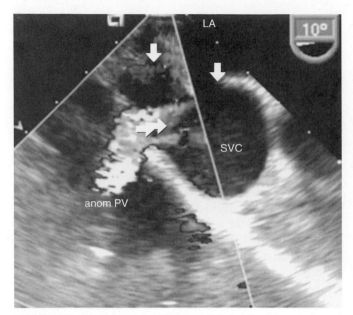

FIGURE 6-7 Sinus venosus atrial septal defect by transesophageal echocardiography with color flow imaging in a horizontal zero-degree plane mid-esophageal view in an adult male. The two arrows point to the ASD gap between the left atrium (LA) and superior vena cava (SVC) and show the anomalous pulmonary vein (anom PV) connecting to the SVC.

atrioventricular valves hinging at the same level (see section on atrioventricular septal defects). A coronary sinus ASD is identified by examination of the entire coronary sinus using inferiorly angulated four-chamber views or serial short and long-axis views. A left superior vena cava commonly coexists.

Because of frequent false-positive echocardiographic dropout in the region of the fossa ovalis on transthoracic echocardiograms in adults, PW Doppler and color flow imaging should be used to identify the shunt. The PW Doppler sample volume is placed in the right atrium adjacent to the suspected defect. Turbulent flow toward the right atrium begins in midsystole, peaks in early diastole, declines briefly but continues into mid-diastole, and is augmented in response to atrial contraction, only to decrease by early systole, at which time there can be minor reversal of the shunt. The width of the color flow image approximates the size of the ASD. In adults, a jet width ≤15 mm identifies a QP:QS less than 2:1. The area or spatial extent of the left-right color flow approximates the magnitude of the shunt. However, shunt size can be overestimated because of admixture of flow from vena cavae, coronary sinus, ASD, and tricuspid regurgitation. Conversely, the shunt can be underestimated because some of the ASD flow is low velocity and falls below the threshold of the filter setting. Nevertheless, in an isolated uncomplicated ASD, an unequivocal color flow jet of more than 1 cm in breadth, particularly on TEE, is associated with a clinically significant left-to-right shunt. For most TTE studies, color flow imaging has replaced contrast echocardiography, which remains a useful adjunct. A negative contrast effect in the right atrium is often detected, together with a small right-to-left shunt after a Valsalva maneuver.

With CW Doppler quantification, RV and pulmonary arterial systolic pressures can be estimated by the modified Bernoulli equation on the basis of a right ventricular-to-right atrial gradient that equals $4\times$ peak velocity.[2,30,31] The CW Doppler beam should be directed into the main tricuspid regurgitant jet using color flow imaging as the guide. In an ostium primum ASD, the tricuspid regurgitant jet converges when the mitral regurgitant jet is directed through the ostium primum ASD into the right atrium. If the CW Doppler beam intersects the jet of mitral regurgitant and records a high velocity, the RV systolic pressure will be overestimated.

TEE plays an important role when an ostium secundum ASD is closed by interventional catheterization.[12,146] TEE determines the size of the defect (assuming that size is constant throughout the cardiac cycle), the maximum occluder device size, the septal rims, placement of the device, and the effectiveness of occlusion.

Because TTE and TEE imaging provide excellent detection and relatively refined hemodynamic estimates of shunt size and pulmonary arterial pressure, preoperative cardiac catheterization is rarely necessary in an uncomplicated ostium secundum ASD except for coronary angiography in older adults.[1-4,176,178] TTE with color flow imaging detects anomalous pulmonary venous connections in about two thirds of children and adolescents but less frequently in adults, whereas TEE is excellent in this regard. The rare coronary sinus ASD should be specifically sought with preoperative or intraoperative TEE. These defects are not well seen via the surgeon's standard approach through the atrial septum and are often accompanied by a left superior vena cava that can have surgical implications. A coronary sinus ASD may first be suspected after a Fontan repair in patients with tricuspid atresia when an increase in right atrial mean pressure results in recurrence of cyanosis.

Partial or total anomalous pulmonary venous connections do not connect to the left atrium.[12] They typically accompany certain forms of ASDs, usually the superior vena caval sinus venosus type, although partial anomalous pulmonary venous connections sometimes occur with an intact atrial septum. It is relatively easy with TTE to image the entrance of the right and left superior veins into the left atrium from a combination of the apical, subcostal, and suprasternal notch views. Failure to identify pulmonary veins does not necessarily mean they connect to another structure.

Scimitar syndrome is characterized by abnormal connection of one or more of right-sided pulmonary veins to the inferior vena cava, the course of which is often seen on chest x-ray and likened to the silhouette of a "scimitar," a Turkish sword.[20] A confident diagnosis can be made by TTE through the subcostal window, showing the right-sided veins entering the inferior vena cava. The remaining veins can be imaged from the suprasternal notch view.[179] TEE is best for echo evaluation of pulmonary venous connections. As a rule, all pulmonary veins are readily imaged, and most abnormal connections can be identified.[2,3] If the diagnosis is inconclusive, MRI or CT angiography usually resolves the problem.

Echocardiographic assessment after ASD closure by device or surgery is concerned with residual shunting, the degree of resolution of right atrial and RV enlargement, and the adequacy of RV systolic function.[1,180-182] Patch leaks are infrequent after closure of an uncomplicated ostium secundum ASD.

Patients with sizable preoperative shunts experience a decrease in but not necessarily normalization of right atrial and RV size.[180] Echocardiographic evidence of cardiac remodeling after device or surgical closure in the adult is common and occurs early, with the full effects usually evident by 6 months. There is no significant difference in the degree of remodeling for different types of closure.[183] 2D and 3D echo assessment of RV volumes, hemodynamics, and brain natriuretic protein levels disclose more rapid improvement after percutaneous device ASD closure than after surgery.[180] The time course of cardiac remodeling can occur within a few weeks after successful device closure.[182] Importantly, there is improvement in both RV and LV function; left atrial volume may also decrease.[181] Three-dimensional echocardiography is useful to establish ASD anatomy and assist during device closure.[68,148,149,167,184]

Repair of a superior vena caval sinus venosus ASD is relatively complex.[10] An autologous pericardial patch baffles the anomalous pulmonary venous connection or connections into the left atrium through the ASD. Intraoperative TEE is mandatory to evaluate the adequacy of patch closure, proper incorporation of the anomalous pulmonary venous connection(s), and the presence or absence of superior vena caval and pulmonary venous obstruction.[2-4,10,24] A 3DE system for real-time tracking and shape analysis of ASDs was recently reported, with the goal of assisting in device closure or during minimally invasive surgery.[185]

Ventricular Septal Defect

The ventricular septum is a complex nonplanar curvilinear partition, the components of which are best defined according to anatomic landmarks on the RV surface.[1,12,20,186] Three major components of the muscular ventricular septum abut the membranous septum and radiate from it. The tricuspid annulus divides the *membranous septum* into an atrioventricular component and an intraventricular component. The *inlet septum* is lightly trabeculated and

limited by tensor attachments of the tricuspid valve. The *outlet* or *infundibular septum* is smooth walled. The *heavily trabeculated* septum lies between the inlet septum and the outlet septum. Accordingly, from the RV aspect, the ventricular septum is divided into three major muscular components—a lightly trabeculated inlet septum, a heavily trabeculated trabecular septum, and an outlet septum devoid of trabeculations. These three muscular components converge on the membranous septum. VSDs vary in size, shape, and location and are classified according to their position adjacent to or within the membranous, inlet, trabecular, or outlet septum.[1,12] VSDs have been grouped into four physiologic categories: (1) small (restrictive) defects with normal RV systolic pressure and normal pulmonary vascular resistance, (2) moderately restrictive defects with RV systolic pressure higher than normal but less than systemic and with variable pulmonary vascular resistance, (3) nonrestrictive defects with equal right and LV systolic pressures but variable pulmonary vascular resistance, and (4) nonrestrictive defects with equal right and LV systolic pressures and pulmonary vascular resistance equal to or greater than systemic.

The most common location of a VSD is perimembranous[1,20,186] (Figs. 6–8 through 6–14). Defects in the inlet septum are a component of an atrioventricular septal malformation. Defects in the muscular septum are rimmed entirely by muscle. Nonmuscular defects are rimmed in part by semilunar or atrioventricular valves. Defects in the

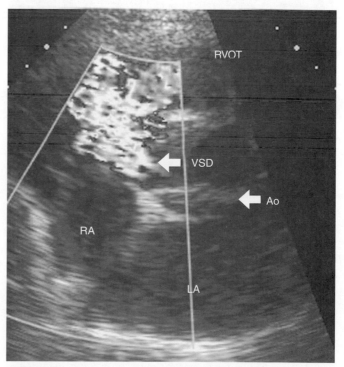

FIGURE 6–8   Perimembranous ventricular septal defect (VSD) in a parasternal short-axis view. Color flow imaging shows the left to right shunt through the VSD at the level of the tricuspid valve. Ao, aorta; LA, left atrium; RA, right atrium; RVOT, right ventricular outflow tract.

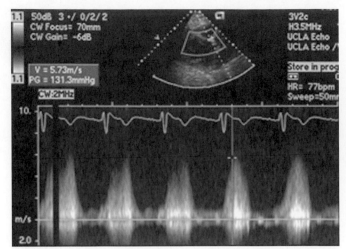

FIGURE 6-9 Ventricular septal defect in the patient referred to in Figure 6-8; continuous-wave Doppler. Systolic velocity of the left-to-right shunt shows a peak instantaneous left ventricle–to–right ventricle systolic gradient of 131 mm Hg. The systemic arterial systolic pressure was 150 mm Hg, indicating a hemodynamically restrictive VSD with a normal right ventricular systolic pressure estimated at 19 mm Hg.

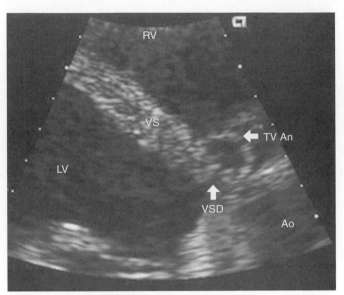

FIGURE 6-11 In the patient referred to in Figure 6-8, a ventricular septal defect (VSD) was partially closed by septal tricuspid valve aneurysm shown from a modified left ventricular (LV) long-axis apical view medially angulated toward the right ventricle (RV) and its inflow tract to display the tricuspid valve aneurysm (TV an).

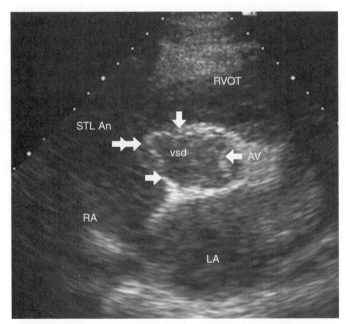

FIGURE 6-10 Ventricular septal defect (VSD) partially closed by a septal tricuspid leaflet aneurysm (STL An) in the same patient and view as in Figure 6-8. AV, aortic valve; LA, left atrium; RA, right atrium; RVOT, right ventricular outflow tract.

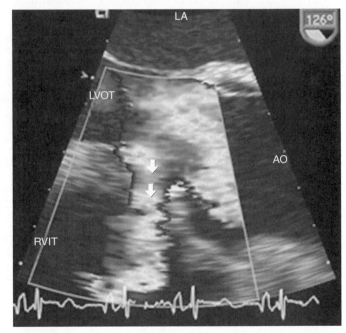

FIGURE 6-12 Perimembranous ventricular septal defect in a transesophageal view of the long axis of the left ventricular outflow tract (LVOT). Magnified view with a left to right shunt (two arrows) by color flow imaging into the right ventricular cavity. AO, aorta; LA, left atrium; RVIT, right ventricular inflow tract.

infundibular septum take the form of malalignment (see later discussion on complex malformations). Infundibular defects may be entirely muscular or rimmed by semilunar valve tissue, which predisposes to aortic regurgitation. The tendency for VSDs—especially perimembranous and trabecular muscular defects—to decrease in size finds its ultimate expression in complete spontaneous closure. Moderate or large defects are easily imaged by 2DE provided all planes are used methodically to examine the entire sep-

tum. When the VSD is large, 2DE reveals the defect, and color flow imaging provides information regarding location, size, and direction of flow. 3DE provides excellent visualization of various types of VSD.[184,186–189] From the LV *en face* projection, the positions, sizes, and shapes of VSDs can be accurately determined by 3DE. Precise imaging by

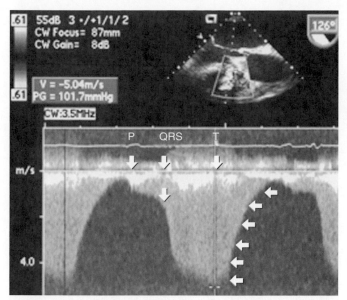

FIGURE 6–13   In the patient referred to in Figure 6–12, a perimembranous ventricular septal defect (VSD) is visualized with a continuous-wave Doppler targeted through the VSD in a transesophageal view of the long axis of the left ventricular outflow tract (LVOT), displaying the spectral profile of the left-to-right shunt throughout the cardiac cycle. A peak systolic velocity of 5.04 m/s reflects a peak instantaneous systolic gradient of 101.7 mm Hg from left ventricle to right ventricle. An anterograde velocity starts just after the P wave of the electrocardiogram, reflecting forward late-diastolic flow. There is a delayed falloff of the early-to-mid diastolic portion of the tracing (well after the T wave). Each of these findings suggests that LV diastolic pressure exceeds diastolic pressure in the right ventricle.

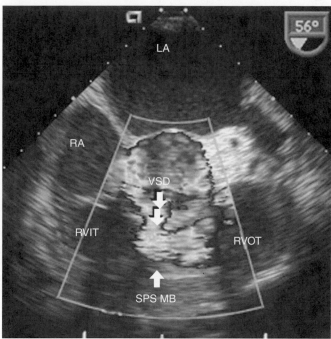

FIGURE 6–14   Double-chambered right ventricle and a perimembranous ventricular septal defect (VSD) on a transesophageal short-axis view in the patient referred to in Figures 6–12 and 6–13. A left-to-right shunt (two arrows, color flow imaging into the right ventricular cavity) affects the contralateral right ventricular wall, causing subpulmonic stenosis (SPS) due to intimal proliferation and an hypertrophied muscular band (MB). LA, left atrium; RA, right atrium; RVIT, right ventricular inflow tract; RVOT, right ventricular outflow tract.

3DE promises to be beneficial for surgical and catheter-based closure of difficult perimembranous and single or multiple muscular VSDs.[184,186–188] VSDs are inherent components of complex malformations such as tetralogy of Fallot, double-outlet right ventricle, and truncus arteriosus in which echocardiographic imaging is necessarily more demanding.[1,3,10,12]

Restrictive perimembranous and muscular defects, particularly multiple, usually require color flow imaging for visualization. Restrictive muscular defects tend to be tortuous and obscured by RV trabeculations, but high velocities make them readily visible with color flow imaging. Importantly, if one or more restrictive muscular defects coexist with a nonrestrictive perimembranous defect, velocity across the muscular defect(s) may be insufficient to permit visualization by color flow imaging. Spectral PW Doppler mapping along the ventricular septum can usually detect the high-velocity jet of a small defect, but without color flow imaging this procedure can be unduly time consuming.

Quantification of volumetric shunt flow ratios (QP:QS) and determination of the size of a VSD have met with mixed success. Most errors have been attributed to measurement of the pulmonary artery diameter, particularly in adults. Alternative methods use proximal isove-locity surface acceleration (PISA) or evaluate the region of color flow convergence into the VSD (particularly with 3D reconstruction) and time velocity integral of the CW Doppler profile.[190–194] The width of the color flow jet across a VSD correlates with but may overestimate the size of the shunt. The ratio of color flow diameter to aortic root diameter corrected for patient size compares well with the QP:QS ratio at cardiac catheterization. The color flow image permits alignment of the CW Doppler beam with the vector of the VSD jet to yield a left-to-right ventricular gradient by applying the modified Bernoulli formula (see Figs. 6–9 through 6–13). An isolated, uncomplicated, restrictive VSD is accompanied by high systolic velocity flow toward the right ventricle. There is usually low-velocity diastolic flow toward the right ventricle, except for a brief decrease or even reversal at the time of isovolumetric relaxation. The presence of this left-to-right shunt in diastole is important reassurance that the pulmonary vascular resistance is likely to be normal. It has been reported that a "sloped" or "M-shaped" Doppler signal of the gradient across the VSD results in underestimation of right-sided pressures.[195,196]

Timing and direction of flow can be assessed with color M-mode. Color flow imaging and CW Doppler identify the initially larger VSD that has been reduced in size owing to partial closure by the septal tricuspid leaflet, occasionally by a septal aneurysm or by prolapse of an aortic cusp into the VSD. The temporal sequence of shunt direction tends to follow a biphasic or triphasic pattern. In a large VSD, the left-to-right shunt occurs chiefly during early systole (isovolumetric contraction) when the rate of pressure rise in the left ventricle exceeds that in the right ventricle; right-to-left shunting occurs during late systole and early diastole (isovolumetric relaxation) when right ventricular systolic pressure falls more slowly than LV systolic pressure. During the ejection phase, systolic pressures in the ventricles are equal, and thus shunting depends on relative resistances in the pulmonary and systemic vascular beds. During mid-to-late diastole, left-to-right shunting occurs if the right ventricle is more compliant than the left ventricle. When an increase in pulmonary vascular resistance results in a right-to-left or bidirectional shunt (Eisenmenger reaction), shunt velocities are relatively low.

Serial analysis of color flow diameter can be used to monitor spontaneous reduction in VSD size and, with identification of anatomic margins and position, can be used to predict the unoperated clinical course. Muscular defects in the mid-to-posterior trabecular septum are most likely to close spontaneously. Perimembranous defects with partial or complete closure are associated with adherent tricuspid tissue or septal aneurysm (see earlier discussion)[20,186,197] (see Figs. 6–8, 6–10, and 6–11). 3DE in particular demonstrates the anatomy of perimembranous VSD aneurysm formation.[166] Tricuspid regurgitation sometimes develops as the septal tricuspid leaflet seals the VSD.[1,12] Rarely, aneurysmal septal tricuspid tissue causes obstruction to right ventricular outflow and, even more rarely, causes left ventricle outflow obstruction owing to prolapse of tricuspid tissue. Aortic valve prolapse into the VSD is also a cause of reduction in size or even closure and can be associated with progressive aortic regurgitation.[1,12,186,198–200] A substantial proportion of isolated perimembranous VSDs that undergo aneurysm formation are associated with left ventricular-to-right atrial shunts because the adherent septal leaflet preferentially directs the VSD jet toward the right atrium. Calculated right ventricular pressure may be falsely high because of the "tricuspid" regurgitant jet, which is actually the high-velocity VSD jet. Perimembranous VSDs have a propensity to develop a subaortic ridge that can progress to stenosis[201–210] and can cause aortic regurgitation by damaging the aortic valve. A small percentage of perimembranous VSDs develop a double-chambered right ventricle[20] because the impact of the VSD jet on the contralateral mid-right ventricular wall causes intimal proliferation and muscular overgrowth (Figs. 6–14 and 6–15). Initially mild subinfundibular obstruction can be progressive, with systolic hypertension confined to the right ventricular inflow tract (see earlier discussion).

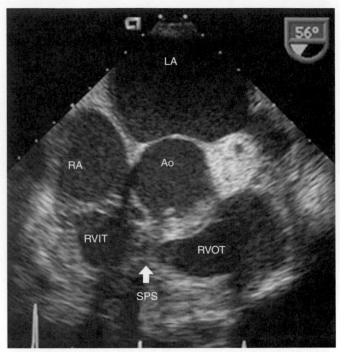

FIGURE 6–15 Double-chambered right ventricle in the same view and patient referred to in Figure 6–14. With the color flow turned off and the view slightly modified, there is better appreciation of the anatomy of the double-chambered right ventricle. Subpulmonic stenosis (SPS) was due to intimal proliferation and a hypertrophied muscular band (MB), which separated the high-pressure RVIT from the lower pressure RVOT. AO, aorta; LA, left atrium; RA, right atrium; RVIT, right ventricular inflow tract; RVOT, right ventricular outflow tract.

Doppler QP:QS ratio can be estimated before and after inspired oxygen or before and after administration of a pulmonary vasodilator to determine the presence and degree of reactivity in patients with elevated pulmonary vascular resistance. Tricuspid regurgitant velocity before and after a pulmonary vasodilator and after exercise is less useful because the pulmonary artery pressure does not predict the pulmonary vascular resistance. Doppler analysis of pulmonary artery velocity acceleration time (corrected and uncorrected for heart rate and right ventricular ejection time) does not reflect pulmonary vascular resistance with sufficient accuracy to preclude cardiac catheterization, although there is a small but significant increase in peak pulmonary artery velocity during vasodilator administration in patients with responsive pulmonary vascular beds.

Echocardiography, especially transesophageal, is useful to establish complete spontaneous, device, or surgical closure of a VSD without residua, and hence with little or no risk of infective endocarditis. Subaortic VSDs risk the development of aortic valve prolapse, aortic regurgitation, or an obstructive subaortic membrane, which are substrates for infective endocarditis.

Most patients with moderately restrictive VSDs and LV enlargement can be safely observed without intervention.[211]

However, surgical or device closure becomes appropriate when the QP:QS is ≥1.7, especially in infants and young children with failure to thrive.

In patients who undergo surgical or device closure, intraoperative or intraprocedure TEE is useful if not imperative to determine residual patch leaks and to evaluate the competence of the aortic valve, especially if valvuloplasty is performed in conjunction with VSD repair. The Amplatzer muscular occluder device is now selected for VSD closure, usually combined with TEE and fluoroscopic guidance.[212-214] TEE is useful during transcatheter device closure, serving to decrease fluoroscopy time, to determine device position relative to the defect and adjacent valves, to detect residual shunting, and to disclose previously unrecognized distal muscular defects. Long-term echocardiographic reassessment is important to detect residual patch or device leaks, to determine the development or progression of aortic regurgitation, and to detect the development of subaortic stenosis (see Chapters 15 and 16).

Shunts from Aorta to Pulmonary Artery or Aorta to Right Side of the Heart

These shunts originate from the aortic root (sinus of Valsalva aneurysm, aortopulmonary window, anomalous origin of a coronary artery from the pulmonary trunk, coronary arterial fistula), from a patent ductus arteriosus (PDA), or from a surgical shunt.[20]

PDA is usually readily recognized in childhood and is only occasionally first diagnosed in adults during TTE or TEE performed for other reasons.[1-3,12,20,215] Isolated PDA in adults falls into two categories: (1) restrictive with a functionally insignificant left-to-right shunt or (2) nonrestrictive with pulmonary vascular disease and reversed shunt[12,20,215] (Figs. 6–16 through 6–19).

Echocardiographic diagnosis of a PDA in adults benefits from high left parasternal and suprasternal notch windows that image the main or proximal left branch of the pulmonary artery and bifurcation, as well as the descending aorta, employing color flow to refine the search[1-4,12] (see Figs. 6–16 through 6–19). Multiplane TEE is helpful when these TTE acoustic windows are poor or cannot be obtained.[3,4]

Continuous high-velocity flow from the aorta emerges immediately to the left of the bifurcation of the main pulmonary artery and typically courses along the lateral wall of the pulmonary trunk, only occasionally along the medial wall. A pulmonary artery pressure curve can be generated from the spectral CW Doppler signal of ductal flow if a complete envelope can be obtained with minimal deviation from a zero-degree angle (i.e., parallel to the flow).[1,215,216] CW Doppler interrogation of the jet reveals high-velocity turbulent flow beginning in early-to-mid systole, peaking in early diastole, then decreasing in velocity by end diastole. Because of

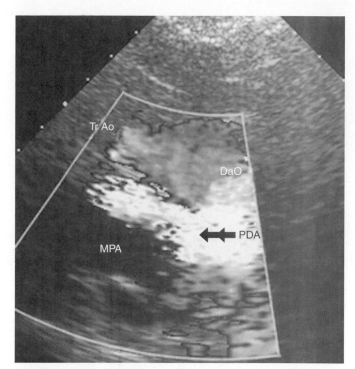

FIGURE 6–16   Patent ductus arteriosus (PDA) in a young adult female patient. Suprasternal notch echo view through the transverse aortic arch (Tr Ao) with color flow imaging shows a left-to-right shunt (double red arrows) from the upper descending aorta (DaO) into the bifurcation main pulmonary artery (MPA).

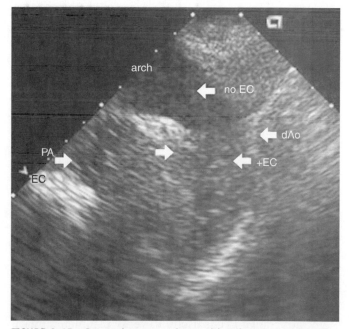

FIGURE 6–17   Patent ductus arteriosus with pulmonary vascular disease. Suprasternal notch echo view in the first two cardiac cycles after agitated saline echo-contrast intravenous injection into an upper extremity right peripheral vein. There is a reversed (right-to-left) shunt from the pulmonary artery (PA) into the descending aorta (dAo; positive echo-contrast signal +EC). Absence of echocontrast (no EC) in the aortic arch proximally indicates that the right-to-left shunt is not intracardiac. The patient exhibited typical differential cyanosis.

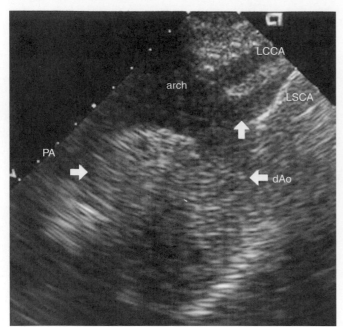

FIGURE 6–18 Patent ductus arteriosus with pulmonary vascular disease and reversed shunt in the patient referred to in Figure 6–17. Suprasternal notch echo view with saline echocontrast after four cardiac cycles. There is the reversed (right-to-left) shunt from the pulmonary artery (PA) into the descending aorta (dAo). The echocontrast (vertical upright arrow) refluxed into the left subclavian artery (LSCA), accounting for some degree of cyanosis of the left hand. No echocontrast reached the left common carotid artery (LCCA) or right subclavian artery. The echocontrast patterns accounted for cyanosis and clubbing of the toes, no cyanosis of the right hand, and an intermediate degree of cyanosis of the left hand.

competitive forward systolic flow from the right ventricle into the pulmonary artery, early-to-mid systolic velocity is often recorded away from the transducer. Sampling near the aortic orifice of the ductus records disturbed systolic and diastolic flow as the jet leaves the aorta and enters the pulmonary artery. Doppler sampling in the ascending and descending aorta remote from the ductus reveals normal systolic forward flow, but in the presence of a large left-to-right shunt, Doppler sampling detects diastolic flow toward the ductus (antegrade in ascending aorta, retrograde in descending aorta). In the presence of a nonrestrictive ductus with suprasystemic pulmonary vascular resistance and reversed shunt, color flow velocity through the ductus is low, but right-to-left flow can be recorded immediately within or adjacent to the ductus. Some left-to-right shunting may occasionally be recorded as well.

Intraoperative TTE is useful to verify complete surgical closure of a patent ductus, especially in older adults with ductal calcification.[3,4] However, for most patients, catheter device closure is routine for an isolated PDA.[215] Ductal closure in adults is usually reserved for small to moderate defects without pulmonary vascular disease (pulmonary vascular resistance < 8U/m²).[215] However, satisfactory results have been reported with transcatheter closure in

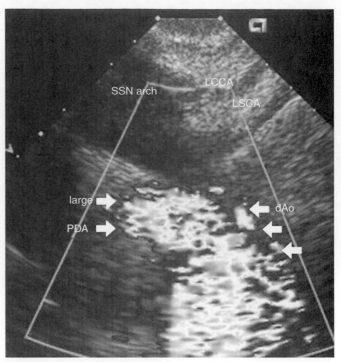

FIGURE 6–19 Patent ductus arteriosus (PDA) with pulmonary vascular disease in the patient referred to in Figures 6–17 and 6–18. Color flow imaging in suprasternal notch aortic arch echo view (SSN arch) shows the right to left shunt via a large PDA into the descending aorta (dAo). LCCA, left common carotid artery; LSCA, left subclavian artery.

adults with pulmonary vascular disease and evidence of reversibility with inhaled oxygen.[217]

Color flow imaging is essential to determine whether the ductus has been completely sealed or whether infective endocarditis prophylaxis is necessary. The effect of percutaneous ductal closure on LV size and function in children was examined in a prospective study using 2DE and 3DE and measurements of serum natriuretic peptides.[218] LV size and pro–brain natriuretic peptide levels decreased by 6 months after the intervention, even in the subgroup that started with a normal LV size.[218] However, LV systolic function 6 months after device closure, although normal, remained lower than that of control subjects. Diastolic function improved and at 6 months was similar to the healthy subjects.[218] A study of the effects on LV volume and systolic function early (within days) and late (≥6 months) after surgical or device PDA closure in adults disclosed that in both groups, LV EF and end-diastolic volume index were significantly decreased immediately after closure, whereas end-systolic volume index did not change.[219] During long-term follow-up, end-systolic as well as end-diastolic volume indices decreased significantly in both groups, and LV EF recovered compared with the immediate post closure state. However, LV EF remained low compared with preclosure.[219]

An *aortopulmonary window* permits adult survival under anatomic and physiologic conditions analogous to those of PDA (see earlier discussion), namely, either a nonrestrictive communication with pulmonary vascular disease and reversed shunt or, more rarely, a restrictive communication.[20] TTE can detect the aortopulmonary window, but false dropout is common.[1] TEE readily confirms the anomaly. The pattern of color flow imaging depends on whether the communication is nonrestrictive with suprasystemic pulmonary vascular resistance and right-to-left shunt or restrictive with left-to-right shunt (see earlier, patent ductus arteriosus).

Sinus of Valsalva aneurysm, ruptured or unruptured, typically expresses itself in male young adults.[20,220] These aneurysms are readily detected by TTE 2D imaging, but TEE provides exquisite anatomic detail[1] (Figs. 6–20 through 6–22). The aneurysm almost always originates in the right or noncoronary sinus. Color flow imaging establishes the shunt from the aortic sinus into the right atrium or right ventricle. A subaortic VSD is occasionally accompanied by late-onset rupture of a sinus of Valsalva aneurysm. TTE color flow imaging in the parasternal short axis with interrogation of the right ventricle adjacent to the septal tricuspid leaflet detects the flow patterns of a restrictive VSD and a coexisting ruptured sinus of Valsalva aneurysm. Long-axis TTE imaging identifies the zone of acceleration of the rupture *above* the aortic annulus, whereas the acceleration associated with the subaortic VSD is *below* the aortic annulus. The characteristic high-systolic/low-diastolic velocity associated with left-to-right shunts through a restrictive VSD (see earlier discussion) differs distinctly from the nearly continuous systole and diastole high-velocity flow in that it characterizes a ruptured sinus of Valsalva aneurysm.

A retrospective study of sinus of Valsalva aneurysms with a systematic overview was reported in 86 patients who underwent repair between 1956 and 2003, representing a 47-year, single-center experience.[220] Echocardiography was the most common diagnostic tool. The most common site of rupture was the right coronary sinus, and the rupture was into the right ventricle in one third of patients.[220] Concomitant repair of VSDs, ASDs, and aortic regurgitation was frequent.[220] Intraoperative TEE is useful to verify complete closure of the rupture and an associated VSD and in evaluating the status of aortic valve repair.[3,4,10]

Congenital anomalies of the coronary arteries most relevant to this section include coronary arterial-to-venous fistulae and anomalous origin of a coronary artery from the pulmonary trunk.[20,221,222] These anomalies can often be detected by 2D TTE but are more readily identified and characterized by TEE with color flow imaging.[1,3,4,223–226] The value of real-time 3DE has been demonstrated in identifying congenital anomalies of the coronary arteries.[172,173]

A *coronary arterial fistula* is accompanied by enlargement of the artery giving rise to the fistulous connection. Color flow and PW Doppler imaging identify increased flow velocity in the fistulous coronary artery. Coronary arteriovenous fistulae cause grapelike dilatation of the coronary sinus when that structure receives the fistulous connection from the left circumflex coronary artery.[13] Disturbed blood flow can be detected in the chamber or vessel receiving the fistulous communication.

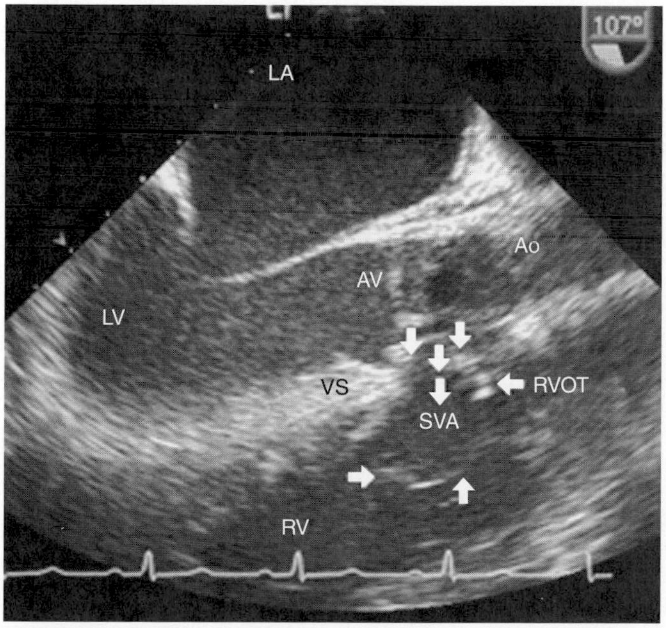

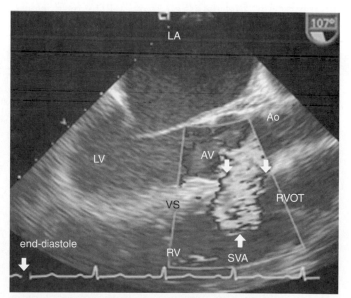

FIGURE 6–20   Transesophageal echocardiogram in the long-axis view of the left ventricular outflow tract showing a sinus of Valsalva aneurysm (SVA, yellow arrows) protruding through the right aortic sinus (double turquoise arrows) above the aortic valve (AV) into the right ventricle (RV) and right ventricular outflow tract (RVOT). AO, aorta; LA, left atrium; LV, left ventricle; VS, ventricular septum.

FIGURE 6–21   In the patient referred to in Figure 6–20, a transesophageal echo shows the sinus of Valsalva aneurysm (SVA) protruding through the right aortic sinus with color flow imaging of the left-to-right shunt at end-diastole in the region above the aortic valve (AV) into the right ventricular outflow tract (RVOT). AO, aorta; LA, left atrium; LV, left ventricle; VS, ventricular septum.

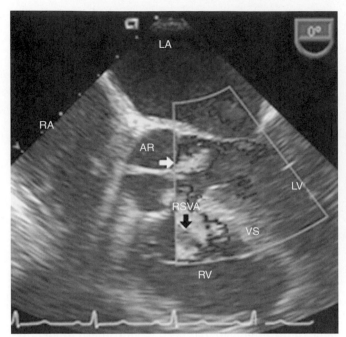

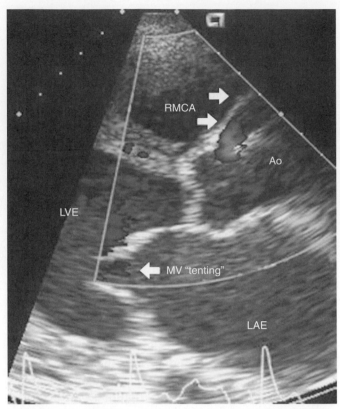

FIGURE 6–22 Sinus of Valsalva aneurysm in the patient referred to in Figures 6–20 and 6–21. Transesophageal echo from a superiorly angulated four-chamber equivalent view in the horizontal zero-degree plane of the ruptured sinus of Valsalva aneurysm (RSVA). The left-to-right shunt is visualized above the aortic valve (AV) into the right ventricle (RV). A small jet of mild aortic regurgitation is directed away from the prolapsing right coronary cusp and RSVA. AO, aorta; LA, left atrium; LV, left ventricle; VS, ventricular septum.

FIGURE 6–23 Left coronary artery to main pulmonary artery fistula. Transthoracic echo parasternal long-axis view at end-diastolic shows a dilatated right main coronary artery (RMCA) arising from the aorta (AO). Color flow is seen in the RMCA (red). The left ventricle is enlarged (LVE), and the estimated LVEF was 30%. The mitral leaflets exhibited apical tenting in systole (not shown). There was mild-to-moderate central mitral regurgitation. The left atrium is enlarged (LAE).

Anomalous origin of a coronary artery, usually the left, from the pulmonary trunk can be diagnosed by echocardiography and distinguished from a PDA by a jet entrance site immediately distal to the pulmonary valve, by absence of a left main coronary artery from its aortic sinus, and by retrograde flow in at least two segments of the left coronary artery[13] (Figs. 6–23 and 6–24). Long-term postoperative follow-up includes echocardiographic interrogation of regional and global LV wall motion and assessment of the presence and degree of mitral regurgitation caused by ischemic papillary muscle dysfunction.

Anomalous origin of a right coronary from the left coronary or coronary cusp has potentially important consequences if a major branch runs an angulated intramural course or passes between the aorta and pulmonary trunk.[20,221,222] In infants and children, coronary origins are usually well seen by TTE when sought by an experienced operator but are more difficult to image in adults. In the echo screening of any young individual, particularly an athlete, the presence of both coronary ostia should be established. Identification of two ostia effectively precludes a single coronary artery, but identification of only one ostium may mean that the second was missed. Multiplane TEE, 3D MRI angiography, multidetector CT, or standard selective radiographic angiography can be used to establish the presence and course of the coronary arteries.[3,4,227–229]

Surgical Aortopulmonary Shunts

The majority of these surgical communications are best visualized with color flow imaging on TTE from suprasternal views.[1] TEE with color flow nicely demonstrates the aortic origin and pulmonary entrance of the shunt. Because flow is from high-pressure aorta to low-pressure pulmonary artery, patency can be evaluated with PW and CW Doppler imaging with nonlaminar flow in both systole and diastole toward the pulmonary artery[3,4] (Fig. 6–25).

TTE imaging of a classic Blalock-Taussig or GORE-TEX® shunt can be achieved using suprasternal and supraclavicular views with color flow imaging. Multiplane TEE permits reliable visualization. Flow is virtually continuous. Because the classic Blalock-Taussig shunt is a narrow curving conduit, precise estimation of pulmonary artery pressure by the method described earlier is not necessarily reliable, but a high-velocity continuous shunt toward the pulmonary artery usually indicates low pulmonary vascular resistance.

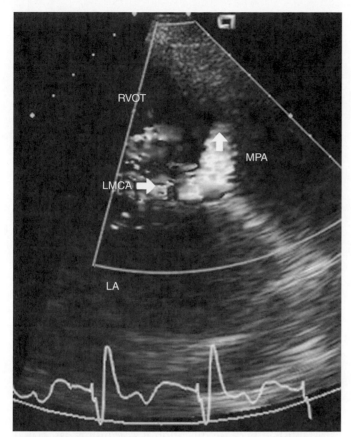

FIGURE 6–24   Left coronary artery to main pulmonary artery fistula from the patient referred to in Figure 6–23. Parasternal short-axis view oriented to display the main axis of the right ventricular outflow tract (RVOT) and main pulmonary artery (MPA). Color shows flow into the proximal MPA via the left main coronary artery (LMCA). The right coronary artery carries flow from the aorta to the myocardium and connects to the left coronary artery system, which drains into the low-pressure MPA, potentially causing myocardial ischemia due to a coronary steal.

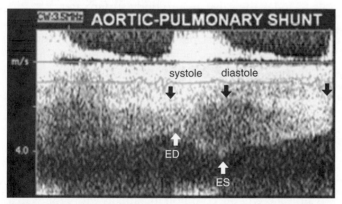

FIGURE 6–25   Blalock-Taussig shunt in a patient with tetralogy of Fallot. Doppler shows continuous high velocity throughout the cardiac cycle, indicating an aorta-to-pulmonary artery pressure gradient in both systole and diastole. The systolic velocity peaks at end-systole (ES) at 4.3 m/s, predicting a peak ES pressure gradient of 74 mm Hg. End-diastolic (ED) velocity was 3.7 m/s, predicting an ED gradient of 55 mm Hg. In the unaffected arm, the sphygmomanometer systemic blood pressure was 110/70, predicting a pulmonary artery (PA) pressure of about 36/15 mm Hg.

Waterston (ascending aorta/right pulmonary artery) and Potts (descending aorta/left pulmonary artery) shunts are best imaged by TEE. Spectral CW Doppler alignment with color flow imaging permits calculation of the gradient by the Bernoulli equation. The pulmonary artery systolic pressure is estimated by subtracting the peak systolic pressure gradient from the brachial arterial peak systolic pressure.

SIMPLE OBSTRUCTIVE AND REGURGITANT LESIONS

Congenital obstruction to left ventricular outflow can be subaortic, valvular, supravalvular, or in the aortic isthmus (coarctation). Echocardiography plays a crucial role in detection and quantification of these lesions.

Bicuspid Aortic Valve and Aortic Root Disease

A bicuspid aortic valve (BAV) is the most frequent congenital malformation of the heart or great arteries[230] (Figs. 6–26 through 6–28). BAVs are present in as much as 2% of the U.S. population with a 2:1 male:female ratio.[14,15,231] In an Italian study of young male conscripts studied with echocardiography, the frequency of BAV was 0.8%.[232] A bicuspid or unicuspid stenotic or regurgitant aortic valve (or both) is the commonest indication for isolated aortic valve replacement.[233,234] Nearly all patients with BAV will require interventional catheterization or surgery,[235] although occasionally, a patient with a functionally normal BAV presents in

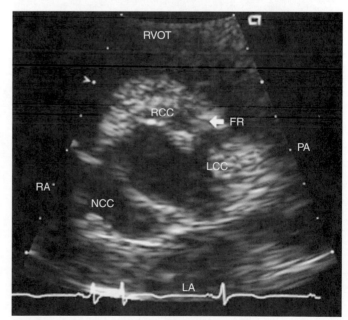

FIGURE 6–26   Short-axis systolic frame of a bicuspid aortic valve showing an oval eccentric opening with the bicommissural line from about 5 to 10 o'clock. The left coronary cusp (LCC) contains a false raphe (FR) at 2 o'clock. NCC, posterior noncoronary cusp; RCC, right coronary cusp.

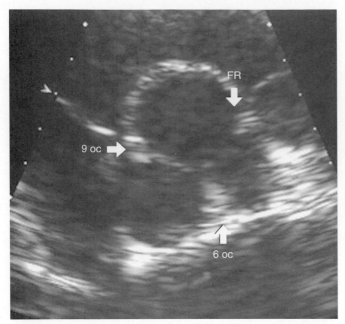

FIGURE 6-27 Bicuspid aortic valve. The diastolic closure frame misleadingly suggests an inverted Mercedes-Benz sign of three-leaflet morphology. The true diastolic closure line is a curvilinear silhouette from 6 to 9 o'clock. The false raphe (FR) is at 2 o'clock.

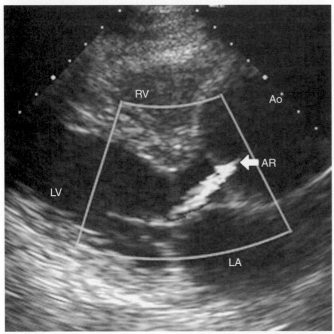

FIGURE 6-28 Bicuspid aortic valve. The aorta (Ao) measured 52 mm at the sinuses with an effaced sinotubular ridge and an ascending aorta of 55 mm. Mild aortic regurgitation (AR) is shown by color flow imaging (arrow). There was no aortic stenosis. (Doppler peak instantaneous gradient 14 mm Hg.) LA, left atrium; LV, left ventricle; RV, right ventricle.

the fourth or fifth decades, with a dilatated ascending aorta or with infective endocarditis.[231,236–239] Inherent medial abnormalities incur the risk of dissection and are coupled with the bicuspid condition of the aortic valve, not its functional state[231,238,240–250] (see Fig. 6–28). Coarctation of the

aorta is a common association. The sinuses of Valsalva and proximal ascending aorta may dilatate at rates as high as 0.5 mm/year and 0.9 mm/year, respectively.[248]

There are two basic types of aortic cusp orientation in bicuspid valves—namely, right-to-left (R-L) or anteroposterior (A-P), with an incidence of 52.5% and 47.5%, respectively.[230] A false raphe usually resides in the larger of the two leaflets. In the R-L variety, the commissural slit is relatively vertical or oblique and separates the cusps into right and left; the false raphe is virtually always in the right cusp.[230] In the A-P type, the commissural plane is horizontal, resulting in a larger anterior cusp. The false raphe is located between the origins of the two coronary arteries.[230] Fusion of the right and left coronary cusps is associated with coarctation of the aorta. Fusion of the right and noncoronary cusps is associated with fibrocalcific degeneration.[251] Awareness of these morphologic features assists in echocardiographic interpretation.

The parasternal short-axis TTE view discloses a single transverse horizontal or vertical diastolic closure line. The presence of a false raphe should not be mistaken for a trileaflet valve[231] (see Figs. 6–26 and 6–27). Error is avoided by careful attention to systolic opening that is characterized by doming of two unequal leaflets with an elliptical orifice, in contrast to the isosceles triangle opening that typifies an open trileaflet aortic valve. The aortic root dimensions must be established because dilatation is commonly associated with intrinsic medial abnormalities, even if the bicuspid valve is functionally normal[240] (see earlier discussion).

Two-dimensional TTE is used to measure the LV outflow tract diameter, PW Doppler is used to measure the LV outflow tract velocity, and CW Doppler is used to establish the mean systolic gradient and peak instantaneous gradient. The effective aortic orifice area must be calculated with the continuity equation, and it is desirable to index the valve area to body surface area.[252]

Planimetric quantification of the aortic valve orifice is feasible by TEE in adults, but in bicuspid aortic stenosis, the technique overestimates the valve area compared with the continuity equation.[253] This is in part due to the "windsock" shape of the stenotic BAV and the difficulty in targeting the echo beam through the true short axis at exactly the tip of the wind sock. There is the tendency to estimate a larger orifice size. The reader is referred to a state-of-the-art publication[254] on valvular aortic stenosis for techniques used to quantify severity, for pitfalls, and for observations on and algorithms for the timing of intervention.

Clinical events are common in patients with BAV.[255] In a study of 51 adults followed for a median of 21 months, 12% underwent aortic valve replacement for stenosis in 2%, regurgitation in 6%, and infective endocarditis in 4%.[256] In a report of 208 patients with BAV, 16% underwent aortic valve replacement over a mean of 24 months, 81% for aortic stenosis, and 19% for aortic regurgitation.[255] One third of the patients had a dilated aortic root for which surgery was performed for aneurysm or dissection in 3%.[255]

The Mayo Clinic surgical pathology study from 1999 reported that 11% of patients with BAVs had evidence of ascending aortic disease, and 0.6% had aortic dissection.[257]

No single measurement of aortic gradient or valve area establishes need for intervention. The 2006 American Heart Association/American College of Cardiology guidelines on management of valvular heart disease is a consensus report on severity.[252] Follow-up echo studies of gradients, valve areas, aortic root size, degree of aortic regurgitation, ventricular size, wall thickness, and ventricular function are essential. Interpretation frequency depends on comparison with the initial assessment.[24-26,252] An appreciable number of patients with BAVs have larger than normal aortic annular sizes (54% were ≥ 23 mm) related to dilatation of the aortic root. The larger annulus per se results in a larger calculated aortic valve area for equivalent velocity estimates of the gradient.

TEE is useful in monitoring balloon catheter valvuloplasty for bicuspid aortic stenosis. When a Ross procedure is performed (pulmonary autograft in the aortic position, heterograft, or homograft in the pulmonary position), TEE is employed preoperatively to measure the size of the pulmonary annulus and aortic annulus to ensure normal structure and function of the pulmonary valve. Intraoperative TEE is used to interrogate the neoaortic valve, patency of the coronary artery reimplantation sites, and LV regional wall motion.

Discrete Subaortic Stenosis (SAS)

The subaortic lesion is represented by a fibrous membrane, a muscular ledge or tunnel, or fibromuscular tissue (Fig. 6–29). In addition to LV outflow tract obstruction per se, the impact of the subaortic jet often damages the aortic valve inducing regurgitation.[3,9-11,13,231] TTE and TEE are the methods of choice for the diagnosis and quantification of both the severity of discrete SAS and the presence and degree of coexisting aortic regurgitation.[231] Intraoperative TEE establishes the efficacy of repair, the degree of postoperative aortic regurgitation, the integrity of the anterior mitral leaflet, and the absence of operative perforation of the ventricular septum.[3,4] Echocardiography is used for postoperative follow-up, including resolution of hypertrophy and surveillance for recurrent subaortic obstruction.[10]

Coarctation of the Aorta

This anomaly is not simply isolated obstruction of the aortic isthmus but is one of a number of coexisting congenital vascular disorders that include abnormalities of proximal and distal paracoarctation aortic media, aneurysms of the circle of Willis, aneurysms of the left subclavian artery and occasionally of intercostals arteries, tortuous retinal arterioles, vascular rings, interruption of the aortic arch, and impaired function of upper extremity conduit arteries.[21] BAV is a frequent association that incurs an

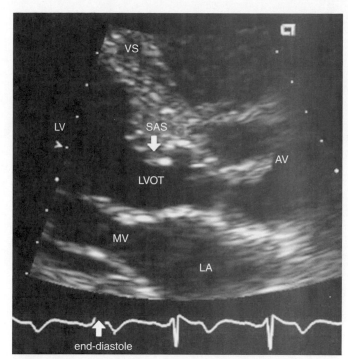

FIGURE 6–29   A fibromuscular ridge narrows the left ventricular outflow tract (LVOT) causing subaortic stenosis. The peak systolic gradient was 60 mm Hg. The aortic valve (AV) is mildly thickened. Aortic regurgitation was mild-to-moderate on color flow imaging. LA, left atrium; LV, left ventricle; MV, open mitral valve; RV, right ventricle.

increased risk of ascending aortic dilatation, aneurysm, and dissection.[258-260] After successful elimination of the coarctation gradient by catheter intervention or surgery, systemic hypertension, premature coronary artery disease, and the previously cited coexisting congenital vascular abnormalities may remain as important residua.[261,262]

Coarctation in young patients is readily imaged by TTE, but imaging in the adult is more difficult.[231] The suprasternal notch window with color flow imaging identifies the coarctation as a localized zone of accelerated flow and provides a target through which the spectral CW Doppler beam can be aligned to determine the gradient (Figs. 6–30 and 6–31). The peak systolic velocity permits estimation of the systolic gradient, and gradually decreasing high-velocity diastolic forward flow (CW Doppler) during elastic recoil of the ascending aorta indicates that the coarctation is hemodynamically significant.[1,3,10,13] The diameter of the color flow image at the coarctation site and the rate of narrowing of the cone of acceleration in the descending aorta proximal to the zone of obstruction coincide with angiographic severity. Multiplane TEE imaging is more effective than TTE for determining the degree and anatomic extent of the coarctation.

Echocardiographic evaluation after repair (suprasternal notch views) determines residual or recurrent obstruction or paracoarctation aneurysm formation.[10] Postoperative exercise echo-Doppler is useful for evaluating gradients and ventricular function. Doppler peak systolic velocity in

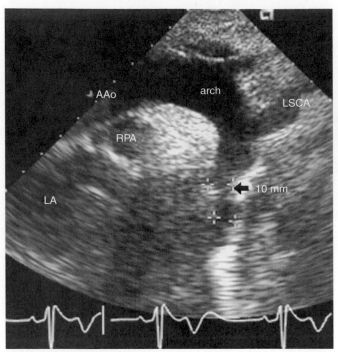

FIGURE 6-30 Coarctation of the aorta. Suprasternal notch transverse aortic arch view shows the narrowed descending aortic coarctation segment of 10 mm. AAo, ascending aorta; LA, left atrium; LSCA, left subclavian artery; RPA, right pulmonary artery.

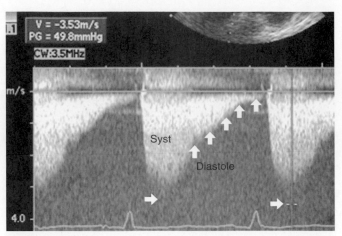

FIGURE 6-31 Aortic coarctation. Continuous-wave Doppler shows a high peak systolic velocity of 3.53 m/s. The diastolic runoff signifies a hemodynamically significant obstruction.

the descending aorta correlates better with residual narrowing of the aortic isthmus or distal aortic arch than does the systolic blood pressure gradient between the upper and lower extremities. A peak velocity of more than 2.5 m/sec establishes narrowing of 25% or more. Prolonged antegrade flow during diastole indicates restenosis or aneurysmal dilatation.

MRI is superior to standard TTE for assessing the aortic isthmus after surgical repair. MRI velocity mapping correlates well with Doppler velocity estimates of the severity of obstruction and can be used when echocardiographic windows are inadequate or when the Doppler beam cannot be aligned with the zone of obstruction.

Balloon catheter dilatation with stenting is now commonly used for native coarctation and frequently for uncomplicated recurrent or residual coarctation. Intravascular echocardiography and TEE during balloon dilatation are useful for precise stent localization, for detection of dissection or aneurysm formation, and to minimize fluoroscopy time.

Congenital Malformations of Left Ventricular Inflow

Congenital malformations of the LV inflow tract can be obstructive, regurgitant, or both. Obstruction can reside in the pulmonary veins (pulmonary venous stenosis), within the left atrium (cor triatriatum), or in the mitral

apparatus (supravalvular stenosing ring, parachute mitral valve, double-orifice mitral valve). Color flow imaging of stenotic jets is best achieved from apical windows. PW Doppler mapping and color flow imaging of the zones of accelerated flow localize the site or sites of stenosis. CW Doppler imaging coupled with color flow establishes severity by recording the velocity profile. The mean pressure gradient and the mitral orifice area are determined from the atrioventricular diastolic pressure half-time as in acquired mitral stenosis. In Lutembacher's syndrome (congenital ASD with acquired rheumatic mitral stenosis), the Doppler pressure half-time method is inaccurate. Planimetry of the mitral orifice area and calculation of the Doppler continuity equation are used instead.

Cor triatriatum is characterized by a membrane that divides the left atrium into a superior chamber that contains the pulmonary veins and an inferior chamber that contains the left atrial appendage. With echocardiographic imaging, the obstructing membrane is seen to attach medially above the fossa ovalis and laterally at the junction between the left superior pulmonary vein and the left atrial appendage (Figs. 6–32 and 6–33). The site of obstruction is identified by a high-velocity color flow jet, and the gradient is established by CW Doppler.

Pulmonary vein stenosis can involve one or all four major pulmonary veins, each of which must be identified.[2–4,263] Normal pulmonary venous flow is laminar irrespective of the amount of pulmonary blood flow and exhibits a biphasic or triphasic pattern reflecting left atrial pressure dynamics.[1,13] Timing of peak flow corresponds to the X and Y troughs, with minimal or reversed flow at the time of the A and V peaks. TEE is usually required for complete pulmonary vein anatomic and hemodynamic evaluation in adults.[2,3]

An isolated *supravalvular mitral ring* is extremely rare in adults. Both TTE and TEE can accurately image the membrane and determine the degree of obstruction.[13] In con-

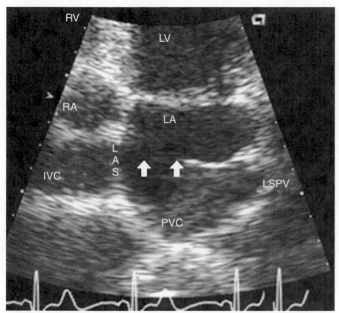

FIGURE 6–32   Cor triatriatum. Transthoracic echo with modified four-chamber apical view focusing on the left atrium. A membrane divides the pulmonary venous confluence (PVC) from the true anatomic left atrium (LA). The double arrows show the residual opening from the PVC to LA, resulting in mild inflow obstruction. IVC, inferior vena cava; LAS, left atrial septum; LSPV, left superior pulmonary vein; LV, left ventricle; RA, right atrium; RV, right ventricle.

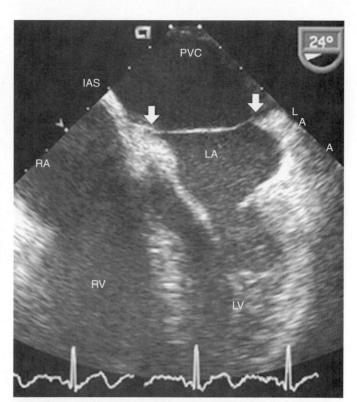

FIGURE 6–33   Transesophageal echo four-chamber view of cor triatriatum in the patient referred to in Figure 6–32. IAS, interatrial septum; LA, left atrium; LAA, left atrial appendage; LV, left ventricle; PVC, pulmonary venous confluence; RA, right atrium; RV, right ventricle.

trast to cor triatriatum (discussed earlier), the supravalvular mitral ring resides immediately above the mitral valve, and the pulmonary veins and left atrial appendage share the same compartment.

Double-orifice mitral valve, a rare malformation, is recognized more frequently since the advent of TTE and TEE.[13] There are three morphologic types: (1) a fibrous bridge that completely divides the orifice into two relatively equal parts that are visible from leaflet edge to valve ring; (2) an incomplete bridge at the leaflet edge, with a single orifice identified when the transducer is tilted superiorly toward the middle and annular portion of the valve; and (3) a larger medial orifice at midleaflet level, with a smaller second orifice laterally, whereas at annular level, there is only a cleft in the anterior mitral leaflet.

Accessory mitral leaflet tissue is a rare disorder usually identified in asymptomatic patients referred for evaluation of a systolic murmur assigned to the left ventricular outflow tract.[13] The echocardiogram identifies a mobile mass connected to the anterior mitral leaflet or chordae, with systolic movement into the left ventricular outflow tract.

Ebstein Anomaly of the Tricuspid Valve

Ebstein's anomaly exhibits a wide spectrum of severity ranging from intrauterine or neonatal death to opportunistic detection during a routine echocardiogram in an older adult.[264,265] Moderate and severe forms are often found in adults.[264] The right side of the heart in Ebstein's anomaly consists of three morphologic components: (1) the right atrium proper, (2) the atrialized right ventricle, which is thin-walled and mechanically integrated with the right atrium, and (3) the trabecular and outlet portions that constitute the right ventricle proper (Figs. 6–34 through 6–37). The anterior tricuspid leaflet, which is attached basally at the level of the atrioventricular sulcus (annulus), is large and potentially mobile (sail-like), but mobility can be compromised by multiple short thick chordae. The basal attachments of the septal and posterior leaflets are apically displaced, and their movement is impaired by short, thickened chordae tendineae.[266] The displaced insertions of these two malformed leaflets allow free communication between the proximal (atrialized) and distal (functional) parts of the right ventricle. Rarely, communication between the atrialized and functional right ventricle is confined to slits or perforations in the anterior leaflet. The thin-walled atrialized right ventricle is typically dilatated, often aneurysmal, and expands paradoxically during ventricular systole. The majority of hearts with Ebstein's anomaly have an interatrial communication that takes the form of a patent foramen ovale or an ostium secundum ASD.

Comprehensive TTE and TEE interrogation of the anatomy and physiology of the Ebstein tricuspid apparatus permit a confident diagnosis of the anomaly and determine

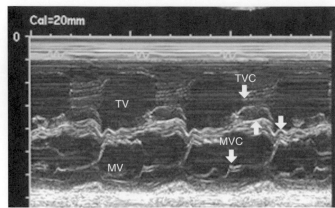

FIGURE 6-34 Ebstein's anomaly. The M-mode tracing shows the tricuspid valve (TV) and the mitral valve (MV) in the same plane due to displacement of the TV toward the RV apex. Tricuspid valve closure (TVC) to mitral valve closure (MVC) was nearly 90 ms because of the characteristically delayed closure of the Ebstein tricuspid valve. There is paradoxical motion of the ventricular septum (turquoise arrows).

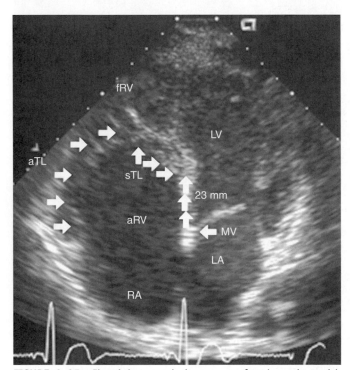

FIGURE 6-35 Ebstein's anomaly in a young female patient with right-sided Wolff-Parkinson-White bypass tract and a small atrial septal defect (see Fig. 6-37) The crux anatomy is abnormal, with the septal tricuspid valve leaflet (sTL) displaced 23 mm apically from the mitral valve (MV) insertion site. An elongated anterior tricuspid leaflet (aTL) in real time was highly mobile. aRV, atrialized right ventricle; fRV, functional RV; LA, left atrium; LV, left ventricle; RA, right atrium.

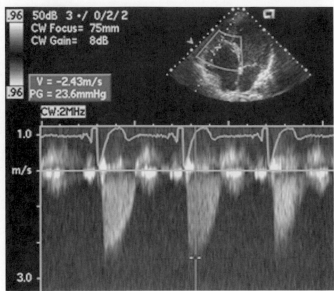

FIGURE 6-36 Ebstein anomaly, same patient referred to in Figure 6-35. Continuous-wave Doppler of tricuspid regurgitation shows an early systolic profile with a peak velocity of 2.43 m/s, typical of Ebstein's anomaly. The mean jugular venous pressure and waveform were normal. The RV systolic pressure was estimated at 29 mm Hg.

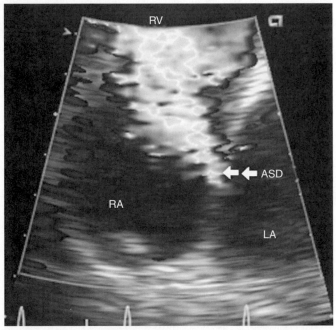

FIGURE 6-37 Ebstein anomaly, same patient referred to in Figures 6-35 and 6-36. Color flow imaging of the four-chamber apical view reveals a left-to-right shunt via a small secundum atrial septal defect (ASD). LA, left atrium; RA, right atrium.

suitability for surgical repair.[1,3,10,12,13,266,267] TTE best evaluates the three leaflets from parasternal short-axis views, whereas the best TEE views are multiplane deep transgastric and mid-esophageal.[1,3,10,13] A long, mobile anterior leaflet sets the stage for operative reconstruction.[12] Evaluation of

the crux anatomy is central to the diagnosis (see Fig. 6-35). In normal hearts, the attachments of the septal tricuspid leaflet are only slightly more apically displaced than the anterior mitral leaflet attachments. The small offset is due to an atrioventricular membrane. In Ebstein anomaly, the distance between the basal tricuspid and mitral attachments is exaggerated because of major apical displacement of the septal and posterior tricuspid insertions. Other volume overload lesions of the right heart can result in small increases in separation of the attachments of the septal tricuspid and anterior mitral leaflets, so a "cutoff" value for septal tricuspid-mitral insertion distance indexed to body surface area has been established. A distance 8 mm/m identifies Ebstein's anomaly at all ages.[266,268] Ebstein's anomaly of the tricuspid valve in the inverted right ventricle of congenitally corrected transposition of the great arteries is discussed later.

Tricuspid regurgitation is usually moderate to severe and is not always in proportion to the degree of anatomic abnormality. Color flow discloses regurgitation emerging from the displaced septal and posterior leaflets. Detection of multiple jets assists in identifying leaflet fenestrations. In uncomplicated Ebstein anomaly, the tricuspid regurgitation by CW Doppler imaging is low pressure/low velocity (see Fig. 6–36). Color flow imaging and agitated saline contrast echocardiography identify a right-to-left shunt through a patent foramen ovale or an ostium secundum ASD (discussed earlier; see Fig. 6–37). Echocardiography also defines left ventricular function that may be reduced at rest or after exercise.[269] A distinction between Uhl's anomaly (parchment right ventricle) and Ebstein anomaly can be made by echocardiography.[270]

Pulmonary Stenosis

Obstruction to RV outflow can be subvalvular, valvular, supravalvular, or in the pulmonary artery or its branches.[1,13,20,271] The common variety is characterized by a thin, mobile, dome pulmonary valve that is readily identified anatomically and functionally by echocardiography. The valve is best seen in short-axis parasternal views. Color flow imaging records a high jet velocity directed along the lateral wall of the pulmonary trunk into the left branch and identifies coexisting pulmonary and tricuspid regurgitation. Multiple transducer positions should be used to establish the highest velocity. CW Doppler quantifies the mean and peak systolic gradients. Right ventricular systolic pressure is determined from the tricuspid regurgitant velocity (discussed earlier). A late-peaking systolic profile of dynamic subvalvular obstruction is sometimes seen within the rounded velocity profile of pulmonary valve stenosis. Identification of multiple sites of RV outflow obstruction requires 2DE and color flow imaging combined with PW and CW Doppler. TEE can be helpful.

Adults and adolescents who have undergone surgical pulmonary valvuloplasty are occasionally encountered, but the current treatment of choice is catheter balloon dilatation. Echocardiographic assessment after surgery or balloon valvuloplasty identifies residual pulmonary valve obstruction, the presence and degree of pulmonary regurgitation, and regression of dynamic hypertrophic subpulmonary stenosis.

Isolated fixed *infundibular pulmonary stenosis* is uncommon in both children and adults. Echocardiography with color flow imaging reveals the site of obstruction, and CW Doppler imaging determines the severity. *Subinfundibular obstruction*, also called *double-chambered right ventricle*, is recognized by 2DE with color flow imaging, which also identifies a commonly associated VSD.

Pulmonary artery banding is surgically induced therapeutic obstruction to RV outflow. Two-dimensional echocardiography and color flow imaging localize the band relative to the pulmonary valve and bifurcation of the pulmonary trunk and quantify the band gradient by aligning the CW Doppler beam with the acceleration of color flow into the zone of obstruction. Because banding is usually performed to reduce pulmonary blood flow and pressure in infants with a nonrestrictive VSD, the proximal pulmonary arterial and RV systolic pressures remain the same as systemic.

ISOLATED LEFT VENTRICULAR NONCOMPACTION

This rare genetic congenital abnormality—Barth syndrome—is characterized by prominent trabeculations and conspicuous intrabecular recesses that penetrate deeply into left ventricular myocardium.[272,273] Intrauterine compaction of the spongy meshwork normally occurs between embryonic weeks 5 to 8 and proceeds from epicardium to endocardium, from base toward apex.[272-276] Hypertrabeculation is most obvious at the apex. The clinical course of LV noncompaction is characterized by progressive heart failure, thromboembolic events, and ventricular arrhythmias.[273,276-278,273,276-278]

The diagnosis can be established with high-quality TTE, although the anomaly is often missed because of lack of familiarity[274-276,279] (Figs. 6–38 through 6–40). The first useful echo description was in 1990.[280] The major diagnostic criteria depend on imaging the intertrabecular recesses and measuring the ratio of noncompacted to compacted (NC/C) myocardium at a site of maximum thickness, with a diagnostic cutoff of NC/C ≥ 2 in systole. Detection is improved by 2DE with color flow imaging and echo-contrast enhancement.[276,278,280] 3D-TTE is a useful supplement to 2D TEE.[281] It has been recommended that the diagnosis be considered simply on the basis of a two-layered myocardium with hypertrabeculation on echocardiography or MRI, even if the NC/C ratio is less than 2:1.[282] MRI assessment of documented LV noncompaction has been compared with results from normal volunteers, from athletes, and from patients with hypertrophic cardiomyopathy or valvular aortic stenosis.[283] In

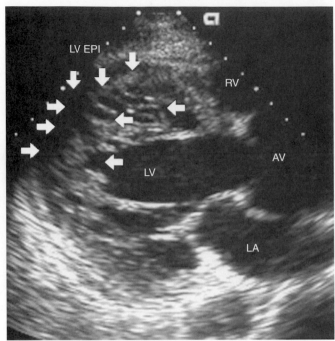

FIGURE 6–38 Left ventricular noncompaction. Parasternal long-axis view shows marked left ventricle (LV) apical hypertrabeculation (multiple arrows) with clefts extending to the LV epicardium (LV EPI). AV, aortic valve; LA, left atrium; RV, right ventricle.

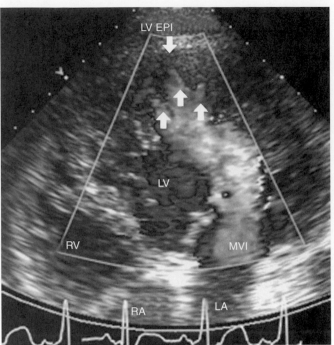

FIGURE 6–40 Left ventricular noncompaction in the patient referred to in Figures 6–38 and 6–39. Color flow imaging in diastole superimposed on the view in Figure 6–40 shows low-velocity flow from endocardium to epicardium into LV apical interstices (LV EPI). LA, left atrium; LV, left ventricle; MVI, mitral valve inflow; RA, right atrium; RV, right ventricle.

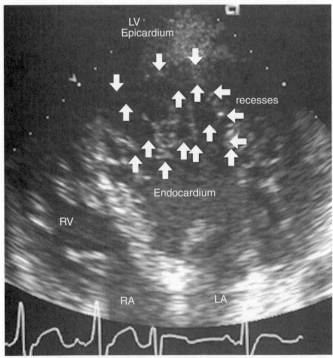

FIGURE 6–39 Left ventricular noncompaction. Apical four-chamber view in the patient referred to in Figure 6-38. Hypertrabeculation is well seen, with deep clefts extending from the endocardium to epicardium of the left ventricle (LV). LA, left atrium; RA, right atrium; RV, right ventricle.

all groups, noncompaction was confined to the apical and lateral segments of the left ventricle rather than the basal or septal walls.[283] The best noncompacted to compacted differentiation was an MRI diastolic NC/C ≥2.3.

COMPLEX MALFORMATIONS

Tetralogy of Fallot (TOF) is the prototype of complex congenital heart disease with which echocardiographic laboratories should be familiar[1,3,10–13,20,271] (Figs. 6–41 through 6–50). Postoperative TOF is among the most common of the complex malformations seen in adults.[21,271,284] TOF with *pulmonary atresia* represents the severest form of the anomaly. Meticulous color flow imaging can identify aortopulmonary collaterals, and 2D imaging with color flow can distinguish TOF with pulmonary atresia from truncus arteriosus.[1] Echocardiography also identifies coexisting congenital malformations such as absent pulmonary valve, absent left pulmonary artery, endocardial cushion defect, and ASD.

In unoperated adolescents and adults, the morphologic and physiologic features of TOF can be identified by TTE supplemented by TEE[1,3,4,9–11,13,285] (see Figs. 6–41 through 6–43). The malaligned VSD and the biventricular aorta are well seen from parasternal and apical views. The rare restrictive malaligned VSD is accompanied by

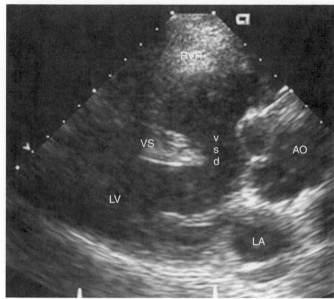

FIGURE 6–41 Unoperated tetralogy of Fallot. Parasternal long-axis view shows the nonrestrictive malaligned ventricular septal defect (VSD) and the biventricular aorta (AO). Right ventricular hypertrophy (RVH) reflects the systemic pressure of the nonrestrictive VSD. LA, left atrium; LV, left ventricle; VS, ventricular septum.

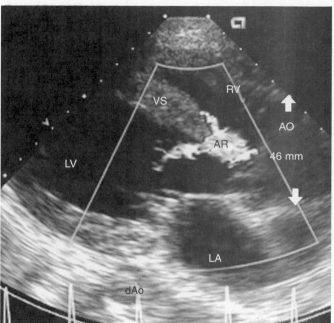

FIGURE 6–43 Tetralogy of Fallot, same patient referred to in Figures 6–41 and 6–42. Parasternal long-axis transthoracic echo with color flow imaging. The aortic root (AO) is dilatated to 46 mm, and a jet of mild aortic regurgitation (AR) affects the crest of the ventricular septum (VS), splaying into both the left (LV) and right ventricle (RV). dAo, descending aorta.

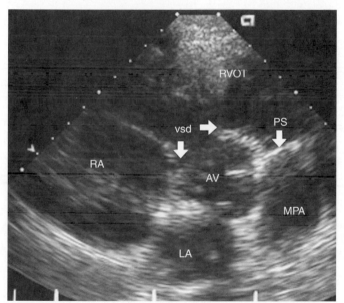

FIGURE 6–42 Tetralogy of Fallot in the patient referred to in Figure 6–41. Parasternal short axis through the level of the aortic valve (AV) and right ventricular outflow tract (RVOT) shows the VSD and thickened pulmonary valve tissue representing valvular pulmonary stenosis (PS). LA, left atrium; MPA, main pulmonary artery; RA, right atrium.

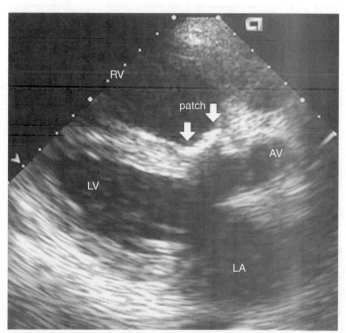

FIGURE 6–44 Tetralogy of Fallot in a 60-year-old woman who had undergone intracardiac repair. She presented with chronic atrial fibrillation and right ventricular failure. Parasternal long-axis view shows the ventricular septal defect patch from the malaligned ventricular septal defect to the overriding aorta. AV, aortic valve; LA, left atrium; LV, left ventricle; RV, right ventricle.

excessive tricuspid valve tissue that partially occludes the defect and by disproportionate septal hypertrophy in response to suprasystemic RV systolic pressure. Additional muscular VSDs are uncommon in adults but should be sought with color flow imaging. Identifying and characterizing the levels of RV outflow obstruction require multiple subcostal and suprasternal views that include

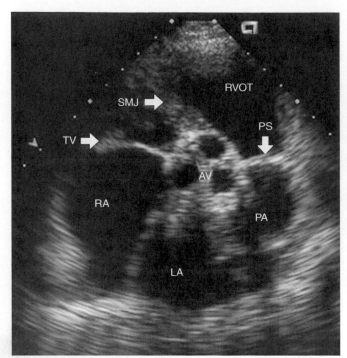

FIGURE 6–45 Tetralogy of Fallot, in the same patient referred to in Figure 6–44. Short-axis view through the right ventricular outflow tract (RVOT) and aortic valve (AV). Residual or recurrent pulmonary valve stenosis (PS) is seen as a band of thickened tissue. There is a prominent septomarginalis junctional muscle band (SMJ) between the septum and the right ventricular free wall. LA, left atrium; PA, pulmonary artery; RA, right atrium; TV, tricuspid valve.

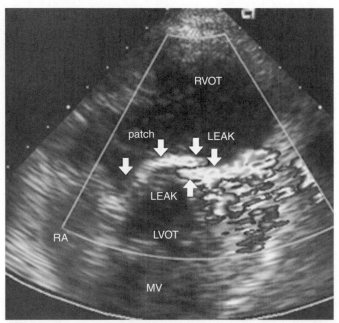

FIGURE 6–46 Tetralogy of Fallot in the patient referred to in Figures 6–44 and 6–45. Short-axis parasternal view with color flow imaging at a slightly inferior plane to that in Figure 6–45 shows a markedly eccentric serpiginous ventricular septal defect patch leak with a left to right color flow jet directed toward the right ventricular outflow tract (RVOT), which is somewhat aneurysmal. LVOT, left ventricular outflow tract; MV, mitral valve; RA, right atrium.

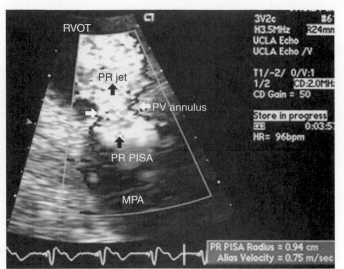

FIGURE 6–47 Tetralogy of Fallot in the patient referred to in Figures 6–44 through 6–46. Diastolic color flow image of the proximal isovelocity surface acceleration (PISA) of the pulmonary regurgitation (PR) jet shows a large PISA radius (0.94 cm), a high aliasing velocity (75 cm/s), and a broad vena contracta into the pulmonary annulus diagnostic of severe pulmonary regurgitation. MPA, main pulmonary artery; RVOT, right ventricular outflow tract.

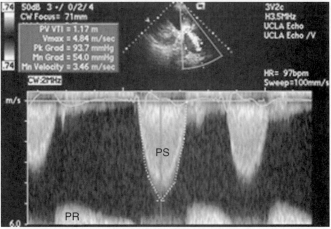

FIGURE 6–48 Tetralogy of Fallot in the same patient referred to in Figures 6–45 through 6–47. Continuous-wave Doppler spectral profile through the pulmonary valve shows a high systolic gradient of severe pulmonary stenosis (PS). The pulmonary regurgitation jet (PR) could not be quantitated on this frame. Peak systolic velocities vary because of the varying R-R intervals of atrial fibrillation.

the subinfundibulum through the pulmonary trunk and its branches. Two-dimensional TTE with color flow imaging and CW Doppler are applied to the sites of obstruction and to the tricuspid regurgitant jet velocity that reflects RV systolic pressure. Multiplane TEE provides the most versatile angles from which to view the RV outflow tract and the pulmonary artery segment. Optimal multiplane angles are from 75 to 90 degrees, combined with appropriate rotation of the probe from right to left,

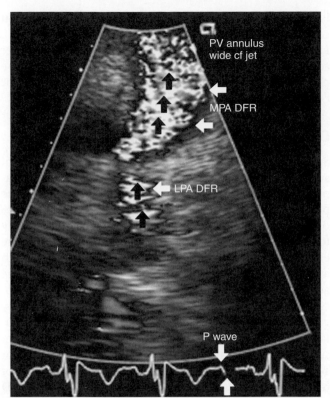

FIGURE 6-49 Tetralogy of Fallot after intracardiac repair. Main pulmonary artery (MPA) and left pulmonary artery (LPA) diastolic flow reversals (DFR) indicate severe pulmonary regurgitation confirmed on magnetic resonance imaging. The broad pulmonary regurgitant jet through the pulmonary valve annulus reflects severe pulmonary regurgitation.

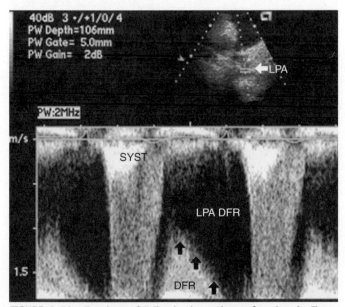

FIGURE 6-50 Tetralogy of Fallot in the patient referred to in Figure 6-49. Pulsed Doppler sample in the left pulmonary artery (LPA) shows the diastolic flow reversal (DFR) of severe pulmonary regurgitation confirmed on magnetic resonance imaging, and disturbed flow and increased velocity of mild branch stenosis. The right pulmonary artery showed the same pattern of DFR without evidence of stenosis, not shown.

individualized for each patient. These angles should be selected from the usual esophageal views, as well as from deep transgastric views. Although TEE can usually image the origins of aortopulmonary collaterals, standard selective angiography, magnetic resonance techniques, and CT angiography are superior.

Echocardiography with color flow imaging and CW Doppler plays a central role in identifying residua and sequelae after repair of TOF[1,3,10,12,13,286] (see Figs. 6-44 through 66-50; see Chapter 20). Major sequelae amenable to echocardiographic delineation include low-pressure pulmonary regurgitation, dilatation, and failure of the right ventricle, tricuspid regurgitation, and incisional aneurysm. Major residua include obstruction to RV outflow (see Figs. 6-45 through 6-48), overlooked VSDs or patch leaks (see Fig. 6-46), aortic regurgitation, aortic root dilatation, and abnormal LV function, usually due to the effects of LV volume overload induced by palliative shunts in childhood.[1,3,10,12,13,286]

Moderate to severe low-pressure pulmonary regurgitation is an important determinant of long-term RV function and also serves as a trigger for the arrhythmogenic substrate of reentrant monomorphic ventricular tachycardia[9-11,13,59,285-290] (see Figs. 6-47 through 6-50). Ventricular tachycardia and sudden cardiac death are more likely in patients with significant pulmonary regurgitation, with a QRS ≥180 ms, and with a positive signal averaged electrocardiogram[291,292] (see Chapter 22). Pulmonary valve replacement eliminates the arrhythmogenic trigger and improves RV function.[293,294]

Echocardiography reliably determines the severity of pulmonary regurgitation (PR)[295] (see Figs. 6-47, 6-49, and 6-50) and has been used with MRI in repaired TOF to measure the width of the PR color flow jet, to establish the Doppler duration of the PR signal, and to calculate the "PR index" (PRi or PR duration divided by the duration of diastole).[296,297] The degree of pulmonary regurgitation is reflected in an MRI regurgitant fraction > 24.5%, a broader color flow PR width, a shorter PR duration, and a lower PRi.[297] Our cardiac MRI laboratory considers a PR regurgitant fraction ≥40% (by MR phase velocity mapping) as indicative of severe pulmonary regurgitation. Our studies by color flow imaging and PW Doppler reveal that diastolic flow reversals (DFR) in the main pulmonary artery (MPA) and branch pulmonary arteries (BPA) are the most reliable indicators of a PR regurgitant fraction ≥40%. Branch pulmonary artery diastolic flow reversal is the most specific and main pulmonary artery diastolic flow reversal the most sensitive echo-Doppler method for detecting severe PR[295] (see Figs. 6-49 and 6-50). We also found that a PRi < 0.77, a CW Doppler pressure half-time < 100 ms, and color flow width > 50% of the pulmonary annulus diameter are reliable indicators of severe PR[295] (see Figs. 6-47 and 6-49).

VSD patch leaks, which are usually eccentric, occur anywhere along the closure line. Because the leaks are usually small, detection and localization require color flow imaging from several angles. Occasionally the patch dehisces sufficiently to permit detection by transthoracic 2D imaging alone. Deep transgastric transesophageal views are helpful because standard midesophageal views can be associated with shadowing of more anterior structures by the VSD patch that may obscure the jet from the patch leak.

The size and function of the right ventricle are assessed from apical and parasternal views. An incisional aneurysm is best imaged from a parasternal short-axis view or with the longitudinal equivalent plane by TEE. LV size and EF are assessed from multiple apical views.

Echocardiography identifies and quantifies aortic regurgitation, which tends to accrue decade by decade and is therefore more common in adults. Aortic regurgitation is usually accompanied by dilatation of the ascending aorta caused by an inherent medial abnormality[240,298–300] (see Fig. 6–45). Central and peripheral arterial stiffness in repaired TOF have also been implicated in the progression of aortic dilatation.[301] The regurgitant volume is imposed on the already afterloaded right ventricle, as well as on the left ventricle, because regurgitant flow is biventricular (see Fig. 6–43). An increase in aortic stiffness with aging compounds the effect of aortic regurgitation on the volume overload left ventricle.

Echocardiographic identification of aortic regurgitation is also important because the lesion is a substrate for infective endocarditis that can result in acute severe augmentation of biventricular regurgitation.[237] The conventional method for measuring the dimension of the aortic regurgitant jet is inaccurate with a malaligned VSD because of the abnormal relationship of the aorta to the LV outflow tract. In unoperated TOF, the regurgitant jet strikes the apex of the trabecular septum and then variably deflects into both ventricles, or in repaired TOF deflects off the crest of the septum, around the patch, and into the left ventricle. The jet impact on the crest of the septum may be associated with the development of a subaortic ledge, which can progress to subaortic stenosis.

A right aortic arch that can be visualized from suprasternal notch views occurs in about 25% of patients with TOF, more often with pulmonary atresia. The origin and course of proximal coronary arteries are surgically important and can be identified in modified parasternal short-axis and suprasternal notch imaging in infants and children but much less adequately in adults.

For delineation of the pulmonary artery branches by TTE, suprasternal views and high parasternal short-axis views are essential and are valuable in patients with aorta/pulmonary shunts. The right branch is often well seen, but the left branch is more difficult to image. TEE or MRI is usually necessary in adults to visualize adequately both branches of the pulmonary artery, aortopulmonary shunts, and aortopulmonary collaterals. TEE

is also useful to identify the origins and proximal courses of the coronary arteries (see earlier discussion). Liberal use of intraoperative TEE immediately after coming off cardiopulmonary bypass minimizes the chance of overlooking important residua, sequelae, or complications.[10]

Complete Transposition of the Great Arteries

Survival to adulthood is the result of atrial or arterial switch operations.[21,302] Two-dimensional echocardiography identifies the aorta anterior and to the right of the posterior and leftward pulmonary trunk, but in 5% to 10% of patients, the aorta is directly anterior and occasionally to the left of the pulmonary trunk.[1] These relationships are easily established from parasternal short-axis views, with attention to the ventricular origin of each great artery. The aorta is identified by the coronary arteries and the brachiocephalic arteries, whereas the main pulmonary artery is identified by its two major proximal branches. Ventricular origins of the great arteries are best established from subcostal and apical windows with careful anteroposterior sweeps of the coronal views and right-to-left sweeps of the oblique and sagittal planes (Fig. 6–51). Mental 3D

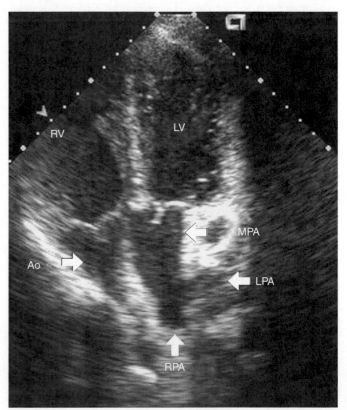

FIGURE 6–51 D-transposition of the great arteries after a Mustard interatrial baffle. Apical four-chamber transthoracic echo shows the great arteries in a superiorly angulated view. The leftward main pulmonary artery (MPA) branches into a right (RPA) and left pulmonary artery (LPA) and arises from the anatomic left ventricle (LV)–ventriculoarterial discordance.

reconstruction is necessary for successful interpretation of 2D-TTE information. Identification of morphologic right and morphologic left ventricles was discussed earlier.

In adults with complete transposition, the sites (levels) of LV outflow obstruction are best determined from parasternal long-axis views, whereas severity is best established by CW Doppler recordings from apical and subcostal views. The location of a given site of outflow obstruction influences surgical planning and, if not properly addressed, contributes to postoperative morbidity and mortality.

The Rastelli repair, applied to patients with complete transposition, VSD, and pulmonary stenosis, consists of an intraventricular conduit that channels left ventricular blood through the VSD into the aorta and an external valved conduit that channels blood from the right ventricle into the pulmonary artery.[10,13,21,302] Echocardiography is central to the clinical recognition of obstruction or regurgitation within the external conduit and for interrogation of a leak or obstruction of the internal conduit that may partially obstruct the right ventricle through which it passes.[10,13]

The Damus-Kaye-Stansel procedure consists of anastomosis of the proximal pulmonary artery to the side of the aorta, oversewing the aortic valve or proximal aorta, patch closure of the VSD, and an external valved conduit from right ventricle to the distal main pulmonary artery. Echocardiography focuses on the presence and degree of pulmonary regurgitation and on the integrity of the VSD patch.

Atrial switch surgery (Mustard or Senning) accounts for why most patients with complete transposition of the great arteries survive to adolescence and young adulthood.[10,13,21,302] Sequelae and complications amenable to echocardiographic interrogation include baffle leaks or obstruction, vena caval and pulmonary venous obstruction, tricuspid regurgitation, aortic regurgitation, and RV dysfunction, the latter a consequence of a subaortic morphologic right ventricle in the systemic location.[10,13] TTE imaging from multiple planes defines the pulmonary venous and systemic venous portions of the atrial compartment and the inferior vena caval to right atrial junction, but the superior vena caval to right atrial region and the pulmonary venous connections are not reliably visualized in adults (Figs. 6–52 and 6–53). Indirect evaluation of superior vena caval obstruction can be achieved with peripheral injection of agitated saline into an arm vein. If there is obstruction, the systemic venous atrium will preferentially fill with echo contrast from the inferior vena cava through azygous venous collaterals. Baffle leaks are identified with color flow imaging or echo contrast. Pulmonary venous obstruction most commonly resides at the isthmus between the posterior and anterior segments where the intraatrial baffle makes a waist in the pulmonary venous atrium. Diastolic flow disturbances within the posterior portion of the pulmonary venous atrium do not necessarily indicate obstructed flow, which is best identified with color flow and 2D imaging that

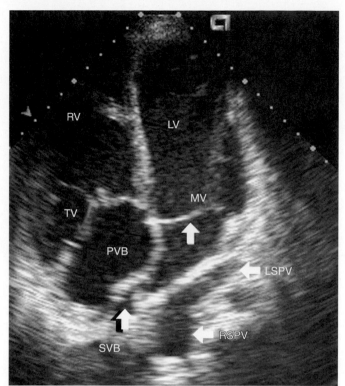

FIGURE 6-52   D-transposition of the great arteries after a Mustard interatrial baffle in the patient referred to in Figure 6–51. This more inferior four-chamber view is angulated to show the course of the systemic venous baffle (SVB) coursing anterior and leftward (arrows) to the mitral valve (MV) and anatomic left ventricle (LV). Portions of the pulmonary venous baffle (PVB) are seen coursing posterior and rightward of the tricuspid valve (TV) and anatomic right ventricle (RV). LSPV, left superior pulmonary vein; RSPV, right superior pulmonary vein.

seek a narrow anatomic area with turbulent biphasic or continuous flow. The systemic venous baffle may be narrowed in its midportion as it crosses the posterior pulmonary venous atrium. TEE with biplane or multiplane probes is required for visualization of all of the Mustard or Senning anatomy and is often necessary for accurate detection of the site(s) of baffle leaks and the entrance sites of all four pulmonary veins and for imaging of the caval junctions, particularly at the level of the inferior systemic venous baffle limb.[10]

Echocardiography is pivotal in the long-term followup of patients with atrial switch repairs, focusing on function of the subaortic morphologic right ventricle and on the presence and degree of aortic and tricuspid regurgitation[21,302] (see Figs. 6–51 through 6–54). TTE assessment of RV function and evaluation of RV volumes is most accurate using the RV inflow tract view in the apical four-chamber projection.[303] Measurement of RV myocardial performance with the Tei Index (see earlier discussion), which is unaffected by geometrically altered ventricles, compared well with MRI quantitation of RV EF.[74]

The *arterial switch* (Jatene repair) is now the operation of choice that was designed to obviate problems that followed

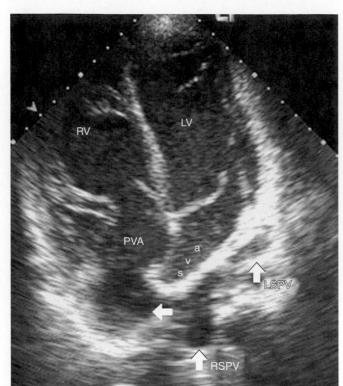

FIGURE 6-53 D-transposition of the great arteries after a Mustard interatrial baffle in the patient referred to in Figures 6–51 and 6–52. Four-chamber view is now rotated to show the pulmonary venous atrium (PVA) coursing posterior to and rightward of the right ventricle (RV). A portion of the systemic venous atrium (SVA) courses anterior to and leftward of the anatomic left ventricle (LV). LSPV, left superior pulmonary vein; RSPV, right superior pulmonary vein.

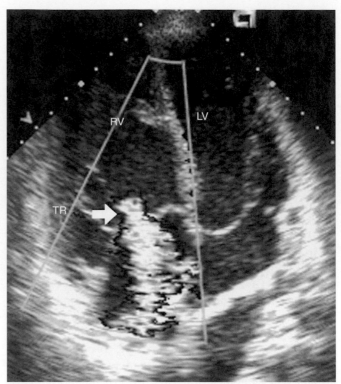

FIGURE 6-54 D-transposition of the great arteries after a Mustard interatrial baffle in the patient referred to in Figures 6–51 through 6–53. There is superimposed color flow imaging of moderate tricuspid regurgitation (TR).

an atrial switch, especially the subaortic morphologic right ventricle. However, the neo-aortic root may progressively dilatate, and neo-aortic regurgitation, although initially mild, requires sequential echocardiographic reevaluation.[21,302] Obstruction is most common at the pulmonary artery anastomosis. Long-term growth and patency of the reimplanted coronary arteries is crucial, and thus preoperative echocardiographic assessment of proximal coronary anatomy in infants must be precise.

Postoperative echocardiography plays an important adjunctive role to angiography in evaluating coronary and great arterial anastomoses and ventricular function. TTE with color flow imaging and Doppler interrogation evaluates the neo-aorta and neo-pulmonary artery. Echocardiographic imaging from parasternal views usually reveals a long segment of narrowing that includes the neo-pulmonary suture lines and the patches that were placed where the coronary arteries and the surrounding button of tissue were removed. Imaging of the proximal segments of the left and right pulmonary arteries is important because distortion may occur where the confluent pulmonary arterial branches were brought anterior to join the aorta. The status of the neo-aortic valve is a long-term concern that echocardiography addresses. Intraop-

erative patency of the proximal coronary arteries can be confirmed by TEE.[10] Myocardial perfusion defects are relatively common after an arterial switch operation. The associated regional wall motion abnormalities are amenable to echocardiographic assessment, and myocardial ischemia can be detected by stress echocardiography.

Congenitally Corrected Transposition of the Great Arteries

This malformation is characterized by a double discordance—atrioventricular and ventriculoarterial—and an L-malposed aorta[20,21,302] (Figs. 6–55 through 6–59). Most commonly associated lesions are VSD, pulmonic or subpulmonic stenosis, and an Ebstein-like malformation of the left-sided tricuspid valve. Long-term concerns in otherwise uncomplicated congenitally corrected transposition of the great arteries include progressive dysfunction of the subaortic systemic RV, progressive left-sided atrioventricular (tricuspid) valve regurgitation, and progressive atrioventricular conduction disturbances.[21,302] Echocardiographic imaging of crux anatomy reveals a *left* atrioventricular valve that is more apically placed than the *right* atrioventricular valve, thus identifying tricuspid and mitral valves, respectively (see Fig. 6–55). Because the morphology of an atrioventricular valve is coupled with the morphology of the ventricle to which it is

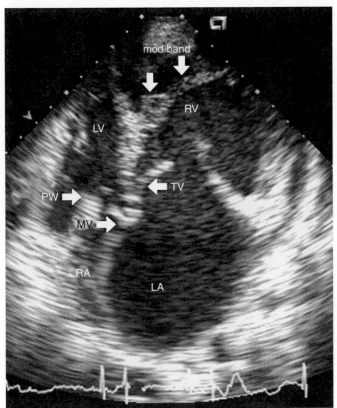

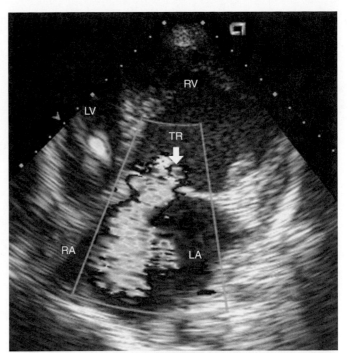

FIGURE 6-56 Congenitally corrected transposition of the great arteries in the patient referred to in Figure 6-55. Apical four-chamber view shows severe tricuspid regurgitation (TR) by color flow imaging. LA, left atrium; LV, left ventricle; RA, right atrium; RV, right ventricle.

FIGURE 6-55 Congenitally corrected transposition of the great arteries. Transthoracic four-chamber apical view in a female patient who developed transient heart failure during pregnancy. The crux anatomy shows the left-sided tricuspid atrioventricular valve more apically positioned than the right-sided mitral valve. The atrioventricular valves follow their concordant morphologic ventricles. The left atrium (LA) connects through the tricuspid valve (TV) to the left-sided anatomic right ventricle (RV). Note the moderator (mod) band. The right atrium (RA) connects through the mitral valve (MV) to the right-sided anatomic left ventricle (LV)—atrioventricular discordance. Right ventricular ejection fraction was 30%.

attached, echocardiographic identification of a tricuspid valve identifies a morphologic *right* ventricle in the subaortic location, and identification of the mitral valve identifies a morphologic *left* ventricle in the subpulmonary location—ventricular inversion—which is the essential morphologic basis of congenitally corrected transposition of the great arteries. The anatomic right ventricle gives rise to an aorta that is leftward and anterior to a rightward and posterior pulmonary trunk, features that can be established with short-axis parasternal views. The aorta exits from the morphologic right ventricle at a broad angle to the inflow tract. A four-chamber apical view shows the pulmonary trunk originating from the morphologic left ventricle at an acute angle from the inflow tract and deeply wedged between the two atrioventricular valves (Fig. 6-59). Echocardiography identifies the malformations most commonly associated with congenitally corrected transposition (discussed earlier). For best delineation of the left-sided Ebstein anomaly, the

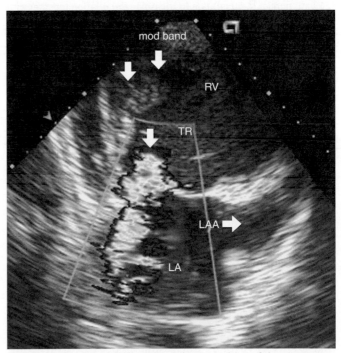

FIGURE 6-57 Congenitally corrected transposition of the great arteries in the patient referred to in Figures 6-55 and 6-56. Modified four-chamber apical view shows the degree of tricuspid regurgitation (TR) and identifies the left-sided atrium as an anatomic left atrium (LA) by the anatomy of the left atrial appendage (LAA), which is dog-eared with a narrow slit-like opening. Connection of the left atrium to a left-sided anatomic right ventricle (RV) constitutes atrioventricular discordance. Note the apical moderator band (MB).

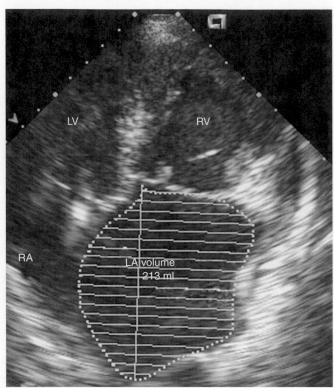

FIGURE 6-58 Congenitally corrected transposition of the great arteries in the patient referred to in Figures 6-55 through 6-57. Apical four-chamber view shows the greatly increased volume of the left atrium (213 ml; normal < 50 ml) due to tricuspid regurgitation together with abnormal diastolic function of the right ventricle (RV). LV, left ventricle; RA, right atrium; RV, right ventricle.

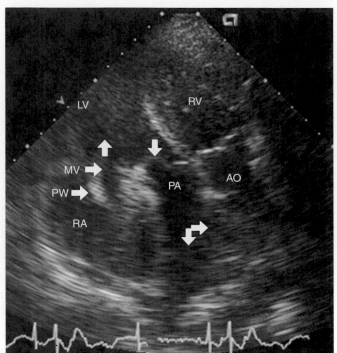

FIGURE 6-59 Congenitally corrected transposition of the great arteries in the patient referred to in Figures 6-55 through 6-58. Apical views are superiorly oriented to visualize the origins and relationships of the great arteries. The pulmonary artery (PA) arises from the morphologic left ventricle (LV) and is identified by its branching pattern (bifurcated arrows). The PA is rightward and posterior to the anterior and leftward aorta (AO), which arises from the outlet of the morphologic right ventricle (RV)—ventriculoarterial discordance. There is the characteristic acute angle (white arrows) between the inflow and outflow tracts of the LV. The connection between right atrium (RA) and LV represent atrioventricular discordance. MV, mitral valve; PW, pacing wire.

examiner must use whichever planes are necessary to image the mural (inferior) leaflet's proximal hinge point, which is consistently displaced inferiorly from the atrioventricular junction when an Ebstein-like malformation is present.

Echocardiography in long-term postoperative follow-up focuses chiefly on the function of the morphologic subaortic right ventricle and on the presence and progression of left atrioventricular valve regurgitation.

Double-Outlet Right Ventricle

Double-Outlet Right Ventricle (DORV) refers to abnormal ventriculoarterial alignments in which both great arteries originate exclusively or predominately (≥50%) from a morphologic right ventricle.[271] It has been argued that DORV is virtually unclassifiable because of its complex and diverse anatomy, but certain gross morphologic features are sufficiently recurrent to serve as a basis for classification—namely,[271] (1) the connections of the great arteries to the ventricles; (2) the location, size, and relationship of an obligatory VSD to the great arteries; and (3) the absence, presence, and degree of pulmonary stenosis. The VSD—usually large—can be committed to the

aorta (subaortic), to the pulmonary artery (subpulmonary), to both great arteries (doubly committed), or to neither great artery.[20,271] The commitment of the VSD governs the streaming characteristics of blood leaving the left ventricle. DORV with a subaortic VSD and pulmonary stenosis resembles TOF. DORV with a nonrestrictive subpulmonary VSD and RV or biventricular origin of pulmonary trunk (Taussig-Bing anomaly) resembles complete transposition of the great arteries.

Echocardiography addresses the spatial relationships of the great arteries, the outflow tract beneath each great artery, the location and type of VSD, and the relationship of the VSD to the two great arteries[1,13] (discussed earlier). The aorta is usually to the right of and lateral to the pulmonary trunk (side by side) and in the same transverse plane. Alternatively, the aorta is to the right or left and anterior to the pulmonary trunk or is normally related to the pulmonary trunk. In the usual form of DORV, the great arteries are at the same level above the ventricles because a conus lies beneath each great artery. Parasternal, apical, and subcostal views disclose the alignment of the great arteries to the morphologic right ventricle and the relationship of the great arteries to each other. That relationship is established by orienting the transducer to display the great arteries side by side or front and back and by noting the orientation of the transducer to the chest wall.[1,13] Although both great arteries are usually supported by a subarterial conus (discussed earlier) that precludes mitral-semilunar valve continuity, occasional resorption of the conus beneath the posterior or leftward semilunar valve results in fibrous continuity between that great artery and the mitral valve.

A VSD is committed to either the aorta or the pulmonary trunk if the orifice of the defect is directed mainly to one of the great arteries as imaged from subcostal, parasternal, and apical long-axis views. The defect is usually subaortic and is imaged beneath the septal limb of the crista superventricularis to the right of the conus septum.[303] A subpulmonary VSD necessarily lies beneath the pulmonary valve and above the septal limb of the crista when the great arteries are side by side (original Taussig-Bing description) and resides below the septal limb if the great arteries are malposed. A doubly committed subarterial VSD lies below the crista and is centered beneath both great arteries. Rarely, the VSD is remote from both the aorta and pulmonary trunk.

Pulmonary stenosis can occur with double-outlet right ventricle and a subaortic VSD and is identified by long- and short-axis sweeps from multiple views in conjunction with color flow imaging for the detection of accelerated flow. The CW Doppler beam is aligned parallel to the outflow tracts from apical or subcostal views to quantify the degree of obstruction. Echocardiography should also search for associated anomalies that include malformations of the aortic arch, especially prevalent with the Taussig-Bing anomaly, subaortic stenosis, and anomalous attachments of atrioventricular valves.[1,3,10,13,302]

The goal of surgery is to achieve a biventricular repair.[271] Commitment of the VSD to the aorta is crucial if kinking or compression of the intraventricular (LV-to-VSD-to-aortic) tunnel is to be avoided. If the tunnel causes RV outflow obstruction, a patch can be placed to enlarge the outflow tract.[271] The Rastelli repair (discussed earlier) applies to DORV with a subaortic VSD and pulmonary stenosis.[1,3,10,13,302] Repair with a subpulmonary VSD is usually accomplished with an arterial switch procedure and VSD patch closure.[271] Intraoperative TEE is especially useful in identifying the intraventricular course of the baffle that joins the VSD to the aorta. A long baffle lends itself to kinking or obstruction (see earlier). Echocardiography should be employed meticulously in DORV of the Fallot type because residual defects in the ventricular septum or adjacent to the patch are relatively frequent.[10] Leaks around the anterior portion of the intraventricular baffle require careful color flow imaging for detection. Echocardiography should seek to identify subaortic stenosis that occasionally develops because of narrowing at the VSD repair.

Atrioventricular Septal Defects

This category of anomalies is characterized by complete or partial absence of the atrioventricular septum, that is, by lack of development of the primitive embryonic endocardial cushion.[12,20,176] The most common arrangement in adults is a defect in the ostium primum portion of the atrial septum with a cleft anterior mitral leaflet and abnormal chordal attachments to the endocardium of the left ventricle outflow tract. The complete form of the malformation—complete common atrioventricular canal—consists of a common atrioventricular valve above and below, which are large interatrial and interventricular communications.[12] Subaortic obstruction may coexist as part of the basic malformation or be a sequel of a repair. Intraoperative TEE should be used to minimize residual postoperative defects.[10]

Total Anomalous Pulmonary Venous Connection

The relatively rare adult with this malformation has an enlarged right atrium and right ventricle, an obligatory ASD, and a confluence of pulmonary veins.[1,12,13,20] Color flow imaging and Doppler interrogation determine the course of the pulmonary veins, the pathway from confluence of pulmonary veins to the right side of the heart, and the presence or absence of obstruction.[12] TEE visualizes the more posterior structures, identifies the confluence of pulmonary veins, and traces the connection of the confluence to right-sided chambers or systemic veins.

Univentricular Heart or Single Ventricle

Nearly a century and a half after Thomas Peacock's description, there is still no consensus regarding terminology for hearts with only *one ventricle*. The terms *univentricular heart* and *single ventricle* are interchangeable and are appropriate when two atria are related entirely or almost entirely to one ventricular compartment that qualifies on purely morphologic grounds as a left, right, or indeterminate ventricle.[20,22,23,304] Univentricular atrioventricular connection or double-inlet ventricle is defined according to the gross morphologic characteristics of the ventricular mass and according to the atrioventricular connections to that mass.[20,22,23,304] Most commonly, the ventricular compartment is a morphologic left ventricle that receives both atrioventricular valves (double inlet) and harbors at its base a rudimentary outlet chamber (Figs. 6–60 and 6–61). Less commonly, a single ventricle with right ventricle morphology receives both atrioventricular valves and harbors a rudimentary posterior trabecular pouch. TTE defines the univentricular atrioventricular connections and has supplanted cardiac catheterization. For the typical double-inlet left ventricle, apical and parasternal TTE short-axis views reveal two atrioventricular valves entering the main

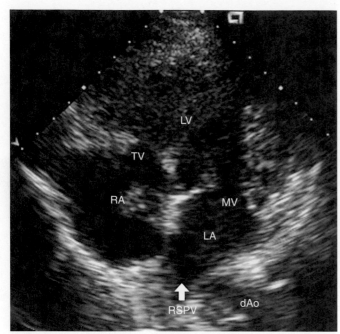

FIGURE 6-60 Double-inlet left ventricle. Apical four-chamber view in mid-diastole shows both the mitral valve (MV) and tricuspid valve (TV) opening directly into the anatomic left ventricle (LV). The aorta arose from a rightward and anterior outlet chamber, and the pulmonary trunk arose from the LV. dAO, descending aorta; LA, left atrium; RA, right atrium; RSPV, right superior pulmonary vein.

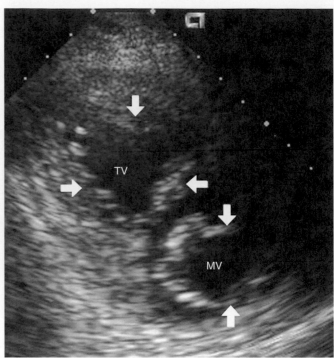

FIGURE 6-61 Double-inlet left ventricle, same patient referred to in Figure 6-60. Short-axis parasternal view shows the leftward and posterior mitral valve (MV, blue arrows) and the rightward and anterior tricuspid valve (TV, yellow arrows).

ventricular chamber, the morphology of which is established as described earlier (see Figs. 6–60 and 6–61). The outlet chamber can be at the right or left basal aspect of the single left ventricle, that is, noninverted or inverted. Echocardiography identifies the pulmonary trunk originating from the main ventricular compartment that is a morphologic left ventricle (ventricular/great arterial discordance) and identifies the aorta originating from the outlet chamber (infundibular remnant). Although the communication between the main ventricular compartment and the outlet chamber is rimmed by muscle that consists of a remnant of trabecular septum inferiorly and outlet septum superiorly, the communication is best called an *outlet foramen* to avoid the contradiction implied by using the term *ventricular septal defect*, which implies two ventricles in hearts that are equipped with only one ventricle.[20] Echocardiography plays an important role in identifying obstruction of the outlet foramen, identifying pulmonary stenosis, and delineating malformations of the atrioventricular valves. Stenosis of the outlet foramen can develop after pulmonary artery banding or cavopulmonary shunting. Sequential measurements of the size of the outlet foramen with Doppler gradients are important parts of routine surveillance.[1,10,13] The presence of obstruction—effectively subaortic stenosis—is detected in part by echocardiographic anatomic sizing from at least two orthogonal planes. Search should seek atrioventricular valve tissue or fibrous tissue encroaching on the outlet

foramen. Because of anticipated color flow acceleration through the outlet foramen, CW Doppler evaluation of a gradient is necessary for hemodynamic quantification. A gradient may be significant only during exercise, and thus hemodynamic assessment may require exercise or dobutamine stress testing in the echo or cardiac catheterization laboratory.

Tricuspid Atresia

Two-dimensional echocardiography reveals a dense band at the right atrioventricular groove, representing absence of an atrioventricular connection between the floor of the right atrium and the ventricular mass[1,3,13] (Fig. 6–62). The only exit from the morphologic right atrium is through an interatrial communication that is usually an ASD and less commonly and less desirably a patent foramen ovale. The type and functional adequacy of the interatrial communication can be determined by echocardiography with color flow imaging and Doppler interrogation. Intraoperative TEE without cardiopulmonary bypass has been used to assist in blade atrial septostomy.[3,4] Echocardiography identifies an interventricular communication that is usually a perimembranous VSD and identifies the ventricular origin of each great artery. A restrictive VSD recognized by color flow imaging and CW Doppler constitutes subpulmonary stenosis when the great arteries are normally related, which is usually the case.

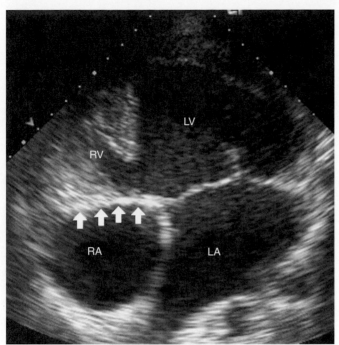

FIGURE 6-62 Tricuspid atresia. Four-chamber apical view shows a muscular ridge at the site of the absent tricuspid valve (four turquoise arrows). This is the common type of tricuspid atresia. The hypoplastic right ventricle (RV) and the restrictive ventricular septal defect can be seen but are not labeled. A large secundum atrial septal defect is not well seen in this frame. LA, left atrium; LV, left ventricle.

Fontan Operation

Surgical construction of a Fontan circulation is employed in complex lesions with low pulmonary vascular resistance in which a biventricular repair is not feasible.[305] There have been many Fontan variations, but each represents a circulation in series without a subpulmonary right ventricle.[305-307] A sizeable number of patients undergo the procedure for the first time as young adults.[308] Applicable to both univentricular hearts and to tricuspid atresia, the Fontan operation requires meticulous preoperative criteria, which include a normal or low pulmonary vascular resistance, normal systemic ventricular systolic and diastolic function, and no significant valvular regurgitation or stenosis.[9-12,103,304,309-312] Echocardiography assists materially in that assessment.[10] In univentricular hearts, the Fontan repair employs either a direct right atriopulmonary connection or total cavopulmonary connection employing a bidirectional Glenn anastomosis with inferior vena caval anastomosis to right pulmonary artery through a lateral tunnel or an extracardiac tube connection. In tricuspid atresia with a well-formed right ventricle, a right atrial to RV anastomosis is sometimes employed. Intraoperative TEE ensures that connections are unobstructed, assists in determining the size of an adjustable ASD, and evaluates ventricular and valvular function. Echocardiography is central to postoperative management. Patch exclusion of the right atrioventricular valve can result in significant regurgitation. Obstruction of the outlet foramen may develop. Complications in the atrial portion of the Fontan circulation should be sought by 2DE with color flow imaging and spectral Doppler velocities that identify cavoatrial shunting, atrial septal shunting, thrombus, pulmonary venous pathway obstruction, and right atrial-to-pulmonary artery obstruction. In high-risk patients, operation includes atrial fenestrations and an adjustable ASD. TEE is often used in the interventional catheterization laboratory to guide closure of the surgically created atrial fenestration or adjustable ASD or is required in the intensive care unit.

Mortality and morbidity have improved because of technical improvements and better postoperative care, but long-term concerns remain.[313-315] Arrhythmias may become less frequent with the current total cavopulmonary anastomosis, and sinus node dysfunction may become more frequent in the extracardiac form than with the lateral tunnel technique.[316] The potential need for a pacemaker and for management of arrhythmias is apparent. Protein-losing enteropathy, coagulopathy, and liver dysfunction remain important issues. Important long-term postoperative concerns amenable to evaluation by echocardiography include systolic and diastolic function of the systemic ventricle, valvular regurgitation, and reassessments of the bulboventricular foramen.[9-11,101,285,312] Right atrial-to-right ventricular and right-atrial-to pulmonary anastomotic sites may be incompletely visualized in adults through standard imaging planes from subcostal and high parasternal or suprasternal notch views. Biplane or multiplane TEE consistently images the Fontan anastomoses, although it may be difficult to achieve alignment that allows accurate spectral Doppler assessment of peak velocity profiles[2-4,10,13] (Fig. 6-63). Thrombus formation remains an issue, particularly in the older atriopulmonary anastomoses, but can occur in each variety of Fontan operation, particularly during atrial arrhythmias. TEE is usually required for adequate evaluation.[2,3,10,13] The typical right-atrial-to pulmonary artery anastomosis is better seen with a vertical plane equivalent, whereas a right atrial-to-right ventricular anastomosis is better seen with a horizontal plane equivalent. Assessment of lateral tunnel procedures requires both planes. Residual shunts are sought by color flow imaging and agitated saline echo contrast.

The Fontan procedure for tricuspid atresia is essentially the same as described earlier but with certain important variations. The repair may incorporate an adequately sized right ventricle. Peculiar to a Fontan repair in some patients with tricuspid atresia is a coronary sinus/left atrial defect or fenestration that may not be recognized even with intraoperative TEE. The surgeon may not see this area well, even with probe exploration. Initially small and slitlike, these defects deliver a right-to-left shunt when right atrial pressure rises and opens the defect after the Fontan repair. Postoperative cyanosis may be the first sign of a coronary sinus atrial defect.

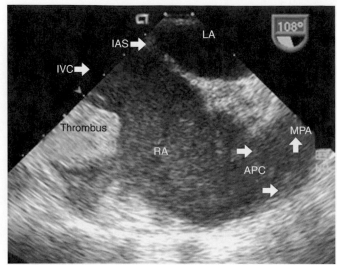

FIGURE 6-63 Atriopulmonary Fontan connection (right atrium-to-pulmonary artery) in a patient with tricuspid atresia who presented with atrial flutter and a right atrial thrombus. Transesophageal echo of a vertical plane equivalent (108 degrees on the multiplane icon) through the enlarged right atrium (RA) and atriopulmonary connection (APC). IAS, interatrial septum; IVC, inferior vena cava; LA, left atrium; MPA, main pulmonary artery.

Glenn Shunt

First used for tricuspid atresia, the classic Glenn shunt (anastomosis of the end of the right superior vena cava to the side of the right pulmonary artery, which is divided from the pulmonary trunk) has been modified and now enjoys a wider application as the bidirectional Glenn operation (superior vena caval to right pulmonary artery anastomosis without dividing the right pulmonary artery from the pulmonary trunk).[10] This modification was designed to improve systemic oxygen saturation without adding volume overload to the subaortic ventricle. Echocardiographic imaging of the bidirectional Glenn connection is achieved from right supraclavicular or suprasternal notch windows with attention to the course of the superior vena cava and to the size of the anastomosis to the right pulmonary artery.[10] TEE imaging in the vertical plane alignment (between 90 and 110 degrees on the multiplane icon) identifies the right atrium and upper stump of the superior vena cava and then, with rotation of the probe rightward, identifies the upper-mid superior vena caval anastomosis to the right pulmonary artery.[2-4,13] A combination of color flow imaging and PW Doppler profiles determines whether the anastomosis is obstructed.

Right lower lobe pulmonary arteriovenous fistulae are adverse sequelae after a classic Glenn shunt. TEE nicely identifies echo contrast returning to the left atrium through right lower lobe pulmonary veins via the pulmonary arteriovenous fistulae.[2-4,13] Prompt appearance of echo contrast in the right atrium implies azygous-venous collateral vessels to the inferior vena cava.

References

1. Child JS. Echo-Doppler and color-flow imaging in congenital heart disease. *Cardiol Clin.* 1990;8:289-313.
2. Child JS. Multiplane transesophageal echocardiography of the atria and related structures. In: Roelandt JR, Pandian N, eds. *Multiplane Transesophageal Echocardiography*. New York: Churchill-Livingstone; 1996:139-154.
3. Child JS. Multiplane transesophageal echocardiography in congenital heart disease. In: Roelandt JR, Pandian N, eds. *Multiplane Transesophageal Echocardiography*. New York: Churchill-Livingstone; 1996:173-198.
4. Marelli AJ, Child JS, Perloff JK. Transesophageal echocardiography in congenital heart disease in the adult. *Cardiol Clin.* 1993;11:505-520.
5. Snider AR, Serwer GA, Ritter SB. *Echocardiography in Pediatric Heart Disease*. 2nd ed. St. Louis: Mosby; 1997.
6. Kimball TR, Meyer RA. Echocardiography. In: Allen HD, Gutgesell HP, Clark EB, Driscoll DJ, eds. *Moss and Adams' Heart Disease in Infants, Children, and Adolescents Including the Fetus and Young Adult*. 6th ed. Philadelphia: Lippincott Williams & Wilkins; 2001:204-233.
7. Rigby ML, Horowitz ES. Cross-sectional echocardiography and Doppler. In: Anderson RH, Baker EJ, Macartney RFJ, et al., eds. *Paediatric Cardiology*. 2nd ed. London: Churchill Livingstone; 2002:379-440.
8. Therrien J. Echocardiography. In: Gatzoulis MA, Webb GD, Daubeney PEF, eds. *Diagnosis and Management of Adult Congenital Heart Disease*. London: Churchill Livingstone; 2003:35-47.
9. Aboulhosn J, Child JS. Congenital heart disease in adults. In: Fuster V, O'Rourke RA, Walsh RA, Poole-Wilson PA, eds. *Hurst's The Heart*. 12th ed. New York: McGraw-Hill; 2008:1922-1948.
10. Child JS. Echocardiographic evaluation of the adult with postoperative congenital heart disease. In: Otto CM, ed. *The Practice of Clinical Echocardiography*. 3rd ed. Philadelphia: W. B. Saunders/Elsevier; 2007:1083-1109.
11. Child JS. Congenital heart disease in the adult. *Harrison's Principles of Internal Medicine*. 17th ed. New York: McGraw-Hill; 2008:1458-1465.
12. Cetta FJ, Seward JB, O'Leary PW. Echocardiography in congenital heart disease: an overview. In: Oh JK, Seward JB, Tajik AJ, eds. *The Echo Manual*. 3rd ed. Philadelphia: Lippincott Williams & Wilkins; 2007:332-367.
13. Child JS. Transthoracic and transesophageal echocardiographic imaging: anatomic and hemodynamic assessment. In: Perloff JK, Child JS, eds. *Congenital Heart Disease in Adults*. 2nd ed. Philadelphia: W.B. Saunders; 1998:91-128.
14. Hoffman JI, Kaplan S, Liberthson RR. Prevalence of congenital heart disease. *Am Heart J*. 2004;147:425-439.
15. Hoffman JI, Kaplan S. The incidence of congenital heart disease. *J Am Coll Cardiol*. 2002;39:1890-1900.
16. Warnes CA, Liberthson R, Danielson GK, et al. Task Force 1: the changing profile of congenital heart disease in adult life. *J Am Coll Cardiol*. 2001;37:1170-1175.
17. Marelli AJ, Mackie AS, Ionescu-Ittu R, et al. Congenital heart disease in the general population: changing prevalence and age distribution. *Circulation*. 2007;115:163-172.
18. Foster E, Graham TP Jr, Driscoll DJ, et al. Task Force 2: special health care needs of adults with congenital heart disease. *J Am Coll Cardiol*. 2001;37:1176-1183.
19. Child JS, Collins-Nakai RL, Alpert JS, et al. Task Force 3: workforce description and educational requirements for the care of adults with congenital heart disease. *J Am Coll Cardiol*. 2001;37:1183-1187.
20. Perloff JK. *The Clinical Recognition of Congenital Heart Disease*. 5th ed. Philadelphia: Saunders/Elsevier; 2003.
21. Warnes CA. The adult with congenital heart disease: born to be bad? *J Am Coll Cardiol*. 2005;46:1-8.
22. Anderson RH. Anatomy. In: Anderson RH, Baker EJ, Macartney RFJ, et al., eds. *Paediatric Cardiology*. 2nd ed. London: Churchill Livingstone; 2002:37-55.

23. Anderson RH. Terminology. In: Anderson RH, Baker EJ, Macartney RFJ, et al., eds. *Paediatric Cardiology*. 2nd ed. London: Churchill Livingstone; 2002:19–36.

24. Cheitlin MD, Alpert JS, Armstrong WF, et al. ACC/AHA Guidelines for the Clinical Application of Echocardiography. A report of the American College of Cardiology/American Heart Association Task Force on Practice Guidelines (Committee on Clinical Application of Echocardiography). Developed in collaboration with the American Society of Echocardiography. *Circulation*. 1997;95:1686–1744.

25. Cheitlin MD, Alpert JS, Armstrong WF, et al. ACC/AHA guidelines for the clinical application of echocardiography: executive summary. A report of the American College of Cardiology/American Heart Association Task Force on practice guidelines (Committee on Clinical Application of Echocardiography). Developed in collaboration with the American Society of Echocardiography. *J Am Coll Cardiol*. 1997;29:862–879.

26. Cheitlin MD, Armstrong WF, Aurigemma GP, et al. ACC/AHA/ASE 2003 guideline update for the clinical application of echocardiography: summary article: a report of the American College of Cardiology/American Heart Association Task Force on Practice Guidelines (ACC/AHA/ASE Committee to Update the 1997 Guidelines for the Clinical Application of Echocardiography). *Circulation*. 2003;108:1146–1162.

27. Lai WW, Geva T, Shirali GS, et al. Guidelines and standards for performance of a pediatric echocardiogram: a report from the Task Force of the Pediatric Council of the American Society of Echocardiography. *J Am Soc Echocardiogr*. 2006;19:1413–1430.

28. Quinones MA, Douglas PS, Foster E, et al. ACC/AHA clinical competence statement on echocardiography: a report of the American College of Cardiology/American Heart Association/American College of Physicians–American Society of Internal Medicine Task Force on clinical competence. *J Am Soc Echocardiogr*. 2003;16:379–402.

29. Douglas PS, Khandheria B, Stainback RF, et al. ACCF/ASE/ACEP/ASNC/SCAI/SCCT/SCMR 2007 appropriateness criteria for transthoracic and transesophageal echocardiography: a report of the American College of Cardiology Foundation Quality Strategic Directions Committee Appropriateness Criteria Working Group, American Society of Echocardiography, American College of Emergency Physicians, American Society of Nuclear Cardiology, Society for Cardiovascular Angiography and Interventions, Society of Cardiovascular Computed Tomography, and the Society for Cardiovascular Magnetic Resonance endorsed by the American College of Chest Physicians and the Society of Critical Care Medicine. *J Am Coll Cardiol*. 2007;50:187–204.

30. Oh JK, Seward JB, Tajik AJ. Doppler echocardiography and color flow imaging: comprehensive noninvasive hemodynamic assessment. In: Oh JK, Seward JB, Tajik AJ, eds. *The Echo Manual*. 3rd ed. Philadelphia: Lippincott Williams & Wilkins; 2007:59–79.

31. Oh JK, Seward JB, Tajik AJ. Pulmonary hypertension and pulmonary vein stenosis. In: Oh JK, Seward JB, Tajik AJ, eds. *The Echo Manual*. 3rd ed. Philadelphia: Lippincott Williams & Wilkins; 2007:143–153.

32. Oh JK, Seward JB, Tajik AJ. Valvular heart disease. In: Oh JK, Seward JB, Tajik AJ, eds. *The Echo Manual*. 3rd ed. Philadelphia: Lippincott Williams & Wilkins; 2007:189–225.

33. Zoghbi WA, Enriquez-Sarano M, Foster E, et al. Recommendations for evaluation of the severity of native valvular regurgitation with two-dimensional and Doppler echocardiography. *J Am Soc Echocardiogr*. 2003;16:777–802.

34. Krivokapich J, Child JS. Role of transthoracic and transesophageal echocardiography in diagnosis and management of infective endocarditis. *Cardiol Clin*. 1996;14:363–382.

35. Click RL, Abel MD, Schaff HV. Intraoperative transesophageal echocardiography: 5-year prospective review of impact on surgical management. *Mayo Clin Proc*. 2000;75:241–247.

36. Click RL, Oh JK. Intraoperative echocardiography. In: Oh JK, Seward JB, Tajik AJ, eds. *The Echo Manual*. 3rd ed. Philadelphia: Lippincott Williams & Wilkins; 2007:368–382.

37. Mathew JP, Glas K, Troianos CA, et al. American Society of Echocardiography/Society of Cardiovascular Anesthesiologists recommendations and guidelines for continuous quality improvement in perioperative echocardiography. *J Am Soc Echocardiogr*. 2006;19:1303–1313.

38. Hansen WH, Gilman G, Finnesgard SJ, et al. The transition from an analog to a digital echocardiography laboratory: the Mayo experience. *J Am Soc Echocardiogr*. 2004;17:1214–1224.

39. Ehler D, Vacek JL, Bansal S, et al. Transition to an all-digital echocardiography laboratory: a large, multi-site private cardiology practice experience. *J Am Soc Echocardiogr*. 2000;13:1109–1116.

40. Mathewson JW, Dyar D, Jones FD, et al. Conversion to digital technology improves efficiency in the pediatric echocardiography laboratory. *J Am Soc Echocardiogr*. 2002;15:1515–1522.

41. Mathewson JW, Perry JC, Maginot KR, Cocalis M. Pediatric digital echocardiography: a study of the analog-to-digital transition. *J Am Soc Echocardiogr*. 2000;13:561–569.

42. Mohler ER 3rd, Ryan T, Segar DS, et al. Comparison of digital with videotape echocardiography in patients with chest pain in the emergency department. *J Am Soc Echocardiogr*. 1996;9:501–507.

43. Pelberg RA, Wei K, Kamiyama N, et al. Potential advantage of flash echocardiography for digital subtraction of B-mode images acquired during myocardial contrast echocardiography. *J Am Soc Echocardiogr*. 1999;12:85–93.

44. Spencer K, Solomon L, Mor-Avi V, et al. Effects of MPEG compression on the quality and diagnostic accuracy of digital echocardiography studies. *J Am Soc Echocardiogr*. 2000;13:51–57.

45. Takeuchi M, Sonoda S, Miura Y, Kuroiwa A. Reproducibility of dobutamine digital stress echocardiography. *J Am Soc Echocardiogr*. 1997;10:344–351.

46. Thomas JD, Adams DB, Devries S, et al. Guidelines and recommendations for digital echocardiography. *J Am Soc Echocardiogr*. 2005;18:287–297.

47. Thomas JD, Greenberg NL, Garcia MJ. Digital echocardiography 2002. Now is the time. *J Am Soc Echocardiogr*. 2002;15:831–838.

48. Umeda A, Iwata Y, Okada Y, et al. A low-cost digital filing system for echocardiography data with MPEG4 compression and its application to remote diagnosis. *J Am Soc Echocardiogr*. 2004;17:1297–1303.

49. Lang RM, Bierig M, Devereux RB, et al. Recommendations for chamber quantification: a report from the American Society of Echocardiography's Guidelines and Standards Committee and the Chamber Quantification Writing Group, developed in conjunction with the European Association of Echocardiography, a branch of the European Society of Cardiology. *J Am Soc Echocardiogr*. 2005;18:1440–1463.

50. Oh JK, Seward JB, Tajik AJ. Assessment of systolic function and quantification of cardiac chambers. In: Oh JK, Seward JB, Tajik AJ, eds. *The Echo Manual*. 3rd ed. Philadelphia: Lippincott Williams & Wilkins; 2007:109–119.

51. Thomas JD, Popovic ZB. Assessment of left ventricular function by cardiac ultrasound. *J Am Coll Cardiol*. 2006;48:2012–2025.

52. Buckberg GD, Weisfeldt ML, Ballester M, et al. Left ventricular form and function: scientific priorities and strategic planning for development of new views of disease. *Circulation*. 2004;110:e333–e336.

53. Sengupta PP, Korinek J, Belohlavek M, et al. Left ventricular structure and function: basic science for cardiac imaging. *J Am Coll Cardiol*. 2006;48:1988–2001.

54. Chuang ML, Hibberd MG, Salton CJ, et al. Importance of imaging method over imaging modality in noninvasive determination of left ventricular volumes and ejection fraction: assessment by two- and three-dimensional echocardiography and magnetic resonance imaging. *J Am Coll Cardiol*. 2000;35:477–484.

55. Hoffmann R, von Bardeleben S, Kasprzak JD, et al. Analysis of regional left ventricular function by cineventriculography, cardiac

magnetic resonance imaging, and unenhanced and contrast-enhanced echocardiography: a multicenter comparison of methods. *J Am Coll Cardiol*. 2006;47:121–128.

56. Sengupta PP, Khandheria BK, Korinek J, et al. Apex-to-base dispersion in regional timing of left ventricular shortening and lengthening. *J Am Coll Cardiol*. 2006;47:163–172.

57. Bleeker GB, Steendijk P, Holman ER, et al. Acquired right ventricular dysfunction. *Heart*. 2006;92(1 Suppl):i14–i18.

58. Bleeker GB, Steendijk P, Holman ER, et al. Assessing right ventricular function: the role of echocardiography and complementary technologies. *Heart*. 2006;92(1 Suppl):i19–i26.

59. Davlouros PA, Niwa K, Webb G, Gatzoulis MA. The right ventricle in congenital heart disease. *Heart*. 2006;92(1 Suppl):i27–i38.

60. Denslow S, Wiles HB. Right ventricular volumes revisited: a simple model and simple formula for echocardiographic determination. *J Am Soc Echocardiogr*. 1998;11:864–873.

61. Joyce JJ, Denslow S, Kline CH, et al. Estimation of right ventricular free-wall mass using two-dimensional echocardiography. *Pediatr Cardiol*. 2001;22:306–314.

62. Voelkel NF, Quaife RA, Leinwand LA, et al. Right ventricular function and failure: report of a National Heart, Lung, and Blood Institute working group on cellular and molecular mechanisms of right heart failure. *Circulation*. 2006;114:1883–1891.

63. Boettler P, Claus P, Herbots L, et al. New aspects of the ventricular septum and its function: an echocardiographic study. *Heart*. 2005;91:1343–1348.

64. Fogel MA, Weinberg PM, Fellows KE, et al. A study in ventricular-ventricular interaction. Single right ventricles compared with systemic right ventricles in a dual-chamber circulation. *Circulation*. 1995;92:219–230.

65. Fogel MA, Weinberg PM, Gupta KB, et al. Mechanics of the single left ventricle: a study in ventricular-ventricular interaction II. *Circulation*. 1998;98:330–338.

66. Geva T, Sandweiss BM, Gauvreau K, et al. Factors associated with impaired clinical status in long-term survivors of tetralogy of Fallot repair evaluated by magnetic resonance imaging. *J Am Coll Cardiol*. 2004;43:1068–1074.

67. Geva T, Powell AJ, Crawford EC, et al. Evaluation of regional differences in right ventricular systolic function by acoustic quantification echocardiography and cine magnetic resonance imaging. *Circulation*. 1998;98:339–345.

68. Li J, Sanders SP. Three-dimensional echocardiography in congenital heart disease. *Curr Opin Cardiol*. 1999;14:53–59.

69. Uebing A, Gibson DG, Babu-Narayan SV, et al. Right ventricular mechanics and QRS duration in patients with repaired tetralogy of Fallot: implications of infundibular disease. *Circulation*. 2007;116:1532–1539.

70. Eidem BW, O'Leary PW, Tei C, Seward JB. Usefulness of the myocardial performance index for assessing right ventricular function in congenital heart disease. *Am J Cardiol*. 2000;86:654–658.

71. Eidem BW, Tei C, O'Leary PW, et al. Nongeometric quantitative assessment of right and left ventricular function: myocardial performance index in normal children and patients with Ebstein anomaly. *J Am Soc Echocardiogr*. 1998;11:849–856.

72. Oh JK, Seward JB, Tajik AJ. Assessment of diastolic function and diastolic heart failure. In: Oh JK, Seward JB, Tajik AJ, eds. *The Echo Manual*. 3rd ed. Philadelphia: Lippincott Williams & Wilkins; 2007:120–142.

73. Perlowski AA, Aboulhosn J, Castellon Y, et al. Relation of brain natriuretic peptide to myocardial performance index in adults with congenital heart disease. *Am J Cardiol*. 2007;100:110–114.

74. Salehian O, Schwerzmann M, Merchant N, et al. Assessment of systemic right ventricular function in patients with transposition of the great arteries using the myocardial performance index: comparison with cardiac magnetic resonance imaging. *Circulation*. 2004;110:3229–3233.

75. Tei C, Dujardin KS, Hodge DO, et al. Doppler index combining systolic and diastolic myocardial performance: clinical value in cardiac amyloidosis. *J Am Coll Cardiol*. 1996;28:658–664.

76. Tei C, Ling LH, Hodge DO, et al. New index of combined systolic and diastolic myocardial performance: a simple and reproducible measure of cardiac function—a study in normals and dilated cardiomyopathy. *J Cardiol*. 1995;26:357–366.

77. Tei C, Nishimura RA, Seward JB, Tajik AJ. Noninvasive Doppler-derived myocardial performance index: correlation with simultaneous measurements of cardiac catheterization measurements. *J Am Soc Echocardiogr*. 1997;10:169–178.

78. Schwerzmann M, Samman AM, Salehian O, et al. Comparison of echocardiographic and cardiac magnetic resonance imaging for assessing right ventricular function in adults with repaired tetralogy of Fallot. *Am J Cardiol*. 2007;99:1593–1597.

79. Pai RG, Bansal RC, Shah PM. Determinants of the rate of right ventricular pressure rise by Doppler echocardiography: potential value in the assessment of right ventricular function. *J Heart Valve Dis*. 1994;3:179–184.

80. Bargiggia GS, Bertucci C, Recusani F, et al. A new method for estimating left ventricular dP/dt by continuous wave Doppler-echocardiography. Validation studies at cardiac catheterization. *Circulation*. 1989;80:1287–1292.

81. Oh JK, Hatle L, Tajik AJ, Little WC. Diastolic heart failure can be diagnosed by comprehensive two-dimensional and Doppler echocardiography. *J Am Coll Cardiol*. 2006;47:500–506.

82. Paulus WJ, Tschope C, Sanderson JE, et al. How to diagnose diastolic heart failure: a consensus statement on the diagnosis of heart failure with normal left ventricular ejection fraction by the Heart Failure and Echocardiography Associations of the European Society of Cardiology. *Eur Heart J*. 2007.

83. Zile MR, Brutsaert DL. New concepts in diastolic dysfunction and diastolic heart failure: part II: causal mechanisms and treatment. *Circulation*. 2002;105:1503–1508.

84. Zile MR, Brutsaert DL. New concepts in diastolic dysfunction and diastolic heart failure: part I: diagnosis, prognosis, and measurements of diastolic function. *Circulation*. 2002;105:1387–1393.

85. Burgess MI, Jenkins C, Sharman JE, Marwick TH. Diastolic stress echocardiography: hemodynamic validation and clinical significance of estimation of ventricular filling pressure with exercise. *J Am Coll Cardiol*. 2006;47:1891–1900.

86. De Keulenaer GW, Brutsaert DL. Diastolic heart failure: a separate disease or selection bias? *Prog Cardiovasc Dis*. 2007;49:275–283.

87. Diwan A, McCulloch M, Lawrie GM, et al. Doppler estimation of left ventricular filling pressures in patients with mitral valve disease. *Circulation*. 2005;111:3281–3289.

88. Gibson DG, Francis DP. Clinical assessment of left ventricular diastolic function. *Heart*. 2003;89:231–238.

89. Hatle L. How to diagnose diastolic heart failure a consensus statement. *Eur Heart J*. 2007;28:2421–2423.

90. Hill JC, Palma RA. Doppler tissue imaging for the assessment of left ventricular diastolic function: a systematic approach for the sonographer. *J Am Soc Echocardiogr*. 2005;18:80–88; quiz 89.

91. Ho CY, Solomon SD. A clinician's guide to tissue Doppler imaging. *Circulation*. 2006;113:e396–398.

92. Isaaz K. Tissue Doppler imaging for the assessment of left ventricular systolic and diastolic functions. *Curr Opin Cardiol*. 2002;17:431–442.

93. Moller JE, Sondergaard E, Seward JB, et al. Ratio of left ventricular peak E-wave velocity to flow propagation velocity assessed by color M-mode Doppler echocardiography in first myocardial infarction: prognostic and clinical implications. *J Am Coll Cardiol*. 2000;35:363–370.

94. Nagueh SF, Kopelen HA, Quinones MA. Assessment of left ventricular filling pressures by Doppler in the presence of atrial fibrillation. *Circulation*. 1996;94:2138–2145.

95. Ommen SR, Nishimura RA. A clinical approach to the assessment of left ventricular diastolic function by Doppler echocardiography: update 2003. *Heart*. 2003;89(3 Suppl):iii18–iii23.

96. Ommen SR, Nishimura RA, Appleton CP, et al. Clinical utility of Doppler echocardiography and tissue Doppler imaging in the estimation of left ventricular filling pressures: a comparative simultaneous Doppler-catheterization study. *Circulation.* 2000;102: 1788–1794.

97. Powell BD, Espinosa RE, Yu C-K, Oh JK. Tissue Doppler imaging, strain imaging, and dyssynchrony assessment. In: Oh JK, Seward JB, Tajik AJ, eds. *The Echo Manual.* 3rd ed. Philadelphia: Lippincott Williams & Wilkins; 2007:80–98.

98. Yu CM, Sanderson JE, Marwick TH, Oh JK. Tissue Doppler imaging a new prognosticator for cardiovascular diseases. *J Am Coll Cardiol.* 2007;49:1903–1914.

99. Abhayaratna WP, Seward JB, Appleton CP, et al. Left atrial size: physiologic determinants and clinical applications. *J Am Coll Cardiol.* 2006;47:2357–2363.

100. Tsang TS, Abhayaratna WP, Barnes ME, et al. Prediction of cardiovascular outcomes with left atrial size: is volume superior to area or diameter? *J Am Coll Cardiol.* 2006;47:1018–1023.

101. DiSessa TG, Child JS, Perloff JK, et al. Systemic venous and pulmonary arterial flow patterns after Fontan's procedure for tricuspid atresia or single ventricle. *Circulation.* 1984;70:898–902.

102. Nagueh SF, Kopelen HA, Zoghbi WA. Relation of mean right atrial pressure to echocardiographic and Doppler parameters of right atrial and right ventricular function. *Circulation.* 1996;93:1160–1169.

103. Tede NH, Child JS. Diastolic dysfunction in patients with congenital heart disease. *Cardiol Clin.* 2000;18:491–499.

104. Sohn DW, Chai IH, Lee DJ, et al. Assessment of mitral annulus velocity by Doppler tissue imaging in the evaluation of left ventricular diastolic function. *J Am Coll Cardiol.* 1997;30:474–480.

105. Sohn DW, Kim YJ, Park YB, Choi YS. Clinical validity of measuring time difference between onset of mitral inflow and onset of early diastolic mitral annulus velocity in the evaluation of left ventricular diastolic function. *J Am Coll Cardiol.* 2004;43:2097–2101.

106. Kasner M, Westermann D, Steendijk P, et al. Utility of Doppler echocardiography and tissue Doppler imaging in the estimation of diastolic function in heart failure with normal ejection fraction: a comparative Doppler-conductance catheterization study. *Circulation.* 2007;116:637–647.

107. Wang M, Yip G, Yu CM, et al. Independent and incremental prognostic value of early mitral annulus velocity in patients with impaired left ventricular systolic function. *J Am Coll Cardiol.* 2005;45:272–277.

108. Brili S, Alexopoulos N, Latsios G, et al. Tissue Doppler imaging and brain natriuretic peptide levels in adults with repaired tetralogy of Fallot. *J Am Soc Echocardiogr.* 2005;18:1149–1154.

109. Sade LE, Gulmez O, Eroglu S, et al. Noninvasive estimation of right ventricular filling pressure by ratio of early tricuspid inflow to annular diastolic velocity in patients with and without recent cardiac surgery. *J Am Soc Echocardiogr.* 2007;20:982–988.

110. Puranik R, Greaves K, Hawker RE, et al. Abnormal right ventricular tissue velocities after repair of congenital heart disease—implications for late outcomes. *Heart Lung Circ.* 2007;16:295–299.

111. Cheung MM, Smallhorn JF, McCrindle BW, et al. Non-invasive assessment of ventricular force-frequency relations in the univentricular circulation by tissue Doppler echocardiography: a novel method of assessing myocardial performance in congenital heart disease. *Heart.* 2005;91:1338–1342.

112. Frigiola A, Redington AN, Cullen S, Vogel M. Pulmonary regurgitation is an important determinant of right ventricular contractile dysfunction in patients with surgically repaired tetralogy of Fallot. *Circulation.* 2004;110(1 Suppl):II153–II157.

113. Hashimoto I, Li XK, Bhat AH, et al. Quantitative assessment of regional peak myocardial acceleration during isovolumic contraction and relaxation times by tissue Doppler imaging. *Heart.* 2005;91:811–816.

114. Vogel M, Cheung MM, Li J, et al. Noninvasive assessment of left ventricular force-frequency relationships using tissue Doppler-derived isovolumic acceleration: validation in an animal model. *Circulation.* 2003;107:1647–1652.

115. Vogel M, Derrick G, White PA, et al. Systemic ventricular function in patients with transposition of the great arteries after atrial repair: a tissue Doppler and conductance catheter study. *J Am Coll Cardiol.* 2004;43:100–106.

116. Vogel M, Schmidt MR, Kristiansen SB, et al. Validation of myocardial acceleration during isovolumic contraction as a novel noninvasive index of right ventricular contractility: comparison with ventricular pressure-volume relations in an animal model. *Circulation.* 2002;105:1693–1699.

117. Hashimoto I, Li X, Hejmadi Bhat A, et al. Myocardial strain rate is a superior method for evaluation of left ventricular subendocardial function compared with tissue Doppler imaging. *J Am Coll Cardiol.* 2003;42:1574–1583.

118. Marwick TH. Measurement of strain and strain rate by echocardiography: ready for prime time? *J Am Coll Cardiol.* 2006;47:1313–1327.

119. Jamal F, Bergerot C, Argaud L, et al. Longitudinal strain quantitates regional right ventricular contractile function. *Am J Physiol Heart Circ Physiol.* 2003;285:H2842–H2847.

120. Weidemann F, Eyskens B, Mertens L, et al. Quantification of regional right and left ventricular function by ultrasonic strain rate and strain indexes after surgical repair of tetralogy of Fallot. *Am J Cardiol.* 2002;90:133–138.

121. Gatzoulis MA, Balaji S, Webber SA, et al. Risk factors for arrhythmia and sudden cardiac death late after repair of tetralogy of Fallot: a multicentre study. *Lancet.* 2000;356:975–981.

122. Vogel M, Sponring J, Cullen S, et al. Regional wall motion and abnormalities of electrical depolarization and repolarization in patients after surgical repair of tetralogy of Fallot. *Circulation.* 2001;103:1669–1673.

123. Helle-Valle T, Crosby J, Edvardsen T, et al. New noninvasive method for assessment of left ventricular rotation: speckle tracking echocardiography. *Circulation.* 2005;112:3149–3156.

124. Notomi Y, Martin-Miklovic MG, Oryszak SJ, et al. Enhanced ventricular untwisting during exercise: a mechanistic manifestation of elastic recoil described by Doppler tissue imaging. *Circulation.* 2006;113:2524–2533.

125. Notomi Y, Srinath G, Shiota T, et al. Maturational and adaptive modulation of left ventricular torsional biomechanics: Doppler tissue imaging observation from infancy to adulthood. *Circulation.* 2006;113:2534–2541.

126. Notomi Y, Lysyansky P, Setser RM, et al. Measurement of ventricular torsion by two-dimensional ultrasound speckle tracking imaging. *J Am Coll Cardiol.* 2005;45:2034–2041.

127. Gotte MJ, Germans T, Russel IK, et al. Myocardial strain and torsion quantified by cardiovascular magnetic resonance tissue tagging: studies in normal and impaired left ventricular function. *J Am Coll Cardiol.* 2006;48:2002–2011.

128. Foster E, Lease KE. New untwist on diastole: what goes around comes back. *Circulation.* 2006;113:2477–2479.

129. Cannesson M, Tanabe M, Suffoletto MS, et al. Velocity vector imaging to quantify ventricular dyssynchrony and predict response to cardiac resynchronization therapy. *Am J Cardiol.* 2006;98:949–953.

130. Rajagopalan N, Dohi K, Simon MA, et al. Right ventricular dyssynchrony in heart failure: a tissue Doppler imaging study. *J Card Fail.* 2006;12:263–267.

131. Suffoletto MS, Dohi K, Cannesson M, et al. Novel speckle-tracking radial strain from routine black-and-white echocardiographic images to quantify dyssynchrony and predict response to cardiac resynchronization therapy. *Circulation.* 2006;113:960–968.

132. Lahmers S, Wu Y, Call DR, et al. Developmental control of titin isoform expression and passive stiffness in fetal and neonatal myocardium. *Circ Res.* 2004;94:505–513.

133. Siedner S, Kruger M, Schroeter M, et al. Developmental changes in contractility and sarcomeric proteins from the early embryonic to the adult stage in the mouse heart. *J Physiol.* 2003;548:493–505.

134. Katz AM, Zile MR. New molecular mechanism in diastolic heart failure. *Circulation.* 2006;113:1922–1925.

135. van Heerebeek L, Borbely A, Niessen HW, et al. Myocardial structure and function differ in systolic and diastolic heart failure. *Circulation.* 2006;113:1966–1973.

136. Senzaki H, Akagi M, Hishi T, et al. Age-associated changes in arterial elastic properties in children. *Eur J Pediatr.* 2002;161:547–551.

137. Safar ME, Levy BI, Struijker-Boudier H. Current perspectives on arterial stiffness and pulse pressure in hypertension and cardiovascular diseases. *Circulation.* 2003;107:2864–2869.

138. Safar ME, Boudier HS. Vascular development, pulse pressure, and the mechanisms of hypertension. *Hypertension.* 2005;46:205–209.

139. O'Rourke MF, Nichols WW. Aortic diameter, aortic stiffness, and wave reflection increase with age and isolated systolic hypertension. *Hypertension.* 2005;45:652–658.

140. Zieman SJ, Melenovsky V, Kass DA. Mechanisms, pathophysiology, and therapy of arterial stiffness. *Arterioscler Thromb Vasc Biol.* 2005;25:932–943.

141. Fellows KE, Fogel M, Weinberg PM. Three-dimensional reconstruction of MR images in congenital heart disease. *Acta Paediatr Suppl.* 1995;410:60–62.

142. Fellows KE, Fogel MA. MR imaging and heart function in patients pre- and post-Fontan surgery. *Acta Paediatr Suppl.* 1995;410:57–59.

143. Fenchel M, Saleh R, Dinh H, et al. Juvenile and adult congenital heart disease: time-resolved 3D contrast-enhanced MR angiography. *Radiology.* 2007;244:399–410.

144. Finn JP, Saleh R, Thesen S, et al. MR imaging with remote control: feasibility study in cardiovascular disease. *Radiology.* 2006;241:528–537.

145. Fogel MA, Gupta KB, Weinberg PM, Hoffman EA. Regional wall motion and strain analysis across stages of Fontan reconstruction by magnetic resonance tagging. *Am J Physiol.* 1995;269:H1132–1152.

146. Oh JK, Hagler DJ, Cabalka A, et al. Transesophageal and intracardiac echocardiography. In: Oh JK, Seward JB, Tajik AJ, eds. *The Echo Manual.* 3rd ed. Philadelphia: Lippincott Williams & Wilkins; 2007:29–58.

147. Oh JK, Seward JB, Tajik AJ. Transthoracic echocardiography: M-mode, two-dimensional, and three-dimensional. In: Oh JK, Seward JB, Tajik AJ, eds. *The Echo Manual.* 3rd ed. Philadelphia: Lippincott Williams & Wilkins; 2007:7–28.

148. Lang RM, Mor-Avi V, Sugeng L, et al. Three-dimensional echocardiography: the benefits of the additional dimension. *J Am Coll Cardiol.* 2006;48:2053–2069.

149. Handke M, Heinrichs G, Moser U, et al. Transesophageal real-time three-dimensional echocardiography methods and initial in vitro and human in vivo studies. *J Am Coll Cardiol.* 2006;48:2070–2076.

150. Corsi C, Lang RM, Veronesi F, et al. Volumetric quantification of global and regional left ventricular function from real-time three-dimensional echocardiographic images. *Circulation.* 2005;112:1161–1170.

151. Grison A, Maschietto N, Reffo E, et al. Three-dimensional echocardiographic evaluation of right ventricular volume and function in pediatric patients: validation of the technique. *J Am Soc Echocardiogr.* 2007;20:921–929.

152. Jaochim Nesser H, Sugeng L, et al. Volumetric analysis of regional left ventricular function with real-time three-dimensional echocardiography: validation by magnetic resonance and clinical utility testing. *Heart.* 2007;93:572–578.

153. Kapetanakis S, Kearney MT, Siva A, et al. Real-time three-dimensional echocardiography: a novel technique to quantify global left ventricular mechanical dyssynchrony. *Circulation.* 2005;112:992–1000.

154. Niemann PS, Pinho L, Balbach T, et al. Anatomically oriented right ventricular volume measurements with dynamic three-dimensional echocardiography validated by 3-Tesla magnetic resonance imaging. *J Am Coll Cardiol.* 2007;50:1668–1676.

155. Lu X, Nadvoretskiy V, Bu L, et al. Accuracy and reproducibility of real-time 3-dimensional echocardiography for assessment of right ventricular volumes and ejection fraction in children. *J Am Soc Echocardiogr.* 2008;20:84–89.

156. Barrea C, Levasseur S, Roman K, et al. Three-dimensional echocardiography improves the understanding of left atrioventricular valve morphology and function in atrioventricular septal defects undergoing patch augmentation. *J Thorac Cardiovasc Surg.* 2005;129:746–753.

157. Espinola-Zavaleta N, Munoz-Castellanos L, et al. Anatomic three-dimensional echocardiographic correlation of bicuspid aortic valve. *J Am Soc Echocardiogr.* 2003;16:46–53.

158. Fukuda S, Saracino G, Matsumura Y, et al. Three-dimensional geometry of the tricuspid annulus in healthy subjects and in patients with functional tricuspid regurgitation: a real-time, 3-dimensional echocardiographic study. *Circulation.* 2006;114(1 Suppl):I492–I498.

159. Garcia-Orta R, Moreno E, Vidal M, et al. Three-dimensional versus two-dimensional transesophageal echocardiography in mitral valve repair. *J Am Soc Echocardiogr.* 2007;20:4–12.

160. Pepi M, Tamborini G, Maltagliati A, et al. Head-to-head comparison of two- and three-dimensional transthoracic and transesophageal echocardiography in the localization of mitral valve prolapse. *J Am Coll Cardiol.* 2006;48:2524–2530.

161. Sharma R, Mann J, Drummond L, et al. The evaluation of real-time 3-dimensional transthoracic echocardiography for the preoperative functional assessment of patients with mitral valve prolapse: a comparison with 2-dimensional transesophageal echocardiography. *J Am Soc Echocardiogr.* 2007;20:934–940.

162. van den Bosch AE, Ten Harkel DJ, McGhie JS, et al. Surgical validation of real-time transthoracic 3D echocardiographic assessment of atrioventricular septal defects. *Int J Cardiol.* 2006;112:213–218.

163. Zamorano J, Cordeiro P, Sugeng L, et al. Real-time three-dimensional echocardiography for rheumatic mitral valve stenosis evaluation: an accurate and novel approach. *J Am Coll Cardiol.* 2004;43:2091–2096.

164. Sinha A, Kasliwal RR, Nanda NC, et al. Live three-dimensional transthoracic echocardiographic assessment of isolated cleft mitral valve. *Echocardiography.* 2004;21:657–661.

165. Khanna D, Vengala S, Miller AP, et al. Quantification of mitral regurgitation by live three-dimensional transthoracic echocardiographic measurements of vena contracta area. *Echocardiography.* 2004;21:737–743.

166. Hsu JH, Wu JR, Dai ZK, Lee MH. Real-time three-dimensional echocardiography provides novel and useful anatomic insights of perimembranous ventricular septal aneurysm. *Int J Cardiol.* 2007;118:326–331.

167. Pepi M, Tamborini G, Bartorelli AL, et al. Usefulness of three-dimensional echocardiographic reconstruction of the Amplatzer septal occluder in patients undergoing atrial septal closure. *Am J Cardiol.* 2004;94:1343–1347.

168. van den Bosch AE, van Dijk VF, McGhie JS, et al. Real-time transthoracic three-dimensional echocardiography provides additional information of left-sided AV valve morphology after AVSD repair. *Int J Cardiol.* 2006;106:360–364.

169. Mehmood F, Vengala S, Nanda NC, et al. Usefulness of live three-dimensional transthoracic echocardiography in the characterization of atrial septal defects in adults. *Echocardiography.* 2004;21:707–713.

170. Lu X, Nadvoretskiy V, Klas B, et al. Measurement of volumetric flow by real-time 3-dimensional Doppler echocardiography in children. *J Am Soc Echocardiogr.* 2007;20:915–920.

171. Baweja G, Nanda NC, Kirklin JK. Definitive diagnosis of cor triatriatum with common atrium by three-dimensional transesophageal echocardiography in an adult. *Echocardiography.* 2004;21:303–306.

172. Ilgenli TF, Nanda NC, Sinha A, Khanna D. Live three-dimensional transthoracic echocardiographic assessment of anomalous origin of left coronary artery from the pulmonary artery. *Echocardiography.* 2004;21:559–562.

173. Miyashita M, Karasawa K, Taniguchi K, et al. Usefulness of real-time 3-dimensional echocardiography for the evaluation of coronary artery morphology in patients with Kawasaki disease. *J Am Soc Echocardiogr.* 2007;20:930–933.

174. Del Pasqua A, Sanders SP, Rinelli G. Three-dimensional echocardiography in criss-cross heart: could a specimen be better? *Circulation.* 2007;116:3414–e3415.

175. Omran AS, Woo A, David TE, et al. Intraoperative transesophageal echocardiography accurately predicts mitral valve anatomy and suitability for repair. *J Am Soc Echocardiogr.* 2002;15:950–957.

176. Webb G, Gatzoulis MA. Atrial septal defects in the adult: recent progress and overview. *Circulation.* 2006;114:1645–1653.

177. Munoz-Castellanos L, Espinola-Zavaleta N, Kuri-Nivon M, et al. Atrial septal defect: anatomoechocardiographic correlation. *J Am Soc Echocardiogr.* 2006;19:1182–1189.

178. Attenhofer Jost CH, Connolly HM, et al. Sinus venosus atrial septal defect: long-term postoperative outcome for 115 patients. *Circulation.* 2005;112:1953–1958.

179. Melduni RM, Mookadam F, Mookadam M, et al. Images in cardiovascular medicine. Scimitar syndrome: complete diagnosis by transthoracic echocardiography. *Circulation.* 2006;114:e373–375.

180. Eerola A, Pihkala JI, Boldt T, et al. Hemodynamic improvement is faster after percutaneous ASD closure than after surgery. *Catheter Cardiovasc Interv.* 2007;69:432–441; discussion 442.

181. Salehian O, Horlick E, Schwerzmann M, et al. Improvements in cardiac form and function after transcatheter closure of secundum atrial septal defects. *J Am Coll Cardiol.* 2005;45:499–504.

182. Pascotto M, Santoro G, Cerrato F, et al. Time-course of cardiac remodeling following transcatheter closure of atrial septal defect. *Int J Cardiol.* 2006;112:348–352.

183. Thilen U, Persson S. Closure of atrial septal defect in the adult. Cardiac remodeling is an early event. *Int J Cardiol.* 2006;108:370–375.

184. Cheng TO, Xie MX, Wang XF, et al. Real-time 3-dimensional echocardiography in assessing atrial and ventricular septal defects: an echocardiographic-surgical correlative study. *Am Heart J.* 2004;148:1091–1095.

185. Linguraru MG, Kabla A, Marx GR, et al. Real-time tracking and shape analysis of atrial septal defects in 3D echocardiography. *Acad Radiol.* 2007;14:1298–1309.

186. Minette MS, Sahn DJ. Ventricular septal defects. *Circulation.* 2006;114:2190–2197.

187. Kardon RE, Cao QL, Masani N, et al. New insights and observations in three-dimensional echocardiographic visualization of ventricular septal defects: experimental and clinical studies. *Circulation.* 1998;98:1307–1314.

188. van den Bosch AE, Ten Harkel DJ, McGhie JS, et al. Feasibility and accuracy of real-time 3-dimensional echocardiographic assessment of ventricular septal defects. *J Am Soc Echocardiogr.* 2006;19:7–13.

189. Mercer-Rosa L, Seliem MA, Fedec A, et al. Illustration of the additional value of real-time 3-dimensional echocardiography to conventional transthoracic and transesophageal 2-dimensional echocardiography in imaging muscular ventricular septal defects: does this have any impact on individual patient treatment? *J Am Soc Echocardiogr.* 2006;19:1511–1519.

190. Sabry AF, Reller MD, Silberbach GM, et al. Comparison of four Doppler echocardiographic methods for calculating pulmonary-to-systemic shunt flow ratios in patients with ventricular septal defect. *Am J Cardiol.* 1995;75:611–614.

191. Moises VA, Maciel BC, Hornberger LK, et al. A new method for noninvasive estimation of ventricular septal defect shunt flow by Doppler color flow mapping: imaging of the laminar flow convergence region on the left septal surface. *J Am Coll Cardiol.* 1991;18:824–832.

192. Karr SS. New Doppler techniques for the evaluation of regurgitant and shunt volumes. *Curr Opin Cardiol.* 1998;13:56–58.

193. Kurotobi S, Sano T, Matsushita T, et al. Quantitative, non-invasive assessment of ventricular septal defect shunt flow by measuring proximal isovelocity surface area on colour Doppler mapping. *Heart.* 1997;78:305–309.

194. Ishii M, Hashino K, Eto G, et al. Quantitative assessment of severity of ventricular septal defect by three-dimensional reconstruction of color Doppler-imaged vena contracta and flow convergence region. *Circulation.* 2001;103:664–669.

195. Lindblade CL, Schamberger MS, Darragh RK, Cordes TM. Use of peak Doppler gradient across ventricular septal defect leads to underestimation of right-sided pressures in a patient with M-shaped Doppler signal: a case report. *J Am Soc Echocardiogr.* 2004;17:1207–1209.

196. Schamberger MS, Farrell AG, Darragh RK, et al. Use of peak Doppler gradient across ventricular septal defects leads to underestimation of right-sided pressures in patients with "sloped" Doppler signals. *J Am Soc Echocardiogr.* 2001;14:1197–1202.

197. Miyake T, Shinohara T, Nakamura Y, et al. Aneurysm of the ventricular membranous septum: serial echocardiographic studies. *Pediatr Cardiol.* 2004;25:385–389.

198. Eroglu AG, Oztunc F, Saltik L, et al. Aortic valve prolapse and aortic regurgitation in patients with ventricular septal defect. *Pediatr Cardiol.* 2003;24:36–39.

199. Saleeb SF, Solowiejczyk DE, Glickstein JS, et al. Frequency of development of aortic cuspal prolapse and aortic regurgitation in patients with subaortic ventricular septal defect diagnosed at <1 year of age. *Am J Cardiol.* 2007;99:1588–1592.

200. Tomita H, Arakaki Y, Ono Y, et al. Impact of noncoronary cusp prolapse in addition to right coronary cusp prolapse in patients with a perimembranous ventricular septal defect. *Int J Cardiol.* 2005;101:279–283.

201. Horta Mda G, Faria CA, Rezende DF, et al. Subaortic stenosis associated with perimembranous ventricular septal defect. Clinical follow-up of 36 patients. *Arq Bras Cardiol.* 2005;84:103–107.

202. Lim DS, Ensing GJ, Ludomirsky A, et al. Echocardiographic predictors for the development of subaortic stenosis after repair of atrioventricular septal defect. *Am J Cardiol.* 2003;91:900–903.

203. Kitchiner D, Jackson M, Malaiya N, et al. Morphology of left ventricular outflow tract structures in patients with subaortic stenosis and a ventricular septal defect. *Br Heart J.* 1994;72:251–260.

204. Kleinert S, Geva T. Echocardiographic morphometry and geometry of the left ventricular outflow tract in fixed subaortic stenosis. *J Am Coll Cardiol.* 1993;22:1501–1508.

205. Gupta SR, Reddy KN, Gupta SK, et al. Subaortic stenosis associated with anomalous right ventricular muscle bundle and ventricular septal defect. *Indian Heart J.* 1989;41:203–205.

206. Freedom RM, Pelech A, Brand A, et al. The progressive nature of subaortic stenosis in congenital heart disease. *Int J Cardiol.* 1985;8:137–148.

207. Chung KJ, Fulton DR, Kreidberg MB, et al. Combined discrete subaortic stenosis and ventricular septal defect in infants and children. *Am J Cardiol.* 1984;53:1429–1432.

208. Vogel M, Freedom RM, Brand A, et al. Ventricular septal defect and subaortic stenosis: an analysis of 41 patients. *Am J Cardiol.* 1983;52:1258–1263.

209. Fisher DJ, Snider AR, Silverman NH, Stanger P. Ventricular septal defect with silent discrete subaortic stenosis. *Pediatr Cardiol.* 1982;2:265–269.

210. Baumstark A, Fellows KE, Rosenthal A. Combined double chambered right ventricle and discrete subaortic stenosis. *Circulation.* 1978;57:299–303.

211. Kleinman CS, Tabibian M, Starc TJ, et al. Spontaneous regression of left ventricular dilation in children with restrictive ventricular septal defects. *J Pediatr.* 2007;150:583–586.

212. Bialkowski J, Szkutnik M, Kusa J, et al. Transcatheter closure of postinfarction ventricular septal defects using Amplatzer devices. *Rev Esp Cardiol.* 2007;60:548–551.

213. Bialkowski J, Szkutnik M, Zembala M. Ventricular septal defect closure—importance of cardiac surgery and transcatheter intervention. *Kardiol Pol.* 2007;65:1022–1024.

214. Szkutnik M, Qureshi SA, Kusa J, et al. Use of the Amplatzer muscular ventricular septal defect occluder for closure of perimembranous ventricular septal defects. *Heart.* 2007;93:355–358.

215. Schneider DJ, Moore JW. Patent ductus arteriosus. *Circulation.* 2006;114:1873–1882.

216. Becker TE, Ensing GJ, Darragh RK, Caldwell RL. Doppler derivation of complete pulmonary artery pressure curves in patent ductus arteriosus. *Am J Cardiol.* 1996;78:1066–1069.

217. Yan C, Zhao S, Jiang S, et al. Transcatheter closure of patent ductus arteriosus with severe pulmonary arterial hypertension in adults. *Heart.* 2007;93:514–518.

218. Eerola A, Jokinen E, Boldt T, Pihkala J. The influence of percutaneous closure of patent ductus arteriosus on left ventricular size and function: a prospective study using two- and three-dimensional echocardiography and measurements of serum natriuretic peptides. *J Am Coll Cardiol.* 2006;47:1060–1066.

219. Jeong YH, Yun TJ, Song JM, et al. Left ventricular remodeling and change of systolic function after closure of patent ductus arteriosus in adults: device and surgical closure. *Am Heart J.* 2007;154: 436–440.

220. Moustafa S, Mookadam F, Cooper L, et al. Sinus of Valsalva aneurysms—47 years of a single center experience and systematic overview of published reports. *Am J Cardiol.* 2007;99:1159–1164.

221. Angelini P. Coronary artery anomalies: an entity in search of an identity. *Circulation.* 2007;115:1296–1305.

222. Gowda RM, Vasavada BC, Khan IA. Coronary artery fistulas: clinical and therapeutic considerations. *Int J Cardiol.* 2006;107:7–10.

223. Krishnamoorthy KM, Rao S. Transesophageal echocardiography for the diagnosis of coronary arteriovenous fistula. *Int J Cardiol.* 2004;96:281–283.

224. Lin FC, Chang HJ, Chern MS, et al. Multiplane transesophageal echocardiography in the diagnosis of congenital coronary artery fistula. *Am Heart J.* 1995;130:1236–1244.

225. Cox ID, Heald SC, Murday AJ. Value of transoesophageal echocardiography in surgical ligation of coronary artery fistulas. *Heart.* 1996;76:181–182.

226. Vitarelli A, De Curtis G, Conde Y, et al. Assessment of congenital coronary artery fistulas by transesophageal color Doppler echocardiography. *Am J Med.* 2002;113:127–133.

227. Chen SJ, Lin MT, Lee WJ, et al. Coronary artery anatomy in children with congenital heart disease by computed tomography. *Int J Cardiol.* 2007;120:363–370.

228. Mavrogeni S, Spargias K, Karagiannis S, et al. Anomalous origin of right coronary artery: magnetic resonance angiography and viability study. *Int J Cardiol.* 2006;109:195–200.

229. Casolo G, Del Meglio J, Rega L, et al. Detection and assessment of coronary artery anomalies by three-dimensional magnetic resonance coronary angiography. *Int J Cardiol.* 2005;103:317–322.

230. Roberts WC. The congenitally bicuspid aortic valve. A study of 85 autopsy cases. *Am J Cardiol.* 1970;26:72–83.

231. Aboulhosn J, Child JS. Left ventricular outflow obstruction: subaortic stenosis, bicuspid aortic valve, supravalvar aortic stenosis, and coarctation of the aorta. *Circulation.* 2006;114:2412–2422.

232. Nistri S, Basso C, Marzari C, et al. Frequency of bicuspid aortic valve in young male conscripts by echocardiogram. *Am J Cardiol.* 2005;96:718–721.

233. Roberts WC, Ko JM. Frequency by decades of unicuspid, bicuspid, and tricuspid aortic valves in adults having isolated aortic valve replacement for aortic stenosis, with or without associated aortic regurgitation. *Circulation.* 2005;111:920–925.

234. Roberts WC, Ko JM, Hamilton C. Comparison of valve structure, valve weight, and severity of the valve obstruction in 1849 patients having isolated aortic valve replacement for aortic valve stenosis (with or without associated aortic regurgitation) studied at 3 different medical centers in 2 different time periods. *Circulation.* 2005;112: 3919–3929.

235. Lewin MB, Otto CM. The bicuspid aortic valve: adverse outcomes from infancy to old age. *Circulation.* 2005;111:832–834.

236. Lamas CC, Eykyn SJ. Bicuspid aortic valve—a silent danger: analysis of 50 cases of infective endocarditis. *Clin Infect Dis.* 2000;30: 336–341.

237. Saw A, Aboulhosn J, Kim PJ, et al. Increased risk of infective endocarditis in adults with tetralogy of Fallot and bicuspid aortic valve disease. *Circulation.* 2007;116:II-463.

238. Ward C. Clinical significance of the bicuspid aortic valve. *Heart.* 2000;83:81–85.

239. Osler W. The bicuspid condition of the aortic valves. *Trans Assoc Am Physicians.* 1886;2:185–192.

240. Niwa K, Perloff JK, Bhuta SM, et al. Structural abnormalities of great arterial walls in congenital heart disease: light and electron microscopic analyses. *Circulation.* 2001;103:393–400.

241. Nkomo VT, Enriquez-Sarano M, Ammash NM, et al. Bicuspid aortic valve associated with aortic dilatation: a community-based study. *Arterioscler Thromb Vasc Biol.* 2003;23:351–356.

242. Cecconi M, Manfrin M, Moraca A, et al. Aortic dimensions in patients with bicuspid aortic valve without significant valve dysfunction. *Am J Cardiol.* 2005;95:292–294.

243. Keane MG, Wiegers SE, Plappert T, et al. Bicuspid aortic valves are associated with aortic dilatation out of proportion to coexistent valvular lesions. *Circulation.* 2000;102(19 Suppl 3):III35–III39.

244. Morgan-Hughes GJ, Roobottom CA, Owens PE, Marshall AJ. Dilatation of the aorta in pure, severe, bicuspid aortic valve stenosis. *Am Heart J.* 2004;147:736–740.

245. Morgan-Hughes GJ, Roobottom CA. Aortic valve calcification on computed tomography predicts the severity of aortic stenosis. *Clin Radiol.* 2004;59:208; author reply 208–209.

246. Ben-Dor I, Sagie A, Weisenberg D, Ben Zekry S, et al. Comparison of diameter of ascending aorta in patients with severe aortic stenosis secondary to congenital versus degenerative versus rheumatic etiologies. *Am J Cardiol.* 2005;96:1549–1552.

247. Nistri S, Sorbo MD, Marin M, et al. Aortic root dilatation in young men with normally functioning bicuspid aortic valves. *Heart.* 1999;82:19–22.

248. Ferencik M, Pape LA. Changes in size of ascending aorta and aortic valve function with time in patients with congenitally bicuspid aortic valves. *Am J Cardiol.* 2003;92:43–46.

249. Alegret JM, Duran I, Palazon O, et al. Prevalence of and predictors of bicuspid aortic valves in patients with dilated aortic roots. *Am J Cardiol.* 2003;91:619–622.

250. Novaro GM, Tiong IY, Pearce GL, et al. Features and predictors of ascending aortic dilatation in association with a congenital bicuspid aortic valve. *Am J Cardiol.* 2003;92:99–101.

251. Beppu S, Suzuki S, Matsuda H, et al. Rapidity of progression of aortic stenosis in patients with congenital bicuspid aortic valves. *Am J Cardiol.* 1993;71:322–327.

252. Bonow RO, Carabello BA, Kanu C, et al. ACC/AHA 2006 guidelines for the management of patients with valvular heart disease: a report of the American College of Cardiology/American Heart Association Task Force on Practice Guidelines (writing committee to revise the 1998 Guidelines for the Management of Patients with Valvular Heart Disease): developed in collaboration with the Society of Cardiovascular Anesthesiologists: endorsed by the Society for Cardiovascular Angiography and Interventions and the Society of Thoracic Surgeons. *Circulation.* 2006;114:e84–e231.

253. Donal E, Novaro GM, Deserrano D, et al. Planimetric assessment of anatomic valve area overestimates effective orifice area in bicuspid aortic stenosis. *J Am Soc Echocardiogr.* 2005;18: 1392–1398.

254. Otto CM. Valvular aortic stenosis: disease severity and timing of intervention. *J Am Coll Cardiol.* 2006;47:2141–2151.

255. Ahmed S, Honos GN, Walling AD, et al. Clinical outcome and echo-cardiographic predictors of aortic valve replacement in patients with bicuspid aortic valve. *J Am Soc Echocardiogr*. 2007;20:998–1003.

256. Pachulski RT, Chan KL. Progression of aortic valve dysfunction in 51 adult patients with congenital bicuspid aortic valve: assessment and follow-up by Doppler echocardiography. *Br Heart J*. 1993;69: 237–240.

257. Sabet HY, Edwards WD, Tazelaar HD, Daly RC. Congenitally bi-cuspid aortic valves: a surgical pathology study of 542 cases (1991 through 1996) and a literature review of 2,715 additional cases. *Mayo Clin Proc*. 1999;74:14–26.

258. Warnes CA. Bicuspid aortic valve and coarctation: two villains part of a diffuse problem. *Heart*. 2003;89:965–966.

259. Roos-Hesselink JW, Scholzel BE, Heijdra RJ, et al. Aortic valve and aortic arch pathology after coarctation repair. *Heart*. 2003;89: 1074–1077.

260. Oliver JM, Gallego P, Gonzalez A, et al. Risk factors for aortic com-plications in adults with coarctation of the aorta. *J Am Coll Cardiol*. 2004;44:1641–1647.

261. Vriend JW, Mulder BJ. Late complications in patients after repair of aortic coarctation: implications for management. *Int J Cardiol*. 2005;101:399–406.

262. Celermajer DS, Greaves K. Survivors of coarctation repair: fixed but not cured. *Heart*. 2002;88:113–114.

263. Latson LA, Prieto LR. Congenital and acquired pulmonary vein stenosis. *Circulation*. 2007;115:103–108.

264. Attie F, Rosas M, Rijlaarsdam M, et al. The adult patient with Eb-stein anomaly. Outcome in 72 unoperated patients. *Medicine (Baltimore)*. 2000;79:27–36.

265. Kapusta L, Eveleigh RM, Poulino SE, et al. Ebstein's anomaly: fac-tors associated with death in childhood and adolescence: a multi-centre, long-term study. *Eur Heart J*. 2007;28:2661–2666.

266. Seward JB. Ebstein's anomaly: ultrasound imaging and hemody-namic evaluation. *Echocardiography*. 1993;10:641–664.

267. Attenhofer Jost CH, Connolly HM, Dearani JA, et al. Ebstein's anomaly. *Circulation*. 2007;115:277–285.

268. Shiina A, Seward JB, Edwards WD, et al. Two-dimensional echo-cardiographic spectrum of Ebstein's anomaly: detailed anatomic assessment. *J Am Coll Cardiol*. 1984;3:356–370.

269. Benson LN, Child JS, Schwaiger M, et al. Left ventricular geometry and function in adults with Ebstein's anomaly of the tricuspid valve. *Circulation*. 1987;75:353–359.

270. Child JS, Perloff JK, Francoz R, et al. Uhl's anomaly (parchment right ventricle): clinical, echocardiographic, radionuclear, hemo-dynamic and angiocardiographic features in 2 patients. *Am J Car-diol*. 1984;53:635–637.

271. Bashore TM. Adult congenital heart disease: right ventricular out-flow tract lesions. *Circulation*. 2007;115:1933–1947.

272. Ritter M, Oechslin E, Sutsch G, et al. Isolated noncompaction of the myocardium in adults. *Mayo Clin Proc*. 1997;72:26–31.

273. Weiford BC, Subbarao VD, Mulhern KM. Noncompaction of the ventricular myocardium. *Circulation*. 2004;109:2965–2971.

274. Ozkutlu S, Ayabakan C, Celiker A, Elshershari H. Noncompaction of ventricular myocardium: a study of twelve patients. *J Am Soc Echocardiogr*. 2002;15:1523–1528.

275. Stollberger C, Finsterer J. Left ventricular hypertrabeculation/noncompaction. *J Am Soc Echocardiogr*. 2004;17:91–100.

276. Jenni R, Oechslin EN, van der Loo B. Isolated ventricular non-compaction of the myocardium in adults. *Heart*. 2007;93:11–15.

277. Murphy RT, Thaman R, Blanes JG, et al. Natural history and famil-ial characteristics of isolated left ventricular non-compaction. *Eur Heart J*. 2005;26:187–192.

278. Oechslin EN, Attenhofer Jost CH, Rojas JR, et al. Long-term fol-low-up of 34 adults with isolated left ventricular noncompaction: a distinct cardiomyopathy with poor prognosis. *J Am Coll Cardiol*. 2000;36:493–500.

279. Kaneda T, Shimizu M, Ino H, et al. Images in cardiovascular medicine. Adult patient with isolated noncompaction of ventricu-lar myocardium. *Circulation*. 2005;112:e96–e97.

280. Chin TK, Perloff JK, Williams RG, et al. Isolated noncompaction of left ventricular myocardium. A study of eight cases. *Circulation*. 1990;82:507–513.

281. Bodiwala K, Miller AP, Nanda NC, et al. Live three-dimensional transthoracic echocardiographic assessment of ventricular non-compaction. *Echocardiography*. 2005;22:611–620.

282. Alhabshan F, Smallhorn JF, Golding F, et al. Extent of myocardial non-compaction: comparison between MRI and echocardio-graphic evaluation. *Pediatr Radiol*. 2005;35:1147–1151.

283. Petersen SE, Selvanayagam JB, Wiesmann F, et al. Left ventricular non-compaction: insights from cardiovascular magnetic resonance imaging. *J Am Coll Cardiol*. 2005;46:101–105.

284. Shinebourne EA, Babu-Narayan SV, Carvalho JS. Tetralogy of Fallot: from fetus to adult. *Heart*. 2006;92:1353–1359.

285. Aboulhosn J, Child JS. Management after childhood repair of tetral-ogy of Fallot. *Curr Treat Options Cardiovasc Med*. 2006;8:474–483.

286. Bouzas B, Kilner PJ, Gatzoulis MA. Pulmonary regurgitation: not a benign lesion. *Eur Heart J*. 2005;26:433–439.

287. Therrien J, Provost Y, Merchant N, et al. Optimal timing for pul-monary valve replacement in adults after tetralogy of Fallot repair. *Am J Cardiol*. 2005;95:779–782.

288. Therrien J, Siu SC, McLaughlin PR, Liu PP, Williams WG, Webb GD. Pulmonary valve replacement in adults late after repair of tetralogy of Fallot: are we operating too late? *J Am Coll Cardiol*. 2000;36:1670–1675.

289. Davlouros PA, Kilner PJ, Hornung TS, et al. Right ventricular func-tion in adults with repaired tetralogy of Fallot assessed with car-diovascular magnetic resonance imaging: detrimental role of right ventricular outflow aneurysms or akinesia and adverse right-to-left ventricular interaction. *J Am Coll Cardiol*. 2002;40:2044–2052.

290. Abd El Rahman MY, Hui W, Yigitbasi M, et al. Detection of left ventricular asynchrony in patients with right bundle branch block after repair of tetralogy of Fallot using tissue-Doppler imaging-derived strain. *J Am Coll Cardiol*. 2005;45:915–921.

291. Ghai A, Silversides C, Harris L, et al. Left ventricular dysfunction is a risk factor for sudden cardiac death in adults late after repair of tetralogy of Fallot. *J Am Coll Cardiol*. 2002;40:1675–1680.

292. Harrison DA, Harris L, Siu SC, et al. Sustained ventricular tachycar-dia in adult patients late after repair of tetralogy of Fallot. *J Am Coll Cardiol*. 1997;30:1368–1373.

293. van Huysduynen BH, van Straten A, Swenne CA, et al. Reduction of QRS duration after pulmonary valve replacement in adult Fallot patients is related to reduction of right ventricular volume. *Eur Heart J*. 2005;26:928–932.

294. van Straten A, Vliegen HW, Lamb HJ, et al. Time course of diastolic and systolic function improvement after pulmonary valve replace-ment in adult patients with tetralogy of Fallot. *J Am Coll Cardiol*. 2005;46:1559–1564.

295. Renella P, Aboulhosn J, Lohan DG, et al. Doppler echocardiogra-phy reliably predicts severe pulmonary regurgitation (PR) as quan-tified by cardiac magnetic resonance (CMR). *Circulation*. 2007;116: II-700.

296. Silversides CK, Veldtman GR, Crossin J, et al. Pressure half-time predicts hemodynamically significant pulmonary regurgitation in adult patients with repaired tetralogy of Fallot. *J Am Soc Echocar-diogr*. 2003;16:1057–1062.

297. Li W, Davlouros PA, Kilner PJ, et al. Doppler-echocardiographic assessment of pulmonary regurgitation in adults with repaired tetralogy of Fallot: comparison with cardiovascular magnetic reso-nance imaging. *Am Heart J*. 2004;147:165–172.

298. Niwa K, Siu SC, Webb GD, Gatzoulis MA. Progressive aortic root dilatation in adults late after repair of tetralogy of Fallot. *Circula-tion*. 2002;106:1374–1378.

299. Tan JL, Davlouros PA, McCarthy KP, et al. Intrinsic histological abnormalities of aortic root and ascending aorta in tetralogy of Fallot: evidence of causative mechanism for aortic dilatation and aortopathy. *Circulation.* 2005;112:961–968.

300. Warnes CA, Child JS. Aortic root dilatation after repair of tetralogy of Fallot: pathology from the past? *Circulation.* 2002;106:1310–1311.

301. Cheung YF, Ou X, Wong SJ. Central and peripheral arterial stiffness in patients after surgical repair of tetralogy of Fallot: implications for aortic root dilatation. *Heart.* 2006;92:1827–1830.

302. Warnes CA. Transposition of the great arteries. *Circulation.* 2006;114:2699–2709.

303. Lissin LW, Li W, Murphy DJ Jr, et al. Comparison of transthoracic echocardiography versus cardiovascular magnetic resonance imaging for the assessment of ventricular function in adults after atrial switch procedures for complete transposition of the great arteries. *Am J Cardiol.* 2004;93:654–657.

304. Khairy P, Poirier N, Mercier LA. Univentricular heart. *Circulation.* 2007;115:800–812.

305. Redington A. The physiology of the Fontan circulation. *Prog Pediatr Cardiol.* 2006;22:179–186.

306. Hsia TY, Khambadkone S, Redington AN, et al. Effects of respiration and gravity on infradiaphragmatic venous flow in normal and Fontan patients. *Circulation.* 2000;102(3 Suppl):III148–153.

307. Mac L, Dervanian MP, Neveux JY, et al. Cardiopulmonary interactions after Fontan operations. *Circulation.* 1999;100:211–214.

308. Gates RN, Laks H, Drinkwater DC Jr, et al. The Fontan procedure in adults. *Ann Thorac Surg.* 1997;63:1085–1090.

309. Aboulhosn J, Child JS. The adult with a Fontan operation. *Curr Cardiol Rep.* 2007;9:331–335.

310. Aboulhosn J, Shavelle DM, Castellon Y, et al. Fontan operation and the single ventricle. *Congen Heart Dis.* 2007;2:2–11.

311. Barber G, Di Sessa T, Child JS, et al. Hemodynamic responses to isolated increments in heart rate by atrial pacing after a Fontan procedure. *Am Heart J.* 1988;115:837–841.

312. Cheung YF, Penny DJ, Redington AN. Serial assessment of left ventricular diastolic function after Fontan procedure. *Heart.* 2000;83:420–424.

313. Giannico S, Hammad F, Amodeo A, et al. Clinical outcome of 193 extracardiac Fontan patients: the first 15 years. *J Am Coll Cardiol.* 2006;47:2065–2073.

314. Mitchell ME, Ittenbach RF, Gaynor JW, et al. Intermediate outcomes after the Fontan procedure in the current era. *J Thorac Cardiovasc Surg.* 2006;131:172–180.

315. d'Udekem Y, Iyengar AJ, Cochrane AD, et al. The Fontan procedure: contemporary techniques have improved long-term outcomes. *Circulation.* 2007;116(11 Suppl):I157–I164.

316. Kumar SP, Rubinstein CS, Simsic JM, et al. Lateral tunnel versus extracardiac conduit Fontan procedure: a concurrent comparison. *Ann Thorac Surg.* 2003;76:1389–1396; discussion 1396–1387.

CHAPTER 7

Cardiac Magnetic Resonance Imaging and Computed Tomography in the Assessment of Adult Congenital Heart Disease

JAMIL ABOULHOSN ▪ HOWARD DINH ▪ JOHN PAUL FINN

The diagnosis and management of congenital heart disease (CHD) are predicated on accurate identification of the anatomy and the functional consequences of the malformations, from simple to complex. The formidable surgical and interventional advancements of the past 50 years have added yet another layer of anatomic and physiologic complexity. Innovative cardiovascular imaging, especially magnetic resonance imaging (MRI) and x-ray computed tomography (CT), are now indispensable modalities in the management of patients with CHD.

BACKGROUND

Four decades after Roentgen's discovery of "a new kind of rays," angiography had its inception with injection of contrast materials into blood vessels of cadavers and animals. In 1937, Castellanos, Pereiras, and Garcia in Havana visualized the right cardiac chambers in infants and children, and George Potts Robb and Israel Steinberg in New York developed angiography in adults, stating, "The internal structure of the living heart had been revealed for the first time." Discovery of piezoelectricity in 1880 by Pierre and Jacques Curie prefigured echocardiography, which was heralded as the diagnostic pathway to the promised land. Although still pivotal in the clinical management of CHD, echocardiography is now supplemented by MRI and CT, which provide noninvasive cross-sectional imaging of intracardiac and extracardiac anatomy and physiology and

are poised to become cornerstones in the assessment of patients with CHD. Dramatic advances in MRI and CT hardware technology have occurred in parallel with enhanced computer performance and software development. As a result, MR and CT imaging have become the tools of choice when detailed morphologic and hemodynamic assessments of complex anatomy are required. CT and MRI are useful in the initial diagnostic workup of pediatric and adult patients with CHD. MRI is preferred in the pediatric population because there is no radiation exposure in contrast to cardiac CT[1] (Table 7–1). Both modalities are useful in postoperative adults as practical means of monitoring residua, sequelae, and complications (Table 7–2). Because of its capacity to quantify blood flow velocities, MRI currently provides more functional information than cardiac CT. A combination of spin-echo and gradient-echo pulse sequences, together with contrast-enhanced MR angiography (MRA), permit precise morphologic assessment of abnormalities, surgically altered anatomy, associated valvular disease, flow patterns, cardiac shunts, and physiological impact.[2,3] The strength of cardiac CT lies in the speed and spatial resolution of current multidetector scanners. Cardiac CT is rapidly replacing invasive cineangiography as the modality of choice for diagnostic coronary angiography.[4,5] Moreover, cardiac CT can be utilized in settings in which MRI is contraindicated, for example, in patients who are pacemaker-dependent.[6] CT is also less prone to artifacts from metallic vascular stents, which are widely used in unoperated,

Table 7-1 Advantages and Disadvantages of MRI Versus CTA in Adult Congenital Heart Disease

	MRI	CTA
Radiation dose	− (no radiation exposure)	++
Ventricular function/volumes	+++	+
Valvular function—quantification of stenosis/regurgitation	+++	+
Coronary artery anatomy	+	+++
Vascular calcification	−	+++
Pulmonary artery angiography	+++	+++
Relative lung perfusion	+++	+
Shunt quantification	+++	++
Stent/device evaluation	+/−	++
Presence of pacemaker/AICD	−	++
Atrial/pulmonary venous anatomy/volumes	++	++
Myocardial fibrosis or fatty infiltration	+++	+
Myocardial ischemia/viability	+++	−
Structure relationship to sternum	++	+++

AICD, automatic implantable cardioverter defibrillator; CTA, computed tomographic angiography; MRI, magnetic resonance imaging.

operated, and postoperative patients with CHD. Contemporary MRI scanners can produce near real-time three-dimensional (3D) images of the first pass of contrast through the heart and great vessels, documenting the functional vascular anatomy and highlighting shunts and collateral pathways.[7,8] This type of time-resolved imaging is not possible with CT, for both technical and radiation-dosimetry reasons. CT is limited to producing images of high spatial resolution at a fixed time, whereas MRI has the potential for spatial and temporal resolution, making it a highly flexible tool for MRA use in adult CHD.[9]

MRI and CT are useful in the noninvasive assessment of patients with CHD because the anatomic abnormality can be visualized and the defect quantified and because the functional significance of the congenital abnormality can be established. Visualization of surrounding structures such as the great arteries, outflow tracts, and coexisting valvular abnormalities can be assessed, and measurements of volumetric parameters such as ejection fraction, stroke volume, diastolic and systolic volumes, and ventricular mass can be achieved.[10] Abnormalities in function may precede the onset of symptoms and signal the need for further investigation

Table 7-2 Congenital Cardiac Malformations Utilizing CTA and MRI

MALFORMATION	UTILITY
ASD	• Determine type, size, rim, 3D geometry, anomalous pulmonary venous connections, atrial and ventricular volumes, shunt quantification • CT useful for post-percutaneous device closure imaging
VSD	• Determination of location and size
Pulmonary stenosis	• MRI useful for valve morphology, PS velocity, PR volume quantification • CT and MR are both useful for evaluating subvalvar or supravalvar PS and pulmonary artery anatomy; determination of RV volume/thickness/ejection fraction
Tetralogy of Fallot	• MRI useful for valve morphology, PS velocity, PR volume quantification, RV EF, volume, and muscle mass quantification
Transpositions (DTGA, CCTGA, complex malpositions)	• CT and MRI both useful for establishing complex anatomic relationships • CTA useful for imagining SVC and pulmonary venous baffles after atrial switch operation • Evaluation of IVC baffle requires lower-extremity injection • MR angiography with time-resolved (early and delayed) imaging useful in evaluating IVC baffle
Fontan operation	• Simultaneous upper- and lower-extremity injections may be necessary for adequate visualization of lateral tunnel or extracardiac Fontan • Time-resolved MRA may be useful
Left ventricular outflow tract obstructions including coarctation	• MRI with velocity quantification can be used to derive functional data • MRI of aortic valve is superior to CTA • CTA is superior in patients with previous coarctation stent or numerous surgical clips
Anomalous coronary anatomy	• CTA is superior for imaging mid- and distal coronary tree
Coronary sinus anatomy	• CTA or MR angiography delayed imaging useful to determine coronary sinus and venous anatomy
Anomalous pulmonary venous connections	• CTA or MRA delayed imaging useful to determine anatomy
Patent ductus arteriosus/systemic arterial to pulmonary arterial collaterals	• CT and MRI both provide excellent images of these connections

ASD, atrial septal defect; CCTGA, congenitally collected transposition of the great arteries; CTA, computed tomographic angiography; DTGA, D-transposition of the great arteries; EF, ejection fraction; IFC, inferior vena cava; MRI, magnetic resonance imaging; PR, pulmonary regurgitation; PS, pulmonary stenosis; RV, right ventricular; SVC, superior vena cava; 3D, three dimensional; VSD, ventricular septal defect.

and early intervention. Phase-contrast MR measurement of flow across a valve or septal defect permits quantification of flow velocity, shunt direction, shunt volume, and Qp:Qs ratio.[3] Shunt quantification can also be secured with cardiac CT.[11,12] CT and MRA identify abnormalities of ventricular wall motion and areas of myocardial ischemia or fibrosis.[13-15] MRI and CT are ideal tools for venous and arterial angiography to identify and quantify luminal stenoses and thromboses. CT accurately quantifies vascular and valvular calcific deposits,[16,17] and MR provides 3D functional angiographic information in a visually attractive format.

CLINICAL EVALUATION OF ADULT CONGENITAL HEART DISEASE

The professional personnel in adult CHD facilities must be well versed in the arcane vocabulary of CHD; they must also understand the diverse ramifications of the disorders, the reparative and palliative surgical procedures, the postoperative residua and sequelae, and the general medical and cardiovascular illnesses that adults with CHD acquire with aging. Infants and children with congenital heart disease have, as a rule, one disorder—their congenital malformation—but this singularity is replaced in the adult by a complex interplay between the preoperative and postoperative congenital cardiac disease and acquired cardiac and noncardiac disease. Pediatric cardiologists for the most part are not trained in acquired heart disease of adults, but cardiologists trained in adult medicine are prepared to assume that responsibility.

Transthoracic echocardiography (TTE) with Doppler and color flow interrogation remains the basic imaging method in the field of adult CHD (see Chapter 6). However, ultrasound waves are reflected by bone and scattered by air, and thus the imaging planes are limited to parasternal, apical, suprasternal, and subcostal windows. The coronary arteries are seldom visualized, and extracardiac vascular anatomy is incompletely assessed. Transesophageal echocardiography (TEE) resolves many of these limitations but cannot be employed routinely. Cardiac catheterization with cineangiography has long been considered the standard for evaluating cardiovascular anatomy and hemodynamics, but it is invasive and carries the small risk of vascular complications. Noninvasive cross-sectional imaging modalities, which are the subjects of this chapter, are ideally suited to bridge this gap between TTE and cardiac catheterization. Spin-echo (SE) sequences have been used in a limited armamentarium of MRI techniques for cardiac and vascular imaging. Major technical advances in cardiac MRI in recent years[18] have largely relegated SE imaging to a secondary role. Among the most useful techniques for the study of adult CHD are *bright blood* cine imaging of the beating heart,[19] phase-sensitive velocity encoding,[20-22] contrast-enhanced MRA,[23,24] and, to a lesser

extent than in ischemic heart disease, delayed myocardial enhancement imaging.[25]

Cardiovascular CT angiography (CTA) depends on electrocardiographic gating for acquisition of thin-slice tomographic axial images. Electron-beam CT (EBCT), also referred to as *EBT* and *Ultrafast-CT,* uses unique technology that permits ultrafast scan acquisition times as fast as 50 ms with minimal motion artifacts and improved contrast-to-noise ratio.[26] EBCT employs a stationary multisource/split-detector combination coupled with a rotating electron beam, and produces serial, contiguous, thin-section tomographic scans synchronous with the heart cycle. EBCT is distinguished by incorporating a scanning electron beam rather than the standard x-ray tube and mechanical rotation device used in current "spiral" single and multiple-detector scanners (MDCT). MDCT physically moves the x-ray tube in a circle about the patient, but with EBCT, only the electron beam is moved.[26] Electrocardiographic (ECG) triggering is during end-systole or early diastole at a time determined from the continuous ECG tracing done during scanning. The current generation of MDCT systems is capable of acquiring 4 to 64 sections of the heart simultaneously with ECG gating in either a prospective or retrospective mode. CTA requires the injection of contrast through a peripheral vein. After determining the transit time required to fully opacify the cardiovascular structures with a pilot injection of iodine-based contrast medium, a mechanical injection is delivered at a preset rate while axial CT images are acquired through the thoracic cavity. The volume of contrast administered ranges from 75 to 150 ml. CTA and MRA images can be reconstructed using 3D software and one or more rendering techniques such as shaded-surface, MIP (maximum intensity projection), and multiplanar reconstruction.

Aortic Arch Disease

Coarctation of the aorta is typically represented by focal narrowing just distal to the origin of the left subclavian artery as originally described by Morgagni in 1760.[27] Less commonly, there is hypoplasia of extended aortic segments (Fig. 7–1, *A*). Severity ranges from mild to complete anatomic obstruction to anatomic interruption of the aortic arch (Fig. 7–2). Aortic coarctation is not simply a focal mechanical disease but is a generalized vascular disorder that includes medial abnormalities of the proximal and distal paracoarctation aorta, abnormalities of the ascending and transverse aorta and conduit arteries, coexisting bicuspid aortic valve, abnormalities of the mitral apparatus, aneurysms of the circle of Willis, abnormalities of the retinal arterioles, and dilatation of proximal coronary arteries with premature atherosclerosis. The presence and extent of arterioarterial collaterals bridging the site of the coarctation are directly correlated with stenosis severity (see Fig. 7–2).

FIGURE 7–1 **(A)** Three-dimensional (3D) surface-rendered reconstruction of magnetic resonance angiogram (MRA) viewed from a left anterior oblique and cranial projection in a 24-year-old woman with a surgically repaired coarctation of the aorta (resection with end-to-end anastomosis). The aortic arch is hypoplastic and has a peaked angular appearance similar to a Gothic arch. There is no residual coarctation, but a peak-to-peak catheter determined gradient of 40 mm Hg was measured at rest between the ascending and descending aorta. The hypoplastic aortic arch was believed to be responsible for this hemodynamically significant stenosis. **(B)** Left anterior oblique projection of 3D-MRA reconstruction in a 36-year-old man with a surgically repaired coarctation (resection with end-to-end anastomosis). The appearance of the aortic arch is rounded, or Romanesque. There is a focal restenosis at the site of surgical repair and dilatation of the distal para-coarctation aorta. The peak-to-peak catheter gradient at rest across the restenosis was 25 mm Hg.

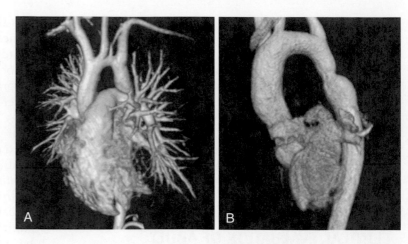

FIGURE 7–2 **(A)** Three-dimensional (3D) surface rendered magnetic resonance angiogram (MRA) of a 41-year-old woman with an unrepaired severe coarctation with near interruption (I) viewed from a right posterior oblique projection. An extensive bypassing collateral network was removed during post-processing and 3D reconstruction to better demonstrate the area of severe coarctation. **(B)** Three-dimensional surface-rendered MRA of the same patient viewed from a left anterior oblique and cranial projection. The extensive arterial collateral network and the dilatated internal mammary arteries (IMA) are typical of unrepaired severe coarctation of the aorta (but not of interrupted aortic arch).

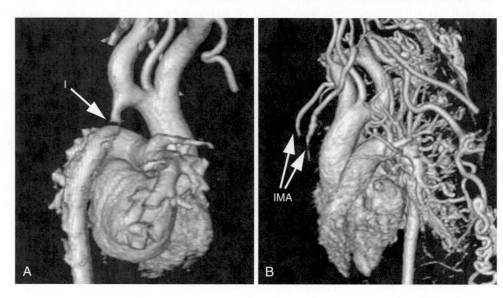

FIGURE 7–3 **(A)** Steady-state free precession (SSFP) cine magnetic resonance image, oblique sagittal slice, in a 59-year-old woman with repaired coarctation of the aorta and an unrepaired moderately stenotic and regurgitant bicuspid aortic valve (BAV). This systolic frame demonstrates the restricted systolic opening of the BAV with fusion of the right and left coronary cusps. Calcium deposits on the leaflet tips appear as black or dark gray on cine MRI. **(B)** Coronal projection demonstrates the characteristic systolic doming of the BAV. The ascending aorta is dilated with effacement of the sinotubular junction, characteristic features that are related to the congenital BAV but not to its functional state.[76]

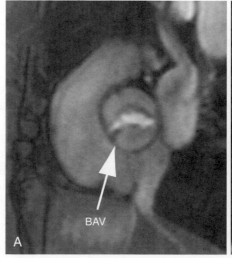
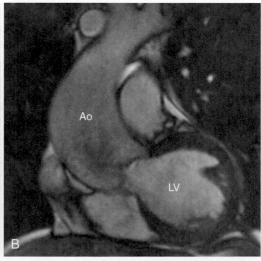

CT and MRI are ideal for imaging of the entire thoracic aorta. Accurate imaging of the ascending aorta, the aortic arch and arteries emerging from it, and the descending thoracic aorta is imperative in both unoperated patients and those who have undergone surgical or transcatheter interventions. The 3D shape of the aortic arch carries prognostic implications; specifically, a "Gothic" angular arch is associated with greater vascular stiffness and exercise-induced hypertension than a "Romanesque" or rounded arch (see Fig. 7–1).[28] The dimensions of the proximal and distal paracoarctation aorta can be accurately measured. CTA and MRA are preferred to cardiac catheterization for delineating collateral arterial anatomy and can be invaluable tools in planning surgical and percutaneous interventions. These cross-sectional imaging modalities can also be used in postoperative and postinterventional follow-up to assess potential complications such as restenosis, dissection, or aneurysm formation (see Figs. 7–1, *B*, and 7–4). MRA can quantify volume and velocity of flow across a narrowed segment, and MRI can assess pulse-wave propagation and determine the degree of stiffness and compliance of the aorta.[29-31] ECG-gated coronary CTA is especially useful because patients with aortic coarctation are prone to premature coronary atherosclerosis (discussed earlier). In addition, MRI and CTA can detect abnormalities of myocardial perfusion secondary to microvascular disease independent of epicardial coronary artery obstruction.[32]

Marfan syndrome is characterized by mutation of the gene that encodes fibrillin-1, a major constituent of microfibrils. Inadequate fibrillin-1 expression in the ascending aorta is responsible for fragmentation of medial elastic fibers, mural attenuation, dilatation, and dissection. The most common cardiovascular features are dilation of the aortic sinuses and mitral valve prolapse (Fig. 7–5). Aortic valve regurgitation, aortic dissection, and mitral regurgitation may require surgical intervention.[33] CT and MRI can be used to image the aorta, but MRI is superior in evaluating mitral valve prolapse and in quantifying valvular regurgitation. Both modalities permit assessment of the origin and extent of a dissecting aneurysm, the dissection flap, whether vital arterial branches are involved and whether they are supplied by the true or false lumen (Fig. 7–6). A characteristic feature of Marfan syndrome is dural ectasia of the lumbar spine, which is readily identified by MRI or CT and is of considerable diagnostic significance (see Fig. 7–6).

Right Ventricular Outflow Malformations

In 1888, Etienne Fallot described a constellation of anatomic findings— right ventricular outflow obstruction, ventricular septal defect (VSD), overriding aorta, and right ventricular hypertrophy—that defined a subset of patients with the what he termed *maladie bleue*. The VSD is malaligned with rightward and anterior deviation of the infundibular septum, and thus the degree of aortic override correlates with the severity of infundibular stenosis. Stenosis or hypoplasia of proximal pulmonary arterial branches frequently coexists. Pulmonary atresia is the extreme form of the malformation in which pulmonary blood flow depends on aortopulmonary collaterals (Fig. 7–7). The surgical options are dictated by the degree of infundibular stenosis and pulmonary

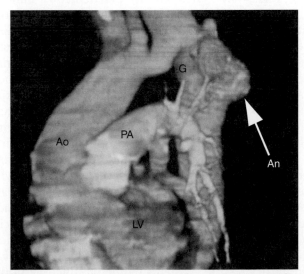

FIGURE 7–4   Three-dimensional (3D) surface-rendered magnetic resonance angiogram in a 59-year-old woman (same patient as in Fig. 7-3) who underwent surgical excision of a focal coarctation with prosthetic tubular graft placement (G). Viewed from a left anterior oblique projection. A large aneurysm (An) arises from the distal anastomosis of the graft (G). AO, ascending aorta; LV, left ventricle; PA, pulmonary artery.

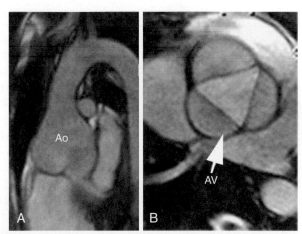

FIGURE 7–5   **(A)** Steady-state free precession cine magnetic resonance image, oblique sagittal slice, of a 22-year-old man with Marfan syndrome. The dilated sinuses of Valsalva (Ao) give the aortic root a characteristic Erlenmeyer flask appearance. **(B)** Axial slice at the level of the trileaflet aortic valve (AV) in systole. The dilatated sinuses of Valsalva prevent systolic apposition of the aortic valve leaflets to the sinotubular junction resulting in the distinctive triangular opening of the aortic valve.

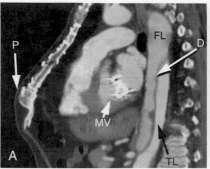
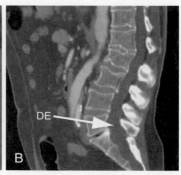

FIGURE 7–6 **(A)** Sixteen-slice multidetector computed to-mographic sagittal images of a 62-year-old man with Marfan syndrome who had undergone a mechanical mitral valve replacement (MV) for mitral valve prolapse and severe mitral regurgitation. The dissection flap (D) in the descending thoracic aorta creates a well-opacified true lumen (TL) and a poorly opacified false lumen (FL). The patient also has a characteristic pectus carinatum (P). **(B)** Abdominopelvic CT angiogram, sagittal projection, demonstrating severe lordosis and characteristic dural ectasia (DE).

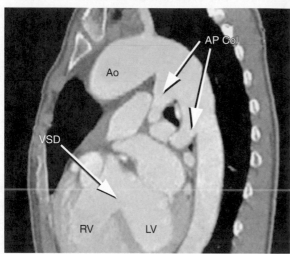

FIGURE 7–7 Computed tomographic angiogram, sagittal projection, of a 36-year-old cyanotic woman with unoperated tetralogy of Fallot, pulmonary atresia, and multiple aortopulmonary collaterals (AP Coll) emerging from the thoracic aorta (Ao). The right ventricle (RV) is enlarged and hypertrophied. A large malaligned ventricular septal defect (VSD) allows nonrestricted communication between the right ventricle (RV) and the left ventricle (LV).

arterial hypoplasia. Patients with hypoplastic pulmonary arteries and pulmonary atresia are often initially palliated with a central shunt (Fig. 7–8). When the pulmonary arteries are confluent and well developed, intracardiac repair is the option, even in infancy. Severe low-pressure pulmonary regurgitation is an immediate sequel of a transannular patch and a delayed sequel of an infundibular incision (Fig. 7–9). Pulmonary regurgitation is a concern because of its hemodynamic effect on the right ventricle and because it serves as a trigger for the slow conduction electrophysiologic substrate of monomorphic ventricular tachycardia (see Chapter 22). Phase-contrast MRI is an accurate means of quantifying pulmonary regurgitant volume and fraction.[34] MRI-determined right ventricular (RV) volume measurements can help guide the timing of pulmonary valve replacement. Therrien et al.[35] reported that pulmonary valve replacement performed when end-diastolic volume > 170 ml/m² or RV end-systolic volume > 85 ml/m² did not result in "normalization" of RV volume at a mean

follow-up of 21 months.[35] RV volume decreases, but ejection fraction does not change.[35,36] Both the inflow and outflow portions of the RV should be included when using the modified Simpson's method for determining systolic and diastolic volumes, especially in the presence of an aneurysmal outflow patch because RV inflow measurements alone can appreciably underestimate the RV volume and overestimate the ejection fraction. CT and MRI provide excellent visualization of the pulmonary arterial and venous systems and can be applied to evaluate pulmonary anatomy (Fig. 7–10). Both modalities can also be used to quantify RV volumes and ejection fraction.[37] Myocardial fibrosis can be detected by late gadolinium enhancement with MR angiography (Fig. 7–11) and correlates with a number of adverse outcomes, including RV dysfunction, elevated brain natriuretic peptide levels, decreased functional capacity, and clinical arrhythmias.[13]

Isolated pulmonary valve stenosis is represented by a mobile doming valve (most common), a dysplastic valve, or a bicuspid valve.[38] Mobile and doming pulmonary valves are amenable to percutaneous balloon valvuloplasty. Calcium deposits are occasionally present at the leaflet tips. The pulmonary trunk and the proximal portions of the right and left pulmonary arteries are typically dilatated. CT and MR angiography are ideal for the anatomic delineation of focal branch pulmonary artery stenosis that may coexist. MRA with phase-contrast imaging quantifies blood flow to the right and left pulmonary arteries, allowing calculation of the relative distribution of blood flow to each lung and helping to guide percutaneous and surgical interventions.[39-41] However, compared with the standard of radionuclide scintigraphy, discrepant results occasionally occur because of MR artifacts and dephasing caused by turbulent flow. MRI velocity encoding permits measurement of transvalvular flow and velocity and can be used to estimate the peak and mean pressure gradients by the modified Bernoulli equation[42] (Fig. 7–12). Care must be taken during data acquisition to be sure that the velocity-encoding plane is perpendicular to the vector of maximum velocity to avoid underestimating the measured pressure gradient.

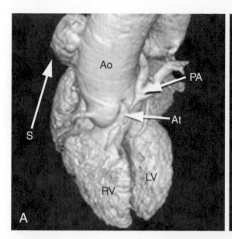
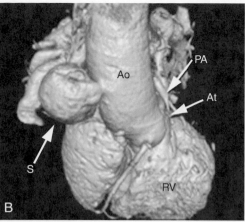

FIGURE 7-8 **(A)** Magnetic resonance angiogram with three-dimensional surface rendering of a patient with tetralogy of Fallot (TOF), pulmonary atresia (At), and hypoplastic main and branch pulmonary arteries (PA) viewed from a left anterior oblique and cranial projection. An aneurysmal central shunt (S) connects the ascending aorta (Ao) to the right pulmonary artery. Dilatation of the ascending aorta is a characteristic finding in TOF and pulmonary atresia (reference Niwa). **(B)** Right anterior oblique and cranial projection. LV, left ventricle; RV, right ventricle.

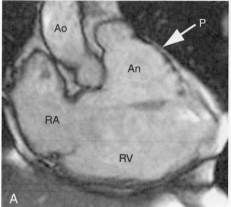
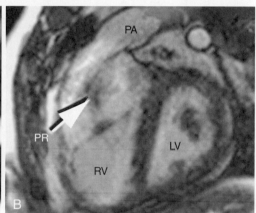

FIGURE 7-9 **(A)** Steady-state free precession cine magnetic resonance image (MRI), coronal projection, in a 48-year-old man with tetralogy of Fallot status post-transannular patch (P) and ventricular septal defect closure at 2 years of age. There was chronic severe pulmonary regurgitation (PR) and marked dilatation of the right ventricle (RV) with an aneurysmal outflow tract (An). The right atrium is enlarged (RA). **(B)** Sagittal projection in mid-diastole demonstrating severe PR into an enlarged RV. The LV is D-shaped, consistent with RV volume overload. Ao, ascending aorta; PA, pulmonary artery.

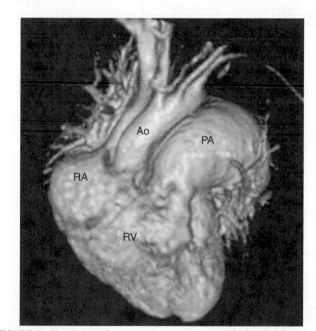

FIGURE 7-10 Magnetic resonance angiogram with three-dimensional surface rendering in a 34-year-old woman with unrepaired tetralogy of Fallot and severe pulmonary stenosis and regurgitation viewed from a right anterior oblique and cranial projection. The pulmonary artery (PA) is markedly dilated. The right ventricle (RV) is mildly dilatated. Ao, aorta; RA, right atrium.

Pulmonary Venous Malformations

Congenital pulmonary vein stenosis is a rare developmental fault of the common pulmonary vein, a structure normally incorporated into the left atrium as four separate venous channels.[43] The abnormality is characterized by hypoplasia of one or more pulmonary veins or by focal narrowing at or near their left atrial junction. Hypoplasia varies from slight narrowing to atresia of individual pulmonary veins or of a common pulmonary vein. Focal narrowing is caused by a circumferential collar of fibrous intimal thickening or by a membranous diaphragm. Focal stenosis, hypoplasia, and atresia may coexist with involvement of most or all pulmonary veins. The management is surgical with pericardial patch enlargement or excision of focal stenoses.[44] More recently, percutaneous catheter-based approaches have come into use.[45] CTA and MRA are useful in the assessment of pulmonary venous stenosis or atresia. Phase-contrast MRI determination of lung perfusion can clarify the functional consequences of pulmonary venous stenosis and help guide intervention. Because of artifact caused by metallic stents, CTA is superior to MRI imaging in assessing pulmonary venous stent patency.[46]

Anomalous pulmonary venous connection can be partial or total. Partial anomalous pulmonary venous

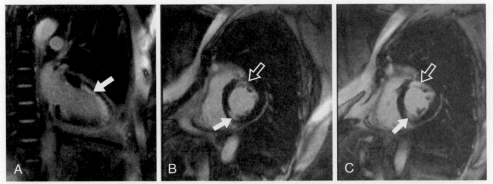

FIGURE 7-11 Myocardial fibrosis. Two-dimensional segmented inversion recovery (IR) TurboFLASH images in vertical long-axis **(A)** and short-axis **(B** and **C)** orientations show subendocardial delayed hyperenhancement (arrows) in the anteroseptal and inferoseptal walls.

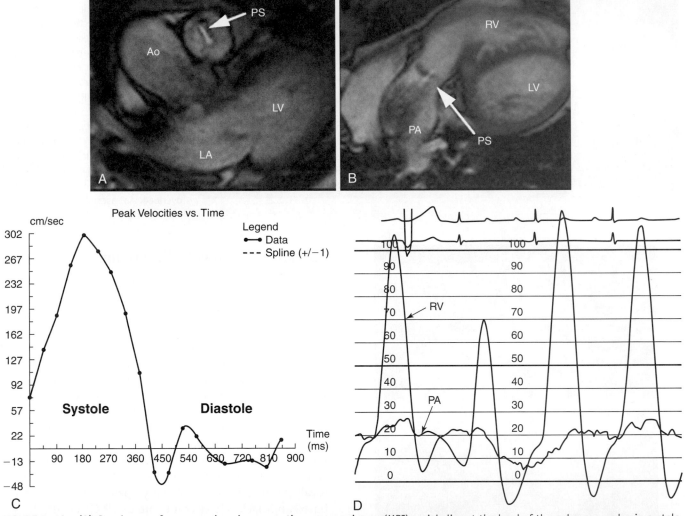

FIGURE 7-12 **(A)** Steady-state free precession cine magnetic resonance image (MRI), axial slice at the level of the pulmonary valve in systole. The opening of the pulmonary valve (PS) is restricted, and the leaflet tips are calcified. Ao, ascending aorta; LA, left atrium; LV, left ventricle. **(B)** Oblique projection showing systolic doming of the stenotic pulmonary valve (PS). There is high-velocity turbulent flow (dark gray) into a dilatated main pulmonary artery (PA). The right ventricle (RV) is hypertrophied. The LV is normal. **(C)** Phase-contrast MRI plot of velocity versus time across the stenotic pulmonary valve. The maximum measured systolic velocity is approximately 3 m/s, which estimates a peak instantaneous gradient of 36 mm Hg across the stenotic pulmonary valve. **(D)** Simultaneous transcatheter pressure measurements in the RV and PA. The maximum pressure gradient is 70 to 80 mm, which far exceeds the estimated peak instantaneous gradient by phase-contrast MRI. Underestimation by MRI was probably because the velocity encoding plane was not truly perpendicular to the PS systolic jet vector during data acquisition, leading to measurement of a submaximal velocity and underestimation of the PS severity.

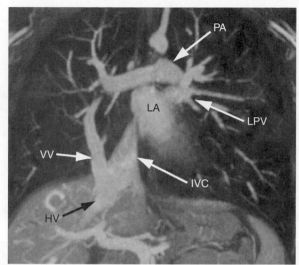

FIGURE 7-13 Magnetic resonance angiogram (MRA), thin maximum intensity projection, coronal plane, in a 16-year-old male adolescent with scimitar syndrome, characterized by connection of the right pulmonary veins to a vertical vein (VV), which drains inferiorly at the juncture of the hepatic vein (HV) and inferior vena cava (IVC). The left pulmonary veins (LPV) connect appropriately to the left atrium (LA). PA, pulmonary artery.

connection exists when one or more than one, but not all, pulmonary veins connect anomalously to the right atrium. Partial anomalous pulmonary venous connection (PAPVC) most often involves the right upper and middle lobe pulmonary veins, may occur with an ostium secundum atrial septal defect (ASD), and usually occurs with a sinus venosus ASD. Isolated PAPVC is rare. The anomalous pulmonary vein(s) connect to the superior vena caval/right atrial junction and directly to the right atrium, inferior vena cava, coronary sinus, or innominate vein through a vertical vein.[47] Scimitar syndrome is a rare anomaly characterized by connection of all of the right pulmonary veins to the inferior vena cava and usually by hypoplasia of the ipsilateral lung and pulmonary artery (Fig. 7-13).

Total anomalous pulmonary venous connection (TAPVC) applies when all four pulmonary veins connect anomalously to a systemic venous tributary of the right atrium or to the right atrium proper but have no connection to the left atrium (Fig. 7-14). Classifications take into account three features:[38] (1) the pathway by which pulmonary venous blood reaches the right atrium, (2) the presence or absence of obstruction along the course of the pathway, and (3) the nature of the interatrial communication. The most widely used clinical classification recognizes supradiaphragmatic connections (three fourths of cases) with or without obstruction and infradiaphragmatic or infracardiac connections that are always obstructed. Except for mixed connections and connections of all four pulmonary veins directly to the right atrium, all varieties of total anomalous pulmonary venous connections incorporate a venous confluence that receives the four pulmonary veins. In the supradiaphragmatic varieties, the confluence joins the coronary sinus or a left vertical vein that ascends to join an innominate bridge to the right superior vena cava and right atrium. Obstruction of the vertical vein results from a hemodynamic vise formed posteriorly by the left bronchus and anteriorly by the pulmonary trunk. Uncommon connections include a venous confluence to the right superior vena cava through a right-sided anomalous venous channel or through the azygous venous system. MRA and CTA are ideal for determining the location, course, and patency of the pulmonary veins[48] (see Fig. 7-14). Surgical repair consists of anastomosing the common pulmonary vein to the left atrium. CTA and MRI can be used in formulating surgical and postoperative management.

Systemic Venous Malformations

Anomalous vena caval connections include a wide range of malformations that vary from minor to major and that occur either in isolation or with coexisting congenital heart disease.[49] Persistent left superior vena cava (LSVC) is the

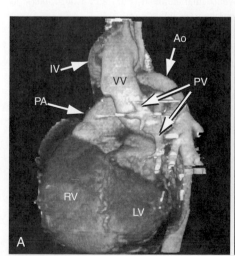

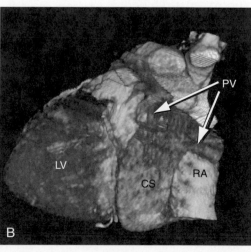

FIGURE 7-14 **(A)** Three-dimensional volume-rendered computed tomography angiogram (CTA) in a 48-year-old cyanotic woman with unrepaired total anomalous pulmonary venous connection (TAPVC) viewed from a left anterior oblique and cranial projection. The pulmonary veins (PV) are connected via a vertical vein (VV) to the innominate vein (IV). The right ventricle (RV) is enlarged, and the main pulmonary artery (PA) is dilatated in contrast to the aorta (Ao). **(B)** Three-dimensional volume-rendered CTA in a 27-year-old cyanotic man with unrepaired TAPVC of the PV to a markedly dilatated coronary sinus (CS), which connects to the right atrium (RA). LV, left ventricle.

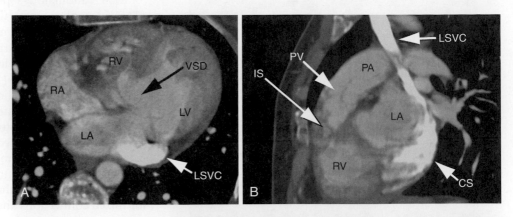

FIGURE 7–15 **(A)** Computed tomography angiogram, axial slice, in a 50-year-old woman with an unrepaired nonrestrictive ventricular septal defect (VSD) and a persistent left superior vena cava (LSVC) that runs along the lateral wall of the left atrium (LA). **(B)** Coronal slice demonstrating the LSVC coursing by the left atrium and draining into a dilatated coronary sinus (CS). The RV is hypertrophied because of stenosis at the ostium of the infundibulum (IS) below the level of the pulmonary valve (PV). LV, left ventricle; RA, right atrium; RV, right ventricle.

most common thoracic venous anomaly, producing no physiologic derangements when it drains harmlessly into the right atrium through the coronary sinus (Fig. 7–15). The coronary sinus sometimes dilates appreciably, especially if there is stenosis or atresia of its right atrial orifice. Less common connections are directly to the left atrium, pulmonary veins, left atrial appendage, or right atrium. An LSVC occurs in isolation or may accompany other congenital cardiovascular anomalies such as ASD or coarctation of the aorta.[50] The LSVC can be readily identified with CTA or MRA, with contrast material injected through a left upper extremity peripheral vein to ensure opacification of the LSVC.

Hearts with Only One Ventricle

Tricuspid Atresia

In tricuspid atresia, the morphologic left ventricle functions as a single pumping chamber. A VSD provides access for pulmonary blood flow when the great arteries are normally related, which is usually the case, and provides access to the aorta when the great arteries are transposed. An interatrial communication is the only outlet for the obstructed right atrium from which unoxygenated blood is shunted into the left atrium through an ASD. CT and MRI[11,51] readily identify the malformation and are ideally suited for defining the atrioventricular and ventriculoarterial connections (Fig. 7–16).

Single Ventricle or the Univentricular Heart

This is a complex malformation in which two atria are related entirely or almost entirely to one ventricular compartment that qualifies on purely morphologic grounds as a left, right, or indeterminate ventricle.[49] Univentricular atrioventricular connections are represented by gross morphologic characteristics of the ventricular mass and according to the atrioventricular connections to that mass. In 80% to 90% of cases, single ventricle as just defined occurs when the ventricular chamber that receives the atrioventricular connec-

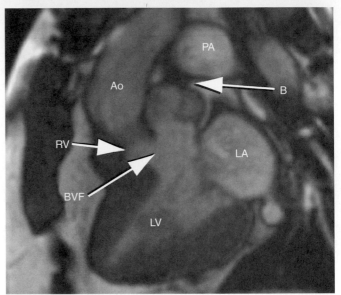

FIGURE 7–16 Steady-state free precession cine magnetic resonance image, sagittal view, in a 32-year-old man with hypoplastic right ventricle (RV) and D-transposition of the great arteries. The pulmonary artery (PA) was surgically banded (B) during a Fontan operation that connected the right atrium to the right pulmonary artery (not shown). The left ventricle (LV) pumps blood into an anteriorly transposed aorta (Ao) through a bulboventricular foramen (BVF) and a hypoplastic RV serving as an outlet chamber. LA, left atrium.

tions has left ventricular morphologic features and incorporates at its base an outlet chamber or infundibular remnant that is remote from the crux of the heart, is anterosuperior, and lies to the right or left of midline. In 10% to 20% of cases, the ventricular chamber that receives the atrioventricular connections has right ventricular morphologic features and incorporates within its mass a rudimentary compartment or trabecular pouch that represents a left ventricular remnant and occupies a posterior, inferior, or lateral position within the ventricular mass. In less than 10% of cases, the single ventricle has intermediate morphologic features and incorporates neither an outlet chamber nor a trabecular pouch. The atrioventricular connections that guard the inlet of a univentricular heart consist of two separate well-formed

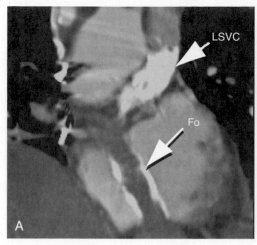
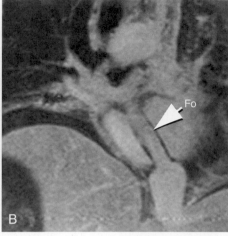

FIGURE 7–17 **(A)** Computed tomography angiogram, coronal view, in a 22-year-old man with tricuspid atresia and a Fontan (Fo) with an intraatrial tunnel. The contrast injection was into a left upper extremity peripheral vein resulting in opacification of a left superior vena cava (LSVC) but no opacification of the Fontan. **(B)** Time-resolved magnetic resonance angiogram, coronal view, demonstrating the well-opacified patent Fontan (Fo).

valves, one well-formed valve with atresia of the other valve, or a common atrioventricular valve.

Many innovative surgical techniques have been developed to address tricuspid atresia. In 1945, Blalock and Taussig described a palliative operation that shunted systemic arterial blood from the subclavian artery to the pulmonary artery.[52] Glenn and Patino in 1954 performed the first systemic venous to pulmonary arterial shunting procedure[53] that prefigured the total cavopulmonary operation of Fontan and Baudet in 1971.[54] During the past 3 decades, this procedure evolved through many modifications[55] (Fig. 7–17). Morphologic and functional assessment of Fontan procedures are feasible with CT.[55,56] In patients with the intraatrial or lateral tunnel, or an extracardiac connection, contrast injection through both an upper and lower extremity vein serves to visualize the entire Fontan connection. Occult pulmonary thrombi and emboli occur in 17% of patients following the Fontan operation.[56] Assessment may be inaccurate if streaming of contrast results in heterogeneous opacification of the pulmonary arterial tree, but dynamic time-resolved MRA overcomes this problem and may be superior to CT for the evaluation of Fontan connections.[57–59]

Great Arterial Malformations

Complete Transposition of the Great Arteries

The term *transposition* is defined as ventriculo–great arterial discordance, that is, a morphologic right ventricle gives rise to the aorta and a morphologic left ventricle gives rise to the pulmonary trunk[49] (Fig. 7–18). In complete or D-transposition (DTGA), the ventricles retain their normal anatomic positions with the right ventricle anterior and medial to the left ventricle. There is atrioventricular concordance with the right atrium anterior and medial and the left atrium posterior and lateral. CTA and MRA readily identify the morphologic features that distinguish a morphologic right atrium from a morpho-

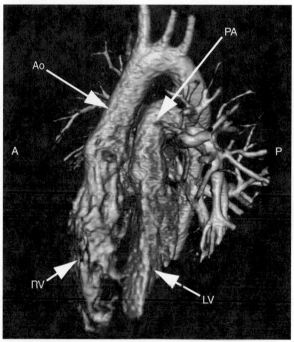

FIGURE 7–18 Magnetic resonance angiogram with three-dimensional surface-rendering viewed from left anterior oblique and cranial projection in a 24-year-old man with D-transposition of the great arteries and a Senning atrial switch operation in infancy. The anterior (A) transposed aorta (Ao) emerges from the right ventricle (RV). The posterior (P) and leftward pulmonary artery (PA) emerges from the left ventricle (LV).

logic left atrium. The suprahepatic inferior vena cava almost always drains into the morphologic right atrium, which is further identified by its broad triangular atrial appendage in contrast to the narrow finger-like left atrial appendage.[60] In the Mustard or Senning atrial switch operations, caval blood is baffled from the superior and inferior vena cavae across the mitral valve into the morphologic left ventricle and into the pulmonary trunk. Pulmonary venous return is baffled across the tricuspid valve into the morphologic right ventricle and into the aorta (Fig. 7–19). CTA and MRA provide excellent

FIGURE 7-19 **(A)** Computed tomography angiogram, axial slice, in a 36-year-old woman with D-transposition of the great arteries status-post Senning atrial switch operation. The pulmonary venous baffle (PB) channels pulmonary venous blood into an hypertrophied enlarged systemic right ventricle (RV). The systemic baffle (SB) channels vena caval blood into the subpulmonic left ventricle (LV). **(B)** Higher axial cut at the level of the left ventricular outflow tract demonstrates a patent stent (St) within the superior arm of the systemic venous baffle. The pulmonary baffle (PB) is well visualized.

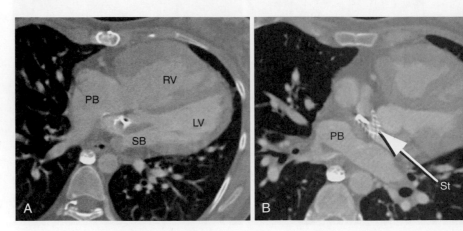

visualization of the baffled circulations and readily identify baffle obstructions or leaks. CTA is particularly useful if a baffle stent is present (see Fig. 7–19). CTA evaluation of the inferior vena caval portion of the baffle benefits from opacification with an upper-extremity contrast injection. MRI-derived ventricular volume parameters, especially end-systolic and end-diastolic volumes of the subaortic morphologic right ventricle, can be correlated with exercise performance in patients who have undergone an atrial switch operation.[61]

Congenitally Corrected Transposition of the Great Arteries

In this malformation, the ventricular–great arterial alignments and the atrioventricular alignments are both are discordant. The double discordance—ventricular-arterial and atrioventricular—physiologically corrects the discordance inherent in each malalignment. Blood from the morphologic right atrium reaches the pulmonary artery albeit across a mitral valve and through a morphologic left ventricle, and blood from the morphologic left atrium reaches the aorta albeit across a tricuspid valve and through a morphologic right ventricle. The ventricles and their respective atrioventricular valves are inverted, but the atria are normally related. The ascending aorta is anterior and leftward, the pulmonary trunk is posterior and rightward, and the great arteries do not cross as in the normal heart. CTA and MRA distinguish the morphologic left ventricle (LV) from the morphologic right ventricle (RV) by (1) the fine trabecular pattern of the LV in contrast to the coarse trabeculae of the RV; (2) the two large papillary muscles of the LV compared with multiple small papillary muscles of the RV; (3) semilunar-atrioventricular fibrous continuity in the LV but not in the RV; and (4) concordance of the morphologic LV with the two morphologic left coronary arteries and concordance of the morphologic right ventricle with a single morphologic right coronary artery (Fig. 7–20). Coexisting anomalies are common, especially a nonrestrictive perimembranous ventricular septal defect, pulmonary

stenosis, Ebstein's anomaly of the left atrioventricular (tricuspid) valve, and atrioventricular conduction defects that anticipate complete heart block.

PHYSIOLOGIC ASSESSMENT OF FUNCTION AND FLOW

CT does not have the capacity for measuring flow and flow velocities, but MRI is robust in assessing both structure and function.

Cardiac Function

CMR is a highly accurate and effective imaging modality in the assessments of global and regional cardiac function and is evolving as the standard for the noninvasive evaluation of cardiac function[62,63] and myocardial muscle mass.[64] Already considered the standard for assessing left ventricular end-diastolic volume (EDV), end-systolic volume (ESV), and ejection fraction (EF), CMR provides accurate and reproducible tomographic, static, and cine images of high spatial and temporal resolution in any desired plane without exposure to ionizing radiation or nephrotoxic contrast agents.[65] Cine CTA is also used for the assessment of ventricular volume, muscle mass, and ejection fraction.[66,67] To achieve adequate MRI resolution images of cardiac function, 7 to 10 separate cine steady-state free precession (SSFP) acquisitions in the short axis and two or three in the long axis are usually required. Segmented SSFP imaging is several times faster than spoiled gradient echo imaging[68] and produces superior blood-myocardial definition.[69]

Magnetic Resonance Flow Imaging

Blood flow through major arteries, veins, cardiac chambers, across valves, and in surgical conduits can be assessed by phase-contrast (velocity-encoded) imaging. Magnetic spins moving along a magnetic gradient at a

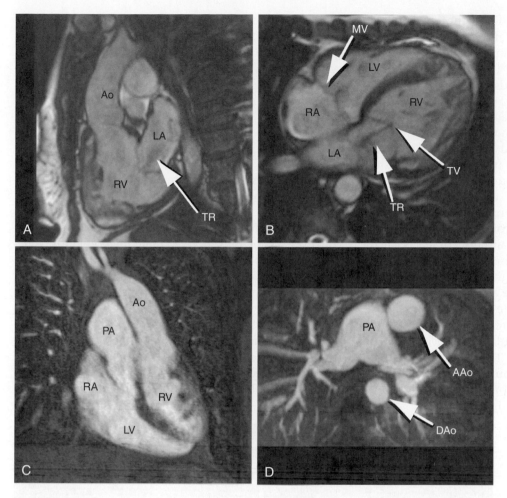

FIGURE 7-20   (A) Steady-state free precession (SSFP) cine magnetic resonance image, sagittal cut, in a 48-year-old woman with congenitally corrected transposition of the great arteries. The left atrium (LA) is connected to an inverted right ventricle (RV) through a tricuspid valve (atrioventricular discordance). TR, mild tricuspid regurgitation. The aorta (Ao) is anterior and originates from the morphologic RV (ventricular–great arterial discordance). **(B)** Axial cut showing inversion of the left (LV) and right ventricle (RV). The tricuspid valve (TV) is apically displacement with mild TR. LA, left atrium; RA, right atrium; RV, right ventricle. **(C)** Time-resolved magnetic resonance angiogram (MRA), coronal view, showing the parallel relationship of the aorta (Ao) and pulmonary artery (PA). **(D)** MRA, axial view, showing the anterior ascending aorta (AAo) and the posterior PA. Dao, descending aorta.

constant velocity accumulate a phase shift proportional to the velocity. Phase maps can be reconstructed so that signal intensity corresponds to the average velocity of each pixel. With the addition of ECG-gating gradient echo sequence, flow-encoding gradients can be prescribed in orthogonal planes perpendicular to the direction of the flow of interest. A region of interest can then be used to assess the flow and velocity over a period of time, and pressure gradients can be derived from the modified Bernoulli equation similar to Doppler echo. Although potential errors stemming from misalignment of the direction of flow, partial volume effects, and low signal-to-noise ratio, phase-contrast imaging has been validated extensively and is now used routinely in the following settings relevant to CHD.

Valvular Disease

Ideal assessment of valvular heart disease addresses the morphology of the valvular apparatus and associated cardiac structures, detection and quantification of stenosis and regurgitation, determination of structural changes of the cardiac chambers and great vessels, and assessment of the functional changes in the ventricles. Visualization of valvular abnormalities can be accomplished with spin-echo (black blood imaging) and gradient echo (GRE; bright blood) images designed to determine the number of leaflets, the degree of excursion, approximate leaflet thickness, and chamber size function.[70] Quantification of the functional consequences of valvular disease is best assessed with phase-contrast sequences. From these data, flow volume, regurgitant fraction, pressure gradients, and valvular area estimates can be derived.[71]

Valvular Regurgitation

Chronic regurgitant flow results in volume overload and ventricular dilatation that anticipate insidious deterioration in ventricular function. Timely detection and quantification of progression set the stage for medical management and timing of surgical treatment. The most widely reported MR modality for assessing the severity of valvular regurgitation is GRE and phase-contrast imaging. The highly disturbed or turbulent flow accompanying GRE technique results in loss of MR signal in the region of the regurgitant stream. The extent of MR signal void corresponds roughly to the area of color Doppler signal by echocardiography.[72,73] The degree and extent of the signal void depends on the severity of the turbulent flow, the direction of regurgitant flow, and acquisition parameters such as echo time, sampling size of the imaged volume element (voxel), and orientation of the imaging plane relative to the flow jet.[74] Signal voids caused by valvular turbulent blood flow indicate regurgitation but not necessarily its severity. The magnitude of regurgitant volume and regurgitant fraction can be determined by measuring right ventricular and left ventricular stroke volumes, assuming that regurgitant lesions involve only one side of the heart. Phase-contrast imaging can also be used to assess the severity of regurgitation, with flow direction encoded by varying the magnetic phases of the blood either in or through an image plane. Information regarding velocity and flow of jets is calculated on the basis of the differences in the magnetic phase of flowing blood. Regurgitant volume and fraction using phase contrast can be assessed by calculating the difference in stroke volume (derived from phase contrast) through the great artery and the difference derived from volumetric calculations based on MR modified Simpson's method. This method assumes only one regurgitant valvular source for the ventricle of interest. Alternatively, phase contrast can be used to assess both forward and reverse flow, the latter of which represents regurgitant volume from which regurgitant fraction can be derived as a percentage of total systolic forward flow. To derive a flow velocity value with MR, the signal must be coherent, and thus the sampling must be sufficiently far from a zone of turbulence.

Valvular Stenosis

GRE imaging is used to estimate the degree of aortic or pulmonic stenosis by observing the extent of turbulent flow (signal loss) in the ascending aorta or pulmonary artery.[75] However, this method is qualitative and provides only a cursory assessment. A more accurate method employs detailed images in the plane of the semilunar valve (with slice thickness reduced to about 2–4 mm) so that planimetry of end-systolic valve opening area can be quantified directly by commonly available software (see Fig. 7–12). The severity of aortic valve stenosis can also be assessed using phase-contrast imaging for flow velocities up to 5 m/s. The severity of stenosis can be assessed more reliably because the pressure gradient across the valve can be computed from the velocity of flow (modified Bernoulli equation).

FIGURE 7–21 Time-resolved magnetic resonance angiogram of a right-to-left shunt (S) through a restrictive perimembranous ventricular septal defect in a patient with congenitally corrected transposition of the great arteries and pulmonary stenosis. **(A)** Contrast opacifies the morphologic right atrium (RA), inverted morphologic left ventricle (LV), and pulmonary arteries (PA; atrioventricular and ventricular great arterial discordance). **(B)** Further opacification showing a right-to-left shunt (S). **(C)** The right-to-left shunt (S) is clearly visualized, with increased opacification of ascending aorta (Ao) before pulmonary venous and left atrial filling. **(D)** Pulmonary venous (PV), left atrial (LA), and left-sided (inverted morphologic right) ventricular filling followed by opacification of the aorta (Ao).

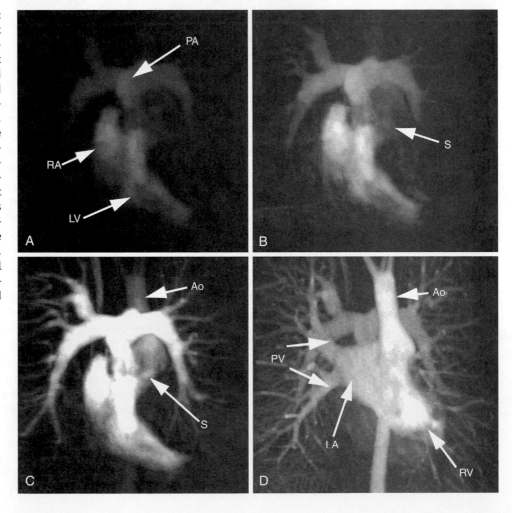

Shunt Analysis

MRI GRE or SSFP sequences are used to assess intracardiac and extracardiac shunts. Cine imaging for cardiac function (discussed earlier) can then be used to assess right and left ventricular stroke volumes. Phase-contrast imaging is helpful to quantify pulmonary and aortic flow, which can then be used to determine the Qp:Qs ratio. Accurate determination of shunt fractions by CTA is also feasible.[11,12] The arterial time-concentration curve produced after intravenous injection of an indicator (iodine) displays a recirculation hump on the downslope with left-to-right shunts or early appearance and hump on the upslope of the curve with right-to-left shunts. The area under the curve reflects the shunt volume. Shunting can be assessed in real time with MRI using time-resolved MRA, which images the first pass of a contrast bolus with subsecond temporal resolution (Fig. 7–21).[7] This method provides a highly visual demonstration of intracardiac or extracardiac shunting, especially right-to-left shunts.[9]

FUTURE OF MAGNETIC RESONANCE IMAGING AND COMPUTED TOMOGRAPHY

The dynamic and evolving fields of cardiac MRI and CT are extremely useful in producing detailed images of cardiac structure and function. MRI-guided interventions such as cardiac biopsy, ablation, and coronary interventions such as placement of MR-compatible coronary stents are currently being investigated. Improved hardware and pulse sequences (e.g., highly parallel acquisition and real-time imaging) are new developments that promise to provide greater flexibility with this once user-unfriendly imaging modality. Higher field magnets (3 or more Tesla) are currently being explored for potentially greater spatial and temporal resolution and better and faster *in vivo* and *ex vivo* imaging.

The future is promising for cardiac CT. The latest generation of multidetector CT systems provides excellent spatial resolution. Development of faster scanners with the capability of imaging thinner slices will permit better visualization of small or thin structures such as valves, the atrial septum, and the membranous ventricular septum. The development of four-dimensional capability promises to be ideal for cardiovascular investigation. The heart is a dynamic organ best understood when studied throughout the cardiac cycle. Photon emission tomography CTA permits evaluation of coronary perfusion, viability, and anatomy and could prove especially useful in simultaneously assessing pulmonary perfusion and arterial anatomy. The coupling of dynamic cross-sectional imaging modalities with software programs capable of 3D reconstruction and "virtual dissection" will promote better understanding of the complex anatomy and physiology of congenital heart disease.

References

1. Moore WH, Bonvento M, Olivieri-Fitt R. Comparison of MDCT radiation dose: a phantom study. *Am J Roentgenol.* 2006;187:W498–502.
2. Wimpfheimer O, Boxt LM. MR imaging of adult patients with congenital heart disease. *Radiol Clin North Am.* 1999;37:421–438, vii.
3. Roest AA, Helbing WA, van der Wall EE, de Roos A. Postoperative evaluation of congenital heart disease by magnetic resonance imaging. *J Magn Reson Imaging.* 1999;10:656–666.
4. Dragu R, Rispler S, Ghersin E, et al. Contrast enhanced multidetector computed tomography coronary angiography versus conventional invasive quantitative coronary angiography in acute coronary syndrome patients-correlation and bias. *Acute Card Care.* 2006;8:99–104.
5. Ghersin E, Litmanovich D, Dragu R, et al. 16-MDCT coronary angiography versus invasive coronary angiography in acute chest pain syndrome: a blinded prospective study. *AJR Am J Roentgenol.* 2006;186:177–184.
6. Goldsher D, Amikam S, Boulos M, et al. Magnetic resonance imaging for patients with permanent pacemakers: initial clinical experience. *Isr Med Assoc J.* 2006;8:91–94.
7. Finn JP, Baskaran V, Carr JC, et al. Thorax: low-dose contrast-enhanced three-dimensional MR angiography with subsecond temporal resolution—initial results. *Radiology.* 2002;224:896–904.
8. Carr JC, Laub G, Zheng J, et al. Time-resolved three-dimensional pulmonary MR angiography and perfusion imaging with ultrashort repetition time. *Acad Radiol.* 2002;9:1407–1418.
9. Fenchel M, Saleh R, Dinh H, et al. Juvenile and adult congenital heart disease: time-resolved 3D contrast-enhanced MR angiography. *Radiology.* 2007;244:399–410.
10. Sugeng L, Mor-Avi V, Weinert L, et al. Quantitative assessment of left ventricular size and function: side-by-side comparison of real-time three-dimensional echocardiography and computed tomography with magnetic resonance reference. *Circulation.* 2006;114:654–661.
11. Aboulhosn J, Oudiz R. Cardiac CT in congenital heart diseases in cardiac CT imaging: diagnosis of cardiovascular disease. In: Budoff MJ, ed. *Cardiac CT Imaging: Diagnosis of Cardiovascular Disease.* Vol. 1. United Kingdom: Springer Publications; 2006:221–238.
12. Funabashi N, Asano M, Sekine T, et al. Direction, location, and size of shunt flow in congenital heart disease evaluated by ECG-gated multislice computed tomography. *Int J Cardiol.* 10 2006;112:399–404.
13. Babu-Narayan SV, Kilner PJ, Li W, et al. Ventricular fibrosis suggested by cardiovascular magnetic resonance in adults with repaired tetralogy of Fallot and its relationship to adverse markers of clinical outcome. *Circulation.* 2006;113:405–413.
14. Bello D, Kipper S, Valderrabano M, Shivkumar K. Catheter ablation of ventricular tachycardia guided by contrast-enhanced cardiac computed tomography. *Heart Rhythm.* 2004;1:490–492.
15. Wong CY, Tatini VR, Bis K. Combined CT-PET criteria for myocardial viability and scar: a preliminary report. *Int J Cardiovasc Imag.* 2004;20:487–491.
16. Aboulhosn J, Castellon YM, Siegerman C, et al. Quantification of pulmonary artery calcium deposits in patients with pulmonary hypertension using computed tomography. Oral abstract presented at the American Foundation for Medical Research Western Convention, 2005.
17. Horiguchi J, Shen Y, Akiyama Y, et al. Electron beam CT versus 16-MDCT on the variability of repeated coronary artery calcium measurements in a variable heart rate phantom. *AJR Am J Roentgenol.* 2005;185:995–1000.
18. Finn JP, Nael K, Deshpande V, et al. Cardiac MR imaging: state of the technology. *Radiology.* 2006;241:338–354.
19. Carr JC, Simonetti O, Bundy J, et al. Cine MR angiography of the heart with segmented true fast imaging with steady-state precession. *Radiology.* 2001;219:828–834.

20. Firmin DN, Nayler GL, Kilner PJ, Longmore DB. The application of phase shifts in NMR for flow measurement. *Magn Reson Med.* 1990;14:230–241.

21. Underwood SR, Firmin DN, Rees RS, Longmore DB. Magnetic resonance velocity mapping. *Clin Phys Physiol Meas.* 1990;11(A Suppl):37–43.

22. Edelman RR, Manning WJ, Gervino E, Li W. Flow velocity quantification in human coronary arteries with fast, breath-hold MR angiography. *J Magn Reson Imaging.* 1993;3:699–703.

23. Prince MR, Narasimham DL, Jacoby WT, et al. Three-dimensional gadolinium-enhanced MR angiography of the thoracic aorta. *AJR Am J Roentgenol.* 1996;166:1387–1397.

24. Nael K, Michaely HJ, Kramer U, et al. Pulmonary circulation: contrast-enhanced 3.0-T MR angiography—initial results. *Radiology.* 2006;240:858–868.

25. Simonetti OP, Kim RJ, Fieno DS, et al. An improved MR imaging technique for the visualization of myocardial infarction. *Radiology.* 2001;218:215–223.

26. Budoff MJ, Achenbach S, Blumenthal RS, et al. Assessment of coronary artery disease by cardiac computed tomography: a scientific statement from the American Heart Association Committee on Cardiovascular Imaging and Intervention, Council on Cardiovascular Radiology and Intervention, and Committee on Cardiac Imaging, Council on Clinical Cardiology. *Circulation.* 2006;114:1761–1791.

27. Aboulhosn J, Child JS. Left ventricular outflow obstruction: subaortic stenosis, bicuspid aortic valve, supravalvar aortic stenosis, and coarctation of the aorta. *Circulation.* 2006;114:2412–2422.

28. Ou P, Mousseaux E, Celermajer DS, et al. Aortic arch shape deformation after coarctation surgery: effect on blood pressure response. *J Thorac Cardiovasc Surg.* 2006;132:1105–1111.

29. Nollen GJ, Groenink M, Tijssen JG, et al. Aortic stiffness and diameter predict progressive aortic dilatation in patients with Marfan syndrome. *Eur Heart J.* 2004;25:1146–1152.

30. Peng HH, Chung HW, Yu HY, Tseng WY. Estimation of pulse wave velocity in main pulmonary artery with phase contrast MRI: preliminary investigation. *J Magn Reson Imaging.* 2006;24:1303–1310.

31. Tran T, Beardslee M, Caruthers S, et al. Aortic characterization in patients with congenital bicuspid aortic valves using MR flow mapping. American Heart Association Scientific Sessions, 2006. 2006;114:II-779, abstract 3649.

32. Cook S, Raman S. Subendocardial ischemia in adults with repaired coarctation: a potential mechanism for early ischemic events. American Heart Association Scientific Sessions, oral abstract presentation. 2006;114:II-408, abstract 2028.

33. Murdoch JL, Walker BA, Halpern BL, et al. Life expectancy and causes of death in the Marfan syndrome. *N Engl J Med.* 1972;286:804–808.

34. Grothoff M, Spors B, Abdul-Khaliq H, et al. Pulmonary regurgitation is a powerful factor influencing QRS duration in patients after surgical repair of tetralogy of Fallot: a magnetic resonance imaging (MRI) study. *Clin Res Cardiol.* 2006;95:643–649.

35. Therrien J, Provost Y, Merchant N, et al. Optimal timing for pulmonary valve replacement in adults after tetralogy of Fallot repair. *Am J Cardiol.* 15 2005;95:779–782.

36. Van Huysduynen B, Henkens I, Swenne C, et al. The effects of pulmonary valve replacement in adult patients with tetralogy of Fallot. American Heart Association Scientific Sessions. 2006;114:II-388, abstract 1943.

37. Elgeti T, Lembcke A, Enzweiler CN, et al. Comparison of electron beam computed tomography with magnetic resonance imaging in assessment of right ventricular volumes and function. *C Comput Assist Tomogr* 2004;28:679–685.

38. Perloff JK. *Clinical Recognition of Congenital Heart Disease.* 5th ed. Philadelphia: W.B. Saunders; 2003.

39. Roman KS, Kellenberger CJ, Farooq S, et al. Comparative imaging of differential pulmonary blood flow in patients with congenital heart disease: magnetic resonance imaging versus lung perfusion scintigraphy. *Pediatr Radiol.* 2005;35:295–301.

40. Roman KS, Kellenberger CJ, Macgowan CK, et al. How is pulmonary arterial blood flow affected by pulmonary venous obstruction in children? A phase-contrast magnetic resonance study. *Pediatr Radiol.* 2005;35:580–586.

41. Martirosian P, Boss A, Fenchel M, et al. Quantitative lung perfusion mapping at 0.2 T using FAIR True-FISP MRI. *Magn Reson Med.* 2006;55:1065–1074.

42. Beekman RP, Beek FJ, Meijboom EJ. Usefulness of MRI for the preoperative evaluation of the pulmonary arteries in tetralogy of Fallot. *Magn Reson Med.* 1997;15:1005–1015.

43. Latson LA, Prieto LR. Congenital and acquired pulmonary vein stenosis. *Circulation.* 2007;115:103–108.

44. Spray TL, Bridges ND. Surgical management of congenital and acquired pulmonary vein stenosis. *Semin Thorac Cardiovasc Surg Pediatr Card Surg Annu.* 1999;2:177–188.

45. Mendelsohn AM, Bove EL, Lupinetti FM, et al. Intraoperative and percutaneous stenting of congenital pulmonary artery and vein stenosis. *Circulation.* 1993;88:II210–II217.

46. Neumann T, Sperzel J, Dill T, et al. Percutaneous pulmonary vein stenting for the treatment of severe stenosis after pulmonary vein isolation. *J Cardiovasc Electrophysiol.* 2005;16:1180–1188.

47. Aboulhosn JA, Criley JM, Stringer WW. Partial anomalous pulmonary venous return: case report and review of the literature. *Catheter Cardiovasc Interv.* 2003;58:548–552.

48. Gulati G, Sharma S. A rare form of supracardiac total anomalous pulmonary venous drainage—evaluation by computed tomography and magnetic resonance imaging. *Clin Radiol.* 2003;58:172–175.

49. Perloff JK. *Clinical Recognition of Congenital Heart Disease.* 5th ed. Philadelphia: W.B. Saunders, 2003.

50. Gonzalez-Juanatey C, Testa A, et al. Persistent left superior vena cava draining into the coronary sinus: report of 10 cases and literature review. *Clin Cardiol.* 2004;27:515–518.

51. Lilje C, Habermann CR, Weil J. Magnetic resonance imaging follow-up of total cavopulmonary connection. *Heart.* 2005;91:395.

52. Blalock A, Taussig HB. Landmark article May 19, 1945. The surgical treatment of malformations of the heart in which there is pulmonary stenosis or pulmonary atresia. By Alfred Blalock and Helen B. Taussig. *JAMA.* 1984;251:2123–2138.

53. Glenn WW, Patino JF. Circulatory by-pass of the right heart. I. Preliminary observations on the direct delivery of vena caval blood into the pulmonary arterial circulation; azygos vein-pulmonary artery shunt. *Yale J Biol Med.* 1954;27:147–151.

54. Fontan F, Baudet E. Surgical repair of tricuspid atresia. *Thorax.* 1971;26:240–248.

55. AboulHosn J, Castellon Y, Shavelle DM, et al. Fontan operation and the single ventricle: patient selection and management. *Congenital Heart Disease: Clinical Studies from Fetus to Adulthood.* 2007;2(1):2–11.

56. Varma C, Warr MR, Hendler AL, Paul NS, Webb GD, Therrien J. Prevalence of "silent" pulmonary emboli in adults after the Fontan operation. *J Am Coll Cardiol.* 18 2003;41(12):2252–2258.

57. de Zelicourt DA, Pekkan K, Parks J, et al. Flow study of an extracardiac connection with persistent left superior vena cava. *J Thorac Cardiovasc Surg.* Apr 2006;131:785–791.

58. Festa P, Ait Ali L, Bernabei M, De Marchi D. The role of magnetic resonance imaging in the evaluation of the functionally single ventricle before and after conversion to the Fontan circulation. *Cardiol Young.* 2005;15 Suppl 3:51–56.

59. Greenberg SB, Morrow WR, Imamura M, Drummond-Webb J. Magnetic resonance flow analysis of classic and extracardiac Fontan procedures: the seesaw sign. *Int J Cardiovasc Imag.* 2004;20:397–405; discussion 407–398.

60. Van Praagh R, Van Praagh S. *Morphologic Anatomy. In Nadas' Pediatric Cardiology.* Philadelphia: Hanley & Belfus; 2006:27–37.

61. LaRocca G, Prakash A, Printz B, et al. MRI predictors of exercise capacity in adult patients after atrial correction for transposition of the great arteries. American Heart Association Scientific Sessions, abstract presentation. 2006:II-727, abstract 3419.
62. Peshock R, Franco F, Chwialkowski M. *Normal Cardiac Anatomy, Orientation, and Function in Cardiovascular Magnetic Resonance.* Edinburgh: Elsevier; 2002:75–96.
63. Peshock RM, Willett DL, Sayad DE, et al. Quantitative MR imaging of the heart. *Magn Reson Imag Clin North Am.* 1996;4:287–305.
64. Fieno DS, Jaffe WC, Simonetti OP, et al. TrueFISP: assessment of accuracy for measurement of left ventricular mass in an animal model. *J Magn Reson Imaging.* 2002;15:526–531.
65. Ioannidis JP, Trikalinos TA, Danias PG. Electrocardiogram-gated single-photon emission computed tomography versus cardiac magnetic resonance imaging for the assessment of left ventricular volumes and ejection fraction: a meta-analysis. *J Am Coll Cardiol.* 2002;39:2059–2068.
66. Dogan H, Kroft LJ, Bax JJ, et al. MDCT assessment of right ventricular systolic function. *AJR Am J Roentgenol.* 2006;186(2 Suppl):S366–370.
67. Dogan H, Kroft LJ, Huisman MV, et al. Right ventricular function in patients with acute pulmonary embolism: analysis with electrocardiography-synchronized multi-detector row CT. *Radiology.* 2006.
68. Atkinson DJ, Edelman RR. Cineangiography of the heart in a single breath hold with a segmented turboFLASH sequence. *Radiology.* 1991;178:357–360.
69. Lee VS, Resnick D, Bundy JM, et al. Cardiac function: MR evaluation in one breath hold with real-time true fast imaging with steady-state precession. *Radiology.* 2002;222:835–842.
70. Schlosser T, Malyar N, Jochims M, et al. Quantification of aortic valve stenosis in MRI-comparison of steady-state free precession and fast low-angle shot sequences. *Eur Radiol.* 17 2006.
71. Weber OM, Higgins CB. MR evaluation of cardiovascular physiology in congenital heart disease: flow and function. *J Cardiovasc Magn Reson.* 2006;8:607–617.
72. Schiebler M, Axel L, Reichek N, et al. Correlation of cine MR imaging with two-dimensional pulsed Doppler echocardiography in valvular insufficiency. *J Comput Assist Tomogr.* 1987;11:627–632.
73. Underwood SR, Klipstein RH, Firmin DN, et al. Magnetic resonance assessment of aortic and mitral regurgitation. *Br Heart J.* 1986;56:455–462.
74. Bryant DJ, Payne JA, Firmin DN, Longmore DB. Measurement of flow with NMR imaging using a gradient pulse and phase difference technique. *J Comput Assist Tomogr.* 1984;8:588–593.
75. de Roos A, Reichek N, Axel L, Kressel HY. Cine MR imaging in aortic stenosis. *J Comput Assist Tomogr.* May-1989;13:421–425.
76. Niwa K, Perloff JK, Bhuta SM, et al. Structural abnormalities of great arterial walls in congenital heart disease: light and electron microscopic analyses. *Circulation.* 2001;103:393–400.

CHAPTER 8

Infective Endocarditis and Congenital Heart Disease

JOHN S. CHILD ▪ DAVID A. PEGUES ▪ JOSEPH K. PERLOFF

Few diseases present greater difficulties in the way of diagnosis than malignant endocarditis. ... In fully one-half of them the diagnosis was made postmortem. ... The protean character..., the latency of the cardiac symptoms, and the close simulation of other disorders, combine to render the detection peculiarly difficult.

—*Osler, 1885*[1]

Infective endocarditis (IE) was almost uniformly fatal before advances in bacteriologic methods in the 19th century and the development of antimicrobials in the 20th century.[2] However, the advances came at a price. In the last 60 years, major achievements in diagnostic, medical, and surgical management of congenital heart disease (CHD) have resulted in survival into adulthood and therefore in many additional decades of exposure to the risk of IE.[3-5] Indwelling catheters permit hemodynamic monitoring, chemotherapy, and parenteral nutrition but are portals of entry for aggressive staphylococci or difficult to treat fungi. Implantable devices, artificial valves, conduits, pacemakers, and defibrillators are sources for infection on either the devices themselves or adjacent endothelial structures.[6,7]

We herein use the term *infective endocarditis* rather than the older term *subacute bacterial endocarditis* because the microorganisms need not be bacterial and the process may be acute, subacute, or chronic. When infection involves a vascular structure (descending aorta in coarctation, pulmonary artery in patent ductus arteriosus), the proper term is *infective endarteritis*. IE was defined by the Task Force on Infective Endocarditis of the European Society of Cardiology Guidelines on Prevention, Diagnosis and Treatment as "an endovascular microbial infection of cardiovascular structures ... including endarteritis of the large intrathoracic vessels ... or of intracardiac foreign bodies ... facing the bloodstream."[8]

HISTORICAL PERSPECTIVE

According to Laennec, necropsy evidence of endocarditis was first described by Lazare Riviere (1589–1655), who identified aortic valve vegetations and stated that "in the left ventricle ... carbuncles ... the larger of which resembled a cluster of hazelnuts and filled up the opening of the aorta."[9] In 1776, Morgagni reported necropsy findings in a 36-year-old man with gonorrhea and valve excrescences of vegetative endocarditis, in addition to a splenic infarct.[9] In 1852, W. S. Kirkes published one of the earliest clinical accounts of endocarditis with embolism.[9] Rudolph Virchow undertook the first detailed microscopic observations of splenic capillary emboli, pointing out that deposits on the valves were new growths and stating that "Ulceration takes place in one of the valves of the heart ... crumbling fragments of the surface of the valve are borne away."[10] Sir Samuel Wilks subsequently related sepsis to endocarditis (1868), and E. F. H. Winge described microorganisms in the endocardial lesions and in the embolic material (1869)—the first proof of the bacterial origin of ulcerative endocarditis.[9]

Clinical and experimental knowledge up to 1885 was summarized by Sir William Osler in his Gulstonian Lectures to the Royal College of Physicians in London. Osler drew on evidence relating microbes to pyemia (Koch) and called attention to the culture of micrococci in endocarditis.[1] However, effective treatment confounded physicians until the advent of penicillin in the 1940s.

EPIDEMIOLOGY

Despite—or perhaps because of—major improvements in health care, the worldwide incidence of IE has changed little if at all over the past 2 decades, with an estimated frequency 1.7 to 6.2 cases per 100,000 person-years.[11-13] One report cited a rising incidence.[14] Gram-positive cocci still predominate. Since the beginning of the 21st century, staphylococcal IE reportedly occurs as frequently as or more frequently than streptococcal IE.[11,13-18]

The clinical setting and presentation of endocarditis have evolved in the past half century in part because of technical advances (cardiac surgery, hemodialysis), prosthetic devices (valves, pacemakers, implantable defibrillators), indwelling lines, injection drug abuse, and evolution of antimicrobial therapy.[11,13,15,16,19-21] The types of patients with IE are changing,[4,11-13,16,21-26] and the emergence of antibiotic-resistant organisms such as methicillin-resistant *Staphylococcus* and vancomycin-resistant *Enterococcus* underscores endocarditis as a protean disease that requires evolving if not novel solutions.

The nature of the disease varies depending on whether the infection is on native valves or prosthetic valves or materials and on whether drugs are legitimate therapy or recreational. (Figs. 8–1 through 8–10). An especially high risk for IE is associated with previous episodes of infection, complex cyanotic CHD, prosthetic valves, conduits, and surgically created shunts.[3,8,21,27-31] (see Figs. 8–5 and 8–7). Except in developing countries where rheumatic heart disease still prevails, IE now occurs chiefly in patients with CHD, prosthetic valves, mitral valve prolapse, and degenerative valvular disease of the elderly. The increased prevalence of obesity and diabetes mellitus contribute to immune deficiency and poorer prognosis.

PATHOGENESIS

IE typically requires a susceptible substrate and a portal of bacterial entry into the bloodstream.[3,11,13,15,20,22,32] Alternatively, endocarditis occurs in the absence of a definable substrate when the infecting organism is sufficiently virulent to cause endothelial damage by adhesins and proteolytic enzymes or by induction of inflammation.[13] The early IE lesion is a variably sized vegetation that includes platelets, fibrin, inflammatory cells, and microorganisms. Lesions progress and cause valvular or vascular destruction, ulceration, erosion, perforation, abscess formation, and fistulous tracts (see Fig. 8–2). Bacteria may bind to platelets in the blood pool and then be deposited at sites of vascular endothelial damage. High-velocity turbulent flow predisposes to endothelial injury either at the site generating the turbulence (increased shear stress) or at the site of the jet impact.[4,33-35] (see Figs. 8–4 and 8–6). The endothelial lesion is usually located at the low-pressure end of an abnormality with a large gradient such as aortic coarctation in which vegetations are usually found downstream in the descending aorta at the high velocity site.[36]

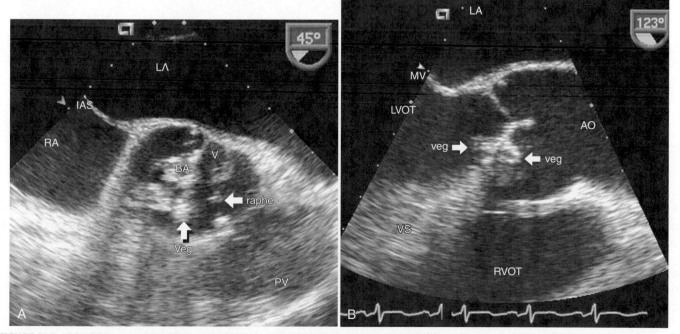

FIGURE 8–1   Bicuspid aortic valve (BAV) vegetation in acute staphylococcal endocarditis with acute severe aortic regurgitation. Transesophageal echocardiograms **(A)** short axis and **(B)** long axis. Patient underwent emergency surgery. AO, aorta; IAS, interatrial septum; LA, left atrium; LVOT, left ventricular outflow tract; RA, right atrium; RV, right ventricle; RVOT, right ventricular outflow tract; PV, pulmonary valve.

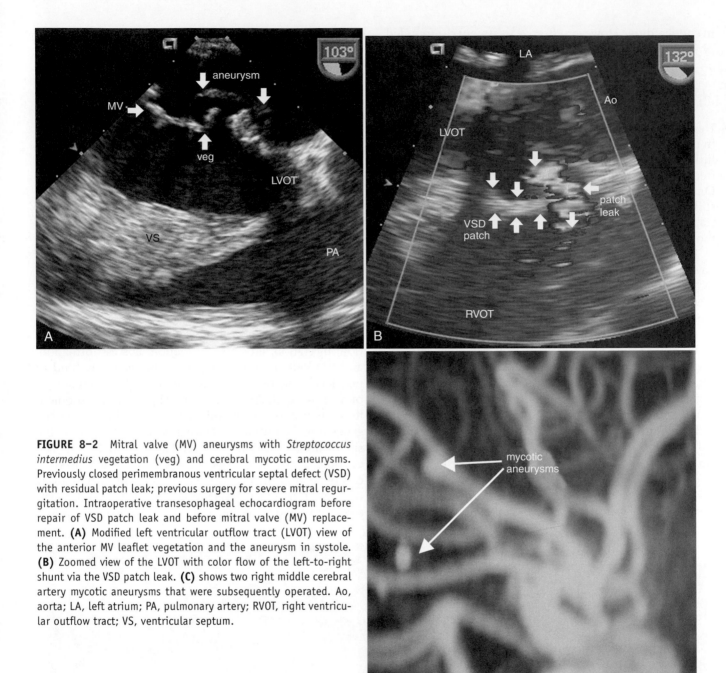

FIGURE 8-2 Mitral valve (MV) aneurysms with *Streptococcus intermedius* vegetation (veg) and cerebral mycotic aneurysms. Previously closed perimembranous ventricular septal defect (VSD) with residual patch leak; previous surgery for severe mitral regurgitation. Intraoperative transesophageal echocardiogram before repair of VSD patch leak and before mitral valve (MV) replacement. **(A)** Modified left ventricular outflow tract (LVOT) view of the anterior MV leaflet vegetation and the aneurysm in systole. **(B)** Zoomed view of the LVOT with color flow of the left-to-right shunt via the VSD patch leak. **(C)** shows two right middle cerebral artery mycotic aneurysms that were subsequently operated. Ao, aorta; LA, left atrium; PA, pulmonary artery; RVOT, right ventricular outflow tract; VS, ventricular septum.

An aortic regurgitant jet or a prolapsing aortic vegetation can affect the anterior mitral leaflet causing a secondary vegetation.

The consequences of the infective vegetation depend on the site or structure involved and on the virulence of the organism. Valvular destruction with acute severe regurgitation causes heart failure. The endarteritis of patent ductus or aortic coarctation can cause aneurysm formation and rupture. Embolizations are responsible for arterial bed obstruction (stroke) and abscess formation. Immunologic reactions trigger glomerulonephritis or vasculitis owing to deposition of circulating immune complexes in the small vessels in skin (Janeway lesions and Osler nodes).[15,19,22,37,38]

CONGENITAL HEART DISEASE AND INFECTIVE ENDOCARDITIS

It is currently estimated that in the United States alone, approximately 1 million adults have CHD, an estimate that exceeds the number of children with CHD[39] (see

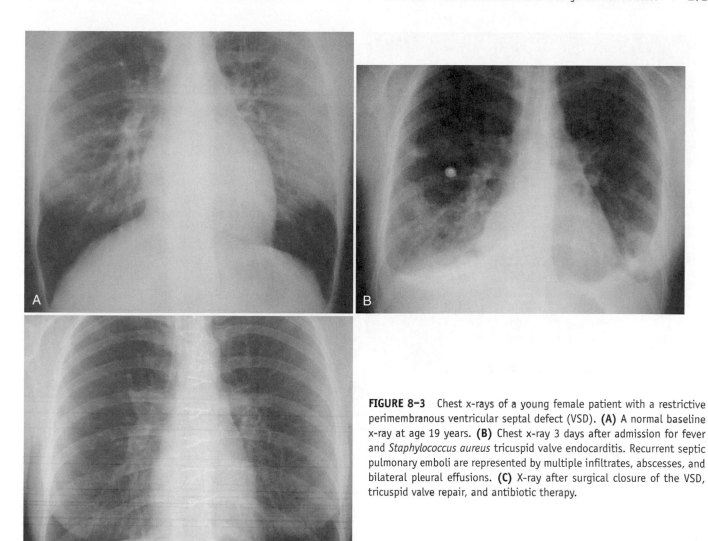

FIGURE 8-3   Chest x-rays of a young female patient with a restrictive perimembranous ventricular septal defect (VSD). **(A)** A normal baseline x-ray at age 19 years. **(B)** Chest x-ray 3 days after admission for fever and *Staphylococcus aureus* tricuspid valve endocarditis. Recurrent septic pulmonary emboli are represented by multiple infiltrates, abscesses, and bilateral pleural effusions. **(C)** X-ray after surgical closure of the VSD, tricuspid valve repair, and antibiotic therapy.

Chapter 1). Because cure in the literal sense is rarely achieved,[5] obligatory postoperative residua and sequelae predispose to or increase the risk of IE[2,29,32,40–42] (see Chapter 20). A study of the cardiac lesions in adults with IE disclosed that in 13% the substrate was CHD.[43] Infective endocarditis accounted for 4% of admissions to a specialized adult CHD service.[29] Unoperated tetralogy of Fallot, transposition of the great arteries, ventricular septal defect (VSD), patent ductus arteriosus, and bicuspid aortic valves were especially well represented,[44] and systemic-to-pulmonary shunts or reparative surgery with prosthetic valves or conduits are major predisposing causes.

Cardiac lesions and their relative susceptibility to IE are listed in Table 8–1. Sixty-two cases of pediatric infective endocarditis from 1977 to 1992 were compared with cases from the 1970s and 1980s.[44] Complex cyanotic CHD represented the highest risk in both groups. Tetralogy of Fallot constituted the largest subgroup in earlier reports, but more recently, complex congenital malformations, palliative

shunts, and valved conduits were the largest categories.[45,46] Repaired tetralogy without residual defects constitutes a relatively low risk. However, long-term survival of children with complex lesions and with surgical repair or palliation results in exposure to the risk of IE for a greater number of patient-years (discussed earlier). Forty-eight episodes of IE in 42 patients with CHD (1970–1990) were compared with a 1953 to 1972 series of 108 cases.[40] In unoperated patients, aortic valve disease was most commonly represented (38%). Three patients had a VSD, and one had tetralogy. Among postoperative patients with IE, two thirds had either repaired tetralogy of Fallot (38%) or aortic valve disease (25%). There was no case of IE in surgically repaired VSDs. Valve replacements including valved conduits accounted for 46%. Early postoperative endocarditis occurred infrequently because of improved management of infection.

The *Second Natural History Study of Congenital Heart Defects* reported the incidence of IE in aortic stenosis,

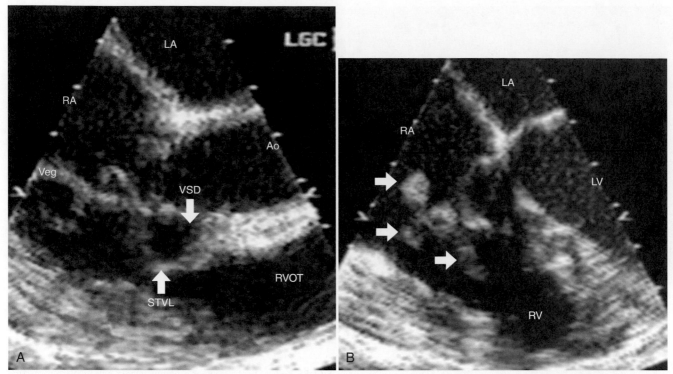

FIGURE 8-4 Perimembranous ventricular septal defect (VSD) and tricuspid valve *Staphylococcus aureus* vegetation (veg). **(A)** Short-axis transesophageal echocardiogram of the VSD showing partial closure by the septal tricuspid valve leaflet (STVL) and the tricuspid vegetation. **(B)** Fourchamber transesophageal echocardiogram showing the multilobular tricuspid valve vegetation (three arrows). In real time, the vegetation was mobile and chaotic. The patient underwent urgent tricuspid valve repair and VSD closure because of recurrent septic pulmonary emboli. Ao, aorta; LA, left atrium; LV, left ventricle; RA, right atrium; RV, right ventricle.

pulmonic stenosis, and VSD.[40] In these patients, by definition unoperated, the incidence of IE was nearly 35 times the population-based rate, with *Streptococcus viridans* as the predominant organism. The prevalence of IE after aortic valvotomy was unchanged because a bicuspid aortic remains bicuspid and therefore retains its susceptibility, with risk apparently related to the peak systolic gradient rather than to aortic regurgitation. Only one case of unoperated pulmonic stenosis appeared in the series. There was no relationship between IE and VSD size. The risk of IE before surgical closure was more than twice the postoperative risk. Aortic regurgitation was an independent risk factor for endocarditis in patients with VSD whether managed medically or surgically. At least 22% of patients who developed IE after VSD repair had a residual defect leak.[40]

In 1998, Li and Somerville[29] reviewed 214 episodes of IE in 185 adults with congenital heart disease. Two time intervals were included—1983 to 1993 and 1993 to 1996. Patients were divided into unoperated or palliated (Group I) and operated with definitive repair or valve repair/replacement (Group II). No cases of IE occurred in ostium secundum ASDs either before or after closure or in closed VSDs, closed patent ductus, isolated PS, unrepaired Ebstein anomaly, or after a Fontan or Mustard operation. In Group I, IE was most commonly associated with VSD (24%) and with lesions of the left ventricular (LV) outflow

tract (17%) and mitral valve (13%). In Group II, IE involved the LV outflow tract (35%), repaired tetralogy of Fallot (19%), and atrioventricular defects (14%). A predisposing event was identified in 41% of IE episodes, including a dental procedure or sepsis in 33% of Group I and cardiovascular surgery in 50% of Group II. IE recurred in 21 of the 185 patients (11%), although specific risk factors were unclear. The time from onset of symptoms to diagnosis of IE differed in the two groups, with a mean of 60 days in Group I and 29 days in Group II.[29] Seven episodes of IE developed in six patients with Eisenmenger syndrome (on the tricuspid valve in three of four with VSD and on all valves in one) and on a truncal valve in two. Four patients with aortic coarctation had IE, one unoperated with severe coarctation and a postcoarctation aneurysm. Tetralogy of Fallot was the malformation in 12 Group I patients, five with Blalock-Taussig shunts, and one with a Waterston shunt. Vegetations were on the Blalock-Taussig shunt in three patients, on the aortic valve in two, and on the tricuspid valve in one. One other patient experienced two episodes of IE in the RVOT after pulmonary valvotomy and infundibular resection.

Among Group II patients with tetralogy of Fallot, IE vegetations were located on the aortic valve in three, on the tricuspid valve in one with a residual VSD, on a Blalock-Taussig shunt in one, on a right ventricular-to-

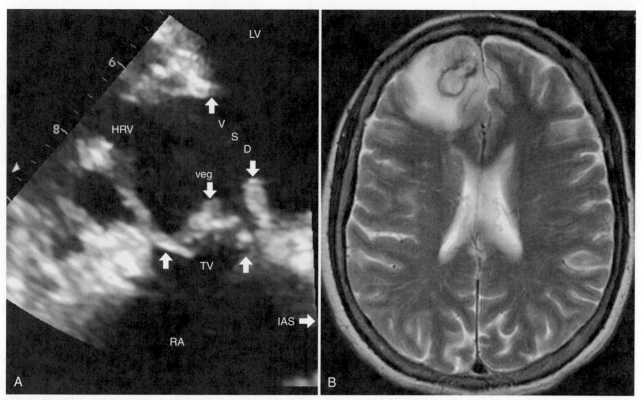

FIGURE 8–5   Eisenmenger ventricular septal defect (VSD) with hypoplastic right ventricle (HRV) and healed tricuspid valve (TV) vegetation (veg). **(A)** A four-chamber transthoracic echocardiogram (zoomed view) showing the vegetation with islands of calcification. In real time, the vegetation was sessile, moving with the motion of the TV. **(B)** Acute headache, altered consciousness, and brain abscess. Magnetic resonance image shows the abscess with peripheral edema and mild compression of adjacent structures. Surgical drainage was followed by a full course of antibiotic therapy and clinical recovery. IAS, interatrial septum; LV, left ventricle; RA, right atrium.

pulmonary conduit in one, on the pulmonary valve in two with infundibular stenosis and a residual VSD, and on a left pulmonary artery stent in one. In 13 patients with congenitally corrected transposition, 20 episodes of IE involved the native left atrioventricular valve, a bioprosthetic left atrioventricular valve, the right atrioventricular valve crossed by a pacemaker lead, the pulmonary valve, and the pulmonary artery bifurcation. Twelve patients with univentricular hearts experienced 15 episodes of IE on the aortic, pulmonary, and atrioventricular valves. Five patients had six episodes of IE on right ventricular to pulmonary artery valved conduits, four on homografts, and one on a pulmonary valve autograft. Deaths included one patient with *Coxiella burneti* infection and another with *Staphylococcus aureus* IE after operation for an obstructed Hancock prosthetic valve.

The incidence of IE after surgery for CHD performed between 1958 and 1998 was reported from the Oregon population-based registry.[30] Patients had undergone surgical repair at age 18 years or younger for 1 of 12 major defects. A decade after operation, the incidence of IE was 1.1% for complete atrioventricular septal defect (ASD), 5.3% for pulmonary atresia with intact ventricular septum, and 6.4% for pulmonary atresia with VSD. Twenty years after surgery, the cumulative incidence of IE for

D-transposition was 4%. Twenty-five years after surgery, the cumulative incidence of IE was 1.3% for tetralogy of Fallot, 2.7% for isolated VSD, 3.5% for aortic coarctation, and 13.3% for aortic valve stenosis. No patient experienced IE after repair of secundum ASD, patent ductus, or pulmonary valve stenosis.

In 2005, Niwa et al.[31] reported data from 66 institutions in a Japanese national multicenter database established to formulate recommendations on the management of IE in CHD. One hundred seventy pediatric patients and 69 adults with CHD experienced 240 admissions for IE between 1997 and 2001. Fifty-nine percent of the patients with IE had undergone surgery, 88 for cyanotic malformations. Most common lesions were VSD, ASD plus VSD or plus PDA (37.5%), tetralogy of Fallot with or without pulmonary atresia (18.1%), single ventricle with heterotaxy (8.8%), double-outlet right ventricle (7.4%), mitral stenosis/regurgitation (6.9%), and aortic stenosis/regurgitation (5.1%). IE was left sided in 46% and right sided in 51%. The most common organisms were streptococci (50%) and staphylococci (37%). Surgery was performed during active IE in 26%, usually for a large vegetation (45%) or heart failure (29%). Complications occurred in 48.5%. Mortality was 8% for medical treatment alone and 11.1% when surgery was employed. In 33.3% of patients, IE was

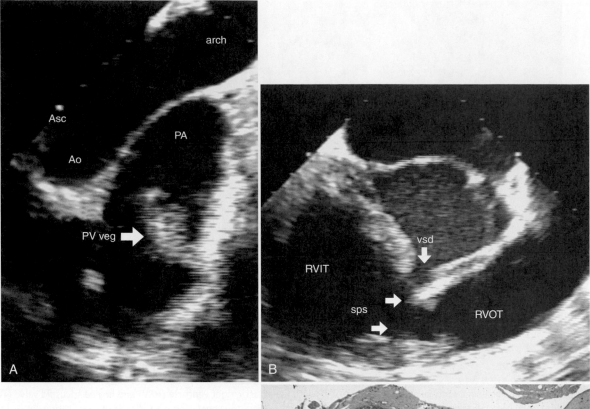

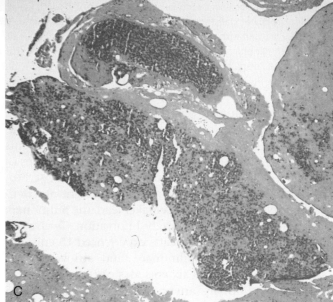

FIGURE 8-6 Pulmonary valve (PV) *Staphylococcus epidermidis* vegetation (veg) in 39-year-old patient with a double-chambered right ventricle, ostial subpulmonic stenosis, and a restrictive perimembranous ventricular septal defect. **(A)** Intraoperative transesophageal echocardiogram (high pulmonary artery view adjacent to the aortic arch, Asc Ao = ascending aorta) showing the pulmonary (PV) vegetation at end-systole. In real time, the vegetation (veg) was mobile, chaotic, and associated with significant pulmonary regurgitation. **(B)** Subpulmonic stenosis (SPS) adjacent to the restrictive ventricular septal defect (vsd), the double-chambered right ventricle with a hypertrophied right ventricular inflow tract (RVIT), and a thin-walled outflow tract (RVOT). **(C)** Resected pulmonary valve vegetation with platelet-fibrin deposits, inflammatory infiltrate, and microorganisms.

associated with a predisposing risk factor—dental procedures (37.2%), cardiovascular surgery (25.6%), and pneumonia (14.1%). Only 28.2% of these patients had received appropriate prophylaxis.

In 2006, Di Filippo et al.[24] reported 153 episodes of IE diagnosed with the revised Duke criteria in patients with CHD. The annual rate increased from 3.5 per year between 1966 and 1989 to 6.0 per year from 1990 to 2001. There were more adults during the second period compared with the first (40% vs. 9%, respectively), with a mean age that increased from 9.6 (± 8.4) years to 16.8

(± 12.1) years. CHD had been recognized before IE in 122 patients and was unrecognized in 31. Of the 153 study patients, 39 had repaired lesions, 35 had palliation usually for complex disease, and 79 were unoperated. The proportion of episodes of IE decreased in tetralogy of Fallot from 12% to 3% and increased from 14% to 28% in complex cyanotic CHD. The proportion associated with unoperated restrictive VSDs and unoperated mitral or aortic valve anomalies also increased. Dental procedures as presumed causes of IE were more common during the 1990 to 2001 period (33% vs. 20%), cutaneous

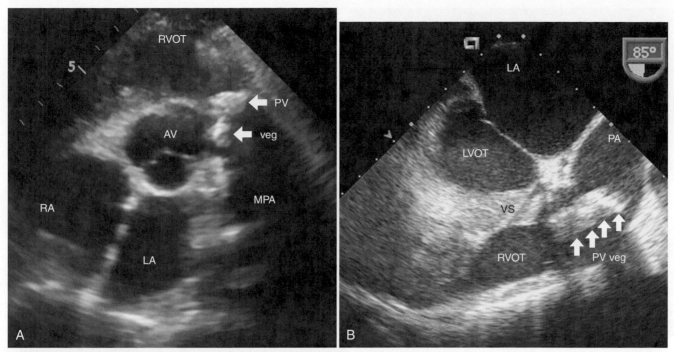

FIGURE 8-7   *Bartonella henselae* endocarditis with pulmonary valve (PV) vegetation (veg) in a patient with tetralogy of Fallot, intracardiac repair, and monocusp pericardial pulmonary valve reconstruction. The diagnosis of infective endocarditis was delayed because of difficulty in identifying an organism. **(A)** Transthoracic short-axis image of the PV vegetation. **(B)** Transesophageal image of the PV vegetation that was long and moderately mobile. AV, aortic valve; LA, left atrium; LVOT, left ventricular outflow tract; MPA, main pulmonary artery; PA, pulmonary artery; RA, right atrium; RVOT, right ventricular outflow tract. While on antibiotic therapy, the patient underwent surgical removal of the vegetation and implantation of a bioprosthetic valve.

infection rose from 5% to 17%, and postoperative infection was less frequent (11% vs. 21%). Streptococci were the most common organisms in both periods followed by staphylococci. The most prevalent substrates were complex cyanotic congenital heart disease, lesions repaired with prosthetic materials, and restrictive VSDs. Prophylaxis targeting dental and skin origins of IE was emphasized.[24]

DIAGNOSIS

Recommendations for the diagnosis and management of IE have appeared in numerous references.[3,8,11,13,][15,19,20,22,24,27,37,47,48] Patients with unexplained fever and with unoperated or operated CHD that predisposes to IE should have at least two sets of blood cultures drawn from different sites before administration of antibiotics.[49] Although the classic Oslerian manifestations of IE—fever, bacteremia, new or worsened murmurs, peripheral emboli, and immunologic vascular abnormalities—are still encountered,[50] presenting features are often atypical and are mistaken for or obscured by coexisting diseases.[51-55] Acute IE involving an aortic valve prosthesis may present as sepsis, stroke (systemic emboli), the sudden murmur of aortic regurgitation, atrioventricular block, and perforation of adjacent structures with a fistulous tract. (see Fig. 8-1).

Clinically suspected IE can be difficult to confirm without blood cultures and echocardiography. The diagnosis may be more difficult in children than in adults, but in both age groups, difficulty is more likely in complex congenital defects, particularly those with surgically created shunts or conduits.[8] Adequate assessment of complex malformations usually requires transesophageal echocardiography (TEE) by an examiner experienced in both TEE and CHD.[56] Even then, the yield tends to be limited unless the diagnosis is clinically suspected.[57]

Duke Criteria

In 1981, Von Reyn et al.[13,57] used strict case criteria to categorize the diagnosis of IE as definite, probable, possible, or rejected. In 1994, the *Duke Criteria* were proposed using two-dimensional transthoracic echocardiography (TTE).[58] The two *major criteria* were a positive echocardiogram and positive blood cultures. A *positive echocardiogram* was based on identification of an oscillating intracardiac mass on a valve or adjacent structure, on a jet impact site, or on prosthetic material, an abscess, or partial dehiscence of a prosthetic valve. Additional evidence included new-onset valvular regurgitation but not a change in a preexisting murmur. *Minor criteria* included a predisposing substrate, fever, vascular and immunologic phenomena, suggestive microbiologic information,

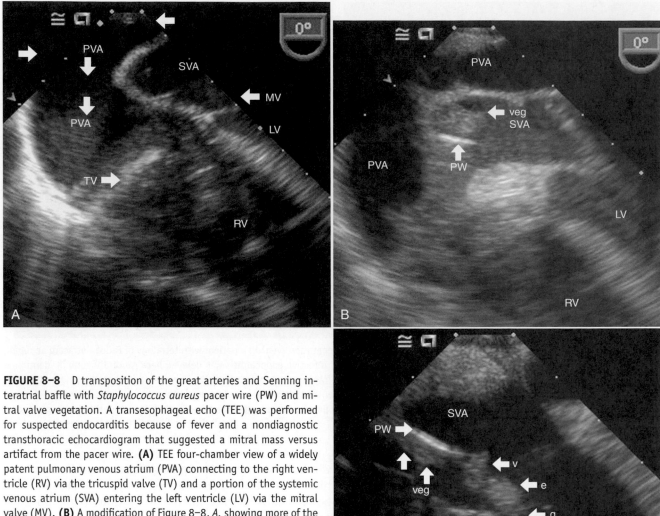

FIGURE 8-8 D transposition of the great arteries and Senning interatrial baffle with *Staphylococcus aureus* pacer wire (PW) and mitral valve vegetation. A transesophageal echo (TEE) was performed for suspected endocarditis because of fever and a nondiagnostic transthoracic echocardiogram that suggested a mitral mass versus artifact from the pacer wire. **(A)** TEE four-chamber view of a widely patent pulmonary venous atrium (PVA) connecting to the right ventricle (RV) via the tricuspid valve (TV) and a portion of the systemic venous atrium (SVA) entering the left ventricle (LV) via the mitral valve (MV). **(B)** A modification of Figure 8–8, *A,* showing more of the SVA. Pacer wire is seen, as is an attached soft homogenous vegetation (veg). **(C)** Further rotation of the TEE probe to show the PW in the SVA via the MV. The pacemaker wire vegetation and MV vegetation are both seen.

and observations consistent with but not meeting the major echocardiographic criteria.

Diagnostic categories for infective endocarditis were divided into *definite* (two major criteria or one major and five minor criteria), *possible* (one major and one minor or three minor criteria), and *rejected* (a firm alternative diagnosis, resolution of the illness, and no evidence of vegetations at surgery or necropsy.)[59] It has been proposed that elevated levels of C-reactive protein be added to the minor diagnostic criteria.[57,60] Compared with von Reyn, the Duke Criteria were more sensitive for the diagnosis of IE, based largely on echocardiographic detection of vegetations.[57,60] However, there was no mention of CHD,[59] infants and young children were not assessed,[49,61,62] and there were only three adults with CHD.[49]

When compared with pathologically confirmed cases of IE, the Duke criteria are sensitive (>80%) and have a high positive and negative predictive value.[3,8,11,13,19,20,48,49,63,64] However, there are shortcomings, particularly the excessively broad category of "possible IE."[51,52,65–67] The Duke Criteria were subsequently refined in an attempt to improve detection of culture negative IE and *S. aureus* bacteremia, to remove suggestive but nondiagnostic minor TTE criteria, and to emphasize use of TEE.[51,52,65–67]

Echocardiography

Delineation of intracardiac and extracardiac anatomy and of flow patterns and hemodynamics by TTE and TEE has revolutionized the diagnosis and management of heart

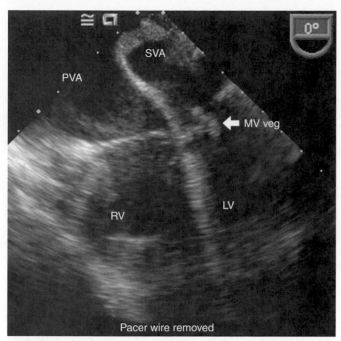

FIGURE 8-9   Pacer wire removed

FIGURE 8–9   Complete transposition of the great arteries after a Senning procedure with mitral vegetation induced by a pacer wire (see Fig. 8–8). Four-chamber transesophageal echo view showing the residual mitral valve (MV) vegetation after pacer lead extraction. LV, left ventricle; PVA, pulmonary venous atrium; RV, right ventricle; SVA, systemic venous atrium.

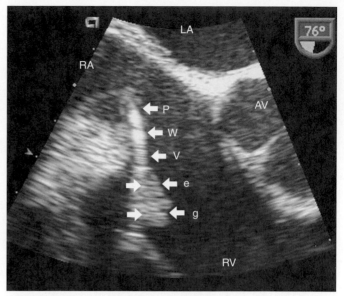

FIGURE 8–10   Transesophageal echocardiogram (TEE) in right-sided *Staphylococcus aureus* endocarditis with pacer wire (PW) vegetation (veg). The TEE was performed for suspected endocarditis because the transthoracic echocardiogram was unrevealing despite fever, bacteremia, and a known foreign body (permanent pacemaker). AV, aortic valve; LA, left atrium; RA, right atrium; RV, right ventricle.

disease.[51–53,55,65,67] Echocardiography is crucial for the diagnosis of IE.[51–53,65,67,68] (see Figs. 8–1 through 8–10). TEE is particularly useful in evaluating congenital cardiovascular malformations, prosthetic valves, palliative shunts, ventricular outflow tracts, valved conduits, the superior vena cava for indwelling catheter or pacer lead vegetations, the thoracic aorta, the paracoarctation aorta, the pulmonary artery, and the ductus arteriosis.[69–73] The recording and interpretation of echocardiography in children and adults require appropriate training, expertise, and experience.[3,8,37,49,59,60,74]

No clinical diagnostic technique is better equipped than echocardiography for visualizing vegetations.[3,27,70,75–78] Inclusion of TTE in the Duke Criteria was a major step forward.[49] Much interest has focused on the merits of TTE versus TEE for low, medium, or high probability IE; when to proceed straightaway with TEE; how best to proceed if the initial examination is negative; and how often a study should be repeated.[3,8,54,55,65,70,72] Modifications of the Duke Criteria proposed in 2000 recommended TEE as the initial diagnostic method in the *possible* category when paravalvular IE or prosthetic valve IE is suspected.[3,8,54,55,65,70,72] A high likelihood of IE clearly warrants an echocardiogram.[78] It is best to proceed first with TTE provided there are no prosthetic materials. In the presence of conduits, prosthetic valves, surgically created shunts, or other connections not well seen by TTE, it is best to proceed initially with TEE.[76] When there is clinical evidence of IE, TEE improves the sensitivity of the Duke Criteria for the diagnosis of *definite IE* and is particularly helpful in the evaluation of *suspected IE* on prosthetic valves. It is appropriate to start with a TEE in patients whose habitus (obesity) or confounding diseases (emphysema) predict suboptimal TTE images. For suspected IE in children, TTE is recommended because the acoustic windows are better than in adults, and TEE in children often requires general anesthesia.

The indications for TTE and TEE are discussed in the American College of Cardiology (ACC)/American Heart Association (AHA)/American Society of Echocardiography (ASE) 2003 Guidelines for the Clinical Application of Echocardiography,[70] in the 2004 ESC endocarditis guidelines,[8] in the 2005 ACC/AHA endocarditis guidelines,[3] in the ACC/AHA valvular heart disease guidelines,[27] and in Chapter 6 of this volume. Echocardiography is useful not only for detecting vegetations but also for identifying pathological and hemodynamic consequences of IE—ventricular dysfunction, valvular regurgitation, perforations, flail or ruptured chords, and abscesses, shunts, and fistulae.[3,11,13,15,27,37,52,54,55,65,66,68–70,72,79–87]   TEE remains more sensitive for detecting vegetations despite advances in TTE imaging technologies such as improved transducers, harmonic imaging, and more powerful microprocessors. The difference in sensitivity is particularly apparent in patients with CHD, prosthetic valves, or prosthetic materials (see Figs. 8–6 through 8–10) and for establishing the presence and severity of complications such as abscesses, perforations, and fistulas [3,15,19,20,27,48,54,55,69–72,88,89] (see Fig. 8–2). Three-dimensional echocardiography has

Table 8–1 Infective Endocarditis: Risk Stratification, Armanson-UCLA Adult Congenital Heart Disease Center

Low-Risk Unoperated (Prophylaxis Not Required)

Uncomplicated secundum atrial septal defect
Ebstein's anomaly
Isolated uncomplicated congenitally corrected transposition of the great arteries
Mild pulmonary valve stenosis
Pulmonary regurgitation
Partial or total anomalous pulmonary venous connection
Pulmonary arteriovenous fistula

Low-Risk Postoperative

Coarctation of the aorta isolated, uncomplicated
Ventricular septal defect isolated, uncomplicated
Patent ductus arteriosus—ligation or division
Cavopulmonary shunt
Fontan operation

Intermediate- to High-Risk Unoperated (Prophylaxis Required)

Prior episode of infective endocarditis
Congenital left atrioventricular valve regurgitation
Bicuspid aortic valve
Coarctation of the aorta
Congenital aortic valve stenosis/regurgitation
Discrete subaortic stenosis
Pulmonary stenosis (moderate to severe)
Ventricular septal defect (restrictive)
Patent ductus arterisus (restrictive)
Tetralogy of Fallot and lesions with tetralogy physiology
Coronary arteriovenous fistula
Truncus arteriosus with truncal valve stenosis/regurgitation

Intermediate- to High-Risk Postoperative

Valvotomy or valvuloplasty for bicuspid aortic valve
Prosthetic valves or external conduits
Surgically constructed systemic arterial-to-pulmonary arterial shunts

Modified from Child JS, Perloff JK: Infective endocarditis: risks and prophylaxis. In: Perloff JK, Child JS: *Congenital Heart Disease in the Adult*. 2nd ed. Philadelphia, WB Saunders, 1998.

not been adequately evaluated in IE but shows promise for improved detection of valve complications.[85] IE is common in patients with *S. aureus* bacteremia (SAB) in which TEE has proved essential for the diagnosis and for determining the duration of therapy.[18,80,90] Echocardiography is also useful in culture-negative IE and for assessing persistent bacteremia, the source of which is unidentified[3,11,13,15,20,27,37,70,72] (see Fig. 8–7). TEE is essential preoperatively and intraoperatively when patients with CHD and IE require surgical intervention (see Figs. 8–2 and 8–6). An operator skilled and experienced with TEE for IE and complex operated CHD is obligatory.[68]

The 2003 update of the 1997 ACC/AHA guidelines on the clinical application of echocardiography includes recommendations for native valve endocarditis (NVE).[69,70]

Class I recommendations for which there is general echocardiographic agreement include the following: (1) detection and characterization of valvular lesions, their hemodynamic severity, and ventricular function; (2) detection and characterization of vegetations and lesions in patients with congenital heart disease; (3) detection of associated abnormalities (abscesses, shunts); (4) reevaluation in complicated endocarditis (virulent organism, severe hemodynamic lesion, aortic valve involvement, persistent fever or bacteremia, clinical change, or symptomatic deterioration); (5) assessment of patients with high clinical suspicion but culture-negative endocarditis (CNE); and (6) use of TEE when TTE is diagnostically equivocal, especially in patients with *Staphylococcus* bacteremia and fungemia of unknown source.

Prosthetic valve endocarditis (PVE), whether mechanical or bioprosthetic, usually starts in the sewing ring and with subsequent erosion, abscess, paravalvular perforation with conduction defects, paravalvular regurgitation, or fistulae to an adjacent chamber.[11,13,19,38,87,88,91–98] Vegetations on prosthetic valves are difficult to detect even with TEE, which is significantly more sensitive than TTE (86%–94% vs. 36%–69%).[27,69,70,72] The 2003 Class I echocardiography guidelines for PVE[70] include the following: (1) detection and characterization of valvular lesions, their hemodynamic severity, and ventricular function; (2) detection of associated abnormalities (abscesses, shunts); (3) reevaluation in complex endocarditis (virulent organism, severe hemodynamic lesion, aortic valve involvement, persistent fever or bacteremia, clinical change, or symptomatic deterioration); (4) evaluation of suspected endocarditis with negative cultures; and (5) evaluation of bacteremia of unknown source.

The 2006 ACC/AHA guidelines for valvular heart disease[27] include the following Class I indications for TEE: (1) to assess the severity of valvular lesions in symptomatic patients with IE when TTE is nondiagnostic; (2) to diagnose IE in valvular heart disease with positive blood cultures if TTE is nondiagnostic; (3) to diagnose complications of IE that potentially impact on prognosis and management (abscesses, perforation, and shunts); (4) as the first-line diagnostic study for prosthetic valve IE and to assess complications; (5) for preoperative evaluation of patients with IE unless the need for surgery is evident on TTE provided imaging does not delay urgently needed surgery; and (6) intraoperative TEE for patients undergoing valve surgery for IE. A Class IIa recommendation argued that TEE is applicable to diagnose possible infective endocarditis in patients with persistent staphylococcal bacteremia of unknown source.[27]

Blood Cultures

Blood cultures should always be obtained to establish a microbiologic etiology before initiating antimicrobial therapy.[3,8,11,13,15,19,20,22,37,48,64,99] Culture-negative endocarditis is often the result of administration of antibiotics before obtaining blood cultures.[3,8,11,13,20,37,48,64] A prospective multicenter survey of medical practice in Europe found that of 159 patients with active IE, only 113 (71%) had blood cultures before the start of antibiotics.[26] The 2006 ACC/AHA Practice Guidelines on the evaluation and management of infective endocarditis in valvular heart disease[27] stated as a Class I recommendation that "Patients at risk for infective endocarditis who have unexplained fever for more than 48 hours should have at least two sets of blood cultures obtained from different sites." Also emphasized was a Class III recommendation that "Patients with known valve disease or a valve prosthesis should not receive antibiotics before blood cultures are obtained for unexplained fever."[27]

Culture-Negative Endocarditis and Unusual or Fastidious Organisms

The most common cause of CNE is the inappropriate administration of antibiotics before blood cultures are obtained. An increasingly common alternative cause of CNE is fastidious bacteria—*Coxiella, Bartonella,* HACEK group (*Hemophilus* species, *Actinobacillus actinometemcomitans, Cardiobacter hominus, Eikenella corrodens, Kingella kingae*), and fungi such as *Candida* or *Aspergillus* species that require for identification specialized culture techniques or modalities.[3,11,13,15,20,22,37,48,64] These fastidious organisms are particularly common on prosthetic valves or conduits,[54] indwelling lines or pacemakers,[6,100,101] or in patients with immunocompromised host defenses or renal failure.[12,14,23,102,103] Many of these microbes are difficult to treat (e.g., *Bartonella* may be intracellular; see Fig. 8–7).

Histological/Immunological/Molecular Diagnosis

Non-culture-based molecular methods substantially improve the diagnostic yield of microbiologic examination of excised heart valves.[106-108] Polymerase chain reaction (PCR) using broad range primers from conserved bacterial and fungal 16S *rRNA* genes can be used to diagnose IE, and direct DNA sequencing of 16sRNA can identify the organism to the species level. PCR improves the diagnosis of IE associated not only with fastidious or slow-growing organisms and difficult-to-culture or nonculturable organisms (e.g., *Bartonella* [Fig. 8–7] and *C. burnetti*) but also with easy-to-culture bacteria such as streptococci and staphylococci.[106] PCR easily becomes contaminated, so control reactions are always required. However, the persistence of bacterial DNA on cardiac valves after treatment does not necessarily indicate the persistence of viable bacteria.[109] Because PCR is most commonly performed on resected valve tissue, it is not useful for the majority of cases of suspected IE in which surgery is neither anticipated nor necessary. Whether PCR techniques

will replace blood cultures is uncertain.[110] Although elevation of these inflammatory markers supports the diagnosis of IE, it does not clarify the microbial etiology or help direct antimicrobial therapy.

Histology is included in the major Duke Criteria—pathologic examination of resected tissue and extracted emboli.[57] The pathology may also guide antimicrobial treatment when the causative microorganism can be identified by special stains or immunohistochemistry.[20,48,64] Serology for *Coxiella burnetti* and *Bartonella* can be diagnostic. Electron microscopy of extracted valvular tissue or vegetations is useful, although expensive and time-consuming.[20] Tissue specimens should be retained for as long as a year after treatment to determine whether another episode of IE is due to a new organism or to recurrence of the prior infection.

To avoid the problem of difficult-to-diagnose organisms, blood culture alternatives have been sought such as cytokines (interleukin-6 and -2R) for diagnosis and monitoring the course of inflammation during treatment.[93] However, chronic heart failure can incur a state of immune activation with endotoxin as a potential trigger for cytokine production. Elevated circulating levels of cytokines (tumor necrosis factor and receptors, interleukins, soluble CD 14 levels) and bacterial endotoxin have been reported in adults with congenital heart disease and systemic ventricular dysfunction but do not resolve the question of predictive value.[104] A prospective study of circulating procalcitonin, another marker of systemic bacterial infection, disclosed negative and positive predictive values of IE in 92% and 72%, respectively.[105] Although elevation in these inflammatory markers may support the diagnosis of IE, they neither clarify the microbial etiology nor help guide antimicrobial therapy.

COMPLICATIONS

IE has been classified clinically as acute or subacute, on native or prosthetic valves, according to responsible organism, in the right or left side of the heart (or both), and as community or nosocomial acquired. Cardiac complications include congestive heart failure (CHF) (often due to acute valvular regurgitation[22]), perforated or flail leaflets, fistulous tracts with large shunts, coronary emboli, and myocarditis. A dreaded complication is perivalvular extension with abscess, perforation, fistula, or conduction defects.[38,88,111] Coronary artery microemboli or embolic arterial obstruction are potential causes of ischemia, infarction, myocarditis, myocardial abscess, or pericarditis.[3,8,11,13,16,19,27,38] Perivalvular extension typically involves the sewing ring or annulus and usually extends to include perivalvular infection, abscess formation, and valve dehiscence.

Risk of embolization tends to be highest shortly after the onset of IE and then declines rapidly following administration of effective antimicrobials. Serious embolic events are rare after 2 to 3 weeks of therapy.[3,27,112] Risk of embolization is greater with mitral valve IE, with echocardiographic evidence of relatively large (> 10–15 mm) mobile vegetations and with *Candida*, *Streptococcus bovis*, or *S. aureus* IE. Left-sided IE is a cause of systemic arterial emboli with neurologic, renal, mesenteric, and splenic involvement (discussed earlier). Right-sided IE can cause pulmonary emboli (see Figs. 8–3 and 8–4), infarction, pneumonitis, or abscess. Persistent sepsis may be due to inadequate therapy but may also reflect abscess formation including mycotic macro-aneurysms or micro-aneurysms or splenic abscess, each of which carries a risk of rupture. Neurologic complications can be devastating (see Chapter 14). Brain injuries usually due to embolization or mycotic aneurysms (see Fig. 8–2) were reported in 20% to 40% of patients during the active phase of IE.[3,11,22,38,113] Systemic emboli tend to be symptomatic, but refined imaging techniques now detect small areas of asymptomatic cerebral involvement (see Chapter 7; see Figs. 8–2 and 8–5). An asymptomatic cerebrovascular episode or a transient ischemic attack carries a relatively good prognosis in contrast to a clinically overt ischemic or hemorrhagic stroke.[11,81,113–115] Cerebrovascular complications increase the risk of cardiac surgery. Prognosis is especially poor with infected mechanical valves or when consciousness is impaired.[115]

Markers that predict early complications of IE or in-hospital death include infection with *S. aureus*, renal insufficiency, diabetes, and a higher APACHE II (Acute Physiology, Age, Chronic Health Evaluation II) score.[81,97,116,117] Prognosis is also affected by the presence and severity of CHF, sepsis, and abnormal mental status.[14,81,93,97,117] Patients who require urgent surgery experience an unfavorable clinical course.[117,118]

TREATMENT OF ENDOCARDITIS

Treatment should be a collaborative effort by cardiologists, infectious disease specialists, and cardiovascular surgeons.[3,8,22] The offending microorganism must be identified and eradicated. Proper treatment depends on prompt, precise, and timely diagnosis by echocardiographic imaging using TEE as indicated, and at least three sets of blood cultures within 1 hour, each sample containing 10 ml of blood from different sites.[3,8,27,55,70,72]

Medical Management

Empiric antimicrobial therapy should be initiated pending the results of blood cultures, especially in patients with acute severe sepsis or CHF. The type of presentation may assist in directing empiric therapy. For example, streptococci or staphylococci are the usual dominant organisms in community-acquired native valve IE. In an intravenous drug user, right-sided IE with *S. aureus* is most likely, but *Candida* or gram-negative organisms including *Serratia* are also encountered.[3,11,19,20,22] The distribution of organisms

in PVE varies substantially according to the time of onset after valve implantation. Early-onset (< 12 months) PVE is most commonly associated with staphylococci (coagulase-negative *S. aureus*), especially within 2 months after surgery.[15,22,23,87,93] Nevertheless, administration of antibiotics best awaits blood culture results, especially if antibiotics had been administered within the previous 2 weeks. After the specific organism has been identified and sensitivity testing performed, an optimal treatment regimen begins. Antimicrobial therapy typically involves bactericidal agents administered parentally at a dose, frequency, and duration sufficient to ensure diffusion of a high concentration of the agent into the vegetation and surrounding tissue to achieve eradication. Surgical intervention is determined by the initial presentation and by evolving events after therapy is begun.

Detailed reviews of antibiotic regimens for all types of organisms in IE appear in the Working Party of the British Society for Antimicrobial Therapy in 2004,[99] in the AHA Scientific Statement in 2005,[3] in the 2004 European Society of Cardiology (ESC) guidelines for IE,[8] in the seventh edition of the Braunwald textbook,[22] and most recently in the 2006 ACC/AHA valvular heart disease guidelines.[27] Because antimicrobial therapy is most commonly administered intravenously, patients with right-to-left shunts (cyanotic CHD) require inline air-bubble/particle filters that minimize iatrogenic air bubble systemic arterial embolism (see Chapter 19).

Tables 8–2 through 8–7 summarize the 2005 AHA Scientific Statement on Infective Endocarditis (Diagnosis, Antimicrobial Therapy, and Management of Complications), therapeutic recommendations for common scenarios (native or prosthetic valve endocarditis due to *viridans* group streptococci, *S. bovis*, or *Staphylococcus*). For more details and for other organisms, the reader is referred to the original reference.[3]

Anticoagulants in patients with mechanical prosthetic valve IE have not clearly been shown to protect against embolic events without risking hemorrhage.[3,11,114] IE with thromboembolism is associated with increased systemic coagulation activation, enhanced platelet activity, and impaired fibrinolysis.[119] Infection-related antiphospholipid antibodies potentially related to endothelial cell activation, thrombin generation, and impairment of fibrinolysis contribute to embolic risk.[120] The role of platelets in the development of vegetations has been well established.[13]

In experimental *S. aureus* IE, aspirin reportedly reduces the indicators of severity and embolic events.[121] Nevertheless, a randomized trial of aspirin in patients already on antibiotic therapy disclosed more bleeding events but no reduction of embolic risk.[111] Lack of effectiveness of aspirin in reducing embolic events in IE may be related in part to interference with platelet-associated antimicrobial activity. Mammalian platelets contain small cationic anti-staphylococcal peptides—thrombin-induced platelet-microbicidal proteins—which appear to play a role in host defense, mitigating the effects of IE as evidenced by reduced

Table 8-2   Therapy for Native Valve Endocarditis Caused by Highly Penicillin-Susceptible Viridans Group Streptococci and *Streptococcus bovis*

REGIMEN	DOSAGE* AND ROUTE	DURATION, WEEKS	STRENGTH OF RECOMMENDATION[†]	COMMENTS
Aqueous crystalline penicillin G sodium	12–18 million U/24 h IV either continuously or in 4 or 6 equally divided doses	4	IA	Preferred in most patients >65 y or patients with impairment of 8th cranial nerve function or renal function
or				
Ceftriaxone sodium	2 g/24 h IV/IM in 1 dose	4	IA	
	Pediatric dose[‡]: penicillin 200,000 U/kg per 24 h IV in 4–6 equally divided doses; ceftriaxone 100 mg/kg per 24 H IV/IM in 1 dose			
Aqueous crystalline penicillin G sodium	12–18 million u/24 h IV either continuously or in 6 equally divided doses	2	IB	2-wk regimen not intended for patients with known cardiac or extracardiac abscess or for those with creatinine clearance of < 20 ml/min, impaired 8th cranial nerve function, or *Abiotrophia, Granulicatella,* or *Gemella* spp. infection; gentamicin dosage should be adjusted to achieve peak serum concentration of < 1 µg/ml when 3 divided doses are used; nomogram used for single daily dosing
or				
Ceftriaxone sodium	2 g/24 h IV/IM in 1 dose	2	IB	
plus				
Gentamicin sulfate[§]	3 mg/kg per 24 h IV/IM in 1 dose	2		
	Pediatric dose: penicillin 200,000 U/kg per 24 h IV in 4–6 equally divided doses; ceftriaxone 100 mg/kg per 24 h IV/IM in 1 dose; gentamicin 3 mg/kg per 24 h IV/IM in 1 dose or 3 equally divided doses[¶]			
Vancomycin hydrochloride[#]	30 mg/kg per 24 h IV in 2 equally divided doses not to exceed 2 g/24 h unless concentrations in serum are inappropriately low	4	IB	Vancomycin therapy recommended only for patients unable to tolerate penicillin or ceftriaxone; vancomycin dosage should be adjusted to obtain peak (1 h after infusion completed) serum concentration of 30–45 µg/ml and a trough concentration range of 10–15 µg/mL
	Pediatric dose: 40 mg/kg per 24 h IV in 2–3 equally divided doses			

IM, intramuscular; IV, intravenous.

*Dosages recommended are for patients with normal renal function.

[†]IA means the benefit greatly exceeds risk; supported by multiple studies. IB means the benefit exceeds the risk; limited studies are available; additional studies are needed.

[‡]Pediatric dose should not exceed a normal adult dose.

[§]Other potentially nephrotoxic drugs (e.g., nonsteroidal anti-inflammatory drugs) should be used with caution in patients receiving gentamicin therapy.

[¶]Data for once-daily dosing of aminoglycosides for children exist, but no data for treatment of IE exist.

[#]Vancomycin dosages should be infused during a course of at least 1 hour to reduce risk of histamine-release "red-man" syndrome.

From Baddour L.M., Wilson W.R., Bayer A.S., et al.: *Circulation* 2005;111:e394–434.

disease progression and lower complication rates in experimental *S. aureus* IE.[122]

Warfarin increases the risk of intracerebral hemorrhage in IE patients who require long-term oral anticoagulation for mechanical heart valves.[123,124] Parenteral unfractionated heparin during the active phase of IE is an alternative,[3,8,11,27,87] in part because of a potential need for urgent surgery.

Surgical Management

Surgical intervention in IE may be needed urgently during the early or late active phase of antibiotic therapy, or it may be performed electively during the postantibiotic phase because of progressive valvular regurgitation.[117] Surgery for IE is mandatory in at least 30% of patients during active IE, and in 20% to 40% of patients during the healed

Table 8-3 Therapy for Native Valve Endocarditis Caused by Strains of *Viridans* Group Streptococci and *Streptococcus bovis* Relatively Resistant to Penicillin

REGIMEN	DOSAGE* AND ROUTE	DURATION, WEEKS	STRENGTH OF RECOMMENDATION[†]	COMMENTS
Aqueous crystalline penicillin G sodium	24 million U/24 h IV either continuously or in 4–6 equally divided doses	4	IB	Patients with endocarditis caused by penicillin-resistant (MIC > 0.5 µg/ml) strains should be treated with regimen recommended for enterococcal endocarditis (see Table 8–7)
or				
Ceftriaxone sodium	2 g/24 h IV/IM in 1 dose	4	IB	
plus				
Gentamicin sulfate[‡]	3 mg/kg per 24 h IV/IM in 1 dose	2		
	Pediatric dose[§]: penicillin 300,000 U/24 h IV, in 4–6 equally divided doses; ceftriaxone 100 mg/kg per 24 h IV/IM in 1 dose; gentamicin 3 mg/kg per 24 h IV/IM in 1 dose or 3 equally divided doses			
Vancomycin hydrochloride[§]	30 mg/kg per 24 h IV in 2 equally divided doses not to exceed 2 g/24 h unless serum concentrations are inappropriately low	4	IB	Vancomycin[¶] therapy recommended only for patients unable to tolerate penicillin or ceftriaxone therapy
	Pediatric dose: 40 mg/kg per 24 h IV in 2 or 3 equally divided doses			

*IM, intramuscular; IV, intravenous; MIC, minimum inhibitory concentration (> 0.12 ug/ml to ≤ 0.5 µg/ml).
*Dosages recommended are for patients with normal renal function.
[†]See Table 8–2.
[‡]See Table 8–2 for appropriate dosage of gentamicin.
[§]Pediatric dose should not exceed that of a normal adult.
[¶]See Table 8–2 for appropriate dosage of vancomycin.
From Baddour L.M., Wilson W.R., Bayer A.S., et al.: *Circulation* 2005;111:e394–434.

phase.[6,8,22,91,125] Complicated left-sided NVE causes significant morbidity and mortality. Surgery reduces 6-month mortality rate from 28% to 15%, particularly in the subgroup with moderate-to-severe CHF (mortality reduction from 51% to 14%).[81,126] An additional advantage of early surgery is a greater likelihood of successful valve repair, especially for an infected mitral valve.[92,127–132]

Surgical intervention is employed in patients with uncontrolled CHF, persistent emboli especially to the central nervous system, uncontrolled infection or sepsis, perivalvular or prosthetic infection, an unstable prosthesis or valvular obstruction, and heart block.[3,8,11,22,27,63,92,125] NVE or PVE with organisms known to be difficult to eradicate (*Bartonella*) or that may be large and bulky (fungal) often dictate the need for surgery[3,8,11,13,19,20,22,27,37,54] (see Fig. 8–7). Infected prosthetic material (pacemaker leads, indwelling catheters) frequently requires extraction of the infected foreign body[3,6–8,15,20,100,101,133] (See Figs. 8–9 and 8–10). Surgery should not be delayed while awaiting a clinical or microbiological response to antibiotics.[3,8,11,19,20,22,37] A TEE is virtually mandatory in the presence of PVE. Otherwise a TEE should be performed when

surgical intervention is necessary to evaluate the anatomic and hemodynamic substrate and to guide the type and extent of surgery. An intraoperative TEE should be performed immediately before and after the surgical intervention.[3,8,15,20,27,55,72]

In patients with PVE, particularly early-onset infection, prompt consultation with a cardiac surgeon is important because of the high in-hospital mortality and significant long-term morbidity.[3,8,11,20,27,92,93] The threshold for surgical intervention in PVE should be low, especially if the vegetation impairs prosthetic valve function. Subgroups that fare better with early surgery include patients with severe CHF, complicated PVE, and infection with *Staphylococcus*. Mortality is high with an in-hospital rate of 25%. Brain embolism and *S. aureus* infection in PVE were independently associated with high in-hospital mortality.[98] Patients with silent cerebrovascular complications have a relatively good prognosis, and surgery may be safely performed with improved survival. By contrast, patients with overt stroke have significantly increased mortality rates, especially in the presence of mechanical PVE or impaired consciousness.[115] PVE is associated with an in-hospital

Table 8–4   Therapy for Endocarditis Caused by Staphylococci in the Absence of Prosthetic Materials

REGIMEN	DOSAGE* AND ROUTE	DURATION, WEEKS	STRENGTH OF RECOMMENDATION[†]	COMMENTS
Oxacillin-susceptable strains				
Nafcillin or oxacillin[‡]	12 g/24 h IV in 4–6 equally divided doses	6 wk	IA	For complicated right-sided IE and for left-sided IE; for uncomplicated right-sided IE, 2 wk
with				
Optional addition of gentamicin sulfate[§]	3 mg/kg per 24 h IV/IM in 2 or 3 equally divided doses	3–5 d		
	Pediatric doses[¶]: nafcillin or oxacillin 200 mg/kg per 24 h IV in 4–6 equally divided doses; gentamicin 3 mg/kg per 24 h IV/IM in 3 equally divided doses			Clinical benefit of aminoglycosides has not been established
For penicillin-allergic (nonanaphylactoid type) patients:				Consider skin testing for oxacillin-susceptible staphylococci and questionable history of immediate-type hypersensitivity to penicillin
Cefazolin	6 g/24 h IV in 3 equally divided doses	6 wk	IB	Cephalosporins should be avoided in patients with anaphylactoid-type hypersensitivity to β-lactams; vancomycin should be used in these cases
with				
Optional addition of gentamicin sulfate	3 mg/kg per 24 h IV/IM in 2 or 3 equally divided doses	3–5 d		Clinical benefit of aminoglycosides has not been established
	Pediatric dose: cefazolin 100 mg/kg per 24 h IV in 3 equally divided doses; gentamicin 3 mg/kg per 24 h IV/IM in 3 equally divided doses			
Oxacillin-resistant strains				
Vancoycin	30 mg/kg per 24 h IV in 2 equally divided doses	6 wk	IB	Adjust vancomycin dosage to achieve 1-h serum concentration of 30–45 µg/ml and trough concentration of 10–15 µg/ml
	Pediatric dose: 40 mg/kg per 24 h IV in 2 or 3 equally divided doses			

IE, infective endocarditis; IM, intramuscular; IV, intravenous.
*Dosages recommended are for patients with normal renal function.
[†]See Table 8–2.
[‡]Penicillin G 24 million U/24 h IV in 4–6 equally divided doses may be used in place of nafcillin or oxacillin if strain is penicillin susceptible (minimum inhibitory concentration ≤ 0.1 g/ml) and does not produce β-lactamase.
[§]Gentamicin should be administered in close temporal proximity to vancomycin, nafcillin, or oxacillin dosing.
[¶]For specific dosing adjustment and issues concerning vancomycin, see Table 8–2 footnotes.
From Baddour L.M., Wilson W.R., Bayer A.S., et al.: *Circulation* 2005;111:e394–434.

mortality of 21%. Among posthospital survivors, late mortality was reported as 26% over a 32-month follow-up and highest in those with CHF, staphylococcal infection, and complicated PVE.[93] The subgroups with staphylococcal PVE and complicated PVE benefited the most from early surgical intervention.[93,98]

The International Collaboration on Endocarditis (ICE) identified the prognostic factors in *S. aureus* PVE.[134] In the merged database of 2212 cases of definite IE, 61 were *S. aureus* PVE with an overall mortality rate of 47.5%. Stroke was associated with increased risk of death.[134] Early valve replacement was not associated with significantly

Table 8-5   Therapy for Endocarditis of Prosthetic Valves or Other Prosthetic Material Caused by *Viridans* Group Streptococci and *Streptococcus bovis*

REGIMEN	DOSAGE* AND ROUTE	DURATION, WEEKS	STRENGTH OF RECOMMENDATION[†]	COMMENTS
Penicillin-susceptible strain (minimum inhibitory concentration ≤ 0.12 µg/ml)				
Aqueous crystalline penicillin G sodium	24 million U/24 h IV either continuously or in 4–6 equally divided doses	6	IB	Penicillin or ceftriaxone together with gentamicin has not demonstrated superior cure rates compared with monotherapy with penicillin or ceftriaxone for patients with highly susceptible strains; gentamicin therapy should not be administered to patients with creatinine clearance of < 30 ml/min
or				
Ceftriaxone sodium	2 g/24 h IV/IM in 1 dose	6	IB	
with or without				
Gentamicin sulfate[‡]	3 mg/kg per 24 h IV/IM in 1 dose *Pediatric dose*[§]: penicillin 300,000 U/kg per 24 h IV in 4–6 equally divided doses; ceftriaxone 100 mg/kg IV/IM once daily; gentamicin 3 mg/kg per 24 h IV/IM in 1 dose or 3 equally divided doses	2		
Vancomycin hydrochloride[¶]	30 mg/kg per 24 h IV in 2 equally divided doses *Pediatric dose*: 40 mg/kg per 24 h IV in 2 or 3 equally divided doses	6	IB	Vancomycin therapy recommended only for patients unable to tolerate penicillin or ceftriaxone
Penicillin relatively or fully resistant to strain (minimum inhibitory concentration > 0.12 µg/ml)				
Aqueous crystalline penicillin sodium	24 million U/24 h IV either continuously or in 4–6 equally divided doses	6	IB	
or				
Ceftriaxone sodium	2 g/24 h IV/IM in 1 dose	6	IB	
plus				
Gentamicin sulfate	3 mg/kg per 24 h IV/IM in 1 dose *Pediatric dose*: penicillin 300,000 U/kg per 24 h IV in 4–6 equally divided doses	6		
Vancomycin hydrochloride	30 mg/kg per 24 h IV in 2 equally divided doses *Pediatric dose*: 40 mg/kg per 24 h IV in 2 or 3 equally divided doses	6	IB	Vancomycin therapy recommended only for patients unable to tolerate penicillin or ceftriaxone

IM, intramuscular; IV, intravenous.

*Dosages recommended are for patients with normal renal function.

[†]See Table 8-2.

[‡]See Table 8-2 for appropriate dosage of gentamicin.

[§]Pediatric dose should not exceed that of a normal adult.

[¶]See Table 8-2 for appropriate dosage of vancomycin.

From Baddour L.M., Wilson W.R., Bayer A.S., et al.: *Circulation* 2005;111:e394–434.

improved survival in the whole study population, but the subgroup with complications and early valve replacement had the lowest mortality rate (28.6%).[134] In a cohort of 91 patients with IE who required surgery, most commonly for intractable CHF, preoperative left bundle branch block predicted the need for permanent pacemaker implantation (24.2%). An LV ejection fraction < 50% predicts in-hospital death (15.4%).[94]

It is generally agreed that more than one embolic episode warrants surgical intervention, the timing of which depends on whether there is cerebral hemorrhage.[3,8,11,22,27,92] Surgery is generally indicated

Table 8-6   Therapy for Prosthetic Valve Endocarditis Caused by Staphylococci

REGIMEN	DOSAGE* AND ROUTE	DURATION, WEEKS	STRENGTH OF RECOMMENDATION[†]	COMMENTS
Oxacillin-susceptable strains				
Nafcillin or oxacillin	12 g/24 h IV in 6 equally divided doses	≥6	IB	Penicillin G 24 million u/24 h IV in 4–6 equally divided doses may be used in place of nafcillin or oxacillin if strain is penicillin susceptible (minimum inhibitory concentration ≤ 0.1 µg/ml) and dose not produce β-lactamase; vancomycin should be used in patients with immediate-type hypersensitivity reactions to β-lactam antibiotics (see table 3 for dosing guidelines); cefazolin may be substituted for nafcillin or oxacillin in patients with non-immediate-type hypersensitivity reactions to penicillins
plus				
Rifampin	900 mg per 24 h IV/PO in 3 equally divided doses	≥6		
plus				
Gentamicin[‡]	3 mg/kg per 24 h IV/IM in 2 or 3 equally divided doses *Pediatric dose[§]*: nafcillin or oxacillin 200 mg/kg per 24 h IV in 4–6 equally divided doses; gentamicin 3 mg/kg per 24 h IV/IM in 3 equally divided doses	2		
Oxacillin-resistant strains				
Vancoycin	30 mg/kg per 24 h IV in 2 equally divided doses	≥6	IB	Adjust vancomycin achieve 1-h serum concentration of 30–45 µg/ml and trough concentration of 10–15 µg/ml
plus				
Rifampin	900 mg per 24 h IV/PO in 3 equally divided doses	≥6		
plus				
Gentamicin	3 mg/kg per 24 h IV/IM in 2 or 3 equally divided doses *Pediatric dose*: vancomycin 40 mg/kg per 24 h IV in 2 or 3 equally divided doses; rifampin 20 mg/kg per 24 h IV/PO in 3 equally divided doses (up to adult dose); gentamicin 3 mg/kg per 24 h IV or IM in 3 equally divided doses	2		

IM, intramuscular; IV, intravenous; PO, per so (oral administration).
*Dosages recommended are for patients with normal renal function.
[†]See Table 8-2.
[‡]Gentamicin should be administered in close proximity to vancomycin, nafcillin, or oxacillin dosing.
[§]Pediatric dose should not exceed that of a normal adult.
From Baddour L.M., Wilson W.R., Bayer A.S., et al.: *Circulation* 2005;111:e394–434.

when there is echocardiographic detection of a large mobile vegetation, especially > 10 mm on the anterior mitral leaflet, a persistent vegetation after embolization, or an increase in vegetation size despite appropriate antimicrobial therapy.[3,8,27,55,69,70,72,73,79,84,97,112] Other surgical indications include acute aortic or mitral regurgitation with LV failure, CHF unresponsive to medical therapy, valve perforation or rupture, perivalvular extension of infection with valve dehiscence, rupture or fistula, heart block, and large abscess or extension of abscess despite appropriate antimicrobial therapy. A secondary mitral vegetation caused by a large aortic valve vegetation prolapsing onto and abutting the anterior mitral leaflet may also be an indication for early surgical intervention.[8] There must be complete debridement or excision of infected tissue. Use of foreign body materials should be minimized while taking into account the need for a credible repair that minimizes the risk of recurrence of infection.[92] When patches are used, autologous pericardium is preferred (see Chapter 16). If the aortic valve requires replacement, a homograft has been advocated, with the Ross procedure an alternative[92] (see Chapter 16).

PREVENTION AND PROPHYLAXIS

Nonchemotherapeutic and chemotherapeutic approaches to IE prophylaxis are essentially the same for congenital and acquired heart disease. A susceptible substrate and a source of entry for the microorganisms must be considered.[3,8,21,22,32,52,74,135] Nonchemotherapeutic methods,

Table 8-7 Therapy for Native Valve or Prosthetic Valve Enterococcal Endocarditis Caused by Strains Susceptible to Penicillin, Gentamicin, and Vancomycin

REGIMEN	DOSAGE* AND ROUTE	DURATION, WEEKS	STRENGTH OF RECOMMENDATION[†]	COMMENTS
Ampicillin sodium	12 g/24 h IV in 6 equally divided doses	4–6	IA	Native vale: 4-wk therapy recommended for patients with symptoms of illness ≤ 3 mo; 6-wk therapy recommended for patients with symptoms > 3 mo
or				
Aqueous crystal-line penicillin G sodium	24 million U/24 h IV either continuously or in 4–6 equally divided doses	4–6	IA	Prosthetic valve or other prosthetic cardiac material: minimum of 6-wk therapy recommended
plus				
Gentamicin sulfate[‡]	3 mg/kg per 24 h IV/IM in 3 equally divided doses *Pediatric dose[§]*: ampicillin 300 mg/kg per 24 h IV in 4–6 equally divided doses; penicillin 300,000 U/kg per 24 h IV in 4–6 equally divided doses; gentamicin 3 mg/kg per 24 h IV/IM in 3 equally divided doses	4–6		
Vancomycin hydrochloride[¶]	30 mg/kg per 24 h IV in 2 equally divided doses	6	IB	Vancomycin therapy recommended only for patients unable to tolerate penicillin or ampicillin
plus				
Gentamicin sulfate	3 mg/kg per 24 h IV/IM in 3 equally divided doses *Pediatric dose*: vancomycin 40 mg/kg per 24 h IV in 2 or 3 equally divided doses, gentamicin 3 mg/kg per 24 h IV/IM in 3 equally divided doses	6		6-wk vancomycin therapy recommended because of decreased activity against enterococci

IM, intramuscular; IV, intravenous.
*Dosages recommended are for patients with normal renal function.
[†]See Table 8–2.
[‡]Dosage of gentamicin should be adjusted to achieve peak serum concentration of 3–4 g/ml and a trough concentration of < 1 g/ml. Patients with creatinine clearance of < 50 ml/min should be treated in consultation with an infectious diseases specialist.
[§]Pediatric dose should not exceed that of a normal adult.
[¶]See Table 8–2 for appropriate dosage of vancomycin.
From Baddour L.M., Wilson W.R., Bayer A.S., et al.: *Circulation* 2005;111:e394–434.

especially skin and gum care, are particularly important.[21] Oral hygiene begins with gum and tooth care. Food (e.g., hard candy) that encourages caries should be avoided. In cyanotic CHD, acne and spongy, friable gums require specific recommendations to reduce the risk of bacteremia[5] (Fig. 8–11). A soft-bristle or electric toothbrush is recommended. Epistaxis is frequent in cyanotic patients, and nasal cautery risks bacteremia. Dental visits that include cleaning and filling are recommended at least twice yearly and must be accompanied by appropriate antibiotic prophylaxis. Meticulous skin care is required, particularly in adolescents and adults with cyanotic heart disease and a predisposition to acne. Nail biting or picking—a compulsive disorder that risks bacteremia—must be aggressively addressed (see Chapter 13). Bites from insects or dogs may become infected.[21] Tattoos and body piercing are proscribed. Injection drug abuse is a well-known high risk factor, especially for acute right-side IE.

A predisposing event has been identified in no more than a minority of cases of IE.[3,4,8,11,13,22,28,74,136–138] Only 30% of children with IE had identifiable predisposing causes, which were, in decreasing order of frequency, cardiovascular surgery; respiratory tract infections; ear-nose-throat procedures; dental procedures; infections of the genitourinary tract, skin, or central nervous system; osteomyelitis; and cardiac catheterization. Predisposing events in 56% of cases were most commonly dental work, open heart surgery, and skin infections.[46] Antecedent events in 32% included dental work without antimicrobial prophylaxis, pharyngitis, sinusitis, enteritis, pelvic inflammatory disease, and cardiac catheterization.[40]

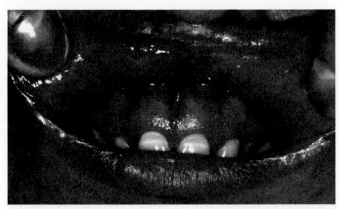

FIGURE 8-11 Cyanotic congenital heart disease and spongy gums as a risk substrate for infective endocarditis. The fingertips show digital clubbing and cyanosis.

Antimicrobial prophylaxis is based on the degree of risk of a susceptible cardiac lesion, the source and type of bacteremia, and drug allergy or sensitivity.[3,8,13,21,27,28,74,135,136] However, there is ongoing controversy because the efficacy of antimicrobial prophylaxis has not been proven in human beings. Instances of IE despite prophylaxis have raised questions. Episodes of IE often occur without exposure to known bacteremia-inducing procedures and thus are technically not preventable. Prophylaxis would not have been prescribed in patients who develop IE without exposure to a known bacteremic risk. A randomized, double-blind, placebo-controlled trial that would require an estimated 6,000 at-risk participants has never been undertaken, and the ethics of doing so are questionable.[28,136]

The connection between oral hygiene and IE was first noted in 1909; "Infection is grafted upon a previously sclerosed endocardium. ... the source of the infecting agent, in most cases, is the mouth."[74,136] Weiss in 1934[140] and Okell and Elliott in 1935[139] confirmed the relationship between oral sepsis and bacteremia in the etiology of IE.[139,140] Oral hygiene—brushing, flossing, mouth rinse, and routine dental care—is a patient responsibility. Education of patients and of health care professionals is the responsibility of the cardiologist. Regular appointments with a dentist or oral hygienist have important implications for prophylaxis.

Perhaps the liveliest focus of discussion during the past 2 decades has been the role of dental procedures in the etiology of IE.[28,136,141,142] It is generally agreed that extractions are accompanied by transient bacteremia that includes microorganisms known to cause endocarditis.[3,8,11,13,21,74,139,140] The presence, duration, and amount of preprocedural bacteremia in large part relates to whether the dental visit is routine in a patient with a normal oral cavity or whether there are abnormalities such as caries, periodontal disease, or periapical abscess. Before a tooth extraction, as many as 86% of patients have positive blood samples using the lysis filtration technique, which is more sensitive than blood cultures.[137,143,144] A recent

randomized, double-blind, controlled trial of 100 children, all of whom had dental caries, and 61% of whom had radiographic abscess formation were compared (placebo vs. amoxicillin prophylaxis) before cleaning and tooth extraction.[145] Cleanings resulted in bacteremia in 20% of the control subjects and 6% of the amoxicillin prophylaxis group.[145] Serial blood cultures before and immediately following single tooth extraction detected bacteremia in 84% of the placebo group versus 33% of the amoxicillin group.[145] Lysis filtration methods showed that detection of bacteremia (mainly genera of *Streptococcus, Actinomyces,* and *Staphylococcus*) was greatest 7.5 minutes after extraction and was negative at 15 minutes.[144]

A major population-based case-controlled study published in 1998 focused on dental and cardiac risk factors for IE.[146] Diagnoses in 273 adults with IE included CHD in 9.5%, mitral valve prolapse in 19%, valvular surgery in 13.6%, rheumatic heart disease in 6.2%, and prior IE in 6.2%. The frequency of dental procedures during the preceding 3 months was no greater in the IE patients than in the control subjects. There was a trend toward increased risk of IE in dentulous versus edentulous patients. A decreased risk with daily flossing suggested that oral hygiene is important.[147] IE patients differed according to important risk factors but not according to the preceding dental work.[147] Another study, by contrast, found that dental work increased the risk of IE fivefold, and prophylaxis prevented 70% of the cases.[148]

With few exceptions, it is our judgment that all adults with CHD—operated or unoperated, simple or complex, cyanotic or acyanotic—should receive IE prophylaxis. Recommendations have evolved significantly over the past decade.[3,8,21,27,28,135,149,150] New Guidelines for the Prevention of Endocarditis: Working Part of the British Society for Antimicrobial Chemotherapy (BSAC) in 2006 are based on local society consensus and not on new data or trials.[99] The AHA 2007 and BSAC 2006 recommend dental prophylaxis only for patients at the highest risk for IE or for significant consequences of IE, with the following indications: prosthetic cardiac valves; previous IE; CHD (unrepaired cyanotic CHD including palliative shunts and conduits; during the first 6 months following repair of CHD with prosthetic materials or devices to allow endothelialization; repaired CHD with residual defects at the site of or adjacent to a prosthetic patch or device that could inhibit endothelialization; or valvulopathy in a cardiac transplantation recipient.[28,150] In a major—indeed, radical—change, the AHA 2007 guidelines no longer recommended prophylaxis for any non-dental procedure. In stark contrast, the BSAC guidelines expanded the at-risk patient list, requiring antimicrobial prophylaxis before nondental potentially bacteremic procedures to include complex CHD (excluding secundum atrial septal defect), complex LV outflow tract malformations (including aortic stenosis and bicuspid aortic valves), acquired valve abnormalities, and mitral valve prolapse in the presence of "substantial leaflet pathology and regurgitation" by echocardiography.[28,150] The AHA 2007 and BSAC 2006 sought to justify these decisions by shifting the emphasis from "procedure-related bacteremia" to "cumulative bacteremia," an untested concept.[28,150] Adverse antibiotic or sensitivity reactions are exceedingly rare, but it has been suggested—without a firm basis—that the risk of anaphylaxis or serious side effects from high-dose penicillin is 5 times the risk of developing IE following dental procedures. These new recommendations are generating a great deal of discussion and controversy, with respondent letters reflecting considerable disagreement between the British Congenital Heart Association and the British Cardiovascular Society[151] and with an editorial aptly titled "Antimicrobial Prophylaxis for Endocarditis: Emotion or Science?"[136] We believe that it is premature to adopt the newer 2006 BSAC recommendations and certainly not the AHA 2007 recommendations, until further evaluations and a broader international consensus are achieved. A quarter-century of experience at the UCLA Adult Congenital Heart Disease Center dictates our policy of liberally extending dental and nondental antimicrobial prophylaxis. We recognize higher or lower risk subgroups, and recommendations are individualized accordingly. Operated patients with residual defects such as aortic regurgitation, VSD patch leak, and left ventricular outflow tract lesions are considered at increased risk, in our opinion and in the opinions of others.[4,8,21,24,27–29,31,42] Based on the studies mentioned in the Congenital Heart Disease section of this chapter, the Fontan or Mustard operations are apparently low risk.[29] Pacer wires have usually not been considered a risk for IE, although vegetations occurred on these wires in the systemic venous baffle in three of our patients with D-transposition and an atrial switch procedure[152] and unpublished personal observations. Isolated uncomplicated secundum atrial septal defect is considered low-to-no risk both before and after closure, although IE prophylaxis is recommended for the first 6 months after patch or device closure, that is, until the foreign body becomes endothelialized. One must be aware of the occasional association of a secundum ASD with true pathologic mitral valve prolapse. Isolated pulmonary valve stenosis, especially mild, is considered low risk. One of our patients with IE had double-chambered right ventricle and a restrictive ventricular septal defect.[21] Ebstein anomaly is regarded as low risk because the tricuspid regurgitation is low velocity. We have yet to encounter IE in isolated uncomplicated Ebstein anomaly, and it is difficult to find a report in the literature.[3,8,27,32,42,49,52] Accordingly, prophylaxis is not recommended for uncomplicated unoperated Ebstein anomaly. However, IE has been encountered when there are pacemaker leads in the right heart.[153]

Until recently, most CHD experts advocated that patients at moderate to high risk for IE should adhere to the 1997 AHA endocarditis guidelines,[21,135] the 2004 European Society of Cardiology recommendations,[8] and the 2006 ACC/AHA valvular heart disease guidelines.[27] De-

vice implantation (pacemaker, intracardiac defibrillator) requires prophylaxis against skin flora. IE is occasionally encountered despite absence of predisposing risk factors, presumably because of the aggressiveness of the offending organism (*S. aureus*) or impaired host immune response or associated diseases such as diabetes, chronic renal disease, and chronic alcoholism.[13,17,18,20]

Another topic in which opinion differs is the significance of bacteremia and the need for prophylaxis during normal vaginal delivery. Guidelines usually state that prophylaxis is unnecessary *unless there is local infection or a complicated delivery*[3,28,135] (see Chapter 9). In a 1980 report of 2165 women with congenital or rheumatic heart disease delivered vaginally in three large Dublin hospitals, there were two (0.09%) cases of endocarditis, neither of which had received prophylaxis. In 83 normal women, 299 blood cultures were drawn immediately after placental separation and up to 30 minutes after vaginal delivery to determine the incidence of asymptomatic puerperal bacteremia. Single blood cultures were positive in three women (3.6% of patients, 1.0% of cultures).[154] It was concluded that IE and puerperal bacteremia after normal vaginal delivery were uncommon, that antibiotic prophylaxis carried a "considerable risk" of drug toxicity and may increase the risk of antibiotic-resistant IE, and that evidence of prophylaxis efficacy was lacking, so "routine peripartum antibiotic prophylaxis is not indicated."[154]

Bacteremia is reportedly common after labor (14% of 119 study patients), especially in primigravidas, in preterm labor, or when there is a positive chorioamnionic-placental culture.[155] Preterm labor with rupture of membranes is associated with a higher rate of postpartum chorioamniitis, urinary tract infection, endometritis, and bacteremia.[156] The study found that the rate of bacteremia was almost twofold higher among 986 woman with preterm labor compared with 4672 women with term delivery (9.4% vs. 5%).[156] Positive blood cultures (asymptomatic bacteremia) occurred in 19% of 235 parturient women and in 25% of their newborns.[157] In 68 cases of pregnancy complicated by IE, maternal mortality was 22%, and fetal mortality was 15%.[157] Four of 486 pregnant women with rheumatic heart disease had IE despite prophylaxis.[158]

The 2006 BSAC guidelines for prevention of endocarditis focused on bacteremia and endocarditis risk.[99] Prophylaxis recommendations for obstetric and gynecologic procedures appeared inconsistent with clinical experience and was not recommended unless infection was suspected or unless there was preterm rupture of membranes.[99] The same report stated that Caesarean delivery is not known to be associated with IE despite a bacteremia rate of 11%, but prophylaxis was recommended.[99] The 2004 comprehensive document by the Task Force on Infective Endocarditis of the European Society of Cardiology Guidelines on Prevention, Diagnosis and Treatment of Infective Endocarditis stated without corroborating data that "Unless infection or infected material is present, normal vaginal delivery or other gynaecologic procedures ... do not require prophylaxis."[8] The 1997 recommendations by the AHA for prevention of bacterial endocarditis did not recommend prophylaxis, arguing that the incidence of bacteremia—usually streptococcal—accompanying "uncomplicated" vaginal delivery is "only" 1% to 5%, and documented cases of endocarditis are "uncommon."[135] However, we agree with the many experts who believe that it is prudent to recommend IE prophylaxis for at-risk patients undergoing vaginal delivery.[21,158-163] It cannot be assumed with a satisfactory degree of certainty that a given vaginal delivery will be uncomplicated. Primigravidas experience relatively long labors, tears are likely, and episiotomy should not be considered uncomplicated. Preterm rupture of membranes increases the risk of infection. IE is accompanied by a significant risk of morbidity and a mortality rate as high as 30%.[74,164] Accordingly, we recommend antibiotic prophylaxis for our CHD gravidas who are at moderate to high risk for IE, including patients with prosthetic heart valves, surgically created shunts or conduits, a previous history of IE, cyanotic congenital heart disease, and probably patients with orthotopic heart transplants on immunosuppressive agents.[163] A substantial number of our patients experienced IE on congenitally incompetent aortic valves, often in conjunction with malformations such as tetralogy of Fallot. These patients routinely receive prophylaxis.

PATIENT AND PHYSICIAN EDUCATION

Education is the most important means of equipping patients for decision making and for ensuring proper prophylaxis.[3,11,13,15,16,19-22,35,135] Despite the numerous guidelines on antibiotic prophylaxis, the worldwide incidence of IE has not been perceptibly reduced (discussed earlier).[165,166] In 1971, less than 50% of patients or families knew about endocarditis prevention or precautions, and even fewer understood why prophylaxis was even indicated.[167] In the intervening years, there has been little progress in the education of patients and their parents. More than two decades later (1995), adults with CHD still had inadequate knowledge about their cardiac lesion, about IE, and about prophylaxis.[168] Educational efforts should be pursued and regularly reinforced.[168]

It is an indictment of the quality of management that so many susceptible cardiac patients are not given prophylaxis before undergoing a risk-generating procedure. Blood cultures are frequently not performed before antibiotics are administered.[166] Only 50% of patients with valvular heart disease are informed of the need for IE prophylaxis, and only 33% schedule regular dental visits. Relatively few patients with a risk-generating procedure in the year proceeding IE had received adequate prophylaxis.[26] It has been suggested that echocardiographic laboratories include in reports to referring physicians a

statement of endocarditis risk to encourage appropriate prophylaxis.[86]

A useful publication for patients seeking in-depth information is the "Cardiology Patient Page" on Bacterial Endocarditis in Circulation in 2003.[47] In the UCLA Adult Congenital Heart Disease Center, it is policy during the first visit to provide patients with a detailed explanation of their diagnosis together with the rationale for IE prevention. An AHA information card is provided, and the recommended regimen for dental procedures is circled. At each subsequent visit, the IE prevention message is reemphasized.[21]

References

1. Osler W. Gulstonian lectures on malignant endocarditis. *Lancet.* 1885;1:415-508.
2. Child JS, ed. *Diagnosis and Management of Infective Endocarditis. Cardiology Clinics.* Philadelphia: W.B. Saunders; 1996. No. 14.
3. Baddour LM, Wilson WR, Bayer AS, et al. Infective endocarditis: diagnosis, antimicrobial therapy, and management of complications: a statement for healthcare professionals from the Committee on Rheumatic Fever, Endocarditis, and Kawasaki Disease, Council on Cardiovascular Disease in the Young, and the Councils on Clinical Cardiology, Stroke, and Cardiovascular Surgery and Anesthesia, American Heart Association: endorsed by the Infectious Diseases Society of America. *Circulation.* 2005;111: e394-434.
4. Dodo H, Child JS. Infective endocarditis in congenital heart disease. *Cardiol Clin.* 1996;14:383-392.
5. Perloff JK, Child JS. *Congenital Heart Disease in Adults.* 2nd ed. Philadelphia: W.B. Saunders; 1998.
6. Baddour LM, Bettmann MA, Bolger AF, et al. Nonvalvular cardiovascular device-related infections. *Circulation.* 2003;108:2015-2031.
7. Schulze MR, Ostermaier R, Franke Y, et al. Images in cardiovascular medicine. Aortic endocarditis caused by inadvertent left ventricular pacemaker lead placement. *Circulation.* 2005;112:e361-363.
8. Horstkotte D, Follath F, Gutschik E, et al. Guidelines on prevention, diagnosis and treatment of infective endocarditis executive summary; the task force on infective endocarditis of the European society of cardiology. *Eur Heart J.* 2004;25:267-276.
9. Major RH. *Classic Descriptions of Disease.* 3rd ed. Springfield, IL: Charles C. Thomas; 1945.
10. Virchow R. *Cellular Pathology.* 2nd ed. London: John Churchill; 1860.
11. Mylonakis E, Calderwood SB. Infective endocarditis in adults. *N Engl J Med.* 2001;345:1318-1330.
12. Tleyjeh IM, Steckelberg JM, Murad HS, et al. Temporal trends in infective endocarditis: a population-based study in Olmsted County, Minnesota. *JAMA.* 2005;293:3022-3028.
13. Moreillon P, Que YA. Infective endocarditis. *Lancet.* 2004;363: 139-149.
14. Hill EE, Herijgers P, Claus P, et al. Infective endocarditis: changing epidemiology and predictors of 6-month mortality: a prospective cohort study. *Eur Heart J.* 2007;28:196-203.
15. Beynon RP, Bahl VK, Prendergast BD. Infective endocarditis. *BMJ.* 2006;333:334-339.
16. Bouza E, Menasalvas A, Munoz P, et al. Infective endocarditis—a prospective study at the end of the twentieth century: new predisposing conditions, new etiologic agents, and still a high mortality. *Medicine (Baltimore).* 2001;80:298-307.
17. Fowler VG Jr, Miro JM, Hoen B, et al. *Staphylococcus aureus* endocarditis: a consequence of medical progress. *JAMA.* 2005;293:3012-3021.

18. Nadji G, Remadi JP, Coviaux F, et al. Comparison of clinical and morphological characteristics of *Staphylococcus aureus* endocarditis with endocarditis caused by other pathogens. *Heart (British Cardiac Society).* 2005;91:932–937.

19. Habib G. Management of infective endocarditis. *Heart.* 2006;92: 124–130.

20. Prendergast BD. The changing face of infective endocarditis. 2006;92:879–885.

21. Child JS, Perloff JK, Kubak B. Infective endocarditis: risks and prophylaxis. In: Perloff JK, Child JS, eds. *Congenital Heart Disease in Adults.* 2nd ed. Philadelphia: W.B. Saunders; 1998:129–143.

22. Karchmer AW. Infective Endocarditis. In: Zipes DP, Libby P, Bonow RO, Braunwald E, eds. *Braunwald's Heart Disease: A Textbook of Cardiovascular Medicine.* 7 ed. Philadelphia: Elsevier Saunders; 2005: 1633–1658.

23. Cecchi E, Imazio M, Trinchero R. The changing face of infective endocarditis. *Heart.* 2006;92:1365–1366.

24. Di Filippo S, Delahaye F, Semiond B, et al. Current patterns of infective endocarditis in congenital heart disease. *Heart.* 2006;92: 1490–1495.

25. Heiro M, Helenius H, Makila S, et al. Infective endocarditis in a Finnish teaching hospital: a study on 326 episodes treated during 1980–2004. *Heart.* 2006;92:1457–1462.

26. Tornos P, Iung B, Permanyer-Miralda G, et al. Infective endocarditis in Europe: lessons from the Euro heart survey. *Heart.* 2005;91:571–575.

27. Bonow RO, Carabello BA, Chatterjee K, et al. ACC/AHA 2006 guidelines for the management of patients with valvular heart disease: a report of the American College of Cardiology/American Heart Association Task Force on Practice Guidelines (writing Committee to Revise the 1998 guidelines for the management of patients with valvular heart disease) developed in collaboration with the Society of Cardiovascular Anesthesiologists endorsed by the Society for Cardiovascular Angiography and Interventions and the Society of Thoracic Surgeons. *J Am Coll Cardiol.* 2006;48: e1–e148.

28. Gould FK, Elliott TS, Foweraker J, et al, Working Party of the British Society for Antimicrobial C. Guidelines for the prevention of endocarditis: report of the Working Party of the British Society for Antimicrobial Chemotherapy. *J Antimicrob Chemother.* 2006;57:1035–1042.

29. Li W, Somerville J. Infective endocarditis in the grown-up congenital heart (GUCH) population. *Eur Heart J.* 1998;19:166–173.

30. Morris CD, Reller MD, Menashe VD. Thirty-year incidence of infective endocarditis after surgery for congenital heart defect. *JAMA.* 1998;279:599–603.

31. Niwa K, Nakazawa M, Tateno S, et al. Infective endocarditis in congenital heart disease: Japanese national collaboration study. *Heart.* 2005;91:795–800.

32. Child JS. Risks for and prevention of infective endocarditis. *Cardiol Clin.* 1996;14:327–343.

33. Weinstein L, Schlesinger JJ. Pathoanatomic, pathophysiologic and clinical correlations in endocarditis (second of two parts). *N Engl J Med.* 1974;291:1122–1126.

34. Weinstein L, Schlesinger JJ. Pathoanatomic, pathophysiologic and clinical correlations in endocarditis (first of two parts). *N Engl J Med.* 1974;291:832–837.

35. Dodo H, Perloff J, Child JS, et al. Are high-velocity tricuspid and pulmonary regurgitation endocarditis risk substrates? *Am Heart J.* 1998;136:109–114.

36. Abbott ME. Coarctation of the aorta of the adult type. II. A statistical and historical retrospect of 200 recorded cases with autopsy, of stenosis or obliteration of the descending arch in subjects above the age of two years. *Am Heart J.* 1928;3:574–628.

37. Bayer AS, Bolger AF, Taubert KA, et al. Diagnosis and management of infective endocarditis and its complications. *Circulation.* 1998;98: 2936–2948.

38. Harris PS, Cobbs CG. Cardiac, cerebral, and vascular complications of infective endocarditis. *Cardiol Clin.* 1996;14:437–450.

39. Warnes CA, Liberthson R, Danielson GK, et al. Task Force 1: the changing profile of congenital heart disease in adult life. *J Am Coll Cardiol.* 2001;37:1170–1175.

40. Gersony WM, Hayes CJ, Driscoll DJ, et al. Bacterial endocarditis in patients with aortic stenosis, pulmonary stenosis, or ventricular septal defect. *Circulation.* 1993;87(2 Suppl):I121–I126.

41. Lankipalli RS, Lax K, Keane MG, et al. Images in cardiovascular medicine. Infected patent ductus arteriosus. *Circulation.* 2005;112: e364–e365.

42. Li W. Infective Endocarditis. In: Gatzoulis MA, Webb GD, Daubeney PEF, eds. *Diagnosis and Management of Adult Congenital Heart Disease.* Philadelphia: Churchill Livingstone; 2003:125–133.

43. McKinsey DS, Ratts TE, Bisno AL. Underlying cardiac lesions in adults with infective endocarditis. The changing spectrum. *Am J Med.* 1987;82:681–688.

44. Saiman L, Prince A, Gersony WM. Pediatric infective endocarditis in the modern era. *J Pediatr.* 1993;122:847–853.

45. Johnson DH, Rosenthal A, Nadas AS. A forty-year review of bacterial endocarditis in infancy and childhood. *Circulation.* 1975;51: 581–588.

46. Awadallah SM, Kavey RE, Byrum CJ, et al. The changing pattern of infective endocarditis in childhood. *Am J Cardiol.* 1991;68:90–94.

47. Cabell CH, Abrutyn E, Karchmer AW. Bacterial endocarditis: the disease, treatment, and prevention. *Circulation.* 2003;107:185e–187e.

48. Prendergast BD. Diagnosis of infective endocarditis. *BMJ.* 2002;325:845–846.

49. Li JS, Sexton DJ, Mick N, et al. Proposed modifications to the Duke Criteria for the diagnosis of infective endocarditis. *Clin Infect Dis.* 2000;30:633–638.

50. Ferrieri P, Gewitz MH, Gerber MA, et al., From the Committee on Rheumatic Fever Endocarditis, and Kawasaki Disease of the American Heart Association Council on Cardiovascular Disease in the Young. Unique features of infective endocarditis in childhood. *Circulation.* 2002;105:2115–2126.

51. Child JS. Echo-Doppler and color-flow imaging in congenital heart disease. *Cardiol Clin.* 1990;8:289–313.

52. Child JS. Transthoracic and transesophageal echocardiographic imaging: anatomic and hemodynamic assessment. In: Perloff JK, Child JS, eds. *Congenital Heart Disease in Adults.* 2nd ed. Philadelphia: W.B. Saunders; 1998:91–128.

53. Child JS, Marelli AJ. The application of transesophageal echocardiography in the adult with congenital heart disease. In: Maurer G, ed. *Transesophageal Echocardiography.* New York: McGraw-Hill; 1994:159–188.

54. Hoffman RM, Aboulhosn J, Child JS, Pegues DA. *Bartonella* endocarditis in complex congenital heart disease. *Congenital Heart Dis.* 2007;2:79–84.

55. Krivokapich J, Child JS. Role of transthoracic and transesophageal echocardiography in diagnosis and management of infective endocarditis. *Cardiol Clin.* 1996;14:363–382.

56. Von Reyn CF, Levy BS, Arbeit RD, et al. Infective endocarditis: an analysis based on strict case definitions. *Ann Intern Med.* 1981;94: 505–518.

57. Durack DT, Lukes AS, Bright DK. New criteria for diagnosis of infective endocarditis: utilization of specific echocardiographic findings. Duke Endocarditis Service. *Am J Med.* 1994;96:200–209.

58. Lamas CC, Eykyn SJ. Suggested modifications to the Duke Criteria for the clinical diagnosis of native valve and prosthetic valve endocarditis: analysis of 118 pathologically proven cases. *Clin Infect Dis.* 1997;25:713–719.

59. Bayer AS, Ward JI, Ginzton LE, Shapiro SM. Evaluation of new clinical criteria for the diagnosis of infective endocarditis. *Am J Med.* 1994;96:211–219.

60. Berlin JA, Abrutyn E, Strom BL, et al. Assessing diagnostic criteria for active infective endocarditis. *Am J Cardiol.* 1994;73:887–891.

61. Bayer AS. Revised diagnostic criteria for infective endocarditis. *Cardiol Clin.* 1996;14:345–350.

62. Dodds GA, Sexton DJ, Durack DT, et al. Negative predictive value of the Duke criteria for infective endocarditis. *Am J Cardiol.* 1996;77:403–407.

63. Butchart EG, Gohlke-Barwolf C, Antunes MJ, et al. Recommendations for the management of patients after heart valve surgery. *Eur Heart J.* 2005;26:2463–2471.

64. Houpikian P, Raoult D. Blood culture-negative endocarditis in a reference center: etiologic diagnosis of 348 cases. *Medicine (Baltimore).* 2005;84:162–173.

65. Child JS. Echocardiographic evaluation of the adult with postoperative congenital heart disease. In: Otto CM, ed. *The Practice of Clinical Echocardiography.* 2nd ed. Philadelphia: W.B. Saunders; 2002:901–921.

66. Deanfield J, Thaulow E, Warnes C, et al. Management of grown up congenital heart disease. *Eur Heart J.* 2003;24:1035–1084.

67. Marelli AJ, Child JS, Perloff JK. Transesophageal echocardiography in congenital heart disease in the adult. *Cardiol Clin.* 1993;11:505–520.

68. Quiñones MA, Douglas PS, Foster E, et al. ACC/AHA clinical competence statement on echocardiography: a report of the American College of Cardiology/American Heart Association/American College of Physicians-American Society of Internal Medicine Task Force on Clinical Competence (Committee on Echocardiography). *J Am Coll Cardiol.* 2003;41:687–708.

69. Cheitlin MD, Alpert JS, Armstrong WF, et al. ACC/AHA guidelines for the clinical application of echocardiography: executive summary. A report of the American College of Cardiology/American Heart Association Task Force on practice guidelines (Committee on Clinical Application of Echocardiography). Developed in collaboration with the American Society of Echocardiography. *J Am Coll Cardiol.* 1997;29:862–879.

70. Cheitlin MD, Armstrong WF, Aurigemma GP, et al. ACC/AHA/ASE 2003 Guideline Update for the Clinical Application of Echocardiography: Summary Article: A Report of the American College of Cardiology/American Heart Association Task Force on Practice Guidelines (ACC/AHA/ASE Committee to Update the 1997 Guidelines for the Clinical Application of Echocardiography). *Circulation.* 2003;108:1146–1162.

71. Chirillo F, Pedrocco A, De Leo A, et al. Impact of harmonic imaging on transthoracic echocardiographic identification of infective endocarditis and its complications. *Heart.* 2005;91:329–333.

72. Evangelista A, Gonzalez-Alujas MT. Echocardiography in infective endocarditis. *Heart.* 2004;90:614–617.

73. Reynolds HR, Jagen MA, Tunick PA, Kronzon I. Sensitivity of transthoracic versus transesophageal echocardiography for the detection of native valve vegetations in the modern era. *J Am Soc Echocardiogr.* 2003;16:67–70.

74. Durack DT. Prevention of infective endocarditis. *N Engl J Med.* 1995;332:38–44.

75. Cabell CH, Fowler VG Jr. Repeated echocardiography after the diagnosis of endocarditis: too much of a good thing? *Heart.* 2004;90:975–976.

76. Greaves K, Mou D, Patel A, Celermajer DS. Clinical criteria and the appropriate use of transthoracic echocardiography for the exclusion of infective endocarditis. *Heart.* 2003;89:273–275.

77. Robles P. Judicious use of transthoracic echocardiography in the diagnosis of infective endocarditis. *Heart.* 2003;89:1283–1284.

78. Vieira ML, Grinberg M, Pomerantzeff PM, et al. Repeated echocardiographic examinations of patients with suspected infective endocarditis. *Heart.* 2004;90:1020–1024.

79. Di Salvo G, Habib G, Pergola V, et al. Echocardiography predicts embolic events in infective endocarditis. *J Am Coll Cardiol.* 2001;37:1069–1076.

80. Fowler VG Jr, Li J, et al. Role of echocardiography in evaluation of patients with Staphylococcus aureus bacteremia: experience in 103 patients. *J Am Coll Cardiol.* 1997;30:1072–1078.

81. Hasbun R, Vikram HR, Barakat LA, et al. Complicated left-sided native valve endocarditis in adults: risk classification for mortality. *JAMA.* 2003;289:1933–1940.

82. Heinle S, Wilderman N, Harrison JK, et al. Value of transthoracic echocardiography in predicting embolic events in active infective endocarditis. Duke Endocarditis Service. *Am J Cardiol.* 1994;74:799–801.

83. Humpl T, McCrindle BW, Smallhorn JF. The relative roles of transthoracic compared with transesophageal echocardiography in children with suspected infective endocarditis. *J Am Coll Cardiol.* 2003;41:2068–2071.

84. Lindner JR, Case RA, Dent JM, et al. Diagnostic value of echocardiography in suspected endocarditis: an evaluation based on the pretest probability of disease. *Circulation.* 1996;93:730–736.

85. Nemes A, Lagrand WK, McGhie JS, ten Cate FJ. Three-dimensional transesophageal echocardiography in the evaluation of aortic valve destruction by endocarditis. *J Am Soc Echocardiogr.* 2006;19:355.e355–355.e356.

86. Sanders GP, Yeon SB, Grunes J, et al. Impact of a specific echocardiographic report comment regarding endocarditis prophylaxis on compliance with American Heart Association Recommendations. *Circulation.* 2002;106:300–303.

87. Tornos P. Management of prosthetic valve endocarditis: a clinical challenge. *Heart.* 2003;89:245–246.

88. Graupner C, Vilacosta I, SanRoman J, et al. Periannular extension of infective endocarditis. *J Am Coll Cardiol.* 2002;39:1204–1211.

89. Vahanian A, Baumgartner H, Bax J, et al. Guidelines on the management of valvular heart disease: The Task Force on the Management of Valvular Heart Disease of the European Society of Cardiology. *Eur Heart J.* 2007;28:230–268.

90. Rosen AB, Fowler VG Jr, et al. Cost-effectiveness of transesophageal echocardiography to determine the duration of therapy for intravascular catheter-associated Staphylococcus aureus bacteremia. *Ann Intern Med.* 1999;130:810–820.

91. Blaustein AS, Lee JR. Indications for and timing of surgical intervention in infective endocarditis. *Cardiol Clin.* 1996;14:393–404.

92. Drinkwater DC Jr, Laks H, Child JS. Issues in surgical treatment of endocarditis including intraoperative and postoperative management. *Cardiol Clin.* 1996;14:451–464.

93. Habib G, Tribouilloy C, Thuny F, et al. Prosthetic valve endocarditis: who needs surgery? A multicentre study of 104 cases. *Heart.* 2005;91:954–959.

94. Jassal DS, Neilan TG, Pradhan AD, et al. Surgical management of infective endocarditis: early predictors of short-term morbidity and mortality. *Ann Thorac Surg.* 2006;82:524–529.

95. Kalra PR, Tang ATM, Morgan JM, Haw MP. Complex and extensive infective endocarditis: a novel surgical approach. *Eur J Cardiothorac Surg.* 2002;21:365–368.

96. Saccente M, Cobbs CG. Clinical approach to infective endocarditis. *Cardiol Clin.* 1996;14:351–362.

97. Thuny F, Di Salvo G, Belliard O, et al. Risk of embolism and death in infective endocarditis: prognostic value of echocardiography: a prospective multicenter study. *Circulation.* 2005;112:69–75.

98. Wang A, Pappas P, Anstrom KJ, et al. The use and effect of surgical therapy for prosthetic valve infective endocarditis: a propensity analysis of a multicenter, international cohort. *Am Heart J.* 2005;150:1086–1091.

99. Elliott TS, Foweraker J, Gould FK, et al. Guidelines for the antibiotic treatment of endocarditis in adults: report of the Working Party of the British Society for Antimicrobial Chemotherapy. *J Antimicrob Chemother.* 2004;54:971–981.

100. Uslan DZ, Baddour LM. Cardiac device infections: getting to the heart of the matter. *Curr Opin Infect Dis.* 2006;19:345–348.

101. Uslan DZ, Sohail MR, Friedman PA, et al. Frequency of permanent pacemaker or implantable cardioverter-defibrillator infection in patients with gram-negative bacteremia. *Clin Infect Dis.* 2006;43:731–736.

102. Duval X, Alla F, Doco-Lecompte T, et al. Diabetes mellitus and infective endocarditis: the insulin factor in patient morbidity and mortality. *Eur Heart J.* 2007;28:59–64.

103. Thilen U, Astrom-Olsson K. Does the risk of infective endarteritis justify routine patent ductus arteriosus closure? *Eur Heart J.* 1997; 18:503–506.

104. Sharma R, Bolger AP, Li W, et al. Elevated circulating levels of inflammatory cytokines and bacterial endotoxin in adults with congenital heart disease. *Am J Cardiol.* 2003;92:188–193.

105. Mueller C, Huber P, Laifer G, et al. Procalcitonin and the early diagnosis of infective endocarditis. *Circulation.* 2004;109:1707–1710.

106. Breitkopf C, Hammel D, Scheld HH, et al. Impact of a molecular approach to improve the microbiological diagnosis of infective heart valve endocarditis. *Circulation.* 2005;111:1415–1421.

107. Grijalva M, Horvath R, Dendis M, et al. Molecular diagnosis of culture negative infective endocarditis: clinical validation in a group of surgically treated patients. *Heart.* 2003;89: 263–268.

108. Imrit K, Goldfischer M, Wang J, et al. Identification of bacteria in formalin-fixed, paraffin-embedded heart valve tissue via 16S rRNA gene nucleotide sequencing. *J Clin Microbiol.* 2006;44: 2609–2611.

109. Rovery C, Greub G, Lepidi H, et al. PCR detection of bacteria on cardiac valves of patients with treated bacterial endocarditis. *J Clin Microbiol.* 2005;43:163–167.

110. Rice PA, Madico GE. Polymerase chain reaction to diagnose infective endocarditis: will it replace blood cultures? *Circulation.* 2005;111:1352–1354.

111. Chan K-L. Early clinical course and long-term outcome of patients with infective endocarditis complicated by perivalvular abscess. *CMAJ.* 2002;167:19–24.

112. Vilacosta I, Graupner C, San Roman JA, et al. Risk of embolization after institution of antibiotic therapy for infective endocarditis. *J Am Coll Cardiol.* 2002;39:1489–1495.

113. Heiro M, Nikoskelainen J, Engblom E, et al. Neurologic manifestations of infective endocarditis: a 17–year experience in a teaching hospital in Finland. *Arch Intern Med.* 2000;160: 2781–2787.

114. Delahaye JP, Poncet P, Malquarti V, et al. Cerebrovascular accidents in infective endocarditis: role of anticoagulation. *Eur Heart J.* 1990;11:1074–1078.

115. Thuny F, Avierinos J-F, Tribouilloy C, et al. Impact of cerebrovascular complications on mortality and neurologic outcome during infective endocarditis: a prospective multicentre study. *Eur Heart J.* 2007;28:1155–1161.

116. Chu VH, Cabell CH, Benjamin DK Jr, et al. Early predictors of in-hospital death in infective endocarditis. *Circulation.* 2004;109: 1745–1749.

117. Revilla A, Lopez J, Vilacosta I, et al. Clinical and prognostic profile of patients with infective endocarditis who need urgent surgery. *Eur Heart J.* 2007;28:65–71.

118. Tleyjeh IM, Ghomrawi HM, Steckelberg JM, et al. The impact of valve surgery on 6–month mortality in left-sided infective endocarditis. *Circulation.* 2007;115:1721–1728.

119. Ileri M, Alper A, Senen K, et al. Effect of infective endocarditis on blood coagulation and platelet activation and comparison of patients with to those without embolic events. *Am J Cardiol.* 2003;91:689–692.

120. Kupferwasser LI, Hafner G, Mohr-Kahaly S, et al. The presence of infection-related antiphospholipid antibodies in infective endocarditis determines a major risk factor for embolic events. *J Am Coll Cardiol.* 1999;33:1365–1371.

121. Kupferwasser LI, Yeaman MR, Shapiro SM, et al. Acetylsalicylic acid reduces vegetation bacterial density, hematogenous bacterial dissemination, and frequency of embolic events in experimental staphylococcus aureus endocarditis through antiplatelet and antibacterial effects. *Circulation.* 1999;99:2791–2797.

122. Kupferwasser LI, Yeaman MR, Shapiro SM, et al. In vitro susceptibility to thrombin-induced platelet microbicidal protein is associated with reduced disease progression and complication rates in experimental *Staphylococcus aureus* endocarditis: microbiological, histopathologic, and echocardiographic analyses. *Circulation.* 2002;105:746–752.

123. Roder BL, Wandall DA, Frimodt-Moller N, et al. Clinical features of *Staphylococcus aureus* endocarditis: a 10-year experience in Denmark. *Arch Intern Med.* 1999;159:462–469.

124. Tornos P, Almirante B, Mirabet S, et al. Infective endocarditis due to *Staphylococcus aureus*: deleterious effect of anticoagulant therapy. *Arch Intern Med.* 1999;159:473–475.

125. Delahaye F, Celard M, Roth O, de Gevigney G. Indications and optimal timing for surgery in infective endocarditis. *Heart.* 2004;90:618–620.

126. Vikram HR, Buenconsejo J, Hasbun R, Quagliarello VJ. Impact of valve surgery on 6-month mortality in adults with complicated, left-sided native valve endocarditis: a propensity analysis. *JAMA.* 2003;290:3207–3214.

127. Aranki SF, Adams DH, Rizzo RJ, et al. Determinants of early mortality and late survival in mitral valve endocarditis. *Circulation.* 1995;92:143–149.

128. de Kerchove L, Vanoverschelde J-L, Poncelet A, et al. Reconstructive surgery in active mitral valve endocarditis: feasibility, safety and durability. *Eur J Cardiothorac Surg.* 2007;31:592–599.

129. Iung B, Rousseau-Paziaud J, Cormier B, et al. Contemporary results of mitral valve repair for infective endocarditis. *J Am Coll Cardiol.* 2004;43:386–392.

130. Livesey SA. Mitral valve reconstruction in the presence of infection. *Heart.* 2006;92:289–290.

131. Ruttmann E, Legit C, Poelzl G, et al. Mitral valve repair provides improved outcome over replacement in active infective endocarditis. *J Thorac Cardiovasc Surg.* 2005;130:765–771.

132. Zegdi R, Debieche M, Latremouille C, et al. Long-term results of mitral valve repair in active endocarditis. *Circulation.* 2005;111: 2532–2536.

133. Maki DG, Kluger DM, Crnich CJ. The risk of bloodstream infection in adults with different intravascular devices: a systematic review of 200 published prospective studies. *Mayo Clin Proc.* 2006; 81:1159–1171.

134. Chirouze C, Cabell CH, Fowler VG Jr, et al. Prognostic factors in 61 cases of Staphylococcus aureus prosthetic valve infective endocarditis from the International Collaboration on Endocarditis merged database. *Clin Infect Dis.* 2004;38:1323–1327.

135. Dajani AS, Taubert KA, Wilson W, et al. Prevention of bacterial endocarditis. Recommendations by the American Heart Association. *Circulation.* 1997;96:358–366.

136. Ashrafian H, Bogle RG. Antimicrobial prophylaxis for endocarditis: emotion or science? *Heart.* 2007;93:5–6.

137. Heimdahl A, Hall G, Hedberg M, et al. Detection and quantitation by lysis-filtration of bacteremia after different oral surgical procedures. *J Clin Microbiol.* 1990;28:2205–2209.

138. Kaplan EL, Rich H, Gersony W, Manning J. A collaborative study of infective endocarditis in the 1970s. Emphasis on infections in patients who have undergone cardiovascular surgery. *Circulation.* 1979;59:327–335.

139. Okell CC, Elliott SD. Bacteremia and oral sepsis with special reference to the aetiology of subacute endocarditis. *Lancet.* 1935; 2:869.

140. Weiss H. Relation of portals of entry to subacute bacterial endocarditis. *Arch Intern Med.* 1934;54:710.

141. van der Meer JT, Thompson J, Valkenburg HA, Michel MF. Epidemiology of bacterial endocarditis in The Netherlands. II. Antecedent procedures and use of prophylaxis. *Arch Intern Med.* 1992;152: 1869–1873.

142. van der Meer JT, Thompson J, Valkenburg HA, Michel MF. Epidemiology of bacterial endocarditis in The Netherlands. I. Patient characteristics. *Arch Intern Med.* 1992;152:1863–1868.

143. Hockett RN, Loesche WJ, Sodeman TM. Bacteraemia in asymptomatic human subjects. *Arch Oral Biol.* 1977;22:91–98.

144. Roberts GJ, Jaffray EC, Spratt DA, et al. Duration, prevalence and intensity of bacteraemia after dental extractions in children. *Heart.* 2006;92:1274–1277.

145. Lockhart PB, Brennan MT, Kent ML, et al. Impact of amoxicillin prophylaxis on the incidence, nature, and duration of bacteremia in children after intubation and dental procedures. *Circulation.* 2004;109:2878–2884.

146. Strom BL, Abrutyn E, Berlin JA, et al. Dental and cardiac risk factors for infective endocarditis. A population-based, case-control study. *Ann Intern Med.* 1998;129:761–769.

147. Strom BL, Abrutyn E, Berlin JA, et al. Risk factors for infective endocarditis: oral hygiene and nondental exposures. *Circulation.* 2000;102:2842–2848.

148. Duval X, Alla F, Hoen B, et al. Estimated risk of endocarditis in adults with predisposing cardiac conditions undergoing dental procedures with or without antibiotic prophylaxis. *Clin Infect Dis.* 2006;42:e102–107.

149. Delahaye F, Wong J, Mills PG. Infective endocarditis: a comparison of international guidelines. *Heart.* 2007;93:524–527.

150. Wilson W, Taubert K, Gewitz M, et al. AHA guideline: prevention of infective endocarditis. *Circulation.* 2007;116:1736–1754

151. Gibbs JL, Cowie M, Brooks N. Comment on: guidelines for the prevention of endocarditis: report of the Working Party of the British Society for Antimicrobial Chemotherapy. *J Antimicrob Chemother.* 2006;58:896; author reply 896–898.

152. Child JS. Echocardiographic evaluation of the adult with postoperative congenital heart disease. In: Otto CM, ed. *The Practice of Clinical Echocardiography.* 3rd ed. Philadelphia: W.B. Saunders; 2007:1083–1107.

153. Bilge AK, Adalet K, Ozyigit T, et al. Tricuspid endocarditis in an adult patient with Ebstein's anomaly who has a residual pacemaker lead. *Int J Cardiovasc Imaging.* 2005;21:641–643.

154. Sugrue D, Blake S, Troy P, MacDonald D. Antibiotic prophylaxis against infective endocarditis after normal delivery—is it necessary? *Br Heart J.* 1980;44:499–502.

155. Boggess KA, Watts DH, Hillier SL, et al. Bacteremia shortly after placental separation during cesarean delivery. *Obstet Gynecol.* 1996;87:779–784.

156. Furman B, Shoham-Vardi I, Bashiri A, et al. Clinical significance and outcome of preterm prelabor rupture of membranes: population-based study. *Eur J Obstet Gynecol Reprod Biol.* 2000;92:209–216.

157. Campuzano K, Roque H, Bolnick A, et al. Bacterial endocarditis complicating pregnancy: case report and systematic review of the literature. *Arch Gynecol Obstet.* 2003;268:251–255.

158. Elkayam U, Bitar F. Valvular heart disease and pregnancy part I: native valves. *J Am Coll Cardiol.* 2005;46(2):223–230.

159. Expert consensus document on management of cardiovascular diseases during pregnancy. *Eur Heart J.* 2003;24:761–781.

160. Connolly HM, Warnes CA. Pregnancy and contraception. In: Gatzoulis MA, Webb G, Daubeney PEF, eds. *Diagnosis and Management of Adult Congenital Heart Disease.* Philadelphia: Churchill Livingstone; 2003:135–144.

161. Gelson E, Johnson M, Gatzoulis M, Uebing A. Cardiac disease in pregnancy. Part 1: congenital heart disease. *Obstetrician Gynaecologist.* 2007;9:15–20.

162. Siu SC, Colman JM. Heart disease and pregnancy. *Heart.* 2001;85:710–715.

163. Thilen U, Olsson SB. Pregnancy and heart disease: a review. *Eur J Obstet Gynecol Reprod Biol.* 1997;75:43–50.

164. Kaplan EL. Bacterial endocarditis prophylaxis. *Pediatr Ann.* 1992;21:249–255.

165. Delahaye F, De Gevigney G. Should we give antibiotic prophylaxis against infective endocarditis in all cardiac patients, whatever the type of dental treatment? *Heart.* 2001;85:9–10.

166. Delahaye F, Rial MO, de Gevigney G, et al. A critical appraisal of the quality of the management of infective endocarditis. *J Am Coll Cardiol.* 1999;33:788–793.

167. Caldwell RL, Hurwitz RA, Girod DA. Subacute bacterial endocarditis in children. Current status. *Am J Dis Child.* 1971;122:312–315.

168. Cetta F, Warnes CA. Adults with congenital heart disease: patient knowledge of endocarditis prophylaxis. *Mayo Clin Proc.* 1995;70:50–54.

CHAPTER 9

Management of Pregnancy and Contraception in Congenital Heart Disease

JOHN S. CHILD ▪ JOSEPH K. PERLOFF ▪ BRIAN KOOS

Animal reproduction is accomplished with inconvenience to the mother, tenacity of the fetus, and cooperative ingenuity between the two.

> —*Burwell and Metcalfe,*
> *Heart Disease and Pregnancy*

HISTORICAL PERSPECTIVE

For the ancient Greeks, pregnancy was part of the natural order and was therefore not considered a condition that warranted medical attention. Accordingly, women in labor were excluded from the sacred sanctuary of Aesclepius.

Virgin births did not originate with Christianity, but in Chinese mythology circa 600 B.C. The offspring were always male. Miraculous births enhanced the stature of ancient dynastic rulers.

It was the conventional wisdom that the mother was not the true parent of the child but instead was a passive repository for growth of the seed (Fig. 9–1), the vital force implanted by the true parent, the father. This ancient belief finds contemporary expression in the practice of *in vitro* fertilization from donor eggs in which the mother is not the true parent of the child but is a passive repository for growth of the implanted seed.

Five hundred years after Aristotle, Galen concluded that the female germ originated in the ovaries and that union with the male sperm took place in the uterus. Yet for the next 15 centuries, there was virtual ignorance of embryology. The very discussion of procreation was considered sacrilegious. Not surprisingly, imagination and fantasy played a prominent role in the folklore of reproduction. In the Middle Ages, fireflies were believed to be the souls of infants who died before baptism. Developmental biology was not a remote consideration. It was taught that at the moment of conception, a fully formed human being existed—an *homunculus* ("little man")—that simply increased in size during gestation. The ancients showed *homunculi* in atypical fetal positions that predicted a difficult delivery, as illustrated in medical miniatures from the *Gynekeia* by Soranus of Ephesus (*Presentation of the fetus in utero. 9–10th centuries.* © Bibliothèque Royale Albert premier, Brussels).

Paradoxically, risk increased when delivery was managed by physicians. Witness the diaries of Ignaz Semmelwei (1818–1865) in which the rate of childbirth fever and death in hospital maternity wards that were attended by physicians was far greater than at home where women were delivered by midwives. Physicians doing autopsies were in the habit of going directly from handling cadavers to handling births. Semmelweis was an example of a prepared mind that unraveled a major clinical problem. In an effort to curtail deaths due to childbed fever, he instituted a strict policy of hand washing with chlorinated lime water before attending deliveries. Mortality rates dropped immediately. Not a single woman died from childbirth in Semmelweis's ward.

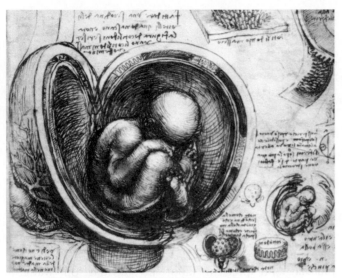

FIGURE 9–1   Leonardo da Vinci's fetus in the womb.

CARDIAC DISEASE AND PREGNANCY—AN OVERVIEW

Approximately 1% of pregnancies are complicated by maternal cardiovascular disease.[1,2] In the United Kingdom, heart disease is the most common cause of maternal death, with cardiomyopathy and pulmonary hypertension the two leading contributors (Fig. 9–2).[2,3] Valvular heart disease is the prevalent form of acquired heart disease,[4–6] but in developed countries, pregnancy is now accompanied by congenital heart disease (CHD) more often than by rheumatic heart disease.[3,7–9] Congenital malformations are responsible for about 80% of cardiac disease in pregnant women.[10]

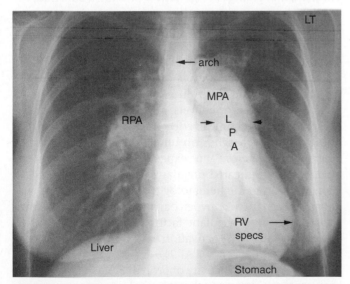

FIGURE 9–2   Chest x-ray of a patient with idiopathic (primary) pulmonary hypertension—a categorical contraindication to pregnancy, which she was counseled to avoid. Contraceptive advice was provided.

Because of the remarkable advances in diagnostic methods and surgical techniques in the last 60 years, more than 85% of infants with CHD are now expected to reach adulthood.[7,9,11,12] In the United States, the number of adults with CHD currently exceeds the number of children, and the number of females reaching childbearing age has increased proportionately.[12,13] Cures, however, are few and far between. Postoperative residua and sequelae are the rule, varying from minor to major and more often than not requiring long-term if not life-long medical care.[14] This relatively new and growing population of women confront the hemodynamic burden of pregnancy superimposed on their postoperative CHD.

Improvements in medical care have significantly increased longevity in Eisenmenger syndrome, which incurs major risks to both mother and fetus. Inherent abnormalities of great arterial walls in CHD increase the risk of rupture because of coexisting gestational changes in aortic media. Some malformations first become evident during pregnancy, such as congenitally corrected transposition of the great arteries that presents with failure of the subaortic morphologic right ventricle. Mechanical valves require anticoagulants to protect the mother but impose risks on the fetus.

Counseling regarding pregnancy in women with CHD is too often scant or incorrect. Patients may never have had a discussion with either their pediatric or medical cardiologist about pregnancy or about the advisability and type of contraception to be used. Physicians are apt to warn against pregnancy simply because of the presence of heart disease without consideration of relative risk. When risks are excessive, the patient should be so informed before conception. If already pregnant, the option of termination versus the risk of continuation must be carefully explained.

This chapter deals with the complex interplay between maternal circulatory and respiratory physiology and maternal CHD, and the effects of this interplay on the fetus. Our goal is to provide timely preconception counseling, information regarding the effects of pregnancy on coexisting CHD, general management principles, and specific issues that bear on genetic transmission of malformations. Prevention of maternal and fetal death and morbidity is the focus in this chapter and requires a clear understanding of risk stratification. Recommendations regarding contraception are also provided.

CARDIOVASCULAR PHYSIOLOGY DURING NORMAL PREGNANCY, LABOR, AND DELIVERY

An appreciation of the potential impact of pregnancy on the gravida with CHD requires an understanding of the circulatory and hematologic changes that occur sequentially during normal gestation, labor, and delivery.[9,10] Pregnancy is characterized by a high-volume, low-resistance physiology. There is an increase in cardiac output and heart rate, a decrease in systemic vascular resistance, and an increase in circulating blood volume in response to hormonal changes, retention of salt and water, release of prostaglandins, and the uteroplacental circulation that acts as a low-resistance shunt. Blood volume begins to rise within the first few weeks after conception and continues to do so until the 28th to 34th week. Red cell mass begins to rise in the 8th week of gestation. Plasma volume expansion outstrips the rise in red cell mass, with peak hemodilution occurring at about 26 weeks. A modest decrease in hematocrit results in "anemia" in an iron-replete state. The physiologic effects of increased intravascular volume and relative anemia are beneficial because a decrease in whole blood viscosity and improved microvascular rheology permits more effective fetal-placental perfusion at lower cardiac work. Peak blood volume and red cell mass at term are about 50% and 30%, respectively, over the nonpregnant state. Salt and water retention together with increased peripheral venous capacitance results in mild peripheral edema, which is expected and should be considered normal. Aggressive use of diuretics acutely reduces maternal blood volume and arterial pressure and decreases uterine blood flow and placental oxygen delivery.

Systemic and pulmonary vascular resistances fall significantly. Diastolic blood pressure falls disproportionately, so that the systemic pulse pressure widens. Cardiac output rises progressively, peaking at 30 weeks. Stroke volume increases 20% to 30%, and heart rate averages 10 to 20 beats over a nonpregnant baseline.[15,16] At about 20 weeks, these effects are modulated by aortocaval compression caused by the enlarging gravid uterus. Preload decreases, particularly in the supine position, can result in hypotension and syncope—the "supine hypotensive syndrome," which is ameliorated by assuming a lateral decubitus position. A slight increase in left ventricular contractility is believed to occur during gestation.[17] Twin pregnancies carry a greater cardiovascular burden, with cardiac output 20% higher than singleton pregnancies.[18] During labor and delivery, cardiac output tends to increase abruptly in response to pain and anxiety, and uterine contractions cause a rise in systemic blood pressure.[11] These adverse effects should be anticipated and modulated by analgesia and epidural anesthesia.[11,16] Hemodynamic effects of a major painful uterine contraction in the supine position include a 25% increase in cardiac output, a 35% increase in stroke volume, and a 10% increase in systemic blood pressure; 300 to 500 cc of blood are expressed into the proximal systemic vascular compartment. The effect of maternal position is pivotal (Fig. 9–3).

Preload suddenly increases after delivery because of autotransfusion of uterine blood entering the circulation and abrupt aortocaval decompression. This preload effect is proportionately modified by blood loss during delivery.[16] Cesarean delivery is reserved for obstetrical indications—cephalopelvic disproportion, breech presentation, placenta

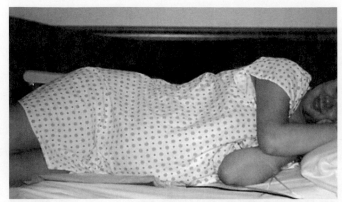

FIGURE 9-3 Lateral decubitus position for labor in a patient with complete transposition of the great arteries and a Mustard procedure.

praevia, and preterm labor in gravidas on warfarin (Coumadin). Blood loss can be twice as great in cesarian compared with vaginal delivery (1000 ml vs. 500 ml, respectively)[8] and is even greater in cyanotic gravida. Complications accompany delayed ambulation, and anesthetic hypotension increases right-to-left shunts.[11,16] The degree of postpartum blood loss competes with increased venous return from autotransfusion (as noted earlier). A sudden increase in preload, filling pressure, and stroke volume can precipitate congestive heart failure.[16] The hemodynamic adaptations to pregnancy usually persist to lesser degrees for several weeks postpartum.[8,16]

Changes in aortic media occur during normally pregnancy.[19,20] Estrogen has been held responsible for interference with collagen turnover, which, in conjunction with elastases, results in fragmentation of the elastic lamellae in the aortic wall media.[9,21] Relaxin is an insulin-like growth factor hormone that is present in serum during pregnancy and causes a decrease in collagen synthesis.[22] These medial changes of gestation provide a substrate for arterial dissection, particularly when superimposed on malformations associated with intrinsic medial disease such as Marfan syndrome, bicuspid aortic valve, and coarctation of the aorta.[11,20]

Respiratory physiology is altered early in pregnancy because of chemically induced hyperventilation due to increased progesterone levels, and later in pregnancy because of the mechanical effects of elevation of the diaphragm that encroaches on lung volume reserve. Breathlessness is therefore an expected accompaniment of normal uncomplicated pregnancy.

In addition to the hematologic changes that accompany normal pregnancy, a hypercoagulable state results from activation of anticoagulant factors (increased factor I, II, V, VIII, X, and XII), activation of fibrinolytic inhibitors (increased PAI-1 and PAI-2), resistance to activated protein C, decreased activity of protein S, stasis, and venous hypertension. These pro-thrombotic features are superimposed on risks for deep venous thrombosis, pulmonary embolism, and thrombosis on prosthetic valves.[16,23–27]

CARDIAC SIGNS AND SYMPTOMS DURING PREGNANCY

Cardiovascular and respiratory changes in a normal pregnancy can mimic signs and symptoms of cardiac disease.[8,9,16] Breathlessness (innocent hyperpnea), easy fatigability, a decrease in exercise tolerance, basal rales that disappear with cough or deep breathing, and peripheral edema are common in normal pregnancy and should not be misconstrued as evidence of heart disese.[11]

Beginning in the first trimester of normal pregnancy, the systemic arterial pulse is characterized by a rapid rise and a brisk collapse (small water hammer). The jugular venous pulse becomes more conspicuous after the 20th week because brisk X and Y descents make the A and V waves more obvious. Mean jugular venous pressure estimated from the superficial jugular vein is usually normal, but with the hypervolemia of pregnancy, it may reach the upper range. The left ventricular impulse is relatively hyperdynamic but not sustained, and the right ventricle may be palpable because, like the left ventricle, it handles a larger blood volume that is ejected against relatively low resistance. As pregnancy progresses, enlargement of the breasts and abdomen makes accurate palpation of the heart difficult.

Auscultatory changes accompanying normal gestation begin in the late first trimester, generally disappear within a week after delivery and include modifications of the heart sounds and the presence of systolic and continuous murmurs. The first heart sound is louder because of the increase in heart rate and left ventricular contractility. The second sound tends to exhibit persistent splitting toward the end of pregnancy, especially when the patient is examined in the left lateral decubitus position. Third heart sounds are common because of the augmented volume and rate of atrioventricular flow, but fourth heart sounds are not normal in pregnancy. Innocent pulmonary outflow tract midsystolic murmurs and normal supraclavicular systolic murmurs are augmented by the gestational increase in cardiac output and stroke volume. Mild tricuspid and mitral regurgitation detected by Doppler echocardiography and color flow imaging do not reach the threshold of audibility and are considered normal. The venous hum is ubiquitous in normal pregnant women. Less common is a systolic or continuous mammary souffle, which is peculiar to pregnancy and is heard over the breasts in late gestation, particularly in lactating women.

ECHOCARDIOGRAPHY

Echocardiograms (see Chapter 6) reveal an increase in chamber sizes due to the increased blood volume (preload) and high-output state. Effects on ventricular contractility during normal pregnancy are controversial, but there is evidence of a slight increase in inotropy.[17]

PRINCIPLES OF GENERAL MANAGEMENT

The cornerstones of management include (1) counseling and risk assessment, especially before conception; (2) preconception or early gestational medication adjustments, catheter intervention, or reparative surgery; (3) maternal and fetal monitoring, including fetal echocardiography at about 18 to 22 weeks and during pregnancy as indicated by risk assessment and changes in maternal clinical status; (4) individualized, coordinated cardiac-obstetrical-anesthesiology plans for labor and delivery; and (5) cardiac monitoring and follow-up in the immediate and early postpartum period, including adjustments of medications.

Pregnancy affects maternal CHD, and CHD affects the gravid female and her fetus. The obstetrician and cardiologist are therefore responsible for the welfare of two patients—the mother and the fetus. Pregnancy in women with CHD should be planned and managed by a multidisciplinary team[2,9,28–31] consisting of a cardiologist experienced in both adult CHD and pregnancy, an expert high-risk obstetrician, and an experienced obstetrical anesthesiologist. Valuable assistance is also provided by a nurse practitioner or clinical nurse specialist, a fetal echocardiographer, a neonatologist, and consultation with a CHD surgeon.[11]

Expectations on the outcome of pregnancy for mother and fetus are predicated on correct assessment of risk. If the patient has symptomatic CHD, a catheter-based or surgical intervention should be employed before conception. If already pregnant, bed rest, medications, hospitalization, and catheter-based intervention are selectively employed. If a patient with a high-risk malformation is pregnant, termination must be considered. Cardiac surgery during pregnancy imposes risks on both mother and fetus. Timing is crucial.

Medications employed during pregnancy, especially regarding effects on the fetus, tend to be judged according to animal studies, small selective human studies, or anecdotal reports.[9] Concerns regarding anticoagulants (oral vitamin K antagonists), angiotensin-converting enzyme (ACE) inhibitors, and amiodarone are well-founded. No anticoagulant regimen provides maximum protection at no maternal or fetal risk. Warfarin embryopathy consists of facial dysmorphism, retarded growth, microcephaly, and mental retardation. Importantly, the brain does not obey the rules of organogenesis nor is it immune from teratogens.

Elective delivery before 39 weeks gestation is usually undertaken after fetal lung maturity is documented by amniocentesis, although in infants delivered near term (around 37 weeks), concerns over timing and control may outweigh concerns about the low risk of respiratory distress syndrome. Intravaginal and intracervical prostaglandins soften and dilatate the cervix. Meperidine and

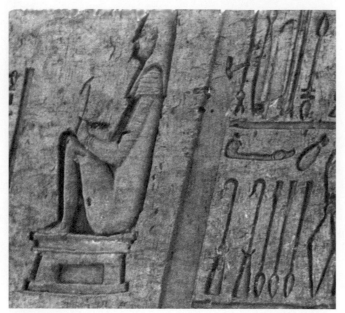

FIGURE 9-4 Stone carving of Twin Temple of Kom Ombro on Nile showing the queen in labor sitting on an obstetric delivery chair. Surgical instruments appear to her right.

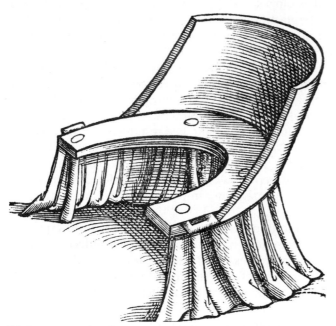

FIGURE 9-5 Medieval birthing chair illustrated in Rueff's *De conceptu et generatione hominis* (1554). *New York Academy of Medicine.*

lumbar epidural anesthesia provide relief of pain and apprehension. The currently preferred lateral decubitus position (see Fig. 9-3) recalls older positions when women were delivered while squatting on two large bricks (Fig. 9-4) or sitting in a chair with the center of the seat removed (Fig. 9-5). Uterine contractions should be unassisted by bearing down to avoid the undesirable effects of the Valsalva maneuver. Vacuum extraction and low forceps are commonly employed. Meticulous leg care

reduces the risk of deep vein thrombophlebitis to which the gravida, especially the multigravida, is prone.

Prophylaxis against infective endocarditis is not included in the 2007 recommendations of the American Heart Association Scientific Statement. The need for antibiotic prophylaxis during routine delivery in pregnant cardiac patients has been questioned because of the low incidence of bacteremia with a normal uncomplicated vaginal delivery—1% to 5% of patients. Rupture of avascular amniotic membranes at term does not pose a risk unless accompanied by chorioamnionitis. It cannot be assumed, however, that a given pregnancy will be uncomplicated. Lacerations of the vagina and perineum commonly occur with a normal vaginal delivery, and episiotomies are frequent. It should not be assumed that a given delivery will be uncomplicated, and strictly speaking, an episiotomy is not "normal." Accordingly, it is our policy that gravidas with a history of infective endocarditis or with cardiac lesions known to be infective endocarditis substrates—a prosthetic heart valve, a surgically created conduit, or an aortopulmonary shunt[2,8,29,30,32,33]—should receive antibiotics beginning at the onset of active labor or rupture of membranes through the first or second postpartum day.

When rupture of membranes occurs well before term (at 24–32 weeks), ampicillin or gentamicin should be administered for 3 to 7 days as prophylaxis against beta *Streptococcus*. Vancomycin and gentamicin are reserved for patients with penicillin sensitivity (see Chapter 8).

PRECONCEPTION EVALUATION AND COUNSELING

Counseling should be obligatory in anticipation of pregnancy. Evaluation begins with a thorough history, including prior cardiac evaluations, diagnostic tests, and therapeutic interventions. Particularly important are interventional or surgical reports and experience with previous pregnancies that serve as a guide to subsequent outcomes. Physical examination establishes the current physiological state. An electrocardiogram and echocardiogram supplement the history and physical and should be routine. Radiologic techniques should be applied selectively and must include proper abdominal shielding. Magnetic resonance imaging is safe and often essential in complex congenital malformations (see Chapter 7).

Prevalence of congenital heart defects in the general population is approximately 4 to 10 per 1000 live births (greater if the bicuspid aortic valve is included)[34,35] (see Chapter 10). The likelihood of a congenital heart defect in the offspring of a mother with CHD is as high as 16%, depending on the maternal lesion.[9,36] If the father has CHD, the chance of recurrence is about one half of that. The chance of transmission is higher if there is a history of familial recurrence of specific lesions.[37,38] Abnormalities transmitted as autosomal dominant such as Marfan syndrome have a 50% probability of recurrence.

Chromosome analysis and FISH (fluorescence *in situ* hybridization) testing for specific deletions are now accepted clinical tools in selected circumstances.[38] If a specific chromosomal abnormality is detected, the family can be counseled on advisability of further pregnancies. An example of the value of this knowledge is in the group of defects related to a 22q11 deletion (tetralogy of Fallot, interrupted aortic arch, truncus arteriosus, etc.).[38-41] The 22q11 deletion tends to be underrecognized in adults with CHD because of absence of characteristic facial dysmorphic features or only subtle phenotypic clues (long narrow face, flat malar bones, small chin, etc).[40,42] Accordingly, prospective parents with certain conotruncal abnormalities benefit from screening that provides evidence of associated extracardiac manifestations and a basis for reproductive counseling.[40] Children born to a parent with 22q11 microdeletion reportedly have a 50% chance of harboring the deletion themselves, with the associated complications.[43,44]

HIGH-RISK CARDIAC DISEASE

Women with cardiovascular disease sometimes experience significant gestational complications despite modern obstetrical and cardiac care.[10] The Cardiac Disease in Pregnancy investigators (CARPREG) developed a scoring system for women with heart disease. The four main predictors of cardiac events (pulmonary edema, arrhythmias, stroke, cardiac arrest, or death) were as follows: (1) New York Heart Association functional class III or IV) or cyanosis, (2) previous cardiac events, (3) mitral or aortic obstruction, and (4) left ventricular ejection fraction < 40%.[45,46] In a 2001 prospective study,[45] one point was assigned for each of the four parameters. Patients with 1 point had relative event rates of 27% versus 75% in patients with scores ≥2 points. When the score was zero, the event rate was 5%. In that prospective study, 74% of pregnancies were in women with CHD, but none had Eisenmenger syndrome. The overall rate of adverse events was 13%, with 55% antepartum occurrence.[45] The predictive value of the 2001 CARPREG risk index was subsequently validated prospectively in 2006 in women who had only CHD (53 women, 90 pregnancies).[47] Adverse events (pulmonary edema, symptomatic arrhythmias, urgent need for invasive intervention) occurred in 25% of the pregnancies.[47] Prediction of adverse outcomes was further improved in patients with a score of 1 point by adding the high-risk presence or low-risk absence of dysfunction of the subpulmonary ventricle or severe pulmonary regurgitation.[47] Neonatal complications occurred in 27.8% of pregnancies in another study,[47] similar to the 20% adverse neonatal outcomes in the 2001 CARPREG report.[45] Importantly, a history of smoking adds to the

likelihood of adverse outcomes.[47,48] Neonatal outcomes are most favorable when the mother with heart disease is between 20 and 35 years of age, does not smoke, does not require anticoagulants, has no obstetrical risk factors, and has a CARPREG score of zero.[48]

A 2007 literature review of English, German, and French publications (1985 or later) of the outcomes of pregnancy in women with CHD provides valuable data.[49] Cardiac complications occurred in 11% of 2491 pregnancies in women with CHD, including 377 (15%) miscarriages and 114 (5%) elective abortions.[49] The most frequent cardiac complication was heart failure (4.8%). Patients with complex CHD (especially Eisenmenger) and palliated or unoperated cyanotic CHD (pulmonary atresia with ventricular septal defect) were at high risk.[49] Significant arrhythmias (4.5%) were usually supraventricular (*n* = 48), with ventricular arrhythmias in nine patients. Arrhythmias were most frequent in gravidas with D-transposition and atrial switch operations, Fontan physiology, or atrioventricular septal defects.[49] There was no increase in prevalence of obstetrical complications, but there were high rates of premature deliveries and of offspring small for gestational age, especially among the more complex CHD cases.[49] Hypertensive disorders were no more prevalent for the group with CHD (8.7%) than for the general population (8%). However, the incidence of hypertension was higher than expected with aortic stenosis (12.8%), aortic coarctation (16%), pulmonic stenosis (14.3%), and transposition of the great arteries (TGA; 16.3%). Preeclampsia occurred in TGA (10.3%), pulmonary atresia with ventricular septal defect (5.9%), pulmonic stenosis (4.9%), and aortic coarctation of the aorta (4.9%) in contrast to a 5% prevalence in the general population of women. Interestingly, no patient with coarctation of the aorta experienced eclampsia. The overall recurrence rate of CHD was 3.5% ranging from 0.6% for TGA to 8% for atrioventricular septal defects. It was emphasized that offspring of women with CHD are at a higher risk of fetal and perinatal mortality. Mortality was 4% throughout the spectrum, greater than the expected < 1% in developed countries, and was chiefly related to the frequency of premature deliveries (16%; before 34 weeks gestation), as well as recurrence of CHD.[49] Eisenmenger syndrome was accompanied by nearly a 65% chance of premature delivery, a 37% chance of a fetus small for gestational age, and nearly 28% offspring mortality.[49]

To summarize, the following conditions pose a high risk of adverse outcomes or the death of the mother or fetus: (1) pulmonary hypertension (pressure greater than three quarters of systemic), (2) maternal cyanosis, (3) systemic ventricular dysfunction, (4) poor maternal functional class, (5) severe left-sided valvular obstruction, (6) dilated aortic root, (7) significant unrepaired defects, and (8) patients with mechanical prosthetic heart valves on oral anticoagulants.[2,4,5,9,10,11,16,28-30,33,45-48,50-63]

In light of the 2006 study, depressed function of the sub-pulmonic ventricle and severe pulmonary regurgitation should be included in this list.[47] Patients with any of these high-risk conditions should be counseled accordingly, and management individualized to determine therapeutic interventions, prohibition of high-risk pregnancy, and selected termination of pregnancy.

LOW-RISK HEART DISEASE

Congenital cardiac diseases that incur little or no gestational risk are addressed in the section on specific lesions. Women with uncomplicated left-to-right shunts, good ventricular function, and no pulmonary hypertension and those with isolated mild to moderate obstructive lesions, asymptomatic regurgitant lesions, and even some complex acyanotic defects with normal systemic ventricular function tolerate pregnancy well.[59] Most women with repaired lesions do well in the absence of significant residua or sequelae or mechanical prosthetic valves that require anticoagulation.[9]

DRUGS DURING PREGNANCY

Cardiovascular drugs for gravidas with CHD fall into four major categories: (1) anticoagulants, (2) antiarrhythmic and (3) antihypertensive agents, and (4) heart failure medications. No drugs should be assumed safe for the fetus. There are three relatively complete published lists of drugs with references on safety.[5,16,54] Anticoagulants are discussed in the section that deals with prosthetic valves.

Heart failure regimens that include ACE inhibitors, angiotensin receptor blockers, or spironolactone antagonists are contraindicated during pregnancy. In a 2006 study of 29,507 infants born between 1985 and 2003, 411 were exposed to an antihypertensive medication in the first trimester, 209 of whom were exposed to ACE inhibitors alone.[64] The adjusted proportion with any major congenital abnormalities was 7.1%, thus demonstrating convincingly that ACE inhibitors during the first trimester incurred a marked increase in the incidence of congenital malformations (cardiovascular system risk ratio 3.72; 95% confidence interval 1.89–7.30 and central nervous system risk ratio 4.39; 95% confidence interval, 1.37–14.02).[64] ACE inhibitors and angiotensin receptor blockers during the second and third trimesters have been associated with oligohydramnios, fetal growth retardation, pulmonary hypoplasia, joint contractures, hypocalvaria, neonatal renal failure, hypotension, and death.[65] Digitalis glycosides are safe for mother and fetus. There is no convincing evidence of an inotropic effect of digitalis on the myometrium with preterm labor or shorter labor. Although digoxin is excreted into breast milk, no adverse effects have been identified in the nursing infant.

Vasodilators such as hydralazine have a long history of safety in pregnancy and are used to treat heart failure and hypertension. Diuretics should not be used for the noncardiac edema of normal pregnancy. Although diuretics in late gestation produce no apparent ill effect, a reduction in maternal plasma volume during early gestation is undesirable and potentially harmful to the fetus.

Beta-blockers are reportedly responsible for intrauterine growth retardation or fetal bradycardia, but there is a long history of relative safety in pregnancy. We have used metoprolol ("class C") for a variety of purposes during pregnancy with no detectable adverse effects. Atenolol reportedly exerts adverse effects, has been classified as a "class D" in pregnancy, and is best avoided. Propranolol increases uterine activity, an effect more pronounced in the nonpregnant than the pregnant uterus. Offspring of propranolol-treated gravidas have not manifested cardiac effects attributable to beta-adrenergic blockade. However, blockade of humeral stimulation of beta-adrenergic receptor sites eliminates a potentially important response of the fetus to acute stress and is therefore undesirable when circumstances demand rapid fetal adaptation.

The use and efficacy of antiarrhythmic agents during pregnancy are similar to their use and efficacy in the nongravid state except for potential placental transfer. Quinidine crosses the placenta and reaches concentrations in fetal serum similar to those in the mother, but there have been no reports of adverse effects. Quinidine diffuses freely into breast milk with a milk-to-plasma ratio of approximately 1.0. An interaction between quinidine and anticoagulants is believed to increase the risk of hemorrhage. Procainamide is best avoided because of its association with antinuclear antibodies, maternal lupus erythematosus, and an increased risk of fetal complete heart block. Lidocaine is considered safe for mother and fetus when used in relatively low doses—just enough to suppress acute ventricular arrhythmias. Verapamil concentrations in the fetus are substantially less than in maternal plasma, but information is incomplete. Information on the safety of disopyramide is not secure enough to warrant a confident recommendation, and disopyramide crosses the placenta and is excreted into breast milk. Data on mexiletine are not adequate to provide a secure basis for judgment. Phenytoin teratogenicity is firmly established and responsible for the fetal hydantoin syndrome, which is characterized by abnormalities in growth and development, craniofacial and limb abnormalities, and occasionally CHD. Amiodarone and its metabolites undergo limited placental transfer. However, there is the large amount of iodine in amiodarone (39% by weight), and iodine readily crosses the placenta, is concentrated in the fetal thyroid as early as the 14th week, and has been associated with neonatal goiter after exposure to comparatively small amounts of the parent compound. Amiodarone is secreted into breast milk in concentrations equivalent to a low maintenance dose. If fetal exposure is to be avoided during the early weeks of pregnancy, amiodarone must be discontinued several months before conception because of its long terminal elimination half-life.

CARDIAC SURGERY DURING PREGNANCY

One of the best ways of simplifying medical management of the gravida is for cardiac surgery to precede conception. It is psychologically damaging for a woman to terminate her pregnancy, undergo heart surgery, and then become pregnant again. Such decisions weigh heavily on both physician and patient. Successful cardiac surgery improves fertility, stabilizes the pregnancy, eliminates the fetal risk of maternal cyanosis, and benefits the subsequent health of mother and child. A major benefit to the fetus of preconception surgery is elimination of maternal cyanosis.[9,58,59]

Cardiac surgery *during* pregnancy is occasionally required in women with CHD.[16] The management of gravida who require cardiopulmonary bypass poses problems that are difficult to resolve. The fetus is at greatest risk early in the pregnancy, whereas the mother is at greatest risk later in the pregnancy. A review of the literature from 1984 to 1996 disclosed that surgery during pregnancy resulted in fetal/neonatal morbidity and mortality of 9% and 30%, respectively, with maternal morbidity and mortality 24% and 6%, respectively.[66] Maternal deaths were reported in 9% of valvular procedures and in 22% of aortic dissection repairs and pulmonary embolectomies.[66] Maternal risks of cardiac surgery during pregnancy are higher than in the nonpregnant state, and fetal/neonatal risks of maternal surgery are high and unpredictable.[66] Operation should be recommended during pregnancy only if strict medical management has failed or if there is an emergency such as aortic dissection or hemodynamically unstable acute severe aortic regurgitation.[16] Importantly, the maternal risks of cardiac surgery are higher when performed at or soon after delivery.[66] Maternal morbidity and mortality of surgery immediately after delivery were 29% and 12%, respectively; surgery later in the postpartum was accompanied by 38% morbidity and 14% mortality.[66] If cardiac surgery is considered essential during early pregnancy, it is best performed at 16 to 20 weeks gestation, a timing that reduces fetal risk and precedes the maximum circulatory demands on the mother.[11] Operation after week 27 was accompanied by significantly poorer maternal outcome.[66]

Fetal risks are related to reduced uteroplacental blood flow during cardiopulmonary bypass and to preterm labor. High-flow (2.5 L/min/m²), high-pressure (mean arterial pressure > 70 mm Hg) are recommended to maintain placental blood flow. The mother should be placed in the left lateral position during surgery to reduce aortocaval compression. The fetal heart rate should be monitored continuously. Fetal bradycardia often responds to an increase in flow rate. Prolonged fetal bradycardia (< 80 beats/min) that is unresponsive to increased pump flow rates is an indication for cesarean delivery.

Animal studies and case reports in pregnant women suggest that hypothermia (to 25°C) does not adversely affect the fetus. However, rewarming tends to increase uterine activity with the risk of preterm labor. Moderate hypothermia (32°C) is probably safe, but the effects on the fetus have not been well established. Because fetal mortality accompanying cardiac surgery during pregnancy is about 15%, operation should be performed only if delay would seriously endanger the mother. Rarely, cesarean delivery has been successfully performed while the mother was on cardiopulmonary bypass. Confronted with the catastrophe of sudden maternal death, immediate postmortem cesarean delivery occasionally retrieves a viable fetus. Approximately 150 postmortem cesarean deliveries have been reported, with an infant survival of approximately 15%.[11]

Anesthetic agents should be carefully selected by an experienced obstetrical anesthesiologist. Heart rate and uterine contractions are monitored continuously during surgery. In the event of emergency cardiac surgery near term, cesarean delivery can be performed in the same operating theater.[16]

LABOR AND DELIVERY

In women with functionally mild unoperated CHD and in those who have undergone successful cardiac surgery, the management of labor and delivery is the same as for normal gravidas except for the selective risk of infective endocarditis[10,11] (see earlier discussion and Chapter 8).

For pregnant women with functionally significant unoperated or operated congenital cardiac disease, planning in anticipation of labor, delivery, and the puerperium are crucial if risk is to be minimized.[10,11] There is a virtual consensus that cesarean delivery is reserved for obstetrical indications— cephalopelvic disproportion, placenta previa, breech presentation, or preterm labor in a gravida on oral anticoagulants. Fetal anticoagulation cannot be reversed. Cesarean delivery reduces the risk of fetal hemorrhagic death. Fresh frozen plasma should be administered to the salvaged neonate.

Cesarean delivery performed with epidural anesthesia incurs the risk of hypotension and tachycardia. General anesthesia incurs hemodynamic risk associated with intubation and the risk of depressing the fetus. Blood loss accompanying Cesarean delivery is about twice as great as with vaginal delivery, in addition to the risks of wound and uterine infection and postoperative complications associated with delayed ambulation, especially thrombophlebitis. However, cesarean delivery is necessarily employed in selected high-risk circumstances such as aortic dissection, aortic root aneurysm larger than 40 mm, preterm labor in a gravida on oral vitamin K antagonists (see earlier), unstable symptomatic heart failure, or severe left ventricular outflow obstruction. Preterm labor is a major risk, especially in a cyanotic gravida with a dysmature fetus (see later discussion). Tocolytic agents for pharmacologic inhibition of uterine contractions include magnesium sulfate and nifedipine, less commonly ritodrine, terbutaline, or other beta-adrenergic agents. The current tendency is to avoid magnesium sulfate because infusion for more than 48 hours may be accompanied by noncardiac pulmonary edema that stands out in bold relief in a gravida with normal ventricular function.

Pregnant women with unoperated or postoperative CHD who are functionally normal or nearly so are allowed to go into labor spontaneously, as in women without heart disease. However, if there is a concern about the functional adequacy of the heart, labor should be induced under controlled conditions. The timing of induction is individualized, taking into account inducibility of the cervix and fetal lung maturity determined by amniocentesis. Long inductions with an unfavorable cervix should be avoided. It is useful to plan the induction so that delivery occurs during the working day when a high-risk obstetrician, neonatologist, and cardiologist are readily available. Induction should not be initiated in women with obstetrical contraindications to vaginal delivery. An elective cesarean delivery should be performed instead.

Induction of labor in gravidas with a favorable cervix usually requires only oxytocin administration and artificial rupture of the membranes. An unfavorable cervix can be ripened with intracervical or intravaginal prostaglandin E_2. Laminaria, which is derived from the stems of the hydrophilic seaweed *Laminaria digitata*, can also be used. The softened, dilatated cervix is more responsive to subsequent induction of labor, permitting the normal physiologic sequence of softening and dilatation before the onset of uterine contractions. After labor is induced, the gravida should be placed in a lateral decubitus position (see Fig. 9–3) to attenuate the hemodynamic fluctuations associated with major uterine contractions in the supine position.

The first obstetrical anesthetic administered in the United States was given on April 7, 1847, in Cambridge, Massachusetts, to Fanny Appleton Longfellow, wife of the famous poet and scholar Henry Wadsworth Longfellow. In the 1970s, natural childbirth was celebrated as an invigorating and transforming experience, but today attitudes are starkly different, with natural childbirth often ridiculed as a primitive ritual. There is a uniform consensus that vaginal delivery in gravida with heart disease should be pain-free. Intramuscular or intravenous narcotics (meperidine, fentanyl) are used to relieve pain and apprehension. Lumbar epidural anesthesia is particularly effective in controlling labor pain and is recommended because it lowers pain-induced elevations of sympathetic activity and exquisitely controls pain without reducing

the strength of uterine contractions, which are monitored together with fetal heart rate (see Fig. 9–8). Venous return can be reduced by epidural anesthesia, which should be used cautiously, if at all, in patients in whom cardiac output is likely to be sensitive to decreases in preload. Narcotic epidural and continuous narcotic spinal anesthesia are safe alternatives, with general anesthesia reserved for cesarean delivery. A reduction in uterine blood flow and placental oxygen delivery accompanies a major uterine contraction. Fetal heart rate slows but rebounds promptly as the uterus relaxes.

The fetus should be allowed to pass through the pelvis in response to the force of uterine contractions alone, unassisted by straining, to avoid the undesirable circulatory effects of the Valsalva maneuver (bearing down). Delivery is assisted by forceps or vacuum extraction when the fetal head has descended to a low station.

Systemic arterial pressure is monitored during labor because lumbar epidural anesthetics may cause hypotension. A flotation catheter for hemodynamic monitoring is not routinely employed. Hemostatic defects in cyanotic CHD increase the risk of bleeding during percutaneous entry of the flotation catheter, and withdrawal of the catheter can be accompanied by bleeding, pulmonary or paradoxical embolization, and death.[39] In patients with Eisenmenger's syndrome, the necessary hemodynamic information is provided by monitoring systemic arterial pressure with an intraarterial line and by fingertip pulse oximetry monitoring of systemic arterial oxygen saturation that varies directly with systemic vascular resistance. Oxygen is often administered intuitively during labor in cyanotic women, but maternal efficacy has not been demonstrated, and it is unclear whether and to what extent maternal oxygen administration increases fetal PaO_2.

After expulsion of the placenta, bleeding is reduced by uterine massage and intravenous oxytocin, which should be infused slowly at less than 2 units/min to avoid hypotension. Meticulous leg care, elastic support stockings, and early ambulation are important preventive measures that reduce the risk of postpartum thromboembolism. In cyanotic gravidas, heparin should not be used because it reinforces intrinsic hemostatic defects and may result in dangerous, if not fatal, hemorrhage.

Breast-feeding as commonly practiced encroaches on cardiac reserve and risks mastitis and bacteremia. Accordingly, breast-feeding should be undertaken selectively in women with CHD, and its duration minimized. Engorgement and suppression of lactation are achieved with binding, cold packs, and analgesics, rather than with bromocriptine, which can cause hypotension.

Misoprostol, a synthetic prostaglandin structurally related to prostaglandin E_1, has been used for the termination of second-trimester pregnancy (12–22 weeks gestation) involving a dead or viable fetus. The method is preferred to mechanical uterine evacuation in high-risk cardiac patients. Intravaginal and intrauterine misoprostol is designed to soften and dilatate the cervix and to initiate uterine contraction (see earlier discussion of prostaglandin E_2). Because of the high concentration of the synthetic prostaglandin, misoprostol is absorbed into the systemic circulation, lowering vascular resistance and augmenting right-to-left shunts. Accordingly, systemic arterial oxygen saturation should be monitored with a pulse oximeter and norepinephrine infused at a rate that supports the diastolic blood pressure, which reflects systemic vascular resistance.

SPECIFIC CONGENITAL CARDIOVASCULAR MALFORMATIONS

Although unoperated malformations often permit survival to childbearing age, gestation after reparative cardiac surgery is one of the most important aspects of heart disease and pregnancy. A prime objective of operation is to increase the safety and success of pregnancy and to preserve the subsequent health of mother and child. There is a uniform consensus that successful surgery can be pivotal in reducing maternal and fetal risks. Operation should therefore be anticipatory. The risk of pregnancy after operation is determined chiefly by the presence, type, and degree of cardiac and vascular residua and sequelae (see Chapters 20 and 21). Operation has no bearing on genetic transmission of maternal CHD. The following remarks deal with some but not all of the anomalies discussed earlier.

Ostium Secundum Atrial Septal Defect

Because unoperated longevity in patients with ostium secundum atrial septal defect spans the reproductive years, and because the majority of patients so affected are female, this malformation is of special importance in the context of CHD and pregnancy. Despite the gestational increase in cardiac output and stroke volume, women with uncomplicated ostium secundum atrial septal defects generally tolerate pregnancy—even multiple pregnancies—with no tangible ill effects. After the fourth decade, however, otherwise uncomplicated secundum defects are accompanied by an increased incidence of supraventricular tachyarrhythmias, especially atrial fibrillation or atrial flutter, that can precipitate right ventricular failure. An important concern is the risk of paradoxical embolization because emboli carried by the inferior vena cava tend to be directed across the atrial septal defect into the systemic circulation. Meticulous leg care minimizes venous stasis. Also important, but less well known, are the deleterious effects of acute blood loss that is accompanied by a rise in systemic vascular resistance and a fall in systemic venous return, a

combination that augments the left-to-right interatrial shunt, sometimes appreciably.

Pulmonary hypertension is seldom a feature of ostium secundum atrial septal defects. However, if pulmonary vascular disease is present, even in the absence of a reversed shunt, there is a significant increase in the risk of pregnancy analogous to the risk in primary pulmonary hypertension.

An asymptomatic woman of reproductive age who has undergone childhood closure of an ostium secundum atrial septal defect can anticipate a risk-free pregnancy. Successful closure of the defect eliminates the hazard of paradoxical embolization. Postoperative residua or sequelae are few and insignificant except for late-onset atrial tachyarrhythmias when operation is performed after childhood.

Patent Ductus Arteriosus

Patency of the arterial duct is of less practical importance as a complication of pregnancy because the clinical diagnosis is simple, and surgical or catheter closure in childhood is routine and curative. An asymptomatic young woman with a small or moderate-sized ductus and normal pulmonary arterial pressure can anticipate an uncomplicated pregnancy, apart from the risk of infective endarteritis during delivery (see earlier discussion and see Chapter 8). One of our patients, a 57-year-old woman with a moderately restrictive patent ductus, endured 20 pregnancies with 12 live births.

The gestational fall in systemic vascular resistance serves to decrease ductal flow, but if the shunt is large, the benefit is unlikely to compensate for the additional hemodynamic burden of pregnancy. Patients with a nonrestrictive patent ductus and reversed shunt are at highest risk, underscoring again the hazard of pulmonary vascular disease. In the presence of fixed pulmonary vascular resistance, the decline in systemic vascular resistance during pregnancy augments the right-to-left shunt, disproportionately increasing the amount of unoxygenated blood delivered to the gravid uterus (differential cyanosis), thus increasing an already high fetal risk. Bearing down during labor imposes a hazard analogous to that in gravidas with other forms of the Eisenmenger syndrome.

There is a single report of spontaneous postpartum rupture of a nonpulmonary hypertensive patent ductus arteriosus without ductal aneurysm. Microscopic examination adjacent to the site of rupture disclosed that the wall of the ductus was composed of elastic tissue with some smooth muscle, but with no evidence of myxoid degeneration.

Closure of a small patent ductus arteriosus in childhood represents one of the few unqualified cures of CHD. Closure of a nonrestrictive patent ductus arteriosus, however, may be followed by incomplete decline in pulmonary vascular resistance or by incomplete functional recovery of the volume-overloaded left ventricle or the pressure-overloaded right ventricle. Postoperative pulmonary vascular disease and depressed ventricular function are important residua that determine gestational risk.

Pulmonary Valve Stenosis

Fifty percent of patients with isolated pulmonary valve stenosis are female. Survival to adulthood is the rule even if there is significant obstruction to right ventricular outflow. Isolated pulmonary valve stenosis reportedly occurs with significant noncardiac maternal complications such as hypertension-related disorders, pre-eclampsia, eclampsia, and thromboembolic events.[67] Preterm delivery and intrauterine or neonatal mortality are not uncommon, with overall offspring mortality 4.8%.[67] There is a 3.7% recurrence rate of CHD, usually concordant.[67]

Mild-to-moderate pulmonary valve stenosis poses little or no maternal risk. Occasionally, even severe pulmonary stenosis is well tolerated despite gestational volume overload imposed on an already pressure-loaded right ventricle.[7,11] Infective endocarditis prophylaxis is advisable during delivery, although the risk with mild pulmonary stenosis is negligible, if not absent, and susceptibility to infective endocarditis is low if not absent after successful valvuloplasty (see Chapter 8). When surgical repair or balloon dilatation leaves behind little or no obstruction and a valve that is competent or nearly so, the mother can anticipate a normal pregnancy and delivery. The salutary effects of balloon dilatation have been a major step forward in reducing the risks of labor, delivery, and the puerperium in gravidas with severe pulmonary valve stenosis, and the procedure has proved successful during pregnancy (Figs. 9–6 and 9–7). The fetal heart rate is monitored (Fig. 9–8).

Coarctation of the Aorta

The malformation occurs chiefly in males, with the sex ratio as high as 3:1, but coarctation is dealt with here because major gestational complications, although uncommon, can be lethal.[7,11] Most of the females with coarctation in our Adult Congenital Heart Disease Center have had some form of surgical repair, and most women with coarctation reach childbearing age.[68] The incidence of toxemia is lower in pregnant women with the hypertension of coarctation than in pregnant women with other forms of hypertension.[7,11] Blood pressure variations are similar in direction to those in normal pregnancy but occur from a higher basal level.

Pregnancy increases the risk of rupture or dissection of the paracoarctation aorta and the ascending aorta above a coexisting bicuspid aortic valve, sites that harbor inherent medial abnormalities that act in concert with the fragmentation of elastic fibers that occur in human aortic media during normal pregnancy.[20]

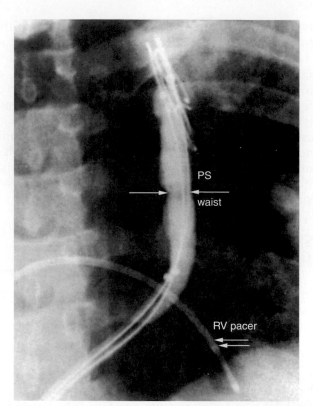

FIGURE 9–6 Percutaneous single-balloon dilatation of severe mobile pulmonary valve stenosis in a symptomatic 18-year-old primigravida near term. Arrows identify the balloon waist. A pacemaker was temporarily placed in the apex of the right ventricle (RV). See Figures 9–7 and 9–8.

Hypertension is not a necessary precondition for cerebral hemorrhage (aneurysm of the circle of Willis) in a gravida with coarctation. Left ventricular failure is exceptional despite the increased volume load imposed on the already pressure-loaded left ventricle. The risk of infective endocarditis is largely determined by a coexisting bicuspid aortic valve. Complete relief of isthmic coarctation, especially in early childhood, favorably influences the probability of long-term normalization of blood pressure and normalization of left ventricular mass, goals that are best achieved by resection with end-to-end anastomosis. Dacron patch aortoplasty carries a risk of aneurysm formation because the procedure necessarily leaves behind segments of the abnormal paracoarctation aorta that harbors inherent medial abnormalities (described earlier). Balloon angioplasty for unoperated coarctation or after patch aortoplasty incurs traumatic injury to the inherently abnormal paracoarctation aorta and accounts for subsequent aneurysm formation. Gestational changes in aortic media then act in concert with the intrinsic paracoarctation medial abnormality, increasing the risk of aortic rupture or dissection. If a bicuspid aortic valve coexists, the inherent connective tissue abnormality that resides in the aortic root is an independent risk (described earlier).

Major cardiovascular complications, although infrequent, continue to be matters of concern in pregnant

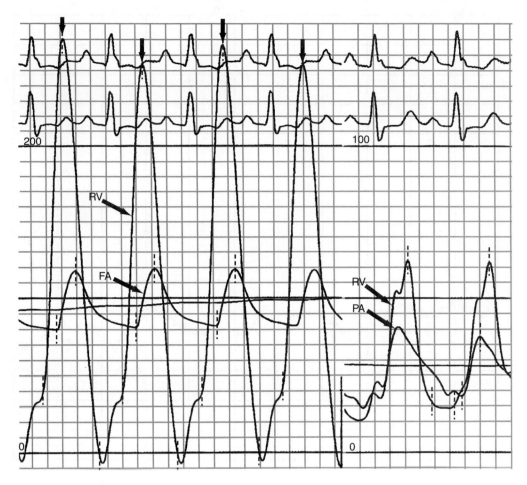

FIGURE 9-7   Pressure tracings in the patient referred to in Figure 9-6 showing a striking increase in right ventricular systolic pressure of 280 mm Hg with right ventricular pulsus alternans, indicating depressed ventricular function. Following balloon dilatation, the right-ventricular-to-pulmonary arterial peak systolic gradient fell from 140 to 22 mm Hg. Vaginal delivery 3 days later was uncomplicated.

women with aortic coarctation.[69] The Mayo Clinic experience with coarctation and pregnancy was reported in 2001 in 50 patients,[69] 30 of whom had repair before pregnancy, 10 had repair after pregnancy, four had repairs before and after pregnancy, and six were unrepaired. The 50 patients experienced 118 pregnancies with 106 live births, 11 miscarriages (9%), 4 preterm deliveries (3%), and 1 early neonatal death. Thirty-eight deliveries (36%) were cesarean. Of the 109 offspring, 4% had CHD. One gravida with Turner syndrome died of an aortic dissection at 36 weeks. Nineteen of the pregnant women (38%) had hemodynamically significant coarctation (gradient ≥20 mm Hg). Fifteen (30%) were hypertensive during their pregnancy, 11 of whom (73%) had hemodynamically significant coarctation (eight with native and three with residual/recurrent coarctation). Systemic hypertension is common and related to a significant coarctation gradient.

In 2005, the CONCOR (CONgenital CORvitia; www.concor.net) national registry on CHD in the Netherlands published a report on pregnancy after coarctation repair.[68] The 54 of 100 women experienced 126 pregnancies that yielded 98 offspring, 22 miscarriages, and 6 abortions. There were 85 vaginal deliveries, 7 with epidural analgesia, 6 caesarean deliveries, and 2 neonatal deaths. Twenty-one

pregnancies in 14 women were complicated by hypertension, and 5 pregnancies in 4 women were complicated by pre-eclampsia. Five patients had an increase in gradient across the coarctation repair ≥15 mm Hg, but only one required reintervention after delivery. Four of the 98 offspring (4%) had a congenital heart defect.[68]

Complete relief of coarctation by resection with end-to-end anastomosis removes the abnormal paracoarctation aorta and eliminates the risk of infective endocarditis at the coarctation site, but the presence of a coexisting bicuspid aortic valve leaves unchanged the risk of infective endocarditis and the risk inherent in the abnormal ascending aortic media[70] (Fig. 9-9). Successful coarctation repair does not reduce the hazard of gestational rupture of an aneurysm of the circle of Willis (discussed earlier).

Functionally Normal Bicuspid Aortic Valve

An isolated functionally normal bicuspid aortic valve is likely to go unrecognized in young women. The clinical index of suspicion is low owing to male prevalence, and the auscultatory signs are subtle.[7] A bicuspid aortic valve may first come to light during gestation because of a dissecting aneurysm of the ascending aorta, or after delivery

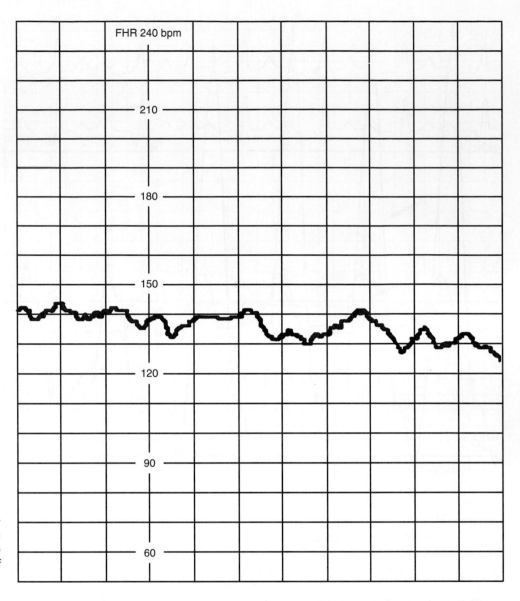

FIGURE 9-8   Fetal heart rate monitor during pulmonary valvuloplasty in the patient referred to in Figures 9-6 and 9-7. There was no evidence of fetal distress.

when fever and acute aortic regurgitation culminate in the diagnosis of infective endocarditis to which the bicuspid aortic valve is susceptible (see Chapter 8).

Congenital Bicuspid or Unicuspid Aortic Stenosis

In patients with severe aortic stenosis, the increased cardiac output of pregnancy is imposed on the pressure-loaded left ventricle.[16,29,30,33,56,71] Most women with aortic stenosis have a congenital aortic valve abnormality.[5,6,11,16] Mild to moderate stenosis tends to be well tolerated during pregnancy because left ventricular systolic function is generally preserved; indeed, the ejection fraction is often above normal. However, severe obstruction encroaches on circulatory reserve. Dyspnea, angina pectoris, or cerebral symptoms that precede conception or appear early in gestation are matters of grave concern.

In 2003, there was a report of 39 women (49 pregnancies) with congenital aortic stenosis in which stenosis was severe in 59% and moderate in 33%.[71] There was a 10% complication rate with a peak gradient > 64 mm Hg or an aortic valve area < 1.0 cm², but no complications occurred in gravida with lesser degrees of stenosis.[71] In the UCLA Adult Congenital Heart Disease Center experience, heart failure or the need for intervention is infrequent when congenital aortic stenosis occurs with a calculated aortic valve area of ≥0.8 cm² (≥0.5 cm²/m²), a mean systolic gradient < 50 mm Hg, and normal or supranormal left ventricular systolic function. An induced vaginal delivery is planned at 37 to 38 weeks gestation, with fetal and maternal monitoring. A flotation pulmonary artery catheter is seldom necessary.

Surgical or interventional relief of peak gradients ≥50 mm Hg appreciably reduces the risk of pregnancy, which is lowest when the peak gradient is ≤25 mm Hg and when left

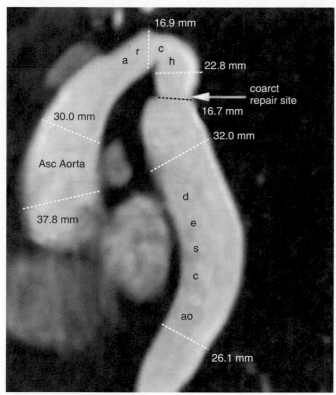

FIGURE 9–9   Magnetic resonance angiography after childhood resection of coarctation of the aorta with end-to-end anastomosis. There was a coexisting functionally normal bicuspid aortic valve, mild dilatation of the proximal ascending aorta (Asc Aorta), and mild aortic arch hypoplasia (see "arch" measurements relative to other segments). The site of anastomosis is slightly narrowed, and the postcoarctation segment is mildly dilatated.

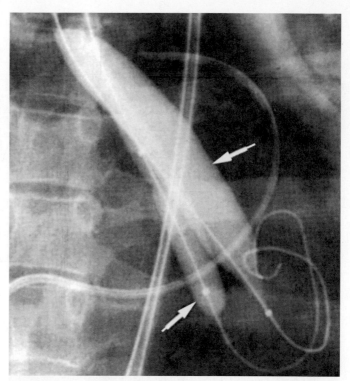

FIGURE 9–10   Still-frame fluoroscopic image of double-balloon aortic valvuloplasty in a 26-year-old gravida with severe bicuspid aortic stenosis in her 36th week of gestation.

ventricular function is normal or supranormal. The least satisfactory procedure in anticipation of pregnancy is valve replacement with a rigid prosthesis that requires anticoagulants (see earlier discussion). Balloon dilatation of a severely stenotic bicuspid aortic valve before or during pregnancy has been a major advance in reducing the hazards of gestation, labor, and delivery (Figs. 9–10 through 9–12). Even in experienced hands, however, percutaneous balloon valvuloplasty incurs the risk of tearing the valve or annulus and inducing acute severe regurgitation. The balloon-dilatated bicuspid aortic valve remains susceptible to infective endocarditis irrespective of its functional state.

Bicuspid Aortic Regurgitation

Moderate, even severe, chronic bicuspid aortic regurgitation is generally well tolerated during pregnancy, provided the adaptive response of the left ventricle permits normal function and functional reserve, which is usually the case. The gestational fall in systemic vascular resistance coupled with the relatively rapid heart rate that shortens diastole serve to decrease regurgitant flow. The risk of infective endocarditis is high, and thus prophylaxis is mandatory (see Chapter 8).

If a woman with moderate to marked aortic regurgitation wishes to become pregnant, it is better to advise her to do so before aortic valve replacement, provided left ventricular functional reserve is normal. If valve replacement is required, an attractive option is the Ross procedure that replaces the aortic valve with the patient's pulmonary valve and replaces the pulmonary valve with a homograft or bioprosthetic tissue valve. It is hoped that the connective tissue changes accompanying gestation will not beset the bioprosthetic tissue valve in the low-pressure pulmonary location or the native pulmonary valve in the aortic location.

Tetralogy of Fallot

The tetralogy is one of the most common cyanotic malformations that permit unoperated survival to reproductive age, and approximately 50% of patients are female. Prevalence is likely to increase because women with successful repairs are now able to conceive and bear children, and the incidence of transmission from the affected mother is about 2% to 5%, which exceeds the 0.8% incidence of CHD in the general population.[39,72] Mild cyanosis and a paucity of symptoms before conception do not ensure a smooth course for either mother or fetus. The gestational decrease in systemic vascular resistance, together with the augmented cardiac output and increased venous return to an obstructed

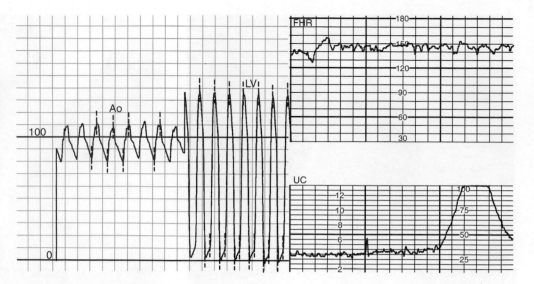

FIGURE 9-11 Results of double-balloon aortic valvuloplasty in the 26-year-old gravida referred to in Figure 9-10. The left panel shows the left ventricular (LV) and aortic (Ao) pressure tracings after balloon dilatation. The peak gradient fell from 100 to 25 mm Hg. The monitored fetal heart rate (FHR) and uterine contractions (UC) shown in the right panels were during a subsequent uncomplicated induced vaginal delivery that yielded a normal neonate.

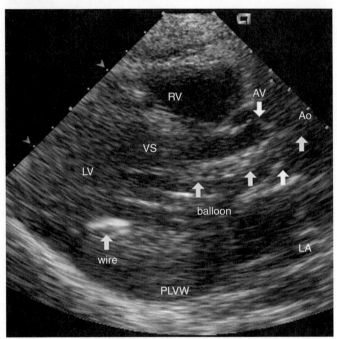

FIGURE 9-12 Percutaneous balloon dilatation of severe bicuspid aortic stenosis with a peak gradient of 139 mm Hg in a 19-year-old symptomatic female in the 27th week of her second pregnancy. Transthoracic echocardiography served to monitor positioning of the balloon catheter and wire system across the doming valve. Dilatation reduced the peak gradient to 27 mm Hg. A focal flail portion of the aortic valve resulted in moderately severe aortic regurgitation. An uncomplicated induced vaginal delivery at 38 weeks gestation yielded a normal neonate. Ao, aorta; AV, aortic valve; LA, left atrium; LV, left ventricle; PLVW, posterior left ventricular wall; RV, right ventricle; VS, ventricular septum.

right ventricle, result in augmentation of the right-to-left shunt and in a fall in systemic arterial oxygen saturation, changes that are particularly detrimental for the fetus. During labor and delivery, a sudden fall in systemic vascular resistance may precipitate intense cyanosis, syncope, and death, and bearing down during labor can abruptly and dangerously reduce systemic, and therefore cerebral, blood flow.

Most patients with the tetralogy have had an intracardiac repair, and a few have had only palliative shunts. Postoperative residua and sequelae range from minor to severe. Surgical relief of cyanosis increases the likelihood of successful conception and substantially improves the stability of the pregnancy and the prospect of normal fetal growth.[39,72,73] Bifascicular block or high-degree heart block are uncommon with current surgical techniques. If a pacemaker is required, pregnancy can proceed. Infective endocarditis remains a concern, even in well-repaired malformations (see Chapter 8).

Pregnancy after successful intracardiac repair of tetralogy of Fallot is accompanied by a justifiable air of optimism—even in patients with pulmonary atresia—especially when there is little or no outflow gradient, no more than mild pulmonary regurgitation, good ventricular function, and neither spontaneous nor exercise-induced disturbances in ventricular rhythm.[39,47,73,74] In the 2004 Mayo Clinic report, mothers did well, but there were a few instances of supraventricular arrhythmias, progressive right ventricular enlargement, right heart failure, and pulmonary embolism.[73] Left ventricular dysfunction, usually related to chronic volume load of a systemic-to-pulmonary shunt or aortic regurgitation, remains a potential problem.[72-74] Right ventricular dysfunction is usually related to outflow tract incisions, scars, patches, residual pulmonary stenosis or regurgitation, or a residual ventricular septal defect.[39,72,73] The tetralogy is accompanied by an increased risk of fetal loss.[39,73,74]

Ventricular Septal Defect

Ventricular septal defect is an example of a congenital cardiac defect that is common in children but infrequent in women of reproductive age. Closure of a moderately restrictive or nonrestrictive ventricular septal defect in early childhood generally precludes the development of pulmonary vascular disease and permits pregnancy to proceed with virtual impunity, provided ventricular function is normal. Major postoperative electrophysiologic sequelae are unusual. The occasional adult female with a small to moderate-sized ventricular septal defect confronts pregnancy with a relatively low risk that is closely related to the magnitude of the left-to-right shunt and to the adaptive response of the left ventricle to the accompanying volume overload. Nonrestrictive ventricular septal defects that permit adult survival almost always do so because a rise in pulmonary vascular resistance reduces the left-to-right shunt and the volume overload of the left ventricle but culminates in an inoperable reversed shunt. The gestational hazards of Eisenmenger to mother and fetus are emphasized once again. Death can occur during gestation, labor, delivery, or the puerperium, with a cumulative risk estimated at 30% to 70%. The gestational fall in systemic vascular resistance increases the right-to-left shunt, further reducing systemic arterial oxygen saturation with adverse effects on both mother and fetus. The fixed pulmonary vascular resistance precludes rapid adaptation to the volatile fluctuations in systemic vascular resistance, cardiac output, and blood volume during labor, delivery, and the puerperium. An abrupt fall in systemic resistance may precipitate intense cyanosis, and bearing down during labor suddenly elevates systemic vascular resistance, depresses systemic and cerebral blood flow, and may provoke fatal syncope.

Congenital Complete Heart Block

High-degree heart block in the neonate can be in response to transplacental transfer of autoantibodies associated with maternal connective tissue disease[75] or in conjunction with CHD, notably congenitally corrected transposition of the great arteries. The isolated form of congenital complete heart block, in which half of patients are female, is an uncommon congenital conduction defect that permits survival to childbearing age. Asymptomatic young women generally experience uneventful pregnancies, provided that the QRS duration is not prolonged and that ventricular function is normal, which is usually the case. However, a Stokes-Adams attack occasionally announces itself for the first time during gestation, and the heart and circulation may not respond adequately to the volatile demands of labor and delivery. When a pacemaker is required, pregnancy can then go forward with relative confidence, especially if the pacemaker is dual chambered. If ventricular function is normal, which is usually the case, a fixed-rate ventricular pacemaker usually suffices.

Ebstein Anomaly

Fifty percent of patients with Ebstein's anomaly of the tricuspid valve are female, and the majority reach adulthood. The functionally inadequate right ventricle, already volume overloaded by tricuspid regurgitation, must cope with the gestational increase in cardiac output. Paroxysmal atrial arrhythmias occur in approximately one third of nongravid women with Ebstein anomaly and are potential hazards during pregnancy. Wolff-Parkinson-White accessory pathways set the stage for excessively rapid ventricular rates in response to atrial fibrillation or atrial flutter, with potentially catastrophic consequences. An additional concern is a pregnancy-related increase in the incidence of supraventricular arrhythmias with the Wolff-Parkinson-White syndrome. Cyanosis associated with a right-to-left shunt at atrial level may first become evident during pregnancy because of a rise in right ventricular filling pressure. In addition, an interatrial communication, including the commonly associated patent foramen ovale, poses a risk of paradoxical embolization, and hypoxemia increases risk to the fetus. Nevertheless, women with Ebstein anomaly usually tolerate pregnancy provided they are acyanotic and in sinus rhythm. The incidence of fetal prematurity and wastage is significant, and birth weights are lowest in infants born to cyanotic mothers. Parental Ebstein's anomaly increases the risk of CHD in offspring.

The preferred surgical repair of Ebstein's anomaly is tricuspid valve reconstruction with resection of the arrhythmogenic atrialized right ventricle. A large, mobile anterior tricuspid leaflet lends itself to reconstruction into a relatively competent unicuspid atrioventricular valve, and catheter ablation or surgical interruption eliminates active or potential bypass tracts. The risk of pregnancy to the mother is then appreciably reduced, if not eliminated. Closure of an interatrial communication resolves the risk of paradoxical embolization. Fetal risk of maternal cyanosis is eliminated, but genetic risk of transmission is necessarily unchanged.

Eisenmenger's Syndrome or Primary Pulmonary Hypertension

Pulmonary hypertension is usually defined as a resting mean pulmonary arterial pressure ≥ 25 mm Hg by cardiac catheterization. A pulmonary arterial systolic pressure ≥ 50 mm Hg, or greater than two thirds systemic, poses an increased gestational risk. In Eisenmenger's syndrome, the pulmonary vascular resistance is systemic or suprasystemic, and the shunt is balanced or reversed. Primary pulmonary hypertension typically becomes overt in young women, with a female-to-male ratio approaching 5:1. The hazards of pregnancy are formidable, and the mortality is prohibitively high.[57,76] We have here in its purest form the gestational risks inherent in pulmonary vascular disease. The fixed pulmonary resistance blunts or precludes adaptive responses to the volatile hemodynamic changes during gestation, labor, delivery, and the puerperium. Patients with Eisenmenger syndrome confront the maternal risk of pulmonary vascular disease in addition to the fetal risk of cyanosis. Contraception should be strict, and pregnancy should be terminated.[8,57] Eisenmenger syndrome and primary pulmonary hypertension are accompanied by a 30% to 50% maternal mortality[57,76,77] (discussed earlier). No treatment or intervention reduces that mortality. Oxygen or a pulmonary arterial flotation catheter are of no value. Anticoagulation serves no useful purpose but instead reinforces the coagulation defects inherent in cyanotic CHD with consequences that can be fatal. Oral sildenafil is efficacious in Eisenmenger syndrome and primary pulmonary hypertension but has not been adequately studied during pregnancy.[78] Death most commonly occurs from the end of the third trimester to 2 weeks postpartum. Sudden death is often due to massive intrapulmonary hemorrhage, and occlusive thromboses of proximal pulmonary arteries cause death by asphyxia.

Complex Congenital Heart Disease

Pregnancy after repair of certain forms of complex cyanotic congenital heart disease is now a practical objective. The following comments focus on patients with Fontan physiology, with D-transposition of the great arteries especially after atrial switch procedures, and with congenitally corrected transposition.

Fontan Physiology

The Fontan operation for single ventricle or tricuspid atresia with pulmonary stenosis creates an atrial-dependent or caval-dependent circulation devoid of a subpulmonary ventricle. A relatively large number of these patients reach childbearing age, and selected adults can undergo the procedure with relatively low morbidity and mortality.[79,80] However, late development of arrhythmias, decreasing ventricular function, or the need for reoperation are serious long-term problems.[79-81] In a 2005 report of long-term results of the Fontan operation for double-inlet left ventricle, 49% of the patients (99 of 203) required additional surgical procedures.[82] Other important late occurring events were atrial flutter or fibrillation (57%), protein-losing enteropathy (9%), and thromboembolism (6%).

Health was considered good or excellent in 84%, fair in 18%, and poor in 12%. Actuarial survival was 80% at 10 years and 69% at 20 years.[82] The 10- and 20-year longevity patterns are matters of concern for long-term maternal care of offspring. These patients have a variety of highly complex anatomic and physiologic substrates.[79,83] Advice and management regarding pregnancy must be individualized. Fertility may be impaired in women with Fontan palliation.[84] There is a litany of potential complications in the 2 decades after the procedure.[83] The most frequent complications are disorders of impulse formation or conduction, particularly atrial arrhythmias and sick sinus syndrome. In gravidas who are pacemaker-dependent, an excessive blood level of magnesium sulfate can raise the pacemaker threshold and impede effectiveness with fatal outcomes.

Despite these misgivings, women who have had a Fontan procedure for tricuspid atresia or univentricular hearts of left ventricular morphology are often in a satisfactory functional class, have adequate ventricular function, and tolerate pregnancy well, although there is an increased rate of miscarriage.[84,85] In response to isotonic exercise, at least a twofold increase in cardiac index can be achieved, and the response to increases in cardiac rate achieved by atrial pacing is similar.[81] The implication of these observations is that women who have undergone successful Fontan repairs and who have satisfactory ventricular function and normal sinus rhythm confront the physiologic burden of pregnancy with circulations that possess adequate hemodynamic reserve.[84] However, the functional adequacy of a univentricular heart of *right* ventricular morphology is not as good as the functional adequacy of a morphologic left ventricle.

D-Transposition of the Great Arteries after Atrial Switch

Until the mid-1980s, most patients with complete transposition of the great arteries underwent palliation with a Mustard or Senning intraatrial baffle. Females who underwent an atrial switch operation in infancy are now reaching reproductive age; some who underwent a Rastelli procedure (ventricular septal defect patch that channels left ventricular blood into the aorta together with a right ventricular-to-pulmonary artery valved conduit) and a few who underwent an arterial switch have reached childbearing age as well. Our experience is chiefly with the Mustard repair. Gestational risks are related to the functional status of the subaortic right ventricle, to the level of pulmonary arterial pressure, and to disturbances in conduction and rhythm. At least 50% of patients with Mustard or Senning repairs have an abnormality of impulse formation or conduction 20 years later, and some have required pacemakers. There are now a few well-performed studies of pregnancy in women after atrial switch operations.[86-89] Many have subclinical right ventricular dysfunction and tricuspid regurgitation.[88] The most common cardiac complication following an intraatrial baffle is an arrhythmia, usually atrial fibrillation or flutter or supraventricular tachycardia, and occasionally nonsustained ventricular tachycardia.[86-88] Maternal death is rare, but some gravida experience failure of the subaortic right ventricle that does not recover its pregestational function.

Pregnancy is usually uneventful provided that exercise capacity is normal, right ventricular ejection fraction is ≥40%, the intraatrial baffles are not obstructed, and the tricuspid valve is not significantly incompetent.[88] If suitability for pregnancy is questionable, a stress echocardiogram and cardiopulmonary stress test quantify cardiopulmonary exercise capacity and right ventricular ejection fraction reserve and determine stress-induced arrhythmias. This group of patients reportedly have a higher incidence of miscarriage, premature labor or rupture of membranes, postpartum hemorrhage, intrauterine growth retardation, premature births, and intrauterine death.[86,87]

Congenitally Corrected Transposition of the Great Arteries

The malformation is characterized by double discordance—atrioventricular and ventricular/great arterial. The long-term durability of a morphologic subaortic right ventricle, incompetence of left-sided (inverted) tricuspid valve, and the accrued risk of high-degree heart block are matters of concern. Most women reach childbearing age, operated or not, but overt failure of the subaortic right ventricle may first become manifest during pregnancy, usually in the third trimester or peripartum (Figs. 9–13 through 9–16).

A Mayo Clinic report included 60 pregnancies in 22 women with congenitally corrected transposition, resulting in 50 live births (83%). None of the 50 offspring had

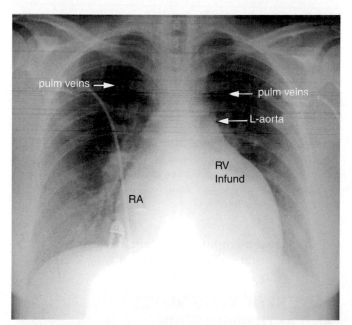

FIGURE 9–13 Chest x-ray from a 32-year-old woman with previously unrecognized congenitally corrected transposition of the great arteries in her second pregnancy. Congestive heart failure had its onset early postpartum. An increased wedge pressure is reflected in the cephalad distribution of pulmonary venous vascularity. The L-transposed aorta originated from the right ventricular (RV) infundibulum. The right atrium (RA) is dilatated. Monitoring electrodes are evident.

CHD.[90] Delivery was vaginal in 88%, with one preterm delivery at 29 weeks.[90] Pregnancy was well tolerated in all but 2 of the 22 women. Nine had some form of prior surgery. One patient with severe tricuspid regurgitation experienced heart failure late in pregnancy and underwent valve replacement in the early postpartum period. Another patient endured 12 pregnancies with multiple pregnancy-related complications (toxemia, heart failure, endocarditis, myocardial infarction with a single coronary artery).

MARFAN SYNDROME

An autosomal-dominant disorder of connective tissue, Marfan syndrome is due to mutation on the fibrillin gene locus of chromosome 15. The characteristic manifestations are ocular, osseous, and cardiovascular.[91,92] Eighty percent of Marfan patients have cardiac involvement.[93] Aortic dilatation usually develops by 5 years of age (35%) and is present in 68% of patients by age 19 years.[94] Beta-blockers are standard medical therapy despite fetal risk,[92] which is highest during the third trimester.[9] A myxomatous mitral valve with prolapse is common. Females with Marfan syndrome reach childbearing age with an inherent medial abnormality—loss of elastic fibers, loss of smooth muscle cells, and an increase in collagen and ground substance—that predisposes to aneurysm, dissection, and progressive aortic regurgitation, risks that are increased by the medial and hemodynamic changes that occur during pregnancy (discussed earlier). There is no aortic root diameter that renders a Marfan patient safe during pregnancy, but risk increases as the root enlarges, especially when the diameter reaches or exceeds 45 to 50 mm.[2,9,29,63,92] Elective aortic root replacement before pregnancy carries a relatively low mortality, whereas the risk of emergency operation for dissection during pregnancy is prohibitive.[95,96] Accordingly, it is prudent to consider elective aortic root surgery and aortic valve repair or replacement when the root size reaches or exceeds 45 to 50 mm or if there is progression of 2 to 5 mm or more within 6 to 12 months, depending on the initial measurement, or when aortic regurgitation is progressive.[5,6,97] The wide pulse pressure of aortic regurgitation accelerates the root abnormality.[98] Women with Marfan syndrome and an aortic root > 40 mm should be cautioned against proceeding with pregnancy. When the aortic root is > 45 mm, we advise preemptive repair before proceeding with a pregnancy; if already pregnant, termination should be strongly considered. If women elect to proceed regardless of advice to the contrary, they should be made aware that their personal risk is compounded by a 50% probability of genetic transmission of the autosomal-dominant disease. Clinical and echocardiographic follow-up each trimester is followed by a planned delivery (vaginal if the aorta is < 40 mm,

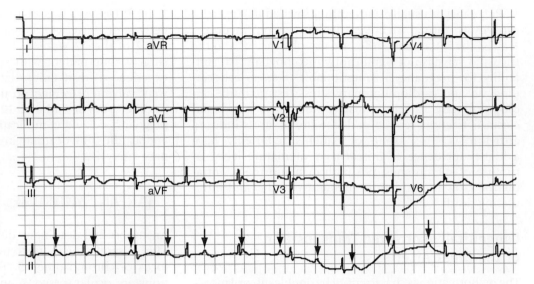

FIGURE 9-14 Electrocardiogram showing complete heart block in the patient with congenitally corrected transposition of the great arteries referred to in Figure 9-13. A pacemaker was subsequently implanted.

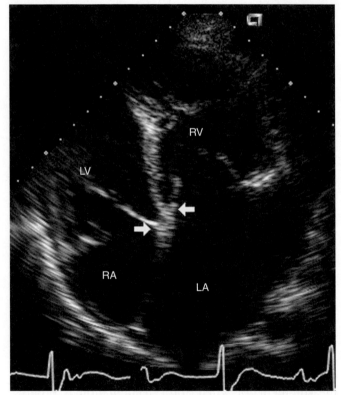

FIGURE 9-15 Transthoracic four-chamber echocardiogram from the patient with congenitally corrected transposition of the great arteries. referred to in Figures 9-13 and 9-14. The crux is inverted. There is a left-sided morphologic right ventricle (RV) and left atrium (LA), and a right-sided morphologic left ventricle (LV) and right atrium (RA). Systolic function of the morphologic subaortic right ventricle was significantly depressed. Color flow imaging disclosed severe regurgitation of the left-sided morphologic tricuspid valve.

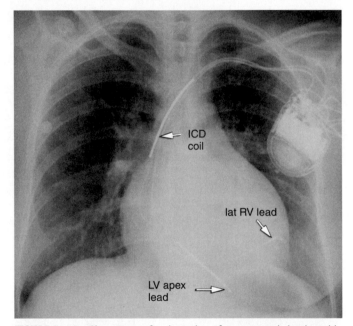

FIGURE 9-16 Chest x-ray after insertion of an automatic implantable defibrillator and biventricular pacemaker in the patient with congenitally corrected transposition of the great arteries referred to in Figures 9-13 to 9-15. Congestive heart failure was refractory. The pacer leads and coil are labeled.

cesarean if the aorta > 44 mm) at 36 to 38 weeks provided there is fetal lung maturity.

In addition to cardiovascular risk, patients with Marfan syndrome have a high rate of obstetrical complications (40%), including miscarriages (20%), preterm delivery (15%), premature rupture of membranes, cervical incompetence, and fetal and neonatal mortality (7.1%).[62]

PROSTHETIC HEART VALVES AND ANTICOAGULATION

Pregnancy is a pro-thrombotic state, and hence a mechanical valve prosthesis poses a significant risk of catastrophic thrombosis, systemic embolism, and death[4,5,9,16,51,99-107] (Figs. 9-17 through 9-20). Anticoagulants can be avoided by valve reconstruction or by

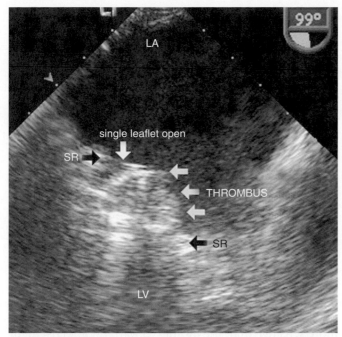

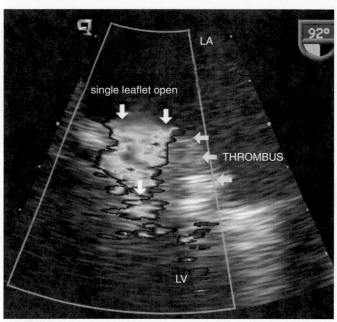

FIGURE 9–17 Mechanical mitral valve prosthetic thrombosis during pregnancy. Thirty-year-old woman with a St. Jude mitral prosthesis admitted at 28 weeks gestation for eclampsia and HELLP (hemolysis, elevated liver enzymes, low platelet count) syndrome. At 32 weeks she underwent a cesarean delivery requiring temporary discontinuation of anticoagulation. Despite restarting her heparin therapy, she developed acute pulmonary edema and hypotension and had an emergency trans-esophageal echocardiogram (shown here). This end-diastolic frame shows the bileaflet valve that has a thrombus completely occuluding one leaflet with reduction of excursion of the other leaflet. LA, left atrium; LV, left ventricle; SR, sewing ring.

FIGURE 9–19 Transesophageal echocardiogram frame with color flow imaging in diastole superimposed on Figures 9–17 and 9–18 showing diastolic inflow through the single restricted leaflet with the large thrombus. LA, left atrium; LV, left ventricle.

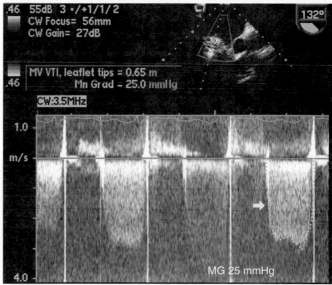

FIGURE 9–20 Continuous-wave Doppler spectral recording of the diastolic mitral inflow gradient (mean 25 mm Hg) in the patient referred to in Figures 9–17 through 9–19. The transducer targeted the transesophageal echocardiogram frame with color flow imaging in diastole through the single opening of the restricted leaflet.

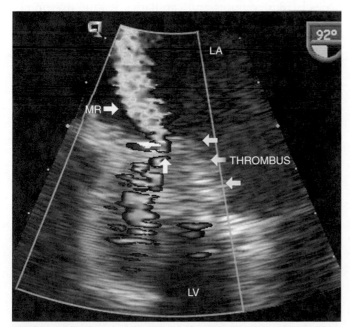

FIGURE 9–18 Transesophageal echocardiogram frame with color flow imaging in systole superimposed on Figure 9–17 showing mitral regurgitation (MR) via the restricted leaflet with the large thrombus. LA, left atrium; LV, left ventricle.

replacement with bioprosthetic heterografts, homografts, or autografts.[5,16,51,108–111] Durability of the bioprosthesis, especially in the right side of the heart, is usually long enough to permit family planning. Evidence suggests that the rate of tissue valve deterioration incurred by pregnancy is only slightly greater than or not significantly different from age-adjusted nonpregnant women.[51,112-114] The Ross procedure is a practical option in selected patients.[4,5,11,16,109,115]

There is a paucity of data on which to base a secure judgment on how best to proceed with anticoagulants in pregnant women with a mechanical valve.[4,5,9,16,51,99,116] No regimen provides equal safety for both mother and fetus. Whatever anticoagulant regimen used, the patient and her spouse should be so advised *before* conception.[2,5,9,11,16,29,33,51,99] Aspirin is questionable as an alternative to oral anticoagulants because of its low efficacy for mechanical prosthetic valves and because of its potential risk for affecting closure of the fetal ductus at higher doses. Maternal thromboembolic mechanical valvular complications tend to be higher when oral anticoagulants are stopped and replaced with heparin.[4,5,9,16,50,51,99,103,104,116,117] Oral anticoagulants protect the mother from potential thromboembolic morbidity and mortality but expose the fetus to the risks of hemorrhage (uteroplacental junction, intracranial), teratogenicity, embryopathy, and developmental delay. It has been proposed that warfarin should be avoided in the first trimester during which organogenesis is completed. However, brain development continues throughout pregnancy, exposing this crucial organ to continued risk. Neurodevelopmental abnormalities were more common in children exposed to maternal coumarins in the second and third trimesters.[118] Women who are on long-term warfarin therapy and who are attempting to conceive should have periodic pregnancy tests. Warfarin is best discontinued *before* conception. An anticoagulant regimen is then carefully planned before pregnancy is achieved. There is no room for a haphazard approach. The pivotal question is how best to proceed. The remainder of this section is devoted to pros and cons for each of three regimens proposed in current guidelines and reviews.[6,8-10,16,51,99,103]

ORAL VITAMIN K ANTAGONISTS

Warfarin, an oral vitamin K antagonist coumarin derivative, is the oral anticoagulant of choice.[117,119] The drug acts through interference with cyclic interconversion of vitamin K and its 2,3 epoxide; vitamin K is a cofactor for carboxylation of glutamine residues to γ-carboxyglutamates (Gla) on vitamin K–dependent proteins including hepatic synthesis of coagulation factors II, VII, IX, and X.[117,119] Warfarin also interferes with epoxide reductase and carboxylation of Gla proteins that play a role in the synthesis of osteocalic and Gla-matrix proteins in formation of bone and cartilage and are possibly involved in central nervous system development, which is relevant because warfarin, with a molecular weight of 1000 daltons, readily crosses the placenta.[120-122] These effects may contribute to first trimester teratogenic bone abnormalities (nasal hypoplasia and chondrodysplasia punctata) and second and third trimester central nervous system abnormalities (optic

atrophy, microcephaly, mental retardation, spasticity, and hypotonia).[117,123,124] The prevalence of warfarin-induced first trimester teratogenicity and embryopathy is unclear, but risk appears to be greatest during gestational weeks 6 to 12 with an incidence of about 4% to 10% that is dose-dependent.[6,9] A dose of ≤ 5 mg per day reportedly reduces the risk of embryopathy and has influenced the selection of an anticoagulation regimen during pregnancy.[9,4,105,106,125]

An extensive review of the literature on anticoagulation in pregnant women with mechanical heart valves reported an incidence of warfarin embryopathy of 6.4% of live births; replacement with heparin between the 6th and 12th week eliminated this risk,[100] but the incidence of valve thrombosis was 9.2%.[100] The regimen with the lowest risk of valve thrombosis (3.9%) was warfarin throughout pregnancy. Embryopathy occurred in 5.5% if the warfarin dosage exceeded 5 mg per day.[106] Immaturity of fetal enzyme systems and relatively low concentration of vitamin K–dependent clotting factors render the fetus more sensitive than the mother to warfarin anticoagulant effects.[99,117] Exposure of the fetus to transplacental warfarin incurs the risk of early abortion and death from intracranial hemorrhage during the trauma of vaginal delivery.[9] This is a particular concern in gravidas with CHD because of unpredictable preterm labor.[16,49,51] Warfarin employed in the second and third trimester should be replaced with heparin around 35 to 36 gestational weeks until culmination of labor and delivery.

Apart from hemorrhagic complications, the most important maternal side effect of warfarin is skin necrosis, a rare but devastating disorder caused by extensive thromboses of skin venules and capillaries within subcutaneous fat, generally between the third and eighth day after administration.[117] After a stable dose of warfarin is established, the complication is unlikely. Etiology is unknown.

Monitoring of warfarin dosage is best achieved with the international normalized ratio (INR) because thromboplastins vary markedly in their responsiveness, depending on tissue of origin and method of preparation.[117,119] Previously employed prothrombin times are unreliable. By converting prothrombin times into an INR, the results are interchangeable. In light of the belief that the risk of warfarin embryopathy is dose related, the anticoagulant should be closely monitored by the INR to achieve a therapeutic response at the lowest possible dose.

For more than 50 years, warfarin has been a mainstay in the treatment of venous and systemic arterial thromboembolism and for prevention of thrombus formation on mechanical prosthetic valves.[99,119] However, the therapeutic window is narrow. There is significant variation in dose response from patient to patient, a changing coagulation cascade during the course of pregnancy, and interactions with drugs and diet. Meticulous laboratory control can be difficult to achieve.[119] Warfarin has nonetheless been advocated throughout pregnancy because of the poor experience with unfractionated heparin for the prevention of thrombus formation on mechanical prosthetic valves.[4,9,99] The following section is devoted to unfractionated heparin versus low-molecular-weight heparin.

HEPARINS

Commonly used commercial preparations of unfractionated heparins (UFH) are mixtures of polysaccharide chains with molecular weights from 5000 to 30,000 daltons, averaging 12,000 to 15,000. Standard UFH with a molecular weight of 12,000 to 15,000 daltons exerts its anticoagulant effect by specific binding to antithrombin III, a naturally occurring inhibitor of coagulation serine proteases such as thrombin and factor XA. UFH binds nonspecifically to plasma proteins in addition to antithrombin III and to proteins of the vascular matrix. There are a number of concerns regarding long-term administration of conventional UFH during pregnancy, especially the relative difficulty in maintaining a stable therapeutic response, the inconvenience of subcutaneous administration, the risk of heparin-induced thrombocytopenia (HIT; estimated occurrence about 1 in 2000 patients), and the risk of osteoporosis, which is believed to be dose related. The thrombocytopenia disappears with discontinuation of heparin. Subcutaneous UFH must be given twice daily and monitored by the activated partial thromboplastin time (aPTT), which is often attenuated during pregnancy because of increased levels of factor VIII and fibrinogen. The midinterval aPTT target now recommended is 2.0× to 2.5× control value for the current low-risk bileaflet aortic valves, and 2.5× to 3.0× control for older aortic valves or mechanical mitral valve prosthesis.[9,51]

Low-molecular-weight heparins (LMWH) are a relatively new class of anticoagulants represented by heparin compounds that possess shorter polysaccharide chains and therefore lower molecular weights (4000 to 6500 daltons), precluding transplacental transfer. The anticoagulant does not affect the fetus and is devoid of teratogenic risk.

LMWH is more cost effective and easier to administer than UFH and causes less *in vitro* clot inhibition while retaining its *in vivo* antithrombotic effect, thus bleeding is less than with UFH. Various forms of LMWH are widely used in Europe, are regarded as safe and effective, and have been approved in North America for treatment of acute coronary syndromes, venous thromboembolism, and deep vein thrombosis. In the United States, the most commonly used derivative is enoxaparin sodium (Lovenox, Aventis Laboratories, Bridgewater, NJ). The various preparations of LMWH are associated with significant reductions in the incidence of thrombocytopenia, osteoporosis, and heparin-induced antiplatelet antibodies.[99,103,107]

Increased bioavailability and longer plasma half-life of LMWH result in a more predictable anticoagulant response to fixed doses administered once or twice daily without the need for frequent laboratory monitoring. Because LMWH is cleared chiefly by the kidneys, the anticoagulant is either contraindicated in renal failure or must be carefully monitored.[99,126,127] Enoxaparin sodium has been approved for intravenous or subcutaneous use in acute coronary syndromes, deep venous thrombosis, and pulmonary embolism.[128] Bioavailability after subcutaneous enoxaparin is 90% of an intravenous dose compared with 15% to 25% bioavailability for an equivalent dose subcutaneous of UFH. However, as pregnancy progresses, coagulation factors change, and most women gain weight, so the volume distribution of LMWH changes.[5,6] To achieve effective anticoagulation, twice-a-day subcutaneous injections and frequent monitoring by anti-Xa activity are strongly advised throughout gestation.[4-6,16,33,99,103,107] There are no adequate trials using LMWH in mechanical valves with or without pregnancy.[5,51,103,107,128] The manufacturer recently commented that "use of Lovenox for thromboprophylaxis in pregnant women with mechanical prosthetic heart valves has not been adequately studied . . . frequent monitoring of peak and trough anti-Xa levels, and adjusting of dosage may be needed."[128]

The duration of LMWH anticoagulant effect is approximately 12 hours. There is no reliable method for reversing the effect,[126,127] and thus LMWH must be discontinued the day before a planned, induced delivery; switched to intravenous UFH; or discontinued 2 weeks before expected spontaneous vaginal delivery. Subcutaneous UFH is then administered until hospital admission, followed by intravenous UFH, which is stopped about 4 to 8 hours before expected delivery. The patient should receive no LMWH heparin within 12 hours or UFH within 4 hours of epidural or spinal analgesia. Risk of bleeding is increased by spinal or epidural indwelling catheters, traumatic or repeated punctures, and drugs that affect hemostasis.[128]

Despite these considerations, UFH has three major advantages over LMWH:[126] (1) the anticoagulant effect can be rapidly and completely neutralized by protamine, (2) UFH is not cleared by the kidneys and is therefore safer in patients with impaired renal function, and (3) UFH is effective in modulating contact activation of the coagulation cascade, which is a potential cause of thrombosis on foreign objects such as catheter tips, stents, and prosthetic valves.[126]

UFH and LMWH are both considered free of risk for the fetus.[5,6,99,127] The Lovenox prescribing information states that "It is not known whether this drug is secreted in human milk. Because many drugs are excreted in human milk, caution should be exercised when Lovenox is administered to nursing women."[128] However, it is generally assumed that LMWH is safe in nursing mothers.[127]

Allergic skin reactions occur rarely with either UFH or LMWH.[5]

RECOMMENDATIONS FOR ANTICOAGULATION OF MECHANICAL HEART VALVES DURING PREGNANCY

The American College of Cardiology/American Heart Association 2006 Guidelines for Valvular Heart Disease state that "all pregnant patients with mechanical prosthetic valves must receive continuous therapeutic anticoagulation with frequent monitoring (Class I-B)."[5,6] Coumadin is considered contraindicated,[11,16,51,99] but neither UFH nor LMWH has been approved by the Federal Drug Administration for use during pregnancy or with mechanical prosthetic valves. Whichever anticoagulant regimen is chosen, dosage must be strictly monitored to maintain the therapeutic response.[5,6,16,51,99] Three regimens have been proposed:[4-6,16,51,99,100,107,117] (1) LMWH (enoxaparin sodium 1 mg/kg) subcutaneously every 12 hours with doses adjusted to achieve an anti-Xa level of about 1.0 IU/ml (optimal range 1.0–1.2 IU/ml) at 4 hours postinjection (this is our preferred regimen); (2) subcutaneous UFH every 12 hours throughout pregnancy with aggressive dose adjustment to achieve a midlevel aPTT ≥2× control levels, or anti-Xa heparin level 0.35–0.70 IU/ml); (3) UFH or LMWH as just described until the 13th week of pregnancy, when warfarin is restarted with a target INR of approximately 3.0 (2.5–3.0 INR for newer bileaflet aortic valves, 3.0–3.5 INR for older aortic valves and all mechanical mitral valves) until mid–third trimester, when UFH or LMWH are reinstituted until shortly before delivery.

For dose adjustment of UFH or LMWH, laboratory tests are initially performed once or twice a week; when a stable response is established, the doses are monitored at intervals of 1 or 2 weeks. An alternative to subcutaneous UFH in regimens 1 and 3 (previous paragraph) is to start with continuous intravenous UFH while warfarin is discontinued, a choice seldom preferred by patients.[16,51,99] If intravenous UFH is selected, the fetal risk is lower, but the maternal risk of prosthetic valve thrombosis, embolization, infection, osteoporosis, and HIT are higher.[5,6] Each of the three regimens requires a switch to intravenous UFH near term. Oral anticoagulation is restarted early postpartum.

Mothers are typically more concerned with a poor fetal outcome than potential harm to themselves. The change from warfarin to heparin is best achieved during a brief hospitalization to establish the therapeutic heparin dose and to provide instructions on subcutaneous self-administration. Sodium heparin has a longer half-life during pregnancy than calcium heparin. The initial dose of sodium heparin is 10,000 units every 12 hours, adjusted to achieve an activated PTT of 2 to 2.5 times the mean of the control determined at the 6th-hour trough. The patient is instructed on the technique of subcutaneous self-administration using a five-eighth-inch, 25- to 26-gauge needle to minimize bruising. An abdominal rather than thigh injection site should be used, and the site should be rotated over the entire abdominal wall. A cleansed skinfold is raised between thumb and index finger, and the injection is made at right angles to the raised skinfold. The needle should be removed slowly. Massaging risks bruising and should be avoided. The majority of patients are readily taught self-administration of heparin, but alternatively, the spouse can be so instructed. After discharge, the PTT is determined at 1- to 2-week intervals throughout the first trimester. The patient must then decide whether she wishes to continue the subcutaneous anticoagulant or switch to warfarin during the second and third trimesters. If heparin is continued, the PTT should be determined at weekly intervals to accommodate the relative hypercoagulability during late pregnancy. Hospitalization is planned for the 36th to 38th week in anticipation of labor. An intravenous infusion of heparin is then initiated and regulated to achieve a PTT of 2 to 2.5× control. The infusion is stopped 4 to 6 hours before epidural placement or vaginal delivery. In practice, intravenous heparin is discontinued when the patient is in the active phases of labor or when cervical dilatation is approximately 4 cm.

Patients who are anticoagulated with UFH until just before the onset of labor generally experience vaginal delivery with no greater blood loss than unanticoagulated gravidas, but cesarean delivery in heparinized patients is accompanied by a significantly greater blood loss than otherwise anticipated. The UFH infusion should be stopped 4 to 6 hours before anticipated delivery, especially before a cesarean. If preterm labor develops in a patient receiving heparin, only the mother is anticoagulated, and protamine sulfate can be used to reverse maternal heparinization. If preterm labor develops in a gravida on warfarin, both mother and fetus are anticoagulated. Vitamin K administration does not achieve immediate reversal of maternal anticoagulation, which may persist for 24 hours. Rapid maternal reversal requires infusion of fresh frozen plasma. Fetal anticoagulation cannot be reversed. A cesarean delivery circumvents hemorrhagic fetal injury or death during vaginal delivery. Fresh frozen plasma should be administered to the salvaged neonate. Maternal subcutaneous heparin is resumed no later than 6 hours after delivery in anticipation of early return to warfarin, which is considered safe for nursing mothers because only an inactive metabolite finds its way into breast milk.

The consequences of mechanical valve thrombosis range from mild interference of function without hemodynamic instability, to life-threatening obstruction or regurgitation.[4,16,51,101] If clinical conditions permit, a transesophageal echocardiogram by an experienced operator is most useful in assessing the anatomic and hemodynamic extent of valve thrombosis. Under less urgent circumstances, a transthoracic echocardiogram or fluoroscopy may be helpful. There is no room for delay in the assessment, however. A mildly malfunctioning valve can quickly become much worse. The objective is prevention of further thrombus formation and valve malfunction and dissolution of the existing thrombus with intravenous UFH. In the event of significant valve malfunction and hemodynamic instability, a choice must be made between intravenous thrombolytic agents or emergency cardiac surgery.

BENEFITS AND RISKS OF CONTRACEPTION

An important aspect of CHD and pregnancy is contraception. Safe hormonal contraception can usually be provided for the growing number of women with CHD who reach reproductive age.[31,129] If thromboembolic risk makes these agents inadvisable, barrier methods, intrauterine devices, or even sterilization are selectively applicable.[129]

Barrier Methods

The condom and diaphragm with spermicide are well-established methods with few cardiac contraindications. The main disadvantages are user-dependency and a significant failure rate even in reliable hands.

An intrauterine device (IUD) is a useful option in acyanotic or mildly cyanotic women. In a monogamous relationship, an IUD probably does not increase the risk of infection, but endometrial irritation is a potential cause of bleeding. During insertion and removal, antibiotic prophylaxis should be considered (see Chapter 8), although after successful stable insertion, the risk of bacteremia is virtually nonexistent. If excessive bleeding occurs during menses, the device should be removed. An IUD is not recommended in cyanotic women with hematocrit levels above 55% because intrinsic hemostatic defects increase the risk of excessive menstrual bleeding (see Chapter 12).

The Mirena® intrauterine system (Bayer HealthCare Pharmaceuticals, Wayne, NJ) uses an IUD impregnated with levonorgestrel. Replacement is required every 5 years. The contraceptive efficacy is as good or better than sterilization.[31] Advantages include oligomenorrhea, in contrast to response to copper coils. A vasovagal response occurs in up to 5% of women at the time of insertion and instrumentation of the cervix.[31] This complication is readily coped with in healthy women, but with a Fontan circulation or with pulmonary hypertension, cardiovascular collapse can be serious if not fatal.[31] The vasovagal response can be mitigated by a paracervical block or by combined spinal and epidural block. A subdermal implant may be preferable in these patients.

Tubal ligation is usually accomplished safely, even in relatively high-risk women. Laparoscopic sterilization includes carbon dioxide insufflation of the abdomen and intermittent head-down position, plus positive pressure ventilation to reduce cardiac output. Despite these precautions, women with a Fontan circulation or pulmonary hypertension tend to tolerate the procedure poorly. Air embolism is a risk in women with right-left shunts. A mini-laparotomy with spinal and epidural anesthesia is safe in skilled hands.[31] An effective new stent-based sterilization product, Essure® (Conceptus Incorporated, Mountain View, CA), is inserted hysteroscopically into the fallopian tubes under sedation and local anesthesia.

Vasectomy for the male is an analogous but less desirable option in light of the divorce rate, or if the husband outlives the wife with heart disease and wishes to remarry and procreate.[31]

Progestin-Only Hormonal Methods

Progestin agents in standard contraceptive doses have few cardiac complications with no thrombogenicity.[31] The various methods and formulations vary in contraceptive efficacy. The main side effect that may prove unacceptable is menstrual irregularity.[31]

Norplant has been taken off the market. The new subdermal implantable system, Implanon® by Organon (Organon USA, Schering-Plough, Kenilworth, NJ), is a 3-year, single-rod implantable contraceptive. Etonogesterol is a third-generation progestin that is slowly released by the rod. Antibiotic prophylaxis is not required if removal is meticulous.

Combined Hormonal Contraceptives

These agents contain both estrogen and progestin, have high contraceptive efficacy,[31] and come as skin patches, oral agents, vaginal rings (NuvaRing®, Organon USA, Schering-Plough, Kenilworth, NJ), and injectable suspensions.[31,129] A potential advantage of the NuvaRing and Implanton is a lower plasma level of hormone(s) compared with oral contraceptives, hence a lower risk. Concerns include thrombogenicity and interactions with warfarin and are best avoided in women with prior thrombotic events or mechanical prosthetic valves that require anticoagulation. Also at risk are women who smoke; who have migraine headache, diabetes, or hypertension; or who are obese. A right-to-left shunt is a concern because of the potential for paradoxical embolization.[31]

Ethinyl estradiol (Loestrin®, Parke-Davis Pharmaceuticals, Morris Plains, NJ) is the lowest estrogen-containing oral contraceptive (20 µg of ethinyl estradiol). The annual failure rate is about 1.5% to 2%. A missed dose is accompanied by a higher failure rate than when higher estrogen forms of contraception are employed. Loestrin is considered safe with a low thrombogenic potential and a low failure rate provided no dose is missed.

GYNECOLOGIC ENDOCRINOLOGY

Gynecologic endocrinology in women with CHD has emerged a focus of attention. Whether ovarian function varies with the type of heart defect or with the absence or presence of cyanosis, and how reparative surgery affects ovarian function remain largely unknown. In cyanotic females, there is delay in establishing menstruation and an increased incidence of abnormally short or long cycle lengths. Dysfunctional bleeding is common, implying an anovulatory nonfertile state with unopposed estrogen production and continuous endometrial stimulation that risks endometrial adenocarcinoma. Important but unknown is the age at which reparative cardiac surgery is followed by normal ovarian function, especially in cyanotic females.

References

1. Thilen U, Olsson SB. Pregnancy and heart disease: a review. *Eur J Obstet Gynecol Reprod Biol.* 1997;75:43–50.
2. Thorne SA. Pregnancy in heart disease. *Heart.* 2004;90:450–456.
3. Steer PJ, Gatzoulis MA, Baker P, eds. *Heart Disease and Pregnancy.* London: RCOG Press; 2006.
4. Vahanian A, Baumgartner H, Bax J, et al. Guidelines on the management of valvular heart disease: The Task Force on the Management of Valvular Heart Disease of the European Society of Cardiology. *Eur Heart J.* 2007;28:230–268.
5. Bonow RO, Carabello BA, Chatterjee K, et al. ACC/AHA 2006 guidelines for the management of patients with valvular heart disease: a report of the American College of Cardiology/American Heart Association Task Force on Practice Guidelines (writing committee to revise the 1998 guidelines for the management of patients with valvular heart disease) developed in collaboration with the Society of Cardiovascular Anesthesiologists endorsed by the Society for Cardiovascular Angiography and Interventions and the Society of Thoracic Surgeons. *J Am Coll Cardiol.* 2006;48:e1–e148.
6. Bonow RO, Carabello BA, Kanu C, et al. ACC/AHA 2006 guidelines for the management of patients with valvular heart disease: a report of the American College of Cardiology/American Heart Association Task Force on Practice Guidelines (writing committee to revise the 1998 Guidelines for the Management of Patients with Valvular Heart Disease): developed in collaboration with the Society of Cardiovascular Anesthesiologists: endorsed by the Society for Cardiovascular Angiography and Interventions and the Society of Thoracic Surgeons. *Circulation.* 2006;114:e84–e231.
7. Perloff JK, Child JS, eds. *Congenital Heart Disease in Adults.* 2nd ed. Philadelphia: W.B. Saunders; 1998.
8. Warnes CA. Pregnancy and contraception. In: Gatzoulis MA, Webb GD, Daubeney PEF, eds. *Diagnosis and Management of Adult Congenital Heart Disease.* Edinburgh: Churchill Livingstone; 2003:135–144.
9. Expert consensus document on management of cardiovascular diseases during pregnancy. *Eur Heart J.* 2003;24:761–781.
10. Koos BJ. Management of uncorrected, palliated, and repaired cyanotic congenital heart disease in pregnancy. *Prog Pediatr Cardiol.* 2004;19:25–45.
11. Perloff JK, Koos B. Pregnancy and congenital heart disease: the mother and the fetus. In: Perloff JK, Child JS, eds. *Congenital Heart Disease in Adults.* 2nd ed. Philadelphia: W.B. Saunders; 1998:144–164.
12. Warnes CA, Liberthson R, Danielson GK, et al. Task force 1: the changing profile of congenital heart disease in adult life. *J Am Coll Cardiol.* 2001;37:1170–1175.
13. Williams RG, Pearson GD, Barst RJ, et al. Report of the National Heart, Lung, and Blood Institute Working Group on research in adult congenital heart disease. *J Am Coll Cardiol.* 2006;47:701–707.
14. Warnes CA. The adult with congenital heart disease: born to be bad? *J Am Coll Cardiol.* 2005;46:1–8.
15. van Oppen AC, Stigter RH, Bruinse HW. Cardiac output in normal pregnancy: a critical review. *Obstet Gynecol.* 1996;87:310–318.
16. Elkayam U. Pregnancy and cardiovascular disease. In: Zipes DP, Libby P, Bonow RO, Braunwald E, eds. *Braunwald's Heart Disease: A Textbook of Cardiovascular Medicine.* 7th ed. Philadelphia: Elsevier Saunders; 2005:1965–1984.
17. Geva T, Mauer MB, Striker L, et al. Effects of physiologic load of pregnancy on left ventricular contractility and remodeling. *Am Heart J.* 1997;133:53–59.
18. Kametas NA, McAuliffe F, Krampl E, et al. Maternal cardiac function in twin pregnancy. *Obstet Gynecol.* 2003;102:806–815.
19. Manalo-Estrella P, Barker AE. Histopathologic findings in human aortic media associated with pregnancy. *Arch Pathol.* 1967;83:336–341.
20. Cavanzo FJ, Taylor HB. Effect of pregnancy on the human aorta and its relationship to dissecting aneurysms. *Am J Obstet Gynecol.* 1969;105:567–568.
21. Immer FF, Bansi AG, Immer-Bansi AS, et al. Aortic dissection in pregnancy: analysis of risk factors and outcome. *Ann Thorac Surg.* 2003;76:309–314.
22. Bryant-Greenwood GD, Schwabe C. Human relaxins: chemistry and biology. *Endocr Rev.* 1994;15:5–26.
23. McColl MD, Ramsay JE, Tait RC, et al. Risk factors for pregnancy associated venous thromboembolism. *Thromb Haemost.* 1997;78:1183–1188.
24. Grandone E, Margaglione M, Colaizzo D, et al. Genetic susceptibility to pregnancy-related venous thromboembolism: roles of factor V Leiden, prothrombin G20210A, and methylenetetrahydrofolate reductase C677T mutations. *Am J Obstet Gynecol.* 1998;179:1324–1328.
25. Gerhardt A, Scharf RE, Beckmann MW, et al. Prothrombin and factor V mutations in women with a history of thrombosis during pregnancy and the puerperium. *N Engl J Med.* 2000;342:374–380.
26. Lockwood CJ. Heritable coagulopathies in pregnancy. *Obstet Gynecol Surv.* 1999;54:754–765.
27. Walker MC, Garner PR, Keely EJ, et al. Changes in activated protein C resistance during normal pregnancy. *Am J Obstet Gynecol.* 1997;177:162–169.
28. Gelson E, Johnson M, Gatzoulis M, Uebing A. Cardiac disease in pregnancy. Part 1: congenital heart disease. *Obstetr Gynaecol.* 2007;9:15–20.
29. Head CE, Thorne SA. Congenital heart disease in pregnancy. *Postgrad Med J.* 2005;81:292–298.
30. Siu SC, Colman JM. Heart disease and pregnancy. *Heart.* 2001;85:710–715.
31. Thorne S, MacGregor A, Nelson-Piercy C. Risks of contraception and pregnancy in heart disease. *Heart.* 2006;92:1520–1525.
32. Wilson W, Taubert KA, Gewitz M, et al. Prevention of infective endocarditis. Guidelines from the American Heart Association. A Guideline from the American Heart Association Rheumatic Fever, Endocarditis, and Kawasaki Disease Committee, Council on Cardiovascular Disease in the Young, and the Council on Clinical Cardiology, Council on Cardiovascular Surgery and Anesthesia, and the Quality of Care and Outcomes Research Interdisciplinary Working Group. *Circulation.* 2007;116:1736–1754.
33. Elkayam U, Bitar F. Valvular heart disease and pregnancy part I: native valves. *J Am Coll Cardiol.* 2005;46:223–230.
34. Hoffman JI, Kaplan S, Liberthson RR. Prevalence of congenital heart disease. *Am Heart J.* 2004;147:425–439.
35. Hoffman JI, Kaplan S. The incidence of congenital heart disease. *J Am Coll Cardiol.* 2002;39:1890–1900.

36. Burn J, Brennan P, Little J, et al. Recurrence risks in offspring of adults with major heart defects: results from first cohort of British collaborative study. *Lancet.* 1998;351:311–316.

37. Calcagni G, Digilio MC, Sarkozy A, et al. Familial recurrence of congenital heart disease: an overview and review of the literature. *Eur J Pediatr.* 2007;166:111–116.

38. Pierpont ME, Basson CT, Benson DW Jr., et al. Genetic basis for congenital heart defects: current knowledge: a scientific statement from the American Heart Association Congenital Cardiac Defects Committee, Council on Cardiovascular Disease in the Young: endorsed by the American Academy of Pediatrics. *Circulation.* 2007;115:3015–3038.

39. Meijer JM, Pieper PG, Drenthen W, et al. Pregnancy, fertility, and recurrence risk in corrected tetralogy of Fallot. *Heart.* 2005;91:801–805.

40. Beauchesne LM, Warnes CA, Connolly HM, et al. Prevalence and clinical manifestations of 22q11. 2 microdeletion in adults with selected conotruncal anomalies. *J Am Coll Cardiol.* 2005;45:595–598.

41. Park IS, Ko JK, Kim YH, et al. Cardiovascular anomalies in patients with chromosome 22q11. 2 deletion: a Korean multicenter study. *Int J Cardiol.* 2007;114:230–235.

42. Cohen E, Chow EW, Weksberg R, Bassett AS. Phenotype of adults with the 22q11 deletion syndrome: a review. *Am J Med Genet.* 1999;86:359–365.

43. Driscoll DA. Prenatal diagnosis of the 22q11.2 deletion syndrome. *Genet Med.* 2001;3:14–18.

44. McDonald-McGinn DM, Tonnesen MK, Laufer-Cahana A, et al. Phenotype of the 22q11.2 deletion in individuals identified through an affected relative: cast a wide FISHing net! *Genet Med.* 2001;3:23–29.

45. Siu SC, Sermer M, Colman JM, et al. Prospective multicenter study of pregnancy outcomes in women with heart disease. *Circulation.* 2001;104:515–521.

46. Siu SC, Sermer M, Harrison DA, et al. Risk and predictors for pregnancy-related complications in women with heart disease. *Circulation.* 1997;96:2789–2794.

47. Khairy P, Ouyang DW, Fernandes SM, et al. Pregnancy outcomes in women with congenital heart disease. *Circulation.* 2006;113:517–524.

48. Siu SC, Colman JM, Sorensen S, et al. Adverse neonatal and cardiac outcomes are more common in pregnant women with cardiac disease. *Circulation.* 2002;105:2179–2184.

49. Drenthen W, Pieper PG, Roos-Hesselink JW, et al. Outcome of pregnancy in women with congenital heart disease: a literature review. *J Am Coll Cardiol.* 2007;49:2303–2311.

50. Elkayam U, Akhter MW, Singh H, et al. Pregnancy-associated cardiomyopathy: clinical characteristics and a comparison between early and late presentation. *Circulation.* 2005;111:2050–2055.

51. Elkayam U, Bitar F. Valvular heart disease and pregnancy: part II: prosthetic valves. *J Am Coll Cardiol.* 2005;46:403–410.

52. Elkayam U, Tummala PP, Rao K, et al. Maternal and fetal outcomes of subsequent pregnancies in women with peripartum cardiomyopathy. *N Engl J Med.* 2001;344:1567–1571.

53. Hameed A, Karaalp IS, Tummala PP, et al. The effect of valvular heart disease on maternal and fetal outcome of pregnancy. *J Am Coll Cardiol.* 2001;37:893–899.

54. Reimold SC, Rutherford JD. Clinical practice. Valvular heart disease in pregnancy. *N Engl J Med.* 2003;349:52–59.

55. Silversides CK, Colman JM, Sermer M, Siu SC. Cardiac risk in pregnant women with rheumatic mitral stenosis. *Am J Cardiol.* 2003;91:1382–1385.

56. Stout KK, Otto CM. Pregnancy in women with valvular heart disease. *Heart.* 2007;93:552–558.

57. Warnes CA. Pregnancy and pulmonary hypertension. *Int J Cardiol.* 2004;97(1 Suppl):11–13.

58. Shime J, Mocarski EJ, Hastings D, et al. Congenital heart disease in pregnancy: short- and long-term implications. *Am J Obstet Gynecol.* 1987;156:313–322.

59. Zuber M, Gautschi N, Oechslin E, et al. Outcome of pregnancy in women with congenital shunt lesions. *Heart.* 1999;81:271–275.

60. Chugh R. Management of pregnancy in patients with congenital heart disease and systemic ventricular failure. *Prog Pediatr Cardiol.* 2004;19:47–60.

61. Mendelson MA. Pregnancy in patients with obstructive lesions: aortic stenosis, coarctation of the aorta and mitral stenosis. *Prog Pediatr Cardiol.* 2004;19:61–70.

62. Meijboom LJ, Drenthen W, Pieper PG, et al. Obstetric complications in Marfan syndrome. *Int J Cardiol.* 2006;110:53–59.

63. Meijboom LJ, Vos FE, Timmermans J, et al. Pregnancy and aortic root growth in the Marfan syndrome: a prospective study. *Eur Heart J.* 2005;26:914–920.

64. Cooper WO, Hernandez-Diaz S, Arbogast PG, et al. Major congenital malformations after first-trimester exposure to ACE inhibitors. *N Engl J Med.* 2006;354:2443–2451.

65. Friedman JM. ACE inhibitors and congenital anomalies. *N Engl J Med.* 2006;354:2498–2500.

66. Weiss BM, von Segesser LK, Alon E, et al. Outcome of cardiovascular surgery and pregnancy: a systematic review of the period 1984–1996. *Am J Obstet Gynecol.* 1998;179:1643–1653.

67. Drenthen W, Pieper PG, Roos-Hesselink JW, et al. Non-cardiac complications during pregnancy in women with isolated congenital pulmonary valvar stenosis. *Heart.* 2006;92:1838–1843.

68. Vriend JW, Drenthen W, Pieper PG, et al. Outcome of pregnancy in patients after repair of aortic coarctation. *Eur Heart J.* 2005;26:2173–2178.

69. Beauchesne LM, Connolly HM, Ammash NM, Warnes CA. Coarctation of the aorta: outcome of pregnancy. *J Am Coll Cardiol.* 2001;38:1728–1733.

70. Plunkett MD, Bond LM, Geiss DM. Staged repair of acute type I aortic dissection and coarctation in pregnancy. *Ann Thorac Surg.* 2000;69:1945–1947.

71. Silversides CK, Colman JM, Sermer M, et al. Early and intermediate-term outcomes of pregnancy with congenital aortic stenosis. *Am J Cardiol.* 2003;91:1386–1389.

72. Child JS. Fallot's tetralogy and pregnancy: prognostication and prophesy. *J Am Coll Cardiol.* 2004;44:181–183.

73. Veldtman GR, Connolly HM, Grogan M, et al. Outcomes of pregnancy in women with tetralogy of Fallot. *J Am Coll Cardiol.* 2004;44:174–180.

74. Neumayer U, Somerville J. Outcome of pregnancies in patients with complex pulmonary atresia. *Heart.* 1997;78:16–21.

75. Jayaprasad N, Johnson F, Venugopal K. Congenital complete heart block and maternal connective tissue disease. *Int J Cardiol.* 2006;112:153–158.

76. Weiss BM, Hess OM. Pulmonary vascular disease and pregnancy: current controversies, management strategies, and perspectives. *Eur Heart J.* 2000;21:104–115.

77. Yentis SM, Steer PJ, Plaat F. Eisenmenger's syndrome in pregnancy: maternal and fetal mortality in the 1990s. *Br J Obstet Gynaecol.* 1998;105:921–922.

78. Chau EM, Fan KY, Chow WH. Effects of chronic sildenafil in patients with Eisenmenger syndrome versus idiopathic pulmonary arterial hypertension. *Int J Cardiol.* 2007;120:301–305.

79. Aboulhosn J, Child JS. The adult with a Fontan operation. *Curr Cardiol Rep.* 2007;9:331–335.

80. Gates RN, Laks H, Drinkwater DC Jr., et al. The Fontan procedure in adults. *Ann Thorac Surg.* 1997;63:1085–1090.

81. Barber G, Di Sessa T, Child JS, et al. Hemodynamic responses to isolated increments in heart rate by atrial pacing after a Fontan procedure. *Am Heart J.* 1988;115:837–841.

82. Earing MG, Cetta F, Driscoll DJ, et al. Long-term results of the Fontan operation for double-inlet left ventricle. *Am J Cardiol.* 2005;96: 291–298.

83. Walker F. Pregnancy and the various forms of the Fontan circulation. *Heart.* 2007;93:152–154.

84. Drenthen W, Pieper PG, Roos-Hesselink JW, et al. Pregnancy and delivery in women after Fontan palliation. *Heart.* 2006;92:1290–1294.

85. Canobbio MM, Mair DD, van der Velde M, Koos BJ. Pregnancy outcomes after the Fontan repair. *J Am Coll Cardiol.* 1996;28: 763–767.

86. Canobbio MM, Morris CD, Graham TP, Landzberg MJ. Pregnancy outcomes after atrial repair for transposition of the great arteries. *Am J Cardiol.* 2006;98:668–672.

87. Drenthen W, Pieper PG, Ploeg M, et al. Risk of complications during pregnancy after Senning or Mustard (atrial) repair of complete transposition of the great arteries. *Eur Heart J.* 2005;26: 2588–2595.

88. Guedes A, Mercier LA, Leduc L, et al. Impact of pregnancy on the systemic right ventricle after a Mustard operation for transposition of the great arteries. *J Am Coll Cardiol.* 2004;44:433–437.

89. Genoni M, Jenni R, Hoerstrup SP, et al. Pregnancy after atrial repair for transposition of the great arteries. *Heart.* 1999;81:276–277.

90. Connolly HM, Grogan M, Warnes CA. Pregnancy among women with congenitally corrected transposition of great arteries. *J Am Coll Cardiol.* 1999;33:1692–1695.

91. Dietz HC, Pyeritz RE. Mutations in the human gene for fibrillin-1 (FBN1) in the Marfan syndrome and related disorders. *Hum Mol Genet.* 1995;(4 Spec No):1799–1809.

92. Dean JC. Management of Marfan syndrome. *Heart.* 2002;88: 97–103.

93. Child AH. Marfan syndrome—current medical and genetic knowledge: how to treat and when. *J Card Surg.* 1997;12(2 Suppl): 131–135; discussion 135–136.

94. Aburawi EH, O'Sullivan J. Relation of aortic root dilatation and age in Marfan's syndrome. *Eur Heart J.* 2007;28:376–379.

95. Gott VL, Greene PS, Alejo DE, et al. Replacement of the aortic root in patients with Marfan's syndrome. *N Engl J Med.* 1999;340: 1307–1313.

96. Treasure T. Cardiovascular surgery for Marfan syndrome. *Heart.* 2000;84:674–678.

97. Groenink M, Lohuis TA, Tijssen JG, et al. Survival and complication free survival in Marfan's syndrome: implications of current guidelines. *Heart.* 1999;82:499–504.

98. Lazarevic AM, Nakatani S, Okita Y, et al. Determinants of rapid progression of aortic root dilatation and complications in Marfan syndrome. *Int J Cardiol.* 2006;106:177–182.

99. Bates SM, Greer IA, Hirsh J, Ginsberg JS. Use of antithrombotic agents during pregnancy: the Seventh ACCP Conference on Antithrombotic and Thrombolytic Therapy. *Chest.* 2004;126(3 Suppl): 627S–644S.

100. Chan WS, Anand S, Ginsberg JS. Anticoagulation of pregnant women with mechanical heart valves: a systematic review of the literature. *Arch Intern Med.* 2000;160:191–196.

101. Choi C, Midwall S, Chaille P, Conti CR. Treatment of mechanical valve thrombosis during pregnancy. *Clin Cardiol.* 2007;30:271–276.

102. De Santo LS, Romano G, Della Corte A, et al. Mitral mechanical replacement in young rheumatic women: analysis of long-term survival, valve-related complications, and pregnancy outcomes over a 3707-patient-year follow-up. *J Thorac Cardiovasc Surg.* 2005; 130:13–19.

103. Ginsberg JS, Chan WS, Bates SM, Kaatz S. Anticoagulation of pregnant women with mechanical heart valves. *Arch Intern Med.* 2003;163:694–698.

104. Ginsberg JS, Hirsh J, Turner DC, et al. Risks to the fetus of anticoagulant therapy during pregnancy. *Thromb Haemost.* 1989;61:197–203.

105. Vitale N, De Feo M, De Santo LS, et al. Dose-dependent fetal complications of warfarin in pregnant women with mechanical heart valves. *J Am Coll Cardiol.* 1999;33:1637–1641.

106. Cotrufo M, De Feo M, De Santo LS, et al. Risk of warfarin during pregnancy with mechanical valve prostheses. *Obstet Gynecol.* 2002;99:35–40.

107. Seshadri N, Goldhaber SZ, Elkayam U, et al. The clinical challenge of bridging anticoagulation with low-molecular-weight heparin in patients with mechanical prosthetic heart valves: an evidence-based

108. comparative review focusing on anticoagulation options in pregnant and nonpregnant patients. *Am Heart J.* 2005;150:27–34.

108. Borger MA, Ivanov J, Armstrong S, et al. Twenty-year results of the Hancock II bioprosthesis. *J Heart Valve Dis.* 2006;15:49–55; discussion 55–46.

109. Dore A, Somerville J. Pregnancy in patients with pulmonary autograft valve replacement. *Eur Heart J.* 1997;18:1659–1662.

110. Smedira NG, Blackstone EH, Roselli EE, et al. Are allografts the biologic valve of choice for aortic valve replacement in nonelderly patients? Comparison of explanation for structural valve deterioration of allograft and pericardial prostheses. *J Thorac Cardiovasc Surg.* 2006;131:558–564.e4.

111. Luciani GB, Favaro A, Casali G, et al. Reoperations for aortic aneurysm after the Ross procedure. *J Heart Valve Dis.* 2005;14:766–772; discussion 772–773.

112. Avila WS, Rossi EG, Grinberg M, Ramires JA. Influence of pregnancy after bioprosthetic valve replacement in young women: a prospective five-year study. *J Heart Valve Dis.* 2002;11:864–869.

113. Jamieson WR, Miller DC, Akins CW, et al. Pregnancy and bioprostheses: influence on structural valve deterioration. *Ann Thorac Surg.* 1995;60(2 Suppl):S282–286; discussion S287.

114. Salazar E, Espinola N, Roman L, Casanova JM. Effect of pregnancy on the duration of bovine pericardial bioprostheses. *Am Heart J.* 1999;137:714–720.

115. Al-Halees Z, Pieters F, Qadoura F, et al. The Ross procedure is the procedure of choice for congenital aortic valve disease. *J Thorac Cardiovasc Surg.* 2002;123:437–441; discussion 441–432.

116. Salazar E, Izaguirre R, Verdejo J, Mutchinick O. Failure of adjusted doses of subcutaneous heparin to prevent thromboembolic phenomena in pregnant patients with mechanical cardiac valve prostheses. *J Am Coll Cardiol.* 1996;27:1698–1703.

117. Hirsh J, Fuster V, Ansell J, Halperin JL. American Heart Association/ American College of Cardiology Foundation guide to warfarin therapy. *J Am Coll Cardiol.* 2003;41:1633–1652.

118. Wesseling J, Van Driel D, Heymans HS, et al. Coumarins during pregnancy: long-term effects on growth and development of school-age children. *Thromb Haemost.* 2001;85:609–613.

119. Ansell J, Hirsh J, Poller L, Bussey H, et al. The pharmacology and management of the vitamin K antagonists: the Seventh ACCP Conference on Antithrombotic and Thrombolytic Therapy. *Chest.* 2004;126(3 Suppl):204S–233S.

120. Hauschka PV, Lian JB, Cole DE, Gundberg CM. Osteocalcin and matrix Gla protein: vitamin K–dependent proteins in bone. *Physiol Rev.* 1989;69:990–1047.

121. Maillard C, Berruyer M, Serre CM, et al. Protein-S, a vitamin K–dependent protein, is a bone matrix component synthesized and secreted by osteoblasts. *Endocrinology.* 1992;130:1599–1604.

122. Price PA. Role of vitamin-K-dependent proteins in bone metabolism. *Annu Rev Nutr.* 1988;8:565–583.

123. Hall JG, Pauli RM, Wilson KM. Maternal and fetal sequelae of anticoagulation during pregnancy. *Am J Med.* 1980;68:122–140.

124. Pettifor JM, Benson R. Congenital malformations associated with the administration of oral anticoagulants during pregnancy. *J Pediatr.* 1975;86:459–462.

125. Ginsberg JS, Greer I, Hirsh J. Use of antithrombotic agents during pregnancy. *Chest.* 2001;119(1 Suppl):122S–131S.

126. Hirsh J, O'Donnell M, Eikelboom JW. Beyond unfractionated heparin and warfarin: current and future advances. *Circulation.* 2007;116:552–560.

127. Hirsh J, Raschke R. Heparin and low-molecular-weight heparin: the Seventh ACCP Conference on Antithrombotic and Thrombolytic Therapy. *Chest.* 2004;126(3 Suppl):188S–203S.

128. Lovenox. Highlights of prescribing information. Available at: http:// products.sanofi-aventis.us/lovenox/lovenox.html. October 2007 ed. Sanofi-Aventis U.S.; 2007.

129. Miner PD. Contraceptive choices for females with congenital heart disease. *Prog Pediatr Cardiol.* 2004;19:15–24.

CHAPTER 10

Genetics, Epidemiology, and Counseling

FABIAN CHEN ▪ EMMANUÈLE DÉLOT ▪ JOSEPH K. PERLOFF

The past decade has witnessed major advances in our understanding of the molecular basis of cardiovascular development and the genetics of congenital heart disease (CHD). Advances in techniques of detection have resulted in identification of even mild examples. Accordingly, the number of new cases of CHD is now thought to be 0.8% to 1.0% per 1000 live births,[1-4] with an annual increase in prevalence of approximately 5% in the United States and a worldwide annual increase of approximately 1.5 million.

The cause(s) of CHD are usually unknown. Familial recurrence suggests a genetic etiology. Exposure to measles, rubella, retinoic acid, or environmental teratogens is held responsible, but more often than not, the mechanism of the presumed teratogenic effect is unknown and not investigated. This chapter focuses on epidemiology, genetic counseling, and family planning, as well as chromosomal, genetic, and environmental factors that contribute to the spectrum of adult CHD. Recent advances in molecular genetics and mutant animal models are highlighted.

EPIDEMIOLOGY

Postnatal Incidence

Congenital heart defects remain the leading cause of death in the neonatal period and early childhood.[5] However, a review of 62 reports discloses large disparities in incidence[1] (Fig. 10-1) that result from differences in identification of mild cases. Ascertainment bias is also responsible for some of the disparities.[1] Some studies are limited to identification of CHD during the first few days of life, and others are limited to the first year of life, thus ignoring defects that are often detected only in adulthood, such as ostium secundum atrial septal defect.[6]

Prenatal Incidence of Congenital Heart Disease

It is generally believed that the prenatal incidence of CHD is higher than the postnatal incidence because cardiac developmental anomalies are responsible for a large number of fetal deaths, and the incidence of CHD is 10 times greater in stillbirths than in live-born infants.[7,8] The incidence in total conceptuses is reportedly five times higher than in live-born children.[3] Although these numbers might appear irrelevant to the topic of CHD in adults, they are in fact crucial when considering etiology. Exclusion of early lethal cases leads to gross underestimation of the influence of teratogens and recurrence risk and to a bias in establishing patterns of genetic inheritance. When providing genetic counseling to CHD patients who themselves are considering pregnancy, it is appropriate to discuss prenatal CHD.

The major limitation in estimating the correct incidence of prenatal CHD is the facility of detecting defects in utero. There is significant variation in the estimated incidence between areas served by specialized pediatric cardiologists and areas not so served.[9] Inclusion of a routine four-chamber view of the heart during fetal ultrasound screening has resulted in increased detection of anomalies such as atrioventricular septal defects (AVSDs). Cardiac malformations are detected more often when associated with noncardiac anomalies that prompt a genetic workup.

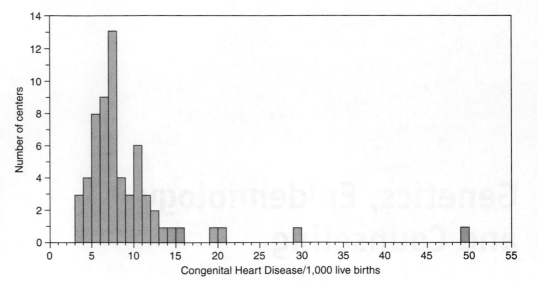

FIGURE 10-1 Histogram of the incidence of congenital heart disease per 1000 live births in 62 reports. The six highest values all came from echocardiographic studies of infants in the newborn nursery. *(Reprinted with permission from Hoffman, J.I., Kaplan, S.: The incidence of congenital heart disease. J Am Coll Cardiol 2002;39:1890.)*

Sex Differences of Incidence Rates

Women with long QT syndrome have a higher risk of syncope and sudden death than men. Women also have a higher incidence of torsades de pointes in drug-induced arrhythmias. The role of hormones in the etiology of these sexual differences is under investigation. There is strong evidence from mouse models that natural estrogens protect females from certain forms of cardiomyopathy.[10] A study of large registries in California, Sweden, and France reported a higher incidence of structural cardiac defects in males than in females (average sex ratio of 1.25).[11] Complex CHD represented by hypoplastic left heart syndrome, D-transposition of the great arteries (D-TGA), and tetralogy of Fallot (TOF) have the highest sex ratio bias with a male:female ratio of 1.45:1, whereas the ratio in mild CHD was 1.09:1, which is not significantly different from normal. Aortic valve stenosis has the highest sex ratio bias of 2.4:1 male:female.[11] The only two defects that were more frequent in females were AVSDs and interrupted aortic arch.[11]

Ethnic Differences

The incidence rate of CHD is stable across geographic and cultural populations except for the effects of regional toxins (discussed later). However, there are marked differences in the types of lesions within populations. Data from the Metropolitan Atlanta Congenital Defects Program disclose statistically significant differences between the Caucasian and African American populations. Caucasians had a higher incidence of D-TGA, truncus arteriosus, Ebstein's anomaly, coarctation of the aorta, and aortic valve stenosis, and African Americans had a higher incidence of peripheral pulmonary stenosis, atrial septal defects (ASDs), and patent ductus arteriosus.[12] The population-based case-control

Baltimore-Washington Infant Study reported similar trends in addition to an excess of pulmonary atresia in Caucasian infants.[13] In Dallas County, Texas, a population-based study after the first year of life disclosed that Caucasian children had the highest incidence of aortic stenosis, atrioventricular septal defects (AVSDs), and ventricular septal defects (VSDs), whereas Mexican Americans had the lowest incidence of hypoplastic left heart syndrome.[14] Socioeconomic factors might account for some of the differences. The cause(s), however, are unknown but are likely to be a combination of genetic and environmental factors.

Prevalence of Congenital Heart Disease

The number of new cases has apparently been constant over a given time course and geographic area, but there has been a steady increase in the prevalence of adults (total number of cases of during a specific time period). The median age of patients with CHD in a Quebec study was 11 years in 1985 and 17 years in 2000 (49% of patients with complex CHD were older than 18 years of age).[3] In the United States, in addition to approximately 3 million adults with bicuspid aortic valves,[15] an estimated 85% of infants with complex CHD undergoing surgical repair now survive to adulthood, resulting in approximately 1 million adult survivors.[16]

Large national registries such as the Wisconsin Pediatric Cardiac Registry[17] and a national registry and DNA bank of patients with CHD in the Netherlands[18] are designed to improve the follow-up of these patients. The Bethesda Task Force estimated that about half of the adult CHD population is at significant risk of complications or premature death and so should be followed regularly in specialized adult CHD facilities[6] (see Chapter 3).

ETIOLOGY

Identification of mutations in humans and in many engineered animal models clearly demonstrates a genetic basis of CHD. The molecular mechanisms causing these genetic defects are varied and include chromosomal alterations, single gene defects, and non-Mendelian genetic inheritance. There are clear examples of CHD caused by environmental influences such as drugs or maternal illnesses, but the molecular and developmental mechanisms are not understood. Interplay between genes (modifier genes, genetic background) or between genes and environment introduces additional levels of complexity that influence the phenotype of CHD.

Our understanding of the molecular and genetic bases of cardiovascular development has been dramatically increased by the ability to alter or mutate genes in animal models such as the mouse, zebrafish, frog, and fruit fly. Mutations that eliminate expression of a gene can be lethal to the embryo because of the critical function of a gene in cardiac development, an observation that has allowed dissection of important pathways that can go awry in CHD. It has also been learned that mutations partially affecting the function of a gene can result in less severe phenotypes than those found with complete elimination of a gene. A mutant protein sometimes has an adverse effect on the normal protein, as is the case with the *FIBRILLIN-1* mutation in Marfan syndrome. Geneticists term this mutation *dominant negative*.

The variability in the phenotype or the manifestation of a gene defect that culminates CHD can be due to the nature or severity of the mutation. Mutations can affect the protein coding sequence, thus affecting the function of the encoded protein. However, many mutations that result in human disease occur in regions of DNA that do not directly encode a protein. These "noncoding" mutations can affect the gene product by affecting the expression level, the alternative RNA splicing, or the timing of gene expression.

It has been learned from animal models of CHD that a cardiac defect does not always occur with a specific gene mutation, an observation referred to as the *penetrance* of the phenotype. Differences in phenotype penetrance are likely due to environmental and genetic background effects. An individual with a gene mutation may inherit specific alleles of other genes that compensate for the defective gene. Environmental effects, such as fetal exposure to teratogens or metabolic stress, are likely to play a role in altered gene expression that results in CHD. Stochastic events may also play a role. A mutation may make the fetus vulnerable because of a cardiac defect, but if the fetus survives that vulnerable stage, other genes that play a redundant role in later stages of development may fully compensate. From a teleological perspective, it is understandable that important biologic functions for development of a system as vital as the cardiovascular system have evolved functional redundancies.

Chromosomal Abnormalities

Chromosomal abnormalities are thought to account for about 5% of CHD cases in live-born children. The spectrum of abnormal chromosomal complement encompasses chromosomes that are entirely missing (Turner syndrome with an XO karyotype), supplementary chromosomes (the trisomy of chromosome 21 in Down syndrome), deleted fragments of chromosomes (the 22q11-deletion syndrome), unbalanced translocations resulting in partial aneuploidy (any genetic material that is not present in two copies in the genome), or balanced translocations that interrupt a gene critical for cardiac development. Most chromosomal abnormalities are de novo events, that is, they originate in the patient and are not inherited. Specific lesions are frequently associated with a particular type of chromosomal abnormality that prompts a specific diagnostic test and focused genetic counseling.

In 17% to 18% of cases, the congenital heart defect is associated with a syndrome or chromosomal abnormality that is considered the "cause" of the cardiac malformation.[4] The proportion of chromosomal anomalies varies greatly according to the type of cardiac defect.[19] Almost 70% of AVSDs are associated with a chromosomal abnormality. Other lesions associated with chromosomal abnormalities are VSDs (18%), AVSDs (32%), and ASDs (27%). In contrast, D-transposition of the great arteries (TGA) and pulmonary atresia with intact ventricular septum are rarely caused by a chromosomal anomaly (0.9% and 2.0%, respectively). Four previously published reports based on high-risk referral practices reported even more dramatic differences, with some form of aneuploidy associated with a 46% incidence of VSD and AVSD, 33% of aortic coarctation, 31% of tetralogy of Fallot (TOF), and 21% of double-outlet right ventricle (DORV), whereas TGA was never associated with a chromosomal abnormality. The many chromosomal abnormalities associated with CHD[9] are summarized in Table 10–1. A few are now described in more detail.

Down Syndrome

On the basis of data from the Baltimore-Washington Infant Study, Down syndrome, which is the second most prevalent birth defect in the United States, accounted for 81% of chromosomal abnormalities in infants with cardiovascular defects.[4] The frequency of Down syndrome ranges from 1.5 per 1000 births in studies from the 1950s to 1.0 per 1000 births in studies from the 1970s,[20] the

Table 10-1 Overall Rate of Aneuploidy (%) for Individual Congenital Cardiac Defects

CARDIAC ANOMALY	OVERALL ANEUPLOID RATE (%)	T 21 (%)	T 18 (%)	T 13 (%)	45X0 (%)	OTHER (%)	22q11 DELETION
AVSD	46	79	13			8	
VSD	46	43	45	2	4	6	10–17
TOF	31	43	29	7		21	6–30
CoA	33	18	24	24	12	22	
CAT	19				25	75	10
IAAb							17–50
APVS	20						
HLHS	7		56	22	11	11	
DORV	21	10	40	20	30		1
Mitral atresia	18						
UVH	15						
PS/PA + IVS	5						
Tricuspid atresia	7				50	50	
TVD	4						
Aortic stenosis	5						
ASD	17						
TGA	0						
cTGA	0						
Tumors	0						
Cardiomyopathy	0						
Cardiosplenic syndromes	0						
DIV	0						

APVS, absent pulmonary valve syndrome; ASD, atrial septal defect; AVSD, atrioventricular septal defect; CAT, common arterial trunk; CoA, coarctation of the aorta; cTGA, corrected transposition of the great arteries; DIV, double inlet ventricle; DORV, double outlet right ventricle; HLHS, hypoplastic left heart syndrome; IAAb, interrupted aortic arch type B; PS/PA + IVS, pulmonary stenosis/pulmonary atresia with intact ventricular septum; TGA, transposition of the great arteries; TOF, tetralogy of Fallot; TVD, tricuspid valve dysplasia; UVH, univentricular heart; VSD, ventricular septal defect.

With permission from Wimalasundera, R.C., Gardiner, H.M.: *Prenat Diag* 2004:24:1116–1122.

difference probably reflecting termination of pregnancy related to increased prenatal diagnosis. The Down phenotype is consistent[21] (Fig. 10–2), but the severity and constellation of clinical expressions can vary with each patient. Cardiac and intestinal malformations, as well as leukemia associated with Down syndrome, have variable expressivity and incomplete penetrance.

CHD is a pivotal feature of Down syndrome, being manifest in at least 40% of patients, many of whom survive to adulthood (see Chapter 4). AVSDs are the most common anomalies, occurring in 60% of Down patients.[4] Less common and in decreasing order of frequency are VSDs, TOF, and patent ductus arteriosus.[4,21,22]

The cause of Down syndrome is an altered dosage of wild-type genes on human chromosome 21. A third copy of chromosome 21 results in altered expression of genes that affect the development of the many organ systems involved in Down syndrome.[23] The mechanism and gene(s) that are primarily responsible for the cardiac defects are currently unknown. Genetic mapping has been used to

identify or localize critical regions on chromosome 21 important for the CHD.[24,25] Despite some candidate genes, there is no single gene or set of genes primarily responsible for the cardiac malformations in Down syndrome. Insights regarding the mechanism of the defect might be gained by examining related genetic disorders, but familial cases of AVSD are rare and have not been linked to chromosome 21. An autosomal-dominant incompletely penetrant transmission of AVSDs was localized to 1p31–p21, but no CHD candidate gene has thus far been identified in this region.[26] A second genetic locus was found on chromosome 3p25 as part of the rare 3p- syndrome.[27,28] At this locus, sequence variants in the gene *CRELD1* were identified and appear to confer susceptibility to AVSD. Missense mutations were found in this gene in two Down syndrome infants, suggesting that the mutations could contribute to the development of AVSD.[29]

Environmental risk factors have not been identified as contributors to the CHD in Down syndrome. A study comparing mothers of trisomy 21 children with or without CHD found no significant association with environmental

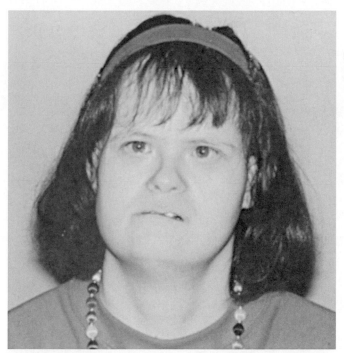

FIGURE 10-2   Facial dysmorphism in a 34-year-old woman with Down syndrome. Her cardiac lesion was unusual—namely, a perforated sinus of Valsalva aneurysm (surgically repaired) rather than an atrioventricular septal defect.

exposures, supporting the notion that the occurrence of CHD in Down syndrome is chiefly genetic.[30] This is in keeping with the Baltimore-Washington study that identified advanced maternal age as the only independent risk factor.[31]

Recent efforts toward a better understanding of this complex disorder have centered on generating a mouse model of Down syndrome. Engineering such a mouse mutant is challenging because of the difference between the mouse and human genomes. Two thirds of the mouse orthologs of the 243 known human chromosome 21 genes reside on mouse chromosome 16, with the remainder residing on mouse chromosomes 10 and 7. It is therefore impossible to make a simple mouse trisomy model of Down syndrome. Alternatively, a mouse that carries an extra copy of human chromosome 21 has been created and recapitulates many of the features of human Down syndrome including congenital heart defects, chiefly VSD.[32]

Despite advances in our knowledge of the genetics of Down syndrome, it remains unclear why cardiac malformations are not uniformly present, nor is it known which genes on chromosome 21 lead to the altered phenotype. A better understanding of the genetic basis of the Down syndrome congenital heart defects is important for genetic counseling and prognosis and will provide insight into how other cardiac malformations occur.

Trisomies 8, 13, and 18

Compared with Down syndrome, less is known about these other three trisomies and the cardiovascular abnormalities that accompany them. The prognosis is poor for trisomies 13 and 18 (Figs. 10-3 and 10-4), but trisomy 8, at least in mosaic form, is compatible with a normal life span. Notable features of trisomy 8, in addition to the characteristic facies, are skeletal anomalies, including

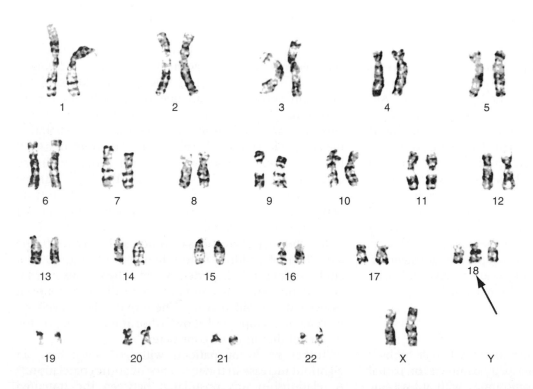

FIGURE 10-3   Karyotype from a female with trisomy 18. The arrow identifies the extra chromosome 18. The patient had patent ductus arteriosus with a ventricular septal defect.

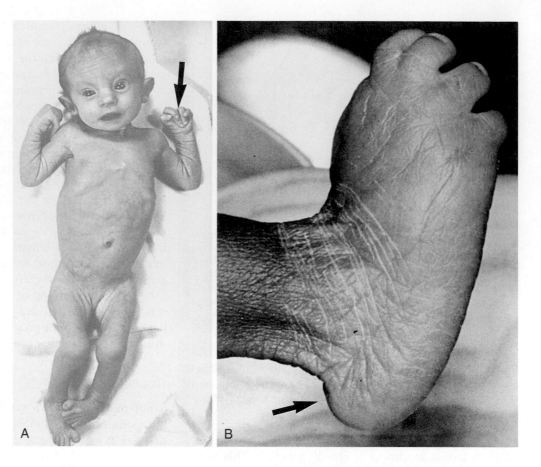

FIGURE 10-4 **(A)** Typical overlapping fingers *(arrow)* and lax skin of a neonate with trisomy 18. The "rocker-bottom feet" cannot be seen. The patient had a patent ductus arteriosus and a ventricular septal defect. **(B)** Typical rocker-bottom heel *(arrow)* of an infant with trisomy 18 and double-outlet right ventricle with a nonrestrictive subaortic ventricular septal defect. *(With permission from Perloff, J.K.: The Clinical Recognition of Congenital Heart Disease. 4th ed. Philadelphia, W.B. Saunders, 1994, pp. 489, 518.)*

scoliosis, abnormal vertebrae, additional ribs, spina bifida, and anomalies of the extremities (Fig. 10–5). Trisomy 8 is rare and highly lethal when, in the pure form, 100% of the cells carry a complete triple set of chromosome 8. Approximately 90% of infants die within the first year of life. However, about 5% of cases are partial trisomies in which only a portion of chromosome 8 is present in triplicate. The phenotypes are variable and seem to depend on the portion of duplicated chromosomes. Another 2% are mosaics that harbor a combination of normal euploid cells and trisomic cells, a mosaicism that is compatible with a longer life span. The degree of mosaicism in trisomy 8 varies in different tissues and also with time.[33] Unfortunately, there is little relationship between the degree of mosaicism in the easily accessible cells (lymphocytes and skin fibroblasts) and the extent of clinical abnormality. The literature is sparse, but a recent survey found VSDs in about half the patients.[34] Also reported are patent ductus arteriosus, pulmonary stenosis, coarctation of the aorta, truncus arteriosus, and total anomalous pulmonary venous connection.[22]

Turner Syndrome

Incidence is approximately 1 per 5000 live female births.[35] Turner syndrome is associated with complete or partial absence of one of the sex chromosomes, with at least one

X chromosome remaining. The classic 45 X karyotype accounts for about 50% of cases.[36] Many patients are mosaics of two cell lines with different karyotypes, including 45X/46XX and 45X/46XY. Rearrangements of the X chromosome and partial deletions of the Y chromosome (Fig. 10–6) also give rise to Turner syndrome, which is characterized by short stature, primary amenorrhea, webbing of the neck, and cubitus valgus (Fig. 10–7).[21] Much of the morbidity and mortality are due to the cardiovascular abnormalities that occur in 15% to 30% of patients.[36,37] The anomalies are primarily left-sided, especially coarctation of the aorta, bicuspid aortic valve, and aortic root disease.[36] Reports suggest an association between Turner syndrome and hypoplastic left heart syndrome, the most extreme form of left-sided obstructive lesions.[38,39] Also described are partial anomalous pulmonary venous connection (13%) and persistent left superior vena cava (13%).[40]

Systemic hypertension is common in Turner syndrome with 30% of children mildly hypertensive and 50% of adults significantly hypertensive.[41,42] There is also an increased incidence of coronary artery disease[43] without associated dyslipidemia.[44,45] The impact of hormone replacement therapy and growth hormone is part of the treatment that must be considered.

Turner syndrome patients with web neck have an eightfold increase in the incidence of aortic coarctation.[46] A relationship was postulated between the impaired

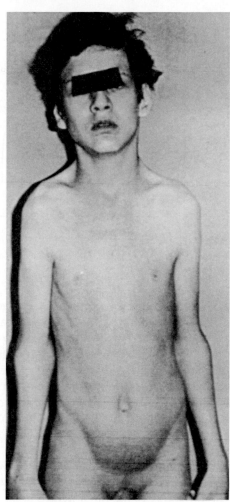

FIGURE 10–5   Seventeen-year-old male patient with trisomy 8. There is a slender trunk, cubitus valgus, flexion deformity of elbows, wide-set nipples, and absence of pubic hair. *(With permission from Lai, C.C., Gorlin, R.J.: Trisomy 8 syndrome.* Clin Orthop *1975;110:239.)*

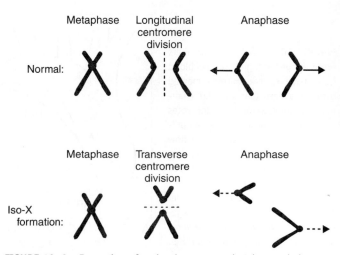

FIGURE 10–6   Formation of an isochromosome by abnormal cleavage of the centromere. *(With permission from Vogel, F., Motulsky, A.G.: Human Genetics. 2nd ed. Berlin, Springer-Verlag, 1986.)*

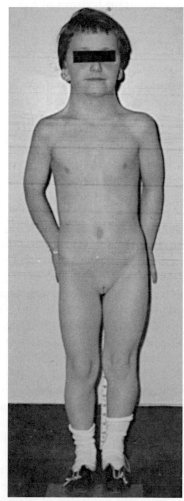

FIGURE 10–7   Thirteen-year-old girl with the typical phenotype of 45,X Turner syndrome and coarctation of the aorta. There is short stature, webbing of the neck, absent pubic hair, wide-set nipples, and a small chin.

lymphatic flow responsible for web neck and the decreased ascending aortic flow associated with coarctation (Fig. 10–8). Seventy-five percent of aborted fetuses with classic Turner phenotype have left-sided obstructive defects,[47] an observation believed to support a relationship among impaired lymphatic flow, decreased ascending aortic flow, web neck, and left-sided obstructive lesions.

Because most Turner are infertile, pregnancy is rare. However, these patients have a uterus and can become pregnant with the help of an egg donor. The recent increase in the number of such pregnancies has disclosed a problem that could have been anticipated. The risk of aortic dissection, already high in Turner syndrome, is dramatically increased because inherent medial abnormalities are reinforced by the medial changes of pregnancy[48] (see Chapter 9).

A recent advance in the understanding of the genetic mechanism of Turner syndrome is the discovery of the short-stature homeobox gene (SHOX) located on both the X and Y chromosomes.[49,50] Haploinsufficiency of

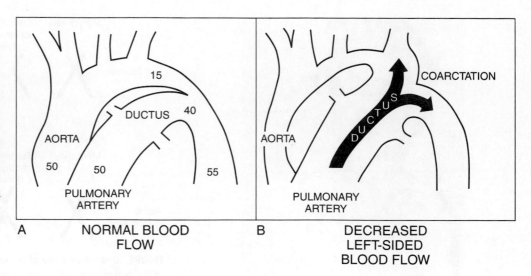

FIGURE 10–8 (A) The numbers represent percentage of normal blood flow (total cardiac output) moving through a particular vascular channel. **(B)** Any event that decreases aortic blood flow and increases pulmonary artery and ductal blood flow may initiate the coarctation sequence. *(With permission from Lacro, R.V., Jones, K.L., Benirschke, K.A.: Coarctation of the aorta in Turner syndrome: A pathologic study of fetuses, with nuchal cystic hygromas, hydrops fetalis and female genitalia. Pediatrics 1988;81:445.)*

SHOX is associated with short stature, skeletal malformations, and deafness. However, this single gene deficiency does not explain the cardiovascular and endocrine abnormalities that are important features of the syndrome.

DiGeorge Syndrome/22q11 Deletion Syndrome

Chromosome band 22q11 contains one or more genes concerned with cardiac morphogenesis,[51] an observation that became evident through the study of small deletions in this region. Syndromes with overlapping phenotypes affecting this area include DiGeorge syndrome, velocardiofacial (Shprintzen) syndrome, and some sporadic and familial cardiac defects. Overlapping features of these disorders have been referred to by the acronym CATCH 22—the letters standing for Cardiac defect, Abnormal facies, Thymic hypoplasia, Cleft palate, Hypocalcemia, and 22q11 deletions.[52] However, the discovery of a common genetic etiology of these overlapping syndromes led to the current nomenclature of *22q11 deletion syndrome* (OMIM#188400; Fig. 10–9).

A characteristic of 22q11 deletion syndrome is its considerable phenotypic variability, both in severity and in type of lesion. For the cardiac features alone, 25% of patients have TOF, 17% type B interrupted aortic arch, 17% VSD, 14% pulmonary atresia with VSD, and 10% persistent truncus arteriosus.[53] No correlations have been found between the size of the deletion and the phenotype,[54] and even discordant monozygotic twins have been reported.[55]

The incidence of 22q11 deletion syndrome is about 1 in 4000 births.[56] Of these, 28% are thought to be familial,[53] but most are sporadic and due to a de novo 22q11 deletion. However, in familial cases, the transmission has an autosomal dominant pattern with variable expressivity and penetrance. Genetic mapping of human DiGeorge patients has identified a critical genomic DNA region that can be manipulated in the mouse, leading to engineering of DNA deletions, homologous to the human 22q11

region deletion in DiGeorge syndrome. Heterozygous mutant mice with this deletion have aortic arch, parathyroid, thymic, and neurobehavioral defects similar to human patients.[57-59] These observations led to further genetic localization and determination that the *TBX1* gene located in this DiGeorge critical region was important for the disease. Mouse mutants deficient for *TBX1* have severe cardiac outflow tract defects.[60-62] In addition, specific *TBX1* mutations were identified in DiGeorge patients who did not harbor a 22q11 deletion.[63] Thus deficiency of *TBX1* is likely to be the primary cause of DiGeorge syndrome, although several yet unknown influences are likely to contribute to the variability of the phenotype.

Our understanding of DiGeorge syndrome has led to improved genetic screening of CHD patients with conotruncal defects. In a study that examined 251 patients with conotruncal defects at the Children's Hospital of Philadelphia, 22q11 deletions were detected in 50% of patients with interrupted aortic arch, 34.5% with truncus arteriosus, and 15.9% with TOF.[64] Knowledge of the genetic defect does not influence health care management but can be important in genetic counseling, as well as in screening family members.

Williams Syndrome

A similar story appears to be evolving for Williams syndrome (OMIM#194050; also called Williams-Beuren syndrome), a developmental disorder involving connective tissue, the central nervous system (mental retardation), visual spatial construction deficit, and an association with supravalvular aortic stenosis[65] (Fig. 10–10). Patients have a characteristic elflike appearance with upturned nose, small chin, and wide mouth. Special features include social gregariousness and perfect pitch, although the patients cannot read music. The syndrome has been associated with a chromosomal deletion greater than 114 kilobases located on chromosome 7q11.23. The area contains the gene for

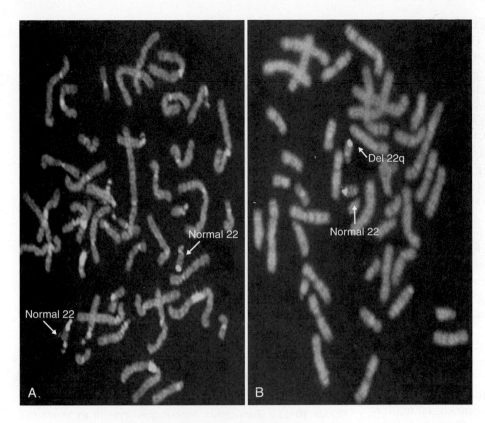

FIGURE 10–9   Diagnosis of a deletion in the chromosome 22q region that causes DiGeorge syndrome is performed using fluorescence *in situ* hybridization (FISH). A deletion of chromosome 22q is detected by absence of the red fluorescent DNA probe signal (Del 22q). The green fluorescent DNA probe signal serves as a control to identify chromosome 22q. *(Courtesy Dr. Nagesh P. Rad, UCLA Cytogenetics Laboratory.)*

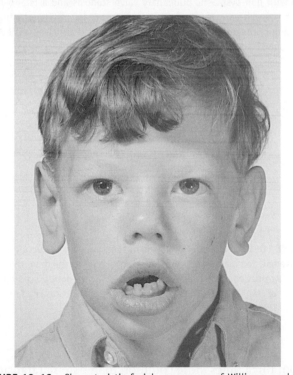

FIGURE 10–10   Characteristic facial appearance of Williams syndrome in a 6-year-old boy with nonfamilial supravalvular aortic stenosis and pulmonary artery stenosis. The patient was mentally retarded and shows the typical large mouth with patulous lips, small chin, baggy cheeks, blunt upturned nose, wide-set eyes, and malformed teeth. *(With permission from Perloff, J.K.: Clinical recognition of aortic stenosis. The physical signs and differential diagnosis of the various forms of obstruction to left ventricular outflow.* Prog Cardiovasc Dis *1968;10:323, Fig. 1.)*

elastin that is defective in familial supravalvular aortic stenosis,[66] suggesting that it is this particular locus within the deleted segment in Williams syndrome that leads to the heart defect. Patients and engineered mouse mutants of the elastin gene have vascular lesions but not the other features of Williams syndrome. Additional genes in the chromosomal deletion are therefore causative for other aspects of Williams syndrome.

The critical region for Williams syndrome on chromosome 7 has 28 known genes. In light of the complex nature of the disorder, it is likely that multiple unknown genes in the region are contributory. Recently, the *GTF2IRD1*,[67] *LIM kinase 1*, and *cytoplasmic linker protein of 115 kDa*[68] genes were identified as important candidate genes. As in the DiGeorge syndrome, a hemizygous state can result in clinical disease. Also as in the DiGeorge syndrome, fluorescent *in situ* hybridization (FISH) technique is routinely used to identify many, if not most, patients with the Williams syndrome deletion.[69]

Single Gene Defects

Unlike the syndromes associated with chromosomal defects, CHDs due to single gene defects typically exhibit Mendelian inheritance and are referred to as monogenic syndromes. The proportion of CHD caused by single gene defects has been estimated at 2%, but the discovery of responsible genes in both human beings and animal models suggests that 2% is a considerable underestimation.[70] It has also become clear that genes important in heart formation play vital roles in the development of other systems, and thus CHD resulting from single gene defects can involve organs other than the heart (see Chapter 14). Mutations in the *JAGGED1* gene causing Alagille syndrome can affect the heart and the liver. Some human mutations cause cardiac-specific lesions, as is the case for mutations in the transcription factor *GATA-4* that were identified as causative in two pedigrees with familial septal defects.[71]

Compared with chromosomal defects, more progress has been made in our understanding of the molecular mechanisms of CHD that result from single gene defects. However, the penetrance or manifestation of the cardiac defect may depend on the capacity of other genes to compensate for the genetic deficiency or on the presence of a "second hit" genetic defect or an environmental exposure. The number of genes that are involved in cardiovascular development and that are potentially important in human CHD is growing rapidly. Some examples of single gene mutations causing CHD are now discussed.

Noonan Syndrome

First recognized in 1963, Noonan syndrome[72] (OMIM# 163950) is the most common nonchromosomal malformation syndrome among children with CHD. Prevalence of Noonan syndrome in children with cardiovascular defects is 1.1% to 1.4%.[47,73] In the general population, prevalence is estimated at 1 in 8000.[74] Cardinal features of the syndrome include short stature, mental retardation, delayed sexual development, broad or web neck, shield chest, inguinal hernia, undescended testes, dystrophic nails, and characteristic facies[75] (Fig. 10–11). Because Noonan and Turner syndromes have some features in common, other names have arisen, including female pseudo-Turner syndrome, the XX and XY Turner phenotype, and the male Turner syndrome. Nevertheless, Noonan syndrome can be distinguished by phenotype, normal karyotype analysis, and the nature of the cardiovascular defect.

A congenital cardiac malformation occurs in approximately two thirds of Noonan patients[22,76,77] and is usually represented by dysplastic pulmonary valve stenosis. Atrial defect coexists in about 25% of patients.[20] Less common are pulmonary artery stenosis and hypertrophic cardiomyopathy. Partial deficiency of coagulation factor XI has been associated with Noonan syndrome.[78]

Family pedigrees indicate that the mode of inheritance is autosomal dominant.[76,79] Figure 10–12 shows the familial inheritance of Noonan syndrome. Dominant inheritance is indicated by the direct (vertical) transmission of the trait. Affected individuals have affected parents. There is roughly an equal incidence of affected and unaffected children. A sex-ratio bias for affected offspring is reflected in a 2:1 male:female ratio, which may be due to a selective effect of the mutation on survival of male embryos. Maternal transmission of Noonan syndrome is

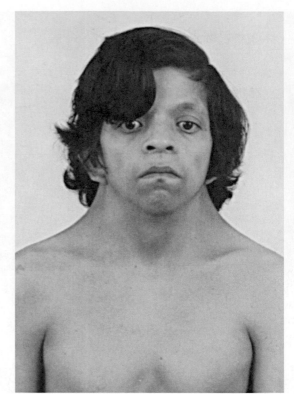

FIGURE 10–11 Characteristic Noonan phenotype in an 18-year-old man with non-dysplastic pulmonary valve stenosis and a left-to-right shunt through an ostium primum atrial septal defect. There is typical webbing of the neck, low-set ears with malformed auricles, small chin, and hypertelorism.

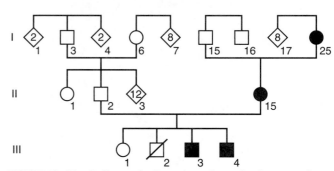

FIGURE 10–12 Pedigree of a Noonan syndrome family supporting an autosomal dominant mode of inheritance as described in the text. *(With permission from Collins, E., Turner, G.: The Noonan syndrome—a review of the clinical and genetic features of 27 cases. J Pediatr 1973;83:941.)*

about three times more common than paternal transmission, probably because of male infertility associated with undescended testes.[75]

Genetic testing was prompted by the discovery that approximately 50% of Noonan syndrome patients have a mutation in the *PTPN11* gene.[80–83] A single mutation that changes an amino acid accounts for one third of cases. The *PTPN11* gene encodes a protein product called Shp2, a tyrosine phosphatase molecule that is ubiquitously expressed and is an important component of intracellular signaling pathways.

Noonan syndrome overlaps phenotypically with three other syndromes: Leopard syndrome (OMIM#151100), Costello syndrome (OMIM#115150), and cardio-facio-cutaneous syndrome (OMIM#218040). Cardiac defects are prominent in Costello syndrome and include pulmonary stenosis (30%) and hypertrophic cardiomyopathy (34%).[84] Mutations in *PTPN11* have also been found in Leopard syndrome, which is therefore an allelic variant of Noonan.[85] It is not understood how different types of mutations in the same gene are responsible for the higher rate of hypertrophic cardiomyopathy in Leopard syndrome compared to Noonan syndrome.[86] Disease-causing mutations have now been found in the gene encoding *HRAS* in Costello syndrome[87] and in four other genes (KRAS, BRAF, MEK1, and MEK2) in cardio-facio-cutaneous syndrome.[88,89] All these gene products interact in the same RAS-MAPK signaling pathway, probably explaining the phenotypic overlap.

In a recently generated mouse model for Noonan syndrome, the heterozygote mutants have VSD, double-outlet right ventricle, and enlarged valve primordia in addition to craniofacial abnormalities, short stature, and myeloproliferative disease.[90] This mouse model provides a framework for understanding the molecular pathogenesis of Noonan syndrome and for developing potential therapies.

Holt-Oram Syndrome

Holt-Oram syndrome (OMIM#142900), described in 1960,[91] is one of a number of syndromes in which congenital cardiac anomalies are associated with upper limb defects.[92,93] The thumb is typically triphalangeal, hypoplastic, or absent (Fig. 10–13); carpals and metacarpals may be absent, hypoplastic, or dysplastic. Radial anomalies vary from minor to complete phocomelia. Radiologic abnormalities of the carpal bones may exist in normal-appearing hands of these patients. All degrees of upper limb defects can be encountered in the same pedigree, and no correlation exists between the severity of the cardiac defect and the skeletal abnormalities.[94] Approximately 70% of patients with Holt-Oram syndrome have CHD. Ostium secundum atrial septal defect is the most common.[91] Other cardiac defects occur without prevailing patterns.[21]

A major advance in understanding Holt-Oram syndrome is the identification of mutations in the *TBX5* gene.[95,96] The protein encoded by this gene is a member of the T-box transcription factor family that is important in regulating gene expression. In addition, a mouse mutant of the *Tbx5* gene has cardiac and forelimb abnormalities similar to the human disease.[97] Identification of the gene defect makes genetic testing possible and permits preimplantation genetic diagnosis of *in vitro* fertilized embryos from affected families.[98]

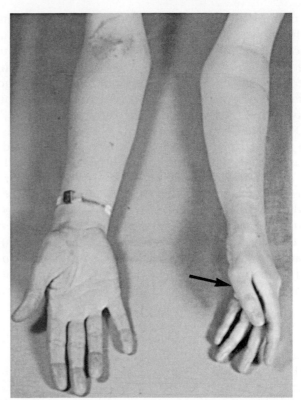

FIGURE 10-13   Forearms and hands of a 34-year-old woman with Holt-Oram syndrome and an ostium secundum atrial septal defect. When the palms are turned up as shown, hypoplasia of the radius prevents full supination of the left hand and the "crooked" appearance of the hypoplastic left thumb becomes apparent *(arrow)*. The fingertips of the right hand are erythematous, owing to a small right-to-left shunt. *(With permission from Lin, A.E., Perloff, J. K.: Upper limb malformations associated with congenital heart disease. Am J Cardiol 1985;55:1576.)*

Laterality Defects and Kartagener Syndrome

Left-right asymmetry is determined early in embryonic development. The heart is the first organ to exhibit asymmetry. The heart as a linear tube begins to loop at embryonic day 23. Three major cardiac malpositions occur in the presence of right/left asymmetry[99]: (1) visceroatrial situs inversus with dextrocardia, (2) visceroatrial situs solitus with dextrocardia, and (3) visceroatrial situs inversus with levocardia. Mesocardia or situs ambiguous is sometimes regarded as a fourth malposition. Cardiac malpositions in the presence of bilateral symmetry are called visceral heterotaxies, which are characterized by bilateral right-sidedness (right isomerism) or bilateral left-sidedness (left isomerism).[100]

Much has been learned in recent years regarding the molecular pathways that determine left-right asymmetry.[101,102] The central organizing structure in the early embryo, the node, is critical for determining laterality. The node has monocilia that are motile and generate laminar leftward flow. A mouse mutant with a defect in the monocilia of the node prevents this leftward flow of fluid surrounding the node, resulting in random laterality of the mutant organism. Supporting this mechanism is artificially generated leftward nodal flow in these mutant mice that can restore normal laterality. It is thought that the leftward flow of fluid around the node results in a mechanosensory signal in the node that is transduced through calcium and signaling molecules to dictate laterality during embryonic development.

Kartagener syndrome (OMIM#244400), a rare disorder with a frequency of 1 in 68,000,[103] is characterized by situs inversus with dextrocardia, bronchiectasis, and sinusitis.[104] The syndrome is now part of a wide spectrum of ciliary dyskinesis that includes immotile cilia of sperm and of the upper respiratory tract.[105,106] Defects in flagella and cilia function result in sperm immotility and result in defective mucociliary transport in the airways. The heart is usually structurally normal despite dextrocardia.

Inheritance is autosomal recessive with incomplete penetrance. The pedigree in Figure 10–14 shows typical horizontal transmission in which only siblings are affected, whereas parents are clinically normal. Males and females are equally involved. For very rare traits such as this, consanguineous mating is common.

The situs inversus mutant mouse model resembles Kartagener syndrome[107,108] but has normal cilia,[107] and thus a different gene or pathway related to or separate from Kartagener syndrome may involved.

Supravalvular Aortic Stenosis

Supravalvular aortic stenosis (SVAS) displays marked heterogeneity in its presentation. Two investigations of large families disclosed an autosomal-dominant pattern

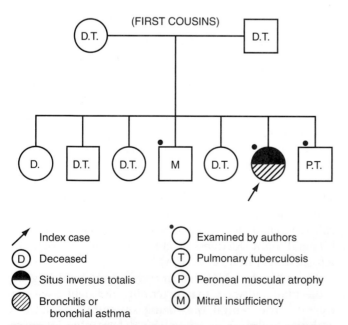

FIGURE 10–14 Pedigree consistent with autosomal recessive inheritance for Kartagener syndrome. *(With permission from Katsuhara, K., Kawamoto, S., Wakabayashi, T., Belsky, J.L.: Sinus inversus totalis and Kartagener's syndrome in a Japanese population. Chest 1972;61:56.)*

of inheritance.[109,110] In both families, the members with supravalvular aortic stenosis exhibited normal intelligence and normal facies that distinguished them from patients with Williams syndrome.[111,112] Echocardiographic assessment of 34 family members revealed that 13 had some degree of supravalvular aortic stenosis that ranged from mild to severe.[109] Judging from the phenotypes and the pattern of inheritance, the trait showed extremely variable expression but complete penetrance. Inheritance was autosomal dominant in a kindred of 80 subjects spanning five generations.[110] Echocardiography identified variable expression of the trait in the pedigree. Eighty-six percent of carriers of the gene had evidence of the aortic root anomaly.

SVAS as a component of Williams syndrome is caused by a mutation of the *ELASTIN* gene that is part of the deleted chromosomal region. Deletions that primarily affect the *ELASTIN* gene result in SVAS, while larger deletions that affect at least 114 kb encompassing the *ELASTIN* gene result in Williams syndrome.

Marfan Syndrome

Marfan syndrome (OMIM#154700) is characterized by skeletal, ocular, and cardiovascular abnormalities. The characteristic cardiovascular abnormality is dilatation of the aortic root due to a defect of the media and valve cusps that predisposes to dissecting aneurysm and aortic regurgitation.[113] Identification of the gene mutations that cause Marfan syndrome resulted from genetic mapping of the Marfan gene to a small region on chromosome 15 and then localizing *FIBRILLIN-1* as a candidate gene in that region. Fibrillin is a large glycoprotein that combines with other proteins to form microfibrils. Molecular analyses have identified more than 30 mutations, with affected families often harboring unique mutations. Screening for mutations is complicated by the great genetic heterogeneity and by the relatively large size of the *FIBRILLIN-1* gene that contains 65 exons and spans approximately 110 kb. Mutations in the *FIBRILLIN-1* gene have also been associated with ascending aortic aneurysm and dissection or ectopia lentis without other manifestations of Marfan syndrome.[114,115] Recent molecular insights regarding fibrillin function offer hope of pharmacologic therapy in Marfan syndrome. Fibrillin has homology to proteins that bind and inhibit the transforming growth factor-β (TGF-β) family and can bind TGF-β and latent transforming growth factor-β-binding proteins (LTBPs), leading to increased TGF-β activity.[116] Loeys and Dietz discovered that mutations in TGF-β receptor (TGFBR1 and TGFBR2) result in a syndrome that overlaps with Marfan syndrome.[116,117] Loeys-Dietz syndrome is characterized by a triad of features including (1) arterial tortuosity and aortic aneurysms, (2) hypertelorism, and (3) bifid uvula or cleft palate. Dietz and colleagues found that the angiotensin II receptor blocker losartan has an antagonistic effect on

TGF-β activity, and a beneficial effect was demonstrated on aortic aneurysm formation in a mouse mutant model of Marfan syndrome.[118] It remains to be determined whether losartan or similar angiotensin II receptor blockers have a beneficial effect in human Marfan patients. This research is a prime example of how advances at the laboratory bench may have an impact on patient care.

Conduction Defects and Arrhythmias

Multiple gene defects can cause conduction defects and arrhythmias such as long QT syndrome, familial heart block, and arrhythmogenic right ventricular dysplasia.[119-122] Considerable progress has been made in understanding the genetics of the long QT (LQT) syndrome, also known as the Romano-Ward syndrome, which appears to be inherited as an autosomal-dominant trait with high penetrance.[123] Affected patients have a corrected QT interval greater than 440 milliseconds, sinus bradycardia, and T wave abnormalities. Symptoms are often triggered by loud noises and emotional stress and tend to occur postpartum. Cardiac arrhythmias are responsible for sudden death. In a study of 193 families observed over a mean of 28 years, 13% died suddenly before age 40 years and before treatment could be initiated.[124] Gene mapping has disclosed at least eight loci associated with the LQT syndrome (Table 10-2),[123] and new genetic loci are likely to be found. Most commonly affected is the *KCNQ1* gene (LQT1), which encodes the I_{KS} potassium channel. Mutations in LQT1 in recessive form cause Jervell-Lange-Nielsen syndrome, which couples LQT with congenital neural deafness.

The *HERG* locus (LQT2) on chromosome 7 codes for a different potassium channel, and the *SCN5A* cardiac sodium channel gene is on the short arm of chromosome 3 (LQT3). Mutations at other LQT loci are less common. Presymptomatic diagnosis may become possible because genes responsible for LQT syndrome continue to be identified and their mutations characterized.

In some pedigrees of familial complete heart block (CHB), there is dominant inheritance and a high incidence of sudden death.[125] Hearts of two neonate siblings from a family with CHB lacked both an AV node

and myocardial fibers in the lower interatrial septum and exhibited areas of inflammation, calcification, and fibrosis.[126,127] CHB may result from a genetically acquired autoimmune response analogous to systemic lupus erythematosus.[128,129]

Arrhythmogenic right ventricular dysplasia (ARVD) is accompanied by ventricular tachycardia/fibrillation and sudden death.[125] The majority of familial cases have an autosomal-dominant inheritance pattern. In an Italian family with ARVD, mutations in the TGF-β receptor 3 (TGFB3) gene were identified as causative.[130,131] Mutations in the cardiac ryanodine receptor (hRYR2) have been associated with a form of ARVD and catecholaminergic-mediated polymorphic ventricular tachycardia.[127] Other variants are caused by mutations in the desmoplakin,[132] desmocollin-2,[133] and desmoglein-2[134] genes that are important components of the desmosomes that interconnect cardiomyocytes. Another desmosome-related molecule, plakoglobin, has been implicated in Naxos disease, a recessively inherited ARVD-like phenotype (OMIM#601414) associated with palmo-plantar keratoderma and woolly hair in families from the Hellenic island of Naxos. In light of the multiple genes that affect desmosome function, it is likely that other gene defects for ARVD will be discovered.

In addition to the examples just discussed, a number of additional congenital heart defects are thought to have a genetic basis, at least in some instances. Familial occurrences of conotruncal malformations include TOF,[135-140] patent ductus arteriosus,[140] ASD,[141-143] total anomalous pulmonary venous connection,[144] tricuspid atresia or annular hypoplasia,[145] discrete subaortic stenosis,[146] and Ebstein's anomaly.[13] The best source for current information is the Online Mendelian Inheritance In Man database available on the Internet (www.ncbi. nlm.nih.gov/Omim).

Left Ventricular Noncompaction

Left ventricular noncompaction (LVNC) is characterized by abnormally prominent trabeculations and deep intertrabecular recesses. The right ventricle is occasionally affected. Severity varies greatly, even in individuals in the same family who can present with congestive heart failure, arrhythmias, and systemic embolization.[147] LVNC is sometimes associated with other congenital cardiac defects including VSD, ASD, and pulmonary stenosis, as well as with neuromuscular disorders.[148]

LVNC has been attributed to an arrest in compaction of the left ventricle, a process that normally occurs between days 30 and 70 of human gestation.[147] Multiple genes and syndromes are associated with LVNC, but the embryonic defect that causes the disorder is unclear. Mutations have been identified in α-dystrobrevin (*DTNA*), G4.5 (*TAZ*), and Cypher (also called LIM-domain-binding protein 3 or ZASP).[149-153]

Table 10-2	Long QT Syndrome Genetic Loci		
LQT SUBTYPE	**GENE**	**CHROMOSOME LOCATION**	**FREQUENCY**
LQT1	KCNQ1	11p15	~50%
LQT2	KCNH2	7q35	30%–40%
LQT3	SCN5A	3p21	5%–10%
LQT4	ANK2	4q25	rare
LQT5	KCNE1	21q22	rare
LQT6	KCNE2	21q22	rare
LQT7	KCNJ2	17q23	rare
LQT8	CACNA1C	12q13	rare

Non-Mendelian Inheritance

Although an increasing proportion of CHD is recognized as inherited in a Mendelian fashion, many cases cannot be attributed to either a single gene defect exhibiting Mendelian inheritance or a chromosomal defect. In this section, two modes of non-Mendelian inheritance patterns are discussed: (1) cytoplasmic or maternal inheritance and (2) the effect of parental imprinting on inheritance of nuclear genes.

Studies of the early 1980s disclosed that the risk of recurrence of CHD is much greater if the mother rather than the father is the affected parent.[154-156] This sex bias applies to some lesions but not to others. Most strikingly, the recurrence risk of aortic stenosis in children of an affected mother was 17.9% compared with 2.8% for a father.[157] Also highly significant was an increased risk from 2.1% to 9.5% when a father rather than a mother was a VSD carrier.

One possible explanation for sexual skewing of inheritance of CHD is parental ascertainment bias. When a female is pregnant, she is securely identified as the mother, but identification of the father is not as secure. The prevalence of false paternity in the general population is estimated at 5% to 10%, thus paternal inheritance could be underestimated. One study of patients with CHD failed to find a difference in the recurrence risk of father compared with mother.[158] Male fertility is reduced in certain congenital disorders, such as Noonan syndrome,[159] which is an interesting example of reverse sexual transmission bias. Studies of sequences of DNA adjacent to de novo disease-causing mutations of the PTPN11 gene demonstrated that all of the mutations ($n = 14$) occurred on the chromosome of paternal origin.[159] The molecular basis for this bias is not understood.

Another hypothesis put forth to account for differences in parental inheritance proposes that the causative DNA mutations are exclusively inherited from the mother. Such sexual skewing of inheritance can be due to mitochondrial DNA in which a paternal contribution is not detected or to nuclear DNA that is subject to genetic imprinting (discussed later). The methylation levels (imprint) of DNA are different in the paternal and maternal gene allele.

Mitochondrial Inheritance

The characteristics of cytoplasmic inheritance derive from the biology of the mitochondrion.[160] Each cell contains hundreds of mitochondria, and each mitochondrion contains several copies of a compact circular mitochondrial DNA (1.65×10^4 base pairs in length). This genome is tiny compared with the nuclear genome (3×10^9 base pairs; approximately 0.3% of cellular DNA is mitochondrial). The genotype of the cell cytoplasm is a composite of the thousands of mitochondrial DNA molecules. At each cell division, the number of mitochondrial DNA molecules doubles, and the organelles segregate randomly into each daughter cell, a phenomenon that leads to mitotic segregation or to changes in genotype during mitotic growth.[161] Changes in phenotype reflect the proportion of normal and mutant mitochondrial DNA molecules. Because mitochondria are cytoplasmic organelles, the genetic material is inherited separately from nuclear DNA—termed *cytoplasmic inheritance*. Mitochondria are almost exclusively inherited from the mother (from the oocyte), although there is evidence that paternal mitochondrial DNA inheritance sometimes occurs.[162]

The mammalian mitochondrial genome is composed of a single circular DNA molecule that contains 37 highly condensed genes. These genes encode for 13 protein components of the respiratory chain and of the oxidation phosphorylation system, 2 ribosomal RNA genes, and 22 transfer RNA genes. Certain sequence changes in mitochondrial DNA are associated with cardiomyopathies, and different mutations in the same gene sometimes result in different disease forms. Heteroplasmy for a A3260G mutation in the gene encoding the tRNA for Leucine has been confirmed as a cause of cardiomyopathy.[163-165] DNA polymorphisms have been identified (and are awaiting confirmation) in other forms of cardiomyopathy and in heteroplasmic or homoplasmic forms (Table 10–3).

Panels for mutation analysis are available, and whole genome sequencing is becoming available, so geneticists can identify mutations in mitochondrial DNA. Mitochondrial inheritance nevertheless remains the most problematic form of disease from the standpoint of genetic counseling. Severity depends largely on the degree of heteroplasmy in the organs at risk, a characteristic that cannot be predicted in the fetus. Examples have been reported in which the mutations were found exclusively in the cardiac tissue. The risk of recurrence ranges from 0% to 100% (if the mother is the carrier) depending on the degree of mitochondrial inheritance of the offspring. Importantly, chemotherapeutic drugs such as doxorubicin or HIV retroviral inhibitors can have a toxic effect on mitochondria, leading to cardiomyopathy. Both genetic and environmental mechanisms exist that result in mitochondrial dysfunction.

Parental Imprinting

Parental imprinting is another mechanism that could account for skewed maternal transmission of certain congenital heart defects.[154-156,166] The hallmark of inheritance of an "imprinted" allele is whether the abnormal gene derives from the maternal or paternal genetic complement. Maternal and paternal genomes do not function equivalently during development. Studies of mouse embryogenesis have shown that embryos with a diploid set of only

Table 10–3   Mitochondrial Cardiomyopathy

SYNDROME	LOCUS	ALLELE	RNA
Mitochondrial myopathy and CM	MTTL1	A3260G (He)	tRNA Leu (UUR)
Mitochondrial myopathy and CM	MTTL1	C3303T (Ho/He)	tRNA Leu (UUR)
Maternally inherited hypertrophic CM	MTTI	A4295G (He)	tRNA Ile
Maternally inherited CM	MTTI	A4300G (He)	tRNA Ile
Cardiomyopathy	MTTK	A8348G (He)	tRNA Lys
Maternally inherited hypertrophic CM	MTTG	T9997C (He)	tRNA Gly
Maternally inherited CM	MTTH	G12192A (Ho)	tRNA His
Dilated cardiomyopathy	MTTL2	T12297C (He)	tRNA Leu (CUN)
Fatal infantile CM plus MELAS	MTTI	A4269G (He)	tRNA Ile
Fatal infantile CM plus MELAS	MTTI	A4317G (nd)	tRNA Ile
Diabetes mellitus, deafness, and CM	MTTK	A8296G (He)	tRNA Lys
Hypertrophic CM	MTCYB	G15243A (He)	
Hypertrophic CM	MTCYB	G15498A (He)	

Mitochondrial DNA polymorphisms associated with forms of cardiomyopathy. CM, cardiomyopathy; He/Ho, heteroplasmy/homoplasmy; MELAS, mitochondrial encephalopathy.

Data from Mitomap [www.mitomap.org], a database of the human mitochondrial genome, including constantly updated lists of disease-causing mutations.

maternal chromosomes (gynogenomes) or with a diploid set of only paternal chromosomes (androgenomes) die *in utero.*[167] Paternally derived zygotes develop predominantly extra embryonic tissues, whereas maternally derived zygotes undergo embryogenesis but experience extremely limited development of trophoblast and other extra embryonic tissues. Mice with Robertsonian translocations have been used to produce offspring with partial disomy of one chromosome. Offspring with identical genotypes have characteristically different phenotypes, depending on whether the disomic chromosomes derive from a maternal or paternal line.[168] Offspring that are paternally nullisomic and maternally disomic for portions of chromosome 11 are smaller than normal littermates. Conversely, offspring that are maternally nullisomic and paternally disomic for chromosome 11 are larger than normal littermates. For other chromosome segments, duplication and deficiency combinations are lethal. These observations strongly imply that there are uniquely male and female genetic contributions that occur during development.

A major mechanism by which imprinting is established is believed to be the degree of DNA methylation.[169,170] The pattern of methylation is consistent with the requirements of imprinting: (1) the pattern persists stably throughout DNA replication and cell division in somatic tissues and (2) the pattern is erased in the germ line and then differentially established once more in sperm and egg genomes.

An example of parental imprinting in human disease is the Beckwith-Wiedeman syndrome, which is characterized by macroglossia, gigantism, umbilical anomalies, and occasionally cardiomyopathy. Microdeletions in a differentially methylated region on chromosome 11 cause the loss of imprinting of the gene coding for the growth factor IGF2, resulting in the mutant phenotype.

Environmental Influences

Well-documented examples of environmental influences that trigger regional increases in CHD are exceptions to the otherwise stable incidence of CHD across geographic and cultural populations. A study from Dallas disclosed a 20% increase in CHD in children of mothers living within 1 mile of a hazardous waste site.[171] The California Birth Defect Registry records an increased incidence of CHD in the heavily polluted Central Valley. Studies of ambient air pollution and risk of birth defects in Southern California disclosed that dose-dependent effects of individual pollutants were associated with increased risk of CHD.[172] Carbon monoxide exposure in the second month of gestation increased the incidence of VSD, whereas exposure to ozone in the second gestational month increased the risk of aortic and other valve defects.[172]

Environmentally caused malformations result from a combination of triggers and the genetic background of the exposed individual. Although knowledge of genes involved in cardiac development and CHD has increased exponentially in recent years, identification of interactions between genes and environmental influences and their consequences continue to evolve.

Table 10–4 illustrates examples in which epidemiology clearly implicates a drug or a maternal disorder as the cause of CHD in the fetus. These examples require little if any genetic predisposition, but the embryological and

Table 10-4 Selected Environmental Factors and Congenital Cardiovascular Defects

ENVIRONMENTAL FACTOR	NO. OF MOTHERS EXPOSED	NO. OF CHILDREN WITH CHD	CHD (%)	RELATIVE RISK*
Thalidomide	471	30	6.4	9.4
Lithium	184	13	7.1	10.4
Alcohol	527	170	32.3	47.4
Oral contraceptives	2591	18	0.7	1.0
Diabetes	13,877	286	2.1	3.0
Phenylketonuria (phenylalanine ≥26 mg/dl)	93	16	17.2	25.3
Rubella—first trimester	58	1	1.7	2.5
Rubella—second trimester	1516	18	1.2	1.7
Rubella—third trimester	714	3	0.4	0.6

CHD, congenital heart disease.

* Relative risk $= \dfrac{\text{Risk of disease among exposed}}{\text{Risk of disease among nonexposed}}$

The risk of disease among nonexposed (baseline risk) was taken to be 0.68%.

All data from Pexieder, T.: Teratogens. In Prerport, M.E.M., and Muller, J.H. (eds): The Genetics of Cardiovascular Disease. Boston, Martinus Nijhoff Publishing. 1987; except for phenylketonuria data, which were taken from Lenke, R.R., and Levy, H.L.: Maternal phenylketonuria and hyperphenylalaninemia. *N Engl J Med* 303:1202–1208, 1980.

molecular mechanisms by which they result in CHD are largely unknown.

Drugs

Thalidomide is a good example of how difficult and lengthy the process can be for establishing the association between congenital malformations and a teratogenic agent. Four years were required (1957–1961) to incriminate thalidomide as the cause of phocomelia.[157] A population study showed that in 6.4% of children, limb defects caused by thalidomide were associated with CHD, most commonly conotruncal anomalies such as TOF and truncus arteriosus. The prevalence was 13.3% when the studies included data derived from cohorts of malformed children.

The spectrum of thalidomide embryopathy defects overlaps significantly with two other syndromes—Holt-Oram syndrome (OMIM#142900) and Okihiro syndrome (OMIM#607323)—which are autosomal-dominant genetic disorders caused by mutations in the genes encoding the transcription factors *TBX5* and *SLL4*, respectively. The phenotypic overlap was recently underscored by the finding that mutations in *SLL4* were present in patients previously labeled as Holt-Oram, as well as in patients previously thought to have thalidomide embryopathy.[173] This observation dramatically changes the assessment of recurrence in the offspring from low population risk (with no further exposure to thalidomide) to 50% (for a dominantly inherited mutation).

Angiotensin-Converting Enzyme Inhibitors

Angiotensin-converting enzyme (ACE) inhibitors have long been recognized as teratogens when taken in the second and third trimester of pregnancy, and, when taken during the first trimester, almost triple the risk of severe CHD.[174] It remains to be determined whether the consequences of these medications represent a teratogenic effect or an effect of altered vascular perfusion.[175]

Lithium

Lithium administered during pregnancy for the treatment of bipolar disorders has been linked to an increase of Ebstein's anomaly.[176] However, a more recent prospective study did not confirm this finding.[177] Lithium in therapeutic doses may not be a significant human teratogen.

Alcohol

Fetal alcohol syndrome is characterized by growth, developmental, and mental retardation and a distinctive facial appearance[178] (Fig. 10–15). Cardiac defects are common, especially VSD and ASD. The effect of alcohol varies in different women, suggesting that genetic factors also come into play.

Oral Contraceptives

In the 1970s, controversy arose following epidemiologic studies that implied an increased risk of congenital heart defects and other teratogenic effects in offspring of women taking progesterone or similar oral contraceptives. The Food and Drug Administration mandated special labeling of oral contraceptive packages. Subsequent studies in animal models and human subjects discounted the risk. In 1999, the Food and Drug Administration removed the warning.[179]

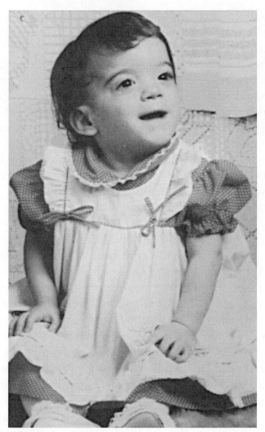

FIGURE 10-15   Physiognomy of a child with fetal alcohol syndrome characterized by micrognathia, absent philtrum, short palpebral fissures, and epicanthal folds.

Retinoic Acid

Deficiency in and excess exposure to vitamin A or its active derivative *retinoic acid* can cause congenital heart defects. A rare pleiotropic syndrome called PAGOD (Pulmonary tract and pulmonary Artery hypoplasia, Agonadism, Omphalocele, Diaphragmatic defect, and Dextrocardia) resembles the malformation complex described in mouse models lacking in retinoic acid during embryogenesis.[180] The syndrome involves genital anomalies, diaphragmatic hernias, and lung hypoplasia with cardiac defects that include hypoplastic ventricles, ASDs and VSDs, and anomalies of the great arteries. In the fetuses of women exposed to isotretinoin (Accutane), the retinoid prescribed for severe acne, a host of malformations occur in addition to conotruncal defects.[181] Exposure to topical tretinoin (Retin-A) during pregnancy does not result in these malformations.[182]

The mechanism by which retinoic acid influences embryonic development is incompletely understood but has been extensively studied in mouse models. In addition, mutations were recently identified in a gene called *STRA6*, a member of the large group of "Stimulated by Retinoic Acid" proteins.[183] Patients harbored a constellation of defects including complex CHD. The function of the *STRA6* gene is unknown but should provide clues regarding the role of retinoic acid in cardiac development.

Noncardiac Maternal Illness

Diabetes

Studies on the complications of diabetes mellitus in pregnancy are numerous. A meta-analysis of 24 studies calculated a 3% relative risk of CHD for children of mothers with diabetes, although the severity of the diabetes and the degree of control can exert a substantial effect on the risk.[2] Whether a specific cardiac lesion is associated with maternal diabetes remains controversial.[19] Fetal ultrasound examinations at 16, 20, and 24 weeks of gestation are recommended during the pregnancy of diabetic mothers.

Phenylketonuria

In uncontrolled phenylketonuria (PKU) with maternal blood levels of phenylalanine above 1.2 mM/L (20 mg/dl), the teratogenic risk of mental retardation is as high as 90%, and the risk of CHD is approximately 15% with TOF and other conotruncal malformations the most common. The risk of CHD is dose-dependent with no adverse effect on women whose phenylalanine blood levels are kept under 360 μM/L.[184] In a study in which the diet was begun postconception, three of six pregnancies resulted in severe or lethal fetal CHD. In contrast, a preconception PKU diet was associated with no CHD in the offspring of 33 of 34 pregnancies,[185] and a larger study disclosed no CHD in offspring of mothers whose levels of phenylalanine were controlled during the first 2 months of pregnancy.[186]

A preconception maternal diet appears to be effective in preventing fetal malformations provided it is started early enough to ensure stabilization of phenylalanine blood level at nonteratogenic levels. However, the special diet is demanding and becomes even more unappealing during the first trimester of pregnancy. Psychosocial support for these mothers is crucial for success.

Infectious Agents: Rubella

Maternal infection with rubella roughly doubles the risk of CHD in the offspring, a risk that decreases with the gestational age at which the infection occurs. First trimester exposure was associated with rubella embryopathy and CHD in 50% to 70% of children. Patent ductus arteriosus and pulmonary artery stenosis were characteristic. Because of widespread vaccination in developed countries, rubella is no longer a significant cause of CHD, but the infection remains an underrecognized public health problem in countries where rubella vaccination is not employed.

Multifactorial Causes of Congenital Heart Disease

The extremely variable expressions of CHD, well represented by the spectrum of anomalies associated with the 22q11 deletion syndrome, have led to underestimation of the contribution of genetic factors to etiology. Although identification of mutations in human subjects and in many engineered animal models have underscored the genetic basis of CHD, it is still not possible to predict the severity of phenotype for a given mutation. The impact of a genetic mutation is influenced by multigenic traits that incur additional contributions to the establishment of disease and by factors that modify gene-environment interactions (genetic susceptibility). Because of genetic diversity and multiple environmental influences, clear examples are yet to be demonstrated in human subjects. However, two examples from mouse models illustrate the methods available for identification of such modifiers. One example is derived from a mouse mutant model of Alagille syndrome, a pleiotropic disorder characterized by defects of the liver, heart (pulmonary stenosis the most frequent), eyes, and brain (OMIM#118450). Most cases of this dominantly inherited disease are caused by mutations in a gene called JAGGED1, which encodes a ligand for the Notch family of cell signaling receptors. Attempts to relate the variability of presentation to a particular type of JAG1 mutation have been unsuccessful,[187] suggesting that there are other influences such as modifier genes. The mouse model in which Jag1 is deleted has eye defects but does not involve the other organs affected in Alagille syndrome.[188] However, a mouse heterozygous for mutations in both Jag1 and its receptor Notch2 exhibits defects in organs similar to those in Alagille patients.[189] Interaction between the Jagged ligand and the Notch2 receptor could explain the variability of the clinical phenotype, but patients with mutations in both Jagged and Notch have not been identified. This observation has led to a search for mutations in the human NOTCH2 gene in Alagille patients who do not harbor a JAGGED1 mutation,[190] demonstrating that heterozygous deficiency of two genes coding for related proteins—the Jagged ligand and Notch receptor—may be important for development of the Alagille syndrome–related phenotype.

Another approach is a blind, genome-wide search without prior assumptions of what the modifier genes might be. In 2002, the first mapping of a genetic locus that influenced the severity of a cardiovascular disorder was reported.[191] Transgenic mice that overexpress calsequestrin, a calcium-binding protein found in the sarcoplasmic reticulum, develop severe dilated cardiomyopathy. Severity and survival rates vary greatly when the same transgene is expressed in different inbred mouse strains. Survival and disease severity both worsened when the mutation was on the C57Bl/6 mouse strain compared with the DBA strain, suggesting that the C57Bl/6 was contributing a dominant susceptibility allele to the cardiomyopathy phenotype.[191] Conversely, another mouse strain, the AKR background, provided a protective effect on the phenotype, increasing survival compared with the DBA strain.[192] Quantitative trait locus mapping is a method that allows identification of linkage of a particular trait, such as severity of cardiomyopathy or lethality, to regions of the genome. A genome-wide search identified two main regions in the C57Bl/6 background, one responsible for decreased survival and the other, on mouse chromosome 3, for decreased survival and heart function.[191] On the other hand, backcrossing DBA/AKR hybrids onto the AKR background has identified two other loci, differing between the AKR and DBA strains, that were each responsible for about 20% of the genetic variability and survival rates. In addition, two more loci were identified; on one locus, the AKR allele provided improved heart function, whereas the other locus conferred increased survival.[192] When the reciprocal backcross (DBA/AKR onto the DBA background) was performed, a locus on which the DBA allele conferred protection for both survival and heart function was identified on chromosome 3.[193] Fine genetic mapping then showed that this locus was overlapping with the locus that conferred susceptibility in the C57Bl/6 strain, suggesting that AKR and C57Bl/6 shared the same ancestral allele. Haplotype sequencing of the overlapping loci identified a smaller region between the two strains that probably contains the causative locus. Thus, the main candidate region was narrowed down to a 2-megabase region that contains only eight candidate genes. The search for differences of expression or genetic polymorphisms in these genes is in progress to identify which one is the cardiomyopathy phenotype modifier.

CLINICAL PRACTICE

Clinical Diagnosis

An important clinical question is whether a congenital heart defect is isolated or part of a syndrome. In the event of a syndrome, knowledge of associated abnormalities is necessarily important. Patients with Marfan syndrome have lenticular dislocation, and patients with Down syndrome can develop premature Alzheimer disease. Knowledge of comorbidities is also important in formulating a diagnosis. Coexistence of pulmonary stenosis and hepatic defects should raise suspicion of Alagille syndrome. Many CHD syndromes are associated with learning disabilities and behavioral abnormalities (see Chapter 13). Behavioral and speech therapy benefit patients with Down, Alagille, and Williams syndrome.

Genetic Diagnosis

DNA mutation analysis can be clinically helpful in two settings. The first involves using the genetic information for prenatal diagnosis. When a specific gene has been established as causative for a specific CHD, DNA mutational analysis can determine whether a particular mutation will be transmitted to the fetus. This information is helpful for parents and physicians and assists in deciding whether to terminate a pregnancy. A second setting in which mutational analysis is clinically useful is in providing a diagnosis when there is phenotypic overlap between two syndromes.

Mutational analysis is currently available for only a few Mendelian conditions. Mutations that cause CHD can occur within a gene or in a noncoding region (discussed earlier). Many genes are large, and the nature of the mutation can vary between individuals. Sequencing the entire gene may be required to identify potential causative mutations. This is seldom practical for a clinical laboratory but can be performed as research. New technologies continue to develop and promise to make mutational analysis feasible. A screen for mutations associated with cardiomyopathies—long unavailable because of the sheer size of the genes to be tested—is now being performed. The test is currently reimbursed by medical insurance on an individual case basis. An invaluable resource for information on the molecular bases of a particular CHD and the available testing is provided by the National Institutes of Health–funded Web site (www.genetests.com) that contains a regularly updated database of laboratory directories, as well as expert-authored disease reviews.

In cases of syndromic CHD, chromosomal testing is available. Most frequently, FISH is used to detect chromosomal anomalies such as trisomies or small deletions (see Fig. 10–9). FISH can be performed with specific probes that identify deletions in the critical 22q11 DiGeorge syndrome region or for the critical Williams syndrome region on chromosome 7. Because of a relative inability to identify the etiology of most CHDs, clinical teams have fallen prey to the "Casablanca syndrome," which calls for rounding of the usual suspects. The genetic equivalent of the usual suspect in any conotruncal anomaly is the cytogenetic test for chromosomal deletion in 22q11. After the introduction of FISH for 22q11 deletion, cause became apparent, and 22q11 deletions were detected in families with recurring CHD.[194] The FISH cytogenetic test for 22q11 deletions is an excellent tool for certain cardiovascular malformations. Fifty percent of patients with interrupted aortic arch, 35% with truncus arteriosus, and 15% with tetralogy of Fallot harbor a 22q11 deletion.[64]

Newer genetic technologies include comparative genomic hybridization (CGH), which might soon render cytogenetics obsolete. Microarray-based CGH allows detection of gene copy numbers, and unlike classical cytogenetics, can detect small chromosomal deletions. CGH was critical in identifying *CHD7* as a gene responsible for CHARGE syndrome that is characterized by Coloboma, Heart Anomaly, choanal atresia, Retardation, Genital, and Ear anomalies[195] (discussed earlier). CGH is faster than FISH, requires a smaller DNA sample, and the price will soon be competitive with cytogenetics. Several commercial companies already offer specialized chips arrayed with DNA probes that permit diagnosis of dozens of rare disorders with a single DNA sample, including Alagille syndrome, DiGeorge syndrome, and X-linked heterotaxy.

Genetic Counseling

As more genes and pathways that have an impact on cardiac development are identified, the role of the geneticist in the care of CHD patients will become more important, especially in syndromic CHD. The geneticist will identify other organs at risk, assist in coordinating follow-up, provide advice regarding reproductive planning, and may recommend genetic or clinical testing of first-degree relatives who are unaware that they harbor CHD. Patients will have information sufficient to provide a basis for judgment on reproductive decisions. The genetics counselor should discuss with the patient the nature, implications, and accuracy of genetic testing. As the life span of patients lengthens, genetic counseling will be directed less to the parents than to the patients themselves.

Risk to the Fetus: Recurrence Risk

In clinical practice, the genetic counselor is likely to quote a 5% recurrence risk to the first-degree relative of a patient. This empirical number is largely the result of an inability to attribute a simple genetic mechanism to CHD, a conclusion that is rapidly changing. Risks are appreciably different depending on the etiology of the CHD. On the basis of purely genetic factors, the risk is 25% for autosomal recessive transmission with the same parents, 50% for autosomal-dominant transmission and, for mitochondrial transmission, 0% to 100% if the mother is the proband, 0% if the father is the proband. At the other end of the spectrum, the risk of transmission may be related solely to environmental factors (population risk). However, most CHDs have multifactorial or multigenic etiologies for which the quantitative contribution of each causative factor cannot be calculated. We must then rely on recurrence risks assessed by population studies showing that rates are dependent on the sex of the proband and the cardiac lesion.[196]

In 2003, a prospective study was performed on a cohort of 6640 fetuses with a first-degree relative who had

CHD.[197] The assessment method was fetal echocardiography to ensure that recurrences were identified even in pregnancies that end in fetal loss (spontaneous or induced abortions). The first-degree relative was the mother in 17% of cases, the father in 6%, and a sibling in 77%. CHD was found in 2.7% of pregnancies, and recurrence risks of 2.9%, 2.7%, and 2.2% were calculated when the proband was the mother, a sibling, or the father, respectively. The lower maternal recurrence risk compared with previous studies was attributed to an ascertainment bias because the study was not population-based. Concordance of the type of lesion present in two members of a family was also assessed. Exact concordance was found in 37% of the cases, and group concordance (lesion thought to have a similar embryological origin) was found in 47%, indicating that in more than half the cases, there was no concordance in members of a same family, underscoring the difficulty in assessment of recurrence risk in CHD. Even in families in which multiple recurrences suggested monogenic inheritance, concordance was not higher than 60% and therefore not predictable. Importantly, the disease can be more severe in recurrences than in the index case or vice versa, with no means of predicting disease severity. This observation illustrates the difficulty confronting geneticists when CHD presents with variable penetrance (whether the disease will be manifest in an individual at risk) and with considerable phenotypic variability even for monogenic disorders.

Recurrence risk varies considerably with the type of lesion (Table 10–5). The different types of left heart obstructive defects (aortic stenosis, hypoplastic left heart syndrome, and coarctation of the aorta) are often segregated in families, suggesting that they are part of a phenotypic spectrum of similar etiology. Familial recurrence was high in this phenotypic spectrum, probably reflecting high genetic contribution with autosomal recessive or dominant inheritance patterns.[197-199] Recurrence risks in 178 fetuses were 38%, 33%, and 13% for aortic stenosis, hypoplastic left heart syndrome, and coarctation of the aorta, respectively. In the phenotypic group of septal defects, exact concordance was found in 80% of atrioventricular septal defects, similar to other studies. Concordance was also high for VSD (55%) but was zero for ASD. In addition, high variability of VSD severity was reflected in cases of recurrence. Similar discrepancies were observed for lesions generally grouped under the "outflow tract defect" label. Recurrence risk was 60% for common arterial trunk, 43% for tetralogy of Fallot, 25% for transposition of the great arteries, but zero for pulmonary atresia with ventricular septal defect. Interestingly, a high recurrence risk (64%) was found for laterality defects (isomerism or inversion), but recurrences could present as TGA or even simple VSD.

Table 10–5   Nonsyndromic Congenital Heart Defect, Implicated Mode of Inheritance, Recurrence Risk, and Genes

CONGENITAL HEART DEFECT	MODE OF INHERITANCE	RECURRENCE RISK	GENES
Atrioventricular canal defect	Multifactorial	3–4%	—
	Autosomal dominant	50%	p93
			CRELD1
			GATA4
			PTPN11
Tetralogy of Fallot	Multifactorial	2.5–3%	—
	Autosomal dominant	50%	NKX2.5
			Jagged 1
			FOG2
	Autosomal recessive	25%	—
	Three-gene model	2.5–3%	—
	Autosomal dominant	50%	CFC1
Transposition of the great arteries	Multifactorial	1–1.8%	—
	Autosomal dominant	50%	CFC1
Congenitally corrected transposition of the great arteries	Multifactorial	5.8%	—
Left-sided obstructions	Multifactorial	3%	—
	Autosomal dominant	50%	NOTCH1
			NKX2.5
	Autosomal recessive	25%	—
Atrial septal defect	Multifactorial	3%	—
	Autosomal dominant	50%	NKX2.5
			GATA4
			MHC6

With permission from Calcagni, G., et al.: *Eur J Pediatr* 2007;166:111–116.

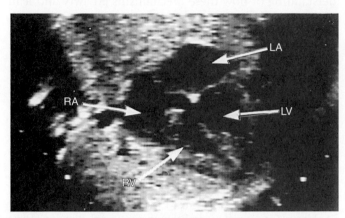

FIGURE 10-16 Fetal echocardiogram of a normal heart. LA, left atrium; LV, left ventricle; RA, right atrium; RV, right ventricle. *(Courtesy of Dr. Stacey E. Drant, Division of Pediatric Cardiology, UCLA Medical Center.)*

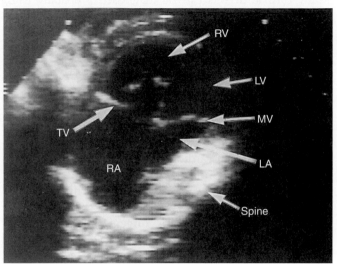

FIGURE 10-18 Fetal echocardiogram of Ebstein's anomaly of the tricuspid valve (TV) with the septal leaflet displaced into the right ventricle (RV). The right atrium (RA) is enlarged. LA, left atrium; LV, left ventricle; MV, mitral valve. *(Courtesy of Dr. Stacey E. Drant, Division of Pediatric Cardiology, UCLA Medical Center.)*

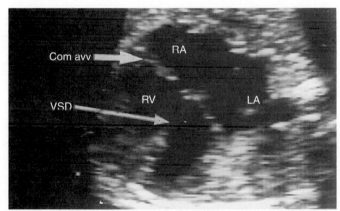

FIGURE 10-17 Fetal echocardiogram of a large-inlet ventricular septal defect (VSD) and the accompanying common atrioventricular valve (Com avv). LA, left atrium; RA, right atrium; RV, right ventricle. *(Courtesy of Dr. Stacey E. Drant, Division of Pediatric Cardiology, UCLA Medical Center.)*

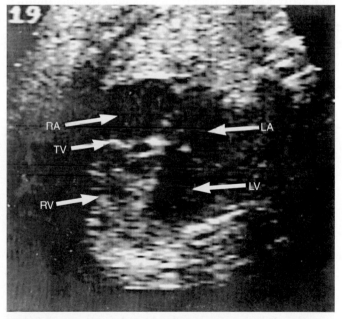

FIGURE 10-19 Fetal echocardiogram of pulmonary atresia with intact ventricular septum, hypoplastic right ventricle (RV), and hypoplastic tricuspid valve (TV). The right atrium (RA) is enlarged. LA, left atrium; LV, left ventricle. *(Courtesy of Dr. Stacey E. Drant, Division of Pediatric Cardiology, UCLA Medical Center.)*

Prenatal Diagnosis of Congenital Heart Disease

Many cardiac defects can be diagnosed prenatally using ultrasonography. A general morphologic survey (high-resolution ultrasound or level II scan) is currently part of the routine prenatal diagnostic regimen. Examination includes a brief cardiac examination in the form of a four-chamber view of the heart (Fig. 10–16) and perhaps a view of the aortic arch. A pregnancy in which CHD is suspected should have an echocardiogram targeted to the fetal heart by a sonographer specially skilled in the technique. The examination includes conventional real-time ultrasonography, M-mode echocardiography, and Doppler interrogation with color flow imaging (see Chapter 6).

With the technology and expertise currently available, it is possible to identify with certainty the intrauterine presence of most of the major congenital heart defects.[200] VSDs (Fig. 10–17), Ebstein's anomaly (Fig. 10–18), and pulmonary atresia with intact ventricular septum (Fig. 10–19) are a few examples. The results are reassuring when the fetus is unaffected. Early identification of a congenital heart defect in the fetus allows the parents to terminate the pregnancy if they consider the malformation unacceptable. The presence of lethal anomalies in the fetus serves to prevent needless interventions that might further jeopardize an already compromised gravida. Early identification of defects also permits mothers with affected fetuses to undergo planned delivery in tertiary care facilities. A cardiac defect in the fetus mandates a rigorous search for associated noncardiac anomalies, even if there is a family history of CHD. The search should include chromosomal analysis, as well as detailed ultrasonography.[201-203]

CONCLUSION

Congenital cardiovascular malformations result from heredity, from environmental exposure, or from genetic-environmental interactions. However, most malformations cannot be assigned to these categories, and many cases of inherited malformations remain unexplained by classic genetics. A significant hindrance to the analysis of inheritance of congenital heart defects is an inability to separate patients into meaningful categories. Current classifications use the anatomic type of lesion, whereas a more useful system classifies the defects into developmental mechanistic groups that reflect pathogenesis. Few families contain a sufficient number of members to permit recurrence risk figures to be generated on the basis of that family alone. Accordingly, average recurrence risks must be used in counseling, despite the many genetic mechanisms and recurrence risks represented in the population.

Genetic diagnosis of the etiology of CHD may have prognostic implications, but there are currently no tailored therapies based on specific gene defects. Nevertheless, a genetic diagnosis improves our ability to counsel CHD patients and their families, to prevent future CHD by family planning, and to reduce environmental risk factors. As our understanding of the genes that orchestrate developmental processes increases, so will our understanding of how these mechanisms go awry and lead to congenital cardiovascular defects. As our understanding of the molecular mechanisms of CHD increases, so will our understanding of acquired and associated heart diseases such as heart failure and arrhythmias.

References

1. Hoffman JI, Kaplan S. The incidence of congenital heart disease. *J Am Coll Cardiol.* 2002;39:1890–1900.
2. Pexieder T. Teratogens. In: Pierpont MEM, Moller JH, eds. *The Genetics of Cardiovascular Disease.* Boston: Martinus Nijhoff, 1987.
3. Marelli AJ, Mackie AS, Ionescu-Ittu R, et al. Congenital heart disease in the general population: changing prevalence and age distribution. *Circulation.* 2007;115:163–172.
4. Ferencz C. Origin of congenital heart disease: reflections on Maude Abbott's work. *Can J Cardiol.* 1989;5:4–9.
5. Allan L. Antenatal diagnosis of heart disease. *Heart.* 2000;83:367.
6. Warnes CA, Liberthson RR, Danielson GKJ, et al. Task Force 1: the changing profile of congenital heart disease in adult life. *J Am Coll Cardiol.* 2001;37:1170–1175.
7. Samanek M. Boy:girl ratio in children born with different forms of cardiac malformation: a population-based study. *Pediatr Cardiol.* 1994;15:53–57.
8. Hoffman JI. Incidence of congenital heart disease: II. Prenatal incidence. *Pediatr Cardiol.* 1995;16:155–165.
9. Wimalasundera RC, Gardiner HM. Congenital heart disease and aneuploidy. *Prenat Diagn.* 2004;24:1116–1122.
10. Xin HB, Senbonmatsu T, Cheng DS, et al. Oestrogen protects FKBP12.6 null mice from cardiac hypertrophy. *Nature.* 2002;416:334–338.
11. Pradat P, Francannet C, Harris JA, Robert E. The epidemiology of cardiovascular defects, Part I: a study based on data from three large registries of congenital malformations. *Pediatr Cardiol.* 2003;24:195–221.
12. Botto LD, Correa A, Erickson JD. Racial and temporal variations in the prevalence of heart defects. *Pediatrics.* 2001;107:E32–.
13. Correa-Villasenor A, Ferencz C, Neill CA, et al. Ebstein's malformation of the tricuspid valve: genetic and environmental factors. The Baltimore-Washington Infant Study Group. *Teratology.* 1994;50:137–147.
14. Fixler DE, Pastor P, Sigman E, Eifler CW. Ethnicity and socioeconomic status: impact on the diagnosis of congenital heart disease. *J Am Coll Cardiol.* 1993;21:1722–1726.
15. Hoffman JI, Kaplan S, Liberthson RR. Prevalence of congenital heart disease. *Am Heart J.* 2004;147:425.
16. Srivastava D. Heart disease: an ongoing genetic battle? *Nature.* 2004;429:819–822.
17. Hanson-Morris KA, Pelech AN. The Wisconsin Pediatric Cardiac Registry: a mechanism for exploring etiologies of congenital heart defects. *WMJ.* 2006;105:45–48.
18. van der Velde ET, Vriend JW, Mannens MM, et al. CONCOR, an initiative towards a national registry and DNA-bank of patients with congenital heart disease in the Netherlands: rationale, design, and first results. *Eur J Epidemiol.* 2005;20:549–557.

19. Harris JA, Francannet C, Pradat P, Robert E. The epidemiology of cardiovascular defects, part 2: a study based on data from three large registries of congenital malformations. *Pediatr Cardiol.* 2003; 24:222-235.

20. Hook EB. Down syndrome: its frequency in human populations and factors pertinent to variation in rates. In: de la Cruz FF, Gerald PS, eds. *Trisomy 21 (Down Syndrome): Research Perspectives.* Baltimore: University Park Press: Baltimore, 1981;3-67.

21. Perloff JK. *The Clinical Recognition of Congenital Heart Disease.* 5th ed. Philadelphia: W.B. Saunders, 2003.

22. Pierpont MEM, Gorlin RJ, Moller JH. Chromosomal abnormalities. In: Pierpont MEM, Moller JH, eds. *Genetics of Cardiovascular Disease.* Boston: Martinus Nijhoff, 1987;13-24.

23. Reeves RH, Baxter LL, Richtsmeier JT. Too much of a good thing: mechanisms of gene action in Down syndrome. *Trends Genet.* 2001;17:83-88.

24. Korenberg JR, Bradley C, Disteche CM. Down syndrome: molecular mapping of the congenital heart disease and duodenal stenosis. *Am J Hum Genet.* 1992;50:294-302.

25. Barlow GM, Chen XN, Shi ZY, et al. Down syndrome congenital heart disease: a narrowed region and a candidate gene. *Genet Med.* 2001;3:91-101.

26. Sheffield VC, Pierpont ME, Nishimura D, et al. Identification of a complex congenital heart defect susceptibility locus by using DNA pooling and shared segment analysis. *Hum Mol Genet.* 1997;6: 117-121.

27. Phipps ME, Latif F, Prowse A, et al. Molecular genetic analysis of the 3p- syndrome. *Hum Mol Genet.* 1994;3:903-908.

28. Green EK, Priestley MD, Waters J, et al. Detailed mapping of a congenital heart disease gene in chromosome 3p25. *J Med Genet.* 2000;37:581-587.

29. Maslen C, Babcock D, Robinson SW, et al. CRELD1 mutations contribute to the occurrence of cardiac atrioventricular septal defects in Down syndrome. *Am J Med Genet.* 2006;140A:2501-2505.

30. Fixler DE, Threlkeld N. Prenatal exposures and congenital heart defects in Down syndrome infants. *Teratology.* 1998;58:6-12.

31. Ferencz C, Correa-Villasenor A, Loffredo CA, Wilson PD. *Genetics and Environmental Risk Factors of Major Cardiovascular Malformations: the Baltimore-Washington Infant Study.* Perspectives in Pediatric Cardiology. Vol. 5. Armonk, NY: Futura, 1997;1981-1989.

32. O'Doherty A, Ruf S, Mulligan C, et al. An aneuploid mouse strain carrying human chromosome 21 with Down syndrome phenotypes. *Science.* 2005;309:2033-2037.

33. Berry AC, Mutton DE, Lewis DG. Mosaicism and the trisomy 8 syndrome. *Clin Genet.* 1978;14:105-114.

34. Tucker ME, Garringer HJ, Weaver DD. Phenotypic spectrum of mosaic trisomy 18: two new patients, a literature review, and counseling issues. *Am J Med Genet.* 2007;143A:505-517.

35. Hook EB, Warburton D. The distribution of chromosomal genotypes associated with Turner's syndrome: livebirth prevalence rates and evidence for diminished fetal mortality and severity in genotypes associated with structural X abnormalities or mosaicism. *Hum Genet.* 1983;64:24-27.

36. Ogata T, Matsuo N. Turner syndrome and female sex chromosome aberrations: deduction of the principal factors involved in the development of clinical features. *Hum Genet* 1995;95: 607-629.

37. Mazzanti L, Prandstraller D, Tassinari D, et al. Heart disease in Turner's syndrome. *Helv Paediatr Acta.* 1988;43:25-31.

38. Natowicz M, Kelley RI. Association of Turner syndrome with hypoplastic left-heart syndrome. *Am J Dis Child.* 1987;141:218-220.

39. van Egmond H, Orye E, Praet M, et al. Hypoplastic left heart syndrome and 45X karyotype. *Br Heart J.* 1988;60:69-71.

40. Ho VB, Bakalov VK, Cooley M, et al. Major vascular anomalies in Turner syndrome: prevalence and magnetic resonance angiographic features. *Circulation.* 2004;110:1694-1700.

41. Elsheikh M, Casadei B, Conway GS, Wass JA. Hypertension is a major risk factor for aortic root dilatation in women with Turner's syndrome. *Clin Endocrinol (Oxf).* 2001;54:69-73.

42. Gravholt CH, Naeraa RW, Nyholm B, et al. Glucose metabolism, lipid metabolism, and cardiovascular risk factors in adult Turner's syndrome. The impact of sex hormone replacement. *Diabetes Care.* 1998;21:1062-1070.

43. Gravholt CH, Juul S, Naeraa RW, Hansen J. Morbidity in Turner syndrome. *J Clin Epidemiol.* 1998;51:147-158.

44. Landin-Wilhelmsen K, Bryman I, Wilhelmsen L. Cardiac malformations and hypertension, but not metabolic risk factors, are common in Turner syndrome. *J Clin Endocrinol Metab.* 2001;86: 4166-4170.

45. Cooley M, Bakalov V, Bondy CA. Lipid profiles in women with 45,X vs 46,XX primary ovarian failure. *JAMA.* 2003;290:2127-2128.

46. Clark EB. Neck web and congenital heart defects: a pathogenic association in 45 X-O Turner syndrome? *Teratology.* 1984;29: 355-361.

47. Lacro RV, Jones KL, Benirschke K. Coarctation of the aorta in Turner syndrome: a pathologic study of fetuses with nuchal cystic hygromas, hydrops fetalis, and female genitalia. *Pediatrics.* 1988;81: 445-451.

48. Gravholt CH. Clinical practice in Turner syndrome. *Nature Clin Pract Endoc Metab.* 2005;1:41-52.

49. Ellison JW, Wardak Z, Young MF, et al. PHOG, a candidate gene for involvement in the short stature of Turner syndrome. *Hum Mol Genet.* 1997;6:1341-1347.

50. Rao E, Weiss B, Fukami M, et al. Pseudoautosomal deletions encompassing a novel homeobox gene cause growth failure in idiopathic short stature and Turner syndrome. *Nat Genet.* 1997;16: 54-63.

51. Demczuk S, Aurias A. DiGeorge syndrome and related syndromes associated with 22q11.2 deletions. A review. *Ann Genet.* 1995;38: 59-76.

52. Wilson DI, Burn J, Scambler P, Goodship J. DiGeorge syndrome: part of CATCH 22. *J Med Genet.* 1998;30:852-856.

53. Ryan AK, Goodship JA, Wilson DI, et al. Spectrum of clinical features associated with interstitial chromosome 22q11 deletions: a European collaborative study. *J Med Genet.* 1997;34:798-804.

54. Lindsay EA, Baldini A. Congenital heart defects and 22q11 deletions: which genes count? *Mol Med Today.* 1998;4:350-357.

55. Yamagishi H, Ishii C, Maeda J, et al. Phenotypic discordance in monozygotic twins with 22q11.2 deletion. *Am J Med Genet.* 1998;78: 319-321.

56. Scambler PJ. Genetics. Engineering a broken heart. *Nature.* 1999;401:335-337.

57. Lindsay EA, Botta A, Jurecic V, et al. Congenital heart disease in mice deficient for the DiGeorge syndrome region. *Nature.* 1999;401: 379-383.

58. Taddei I, Morishima M, Huynh T, Lindsay EA. Genetic factors are major determinants of phenotypic variability in a mouse model of the DiGeorge/del22q11 syndromes. *Proc Natl Acad Sci USA.* 2001;98: 11428-11431.

59. Paylor R, McIlwain KL, McAninch R, et al. Mice deleted for the DiGeorge/velocardiofacial syndrome region show abnormal sensorimotor gating and learning and memory impairments. *Hum Mol Genet.* 2001;10:2645-2650.

60. Jerome LA, Papaioannou VE. DiGeorge syndrome phenotype in mice mutant for the T-box gene, Tbx1. *Nat Genet.* 2001;27: 286-291.

61. Merscher S, Funke B, Epstein JA, et al. TBX1 is responsible for cardiovascular defects in velo-cardio-facial/DiGeorge syndrome. *Cell.* 2001;104:619-629.

62. Lindsay EA, Vitelli F, Su H, et al. Tbx1 haploinsufficiency in the DiGeorge syndrome region causes aortic arch defects in mice. *Nature.* 2001;410:97-101.

63. Yagi H, Furutani Y, Hamada H, et al. Role of TBX1 in human del22q11.2 syndrome. *Lancet.* 2003;362:1366–1373.

64. Goldmuntz E, Clark BJ, Mitchell LE, et al. Frequency of 22q11 deletions in patients with conotruncal defects. *J Am Coll Cardiol.* 1998;32:492–498.

65. Jalal SM, Crifasi PA, Karnes PS, Michels VV. Cytogenetic testing for Williams syndrome. *Mayo Clin Proc.* 1996;71:67–68.

66. Olson TM, Michels VV, Urban Z, et al. A 30 kb deletion within the elastin gene results in familial supravalvular aortic stenosis. *Hum Mol Genet.* 1995;4:1677–1679.

67. Tassabehji M, Hammond P, Karmiloff-Smith A, et al. GTF2IRD1 in craniofacial development of humans and mice. *Science.* 2005;310:1184–1187.

68. Hoogenraad CC, Akhmanova A, Galjart N, De Zeeuw CI. LIMK1 and CLIP-115: linking cytoskeletal defects to Williams syndrome. *Bioessays.* 2004;26:141–150.

69. Borg I, Delhanty JD, Baraitser M. Detection of hemizygosity at the elastin locus by FISH analysis as a diagnostic test in both classical and atypical cases of Williams syndrome. *J Med Genet.* 1995;32:692–696.

70. Gelb BD. Genetic basis of congenital heart disease. *Curr Opin Cardiol.* 2004;19:110–115.

71. Garg V, Kathiriya IS, Barnes R, et al. GATA4 mutations cause human congenital heart defects and reveal an interaction with TBX5. *Nature* .2003;424:443–447.

72. Noonan JA, Ehmke DA. Associated cardiac malformations in children with congenital heart disease. *Midwest Soc Pediatr Res.* 1963;63:468.

73. Kramer HH, Majewski F, Trampisch HJ, et al. Malformation patterns in children with congenital heart disease. *Am J Dis Child.* 1987;141:789–795.

74. Miller M, Motulsky AC. Noonan syndrome in an adult family presenting with chronic lymphedema. *Am J Med.* 1978;65:379–383.

75. Allanson JE. Noonan syndrome. *J Med Genet.* 1987;24:9–13.

76. Mendez HM, Opitz JM. Noonan syndrome: a review. *Am J Med Genet.* 1985;21:493–506.

77. Pearl W. Cardiovascular anomalies in Noonan's syndrome. *Chest.* 1977;71:677–679.

78. Kitchens CS, Alexander JA. Partial deficiency of coagulation factor XI as a newly recognized feature of Noonan syndrome. *J Pediatr.* 1983;102:224–227.

79. Nora JJ, Fraser FC. *Medical Genetics: Principles and Practice.* 3rd ed. Philadelphia: Lea & Ferbiger, 1989.

80. Tartaglia M, Mehler EL, Goldberg R, et al. Mutations in PTPN11, encoding the protein tyrosine phosphatase SHP-2, cause Noonan syndrome. *Nat Genet.* 2001;29:465–468.

81. Kosaki K, Suzuki T, Muroya K, et al. PTPN11 (protein-tyrosine phosphatase, nonreceptor-type 11) mutations in seven Japanese patients with Noonan syndrome. *J Clin Endocrinol Metab.* 2002;87:3529–3533.

82. Maheshwari M, Belmont J, Fernbach S, et al. PTPN11 mutations in Noonan syndrome type I: detection of recurrent mutations in exons 3 and 13. *Hum Mutat.* 2002;20:298–304.

83. Tartaglia M, Kalidas K, Shaw A, et al. PTPN11 mutations in Noonan syndrome: molecular spectrum, genotype-phenotype correlation, and phenotypic heterogeneity. *Am J Hum Genet.* 2002;70:1555–1563.

84. Lin AE, Grossfeld PD, Hamilton RM, et al. Further delineation of cardiac abnormalities in Costello syndrome. *Am J Med Genet.* 2002;111:115–129.

85. Sarkozy A, Conti E, Digilio MC, et al. Clinical and molecular analysis of 30 patients with multiple lentigines LEOPARD syndrome. *J Med Genet.* 2004;41:e68.

86. Noonan JA. Noonan syndrome and related disorders: alterations in growth and puberty. *Rev Endoc Metab Disord.* 2006;7:251–255.

87. Aoki Y, Niihori T, Kawame H, et al. Germline mutations in HRAS proto-oncogene cause Costello syndrome. *Nature Genet.* 2005;37:1038–1040.

88. Niihori T, Aoki Y, Narumi Y, et al. Germline KRAS and BRAF mutations in cardio-facio-cutaneous syndrome. *Nat Genet.* 2006;38:294–296.

89. Rodriguez-Viciana P, Tetsu O, Tidyman WE, et al. Germline mutations in genes within the MAPK pathway cause cardio-facio-cutaneous syndrome. *Science.* 2006;311:1287–1290.

90. Araki T, Mohi MG, Ismat FA, et al. Mouse model of Noonan syndrome reveals cell type- and gene dosage-dependent effects of Ptpn11 mutation. *Nat Med.* 2004;10:849–857.

91. Holt M, Oram S. Familial heart disease with skeletal malformations. *Br Heart J.* 1960;22:236–242.

92. Lin AE, Perloff JK. Upper limb malformations associated with congenital heart disease. *Am J Cardiol.* 1985;55:1576–1583.

93. Smith AT, Sack GH Jr, Taylor GJ. Holt-Oram syndrome. *J Pediatr.* 1979;95:538.

94. Basson CT, Cowley GS, Solomon SD, et al. The clinical and genetic spectrum of the Holt-Oram syndrome (heart-hand syndrome). *N Engl J Med.* 1994;330:885–891.

95. Basson CT, Bachinsky DR, Lin RC, et al. Mutations in human TBX5 [corrected] cause limb and cardiac malformation in Holt-Oram syndrome. *Nat Genet.* 1997;15:30–35.

96. Li QY, Newbury-Ecob RA, Terrett JA, et al. Holt-Oram syndrome is caused by mutations in TBX5, a member of the Brachyury (T) gene family. *Nat Genet.* 1997;15:21–29.

97. Bruneau BG, Nemer G, Schmitt JP, et al. A murine model of Holt-Oram syndrome defines roles of the T-box transcription factor Tbx5 in cardiogenesis and disease. *Cell.* 2001;106:709–721.

98. McDermott DA, Bressan MC, He J, et al. TBX5 genetic testing validates strict clinical criteria for Holt-Oram syndrome. *Pediatr Res.* 2005;58:981–986.

99. Bowers PN, Brueckner M, Yost HJ. The genetics of left-right development and heterotaxia. *Semin Perinatol.* 1996;20:577–588.

100. Casey B. Two rights make a wrong: human left-right malformations. *Hum Mol Genet.* 1998;7:1565–1571.

101. Belmont JW, Mohapatra B, Towbin JA, Ware SM. Molecular genetics of heterotaxy syndromes. *Curr Opin Cardiol.* 2004;19:216–220.

102. Bisgrove BW, Morelli SH, Yost HJ. Genetics of human laterality disorders: insights from vertebrate model systems. *Annu Rev Genomics Hum Genet.* 2003;4:1–32.

103. Miller RD, Divertie MB. Kartagener's syndrome. *Chest.* 1972;62:130–135.

104. Kartagener M, Stucki P. Bronchiectasis with situs inversus. *Arch Pediatr.* 1962;79:193–207.

105. Afzelius BA, Eliasson R, Johnsen O, Lindholmer C. Lack of dynein arms in immotile human spermatozoa. *J Cell Biol.* 1975;66:225–232.

106. Eliasson R, Mossberg B, Camner P, Afzelius BA. The immotile-cilia syndrome. A congenital ciliary abnormality as an etiologic factor in chronic airway infections and male sterility. *N Engl J Med.* 1977;297:1–6.

107. Layton WM Jr. Random determination of a developmental process: reversal of normal visceral asymmetry in the mouse. *J Hered.* 1976;67:336–338.

108. Layton WM Jr. Heart malformations in mice homozygous for a gene causing situs inversus. *Birth Defects Orig Artic Ser.* 1978;14:277–293.

109. Ensing GJ, Schmidt MA, Hagler DJ, et al. Spectrum of findings in a family with nonsyndromic autosomal dominant supravalvular aortic stenosis: a Doppler echocardiographic study. *J Am Coll Cardiol.* 1989;13:413–419.

110. Chiarella F, Bricarelli FD, Lupi G, et al. Familial supravalvular aortic stenosis: a genetic study. *J Med Genet.* 1989;26:86–92.

111. Williams JC, Barratt-Boyes BG, Lowe JB. Supravalvular aortic stenosis. *Circulation.* 1961;24:1311–1318.

112. Beuren AJ, Schulze C, Eberle P, et al. The syndrome of supravalvular aortic stenosis, peripheral pulmonary stenosis, mental

retardation and similar facial appearance. *Am J Cardiol.* 1964;13: 471–483.

113. Niwa K, Perloff JK, Bhuta SM, et al. Structural abnormalities of great arterial walls in congenital heart disease: light and electron microscopic analyses. *Circulation.* 2001;103:393–400.

114. Francke U, Berg MA, Tynan K, et al. A Gly1127Ser mutation in an EGF-like domain of the fibrillin-1 gene is a risk factor for ascending aortic aneurysm and dissection. *Am J Hum Genet.* 1995;56:1287–1296.

115. Kainulainen K, Karttunen L, Puhakka L, et al. Mutations in the fibrillin gene responsible for dominant ectopia lentis and neonatal Marfan syndrome. *Nat Genet.* 1994;6:64–69.

116. Isogai Z, Ono RN, Ushiro S, et al. Latent transforming growth factor beta-binding protein 1 interacts with fibrillin and is a microfibril-associated protein. *J Biol Chem.* 2003;278:2750–2757.

117. Loeys BL, Chen J, Neptune ER, et al. A syndrome of altered cardiovascular, craniofacial, neurocognitive and skeletal development caused by mutations in TGFBR1 or TGFBR2. *Nat Genet.* 2005;37:275–281.

118. Habashi JP, Judge DP, Holm TM, et al. Losartan, an AT1 antagonist, prevents aortic aneurysm in a mouse model of Marfan syndrome. *Science.* 2006;312:117–121.

119. Keating MT, Sanguinetti MC. Molecular genetic insights into cardiovascular disease. *Science.* 1996;272:681–685.

120. Towbin JA. New revelations about the long-QT syndrome. *N Engl J Med.* 1995;333:384–385.

121. Towbin JA, Li H, Taggart RT, et al. Evidence of genetic heterogeneity in Romano-Ward long QT syndrome. Analysis of 23 families. *Circulation.* 1994;90:2635–2644.

122. Towbin, JA. Molecular genetic aspects of the Romano-Ward long QT syndrome. *Tex Heart Inst J* 1994;21:42–47.

123. Modell SM, Lehmann MH. The long QT syndrome family of cardiac ion channelopathies: a HuGE review. *Genet Med.* 2006;8: 143–155.

124. Priori SG, Schwartz PJ, Napolitano C, et al. Risk stratification in the long-QT syndrome. *N Engl J Med.* 2003;348:1866–1874.

125. Johnson MC, Payne RM, Grant JW, Strauss AW. The genetic basis of paediatric heart disease. *Ann Med.* 1995;27:289–300.

126. Crittenden IH, Latta H, Ticinovich DA. Familial congenital heart block. *Am J Dis Child.* 1964;108:104–108.

127. Tiso N, Stephan DA, Nava A, et al. Identification of mutations in the cardiac ryanodine receptor gene in families affected with arrhythmogenic right ventricular cardiomyopathy type 2 (ARVD2). *Hum Mol Genet.* 2001;10:189–194.

128. McCue CM, Mantakas ME, Tingelstad JB, Ruddy S. Congenital heart block in newborns of mothers with connective tissue disease. *Circulation.* 1977;56:82–90.

129. Behan WM, Behan PO, Reid JM, et al. Family studies of congenital heart block associated with Ro antibody. *Br Heart J.* 1989;62: 320–324.

130. Rampazzo A, Beffagna G, Nava A, et al. Arrhythmogenic right ventricular cardiomyopathy type 1 (ARVD1): confirmation of locus assignment and mutation screening of four candidate genes. *Eur J Hum Genet.* 2003;11:69–76.

131. Beffagna G, Occhi G, Nava A, et al. Regulatory mutations in transforming growth factor-beta3 gene cause arrhythmogenic right ventricular cardiomyopathy type 1. *Cardiovasc Res.* 2005; 65:366–373.

132. Rampazzo A, Nava A, Malacrida S, et al. Mutation in human desmoplakin domain binding to plakoglobin causes a dominant form of arrhythmogenic right ventricular cardiomyopathy. *Am J Hum Genet.* 2002;71:1200–1206.

133. Syrris P, Ward D, Evans A, et al. Arrhythmogenic right ventricular dysplasia/cardiomyopathy associated with mutations in the desmosomal gene desmocollin-2. *Am J Hum Genet.* 2006;79:978–984.

134. Pilichou K, Nava A, Basso C, et al. Mutations in desmoglein-2 gene are associated with arrhythmogenic right ventricular cardiomyopathy. *Circulation.* 2006;113:1171–1179.

135. Rein AJ, Sheffer R. Genetics of conotruncal malformations: further evidence of autosomal recessive inheritance. *Am J Med Genet.* 1994;50:302–303.

136. Wulfsberg EA, Zintz EJ, Moore JW. The inheritance of conotruncal malformations: a review and report of two siblings with tetralogy of Fallot with pulmonary atresia. *Clin Genet.* 1991;40:12–16.

137. Digilio MC, Marino B, Giannotti A, et al. Recurrence risk figures for isolated tetralogy of Fallot after screening for 22q11 microdeletion. *J Med Genet.* 1997;34:188–190.

138. Pacileo G, Musewe NN, Calabro R. Tetralogy of Fallot in three siblings: a familial study and review of the literature. *Eur J Pediatr.* 1992;151:726–727.

139. Amati F, Mari A, Digilio MC, et al. 22q11 deletions in isolated and syndromic patients with tetralogy of Fallot. *Hum Genet.* 1995;95:479–482.

140. Sletten LJ, Pierpont ME. Familial occurrence of patent ductus arteriosus. *Am J Med Genet.* 1995;57:27–30.

141. Macdonald IL, McMurtry TJ, Dodek A. Atrial septal defect in adult identical twins: a variation in theme. *Clin Cardiol.* 1983;6: 507–510.

142. Li Volti S, Distefano G, Garozzo R, et al. Autosomal dominant atrial septal defect of ostium secundum type. Report of three families. *Ann Genet.* 1991;34:14–18.

143. Lynch HT, Bachenberg K, Harris RE, Becker W. Hereditary atrial septal defect. Update of a large kindred. *Am J Dis Child.* 1978;132:600–604.

144. Bleyl S, Ruttenberg HD, Carey JC, Ward K. Familial total anomalous pulmonary venous return: a large Utah-Idaho family. *Am J Med Genet.* 1994;52:462–466.

145. Kumar A, Victorica BE, Gessner IH, Alexander JA. Tricuspid atresia and annular hypoplasia: report of a familial occurrence. *Pediatr Cardiol.* 1994;15:201–203.

146. Abdallah H, Toomey K, O'Riordan AC, et al. Familial occurrence of discrete subaortic membrane. *Pediatr Cardiol.* 1994;15:198–200.

147. Chin TK, Perloff JK, Williams RG, et al. Isolated noncompaction of left ventricular myocardium. A study of eight cases. *Circulation.* 1990;82:507–513.

148. Stollberger C, Finsterer J, Blazek G. Left ventricular hypertrabeculation/noncompaction and association with additional cardiac abnormalities and neuromuscular disorders. *Am J Cardiol.* 2002; 90:899–902.

149. Ichida F, Tsubata S, Bowles KR, et al. Novel gene mutations in patients with left ventricular noncompaction or Barth syndrome. *Circulation.* 2001;103:1256–1263.

150. Chen R, Tsuji T, Ichida F, et al. Mutation analysis of the G4.5 gene in patients with isolated left ventricular noncompaction. *Mol Genet Metab.* 2002;77:319–325.

151. Kenton AB, Sanchez X, Coveler KJ, et al. Isolated left ventricular noncompaction is rarely caused by mutations in G4.5, alpha-dystrobrevin and FK Binding Protein-12. *Mol Genet Metab.* 2004;82:162–166.

152. Vatta M, Mohapatra B, Jimenez S, et al. Mutations in Cypher/ZASP in patients with dilated cardiomyopathy and left ventricular noncompaction. *J Am Coll Cardiol.* 2003;42:2014–2027.

153. Bione S, D'Adamo P, Maestrini E, et al. A novel X-linked gene, G4.5. is responsible for Barth syndrome. *Nat Genet.* 1996;12:385–389.

154. Nora JJ, Nora AH. Maternal transmission of congenital heart diseases: new recurrence risk figures and the questions of cytoplasmic inheritance and vulnerability to teratogens. *Am J Cardiol.* 1987;59:459–463.

155. Rose V, Gold RJ, Lindsay G, Allen M. A possible increase in the incidence of congenital heart defects among the offspring of affected parents. *J Am Coll Cardiol.* 1985;6:376–382.

156. Ferencz C. Offspring of fathers with cardiovascular malformations. *Am Heart J.* 1986;111:1212–1213.

157. Steinberg AG, Bearn AG, Motulsky AG, Childs, B, eds. *Genetics of Cardiovascular Disease.* Philadelphia: W.B. Saunders, 1983.

158. Whittemore R, Wells JA, Castellsague X. A second-generation study of 427 probands with congenital heart defects and their 837 children. *J Am Coll Cardiol.* 1994;23:1459–1467.

159. Tartaglia M, Cordeddu V, Chang H, et al. Paternal germline origin and sex-ratio distortion of PTPN11 mutations in Noonan syndrome. *Am J Hum Genet.* 2004;75:492–497.

160. Zeviani M, Bonilla E, DeVivo DC, DiMauro S. Mitochondrial diseases. *Neurol Clin.* 1989;7:123–156.

161. Wallace DC. Mitotic segregation of mitochondrial DNAs in human cell hybrids and expression of chloramphenicol resistance. *Somat Cell Mol Genet.* 1986;12:41–49.

162. Hiendleder S, Wolf E. The mitochondrial genome in embryo technologies. *Reprod Domest Anim.* 2003;38:290–304.

163. Zeviani M, Gellera C, Antozzi C, et al. Maternally inherited myopathy and cardiomyopathy: association with mutation in mitochondrial DNA tRNALeu(UUR). *Lancet.* 1991;338:143–147.

164. Sweeney MG, Brockington M, Weston MJ, et al. Mitochondrial DNA transfer RNA mutation Leu(UUR) A-G 3260. a second family with myopathy and cardiomyopathy. *Q J Med.* 1993;86:435–438.

165. Mariotti C, Tiranti V, Carrara F, et al. Defective respiratory capacity and mitochondrial protein synthesis in transformant cybrids harboring the tRNALeu(UUR) mutation associated with maternally inherited myopathy and cardiomyopathy. *J Clin Invest.* 1994;93:1102–1107.

166. Hoffman M. How parents make their mark on genes. *Science.* 1991;252:1250–1251.

167. Surani MAH. Evidences and consequences of differences between maternal and paternal genomes during embryogenesis in the mouse. In: Rossant J, Pedersen RA, eds. *Experimental Approaches to Mammalian Development.* Cambridge: Cambridge University Press, 1986.

168. Solter D. Differential imprinting and expression of maternal and paternal genomes. *Annu Rev Genet.* 1988;22:127–146.

169. Jaenisch R, Bird A. Epigenetic regulation of gene expression: how the genome integrates intrinsic and environmental signals. *Nat Genet.* 2003;33(Suppl):245–254.

170. Delaval K, Feil R. Epigenetic regulation of mammalian genomic imprinting. *Curr Opin Genet Dev.* 2004;14:188–195.

171. Malik S, Schecter A, Caughy M, Fixler DE. Effect of proximity to hazardous waste sites on the development of congenital heart disease. *Arch Environ Health.* 2004;59:177–181.

172. Ritz B, Yu F, Fruin S, et al. Ambient air pollution and risk of birth defects in Southern California. *Am J Epidemiol.* 2002;155:17–25.

173. Kohlhase J, Schubert L, Liebers M, et al. Mutations at the SALL4 locus on chromosome 20 result in a range of clinically overlapping phenotypes, including Okihiro syndrome, Holt-Oram syndrome, acro-renal-ocular syndrome, and patients previously reported to represent thalidomide embryopathy. *J Med Genet.* 2003;40:473–478.

174. Cooper WO, Hernandez-Diaz S, Arbogast PG, et al. Major congenital malformations after first-trimester exposure to ACE inhibitors. *N Engl J Med.* 2006;354:2443–2451.

175. Quan A. Fetopathy associated with exposure to angiotensin converting enzyme inhibitors and angiotensin receptor antagonists. *Early Hum Dev.* 2006;82:23–28.

176. Nora J, Nora AH, Toews WH. Lithium, Ebstein's anomaly, and other congenital heart defects. *Lancet.* 1974;2:594–595.

177. Jacobson SJ, Jones K, Johnson K, Ceolin L, et al. Prospective multicentre study of pregnancy outcome after lithium exposure during first trimester. *Lancet.* 339:530–533.

178. Streissguth AP, Clarren SK, Jones KL. Natural history of the fetal alcohol syndrome: a 10-year follow-up of eleven patients. *Lancet.* 1985;2:85–91.

179. Brent RL. Congenital malformations following exposure to progestational drugs: the last chapter of an erroneous allegation. *Birth Defects Res A Clin Mol Teratol.* 2005;73:906–918.

180. Macayran JF, Doroshow RW, Phillips J, et al. PAGOD syndrome: eighth case and comparison to animal models of congenital vitamin A deficiency. *Am J Med Genet.* 2002;108:229–234.

181. Lammer EJ, Chen DT, Hoar RM, et al. Retinoic acid embryopathy. *N Engl J Med.* 1985;313:837–841.

182. Loureiro KD, Kao KK, Jones KL, et al. Minor malformations characteristic of the retinoic acid embryopathy and other birth outcomes in children of women exposed to topical tretinoin during early pregnancy. *Am J Med Genet. A* 2005;136:117–121.

183. Pasutto F, Sticht H, Hammersen G, et al. Mutations in STRA6 cause a broad spectrum of malformations including anophthalmia, congenital heart defects, diaphragmatic hernia, alveolar capillary dysplasia, lung hypoplasia, and mental retardation. *Am J Hum Genet.* 2007;80:550–560.

184. Rouse B, Azen C, Koch R, et al. Maternal phenylketonuria collaborative study (MPKUCS) offspring: facial anomalies, malformations, and early neurological sequelae. *Am J Med Genet.* 1997;69:89–95.

185. Brenton DP, Lilburn M. Maternal phenylketonuria: a study from the United Kingdom. *Eur J Pediatr.* 1996;155(Suppl):177–180.

186. Rouse B, Matalon R, Koch R, et al. Maternal phenylketonuria syndrome: congenital heart defects, microcephaly, and developmental outcomes. *J Pediatr.* 2000;136:57–61.

187. McElhinney DB, Krantz ID, Bason L, et al. Analysis of cardiovascular phenotype and genotype-phenotype correlation in individuals with a *JAG1* mutation and/or Alagille syndrome. *Circulation.* 2002;106:2567–2574.

188. Xue Y, Gao X, Lindsell CE, et al. Embryonic lethality and vascular defects in mice lacking the Notch ligand Jagged1. *Hum Mol Genet.* 1999;8:723–730.

189. McCright B, Lozier J, Gridley T. A mouse model of Alagille syndrome: Notch2 as a genetic modifier of Jag1 haploinsufficiency. *Development.* 2002;129:1075–1082.

190. McDaniel R, Warthen DM, Sanchez-Lara PA, et al. NOTCH2 mutations cause Alagille syndrome, a heterogeneous disorder of the notch signaling pathway. *Am J Hum Genet.* 2006;79:169–173.

191. Suzuki M, Carlson KM, Marchuk DA, Rockman HA. Genetic modifier loci affecting survival and cardiac function in murine dilated cardiomyopathy. *Circulation.* 2002;105:1824–1829.

192. Le Corvoisier P, Park H.-Y, Carlson KM, et al. Multiple quantitative trait loci modify the heart failure phenotype in murine cardiomyopathy. *Hum Mol Genet.* 2003;12:3097–3107.

193. Wheeler FC, Fernandez L, Carlson KM, et al. QTL mapping in a mouse model of cardiomyopathy reveals an ancestral modifier allele affecting heart function and survival. *Mamm Genome.* 2005;16:414–423.

194. Wilson DI, Cross IE, Goodship JA, et al. A prospective cytogenetic study of 36 cases of DiGeorge syndrome. *Am J Hum Genet.* 1992;51:957–963.

195. Vissers LE, van Ravenswaaij CM, Admiraal R, et al. Mutations in a new member of the chromodomain gene family cause CHARGE syndrome. *Nature Genet.* 2004;36:955–957.

196. Burn J, Brennan P, Little J, et al. Recurrence risks in offspring of adults with major heart defects: results from first cohort of British collaborative study. *Lancet.* 1998;351:311–316.

197. Gill HK, Splitt M, Sharland GK, Simpson JM. Patterns of recurrence of congenital heart disease: an analysis of 6,640 consecutive pregnancies evaluated by detailed fetal echocardiography. *J Am Coll Cardiol.* 2003;42:923–929.

198. McBride KL, Pignatelli R, Lewin M, et al. Inheritance analysis of congenital left ventricular outflow tract obstruction malformations: segregation, multiplex relative risk, and heritability. *Am J Med Genet A.* 2005;134:180–186.

199. Calcagni G, Digilio MC, Sarkozy A, et al. Familial recurrence of congenital heart disease: an overview and review of the literature. *Eur J Pediatr.* 2007;166:111–116.

200. Ferrazzi E, Fesslova V, Bellotti M, et al. Prenatal diagnosis and management of congenital heart disease. *J Reprod Med.* 1989;34: 207–214.

201. Copel JA, Cullen M, Green JJ, et al. The frequency of aneuploidy in prenatally diagnosed congenital heart disease: an indication for fetal karyotyping. *Am J Obstet Gynecol.* 1988;158:409–413.

202. Wladimiroff JW, Stewart PA, Sachs ES, Niermeijer MF. Prenatal diagnosis and management of congenital heart defect: significance of associated fetal anomalies and prenatal chromosome studies. *Am J Med Genet.* 1985;21:285–290.

203. Berg KA, Clark EB, Astemborski JA, Boughman JA. Prenatal detection of cardiovascular malformations by echocardiography: an indication for cytogenetic evaluation. *Am J Obstet Gynecol.* 1988;159:477–481.

Exercise and Athletics in Adults with Congenital Heart Disease

JAMIL ABOULHOSN ▪ JOSEPH K. PERLOFF

It seems intuitive that cardiovascular reserve would be encroached upon in patients with congenital heart disease (CHD)—unoperated or postoperative. This chapter focuses on the type, intensity, and degree of exercise that is permissible, indeed, desirable in these patients. Ill-advised exercise incurs risk, but intermediate levels are tolerated and generally beneficial. An important additional factor is the effect of deconditioning that results from overprotection of well-meaning but misguided parents and physicians.

The 26th Bethesda Conference provided recommendations for participation in competitive sports by patients with various types of cardiovascular abnormalities,[1] and the American Heart Association provided recommendations for patients with CHD.[2] Exercise has been classified according to the degree of isometric or isotonic stress and according to whether the exercise is competitive or recreational. Recommendations take into account the nature of the congenital cardiovascular abnormality, the physiologic consequences of various types of exercise, and the risk of inducing an arrhythmia.

COMPETITIVE AND RECREATIONAL ATHLETICS

The distinction between competitive or recreational is less than categoric, so overlap is common.[3] *Competitive athletics* require vigorous, disciplined, systematic training that is physically and emotionally demanding (Table 11–1). Because high achievement and the desire to win are stated objectives, competitive athletics necessarily place greater demands on the cardiovascular system. *Recreational athletics* are less demanding because they require much less systematic training and are engaged in for pleasure, relaxation, and maintenance of weight and fitness rather than for high achievement and an unbridled desire to win[4] (see Table 11–1). However, pleasure and relaxation can become competitive.

Patients with CHD should be carefully advised regarding exercise and athletics.[4,5] Objective testing discloses limitations even among patients who consider themselves asymptomatic.[6,7] Simple measures of chronotropic competence and heart rate variability identify patients who are at risk.[8] Cardiopulmonary exercise testing defines maximal functional capacity and hemodynamic and electrophysiologic responses and is of prognostic importance.[3,5,7,9,10] In addition to the sometimes overly simplistic distinctions between competitive and recreational athletics, a number of other considerations determine recommendations for athletics: (1) the type, intensity, and duration of exercise; (2) the risk of bodily collision inherent in a given type of athletic activity; (3) the training (conditioning) required for a given athletic activity; (4) the emotional response (stress, anxiety) that the participant experiences in anticipation of or during a particular athletic activity; (5) the risk of bodily injury to the participant or to spectators or bystanders if the athletic activity is accompanied by loss of consciousness; and (6) locomotor factors affecting exercise (Table 11–2). Cardiovascular exercise assessments change over time and are influenced by training, but exercise testing is nevertheless important in overall risk stratification of adults with CHD (Fig. 11–1).

Table 11-1 Classification of Sports Based on Peak Isometric and Isotonic Components Incurred During Competition

	LOW ISOTONIC (<40% MAX O2)	MODERATE ISOTONIC (40-70% MAX O2)	HIGH ISOTONIC (>70% MAX O2)
I. Low isometric (<20% MVC)	Billiards Bowling Cricket Golf Riflery	Baseball Softball Table tennis Tennis (doubles) Volleyball	Badminton Cross-country skiing (classic) Field hockey[*] Race walking Racquetball Running (long distance) Soccer[*] Squash Tennis (singles)
II. Moderate isometric (20%-50% MVC)	Archery Auto racing[*†] Diving[*†] Equestrian[*†] Motorcycling[*†]	Fencing Field events (jumping) Figure skating[*] Football (American)[*] Rodeo[*†] Rugby[*] Running (sprint) Surfing[*†] Synchronized swimming[†]	Basketball[*] Ice hockey[*] Cross-country skiing (skating) Football (Australian rules)[*] Lacrosse[*] Running (middle distance) Swimming Team handball
III. High Isometric (>50% MVC)	Bobsledding[*†] Field events (throwing) Gymnastics[*†] Karate/judo[*] Sailing Rock climbing[*†] Waterskiing[*†] Weight lifting[*†] Windsurfing[*†]	Body building[*†] Downhill skiing[*†] Wrestling[*]	Boxing[*] Canoeing/kayaking Cycling[*†] Decathlon Rowing Speed skating

The isometric component is defined as the percent of maximal voluntary contraction (MVC) that results in an increased blood pressure load. The isotonic component is defined as the percent of maximal oxygen consumption (MaxO₂) that contributes to cardiac output.
[*]Danger of bodily collision.
[†]Increased risk if syncope occurs.

Table 11-2 Considerations That Determine Recommendations for Athletics

1. Type, intensity, and duration of exercise
2. Risk of bodily collision inherent in a given type of athletic activity
3. Training conditioning required for a given athletic activity
4. Emotional response stress that the participant experiences in anticipation of or during a particular athletic activity
5. Risk of bodily injury to the participant or to spectators or bystanders if the activity is accompanied by loss of consciousness
6. Locomotor factors affecting exercise

TYPES OF EXERCISE

Isotonic (dynamic) exercise is associated with changes in muscle length and rhythmic muscular contraction that develops comparatively small force.[4] A steady state can be achieved. *Isometric (static) exercise* is associated with sudden development of a comparatively large force with little or no change in muscle length.[4] A steady state cannot be achieved, even temporarily. Some forms of exercise are chiefly isotonic (jogging, swimming), whereas others are chiefly isometric (weight lifting). Purely isometric or isotonic exercises represent the two ends of a continuous spectrum with most activities combining various degrees of both.[4] Isotonic exercise results in volume overload of the heart, whereas isometric exercise results in pressure overload.[11] The adaptive responses of the ventricles to these loading conditions differ in both mass and geometry[11-13] (see Chapter 23). Steady-state isotonic exercise is accompanied by an increase in oxygen consumption, stroke volume, cardiac output, and systolic blood pressure, whereas diastolic and mean pressures remain relatively unchanged as peripheral resistance falls (Fig. 11-2). Isometric exercise is accompanied by a sudden, marked increase in systolic, diastolic, and mean arterial pressures but by a relatively small increment in oxygen consumption and cardiac output.

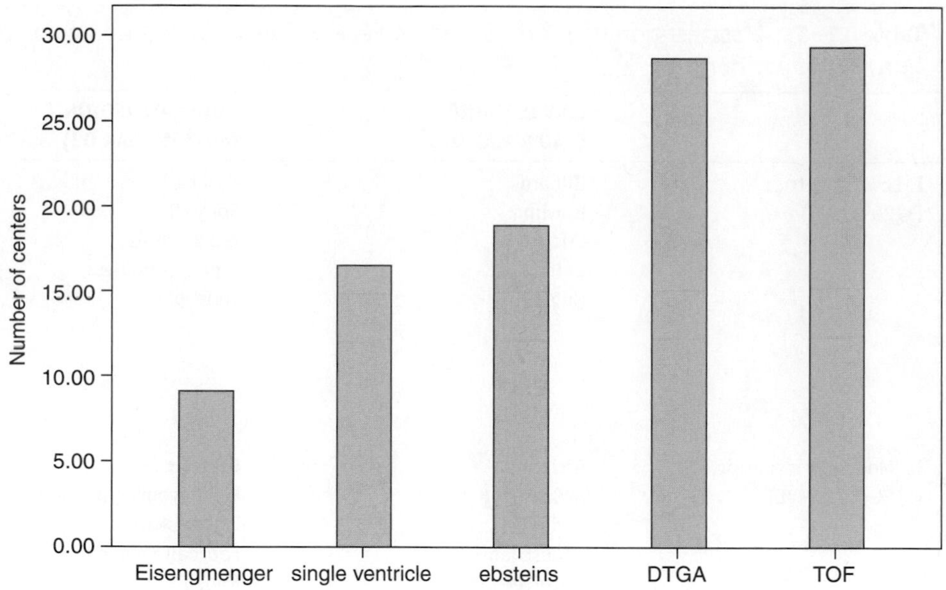

FIGURE 11-1 Maximal oxygen consumption (VO2 max) in 88 adults with various congenital cardiac defects at the Ahmanson/UCLA Adult Congenital Heart Disease Center. Patients with the Eisenmenger syndrome had the lowest VO2 max and were generally the most limited. Patients with repaired tetralogy of Fallot (TOF) and D-transposition of the great arteries (DTGA) status post–atrial switch had significantly higher VO2 max compared with the other subsets.

Steady-state isotonic exercise is amenable to the participant's control (although control is not always exercised), whereas isometric exercise is not amenable to control because of the sudden imposition of physical stress, especially strenuous. Irrespective of the relative proportions of isometric versus isotonic exercise, most competitive athletes have an increase in left ventricular mass compared with sedentary individuals.[11] However, predominantly *isotonic* endurance athletes develop increased right and left ventricular volumes, whereas athletes predominantly involved in *isometric* exercise develop an increase in left ventricular mass (hypertrophy)[11,14] (see Chapter 23). Furthermore, the hearts of endurance athletes have improved diastolic performance as indicated by increased early diastole biventricular filling.[11,15-18] Right ventricular diastolic function is an independent predictor of left ventricular stroke volume and maximal exercise capacity in athletes.[11]

Aerobic and *anaerobic* exercises refer to the type of evoked muscle metabolism, which is dependent on the type, intensity, and duration of exercise. The *intensity* of isotonic and isometric exercise can be low, medium, or high, and the *duration* can be brief or protracted (endurance). Dynamic exercise lasting for just a few minutes is performed aerobically, whereas high-intensity exercise of longer duration is performed anaerobically. Low to moderate intensity isotonic exercise of limited duration is, as a rule, not only permissible but desirable, whereas high-intensity isotonic exercise of prolonged duration is selectively authorized by physician approval. Isometric exercise of low intensity and brief duration is usually permissible, but strenuous isometric exercise is only occasionally permissible and seldom desirable.

The cardiovascular response to training (conditioning) improves exercise performance so that a given level of exercise can be achieved with less expenditure of energy. Supervised conditioning is one of the major roles of cardiac rehabilitation programs, and patients with CHD are no exception.[19-21] After certain types of reparative surgery, conditioning improves physical performance and permits normal or near-normal levels of activity. Ancient Chinese mind-body relaxation exercises (such as *tai chi*) incur a number of beneficial effects on cardiovascular function, including systemic blood pressure reduction, improvement in lipid profile, enhanced microcirculatory function, and endothelium-dependant vasodilatation.[22] When patients are advised about competitive athletics, it should be made clear that the risk of training may equal or exceed the risk of the competitive event for which training sets the stage.[4] The hazards of bodily collision are not confined to patients taking anticoagulants. Emotional stress before or during an athletic event can trigger a disturbance in cardiac rhythm with loss of consciousness, putting participant and bystanders at risk of bodily injury.

EFFECTS OF EXERCISE ON SPECIFIC TYPES OF CONGENITAL HEART DISEASE

Central to this discussion are the types and severity of congenital malformations and the outcomes of medical, surgical, interventional, and electrophysiologic management. The following remarks deal with highlights. No attempt is made to be all-inclusive.

Congenital Complete Heart Block

This rare congenital conduction defect is associated with maternal lupus.[23] Forty percent of patients have associated congenital cardiac malformations, especially left isomerism and congenitally corrected transposition of the great arteries.[24] Normal resting cardiac output is maintained by an increase in stroke volume (end-diastolic volume) rather than by an increase in ejection fraction. An exercise-induced increment in cardiac output is almost exclusively

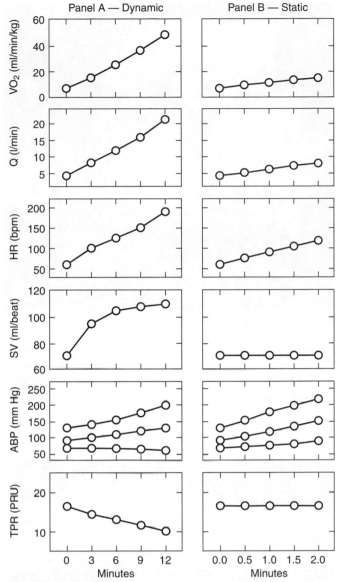

FIGURE 11-2 Cardiac response to exercise. Panel A shows response of progressively increasing workloads of dynamic exercise versus maximal oxygen consumption. Panel B shows response to a static handgrip contraction at 30% maximal voluntary contraction. ABP (arterial blood pressures), systolic, mean and diastolic; HR (bpm), heart rate (beats/min); Q (L/min), cardiac output (L/min); SV (ml/beat), stroke volume; TPR (PRU), total peripheral resistance in peripheral resistance units; VO_2 (ml/min/kg), oxygen consumption (ml/min × body weight in kg). *(With permission from Mitchell J.H., Raven, P.B. Cardiovascular adaptation to physical activity," In: C. Bouchard, ed. Physical Activity, Fitness and Health: International Proceedings and Consensus Statement. Champaign, IL, Human Kinetics, 1994.)*

due to acceleration of ventricular rate rather than to augmentation of stroke volume or ejection fraction.[25] The increase in ventricular rate during isotonic exercise is not necessarily related to the resting pulse rate. Moderate isotonic exercise provokes an appropriate increase in ventricular rate and cardiac output, but higher isotonic workloads are accompanied by blunted or frankly abnormal responses. Tolerance to isotonic exercise is best determined by stress testing, which is accompanied by an acceleration

in atrial rate but by a ventricular response that is of less magnitude and occasionally absent or nearly absent. Although patients with congenital complete heart block sometimes perform well, prolonged high-intensity *isotonic* exercise is ill advised, and strenuous *isometric* exercise is decidedly ill advised. Electronic pacemakers permit isotonic or isometric exercise within the limits of sensible moderation but with awareness of potential accidental contact injury to the pacemaker battery system. Although dual-chamber pacing improves cardiac function by restoring physiological heart rate and atrioventricular synchrony, prolonged ventricular dyssynchrony induced by apical right ventricular pacing leads to progressive left ventricular dilatation, asymmetric hypertrophy, ventricular dysfunction, and reduced exercise capacity.[26-29] Multisite ventricular pacing is an alternative for maintenance of ventricular synchrony. A multicenter study of resynchronization therapy in pediatric CHD included 14 patients with congenital complete heart block, most of whom experienced improved left ventricular ejection fraction and decreased QRS duration when changed from single site to multisite ventricular pacing.[30]

Congenitally Corrected Transposition of the Great Arteries

Durability of the inverted morphologic right ventricle in the systemic location is a long-term matter of concern.[25,26,31] Subpulmonary left ventricular dysfunction is less common (approximately 20% of patients). The ejection fraction of an inverted morphologic right ventricle in the subaortic location is the same as a noninverted morphologic right ventricle in the subpulmonary location[27] (Fig. 11-3). The end-diastolic volume of a normal subpulmonary right ventricle is greater than the end-diastolic volume of a normal subaortic left ventricle,[27] and an inverted right ventricle maintains a normal stroke volume at a lower ejection fraction without implying abnormal function. The inverted right ventricle responds to hemodynamic loads in a manner similar, if not identical, to that of a normal subaortic left ventricle[27] (see Fig. 11-3, A).

Interestingly, the response to exercise of the inverted left ventricle in congenitally corrected transposition is comparable to the response of a normal subpulmonary right ventricle.[27] The exercise response may be limited by complete atrioventricular block, which accrues at a rate of about 2% per year. Patients with isolated uncomplicated congenitally corrected transposition of the great arteries and normal atrioventricular conduction are permitted moderate-intensity isotonic or isometric exercise but should not engage in prolonged high-intensity exercise. The two-dimensional echocardiogram and exercise stress testing provide a satisfactory basis for judging the functional adequacy of the subaortic morphologic right ventricle. Aerobic capacity and lung function in these patients are significantly diminished compared with healthy control subjects,[28] and peak exercise blood pressure,

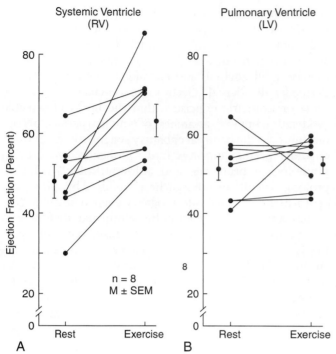

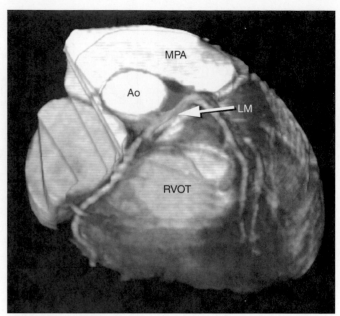

FIGURE 11-3 Radionuclide ejection fractions at rest and in response to supine exercise in isolated congenitally corrected transposition of the great arteries. **(A)** Normal exercise response of the inverted systemic morphologic right ventricle. **(B)** Blunted exercise response of the subpulmonary morphologic left ventricle. *(With permission from Benson, L.N., Burns, R., Shwaiger, M., et al.: Radionuclide angiographic evaluation of ventricular function in isolated congenitally corrected transposition of the great arteries. Am J Cardiol 58:319; 1986.[34])*

FIGURE 11-4 Electrocardiogram-gated coronary computed tomography angiogram with three-dimensional volume rendering demonstrating anomalous origin of the left main (LM) coronary artery from the right coronary cusp. The anomalous coronary courses between the aortic root (Ao) and the right ventricular outflow tract (RVOT). MPA, main pulmonary artery.

heart rate, and oxygen saturation are reduced. Myocardial fibrosis as determined by magnetic resonance imaging (MRI) late gadolinium enhancement is common in the systemic right ventricle and associated with ventricular dysfunction, increased ventricular wall stress, and decreased exercise capacity[30] (see Chapter 7). Myocardial fibrosis is the result of reduced right ventricular coronary flow reserve due to an increase in oxygen demand of a systemic right ventricle that is perfused by a concordant morphologic right coronary artery.[32,33]

Aberrant Coronary Artery between Aorta and Right Ventricular Outflow Tract

Angina pectoris, myocardial infarction, and sudden death are potential risks when an aberrant coronary artery runs between the aorta and pulmonary trunk.[25,31] The risk is believed to be greatest when the left coronary artery arises from the right aortic sinus and passes between the aorta and the right ventricular outflow tract (Fig. 11-4), especially in males.[34] Sudden death also occurs but less commonly in patients with anomalous right coronary arteries[37-38] (Fig. 11-5) and is most likely during or immediately after strenuous exercise. The mechanism is believed to be stress-induced compression of the aberrant coronary

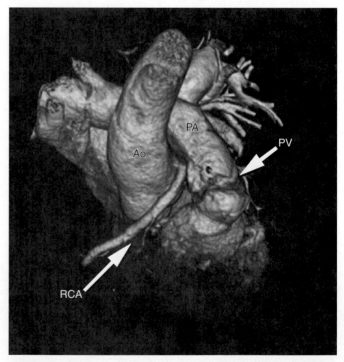

FIGURE 11-5 Electrocardiogram-gated coronary computed tomography angiogram with three-dimensional volume rendering demonstrating anomalous origin of the right coronary artery (RCA) from the left coronary cusp in a patient with repaired tetralogy of Fallot. PV, prosthetic pulmonary valve. The RCA courses between the aortic root (Ao) and the pulmonary artery (PA).

artery together with an increase in the inherently acute angulation of its origin.[39,40] Intravascular ultrasound reveals intramural proximal intussusception of the anomalous coronary artery within the aortic wall.[41] The lumen of the intramural arterial segment is characteristically ovoid and is compromised during systole when the pulsatile aortic root compresses the vessel, which is also compromised during pharmacologic simulation of exercise.[41] If the anomaly is identified and surgically or percutaneously repaired, athletic activity is not restricted provided that coronary flow is demonstrably unobstructed and myocardial perfusion is demonstrably normal.[42]

Anomalous Origin of the Left Coronary Artery from the Pulmonary Trunk

Extensive coronary artery collaterals occasionally permit relatively asymptomatic adult survival. Ten percent to 15% of these patients are believed to reach adulthood when the anomaly may announce itself with angina, heart failure, or sudden death.[25] The permissible level of exercise in surviving adults depends on the presence and degree of myocardial ischemia, the degree of mitral regurgitation (papillary muscle dysfunction), and the adequacy of left ventricular function. Even under the best of circumstances, high-intensity isotonic or isometric exercise should be avoided, and surgery should be recommended, with few exceptions. The original operation of ligation of the anomalously arising left coronary artery[43] has been superseded by aortic implantation or bypass of the left coronary artery. Even so, residual myocardial scarring is frequent.[44] The level of ex-

ercise permitted after operation depends on the adequacy of revascularization, the performance of the left ventricle, and the absence of significant arrhythmias in response to treadmill isotonic stress.

Congenital Coronary Arteriovenous Fistula

The physiologic consequences of this anomaly are determined by the volume of blood flowing through the fistula, the chamber or vessel into which the fistula drains, and myocardial ischemia that can result from the fistulous bypass (steal).[25,35] Symptoms and complications increase with age, and recommendations regarding exercise must be modified accordingly. The majority of adults are asymptomatic when first seen, but high-intensity isotonic or isometric exercise should be avoided unless the fistulous communication is small. In a Dutch national survey of 51 patients with solitary coronary arteriovenous fistulas, obstructive coronary artery disease occurred in approximately half, and myocardial infarction was identified in 18%.[42] Twenty-nine percent had demonstrable aneurysm formation (Fig. 11–6), and there were rare examples of spontaneous rupture with cardiac tamponade.[36-38] Surgical repair or percutaneous closure (see Chapter 18) is recommended especially in the setting of inducible ischemia.[45] If inducible myocardial ischemia is subsequently absent and left ventricular function is normal, the level of exercise is not restricted.

Distal coronary-to-left ventricular microfistulae are rare anomalies that manifest themselves in adults by angina and exercise-induced ischemia.[46] Transcatheter

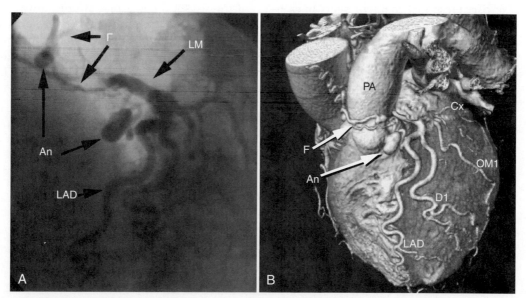

FIGURE 11–6   Coronary arteriovenous fistula from the left anterior descending (LAD) to the pulmonary artery (PA) in a 66-year-old man with hypertension, hypercholesterolemia, and an abnormal resting electrocardiogram (ECG; inferolateral ST depression) but normal functional capacity and absence of ischemic changes with exercise. **(A)** Selective left coronary angiography (LAO cranial projection) demonstrating an unobstructed left coronary system. Left main (LM) and left anterior descending (LAD) coronary arteries are labeled. There is an arteriovenous fistula (F) from the LAD to the pulmonary artery. Two saccular aneurysms (An) are clearly visualized. **(B)** Sixty-four slice ECG gated computed tomography angiogram with three-dimensional volume rendering demonstrating the fistula (F) from the LAD to the PA. The proximal aneurysm (An) is clearly visible.

delivery of microcoils may prove useful in closing these small distal communications.

Congenital Aneurysm of a Sinus of Valsalva

A sinus aneurysm with a small, gradually developing perforation is compatible with asymptomatic adult survival.[25] High-intensity isometric exercise is best avoided to minimize the risk of rupture or aortic regurgitation. High-intensity isotonic exercise incurs an unknown risk. Rarely, an aneurysm compresses a coronary artery, causing myocardial infarction.[47] A sudden large rupture demands urgent surgical closure, although percutaneous device closure has been successfully employed.[48,49] The recommended level of isotonic exercise then depends on postoperative biventricular function. Although aortic sinus aneurysms tend to be single, occasionally more than one sinus is involved, and thus high-intensity isometric exercise is ill advised after successful repair of a single perforation.

Coarctation of the Aorta

The distensibility characteristics of the aorta proximal to the coarctation and the sensitivity or "set" of carotid sinus baroreceptors are important determinants of the systolic hypertension of coarctation.[25] Because the precoarctation aorta is more rigid (less compliant) than the aorta distal to the coarctation, the carotid sinus baroreceptors are set to operate at higher pressures,[50,51] accounting in part for the disproportionate elevation in systolic blood pressure.[50,52-54] Residual coarctation or recoarctation is therefore associated with an excessive rise in proximal aortic systolic pressure during isotonic exercise, a response that represents an exaggeration of the disproportionate upper extremity systolic hypertension in the resting state.[53] Increased flow across the stenotic coarctation segment augments flow velocity and magnifies the basal systolic pressure gradient with

occasional emergence of a diastolic gradient[25,55] (Fig. 11–7). Excessive exercise-induced systolic hypertension after repair devoid of residual coarctation or recoarctation is in large part related to older age at the time of operation, angulated (Gothic) arch anatomy[54,56-59] (see Chapter 7), impaired systemic vascular reactivity, resetting of the carotid baroreceptors, and reduced aortic distensibility.[51,60-65] An additional concern is the normotensive patient who experiences a hypertensive response to exercise after successful repair. The response is not due to sympathetic overdrive or to disorders of the angiotensin-aldosterone system, but instead probably reflects baroreceptor abnormalities or structural (compliance) alterations in the precoarctation aorta.

Residual functional vascular changes after successful repair include elevated resistance in the hands and increased vascular reactivity in the forearms with normal reactivity in the legs.[64,66] Peripheral blood flow kinetics disclose impaired lower limb flow during strenuous dynamic exercise.[67] Echocardiography with measurement of resting and exercise upper and lower extremity blood pressure is useful to determine maximal exercise capacity, blood pressure response to exercise, response of the left ventricle, and basal and exercise gradient across the coarctation segment (see Fig. 11–7). An exaggerated hypertensive response during stress testing warns against high levels of isotonic and isometric exercise.

Aortic Valve Stenosis

Unoperated adults with bicuspid aortic valves (BAV) that are functionally normal or near normal should avoid sudden, strenuous isotonic or isometric exercise because of the risk of a coexisting abnormality of the ascending aortic media.[68-71] Moderately elevated basal velocities across a BAV can increase dramatically with exercise and represent an important variable in determining the recommended levels of exercise (Fig. 11–8). Left ventricular

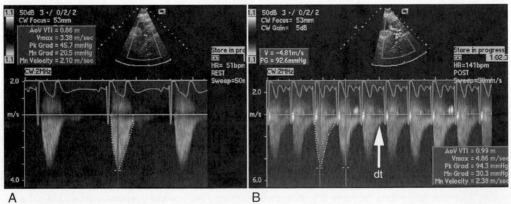

FIGURE 11–7 Thirty-two-year-old woman with recoarctation of the aorta after surgical resection with end-to-end anastomosis at 4 years of age. **(A)** Continuous wave Doppler through the site of recoarctation (supra-sternal notch view) at rest (heart rate 51 bpm) demonstrating increased systolic flow velocity and an estimated peak instantaneous pressure gradient of 46 mm Hg. **(B)** Continuous-wave Doppler profile during exercise (141 bpm) demonstrating a doubling of the peak gradient and the appearance of a "diastolic tail" (dt) indicating magnification of the diastolic pressure gradient. Blood pressure at rest in the right upper extremity was 161/76 mm Hg and 112/65 mm Hg in the right lower extremity. At peak exercise, the right upper extremity pressure increased to 211/95 mm Hg, whereas the right lower extremity pressure was 129/70 mm Hg.

ejection is not only preserved but often supranormal and increases further with exercise (see Chapter 23). Fibrocalcific degeneration of a functionally normal bicuspid aortic valve is accompanied by a normal but not a supranormal ejection fraction (see Chapter 23). Echocardiographic stress testing establishes transvalvular velocities, ventricular function, blood pressure and heart rate responses, and exercise-induced arrhythmias. Increased transvalvular velocities with decreased exercise capacity identify patients at high risk.[72] Exercise testing is safe when protocols with high and unequal work increments are avoided.[73] The severity of aortic stenosis remains the important variable in determining exercise restrictions. Older adults with progressive BAV stenosis may have limited circulatory reserve because of coexisting coronary artery disease.

The American Heart Association and American College of Cardiology guidelines classify aortic stenosis as *mild* when the valve area is ≥1.5 cm², when the mean resting gradient is 25 mm Hg or less, and when the maximum Doppler velocity is <3 m/sec. Aortic stenosis is considered *moderate* when the valve area is between 1.0 and 1.5 cm², an area that coincides with a resting mean gradient of 25 to 40 mm Hg and a Doppler velocity between 3 and 4 m/sec. Aortic stenosis is considered *severe* when the valve area is <1.0 cm², an area that coincides with a resting gradient in excess of 40 mm Hg and a Doppler velocity >4 m/sec.[74] Severity can be accurately assessed by transthoracic echocardiography, with cardiac catheterization reserved for the few exceptions. Mild aortic stenosis requires exercise restrictions because of the risk of the ascending aortic medial abnormality rather than because of the obstruction per se[75] (discussed earlier). The abnormal ascending aorta is an important consideration in determining eligibility for competitive sports.[76] Isometric exercise suddenly increases aortic root pressure. Patients with moderate aortic stenosis and normal or supranormal left ventricular function are advised to restrict themselves to low-intensity isotonic exercise.

Severe aortic stenosis precludes high-intensity isotonic or isometric exercise or competitive sports.

The risk of sudden death is a legitimate concern in establishing exercise limitations in all but mild bicuspid aortic stenosis. Malignant ventricular arrhythmias seldom initiate the syncope that precedes sudden death but are the chief causes of death after loss of consciousness. Left ventricular baroreceptors are activated in response to an exercise-induced increase in left ventricular pressure (stretch), which causes reflex vasodilatation in skeletal muscle followed by systemic hypotension and syncope.[73,77] Although exercise-induced syncope is more likely to provoke electrical ventricular instability and sudden death in adults with acquired fibrocalcific bicuspid aortic stenosis and coexisting coronary artery disease, young patients with severe aortic stenosis and left ventricular hypertrophy have subendocardial ischemia.

Assuming optimal results of surgical valvotomy or balloon valvuloplasty, the bicuspid valve remains bicuspid.[78] Like its unoperated functionally normal counterpart, the valve remains susceptible to infective endocarditis (see Chapter 8), progressive acquired obstruction, and the risk of the medial abnormality of the Marfan-like aortic root. Periodic reassessments with Doppler echocardiography are obligatory.

If postinterventional or postoperative stenosis is moderate or severe, athletic activity should be limited to low or moderate intensity, especially if left ventricular end diastolic dimensions are increased, aortic regurgitation is more than mild, the electrocardiogram has repolarization abnormalities at rest or with exercise, or disturbances in ventricular rhythm occur at rest, with exercise, or on a 24-hour ambulatory electrocardiogram.

Bicuspid aortic stenosis beyond the third decade is typically fibrocalcific and requires surgical valve replacement. The choice of a mechanical or a bioprosthetic valve[74,79,80] is dealt with in Chapter 16. The hemodynamic performance of prosthetic aortic valves at rest and with exercise

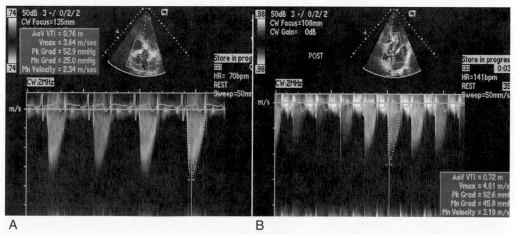

FIGURE 11-8   **(A)** Resting continuous-wave Doppler profile across a moderately stenotic bicuspid aortic valve (apical four-chamber view). **(B)** Doubling of heart rate immediately following peak exercise is accompanied by near doubling of the estimated pressure gradient. The arm cuff blood pressure measurement at peak exercise was 132/75 mm Hg, indicating that the left ventricular systolic pressure exceeded 220 mm Hg.

is determined principally by prosthesis size. When a small size is indicated, bileaflet mechanical valves are superior to monoleaflet valves, and bovine bioprostheses are superior to porcine.

Pulmonary Valve Stenosis

Stenosis of a typical thin mobile pulmonary valve[74,81-84] is considered *mild* if the valve area is 1.0 cm²/m² of body surface, which usually corresponds to a peak-to-peak resting catheter gradient ≤ 25 mm Hg. *Moderate* pulmonary stenosis is so designated when the valve area is 0.5 to 1.0 cm²/m² of body surface, with gradients between 25 and 49 mm Hg. *Moderately severe* pulmonary stenosis defines a valve area < 0.5 cm²/m² of body surface and a gradient in excess of 50 mm Hg. A peak-to-peak resting gradient > 80 mm Hg is considered *severe*.

Patients with mild pulmonary valve stenosis are permitted unrestricted athletic activity.[85] When obstruction is moderate, high-intensity competitive sports may be tolerated but are unwise because right ventricular systolic pressure rises appreciably.[25,84,86] When the resting peak systolic gradient is 50 mm Hg or greater, especially if there is echocardiographic or radionuclide evidence of impaired right ventricular function, isotonic athletic activity should be limited to mild intensity and short duration. These constraints are appropriate despite the occasional tolerance of strenuous isotonic exercise in patients with severe pulmonary valve stenosis.[25]

Because of the salutary results of balloon valvuloplasty or surgical valvotomy, especially when performed before age 21 years, most if not all of these patients are unrestricted and can safely participate in high-intensity competitive athletics. *Secondary* hypertrophic subpulmonary stenosis regresses with time. The type of athletic activity then permitted depends on the degree of regression and on right ventricular function. If obstruction to right ventricular outflow remains moderate or more, athletic activity should be limited to noncompetitive low-intensity or moderate-intensity isotonic exercise, especially if right ventricular dimensions are increased and systolic function is abnormal. In 90 patients who had undergone surgical repair of isolated pulmonary valve stenosis in childhood,[87] exercise capacity was mildly reduced but unrelated to basal transvalvular gradients. Moderate to severe pulmonary regurgitation was present in 37% of these patients, especially if a transannular patch was employed in the original repair. Severe pulmonary regurgitation with right ventricular dilatation incurred a significant reduction in exercise capacity.

Congenital Pulmonary Valve Regurgitation

The functional consequences of this malformation depend on the degree of regurgitant flow and the adaptive response of the right ventricle to volume overload.[25] As a low-pressure

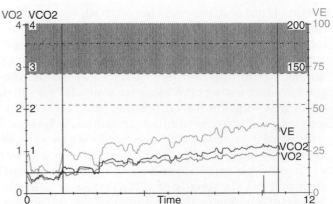

FIGURE 11-9 Results of a modified Bruce treadmill cardiopulmonary exercise test in a 43-year-old man with Noonan's syndrome and pulmonary valve stenosis. Surgical pulmonary valvotomy in childhood resulted in chronic severe pulmonary regurgitation. The exercise capacity was severely reduced. The maximum oxygen consumption (VO2 max) was 14.8 ml/kg/min (38% predicted). The patient had a reduced VO2 and reduced anaerobic threshold. VO2 and VCO2 kinetics are slow. Minute ventilation (VE) increased dramatically at the start of exercise and then rose gradually. Chronic atrial fibrillation was treated with a beta-blocker.

pump, the mature right ventricle readily adapts to increased volume. Accordingly, mild to moderate congenital pulmonary valve regurgitation is usually well tolerated, but severe regurgitation is accompanied by right ventricular dilatation and reduced exercise capacity[87] (Fig. 11-9).

In patients with no more than moderate regurgitation, athletic activities are not restricted. However, the degree of regurgitation tends to increase with age, and thus long-term reassessments with Doppler echocardiography or MRI are required to establish the comparative degrees of regurgitant flow, the changes in right ventricular dimensions, the adequacy of right ventricular function, and the recommended level of physical activity.

Ostium Secundum Atrial Septal Defect

Unrepaired young adults are usually asymptomatic and tolerate high-intensity exercise.[25] As long as pulmonary vascular resistance remains normal or low (which is usually the case), exercise is not restricted, but repair is still advised. When the shunt is abolished in early childhood, long-term outlook is excellent, and athletic activity is unrestricted, assuming that sinus node and atrioventricular conduction are normal and right atrial and right ventricular volumes normalize[88,89] (see Chapter 5). In patients who undergo closure in their late teens or early 20s without residua, exercise restrictions are not imposed. However, athletic activity should be limited to low intensity if mean resting pulmonary arterial pressure exceeds 20 mm Hg, right ventricular internal dimensions exceed two standard deviations from normal, there is sinus node dysfunction or abnormal atrioventricular conduction, or atrial tachyarrhythmias develop or recur.[90] When an ostium secundum atrial septal defect with a large left-to-right shunt remains unrepaired beyond young adulthood, volume overload impairs right ventricular systolic function, and leftward deviation of the ventricular septum may impair left ventricular diastolic function[6,89] (see Chapter 5).

Ventricular Septal Defect

The physiologic consequences of an isolated ventricular septal defect depend chiefly on the size of the defect and the pulmonary vascular resistance.[25] Both variables may change with time, and the physiologic and clinical manifestations change accordingly.

Ventricular septal defects are grouped into four anatomic/physiologic categories[25]: (1) small defects with normal pulmonary vascular resistance (<1.2 Wood units) and pulmonary/systemic flow ratios of 1.5:1 or less; (2) moderately restrictive defects with low but variable pulmonary vascular resistance and shunts between 1.5:1 and 2.0:1; (3) nonrestrictive defects with elevated but variable pulmonary vascular resistance and shunts in excess of 2:1; and (4) nonrestrictive defects with pulmonary vascular resistance equal to or greater than systemic and reversed shunts (see Chapter 4). In small defects, the minimal shunting is not significantly increased by exercise, and functional capacity is normal, thus physical activity is unrestricted.[88,91] A caveat is a defect that is small because of partial closure by the septal tricuspid leaflet. A sudden rise in left ventricular systolic pressure induced by strenuous isometric exercise can cause rightward displacement of the septal leaflet, an increase in effective defect size, and an increase in left-to-right shunt. Patients with moderately restrictive ventricular septal defects participate safely in isotonic exercise of mild intensity and limited duration, but isometric exercise should be curtailed because the accompanying increase in left ventricular systolic pressure suddenly augments the shunt. Eisenmenger syndrome is discussed later in the section on pulmonary vascular disease.

A variation on the theme is the adult with a moderately restrictive perimembranous ventricular septal defect that has decreased in size or closed spontaneously. Such patients are physiologically normal and are permitted unrestricted activity. There is no evidence that unrestricted athletic activity risks interrupting the integrity of the spontaneously closed defect, but it is prudent to be aware of the morphologic substrate accompanying spontaneous closure. Echocardiography or MRI should be performed to determine whether the defect has sealed with formation of a septal aneurysm.

Recommendations regarding physical activity and competitive sports after surgical or transcatheter closure of a moderate to large ventricular septal defect depend on the pulmonary artery pressure, the absence or presence of ventricular arrhythmias during maximal exercise stress testing and during 24-hour ambulatory electrocardiography, and echocardiographic evidence with color flow imaging showing that the ventricular septum is intact, left atrial size is normal, and left ventricular size and function are normal.[78] It is also desirable that the scalar electrocardiogram shows no signs of residual left ventricular volume overload or right ventricular pressure overload. If these criteria are met, patients are permitted unrestricted high-intensity isotonic and isometric exercise.[35] Persistent elevation of pulmonary arterial systolic pressure, especially if accompanied by exercise-induced right ventricular ectopic rhythms, mandates that physical activity be limited to low intensity and short duration.

Patent Ductus Arteriosus

A restrictive patent ductus arteriosus with normal pulmonary arterial pressure and a pulmonary:systemic flow ratio of 1.5:1 or less is of little hemodynamic consequence, and thus physical activity is not limited. A moderately restrictive patent ductus with a large left-to-right shunt and elevated but less than systemic pulmonary arterial pressure mandates that physical activity be restricted to low-intensity isotonic exercise. When a nonrestrictive patent ductus is accompanied by suprasystemic pulmonary vascular resistance and reversed shunt (Eisenmenger syndrome), exercise is limited to low intensity and brief duration. See the following section on pulmonary vascular disease.

Division of an isolated restrictive patent ductus arteriosus in childhood represents one of the few surgical cures of CHD, and there are no restrictions on athletic activity after repair. After closure of a moderately restrictive patent ductus with a large left-to-right shunt and variable elevations of pulmonary arterial pressure, exercise recommendations are similar to those for moderately restrictive ventricular septal defects that have undergone closure (see previous section).

Pulmonary Vascular Disease

Idiopathic (primary) pulmonary hypertension represents the purest expression of an increase in pulmonary vascular resistance. Effort syncope is an ominous feature that heralds sudden death. Exercise-induced systemic vasodilatation provokes a fall in blood pressure and in cerebral perfusion because the elevated pulmonary resistance does not permit the fall in systemic vascular resistance to be countered by an appropriate increase in venous return to the systemic circulation. Cardiac output falls farther if acute right ventricular failure is induced by exercise. Accordingly, patients with idiopathic pulmonary hypertension should confine themselves strictly to the mildest isotonic exercise of brief duration. Isometric exercise should be wholly avoided. Physical activity and training, even when monitored, are disputed.[22,92] Exercise of any type should cease promptly with the earliest onset of symptoms.

Pulmonary vasodilatators have had a positive impact on maximal and submaximal exercise capacity in patients with idiopathic pulmonary hypertension.[93-95] The vasodilatators include prostacyclins (intravenous, inhaled, or subcutaneous), the endothelin receptor antagonist bosentan, and the phosphodiesterase type 5 inhibitors sildenafil and tadalafil. Thirty patients with idiopathic pulmonary hypertension were treated with one or a combination of these medications and randomized to a 15-week supervised monitored low-isometric (10–60 watt) daily bicycle ergometer or low isometric weight training.[21] Both groups manifested significant improvement in 6-minute walk distance, improved quality of life, and improved peak oxygen consumption with no exercise-related adverse events. The combination of medical therapy and monitored low isometric and isotonic exercise training may be beneficial.

For patients with Eisenmenger syndrome, even low levels of isotonic exercise tend to be accompanied by tissue lactic acidosis and marked decrements in systemic arterial oxygen content. The exercise-induced increase in right-to-left shunt poses a special problem for the elimination of metabolically produced carbon dioxide, resulting in high ventilatory requirements—subjective dyspnea—and occasionally in respiratory acidosis.[96] Patients invariably have decreased exercise tolerance and low maximal oxygen consumption.[96-99] The maximal oxygen consumption measured in the lungs does not reflect the tissue oxygen consumption because the intracardiac right-to-left shunt prevents an appropriate increase in oxygen consumption in response to increasing tissue oxygen demand with exercise (Fig. 11–10). Patients with Eisenmenger syndrome appear to derive benefits from pulmonary arterial vasodilatator therapies similar to the benefits derived by patients with idiopathic pulmonary hypertension with measurable improvements in functional class and submaximal and maximal exercise capacity.[100-103]

The response to isotonic exercise in patients with pulmonary vascular disease and reversed shunts is, in part, related to the site (level) of venoarterial mixing—atrial, ventricular, or great arterial. In the presence of a nonrestrictive ventricular septal defect, the exercise-induced increase in right-to-left shunt is distributed equally throughout the systemic circulation, thus the respiratory center and carotid receptors are exposed equally to the changes in blood gas composition and pH. However, in the presence of a nonrestrictive patent ductus arteriosus with suprasystemic pulmonary vascular resistance and reversed flow, shunted blood is delivered distal to the left subclavian artery and therefore distal to the vital centers of the head and neck,[25] thus exercise is not accompanied by breathlessness.

Exercise-induced syncope in patients with suprasystemic pulmonary vascular resistance differs according to the level of the right-to-left shunt. In the presence of an ostium secundum atrial septal defect, right ventricular systolic pressure can exceed systemic because the ventricular septum is intact. Effort syncope occurs because the exercise-induced increase in right-to-left shunt is not sufficient

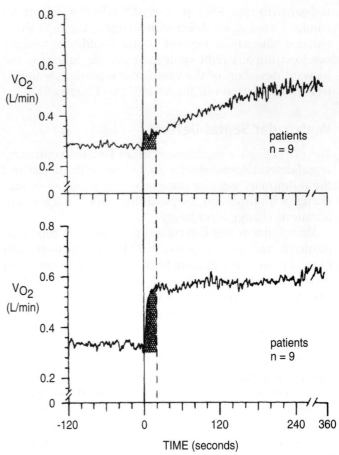

FIGURE 11-10 Oxygen consumption (VO2) response to exercise in patients with Eisenmenger syndrome and in normal subjects. Data from six transitions from each of nine patients and nine control subjects were averaged. Exercise began at time 0. The shaded area indicates the VO2 response in the first 20 seconds of exercise (Phase 1). The increase in VO2 during phase 1 is severely diminished in the patients, reflecting the immediate increase in right-to-left shunting with exercise.[110] *(With permission from Sietsema, K., Cooper, D.M., Perloff, J.K., et al.: Dynamics of oxygen uptake during exercise in adults with cyanotic congenital heart disease.* Circulation 1986;6: 1137–1144.)

to maintain left ventricular stroke volume and cerebral blood flow. Conversely, exercise-induced syncope is not a feature of a nonrestrictive ventricular septal defect or patent ductus arteriosus with reversed shunt because systemic blood flow, including cerebral, is adequately augmented, albeit at the expense of increased hypoxemia.

Tetralogy of Fallot

The physiologic consequences of tetralogy of Fallot depend chiefly on the degree of obstruction to right ventricular outflow and, to a lesser extent, on systemic vascular resistance.[25] Right ventricular outflow obstruction is fixed, but systemic resistance is variable. During isotonic exercise, a fall in systemic resistance coincides with an increase in venous return to a right ventricle with fixed obstruction to outflow, resulting in an obligatory increase in right-to-left shunt. The sensation of breathlessness is triggered by the response of the respiratory center and carotid receptors to the sudden change in blood gas composition and pH. Squatting, a time-honored hallmark for relief of exercise-induced breathlessness in children with the tetralogy, exerts its salutary effect by increasing systemic vascular resistance, which diverts the amount of low oxygen content inferior vena caval return from the biventricular aorta into the pulmonary circulation.[25,35]

The risk of isometric exercise in tetralogy of Fallot is dramatically illustrated by straining (bearing down) during labor. Strenuous isometric exercise abruptly increases systemic vascular resistance and reduces flow from the right ventricle into the aorta, thus systemic blood flow falls precipitously, inducing syncope and rarely causing sudden death. All but low-intensity isometric exercise should therefore be avoided in unrepaired tetralogy of Fallot.

The level of physical activity permitted after intracardiac repair depends on the presence and degree of postoperative residua and sequelae and on patient age at operation.[35,104–108] Repairs performed in early childhood permit participation in high-intensity sports with minimal evident risk. Although the relationship between age at operation and exercise capacity is not linear, the response to exercise is less adequate if reparative surgery is initially undertaken in older children or young adults. When patient age at repair averaged 19.5 years, maximal oxygen uptake during exercise was only 30% to 40% of normal.[104,105] The response to exercise is poorer if surgery is undertaken in older, even asymptomatic adults in whom right ventricular ejection fraction may not increase normally with exercise.

Adults should undergo postoperative two-dimensional echocardiography with Doppler interrogation and color flow imaging together with exercise stress testing. If obstruction to right ventricular outflow is absent or mild, pulmonary regurgitation is moderate or less, there is minimal or no residual shunt, there are no exercise-induced disturbances in ventricular rhythm, and ventricular size and function are normal, no limitations are imposed on isotonic or isometric exercise.[104–106,108]

Cardiopulmonary exercise testing is especially useful in patients with repaired tetralogy of Fallot. Those with peak oxygen consumption less than 36% of predicted and with a steep slope of ventilation per unit of carbon dioxide production (> 39) are at increased risk.[108] Postoperative bifascicular block is uncommon with current surgical techniques, and its isolated occurrence does not necessarily imply a risk of exercise-induced high-degree heart block. In patients with tetralogy of Fallot and absent pulmonary valve, postoperative cardiopulmonary response to exercise is similar to that of patients with a transannular patch.[109] Severe pulmonary regurgitation is not only accompanied by right ventricular dilatation and decreased exercise capacity but serves as a trigger for monomorphic ventricular tachycardia in patients with slowed conduction reentrant arrhythmogenic substrates[92,107,110,111] (see Chapter 22).

Palliative Shunts

Palliative shunts are designed to increase systemic oxygen saturation in patients with deficient pulmonary blood flow. The majority of these patients can anticipate relatively early reparative surgery, but an occasional patient who underwent a shunt in childhood presents as an adult. Some of these palliated adults claim to be asymptomatic, but exercise testing usually discloses markedly decreased exercise capacity.[112] Other shunted patients have depressed function of their volume-overloaded left ventricle or, less commonly, shunt-induced pulmonary vascular disease and are symptomatic with low-intensity exercise.

Ebstein's Anomaly of the Tricuspid Valve

In unoperated patients with Ebstein's anomaly, physiologic reserve is limited by the functional inadequacy inherent in an atrialized right ventricle that is beset by the volume overload of tricuspid regurgitation, restrictive diastolic filling, the presence and degree of a right-to-left atrial shunt, and paroxysmal or chronic disturbances in atrial rhythm, especially but not necessarily associated with accessory pathways. Despite these qualifications, there are legendary accounts of impressive exercise tolerance in patients with Ebstein's anomaly.[25] A 75-year-old man in whom Ebstein's anomaly was discovered at necropsy had been a lumberjack as a young man and was reportedly asymptomatic until his 50s, when he succeeded in outrunning an irate female bear. As a rule, however, physical activity is limited by lesion severity, especially in cyanotic patients.[113] Successful reconstruction of the Ebstein tricuspid valve with closure of an interatrial communication and elimination of accessory pathways by radiofrequency ablation or at operation materially improves physiologic reserve, permitting at least moderate isotonic exercise.

Complete Transposition of the Great Arteries

Postoperative data on the physiologic status and exercise tolerance in adults with this malformation are derived chiefly from patients who have undergone Mustard or Senning atrial switch operations in childhood.[114,115] The majority are asymptomatic with activities of daily living but have objective evidence of reduced exercise capacity.[116] A morphologic right ventricle in the systemic location is an inherent limitation that worsens with age.[36,103,117] Aortic and tricuspid regurgitation impose volume load, obstruction or leaks of the intraatrial baffle are problematic, and sinus node dysfunction, atrial tachyarrhythmias, and abnormal atrioventricular conduction loom as undesirable electrophysiologic sequelae. Pharmacologic attempts to improve the function of a morphologic subaortic left ventricle cannot necessarily be extrapolated to the morphologic subaortic right ventricle of complete transposition.

Patients who have undergone arterial switch operations are now reaching adulthood and require assessment regarding physical activity. An air of cautious optimism assumes no obstruction of the relocated coronary arteries, no stenosis of the neoaorta, and little or no stenosis or incompetence of the neoaortic valve (see Chapter 5). Nearly two thirds of these patients have impaired left ventricular function at rest and reversible myocardial perfusion defects,[118] although in the majority, exercise capacity is near the normal predicted for age.[119]

Fontan Operation

Modifications of the original Fontan operation leave unchanged a circulation in series devoid of a functional subpulmonary ventricle. Only one ventricle serves the systemic circulation whether the operation is performed for tricuspid atresia or a univentricular heart. In tricuspid atresia, that ventricle is necessarily a morphologic left

ventricle in which systolic function is usually within normal range. When a univentricular heart is characterized by a morphologic left ventricle, function of the single ventricle is usually less than that of the left ventricle of tricuspid atresia. Ventricular function is poorest in the presence of a single morphologic right ventricle.

Postoperative exercise performance improves after a Fontan repair but, not surprisingly, remains subnormal.[120,121] Patients may experience few or no symptoms and minimal abnormalities of ventricular function at rest, but during exercise tend to have limited inotropic and chronotropic capacity, poorer diastolic filling, and higher venous pressure.[122] The hemodynamic response to isotonic exercise differs fundamentally from normal. Aerobic capacity or maximal oxygen consumption at peak exercise is approximately 50% of predicted values,[120,123,124] and heart rate at peak exercise is usually reduced.[8,121,123,124] (Fig. 11–11). The blunted chronotropic response has been attributed to autonomic impairment or sinus node dysfunction.[125,126] Postoperative hypoxemia has been ascribed to persistent intracardiac right-to-left shunt,

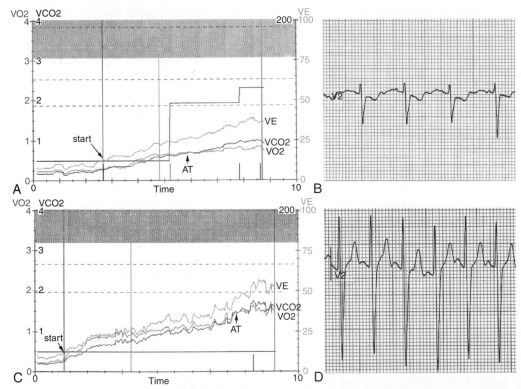

FIGURE 11–11 Results of cardiopulmonary exercise test after Fontan operation in two patients with single ventricle physiology. The patient whose data are shown in the upper panels **(A and B)** was a sedentary 29-year-old woman who underwent a right atrial-to-pulmonary artery Fontan operation in childhood for a hypoplastic right ventricle. **(A)** Poor exercise performance is indicated by the short duration of exercise (Bruce protocol) of 6 minutes, achieving a maximum oxygen consumption (VO2) of 13.6 ml/kg/min (38% of predicted). The anaerobic threshold (AT) was reached early in exercise (<4 minutes). **(B)** Maximum heart rate achieved was only 110 bpm (58% of predicted), indicating poor heart rate reserve. The patient whose data are presented in the lower panels **(C and D)** was a very active 21-year-old woman (three-time high school national dance champion) with double-inlet left ventricle and a lateral tunnel Fontan performed in childhood. Her father was an Olympic gold medalist in track and field. **(C)** Good exercise tolerance, achieving a VO2 max of 29 ml/kg/min (72% predicted), and exercising for 12 minutes (Bruce). The AT is reached nearly 10 minutes into the protocol. **(D)** Maximum heart rate was 155 bpm (77% of predicted), indicating adequate but subnormal heart rate reserve.

diversion of coronary sinus blood into the left atrium, or abnormal ventilation-perfusion.[59] Cardiac index increases with exercise but seldom more than twofold.[51,54,55,60] This subnormal cardiac output results from blunted chronotropic response together with impaired function of the single subaortic ventricle.[61] Abnormalities of skeletal muscle metabolism contribute further to the decrease in exercise capacity. [127]

Conversion from a right atrial/pulmonary artery Fontan to a lateral tunnel or extracardiac Fontan improves survival, lowers the incidence of arrhythmias, and improves exercise capacity[128-130] (see Fig. 11–11). Irrespective of the type of Fontan modification, exercise performance remains below normal[128] and usually decreases further in the long term, a change that has been attributed at least in part to a more blunted rate response, probably because of sinus node dysfunction.[131] Monitored exercise training appears to improve functional capacity[127] (see Fig. 11–11). Pharmacologic afterload reduction is designed to increase the functional reserve of the subaortic ventricle and preserve, if not increase, exercise performance.

References

1. Maron BJ, Mitchell JH. Revised eligibility recommendations for competitive athletes with cardiovascular abnormalities. *J Am Coll Cardiol.* 1994;24:848–850.
2. Gutgesell HP, Gessner IH, Vetter VL, et al. Recreational and occupational recommendations for young patients with heart disease. A Statement for Physicians by the Committee on Congenital Cardiac Defects of the Council on Cardiovascular Disease in the Young, American Heart Association. *Circulation.* 1986;74:1195A–1198A.
3. Mitchell JH, Haskell W, Snell P, Van Camp SP. Task Force 8: classification of sports. *J Am Coll Cardiol.* 2005;45:1364–1367.
4. Freed MD. Recreational and sports recommendations for the child with heart disease. *Pediatr Clin North Am.* 1984;31:1307–1320.
5. Thaulow E, Fredriksen PM. Exercise and training in adults with congenital heart disease. *Int J Cardiol.* 2004;97(1 Suppl):35–38.
6. Brochu MC, Baril JF, Dore A, et al. Improvement in exercise capacity in asymptomatic and mildly symptomatic adults after atrial septal defect percutaneous closure. *Circulation.* 2002;106:1821–1826.
7. Diller GP, Dimopoulos K, Okonko D, et al. Exercise intolerance in adult congenital heart disease: comparative severity, correlates, and prognostic implication. *Circulation.* 2005;112:828–835.
8. Diller GP, Dimopoulos K, Okonko D, et al. Heart rate response during exercise predicts survival in adults with congenital heart disease. *J Am Coll Cardiol.* 2006;48:1250–1256.
9. Aboulhosn J, Castellon Y, Rao S, et al. Serum brain natriuretic peptide predicts adverse clinical events in adults with Eisenmenger syndrome. Chicago: American Heart Association Scientific Sessions, oral abstract presentation, 2006.
10. Dimopoulos K, Okonko DO, Diller GP, et al. Abnormal ventilatory response to exercise in adults with congenital heart disease relates to cyanosis and predicts survival. *Circulation.* 2006;113:2796–2802.
11. D'Andrea A, Caso P, Scarafile R, et al. Biventricular myocardial adaptation to different training protocols in competitive master athletes. *Int J Cardiol.* 2007;115:342–349.
12. Huston TP, Puffer JC, Rodney WM. The athletic heart syndrome. *N Engl J Med.* 1985;313:24–32.
13. Henriksen E, Landelius J, Kangro T, et al. An echocardiographic study of right and left ventricular adaptation to physical exercise in elite female orienteers. *Eur Heart J.* 1999;20:309–316.
14. D'Andrea A, Zeppilli P, Caso P, et al. Doppler myocardial imaging in the evaluation of the athlete's heart. *Ital Heart J Suppl.* 2003;4:635–644.
15. Pluim BM, Zwinderman AH, van der Laarse A, van der Wall EE. The athlete's heart. A meta-analysis of cardiac structure and function. *Circulation.* 2000;101:336–344.
16. Pelliccia A, Culasso F, Di Paolo FM, Maron BJ. Physiologic left ventricular cavity dilatation in elite athletes. *Ann Intern Med.* 1999;130:23–31.
17. D'Andrea A, Caso P, Severino S, et al. Effects of different training protocols on left ventricular myocardial function in competitive athletes: a Doppler tissue imaging study. *Ital Heart J.* 2002;3:34–40.
18. D'Andrea A, Limongelli G, Caso P, et al. Association between left ventricular structure and cardiac performance during effort in two morphological forms of athlete's heart. *Int J Cardiol.* 2002;86:177–184.
19. Goldberg B, Fripp RR, Lister G, et al. Effect of physical training on exercise performance of children following surgical repair of congenital heart disease. *Pediatrics.* 1981;68:691–699.
20. Ruttenberg HD, Adams TD, Orsmond GS, et al. Effects of exercise training on aerobic fitness in children after open heart surgery. *Pediatr Cardiol.* 1983;4:19–24.
21. Mereles D, Ehlken N, Kreuscher S, et al. Exercise and respiratory training improve exercise capacity and quality of life in patients with severe chronic pulmonary hypertension. *Circulation.* 2006;114:1482–1489.
22. Cheng TO. Tai Chi: the Chinese ancient wisdom of an ideal exercise for cardiac patients. *Int J Cardiol.* 2007;117:293–295.
23. Verdier F, Jimenez M, Chevalier JM, et al. Outcome of 30 congenital atrio-ventricular blocks. *Arch Mal Coeur Vaiss.* 2005;98:513–518.
24. Jaeggi ET, Hornberger LK, Smallhorn JF, Fouron JC. Prenatal diagnosis of complete atrioventricular block associated with structural heart disease: combined experience of two tertiary care centers and review of the literature. *Ultrasound Obstet Gynecol.* 2005;26:16–21.
25. Perloff JK. *The Clinical Recognition of Congenital Heart Disease.* Philadelphia: W.B. Saunders, 2003.
26. Puley G, Siu S, Connelly M, et al. Arrhythmia and survival in patients >18 years of age after the mustard procedure for complete transposition of the great arteries. *Am J Cardiol.* 1999;83:1080–1084.
27. Benson LN, Burns R, Schwaiger M, et al. Radionuclide angiographic evaluation of ventricular function in isolated congenitally corrected transposition of the great arteries. *Am J Cardiol.* 1986;58:319–324.
28. Fredriksen PM, Chen A, Veldtman G, et al. Exercise capacity in adult patients with congenitally corrected transposition of the great arteries. *Heart.* 2001;85:191–195.
29. Giardini A, Lovato L, Donti A, et al. Relation between right ventricular structural alterations and markers of adverse clinical outcome in adults with systemic right ventricle and either congenital complete (after Senning operation) or congenitally corrected transposition of the great arteries. *Am J Cardiol.* 2006;98:1277–1282.
30. Dubin AM, Janousek J, Rhee E, et al. Resynchronization therapy in pediatric and congenital heart disease patients: an international multicenter study. *J Am Coll Cardiol.* 2005;46:2277–2283.
31. Angelini P. Coronary artery anomalies: an entity in search of an identity. *Circulation.* 2007;115:1296–1305.
32. Hauser M, Bengel FM, Hager A, et al. Impaired myocardial blood flow and coronary flow reserve of the anatomical right systemic ventricle in patients with congenitally corrected transposition of the great arteries. *Heart.* 2003;89:1231–1235.
33. Singh TP, Humes RA, Muzik O, et al. Myocardial flow reserve in patients with a systemic right ventricle after atrial switch repair. *J Am Coll Cardiol.* 2001;37:2120–2125.
34. Barth CW 3rd, Roberts WC. Left main coronary artery originating from the right sinus of Valsalva and coursing between the aorta and pulmonary trunk. *J Am Coll Cardiol.* 1986;7:366–373.
35. Perloff J, Child J. *Congenital Heart Disease in Adults.* Philadelphia: WB Saunders, 1998:393.

36. Said SA, van der Werf T. Dutch survey of coronary artery fistulas in adults: congenital solitary fistulas. *Int J Cardiol*. 2006;106: 323–332.

37. Choh S, Orime Y, Tsukamoto S, et al. Successful surgical treatment of rupture of coronary arteriovenous fistula with unconsciousness after chest and back pain. *Ann Thorac Cardiovasc Surg*. 2005;11: 190–193.

38. Kimura S, Miyamoto K, Ueno Y. Cardiac tamponade due to spontaneous rupture of large coronary artery aneurysm. *Asian Cardiovasc Thorac Ann*. 2006;14:422–424.

39. Cheitlin MD, De Castro CM, McAllister HA. Sudden death as a complication of anomalous left coronary origin from the anterior sinus of Valsalva, a not-so-minor congenital anomaly. *Circulation*. 1974;50:780–787.

40. Maron BJ, Roberts WC, McAllister HA, et al. Sudden death in young athletes. *Circulation*. 1980;62:218–229.

41. Angelini P, Velasco JA, Ott D, Khoshnevis GR. Anomalous coronary artery arising from the opposite sinus: descriptive features and pathophysiologic mechanisms, as documented by intravascular ultrasonography. *J Invasive Cardiol*. 2003;15:507–514.

42. McNamara DG, Bricker JT, Galioto FM Jr, et al. Cardiovascular abnormalities in the athlete: recommendations regarding eligibility for competition. Task Force I: congenital heart disease. *J Am Coll Cardiol*. 1985;6:1200–1208.

43. Kececioglu D, Voth E, Morguet A, et al. Myocardial ischemia and left-ventricular function after ligation of left coronary artery (Bland-White-Garland syndrome): a long-term follow-up. *Thorac Cardiovasc Surg*. 1992;40:283–287.

44. Moodie DS, Cook SA, Gill CC, Napoli CA. Thallium-20 1 myocardial imaging in young adults with anomalous left coronary artery arising from the pulmonary artery. *J Nucl Med*. 1980;21:1076–1089.

45. Sato F, Koishizawa T. Stress/rest (99m)Tc-MIBI SPECT and 123I-BMIPP scintigraphy for indication of surgery with coronary artery to pulmonary artery fistula. *Int Heart J*. 2005;46:355–361.

46. Said SA, van der Werf T. Dutch survey of congenital coronary artery fistulas in adults: coronary artery-left ventricular multiple microfistulas multi-center observational survey in the Netherlands. *Int J Cardiol*. 2006;110:33–39.

47. Ferreira AC, de Marchena E, Mayor M, Bolooki H. Sinus of Valsalva aneurysm presenting as myocardial infarction during dobutamine stress test. *Cathet Cardiovasc Diagn*. 1996;39:400–402.

48. Onorato E, Casilli F, Mbala-Mukendi M, et al. Sudden heart failure due to a ruptured posterior Valsalva sinus aneurysm into the right atrium: feasibility of catheter closure using the Amplatzer duct occluder. *Ital Heart J*. 2005;6:603–607.

49. Lin CY, Hong GJ, Lee KC, et al. Ruptured congenital sinus of valsalva aneurysms. *J Card Surg*. 2004;19:99–102.

50. Sehested J, Baandrup U, Mikkelsen E. Different reactivity and structure of the prestenotic and poststenotic aorta in human coarctation. Implications for baroreceptor function. *Circulation*. 1982;65: 1060–1065.

51. Johnson D, Perrault H, Vobecky SJ, et al. Resetting of the cardiopulmonary baroreflex 10 years after surgical repair of coarctation of the aorta. *Heart*. 2001;85:318–325.

52. Clarkson PM, Nicholson MR, Barratt-Boyes BG, et al. Results after repair of coarctation of the aorta beyond infancy: a 10 to 28 year follow-up with particular reference to late systemic hypertension. *Am J Cardiol*. 1983;51:1481–1488.

53. Maron BJ, Humphries JO, Rowe RD, Mellits ED. Prognosis of surgically corrected coarctation of the aorta. A 20-year postoperative appraisal. *Circulation*. 1973;47:119–126.

54. Ou P, Celermajer DS, Mousseaux E, et al. Vascular remodeling after "successful" repair of coarctation: impact of aortic arch geometry. *J Am Coll Cardiol*. 2007;49:883–890.

55. Aboulhosn J, Child JS. Left ventricular outflow obstruction: subaortic stenosis, bicuspid aortic valve, supravalvar aortic stenosis, and coarctation of the aorta. *Circulation*. 2006;114:2412–2422.

56. James FW, Kaplan S. Systolic hypertension during submaximal exercise after correction of coarctation of aorta. *Circulation*. 1974;50: II27–II34.

57. Cohen M, Fuster V, Steele PM, et al. Coarctation of the aorta. Long-term follow-up and prediction of outcome after surgical correction. *Circulation*. 1989;80:840–845.

58. Ou P, Mousseaux E, Celermajer DS, et al. Aortic arch shape deformation after coarctation surgery: effect on blood pressure response. *J Thorac Cardiovasc Surg*. 2006;132:1105–1111.

59. De Caro E, Trocchio G, Smeraldi A, et al. Aortic arch geometry and exercise-induced hypertension in aortic coarctation. *Am J Cardiol*. 2007;99:1284–1287.

60. de Divitiis M, Pilla C, Kattenhorn M, et al. Ambulatory blood pressure, left ventricular mass, and conduit artery function late after successful repair of coarctation of the aorta. *J Am Coll Cardiol*. 2003;41:2259–2265.

61. de Divitiis M, Pilla C, Kattenhorn M, et al. Vascular dysfunction after repair of coarctation of the aorta: impact of early surgery. *Circulation*. 2001;104:I165–I170.

62. Gardiner HM, Celermajer DS, Sorensen KE, et al. Arterial reactivity is significantly impaired in normotensive young adults after successful repair of aortic coarctation in childhood. *Circulation*. 1994;89:1745–1750.

63. Simsolo R, Grunfeld B, Gimenez M, et al. Long-term systemic hypertension in children after successful repair of coarctation of the aorta. *Am Heart J*. 1988;115:1268–1273.

64. Gidding SS, Rocchini AP, Moorehead C, et al. Increased forearm vascular reactivity in patients with hypertension after repair of coarctation. *Circulation*. 1985;71:495–499.

65. Barton CH, Ni Z, Vaziri ND. Enhanced nitric oxide inactivation in aortic coarctation-induced hypertension. *Kidney Int*. 2001;60: 1083–1087.

66. Guenthard J, Wyler F. Exercise-induced hypertension in the arms due to impaired arterial reactivity after successful coarctation resection. *Am J Cardiol*. 1995;75:814–817.

67. Johnson D, Bonnin P, Perrault H, et al. Peripheral blood flow responses to exercise after successful correction of coarctation of the aorta. *J Am Coll Cardiol*. 1995;26:1719–1724.

68. Niwa K, Perloff JK, Bhuta SM, et al. Structural abnormalities of great arterial walls in congenital heart disease: light and electron microscopic analyses. *Circulation*. 2001;103:393–400.

69. Fedak PWM, Verma S, David TE, et al. Clinical and pathophysiological implications of a bicuspid aortic valve. *Circulation*. 2002;106: 900–904.

70. Bauer M, Pasic M, Meyer R, et al. Morphometric analysis of aortic media in patients with bicuspid and tricuspid aortic valve. *Ann Thorac Surg*. 2002;74:58–62.

71. Gurvitz M, Chang RK, Drant S, Allada V. Frequency of aortic root dilation in children with a bicuspid aortic valve. *Am J Cardiol*. 2004;94:1337–1340.

72. Lancellotti P, Lebois F, Simon M, et al. Prognostic importance of quantitative exercise Doppler echocardiography in asymptomatic valvular aortic stenosis. *Circulation*. 2005;112:I377–I382.

73. Atwood JE, Kawanishi S, Myers J, Froelicher VF. Exercise testing in patients with aortic stenosis. *Chest*. 1988;93:1083–7.

74. Bonow RO, Carabello BA, Kanu C, et al. ACC/AHA 2006 guidelines for the management of patients with valvular heart disease: a report of the American College of Cardiology/American Heart Association Task Force on Practice Guidelines (writing committee to revise the 1998 Guidelines for the Management of Patients with Valvular Heart Disease): developed in collaboration with the Society of Cardiovascular Anesthesiologists: endorsed by the Society for Cardiovascular Angiography and Interventions and the Society of Thoracic Surgeons. *Circulation*. 2006;114: e84–e231.

75. James FW, Schwartz DC, Kaplan S, Spilkin SP. Exercise electrocardiogram, blood pressure, and working capacity in young patients

with valvular or discrete subvalvular aortic stenosis. *Am J Cardiol.* 1982;50:769–775.

76. Scharhag J, Meyer T, Kindermann I, et al. Bicuspid aortic valve: evaluation of the ability to participate in competitive sports: case reports of two soccer players. *Clin Res Cardiol.* 2006;95:228–234.

77. Mark AL, Abboud FM, Schmid PG, Heistad DD. Reflex vascular responses to left ventricular outflow obstruction and activation of ventricular baroreceptors in dogs. *J Clin Invest.* 1973;52:1147–1153.

78. Graham TP Jr. Ventricular performance in adults after operation for congenital heart disease. *Am J Cardiol.* 1982;50:612–620.

79. Eichinger WB, Botzenhardt F, Wagner I, et al. Hemodynamic evaluation of the Sorin Soprano bioprosthesis in the completely supra-annular aortic position. *J Heart Valve Dis.* 2005;14:822–827.

80. Ali NF, Mahadevan VS, Muir A, et al. The influence of prosthesis size and design on exercise dynamics after aortic valve replacement. *J Heart Valve Dis.* 2006;15:755–762.

81. Moller JH, Adams P Jr. A simplified method for calculating the pulmonary valvular area. *Am Heart J.* 1966;72:463–465.

82. Nugent EW, Freedom RM, Nora JJ, et al. Clinical course in pulmonary stenosis. *Circulation.* 1977;56:I38–I47.

83. Moller JH, Adams P Jr. The natural history of pulmonary valvular stenosis. Serial cardiac catheterizations in 21 children. *Am J Cardiol.* 1965;16:654–664.

84. Krabill KA, Wang Y, Einzig S, Moller JH. Rest and exercise hemodynamics in pulmonary stenosis: comparison of children and adults. *Am J Cardiol.* 1985;56:360–365.

85. Driscoll DJ, Wolfe RR, Gersony WM, et al. Cardiorespiratory responses to exercise of patients with aortic stenosis, pulmonary stenosis, and ventricular septal defect. *Circulation.* 1993;87:I102–I113.

86. Moller JH, Rao S, Lucas RV Jr. Exercise hemodynamics of pulmonary valvular stenosis. Study of 64 children. *Circulation.* 1972;46:1018–1026.

87. Roos-Hesselink JW, Meijboom FJ, Spitaels SE, et al. Long-term outcome after surgery for pulmonary stenosis (a longitudinal study of 22–33 years). *Eur Heart J.* 2006;27:482–488.

88. Fratellone PM, Steinfeld L, Coplan NL. Exercise and congenital heart disease. *Am Heart J.* 1994;127:1676–1680.

89. Bonow RO, Borer JS, Rosing DR, et al. Left ventricular functional reserve in adult patients with atrial septal defect: pre- and postoperative studies. *Circulation.* 1981;63:1315–1322.

90. Reybrouck T, Bisschop A, Dumoulin M, van der Hauwaert LG. Cardiorespiratory exercise capacity after surgical closure of atrial septal defect is influenced by the age at surgery. *Am Heart J.* 1991;122:1073–1078.

91. Gabriel HM, Heger M, Innerhofer P, et al. Long-term outcome of patients with ventricular septal defect considered not to require surgical closure during childhood. *J Am Coll Cardiol.* 2002;39:1066–1071.

92. van den Berg J, Wielopolski PA, Meijboom FJ, et al. Diastolic function in repaired tetralogy of Fallot at rest and during stress: assessment with MR imaging. *Radiology.* 2007;243:212–219.

93. Galie N, Torbicki A, Barst R, et al. Guidelines on diagnosis and treatment of pulmonary arterial hypertension. The Task Force on Diagnosis and Treatment of Pulmonary Arterial Hypertension of the European Society of Cardiology. *Eur Heart J.* 2004;25:2243–2278.

94. Humbert M, Sitbon O, Simonneau G. Treatment of pulmonary arterial hypertension. *N Engl J Med.* 2004;351:1425–1436.

95. Galie N, Ghofrani HA, Torbicki A, et al. Sildenafil citrate therapy for pulmonary arterial hypertension. *N Engl J Med.* 2005;353:2148–2157.

96. Sietsema KE, Cooper DM, Perloff JK, et al. Dynamics of oxygen uptake during exercise in adults with cyanotic congenital heart disease. *Circulation.* 1986;73:1137–1144.

97. Sietsema KE. Cyanotic congenital heart disease: dynamics of oxygen uptake and ventilation during exercise. *J Am Coll Cardiol.* 1991;18:322–323.

98. Sietsema KE, Cooper DM, Perloff JK, et al. Control of ventilation during exercise in patients with central venous-to-systemic arterial shunts. *J Appl Physiol.* 1988;64:234–242.

99. Strieder DJ, Mesko ZG, Zaver AG, Gold WM. Exercise tolerance in chronic hypoxemia due to right-to-left shunt. *J Appl Physiol.* 1973;34:853–858.

100. Galie N, Beghetti M, Gatzoulis MA, et al. Bosentan therapy in patients with Eisenmenger syndrome: a multicenter, double-blind, randomized, placebo-controlled study. *Circulation.* 2006;114:48–54.

101. Mukhopadhyay S, Sharma M, Ramakrishnan S, et al. Phosphodi-esterase-5 inhibitor in Eisenmenger syndrome: a preliminary observational study. *Circulation.* 2006;114:1807–1810.

102. Gatzoulis MA, Rogers P, Li W, et al. Safety and tolerability of bosentan in adults with Eisenmenger physiology. *Int J Cardiol.* 2005;98:147–151.

103. Roos-Hesselink JW, Meijboom FJ, Spitaels SE, et al. Decline in ventricular function and clinical condition after Mustard repair for transposition of the great arteries (a prospective study of 22–29 years). *Eur Heart J.* 2004;25:1264–1270.

104. James FW, Kaplan S, Schwartz DC, et al. Response to exercise in patients after total surgical correction of tetralogy of Fallot. *Circulation.* 1976;54:671–679.

105. Wessel HU, Cunningham WJ, Paul MH, et al. Exercise performance in tetralogy of Fallot after intracardiac repair. *J Thorac Cardiovasc Surg.* 1980;80:582–593.

106. Garson A Jr, Gillette PC, Gutgesell HP, McNamara DG. Stress-induced ventricular arrhythmia after repair of tetralogy of Fallot. *Am J Cardiol.* 1980;46:1006–1012.

107. Giardini A, Specchia S, Coutsoumbas G, et al. Impact of pulmonary regurgitation and right ventricular dysfunction on oxygen uptake recovery kinetics in repaired tetralogy of Fallot. *Eur J Heart Fail.* 2006;8:736–743.

108. Giardini A, Specchia S, Tacy TA, et al. Usefulness of cardiopulmonary exercise to predict long-term prognosis in adults with repaired tetralogy of Fallot. *Am J Cardiol.* 2007;99:1462–1467.

109. Mulla N, Paridon SM, Pinsky WW. Cardiopulmonary performance during exercise in patients with repaired tetralogy of Fallot with absent pulmonary valve. *Pediatr Cardiol.* 1995;16:120–126.

110. van den Berg J, de Bie S, Meijboom FJ, et al. Changes during exercise of ECG intervals related to increased risk for ventricular arrhythmia in repaired tetralogy of Fallot and their relationship to right ventricular size and function. *Int J Cardiol.* 2007, April 10 [Epub ahead of print].

111. Trojnarska O, Szyszka A, Gwizdala A, et al. The BNP concentrations and exercise capacity assessment with cardiopulmonary stress test in patients after surgical repair of Fallot's tetralogy. *Int J Cardiol.* 2006;110:86–92.

112. Dimopoulos K, Okonko DO, Diller GP, et al. Abnormal ventilatory response to exercise in adults with congenital heart disease relates to cyanosis and predicts survival. *Circulation.* 2006;113:2796–2802.

113. Trojnarska O, Szyszka A, Gwizdala A, et al. Adults with Ebstein's anomaly—cardiopulmonary exercise testing and BNP levels exercise capacity and BNP in adults with Ebstein's anomaly. *Int J Cardiol.* 2006;111:92–97.

114. Mathews RA, Fricker FJ, Beerman LB, et al. Exercise studies after the Mustard operation in transposition of the great arteries. *Am J Cardiol.* 1983;51:1526–1529.

115. Hesslein PS, Gutgesell HP, Gillette PC, McNamara DG. Exercise assessment of sinoatrial node function following the Mustard operation. *Am Heart J.* 1982;103:351–357.

116. De Bleser L, Budts W, Sluysmans T, et al. Self-reported physical activities in patients after the Mustard or Senning operation: comparison with healthy control subjects. *Eur J Cardiovasc Nurs.* 2007;6:247–251.

117. Budts W, Scheurwegs C, Stevens A, et al. The future of adult patients after Mustard or Senning repair for transposition of the great arteries. *Int J Cardiol.* 2006;113:209–214.

118. Hui L, Chau AK, Leung MP, et al. Assessment of left ventricular function long term after arterial switch operation for transposition of the great arteries by dobutamine stress echocardiography. *Heart.* 2005;91:68–72.

119. Reybrouck T, Eyskens B, Mertens L, et al. Cardiorespiratory exercise function after the arterial switch operation for transposition of the great arteries. *Eur Heart J.* 2001;22:1052–1059.

120. Driscoll DJ, Danielson GK, Puga FJ, et al. Exercise tolerance and cardiorespiratory response to exercise after the Fontan operation for tricuspid atresia or functional single ventricle. *J Am Coll Cardiol.* 1986;7:1087–1094.

121. Barber G, Di Sessa T, Child JS, et al. Hemodynamic responses to isolated increments in heart rate by atrial pacing after a Fontan procedure. *Am Heart J.* 1988;115:837–841.

122. Senzaki H, Masutani S, Ishido H, et al. Cardiac rest and reserve function in patients with Fontan circulation. *J Am Coll Cardiol.* 2006;47:2528–2535.

123. Grant GP, Mansell AL, Garofano RP, et al. Cardiorespiratory response to exercise after the Fontan procedure for tricuspid atresia. *Pediatr Res.* 1988;24:1–5.

124. Zellers TM, Driscoll DJ, Mottram CD, et al. Exercise tolerance and cardiorespiratory response to exercise before and after the Fontan operation. *Mayo Clin Proc.* 1989;64:1489–1497.

125. Eckberg DL, Drabinsky M, Braunwald E. Defective cardiac parasympathetic control in patients with heart disease. *N Engl J Med.* 1971;285:877–883.

126. Goldstein RE, Beiser GD, Stampfer M, Epstein SE. Impairment of autonomically mediated heart rate control in patients with cardiac dysfunction. *Circ Res.* 1975;36:571–578.

127. Brassard P, Bedard E, Jobin J, et al. Exercise capacity and impact of exercise training in patients after a Fontan procedure: a review. *Can J Cardiol.* 2006;22:489–495.

128. Rosenthal M, Bush A, Deanfield J, Redington A. Comparison of cardiopulmonary adaptation during exercise in children after the atriopulmonary and total cavopulmonary connection Fontan procedures. *Circulation.* 1995;91:372–378.

129. Giardini A, Napoleone CP, Specchia S, et al. Conversion of atriopulmonary Fontan to extracardiac total cavopulmonary connection improves cardiopulmonary function. *Int J Cardiol.* 2006;113: 341–344.

130. Mavroudis C, Deal BJ, Backer CL. The beneficial effects of total cavopulmonary conversion and arrhythmia surgery for the failed Fontan. *Semin Thorac Cardiovasc Surg Pediatr Card Surg Annu.* 2002;5:12–24.

131. Nir A, Driscoll DJ, Mottram CD, et al. Cardiorespiratory response to exercise after the Fontan operation: a serial study. *J Am Coll Cardiol.* 1993;22:216–220.

CHAPTER 12

Cyanotic Congenital Heart Disease: A Multisystem Disorder

JOSEPH K. PERLOFF

Cyanotic congenital heart disease in adults is a multisystem disorder that includes hematologic issues, the systemic and coronary vascular beds, bilirubin kinetics, the kidneys, the digits and long bones, the lungs, the central nervous system, and gynecologic endocrinology (Fig. 12–1).

HEMATOLOGIC ISSUES

Red Blood Cell Mass

There is a clear distinction between *polycythemia* and *erythrocytosis*. Clinical decisions based on an analogy between polycythemia and the erythrocytosis of cyanotic congenital heart disease (CHD) are erroneous.[1,2] Polycythemia rubra vera is a malignant clonal stem cell disorder characterized by excessive proliferation of all three hematopoietic cell lines—erythroid, myeloid, and megakaryocytic—resulting in an increase in red blood cells, an increase in plasma volume, and an increase in platelets and granulocytes.[3-5] By contrast, *erythrocytosis* refers to an isolated increase in the number of red blood cells.[4] *Primary* erythrocytosis refers to an isolated increase in red cell mass in the absence of a definable cause, whereas *secondary* erythrocytosis refers to an isolated increase in red cell mass in response to a definable stimulus such as low systemic arterial oxygen saturation of cyanotic CHD[4] or high altitude.[6] Platelet counts are in the low range of normal or thrombocytopenic,[7] and granulocyte counts are normal.

The essential function of erythrocytes is the transport of oxygen to metabolizing tissues. In cyanotic CHD, erythrocytosis is a desirable and altogether appropriate adaptive response to arterial hypoxemia and decreased tissue oxygenation.[4]

Importantly, employment of phlebotomy in the treatment of polycythemia vera is accompanied by a significant *increase* in the incidence of thrombosis—including cerebral—and the incidence increases as the phlebotomy rate increases.[3,5] In cyanotic CHD, phlebotomy as a means of reducing a presumed risk of cerebral arterial thrombosis has no rationale (see later).[1] In polycythemia rubra vera and in cyanotic CHD, anticoagulants or antiplatelet agents are of no established benefit but significantly increase the risk of hemorrhage.

Erythrocyte mass is determined chiefly by factors that affect tissue oxygenation. Erythrocytosis in response to the chronic hypoxemia of cyanotic CHD is essential for maintaining systemic oxygen transport.[8] Tissue oxygenation depends on a number of variables, including the availability of oxygen to erythrocytes during their pulmonary transit, the transport of erythrocytes to metabolizing tissues, the amount of hemoglobin available for oxygen transport, and luminal diffusion of endothelial nitric oxide.[9]

The position of the oxygen-hemoglobin dissociation curve is normal or shifted slightly to the right in cyanotic CHD.[10,11] Because erythrocytosis is a desirable adaptive response that offsets the deficit in tissue oxygenation, appropriate equilibrium conditions are usually established at elevated hematocrit levels.

Erythropoietin is a sialoglycoprotein that is the major regulator of red blood cell production.[12] Tissue hypoxemia stimulates release of erythropoietin from specialized interstitial cells in the renal cortex, which is the major site of production.[12,13] The hypoxemic stimulus of cyanotic CHD provokes renal cortical release of erythropoietin, which stimulates proliferation and differentiation of erythroid elements in the bone marrow, an increase in the number of circulating red blood cells,

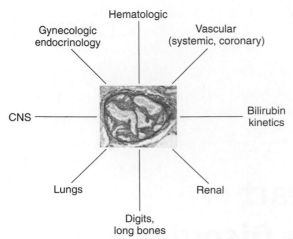

Hematologic

Gynecologic endocrinology

Vascular (systemic, coronary)

CNS

Bilirubin kinetics

Lungs

Renal

Digits, long bones

FIGURE 12-1 Schematic illustration of cyanotic congenital heart disease (CCHD) as a multisystem systemic disorder—hematologic, vascular, bilirubin kinetics, renal, digits and long bones, lungs, central nervous system (CNS), and gynecologic endocrinology.

and an increase in hemoglobin concentration. When the rise in red cell mass and the hemoglobin concentration are adequate to offset tissue hypoxemia, the serum erythropoietin levels normalize.[12,13] The erythrocytosis is therefore compensatory, that is, it is a physiologically appropriate adaptive response to increased erythropoietin production prompted by tissue hypoxemia.[2] Occasionally, tissue oxygen concentration fails to reach the threshold of renal cortical oxygen sensors. Erythrocyte mass then exceeds the range at which blood viscosity per se becomes a limiting factor in tissue oxygen delivery, and equilibrium conditions are not achieved. An increase in erythropoietin secretion and an increase in erythrocyte mass continue despite potentially detrimental effects.[4,14]

Whole blood viscosity is determined by a complex interplay of a number of variables including red cell mass, red cell morphology and deformability, plasma viscosity, plasma protein morphology and concentration, aggregation and dispersion of cellular elements, shear rate, temperature, and vascular walls (bore).[15] In cyanotic CHD, oxygen delivery is facilitated by a combination of systemic vasodilatation and enhanced oxygen transfer from red cells to tissue.[16] Increased endothelial shear stress provoked by erythrocytosis stimulates release of nitric oxide (NO). The molecule diffuses abluminally to regulate blood flow by activating soluble guanylate cyclase in medial smooth muscle and diffuses luminally where the extremely high reaction rate with red blood cell hemoglobin effectively reduces the concentration to zero.[9] In light of enhanced NO production prompted by the increased endothelial shear stress of erythrocytosis, it was anticipated that HbNO concentration would increase in proportion to nitrate concentration. The formation of HbNO might serve as a pivotal mechanism by which red cells in hypoxemic patients compensate for reduced oxygen content by increasing the rate of transfer of oxygen to tissues.[9] The normal biconcave erythrocyte

(Fig. 12-2, *A*) is an infinitely deformable membrane partially filled with a viscous, noncompressible hemoglobin solution. Iron-deficiency changes the shape of red blood cells from deformable biconcave discs to microspherocytes (see Fig. 12-2, *B*) that resist deformation.[15,17-22]

At high shear rates in larger conductance vessels, normal biconcave red cells alter their shapes into prolate ellipsoids with major axes parallel to the direction of flow.[22] Microspherocytes cannot alter their shape, even at high shear rates. Red blood cells pass single file through capillary beds where viscosity depends on membrane flexibility.[23] In the microcirculation, capillary diameter is significantly smaller than red cell diameter, a mismatch that is responsible for increased viscosity at capillary level.[19]

The normal biconcave erythrocyte is 2 μm in width and 8 μm in diameter but, because of deformability, traverses a 14-μm long channel that is only 2.8 μm in width and can squeeze through 0.5-μm openings between cells.[19] Because microspherocytes resist deformability in the capillary bed, resistance appreciably increases.

Repeated phlebotomy causes iron deficiency with microcytosis and the undesirable effects just described, in addition to the negative effects of iron deficiency on exercise performance and muscle strength.[18-22,24-26] In infants and children, iron deficiency is usually dietary. In adults, the chief cause is injudicious phlebotomy, although hemoptysis, epistaxis, and menorrhagia sometimes contribute. Immediately following an isovolumetric phlebotomy in an erythrocytotic cyanotic adult, stroke volume, systemic blood flow, and oxygen transport improve,[27] but these benefits are short-lived because elaboration of erythropoietin rapidly returns the red cell mass to prephlebotomy levels. Pentoxifylline (Trental), a theobromine derivative of methylxanthine, increases red blood

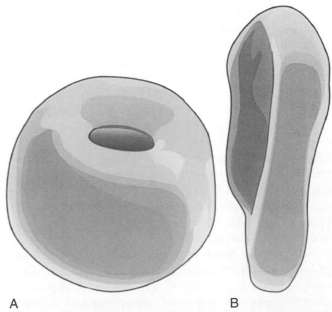

A

B

FIGURE 12-2 Illustration of a rigid, nondeformable microspherocyte **(A)** compared with an infinitely deformable biconcave disk **(B).**

cell deformability and decreases resistance to flow in the microcirculation. The moderate clinical improvement in hyperviscosity symptoms must be weighed against a risk of bleeding.[28]

Erythrocytosis in cyanotic CHD has been classified as *compensated* and *decompensated.*[11] Compensated erythrocytosis represents an appropriate adaptive response to tissue hypoxemia, with equilibrium hematocrit established in an iron-replete state (discussed earlier). Decompensated erythrocytosis represents a maladaptive response to tissue hypoxemia characterized by failure to establish equilibrium conditions in an iron-replete state, together with moderate to severe hyperviscosity symptoms.[11,29] Total blood volume and erythrocyte mass may reach three times normal, but the magnitude of the increase does not predict whether a given response will be compensated or decompensated.[11]

The Cyanotic Congenital Heart Disease Questionnaire (Table 12–1) serves as a basis for assessing the presence and degree of hyperviscosity symptoms. Myalgias and muscle weakness occur with iron-deficient and iron-replete erythrocytosis, but when hematocrit levels are below 65%, these symptoms almost always reflect iron deficiency rather than hyperviscosity (discussed later). Iron is an integral part of myoglobin and of certain mitochondrial enzymes and plays an important role in oxidative metabolism. Iron deficiency, even when mild, impairs muscle performance in occupations requiring heavy expenditures of energy[30] and augments exercise-induced increases in blood lactate levels.[31] Iron-deficient microcytic erythrocytes exhibit decreased oxygen-carrying capacity because of reduced mean corpuscular hemoglobin concentration and because of less effective oxygen release during the capillary transit because of reduced deformability.[9]

A reduction in cerebral blood flow has been reported in human subjects with hematocrits in the upper range of normal.[32] However, venous hematocrit is higher than hematocrit in the microcirculation, and whole blood viscosity per se has comparatively little effect on microcirculatory flow rate, a point relevant to the cerebral circulation in which flow rate is determined by vessels that are of comparatively small caliber. Cerebral thrombosis reported in "smoker's erythrocytosis" is associated with an increase in carboxyhemoglobin and normal or reduced plasma volume.[33] There is a direct relationship between the number of cigarettes smoked per day and hematocrit levels in otherwise normal persons.[34] Tobacco products in patients with cyanotic CHD cause carboxyhemoglobinemia, which impairs red cell oxygen-carrying capacity and promotes erythrocytosis. Cyanotic patients should avoid both active and passive inhalation of tobacco products.

The low incidence of stroke at high altitudes despite elevated hematocrit levels calls into question a proposed relationship between hematocrit, viscosity, and stroke.[35] Although a thrombotic predisposition, including a relatively high incidence of cerebral thrombosis, is a feature of polycythemia rubra vera,[3,5] the differences between polycythemia vera and the secondary erythrocytosis of cyanotic CHD have been underscored (discussed earlier). Importantly, iron-deficient erythrocytosis in cyanotic children younger than 4 years predisposes to cerebrovascular accidents, but the offending thromboses are in intracranial venous sinuses and veins[21,36-38] (Fig. 12–3).

Table 12–1   Cyanotic Congenital Heart Disease Questionnaire
Presence and Degree of Symptoms
Absent—asymptomatic
Mild—symptoms are present but do not interfere with normal activities
Moderate—symptoms interfere with some but not most activities
Marked to Severe—interferes with most if not all activities
Erythrocytosis
Headache
Faintness, dizziness, lightheadedness
Slow mentation, impaired alertness, irritability, a sense of distance or dissociation
Blurred or double vision, scotoma
Paresthesias of fingers, toes, or lips
Tinnitus
Fatigue, lassitude, lethargy
Myalgias, muscle weakness
Do you take over-the-counter drugs that contain iron?
Hemorrhagic Diathesis
Do you take aspirin or over-the-counter anti-inflammatory drugs?
Easy bruising (fragile skin)
Gingival bleeding (fragile gums)
Epistaxis (fragile nasal mucous membranes)
Pulmonary hemorrhage (hemoptysis, intrapulmonary)
Menorrhagia
Traumatic bleeding (accidental injury, surgery)
Urate Metabolism
Gouty arthritis
Osteoarthropathy—long-bone pain and tenderness

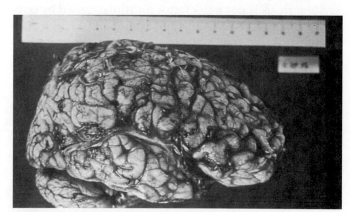

FIGURE 12–3   The brain of an 18-month-old cyanotic, erythrocytotic, iron-deficient infant who died after a transverse (lateral) cerebral venous sinus thrombosis.

Dehydration accompanying diarrhea or vomiting in these children is an aggravating cause of cerebral venous thromboses. Neonatal erythrocytosis attributed to delayed umbilical cord clamping, cord stripping, or chronic intrauterine hypoxemia results in increased hematocrit levels and multiple small cerebral occlusions.[39] Most relevant here is whether erythrocytosis in adults with cyanotic CHD incurs the risk of stroke caused by cerebral arterial thrombosis. In a study of more than 100 adults with cyanotic CHD[40] (748 patient-years) in whom independent risk factors for embolic or vasospastic stroke were excluded, no patient experienced stroke due to cerebral arterial thrombosis irrespective of hematocrit level, iron stores, the degree or recurrence of cerebral hyperviscosity symptoms or whether erythrocytosis was compensated or decompensated. The therapeutic implications of these observations are dealt with later.

Laboratory Precautions

Routine clinical hematologic assessment should include hematocrit level, hemoglobin concentration, and red cell indices, particularly mean corpuscular volume and mean corpuscular hemoglobin concentration. Because microhematocrit centrifugation in the presence of erythrocytosis results in plasma trapping and falsely elevated hematocrit levels, inaccuracies are incurred unless determinations are made by automated electronic particle counts.[41] Increased plasma levels of homocysteine are accompanied by hyperchromia and macrocytosis that may mask hypochromia and microcytosis.[42]

Blood glucose levels may be reported as dramatically reduced in erythrocytotic patients, but the "hypoglycemia" is artifactual because increased *in vitro* glycolysis results from the greater than normal number of erythrocytes. Accurate blood glucose determinations require the addition of sodium fluoride to the tube to prevent red cell glycolysis and to prevent spurious erythrocytotic hypoglycemia.

Phlebotomy

Erythrocytosis is not a risk factor for stroke caused by cerebral arterial thrombosis in adults with cyanotic CHD (discussed above).[40] The circulatory effects of phlebotomy are transient,[1,11,27,43] and phlebotomy-induced iron deficiency has adverse consequences already mentioned. Phlebotomy should therefore not be based on hematocrit irrespective of level but should be employed selectively for temporary relief of intrusive hyperviscosity symptoms (see Table 12–1). Dehydration caused by heat, humidity, fever, diarrhea, vomiting, and commercial air travel provokes a rise in hematocrit level and symptomatic hyperviscosity.[1] The treatment is volume repletion, not phlebotomy.[2] Hyperviscosity symptoms in an iron-replete state rarely occur unless the hematocrit exceeds 65%.[11] When symptoms occur with hematocrit levels less than 65%, the cause is almost always

iron deficiency. Phlebotomy further depletes iron stores and aggravates rather than alleviates the symptoms that respond to iron.[11,29] Preoperative phlebotomy for its hemostatic effect is dealt with later.

Let us now focus on the clinical setting in which phlebotomy is appropriate, including the amount of blood removed, the method of removal, and the vehicle for volume repletion.[2] A comparatively simple, safe outpatient method for adults is withdrawal of 500 ml of blood followed by quantitative volume replacement.[2] Phlebotomy without volume repletion may provoke a transient decrease in systemic blood flow, oxygen delivery, and cerebral perfusion.[27] For routine purposes, an equivalent volume of isotonic saline suffices. Should saline administration be clinically inappropriate, 5% dextrose (Dextran 40) contains no sodium but risks allergic or bleeding side effects. Cuff blood pressure should be recorded before phlebotomy with the patient in the supine, sitting, and standing positions and at 15-minute intervals after the procedure until the pressure stabilizes.[29] The beneficial effects are usually evident within 24 hours and reflect an increase in systemic blood flow induced by the isovolumetric reduction in red cell mass.[27,38,44] Pulmonary arterial blood flow and pulmonary alveolar oxygen uptake play little or no role in the symptomatic response[45,46] (Fig. 12–4).

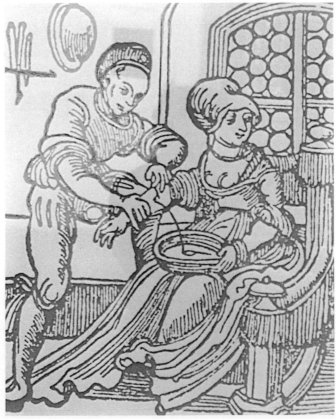

FIGURE 12–4 Illustration of venisection (phlebotomy) as displayed in the window of a Swiss apothecary. (*Photograph by the author, Zurich, 1990.*)

OTHER THERAPEUTIC RECOMMENDATIONS

Because erythropoietin levels are elevated in patients with iron-deficient erythrocytosis,[13] administration of iron results in a rapid increase in red cell mass.[11,29,47] The dose should therefore be small (325 mg of ferrous sulfate, which is 65 mg of elemental iron) once daily.[1,20] Monitoring must be frequent, and iron is discontinued at the first discernible rise in hematocrit level, which is usually within a week. Patients with cyanotic CHD, especially those with decompensated erythrocytosis, should be cautioned against using over-the-counter preparations that contain nonprescribed iron. When there is intolerance to oral ferrous sulfate, a carbohydrate preparation (Niferex) may be acceptable. For the occasional patient who is intolerant of any oral iron preparation, intravenous iron Dextran can be used but with caution to avoid extravasation. Intravenous iron results in alleviation of myalgias and muscle weakness before an erythrocytotic response is detectable, an observation in accord with data that iron deficiency per se has an independent negative effect on exercise performance.[24]

Hydroxyurea, an antitumor agent, reduces cell proliferation and suppresses erythrocytosis in cyanotic patients who exceed a physiologically adaptive increase in red cell mass in an iron-replete state (decompensated erythrocytosis).[48] The drug has also been successful in countering the erythrocytotic rebound induced by phlebotomy.[48] Hydroxyurea together with oral iron has been employed in the uncommon, if not rare, cyanotic patient with refractory hypochronic erythrocytosis, which is, by definition, unresponsive to iron alone, even intravenous iron.[11,29] The thrombocytopenia and neutropenia occasionally caused by hydroxyurea disappear rapidly when the drug is discontinued. The mechanism responsible for an increase in fetal hemoglobin induced by hydroxyurea has not been established.[48]

It seems intuitive that inhaled oxygen should benefit patients with decreased arterial oxygen saturation. There is a general consensus, however, that the benefits of oxygen reported by cyanotic patients have a psychologic rather than physiologic basis. High levels of inhaled oxygen raise systemic arterial oxygen saturation in the presence of a right-to-left shunt because of an increase in oxygenation of alveolar blood.[49,50] In cyanotic congenital disease, however, systemic venous blood is shunted into the systemic arterial circulation before reaching the alveoli, so inhaled oxygen cannot significantly affect the saturation of shunted blood unless there is a ventilation-perfusion mismatch. Extended administration of oxygen risks potential pulmonary toxicity. The drying effect of oxygen on nasal mucous membranes provokes epistaxis, which is aggravated by increased nasal tissue vascularity and the inherent

hemostatic defects in cyanotic patients (discussed later). Oxygen administration, especially at night, dries the tracheobronchial mucous membranes, provoking cough, interfering with sleep, and occasionally provoking hemoptysis. If used at all, oxygen should be humidified.

Hemostasis

A bleeding tendency has been recognized in CHD patients since the 1950s, especially in those who are cyanotic.[51-61] The increased endothelial shear stress inherent in the erythrocytotic perfusate of cyanotic CHD stimulates release of endothelial-derived nitric oxide and prostaglandins that induce arteriolar dilatation. The increase in tissue vascularity acts in concert with intrinsic hemostatic defects to increase the bleeding tendency (see Systemic Vascular Bed). Bleeding is characterized by easy bruising, gingival bleeding induced by brushing the teeth, excessive bleeding during dental work or oral surgery, epistaxis, menorrhagia, traumatic bleeding (accidental, perioperative), and pulmonary hemorrhage.

The von Willebrand factor is a multimeric glycoprotein that is a major adhesive link between exposed vascular subendothelium and platelets.[61] Depletion of the largest von Willebrand multimers in adults with CHD contributes to the bleeding diathesis[61] (Fig. 12-5). Cyanosis, pulmonary vascular disease, and turbulent blood flow are major determinants of the von Willebrand abnormality, which normalizes after reparative surgery, indicating that the reversible defect is acquired.

Platelet counts in cyanotic CHD are typically in the low range of normal or thrombocytopenic[3] and vary inversely with hematocrit levels.[7,14,54,57,61-63] Platelet production is decreased because of ineffective thrombopoiesis, not because of increased platelet destruction or activation.[7] Low platelet counts typically increase immediately after phlebotomy, providing a rationale for preoperative phlebotomy to improve hemostasis.[57] In anticipation of surgery, whole blood should be removed isovolumetrically in daily amounts of 500 ml to reduce the hematocrit to just below 65%. Within hours after the initial phlebotomy, platelet counts increase and platelet aggregation and hemostasis improve.[7] Remember, however, that cardiopulmonary bypass per se is associated with a reduction in platelet counts and platelet dysfunction.

Pulmonary hemorrhage is manifested by external bleeding—hemoptysis (Gr. *haima* = blood; *ptyein* = to spit; Fig. 12-6)—and intrapulmonary hemorrhage, which by definition is internal (Figs. 12-7 and 12-8). The presence and degree of intrapulmonary hemorrhage cannot be determined from the presence and degree of hemoptysis. Intrapulmonary hemorrhage,

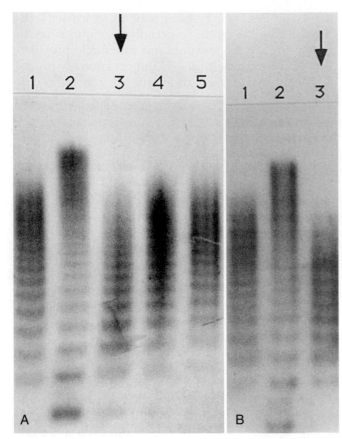

FIGURE 12–5 Agarose gel electrophoresis for identification of the largest von Willebrand multimers. **(A)** Lane 1 is normal plasma. Lane 2 is normal plasma with endothelial cell supernate. Lane 3 is from a cyanotic patient with pulmonary vascular disease. There is a significant decrease in the largest von Willebrand multimers. Lane 4 is normal plasma. Lane 5 is from an acyanotic patient with normal pulmonary vascular resistance, no turbulent blood flow, and normal von Willebrand multimer concentrations. **(B)** Lane 1 is normal plasma. Lane 2 is normal plasma with endothelial cell supernate. Lane 3 is from a cyanotic patient with turbulent flow and normal pulmonary vascular resistance. The largest von Willebrand multimers are absent.

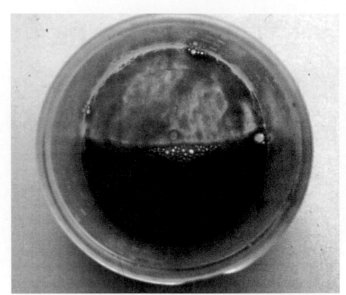

FIGURE 12–6 Hemoptysis (external pulmonary hemorrhage) as judged by the amount of blood coughed into a plastic measuring cup.

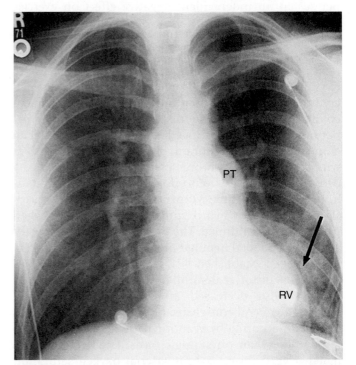

FIGURE 12–7 Chest radiograph from a 26-year-old cyanotic man with a nonrestrictive ventricular septal defect and pulmonary vascular disease. Brisk hemoptysis was associated with intrapulmonary hemorrhage that caused the infiltrate in the left lower lobe *(arrow)*. PT, pulmonary trunk; RV, right ventricle.

which varies from mild and occasional to copious, recurrent, massive, and fatal (see Fig. 12–8), is the most serious type of bleeding in Eisenmenger syndrome and the most common cause of sudden death.[64] Recall the 32-year-old man reported by Victor Eisenmenger in 1897 who "died more or less suddenly . . . following a large hemoptysis."[65]

There is a seeming paradox between a bleeding tendency—abnormal hemostasis—on one hand and a thrombotic predisposition in specific vascular beds on the other. *In situ* upper lobe thrombosis occasionally occurs in cyanotic patients with pulmonary vascular disease[29] (Fig. 12–9). Far more ominous is the tendency for large laminated thrombi to form in the dilatated pulmonary trunk and proximal arteries of these patients[2] (Figs. 12–10 through 12–12). The proximal thrombotic material is prone to embolize into distal pulmonary arteries (artery-to-artery intrapulmonary embolus), resulting in pulmonary infarction. The coexisting hemostatic defects convert these pulmonary infarcts into zones of intrapulmonary hemorrhage and hemorrhagic pleural effusion (Fig. 12–13).

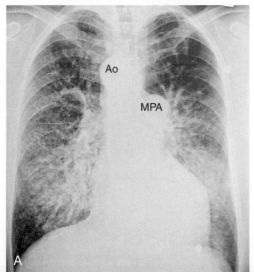

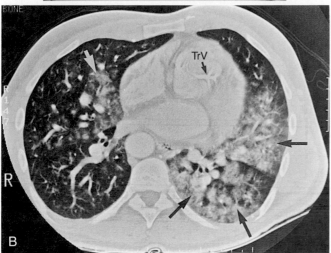

FIGURE 12–8 **(A)** Chest radiograph from a 46-year-old cyanotic man with truncus arteriosus and pulmonary vascular disease. Bilateral pulmonary infiltrates represent extensive intrapulmonary hemorrhage that accompanied moderate hemoptysis. Ao, right aortic arch; MPA, main pulmonary artery. **(B)** Computed tomographic scan from the same patient showing extensive intrapulmonary hemorrhage in the left lung *(black arrows)*, and less extensive hemorrhage in the right lung *(white arrow)*. TrV, calcified truncal valve.

OTHER HEMATOLOGIC DISORDERS

Two additional hematologic disorders accompanying CHD warrant comment—neutrophil degranulation in cyanotic patients[66] and leukemia in Down syndrome.[67-69] Increased plasma neutrophil elastase levels in cyanotic patients indicate degranulation, which is a reliable index of neutrophil activation.[66] Activated neutrophils release vasoconstrictors and proteolytic enzymes that cause endothelial injury and activation of platelets and coagulation pathways.[66] Down syndrome, a chromosomal abnormality (see Chapter 10), is associated with an increased incidence of leukemia.[67-69] Among children with acute leukemia, Down syndrome is disproportionately represented—20 times greater than would otherwise be expected.[69] Leukemia in Down

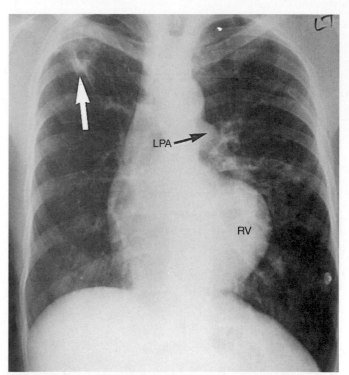

FIGURE 12–9   Chest radiograph from a 31-year-old cyanotic man who developed pulmonary vascular disease after a left Blalock-Taussig shunt for tetralogy of Fallot. White arrow points to an *in situ* right upper lobe pulmonary infarct. LPA, dilatated left pulmonary artery; RV, boot-shaped right ventricle that occupies the apex.

syndrome is usually myeloblastic, less commonly lymphoblastic.[69]

Laboratory Precautions

The standard amount of citrate anticoagulant added to blood samples of patients with normal hematocrit is excessive for patients with erythrocytosis because plasma volume is diminished in erythrocytotic whole blood. Failure to adjust the citrate concentration when hematocrit levels are above 55% leads to spurious results in routinely performed coagulation tests. Overdilution of plasma by anticoagulant must be avoided when assessing coagulation parameters in erythrocytotic patients. The volume of Wares anticoagulant should be down-adjusted as follows: Volume of Anticoagulant per Milliliter of Blood = $(100 - \text{Hct}) \div (595 - \text{Hct})$.

Precautions

The hemorrhagic predisposition in cyanotic CHD is sometimes appreciably reinforced by ill-advised use of antiplatelet agents, nonsteroidal anti-inflammatory agents that inhibit platelet aggregation, and warfarin or heparin anticoagulants. Fragile, spongy gums (Fig. 12–14) bleed easily when a hard-bristle toothbrush is used vigorously and during routine dental work or oral surgery. Brushing teeth should be gentle, employing a toothbrush with soft

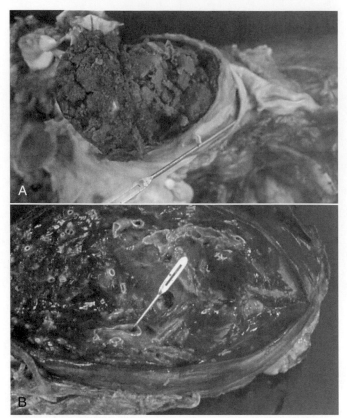

FIGURE 12–10 Necropsy specimens from a 43-year-old cyanotic man with a nonrestrictive ventricular septal defect and pulmonary vascular disease. **(A)** The dilatated right pulmonary artery is filled with massive thrombus. **(B)** Cross-section of the right lung showing massive intra-pulmonary hemorrhage that resulted in sudden death. Note thickened raised cross sections of intrapulmonary arteries typical of pulmonary vascular disease.

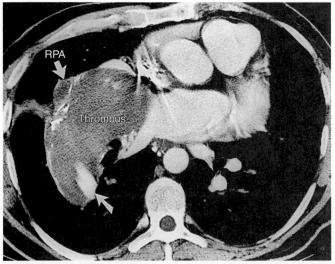

FIGURE 12–11 Images from a 54-year-old cyanotic man with a non-restrictive ventricular septal defect, pulmonary vascular disease, an enlarged pulmonary trunk, and aneurysmal dilatation of the right pulmonary artery. Computed tomographic scan showing a massive thrombus in the aneurysmally dilatated right pulmonary artery (RPA). Lower arrow identifies the remnant of a lumen.

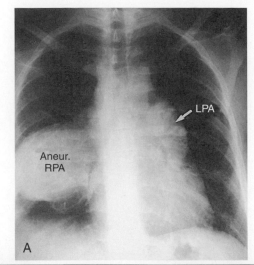

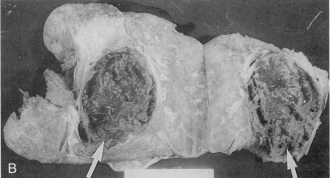

FIGURE 12–12 **(A)** Chest radiograph from a 30-year-old cyanotic woman with a univentricular heart, pulmonary atresia, left Blalock-Taussig shunt, pulmonary vascular disease in the left lung with dilatation of the left pulmonary artery (LPA), and aneurysmal dilatation of the right pulmonary artery (Aneur. RPA) distal to a zone of stenosis. **(B)** Extirpated specimen (heart/lung transplantation) shows massive thrombus *(arrows)* in the aneurysm of the right pulmonary artery.

bristles or, better still, an electric toothbrush. Epistaxis induced by drying of nasal mucous membranes with inhaled oxygen can be controlled by a humidifier or, better still, by cessation of oxygen (discussed earlier).

The most serious type of spontaneous bleeding is pulmonary hemorrhage (discussed earlier). The first necessity is to avoid bronchoscopy, which incurs risk without providing therapeutically useful information. It should be re-emphasized that *hemoptysis* is *external* (Fig. 12–15) and does not necessarily reflect the extent of hemorrhage that may be principally or entirely intrapulmonary (see Fig. 12–8). If a technically good chest x-ray discloses pulmonary infiltrates, a computed tomographic scan should be employed to determine the degree of intrapulmonary hemorrhage (see Figs. 12–8 and 12–10). Pulmonary neovascularity[70] can be mistaken for the infiltrates of intrapulmonary hemorrhage (Fig. 12–16, *A* and *B*), a distinction readily made by computed tomography. If a technically good chest x-ray shows no infiltrates and if hemoptysis is mild to moderate, expectant observation is in order.

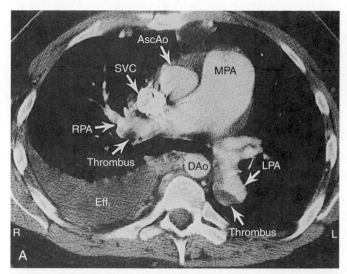

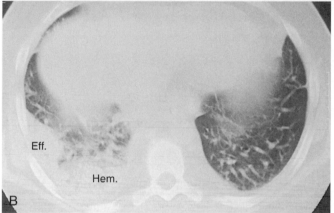

FIGURE 12–13 **(A)** Magnetic resonance image from a 39-year-old cyanotic man with Down syndrome, an atrioventricular septal defect, and pulmonary vascular disease. The main pulmonary artery (MPA) is markedly dilatated. There is thrombus in the proximal branches of left (LPA) and right pulmonary arteries (RPA). A hemorrhagic pleural effusion (Eff.) is present on the right. Asc Ao, ascending aorta; DAo, descending aorta; SVC, superior vena cava. **(B)** Computed tomographic scan shows intrapulmonary hemorrhage (Hem.) and the hemorrhagic pleural effusion (Eff.) due to a pulmonary infarct caused by an embolus from the thrombus in the right pulmonary artery.

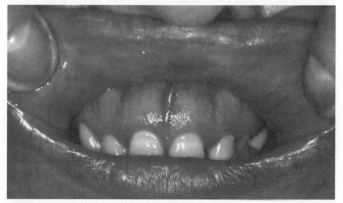

FIGURE 12–14 Spongy, fragile gums in a 32-year-old cyanotic woman with tricuspid atresia, pulmonary stenosis, and a bidirectional Glenn shunt. Note clubbing of the fingers and the cyanotic everted upper lip.

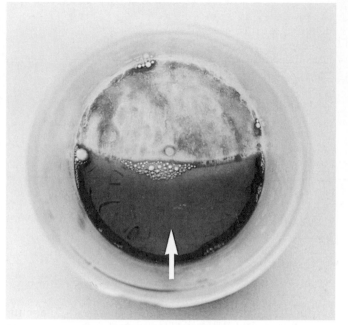

FIGURE 12–15 Hemoptysis (external pulmonary hemorrhage) as judged by the amount of blood *(arrow)* coughed into a plastic measuring cup.

Patients should be questioned regarding use of antiplatelet or nonsteroidal anti-inflammatory agents, especially if hemoptysis is copious and if intrapulmonary hemorrhage is radiologically extensive. A therapeutic attempt should be made to curtail pulmonary hemorrhage with fresh frozen plasma or cryoprecipitate or with platelet transfusion to correct thrombocytopenia or to counter recent exposure to antiplatelet agents.

Cyanotic CHD incurs a significant risk of bleeding in response to accidental trauma or the intentional trauma of cardiac and noncardiac surgery (see Chapter 19). Reduction in red cell mass by preoperative phlebotomy improves hemostasis,[14,55] as pointed out earlier. An initial 500 ml isovolumetric phlebotomy should be followed by a subsequent withdrawal in 24 hours and then repeated until the hematocrit level is just below 65%. Low platelet counts rise promptly as the hematocrit falls (discussed earlier). Phlebotomized units should be reserved for potential perioperative autologous transfusion.

Now let us turn to a therapeutic dilemma in Eisenmenger syndrome—namely, pulmonary arterial thromboses that vary from segmental (see Fig. 12–13) to massive and occlusive (see Figs. 12–10 through 12–12). Oral anticoagulants cause hemorrhage rather than reduce the thrombus. Intrapulmonary infusion of thrombolytic agents is ineffective because the central pulmonary thrombi are not fresh. When a proximal thrombus gives rise to an intrapulmonary embolus, the pulmonary infarction is often hemorrhagic with hemorrhagic pleural effusion (see Fig. 12–13 and earlier discussion) reinforced by anticoagulants.

If an oral anticoagulant is considered necessary in a patient with cyanotic CHD—atrial fibrillation with cerebral embolus, for example—the INR (International

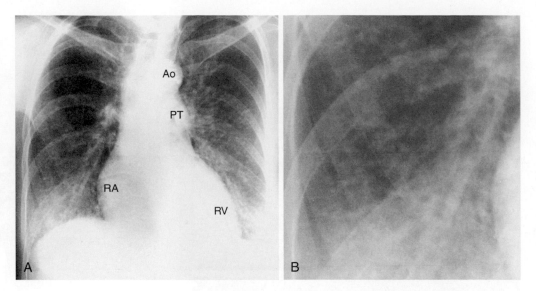

FIGURE 12–16 Images from a 22-year-old cyanotic woman with pulmonary vascular disease, a nonrestrictive patent ductus arteriosus, and an ostium secundum atrial septal defect. **(A)** The chest radiograph shows bilateral lacy, punctuate radiodensities that are more apparent in the lower lobes because of soft tissue breast attenuation. Ao, transverse aorta; PT, dilated pulmonary trunk; RA and RV, right atrium and right ventricle. **(B)** Close-up of the right lower lobe shows the mottled densities in greater detail.

Normalized Ratio) best determines the safest therapeutic dose. Low-molecular-weight heparin has high bioavailability and less *in vitro* clot inhibition, while retaining an *in vivo* antithrombotic effect (see Chapter 9). Because its anticoagulant effect is not readily reversible, unfractionated heparin may be preferable in this setting.

SYSTEMIC VASCULAR BED

Cardiac surgeons have long been aware that increased tissue vascularity promotes perioperative bleeding in cyanotic patients. The increased shear stress of the erythrocytotic perfusate provokes release of endothelial nitric oxide that diffuses according to Fickian principles.[9,71–74] Abluminal diffusion regulates blood flow and promotes systemic vasodilatation by activating soluble guanylate cyclase in medial smooth muscle cells.[9] However, a significant fraction of NO diffuses luminally and is regulated by a high reaction rate with red cell hemoglobin while promoting delivery of oxygen from oxyhemoglobin to metabolizing tissues.[9]

Cyanotic CHD sets the stage for paradoxical emboli delivered into the systemic vascular bed via right-to-left shunts. Paradoxical emboli result in clinically occult infarcts discovered at necropsy (Fig. 12–17), can lodge in the cerebral circulation and announce themselves as strokes (see Chapter 14), or rarely can enter the coronary circulation and cause an acute myocardial infarction.[75]

Syncope in cyanotic patients can be prompted by inappropriate systemic vasodilatation. When a cyanotic patient with pulmonary vascular disease stands in a hot shower or stands after immersion in a hot bath, the gravitational effect of the upright position together with heat-induced peripheral vasodilatation induce hypotension, increased cyanosis, decreased cerebral blood flow, and syncope. Hot showers, hot baths, saunas, and Jacuzzis should therefore be avoided.

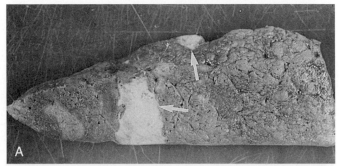

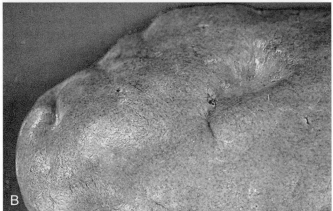

FIGURE 12–17 Clinically occult paradoxical emboli identified at necropsy. **(A)** Splenic infarcts *(arrows)* and **(B)** a renal infarct in two cyanotic adults, one with tricuspid atresia and pulmonary stenosis, the other with a nonrestrictive ventricular septal defect and pulmonary vascular disease.

CORONARY CIRCULATION

The response of the coronary circulation in cyanotic CHD includes dilatation and tortuosity of the extramural coronary arteries, basal coronary blood flow and flow reserve, the coronary microcirculation, and the paucity of atherosclerosis.[76–81] The extramural coronary arteries are typically dilatated, tortuous, or ectatic (Figs. 12–18 and 12–19).

Increased shear stress accompanying erythrocytosis initiates vasodilatation in response to elaboration of endothelial NO and prostaglandins,[16,73,82,83] but dilatation usually exceeds the anticipated vasodilatator response because coexisting structural abnormalities of the media—loss of smooth muscle, increased collagen, and duplication of internal elastic lamina—attenuate the coronary arterial walls[84] (Fig. 12–20). Basal blood flow is appreciably increased in the dilatated extramural coronary arteries of cyanotic CHD[81,82,85] (see Fig. 12–20), and maximal oxygen extraction is demanded by myocardial nutritional requirements. Accordingly, preservation of flow reserve cannot be attributed to further dilatation of the extramural coronaries or further oxygen extraction but must reside in the coronary microcirculation that remodels as it does in hypoxemic erythrocytotic residents acclimatized to high altitude.[86] Remodeling of the microcirculation characterized by greater diameter of the terminal arterioles and supplemented by enhanced vasodilatatory capacity is the key mechanism that accounts for preservation of flow reserve in cyanotic CHD.[86]

The paucity of coronary atherosclerosis in cyanotic CHD is the result of five independent but coexisting variables: hypocholesterolemia,[87] hypoxia, upregulated nitric oxide,[9] low platelet counts,[7] and hyperbilirubinemia.[88,89]

Hypoxemic erythrocytotic residents acclimatized to high altitude are hypocholesterolemic.[90] The incidence of clinical coronary artery disease is negligible, and in 300 necropsies of adults who resided in the Peruvian Andes, there was no evidence of coronary atherosclerosis.[90,91] By analogy, approximately 60% of hypoxemic erythrocytotic adults with cyanotic CHD have total nonfasting cholesterol levels < 160 mg/dl,[87,92] and of those who were hypocholesterolemic before being rendered acyanotic by

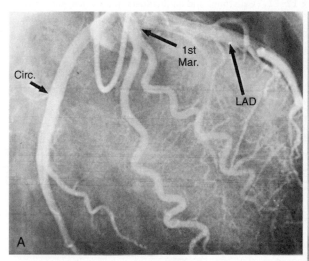
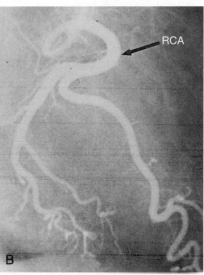

FIGURE 12–18   Selective coronary arteriograms from a 50-year-old cyanotic man with a nonrestrictive ventricular septal defect and pulmonary vascular disease. **(A)** The left coronary arterial system is enlarged, and its branches are tortuous, especially the first marginal (1st Mar.). Circ., circumflex artery; LAD, left anterior descending artery. **(B)** The right coronary artery (RCA) is large and its branches are tortuous.

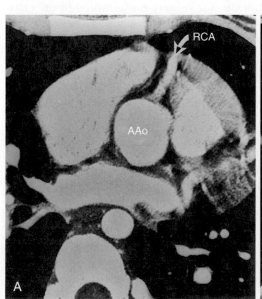
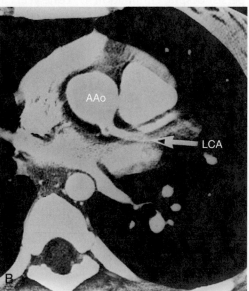

FIGURE 12–19   **(A and B)** Computed tomographic scans from a 31-year-old cyanotic woman with a nonrestrictive ventricular septal defect, patent ductus arteriosus, and pulmonary vascular disease. The right coronary artery (RCA) and the left coronary artery (LCA) are considerably dilatated. AAo, ascending aorta.

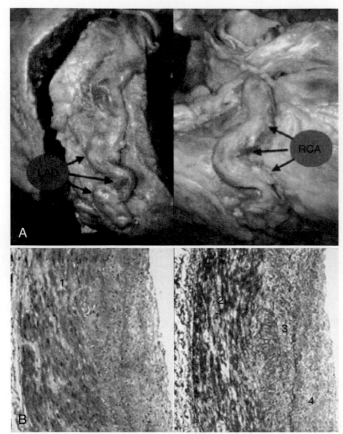

FIGURE 12-20   (A) Dilatation is in excess of the vasodilator effect because coexisting mural structural abnormalities cause mural attenuation. **(B)** 1, loss of medial smooth muscle cells (SMCs); 2, increase medial collagen; 3, duplication of internal elastic lamina (IEL); 4, fibromuscular intimal hyperplasia.

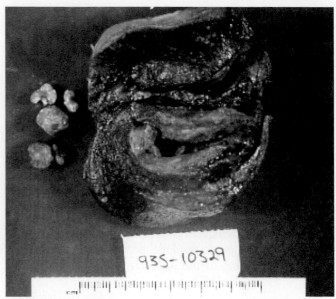

FIGURE 12-21   Gallstones and gallbladders in a 44-year-old cyanotic man with a nonrestrictive ventricular septal effect, pulmonary vascular disease, and acute cholecystitis.

surgery, only 11% experienced a postoperative rise in total cholesterol levels ≥160 mg/dl.[87,92] Persistence of hypocholesterolemia after surgical elimination of cyanosis/hypoxemia suggests induction or suppression of gene(s) that leads to a reduction in cholesterol. After the gene(s) are expressed, their effects may persist despite elimination of the provoking stimulus. The hypocholesterolemia primarily reflected reductions in low-density lipoprotein (LDL) cholesterol.

Hypoxemia is associated with a reduction in oxidized plasma LDL and a reduction in intimal oxidized LDL, which are atherogenic.[87] Nitric oxide, the ubiquitous signaling molecule synthesized from L-arginine and oxygen, is upregulated in cyanotic congenital heart disease (CHD)[9] and is antiatherogenic because it opposes platelet adherence and aggregation, stimulates disaggregation of preformed platelet aggregates, and inhibits monocyte adherence and infiltration.[87] Low platelet counts are antiatherogenic, and platelet counts are typically in the lower range of normal or thrombocytopenic in CHD.[7] Bilirubin is formed from the breakdown of heme, a process that is excessive in cyanotic CHD because the increased red cell mass results in a substantial increase in unconjugated bilirubin, which is a natural antioxidant that protects LDL cholesterol from oxidation.[87] Gilbert's disease, a benign disorder of bilirubin metabolism, is accompanied by increased levels of unconjugated bilirubin and a relative immunity from coronary atherogenesis.[88,89] Another aspect of bilirubin metabolism is not so favorable. More than 95% of bilirubin in bile is conjugated to glucuronic acid and is water soluble. Unconjugated bilirubin is virtually water *insoluble* at physiologic pH. When the concentration of insoluble unconjugated bilirubin in the bile is increased, calcium bilirubinate gallstones are formed (Fig. 12-21). Acute cholecystitis caused by pigment stones is relatively common in cyanotic CHD, and occult pigment stones may announce themselves as biliary colic years after cardiac surgery has eliminated the causative cyanosis and erythrocytosis (Fig. 12-22).

RENAL INVOLVEMENT

Both functional and structural disorders of the kidneys occur in cyanotic CHD. Functional disorders include urate clearance, which is dealt with in the section on digits and long bones, and proteinuria, which is a common functional glomerular abnormality. Plasma macromolecules such as proteins are impeded from crossing the glomerular capillary wall because of molecular size, shape, and charge.[93] The erythrocytotic perfusate entering the afferent glomerular arteriole in cyanotic CHD, together with obligatory ultrafiltration from afferent to efferent arteriole, materially increase glomerular hydraulic pressure and account for most of the proteinuria.[93]

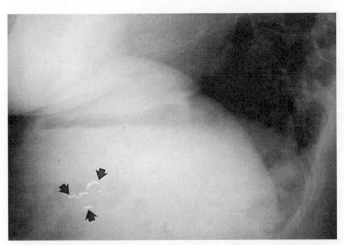

FIGURE 12–22 Lateral chest radiograph (infradiaphragmatic view) from a 38-year-old woman who had undergone intracardiac repair for cyanotic tetralogy of Fallot 4 years earlier. Arrows point to surgical clips of cholecystectomy for acute cholecystitis caused by calcium bilirubinate gallstones that developed 2 years after cardiac surgery had eliminated the cyanosis.

Negatively charged proteins are more restricted from passage into tubular fluid than neutral or cationic proteins because the glomerular capillary wall is also negatively charged.[93] Angiotensin-converting enzyme inhibitors decrease glomerular capillary hydraulic pressure in experimental animals and decrease proteinuria[93,94] but have not been tested in cyanotic adults with proteinuria. Phlebotomy is followed by a temporary rise in effective renal plasma flow and glomerular filtration rate, a substantial fall in filtration fraction, and a decrease in fractional excretion of albumin.[95]

Now let us turn to structural abnormalities of the kidney, focusing on the glomerulus.[96] Renal lesions were reported in more than 400 CHD patients from the 1948 to 1958 necropsy files of the Johns Hopkins Hospital.[97] In the 288 cyanotic patients, the striking changes were in the glomeruli, which were enlarged, congested, and hypercellular. Capillary dilatation was sometimes extreme, together with dilatation of hilar arterioles and prominence of the juxtaglomerular apparatus and mesangium.[97] These early observations[96,97] were confirmed by Bauer and Rosenberg in the United States[98] and Serapio and Labio in Brazil.[99] There are two distinct glomerular abnormalities—*vascular* (dilatation of capillary and hilar arterioles; (Fig. 12–23) and *nonvascular* (increased mesangial matrix and glomerular cellular elements; Fig. 12–24) that result from two distinct pathogenetic mechanisms.[100,101] The vascular and nonvascular disorders of the kidney usually leave renal function relatively intact. Exceptionally, adults with cyanotic CHD develop renal failure.[102]

The vascular abnormality—dilatation and engorgement of glomerular capillaries and hilar arterioles—is in response to nitric oxide elaborated from capillary and juxtamedullary endothelial cells and from the cytosol of glomerular mesangial cells (Fig. 12–25).[101,103,104] Nitric oxide plays a major role in the regulation of renal and glomerular blood flow[104,105] and functions as an autocrine hormone that modulates the glomerular vascular response to the increased shear stress of erythrocytosis. Hilar afferent and efferent arterioles and glomerular capillaries dilate and elongate, resulting in a considerable increase in glomerular blood flow.[74] The enlarged, dilatated, hypervascular glomeruli may double glomerular mass and renal cortical vascularity that can be detected as an increase in cortical echogenicity (Fig. 12–26).

The *nonvascular* glomerular abnormalities are characterized by an increase in juxtaglomerular cellularity and an increase in mesangial cells and mesangial matrix, the pathogenesis of which is distinct from that of the glomerular vascular disorder. A significant portion of megakaryocytes in bone marrow sinusoids (Fig. 12–27) normally enter the systemic venous circulation and are carried into the pulmonary circulation where platelets are formed by physical fragmentation of megakaryocytic cytoplasm.[106,107] The right-to-left shunts in cyanotic CHD deliver whole megakaryocytes from the systemic venous circulation into the systemic arterial circulation (see Figs. 12–23 and 12–24 and the following section on digits and long bones). These large formed elements affect glomeruli and release from their cytoplasm platelet-derived growth factor and transforming growth factor beta cytokines and mitogens that are responsible for the nonvascular glomerular abnormalities described earlier[101] (see Fig. 12–24).

DIGITS AND LONG BONES

Acute gouty arthritis is less common than would be expected from the relatively high prevalence of elevated uric acid levels in contrast to the positive correlation in other forms of secondary hyperuricemia.[1,11,108] Hyperuricemia occurs in cyanotic infants, increases in prevalence with age,[108–110] and is common in adolescents and adults with cyanotic CHD.[108,109] Renal clearance of uric acid involves filtration, reabsorption, and excretion.[108] Hyperuricemia in cyanotic infants has been ascribed to uric acid overproduction from red blood cell nucleoprotein, together with impaired urate clearance.[109] In cyanotic adults, high plasma uric acid levels are ascribed to enhanced urate reabsorption that results from renal hypoperfusion reinforced by a high filtration fraction.[108] Hyperuricemia in cyanotic CHD appears to exert little or no deleterious effect on renal function, and it is doubtful that urate deposits cause clinically significant renal disease.[1] Deposition of uric acid crystals in collecting tubules occurs when uric acid is overproduced or overexcreted, but among the 300 or more cyanotic patients in the UCLA Adult Congenital Heart Disease Center Registry, only one had a uric acid kidney stone.[29]

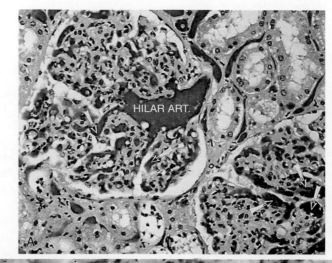

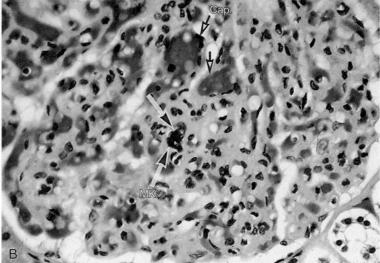

FIGURE 12-23 **(A)** Glomerular histology (necropsy specimen) in a 36-year-old man with cyanotic congenital heart disease. There is striking dilatation of hilar arterioles (HILAR ART.) and dilatation of capillaries within both glomeruli *(arrows)*, in addition to an increase in mesangial matrix and cellularity. **(B)** High-power view showing an increase in mesangial matrix and cellularity and dilated, engorged capillaries (Cap., *small open black arrows*). Note the typical lobulated nucleus of a megakaryocyte (MK, *large black-on-white arrows*).

Clinical manifestations of gout in cyanotic patients are similar to those of primary gout and to gout due to other forms of secondary hyperuricemia except for the presence of tophi in the former. Soft tissue urate deposits are exceptional in the hyperuricemia of cyanotic CHD (Fig. 12–28), even with high uric acid levels. Joint effusions (inflammatory arthropathy) are uncommon, especially large effusions.

Management of hyperuricemia and gout in cyanotic CHD differs somewhat from the management of primary gout. Because secondary hyperuricemia per se appears to exert little or no ill effect on renal function (discussed earlier) and because urate deposits seldom cause clinically overt renal disease, asymptomatic hyperuricemia in cyanotic adults is not routinely treated. Acute gouty arthritis responds to colchicine, but a major limitation is dehydration caused by vomiting and diarrhea, which are frequent gastrointestinal side effects of oral colchicine in full therapeutic doses.[1] The undesirable hemoconcentration and rise in hematocrit associated with dehydration are obviated by intravenous administration of colchicine diluted in 0.9%

sodium chloride or sterile water and infused through tubing rather than by direct intravenous injection to avoid severe local irritation caused by extravasation. The initial intravenous dose is usually 2 mg over 2 to 5 minutes followed by 0.5 mg every 6 hours until a satisfactory symptomatic response is achieved, with the total dose not to exceed 4 mg in 24 hours. If gouty pain recurs, 1 to 2 mg can be given intravenously for several days followed by oral colchicine. After resolution of acute gouty arthritis, prophylaxis is achieved in 75% to 90% of patients with a maintenance dose of 0.6 mg of oral colchicine once daily, a regimen that is usually well tolerated. Patients should be instructed to take an additional 0.6-mg tablet at the onset of a gouty recurrence, and the dose should then be increased to 0.6 mg twice daily. Nonsteroidal anti-inflammatory drugs are less effective for prophylaxis and tend to reinforce the hemostatic defects of cyanotic CHD as noted earlier.

When gouty arthritis recurs despite these recommendations, treatment is with probenecid or sulfinpyrazone (uricosuric agents), allopurinol (the only available agent that decreases uric acid synthesis), or a combination of these

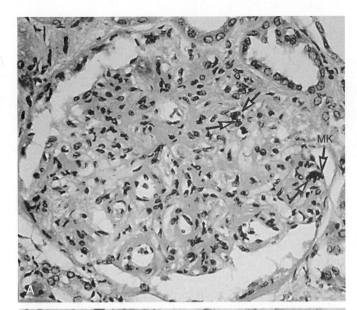

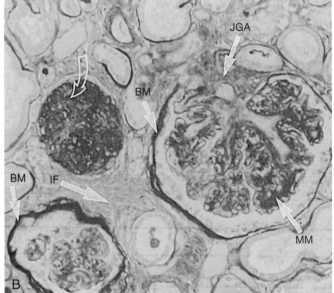

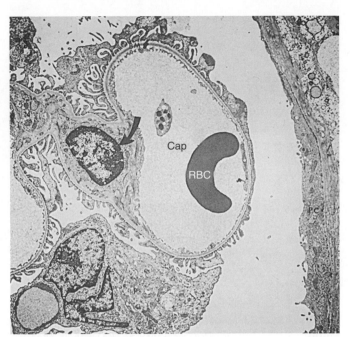

FIGURE 12–25 Electron microscopic image of a glomerular capillary (Cap) containing a red blood cell (RBC). A mesangial cell *(curved black arrow)* abuts the capillary on its left. *(From Latta, H.: An approach to the structure and function of the glomerular mesangium.* J Am Soc Nephrol *1992;2:565.)*

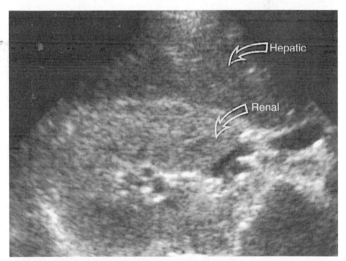

FIGURE 12–26 Sonographic image of the right upper quadrant of the abdomen showing renal cortical echogenicity markedly greater than that of hepatic echogenicity in a 32-year-old cyanotic woman with a univentricular heart and pulmonary vascular disease.

FIGURE 12–24 **(A)** Glomerular histology (necropsy) from a 45-year-old woman with cyanotic congenital heart disease. Paired arrows identify the large, multilobulated nuclei of two megakaryocytes (MK). There is a marked increase in mesangial matrix and cellularity. **(B)** Three glomeruli from the necropsy specimen of a 58-year-old woman with cyanotic congenital heart disease and chronic renal failure. The glomerulus on the right has reduced cellular elements but increased mesangial matrix (MM). The basement membrane (BM) of Bowman's capsule is segmentally thickened. The lower left glomerulus (smaller because of a tangential cut) exhibits reduced cellular elements, moderately increased mesangial matrix, and a thickened basement membrane (BM). The upper left glomerulus *(open arrow)* is entirely sclerotic. IF, interstitial fibrosis; JGA, juxtaglomerular apparatus.

drugs. In selected patients, intraarticular corticosteroids are useful. Thiazide diuretics suppress renal tubular excretion of urate, and thus hyperuricemia increases. Salicylates are best avoided because uric acid levels increase even at low doses and because the effect on hemostasis is adverse.

Salsalate, a nonacetylated anti-inflammatory analog of aspirin that is not an antiplatelet agent, is sometimes useful in treating arthralgias.[111]

In the fifth century B.C., Hippocrates observed that in patients with empyema, "the fingernails become curved and the fingers become warm, especially at their tips."[112] The term *hippocratic fingers* was used in early writings to refer to what is now called *clubbing*.[113] The initial changes in digital clubbing consist of an increase in thickness of

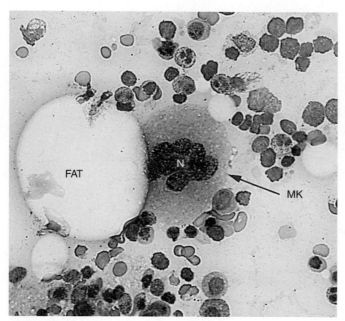

FIGURE 12-27 Bone marrow megakaryocyte (MK) with its cytoplasm and its typical multilobated nucleus (N). Compare size with other formed elements.

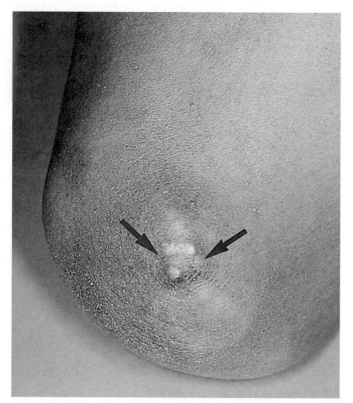

FIGURE 12-28 Urate deposits *(arrows)* in the elbow of a 28-year-old man with complex cyanotic congenital heart disease, hyperuricemia, and gouty arthritis.

the nail bed and soft tissues of the volar surface followed by connective tissue proliferation, collagen deposition, capillary dilatation, and infiltration with lymphocytes and plasma cells.[114-116] Digital clubbing is asymptomatic except for occasional dysesthesia.

Hypertrophic osteoarthropathy, which is seemingly unrelated to clubbing, occurs in upwards of one third of patients with cyanotic CHD.[117] The disorder begins at the distal ends of metacarpal, metatarsal, and long bones of the forearms and legs. The earliest histologic changes are edema and round cell infiltration of periosteum, synovial membrane, articular capsule, and contiguous subcutaneous tissues, with lifting of the periosteum (Fig. 12-29). New bone formation coexists with accelerated reabsorption. Symptoms consist of mild to moderate and occasionally marked aching, tenderness, and pain in long bones of the forearms and legs.

Until relatively recently, the pathogenesis of clubbing of the digits excited little attention,[112,118,119] but it is now held that clubbing of the fingers and toes and hypertrophic osteoarthropathy share a common pathogenesis.[112,117-119] The avidity for technetium 99m is the same in clubbed digits (Fig. 12-30) and in periosteum of long bones (see Fig. 12-29). Dickinson and Martin proposed that the cellular and connective tissue abnormalities in digital clubbing and hypertrophic osteoarthropathy are largely responses to platelet-derived growth factor and transforming growth factor-beta delivered to the capillaries of the digits and periosteum in the cytoplasm of megakaryocytes that are carried into the systemic arterial circulation through the right-to-left shunts of cyanotic CHD (see the section on renal involvement).[105,106,112,117,120,121] Whole megakaryocytes have been identified at necropsy in the clubbed fingers of patients with cyanotic CHD.[112] Platelet-derived growth factor is a powerful mitogen that binds with high affinity to responsive cells and exerts its action locally because of an extremely short half-life. It is a growth factor for mesenchymally derived cells such as fibroblasts and smooth muscle cells and promotes protein synthesis, connective tissue formation, and cell proliferation.[120] Transforming growth factor-beta is a key cytokine that acts as a potent regulator of tissue repair; is chemotactic for neutrophils, T cells, monocytes, and fibroblasts; and enhances deposition of extracellular matrix.[120]

LUNGS—RESPIRATION, OXYGEN CONSUMPTION, AND VENTILATION

In normal subjects in steady-state resting conditions, cardiac output and ventilation are maintained at levels that provide adequate oxygen to metabolizing tissues and remove carbon dioxide as it is produced. A constant isotonic exercise work rate is accompanied by an unsteady state during which the cardiovascular and respiratory systems accommodate to the need for increased gas exchange between metabolically active tissues and the atmosphere. For moderate-intensity isotonic exercise that can be maintained for a prolonged period of time without a sustained increase in blood levels of lactic acid, these adaptive responses are normally completed within a few minutes and are characterized by close coupling of

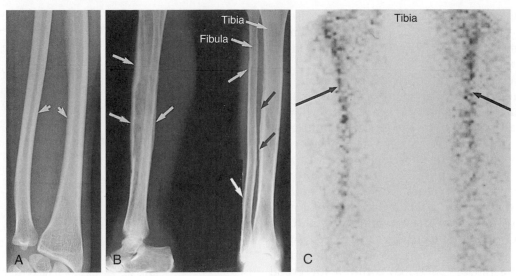

FIGURE 12-29   **(A)** Radiograph of radius and ulna illustrating normal long-bone periosteum *(arrows)*. **(B)** Radiograph of the tibia and fibula of a 44-year-old cyanotic woman with complete transposition of the great arteries, ventricular septal defect, and pulmonary stenosis. Arrows point to zones of typical hypertrophic osteoarthropathy with raised, thickened, irregular periosteum. **(C)** Radionuclide bone scan (intravenous technetium 99m) from a 23-year-old cyanotic man with complete transposition of the great arteries, ventricular septal defect, and pulmonary stenosis. Increased tracer concentrations identify hypertrophic osteoarthropathy *(arrows)* extending from the infrapatellar area along the lateral cortices of the tibia. *(B courtesy of Dr. Gordon Danielson, Mayo Clinic, Rochester, Minnesota.)*

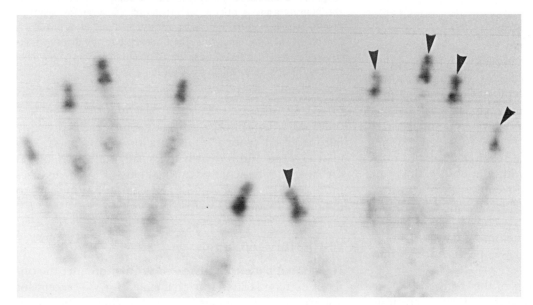

FIGURE 12-30   Radionuclide bone scan (intravenous technetium 99m) showing increased tracer concentrations in the clubbed distal phalanges *(arrowheads,* right hand) of the 23-year-old cyanotic man referred to in Figure 12-29.

blood transport function and pulmonary ventilation, so only trivial perturbations of levels of respiratory gases can be detected in circulating blood.[122,123]

The rate at which new steady states of gas exchange are achieved provides information regarding the adequacy of the hemodynamic response to the metabolic stress of exercise and to the character and duration of non-steady-state conditions incurred during the transition from one metabolic state to another. These observations afford insight into the functional impact of disease and on how disease encroaches on the physical activities of daily living. The following remarks deal with the cardiovascular and ventilatory responses of normal subjects to moderate intensity constant work rate exercise and with

alterations in these responses in patients with right-to-left shunts of cyanotic CHD.

Cardiovascular Responses to Step Exercise

The heart rate, stroke volume, and cardiac output increase abruptly when isotonic exercise in a normal upright subject begins from a background of rest.[124,125] The increase in stroke volume for a given work rate is largely accomplished within the first few seconds of exercise, with only moderate additional increments.[124,125] Further increases in cardiac output are then accomplished primarily by an acceleration in heart rate that rises to a steady state over a period of minutes. When equivalent exercise is performed supine, the magnitude of changes from rest to exercise are attenuated because resting stroke volume and cardiac output are higher in the horizontal position than in the upright position.[124]

The initial exercise-induced increase in cardiac output is associated with displacement of blood from peripheral venous pools toward the heart[126] and with increases in heart rate and in the force of ventricular contraction.[124,125] As exercise proceeds, a change occurs in the relative contributions of various vascular beds to mixed venous blood composition, so a greater proportion of venous effluent comes from skeletal muscle venous pools that contain a relatively low partial pressure of oxygen. The central arteriovenous oxygen difference $C(a - v)O_2$ therefore increases early in exercise.[127] (C = oxygen content, $a - v$ = arteriovenous difference). Further widening of $C(a - v)O_2$ may continue for several minutes as blood returning from exercising muscles becomes progressively more desaturated until a steady state is reached or until exercise ends.

Dynamics of Oxygen Uptake

In the steady state, oxygen uptake by the lungs (VO_2) is equal to oxygen consumption at the cellular level. During the dynamic period between steady states, oxygen consumption by tissues increases. VO_2 is dependent on the time course of change of tissue oxygen consumption and on the circulatory responses that link cellular respiration and external gas exchange. The mass balance of oxygen at any time during this process is summarized by the Fick relationship: $VO_2 = Q \times C(a - v)O_2$. When VO_2 is measured by analysis of respired gases, Q in the Fick relationship represents pulmonary blood flow, and $C(a - v)O_2$ represents the arteriovenous difference across the pulmonary circulation. The rate and pattern of change of VO_2 in response to a constant work rate of dynamic exercise are therefore immediate reflections of changes in blood flow and composition of pulmonary blood.

The normal rate and pattern of the increased VO_2 response to moderate intensity exercise[123,128,129] are illustrated in Figure 12–31. The response is characterized by three phases: (1) In Phase I, there is an abrupt increase in VO_2 immediately after the onset of exercise. (2) In Phase II, about 15 to 20 seconds later, VO_2 begins a more gradual, exponential increase toward a steady state, which is normally attained within 3 minutes. (3) Phase III is the exercise steady state.

An increase in VO_2 above resting levels requires an increase in the amount of desaturated hemoglobin entering the pulmonary circulation. The earliest cardiovascular response to a step workload includes abrupt increases in stroke volume and heart rate as stated earlier. Most of the increase in Phase I VO_2 has thus been attributed to the accompanying increase in pulmonary blood flow.[130] The

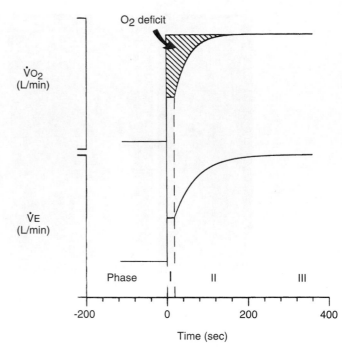

FIGURE 12–31 Idealized representation of normal oxygen uptake (VO_2) and ventilation ($\dot{V}E$) in response to constant work rate of moderate intensity exercise from a background of rest. Exercise begins at time 0, as indicated by the solid vertical line. The end of phase I is denoted by the interrupted line. The O_2 deficit brought about by exercise is shown in the shaded area. (Based on our data from nine normal healthy subjects performing 100-W cycling exercise.)

other factor contributing to Phase I increase is the early fall in central venous VO_2 saturation.[127] Except for very light exercise during which the steady-state level of gas exchange may be achieved during Phase I,[131] VO_2 increases in Phase II as cardiac output and $C(a - v)O_2$ increase to their exercise levels.[124,125,128]

Ventilatory Dynamics

The normal pattern of increased ventilation after the onset of exercise is similar to that stated for VO_2 except for a slower time course (see Fig. 12–31). There is close coupling of ventilatory kinetics to carbon dioxide output kinetics.[123] Accordingly, arterial PCO_2 levels are maintained within a narrow range in normal subjects, even during the unsteady state of exercise.[122]

Dynamics of Cardiorespiratory Responses to Constant Work Rate Exercise in Patients with Right-to-Left Shunts

Dynamics of Oxygen Uptake

A fundamental physiologic fault in patients with cyanotic CHD is the diversion of systemic venous blood into the systemic arterial circulation. Exercise significantly increases the degree of venoarterial mixing and materially influences the dynamics of VO_2 and ventilation. Patients with cyanotic CHD exhibit marked abnormalities in attaining a steady state for VO_2 after the onset of exercise.[46] Figure 12–32 illustrates the VO_2 response to low-level (unloaded) upright cycle ergometry in adults with right-to-left shunts. During Phase I, no patient experienced a normal increase in VO_2, and several had no VO_2 increase at all during this phase. Increases in VO_2 may be delayed for 20 to 30 seconds after exercise commences, probably corresponding to the time required for central venous VO_2 to decrease because of greater extraction in skeletal muscles. The Phase I VO_2 response correlates strongly with functional capacity,[46] a correlation that probably reflects the degree to which pulmonary blood flow is constrained at the onset of exercise and is consistent with the observation that pulmonary flow correlates with maximum exercise capacity in the presence of right-to-left or bidirectional shunts.[132]

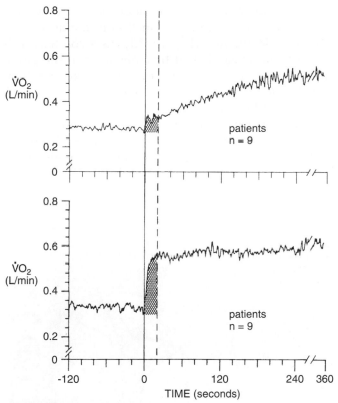

FIGURE 12–32 Oxygen uptake ($\dot{V}O_2$) response to unloaded cycle ergometric exercise in nine adults with cyanotic congenital heart disease **(top panel)** and nine normal control subjects **(bottom panel).** Each response represents the average of six rest to exercise transitions for each of the nine subjects. Exercise begins at time 0. Phase I is indicated by shading of the increment of $\dot{V}O_2$, which occurred within the first 20 seconds of exercise. The patients have a smaller $\dot{V}O_2$ increase in phase I and a slower increase toward the steady state $\dot{V}O_2$ requirement. *(From Sietsema, K.E., Cooper, D.M., Perloff, J.K., et al.: Dynamics of O_2 uptake during exercise in adults with cyanotic congenital heart disease. Circulation 1986;73:1137, by permission from the American Heart Association, Inc.)*

Attainment of the steady state for VO_2 is prolonged in patients with right-to-left shunts. Some patients do not achieve a steady state even when the levels of exercise are low.[46] Low VO_2 kinetics reflect the accumulation of a large exercise-associated "oxygen deficit." With respect to muscle bioenergetics, the oxygen deficit is attributed to work that is accomplished by using preformed energy stores such as phosphocreatine and adenosine triphosphate, stored oxygen from venous blood sources, or nonaerobic glycolytic metabolism.[133] In cyanotic CHD, the low oxygen content in shunted blood cannot be re-oxygenated by pulmonary gas exchange, so oxygen stores in systemic arterial blood decline as more markedly desaturated venous blood contributes to shunt flow. This depletion of systemic oxygen stores is accelerated when the shunt fraction increases in response to exercise.[134] At the end of exercise, VO_2 normally decreases exponentially with a time course similar to that required to reach the steady state after the onset of exercise.[123,127] As a result, the oxygen deficit incurred at the onset of exercise is "repaid" by a similar volume of oxygen supplied during the recovery time as VO_2 returns to the original resting state. The recovery time is prolonged in children with cyanotic CHD,[135] which mirrors the prolonged onset kinetics in adults.[46] The recovery dynamics for resynthesis of phosphocreatine after cessation of exercise, as estimated from magnetic resonance spectroscopy with phosphorus-31 of skeletal muscle, are prolonged in patients with cyanotic CHD compared with control subjects.[136]

The prolonged onset and recovery of VO_2 kinetics result in large oxygen deficits and hypoxemia even with low levels of exercise, and together with the associated hypoxemia, suggest that patients with significant right-to-left shunts rely to an unusual degree on anaerobic metabolism to perform exercise. Studies of lactate in patients with cyanotic CHD have identified normal blood levels at rest,[50,134,137,138] although elevated levels of the lactate/pyruvate ratio have occasionally been reported.[138] Lactate levels that are reached during exercise are not especially high when compared with values that accompany maximum exercise in normal subjects,[50,134,139] an observation that does not imply that hypoxemia is physiologically unimportant in cyanotic CHD. Skeletal muscle biopsy specimens obtained during exercise in patients with tetralogy of Fallot contain high tissue levels of lactate, despite only mild elevations of blood levels.[137] Similarly, magnetic resonance spectroscopy with phosphorus-31 demonstrates a decrease in intramuscular pH that is greater in patients with cyanotic CHD than in age-matched control subjects during similar exercise.[136] The metabolic state of tissues is apparently not well reflected in blood lactate levels in cyanotic patients. Tissue hypoxemia is probably the major limiting factor in exercise tolerance.

Ventilatory Dynamics

Patients with cyanotic CHD tend to exhibit higher than normal levels of ventilation at rest and lower levels of resting arterial PCO_2, which indicate chronic alveolar hyperventilation.[49,134,139,140] The resting alveolar hyperventilation tends to be coupled with a blunted respiratory sensitivity to the superimposition of acute hypoxemia.[141-143] The blunted response may[141,142] or may not[143] be reversed when reparative surgery eliminates the cyanosis and hypoxemia. The ventilatory response to acute hypoxemia reflects the sensitivity or insensitivity of the respiratory control system, a response that includes a complex interplay between neurotransmitters in the central nervous system and the carotid body, which is a 4- to 5-mm nodule of chemoreceptor tissue located at the bifurcation of the common carotid artery just above the carotid sinus.[144] The cells of the carotid body respond to hypoxemia, acidosis, hypotension, hypercarbia, and hyperthermia. Chemoreflex ventilatory responses to hypoxic adaptation in natives of high altitude are characterized by an increase in ventilation and blunted ventilatory response to inhaled oxygen and hypoxia. Sea-level natives residing at high altitude do not lose their hypoxic sensitivity, and subjects born and raised at sea level but of high altitude ancestry have normal hypoxic sensitivity. Hypoxia provokes a hyperplastic response of the carotid body. Carotid tumors are most common in individuals chronically exposed to low partial pressures of oxygen by living at high altitude. The carotid bodies are enlarged in cyanotic CHD and are responsible for the bulk of the increased ventilatory response to hypoxemia.[145]

Table 12-2 UCLA Congenital Heart Disease Functional Class

Presence and Degree of Symptoms

Class 1. Asymptomatic
Class 2. Symptoms present but do not interfere with normal activities
Class 3. Symptoms interfere with some but not most activities
Class 4. Symptoms interfere with most if not all activities

During exercise, patients with right-to-left shunts have a greater increase in ventilation than normal subjects.[45,49,50,139,146,147] The exercise-induced hyperventilation is subjectively perceived as "dyspnea," a prominent clinical complaint that is taken into account in the Functional Classification of Congenital Heart Disease (Table 12-2) and that was accurately described in 1958 by Paul Wood:[65] "The lack of symptoms in patent ductus with reversed shunt is attributed to the relatively normal oxygen tension of blood going to the head and neck; in most cases only the blood passing down the descending aorta below the junction of the duct is appreciably desaturated (Fig. 12-33). As a corollary, this explanation demands that breathlessness in the Eisenmenger syndrome is due to a low arterial oxygen saturation in blood passing through the chemoreceptors of the head and neck."

Ventilatory stimuli that potentially come into play during exercise coincide with an increase in right-to-left shunt, an increase in hypoxemia, an increase in shunting of carbon dioxide into the systemic arterial circulation, and the development of metabolic acidosis. Compared with normal subjects, patients with cyanotic CHD exhibit large

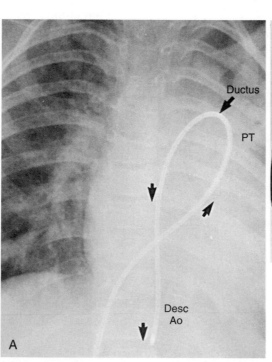
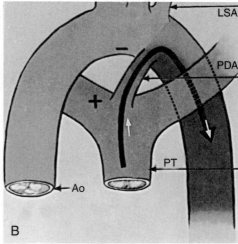

FIGURE 12-33 **(A)** Femoral venous catheter in a patient with a nonrestrictive patent ductus, suprasystemic pulmonary vascular resistance, and differential cyanosis. The catheter traces the pathway of unoxygenated blood *(arrows)* through the patent ductus into descending thoracic aorta (Desc Ao). **(B)** Schematic illustration of reversed flow from pulmonary trunk (PT) distal to the left subclavian artery (LSA) through a patent ductus arteriosus (PDA) into the descending aorta. Ao, ascending aorta.

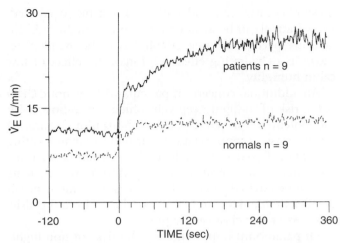

FIGURE 12–34   The increase in ventilation in response to unloaded cycle ergometric exercise in nine adults with right-to-left shunts and nine normal subjects. The patients had higher minute ventilation both at rest and in response to exercise. *(With permission from Sietsema, K.E., Cooper, D.M., Perloff, J.K., et al.: Control of ventilation during exercise in patients with central venous to systemic arterial shunts. J Appl Physiol 1988;64:234.)*

increases in ventilation in Phase I and more rapid increases in ventilation in Phase II (Fig. 12–34).[45] End-tidal PCO_2 values decrease at the onset of exercise and remain depressed throughout the period of exercise (Fig. 12–35), a response that implies alveolar hyperventilation and that has been characterized as hyperventilatory.[49,132,147,148] However, blood gas analysis indicates that arterial PCO_2 either remains constant or increases somewhat during constant work rate exercise in cyanotic patients.[45,50,139] Accordingly, the response is not hyperventilation because it is not in excess of what is required to maintain eucapnia. The maintenance of arterial PCO_2 near resting values during the exercise transition, despite large changes in ventilation, implies that mechanisms controlling ventilation in cyanotic CHD are acting to defend arterial acid-base homeostasis, as in normal subjects.[149]

In patients with large right-to-left shunts, especially during heavy-intensity exercise or rapidly increasing levels of exercise, the arterial PCO_2 often rises above resting levels, resulting in respiratory acidosis with or without associated metabolic (lactic) acidosis.[45,49,134,137,139] Clearance of metabolic carbon dioxide under these circumstances may require extraordinary levels of ventilation (discussed later), subjectively sensed as marked dyspnea.

Because patients with right-to-left shunts have high minute ventilation for a given level of carbon dioxide production[45,49,132,134,135,139,146,148] and because they may develop respiratory acidosis despite a greater than normal increase in ventilation, inefficient gas exchange caused by abnormally high alveolar dead space has been postulated.[49,146,150,151] However, for *hypocapnia* in the pulmonary circulation to compensate for the *hypercapnia* of shunted blood mixed in the systemic arterial circulation, ventilation

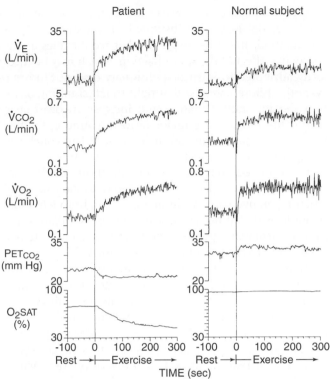

FIGURE 12–35   The changes in oxygen uptake (VO₂), carbon dioxide output (VCO₂), ventilation (VE), end-tidal PCO₂ (PETCO₂), and arterial oxygen saturation (O₂SAT) in one representative patient with cyanotic congenital heart disease characterized by single-ventricle, pulmonary atresia and Blalock-Taussig anastomosis are shown in the left panel and those for one normal control subject are shown in the right panel. The subjects were matched for age, sex, and size, and each performed exercise that resulted in similar increases in VO₂ (15- and 20-W cycling for the patient and the normal subject, respectively). Data are scaled identically for patient and control. The patient had slower kinetics of VO₂ and VCO₂ than the normal subject and a greater increase in ventilation. End-tidal PCO₂ decreased during exercise in the patient, in contrast to an increase in the normal subject. The decrease in arterial O₂ saturation (oximetry) began immediately at the onset of exercise, consistent with an abrupt increase in shunt fraction. *(With permission from Sietsema, K.E., Cooper, D.M., Perloff, J.K., et al.: Control of ventilation during exercise in patients with central venous to systemic arterial shunts. J Appl Physiol 1988;64:234.)*

must be sufficiently high to reduce alveolar PCO_2 to low levels.[45,50,134,139,150] If both systemic venous carbon dioxide concentration and the shunt fraction increase with exercise, the PCO_2 of pulmonary capillary blood must be reduced even further to maintain a constant arterial PCO_2. The hyperbolic relationship between alveolar ventilation and alveolar PCO_2 therefore results in an extremely high ventilatory cost for eliminating even a small increment of carbon dioxide production in patients with right-to-left shunts.

Separation of the effects of increased alveolar dead space and the inefficiency of the gas exchange that is induced when carbon dioxide–rich blood bypasses the lung is difficult because calculation of the former requires knowledge of alveolar PCO_2. Computation of *physiologic* rather than *alveolar* dead space employs a modified Bohr equation in which arterial PCO_2 is substituted for alveolar PCO_2. By this method, the physiologic dead space includes a dead space–like effect of the shunt fraction, which may be incorrectly attributed to intrinsic pulmonary disease. Studies in cyanotic children suggest that right-to-left shunting of carbon dioxide, rather than a true increase in dead space within the lung, is the major factor accounting for high ventilatory requirements during exercise.[50] This conclusion is supported by observations that ventilatory equivalents (ventilation required for a given metabolic rate[148]) and physiologic dead space[151] are reduced to normal levels when reparative surgery eliminates the right-to-left shunt. In adults with pulmonary vascular disease, ventilation-perfusion mismatching within the lung may contribute relatively more to high ventilatory requirements.

Analysis of the dynamics of cardiorespiratory responses to exercise levels that are commensurate with the requirements of daily living indicate that patients with cyanotic CHD have impaired rates of gas exchange in the lung in response to increased needs for oxygen delivery. There are prolonged periods in which external gas exchange lags behind cellular requirements. Low levels of physical activity may therefore be accompanied by profound decrements in arterial oxygen content and by tissue lactic acidosis. In addition, the exercise-induced increase in right-to-left shunt creates a unique challenge for the elimination of metabolically produced carbon dioxide resulting in high ventilatory requirements and occasionally in respiratory acidosis.

Commercial Air Travel

Concern is often expressed that in-flight atmospheric conditions aboard a commercial jet aircraft incur risks in cyanotic patients who are sometimes advised to use supplementary oxygen or even to avoid flying because of fear that a reduction of in-flight partial pressure of oxygen might induce dangerous hypoxemia.[2] Cabin atmospheric conditions in a commercial jet aircraft are altitude equivalents of 6000 to 8000 feet,[152] which in normal individuals results in a marked decrease in arterial PO_2 but only a mild decrease in arterial oxygen saturation, changes of which passengers are usually unaware except for drowsiness.[153] During commercial air travel, cyanotic patients incur little or no risk of a hazardous decrease in either PO_2 or oxygen saturation.[153] Accordingly, cyanotic patients need not be discouraged from flying, nor should they be advised that in-flight supplemental oxygen must be available.

After a cyanotic patient is safely and comfortably seated in the aircraft, the flight itself can be anticipated with relative safety.[153] Nevertheless, there are certain concerns. The low in-flight humidity in a pressurized jet aircraft is dehydrating, and dehydration can result in undesirable hemoconcentration in cyanotic erythrocytotic patients. Thirst is a poor indicator of dehydration under these circumstances, and patients must be so advised. Dehydration can be avoided by ample in-flight fluid intake irrespective of thirst. Alcohol is to be avoided because its dehydrating effect reinforces the effect of low cabin humidity.

An additional concern in patients with cyanotic CHD is the risk of in-flight deep vein phlebothrombosis with the potential for paradoxical embolization. Cramped tourist class accommodations virtually demand sitting with knees flexed and legs dependent for hours at a time, predisposing to venous stasis and thrombosis. Patients should be advised to extend their legs in so far as possible, flex their ankles, and take periodic walks in the aisle. Business or first class can be preventive.

Of paramount importance are the risks of non-flight-related stress[153] and the accompanying travel fatigue. These risks should be anticipated and minimized if not obviated by preparatory arrangements immediately before and after the flight. Rushing at the last minute, flying at peak periods, and transferring from one aircraft to another in large airports are ill advised. Transportation to and from the airport should be planned and advantage taken of special services for luggage (which should not be lifted) and for a wheelchair or minibus from curb to gate and on arrival at destination from gate to curb.

References

1. Perloff JK. Systemic complications of cyanosis in adults with congenital heart disease. Hematologic derangements, renal function, and urate metabolism. *Cardiol Clin.* 1993;11:689–699.
2. Diller GP, Gatzoulis MA. Pulmonary vascular disease in adults with congenital heart disease. *Circulation.* 27 2007;115:1039–1050.
3. Berk PD, Goldberg JD, Donovan PB, et al. Therapeutic recommendations in polycythemia vera based on Polycythemia Vera Study Group protocols. *Semin Hematol.* 1986;23:132–143.
4. Golde DW, Hocking WG, Koeffler HP, Adamson JW. Polycythemia: mechanisms and management. *Ann Intern Med.* 1981;95:71–87.
5. Wasserman LR, Balcerzak SP, Berk PD, et al. Influence of therapy on causes of death in polycythemia vera. *Trans Assoc Am Physicians.* 1981;94:30–38.
6. Penaloza D, Arias-Stella J. The heart and pulmonary circulation at high altitudes: healthy highlanders and chronic mountain sickness. *Circulation.* 2007;115:1132–1146.
7. Lill MC, Perloff JK, Child JS. Pathogenesis of thrombocytopenia in cyanotic congenital heart disease. *Am J Cardiol.* 2006;98:254–258.
8. Gidding SS, Bessel M, Liao YL. Determinants of hemoglobin concentration in cyanotic heart disease. *Pediatr Cardiol.* 1990;11:121–125.
9. Han TH PJ, Perloff JK, Lia JC. Nitric oxide metabolism in adults with cyanotic congenital heart disease. *Am J Cardiol.* 2007;99:691–695.
10. Berman W Jr, Wood SC, Yabek SM, et al. Systemic oxygen transport in patients with congenital heart disease. *Circulation.* 1987;75:360–368.
11. Rosove MH, Perloff JK, Hocking WG, et al. Chronic hypoxaemia and decompensated erythrocytosis in cyanotic congenital heart disease. *Lancet.* 1986;2:313–315.
12. Tyndall MR, Teitel DF, Lutin WA, et al. Serum erythropoietin levels in patients with congenital heart disease. *J Pediatr.* 1987;110:538–544.
13. Gidding SS, Stockman JA 3rd. Erythropoietin in cyanotic heart disease. *Am Heart J.* 1988;116:128–132.
14. Colon-Otero G, Gilchrist GS, Holcomb GR, et al. Preoperative evaluation of hemostasis in patients with congenital heart disease. *Mayo Clin Proc.* 1987;62:379–385.

15. Wells R. Syndromes of hyperviscosity. *N Engl J Med.* Jul 23 1970; 283:183–186.

16. Koller A, Sun D, Kaley G. Role of shear stress and endothelial prostaglandins in flow- and viscosity-induced dilation of arterioles in vitro. *Circ Res.* 1993;72:1276–1284.

17. Dintenfass L. Inversion of the Fahraeus-Lindqvist phenomenon in blood flow through capillaries of diminishing radius. *Nature.* 1967;215:1099–1100.

18. Gidding SS, Stockman JA 3rd. Effect of iron deficiency on tissue oxygen delivery in cyanotic congenital heart disease. *Am J Cardiol.* 1988;61:605–607.

19. Grotta JC, Manner C, Pettigrew LC, Yatsu FM. Red blood cell disorders and stroke. *Stroke.* 1986;17:811–817.

20. Hutton RD. The effect of iron deficiency on whole blood viscosity in polycythaemic patients. *Br J Haematol.* 1979;43:191–199.

21. Linderkamp O, Klose HJ, Betke K, et al. Increased blood viscosity in patients with cyanotic congenital heart disease and iron deficiency. *J Pediatr.* 1979;95:567–569.

22. Schmid-Schonbein H, Wells R, Goldstone J. Influence of deformability of human red cells upon blood viscosity. *Circ Res.* 1969;25:131–143.

23. Broberg CS, Bax BE, Okonko DO, et al. Blood viscosity and its relationship to iron deficiency, symptoms, and exercise capacity in adults with cyanotic congenital heart disease. *J Am Coll Cardiol.* 2006;48:356–365.

24. Finch CA, Miller LR, Inamdar AR, et al. Iron deficiency in the rat. Physiological and biochemical studies of muscle dysfunction. *J Clin Invest.* 1976;58:447–453.

25. Johnson JA, Willis WT, Dallman PR, Brooks GA. Muscle mitochondrial ultrastructure in exercise-trained iron-deficient rats. *J Appl Physiol.* 1990;68:113–118.

26. Willis WT, Gohil K, Brooks GA, Dallman PR. Iron deficiency: improved exercise performance within 15 hours of iron treatment in rats. *J Nutr.* 1990;120:909–916.

27. Rosenthal A, Nathan DG, Marty AT, et al. Acute hemodynamic effects of red cell volume reduction in polycythemia of cyanotic congenital heart disease. *Circulation.* 1970;42:297–308.

28. Berman W, Jr., Berman N, Pathak D, Wood SC. Effects of pentoxifylline (Trental) on blood flow, viscosity, and oxygen transport in young adults with inoperable cyanotic congenital heart disease. *Pediatr Cardiol.* 1994;15:66–70.

29. Perloff JK, Rosove MH, Child JS, Wright GB. Adults with cyanotic congenital heart disease: hematologic management. *Ann Intern Med.* 1988;109:406–413.

30. Viteri FE TB. Anemia and physical work capacity *Clin Hematol* 1982;3:609.

31. Schoene RB, Escourrou P, Robertson HT, et al. Iron repletion decreases maximal exercise lactate concentrations in female athletes with minimal iron-deficiency anemia. *J Lab Clin Med.* 1983;102:306–312.

32. Thomas DJ, Marshall J, Russell RW, et al. Effect of haematocrit on cerebral blood-flow in man. *Lancet.* 1977;2:941–943.

33. Doll DC, Greenberg BR. Cerebral thrombosis in smokers' polycythemia. *Ann Intern Med.* 1985;102:786–787.

34. Buhler FR, Vesanen K, Watters JT, Bolli P. Impact of smoking on heart attacks, strokes, blood pressure control, drug dose, and quality of life aspects in the International Prospective Primary Prevention Study in Hypertension. *Am Heart J.* 1988;115:282–288.

35. Gordon RS, Jr., Kahn HA, Forman S. Altitude and CBVD death rates show apparent relationship. *Stroke.* 1977;8:274.

36. Amitai Y, Blieden L, Shemtov A, Neufeld H. Cerebrovascular accidents in infants and children with congenital cyanotic heart disease. *Isr J Med Sci.* 1984;20:1143–1145.

37. Phornphutkul C, Rosenthal A, Nadas AS, Berenberg W. Cerebrovascular accidents in infants and children with cyanotic congenital heart disease. *Am J Cardiol.* 1973;32:329–334.

38. West DW, Scheel JN, Stover R, et al. Iron deficiency in children with cyanotic congenital heart disease. *J Pediatr.* 1990;117:266–268.

39. Amit M, Camfield PR. Neonatal polycythemia causing multiple cerebral infarcts. *Arch Neurol.* 1980;37:109–110.

40. Perloff JK, Marelli AJ, Miner PD. Risk of stroke in adults with cyanotic congenital heart disease. *Circulation.* 1993;87:1954–1959.

41. England JM, Walford DM, Waters DA. Re-assessment of the reliability of the haematocrit. *Br J Haematol.* 1972;23:247–256.

42. Kaemmerer H, Fratz S, Braun SL, et al. Erythrocyte indexes, iron metabolism, and hyperhomocysteinemia in adults with cyanotic congenital cardiac disease. *Am J Cardiol.* 2004;94:825–828.

43. Oldershaw PJ, Sutton MG. Haemodynamic effects of haematocrit reduction in patients with polycythaemia secondary to cyanotic congenital heart disease. *Br Heart J.* 1980;44:584–588.

44. Beekman RH, Tuuri DT. Acute hemodynamic effects of increasing hemoglobin concentration in children with a right to left ventricular shunt and relative anemia. *J Am Coll Cardiol.* 1985;5:357–362.

45. Sietsema KE, Cooper DM, Perloff JK, et al. Control of ventilation during exercise in patients with central venous-to-systemic arterial shunts. *J Appl Physiol.* 1988;64:234–242.

46. Sietsema KE, Cooper DM, Perloff JK, et al. Dynamics of oxygen uptake during exercise in adults with cyanotic congenital heart disease. *Circulation.* 1986;73:1137–1144.

47. Erslev AJ, Caro J. Pure erythrocytosis classified according to erythropoietin titers. *Am J Med.* 1984;76:57–61.

48. Triadou P, Maier-Redelsperger M, Krishnamoorty R, et al. Fetal haemoglobin variations following hydroxyurea treatment in patients with cyanotic congenital heart disease. *Nouv Rev Fr Hematol.* 1994;36:367–372.

49. Gold WM, Mattioli LF, Price AC. Response to exercise in patients with tetralogy of Fallot with systemic-pulmonary anastomoses. *Pediatrics.* 1969;43:781–793.

50. Strieder DJ, Mesko ZG, Zaver AG, Gold WM. Exercise tolerance in chronic hypoxemia due to right-to-left shunt. *J Appl Physiol.* 1973;34:853–858.

51. Bahnson HT, Ziegler RF. A consideration of the causes of death following operation for congenital heart disease of the cyanotic type. *Surg Gynecol Obstet.* 1950;90:60–76.

52. Ekert H, Gilchrist GS, Stanton R, Hammond D. Hemostasis in cyanotic congenital heart disease. *J Pediatr.* 1970;76:221–230.

53. Hartmann RC. A hemorrhagic disorder occurring in patients with cyanotic congenital heart disease. *Bull Johns Hopkins Hosp.* 1952;91:49–67.

54. Henriksson P, Varendh G, Lundstrom NR. Haemostatic defects in cyanotic congenital heart disease. *Br Heart J.* 1979;41:23–27.

55. Jackson DP. Hemorrhagic diathesis in patients with cyanotic congenital heart disease: preoperative management. *Ann N Y Acad Sci.* 1964;115:235–251.

56. Jacobson RJ, Rath CE, Perloff JK. Intravascular haemolysis and thrombocytopenia in left ventricular outflow obstruction. *Br Heart J.* 1973;35:849–854.

57. Maurer HM, McCue CM, Robertson LW, Haggins JC. Correction of platelet dysfunction and bleeding in cyanotic congenital heart disease by simple red cell volume reduction. *Am J Cardiol.* 1975;35:831–835.

58. Peters AM, Rozkovec A, Bell RN, et al. Platelet kinetics in congenital heart disease. *Cardiovasc Res.* 1982;16:391–397.

59. Somerville J, McDonald L, Edgill M. Post-operative haemorrhage and related abnormalities of blood coagulation in cyanotic congenital heart disease. *Br Heart J.* 1965;27:440–448.

60. Wedemeyer AL, Edson JR, Krivit W. Coagulation in cyanotic congenital heart disease. *Am J Dis Child.* 1972;124:656–660.

61. Territo MC PJ, Rosove MH, Moake J, Runge A. Acquired von Willebrand factor abnormality in adults with congenital heart disease. *Clin Appl Thrombosis/Hemostasis.* 1998;4:257.

62. Gross S, Keefer V, Liebman J. The platelets in cyanotic congenital heart disease. *Pediatrics.* 1968;42:651–658.

63. Waldman JD, Czapek EE, Paul MH, et al. Shortened platelet survival in cyanotic heart disease. *J Pediatr.* 1975;87:77–79.

64. Niwa K, Perloff JK, Kaplan S, et al. Eisenmenger syndrome in adults: ventricular septal defect, truncus arteriosus, univentricular heart. *J Am Coll Cardiol.* 1999;34:223–232.

65. Wood P. The Eisenmenger syndrome or pulmonary hypertension with reversed central shunt. *Br Med J.* 1958;2:755–762.

66. McLeod KA, Martin P, Williams G, Walker DR. Neutrophil activation and morbidity in young adults with cyanotic congenital heart disease. *Blood Coagul Fibrinolysis.* 1994;5:17–22.

67. DeMayo AP, Kiossoglou KA, Erlandson ME, et al. A marrow chromosomal abnormality preceding clinical leukemia in Down's syndrome. *Blood.* 1967;29:233–241.

68. Miller RW. Relation between cancer and congenital defects in man. *N Engl J Med.* 1966;275:87–93.

69. Wald N BW, Li CC, Turner JH, Harnois MC. Leukemia associated with mongolism. *Lancet.* 1961;1:1228.

70. Sheehan R, Perloff JK, Fishbein MC, et al. Pulmonary neovascularity: a distinctive radiographic finding in Eisenmenger syndrome. *Circulation.* 2005;112:2778–2785.

71. Buga GM, Gold ME, Fukuto JM, Ignarro LJ. Shear stress-induced release of nitric oxide from endothelial cells grown on beads. *Hypertension.* 1991;17:187–193.

72. Jia L, Bonaventura C, Bonaventura J, Stamler JS. S-nitrosohaemoglobin: a dynamic activity of blood involved in vascular control. *Nature.* 1996;380:221–226.

73. Koller A, Kaley G. Role of endothelium in reactive dilation of skeletal muscle arterioles. *Am J Physiol.* 1990;259:H1313–H1316.

74. Wilcox CS, Deng X, Doll AH, et al. Nitric oxide mediates renal vasodilation during erythropoietin-induced polycythemia. *Kidney Int.* 1993;44:430–435.

75. Gerber RS, Sherman CT, Sack JB, Perloff JK. Isolated paradoxical embolus to the right coronary artery. *Am J Cardiol.* 1992;70:1633–1635.

76. Bjork L. Ectasia of the coronary arteries. *Radiology.* 1966;87:33–34.

77. Leung WH, Stadius ML, Alderman EL. Determinants of normal coronary artery dimensions in humans. *Circulation.* 1991;84:2294–2306.

78. MacAlpin RN, Abbasi AS, Grollman JH Jr, Eber L. Human coronary artery size during life. A cinearteriographic study. *Radiology.* 1973;108:567–576.

79. Perloff JK, Urschell CW, Roberts WC, Caulfield WH Jr. Aneurysmal ilatation of the coronary arteries in cyanotic congenital cardiac disease. Report of a forty year old patient with the Taussig-Bing complex. *Am J Med.* 1968;45:802–810.

80. Vieweg WV, Alpert JS, Hagan AD. Caliber and distribution of normal coronary arterial anatomy. *Cathet Cardiovasc Diagn.* 1976;2:269–280.

81. Villari B, Hess OM, Meier C, et al. Regression of coronary artery dimensions after successful aortic valve replacement. *Circulation.* 1992;85:972–978.

82. Brunken RC, Perloff JK, Czernin J, et al. Myocardial perfusion reserve in adults with cyanotic congenital heart disease. *Am J Physiol Heart Circ Physiol.* 2005;289:H1798–H1806.

83. Koller A, Kaley G. Prostaglandins mediate arteriolar dilation to increased blood flow velocity in skeletal muscle microcirculation. *Circ Res.* 1990;67:529–534.

84. Chugh R, Perloff JK, Fishbein M, Child JS. Extramural coronary arteries in adults with cyanotic congenital heart disease. *Am J Cardiol.* 2004;94:1355–1357.

85. Iida H, Rhodes CG, Araujo LI, et al. Noninvasive quantification of regional myocardial metabolic rate for oxygen by use of 15O2 inhalation and positron emission tomography. Theory, error analysis, and application in humans. *Circulation.* 1996;94:792–807.

86. Dedkov EI, Perloff JK, Tomanek RJ, et al. The coronary microcirculation in cyanotic congenital heart disease. *Circulation.* 2006;114: 196–200.

87. Fyfe A, Perloff JK, Niwa K, et al. Cyanotic congenital heart disease and coronary artery atherogenesis. *Am J Cardiol.* 2005;96:283–290.

88. Madhavan M, Wattigney WA, Srinivasan SR, Berenson GS. Serum bilirubin distribution and its relation to cardiovascular risk in children and young adults. *Atherosclerosis.* 1997;131:107–113.

89. Vitek L, Jirsa M, Brodanova M, et al. Gilbert syndrome and ischemic heart disease: a protective effect of elevated bilirubin levels. *Atherosclerosis.* 2002;160:449–456.

90. Arias-Stella J, Topilsky, M. Anatomy of the coronary artery circulation at high altitude. *High Altitude Physiology.* Edinburgh: Churchill Livingstone, 1971.

91. Mortimer EA Jr, Monson RR, MacMahon B. Reduction in mortality from coronary heart disease in men residing at high altitude. *N Engl J Med.*1977;296:581–585.

92. Perloff JK. The coronary circulation in cyanotic congenital heart disease. *Int J Cardiol.* 2004;97(1 Suppl):79–86.

93. Larson TS. Evaluation of proteinuria. *Mayo Clin Proc.* 1994;69: 1154–1158.

94. Maschio G, Alberti D, Janin G, et al. Effect of the angiotensin-converting-enzyme inhibitor benazepril on the progression of chronic renal insufficiency. The Angiotensin-Converting-Enzyme Inhibition in Progressive Renal Insufficiency Study Group. *N Engl J Med.* 1996;334:939–945.

95. de Jong PE, Weening JJ, Donker AJ, van der Hem GK. The effect of phlebotomy on renal function and proteinuria in a patient with congenital cyanotic heart disease. *Nephron.* 1983;33:225–226.

96. Meessen H, Litton MA. Morphology of the kidney in morbus caeruleus. *AMA Arch Pathol.* 1953;56:480–487.

97. Spear GS. The glomerular lesion of cyanotic congenital heart disease. *Johns Hopkins Med J.* 1977;140:185–188.

98. Bauer WC, Rosenberg BF. A quantitative study of glomerular enlargement in children with tetralogy of Fallot. A condition of glomerular enlargement without an increase in renal mass. *Am J Pathol.* 1960;37:695–712.

99. Serapio CJ, Labio M. Aspectos histologicos de los glomerulos en pacientes portadores de cardiopatias congenitas cianoticas. *Hospital (Rio).* 1962;51:543.

100. Imai M. Pathological morphology of morbus caeruleus. *Tokyo Woman's Med Coll J.* 1960;30:149.

101. Perloff JK, Latta H, Barsotti P. Pathogenesis of the abnormal glomerulus in cyanotic congenital heart disease. *Am J Cardiol.* 2000;86: 1198–2004.

102. Flanagan MF, Hourihan M, Keane JF. Incidence of renal dysfunction in adults with cyanotic congenital heart disease. *Am J Cardiol.* 1991;68:403–406.

103. Latta H. An approach to the structure and function of the glomerular mesangium. *J Am Soc Nephrol.* 1992;2(10 Suppl):S65–S73.

104. Nicolson AG, Haites NE, McKay NG, et al. Induction of nitric oxide synthase in human mesangial cells. *Biochem Biophys Res Commun.* 1993;193:1269–1274.

105. Imig JD, Roman RJ. Nitric oxide modulates vascular tone in preglomerular arterioles. *Hypertension.* 1992;19:770–774.

106. Dickinson CJ, Martin JF. Megakaryocytes and platelet clumps as the cause of finger clubbing. *Lancet.* 1987;2:1434–1435.

107. Trowbridge EA, Martin JF, Slater DN. Evidence for a theory of physical fragmentation of megakaryocytes, implying that all platelets are produced in the pulmonary circulation. *Thromb Res.* 1982;28:461–475.

108. Ross EA, Perloff JK, Danovitch GM, et al. Renal function and urate metabolism in late survivors with cyanotic congenital heart disease. *Circulation.* 1986;73:396–400.

109. Hayabuchi Y, Matsuoka S, Akita H, Kuroda Y. Hyperuricaemia in cyanotic congenital heart disease. *Eur J Pediatr.* 1993;152: 873–876.

110. Young D. Hyperuricemia in cyanotic congenital heart disease. *Am J Dis Child.* 1980;134:902–903.

111. Estes D, Kaplan K. Lack of platelet effect with the aspirin analog, salsalate. *Arthritis Rheum.* 1980;23:1303–1307.

112. Dickinson CJ. The aetiology of clubbing and hypertrophic osteoarthropathy. *Eur J Clin Invest.* 1993;23:330–338.

113. Jones WHS. *Hippocrates Collected Works.* Cambridge: Harvard University Press; 2006.

114. Bigler FC. The morphology of clubbing. *Am J Pathol.* 1958;34:237-261.

115. Currie AE, Gallagher PJ. The pathology of clubbing: vascular changes in the nail bed. *Br J Dis Chest.* 1988;82:382-385.

116. Lovell RHH. Observations on the structure of clubbed fingers. *Clin Sci* 1950;9:299.

117. Martinez-Lavin M. Pathogenesis of hypertrophic osteoarthropathy. *Clin Exp Rheumatol.* 1992;10(7 Suppl):49-50.

118. Pineda CJ, Guerra J Jr, Weisman MH, et al. The skeletal manifestations of clubbing: a study in patients with cyanotic congenital heart disease and hypertrophic osteoarthropathy. *Semin Arthritis Rheum.* 1985;14:263-273.

119. Vazquez-Abad D, Martinez-Lavin M. Macrothrombocytes in the peripheral circulation of patients with cardiogenic hypertrophic osteoarthropathy. *Clin Exp Rheumatol.* 1991;9:59-62.

120. Border WA, Noble NA. Transforming growth factor beta in tissue fibrosis. *N Engl J Med.* 1994;331:1286-1292.

121. Tavassoli M, Aoki M. Migration of entire megakaryocytes through the marrow—blood barrier. *Br J Haematol.* 1981;48:25-29.

122. Forster HV, Pan LG, Funahashi A. Temporal pattern of arterial CO2 partial pressure during exercise in humans. *J Appl Physiol.* 1986;60:653-660.

123. Whipp BJ, Ward SA, Lamarra N, Davis JA, Wasserman K. Parameters of ventilatory and gas exchange dynamics during exercise. *J Appl Physiol.* 1982;52:1506-1513.

124. Loeppky JA, Greene ER, Hoekenga DE, et al. Beat-by-beat stroke volume assessment by pulsed Doppler in upright and supine exercise. *J Appl Physiol.* 1981;50:1173-1182.

125. Miyamoto Y, Hiura T, Tamura T, et al. Dynamics of cardiac, respiratory, and metabolic function in men in response to step work load. *J Appl Physiol.* 1982;52:1198-1208.

126. Bevegard S, Holmgren A, Jonsson B. The effect of body position on the circulation at rest and during exercise, with special reference to the influence on the stroke volume. *Acta Physiol Scand.* 1960;49:279-298.

127. Casaburi R, Daly J, Hansen JE, Effros RM. Abrupt changes in mixed venous blood gas composition after the onset of exercise. *J Appl Physiol.* 1989;67:1106-1112.

128. Cerretelli P, Sikand R, Farhi LE. Readjustments in cardiac output and gas exchange during onset of exercise and recovery. *J Appl Physiol.* 1966;21:1345-1350.

129. Pearce DH, Milhorn HT Jr. Dynamic and steady-state respiratory responses to bicycle exercise. *J Appl Physiol.* 1977;42:959-967.

130. Weissman ML, Jones PW, Oren A, et al. Cardiac output increase and gas exchange at start of exercise. *J Appl Physiol.* 1982;52:236-244.

131. Sietsema KE, Daly JA, Wasserman K. Early dynamics of O_2 uptake and heart rate as affected by exercise work rate. *J Appl Physiol.* 1989;67:2535-2541.

132. Barber G, Danielson GK, Heise CT, Driscoll DJ. Cardiorespiratory response to exercise in Ebstein's anomaly. *Am J Cardiol.* 1985;56:509-514.

133. di Prampero PE. Energetics of muscular exercise. *Rev Physiol Biochem Pharmacol.* 1981;89:143-222.

134. Davies H, Gazetopoulos N. Dyspnoea in cyanotic congenital heart disease. *Br Heart J.* 1965;27:28-41.

135. Drakonakis AC, Halloran KH. Oxygen consumption during recovery from exercise in children with congenital heart disease. *Am J Dis Child.* 1974;128:651-656.

136. Adatia I, Kemp GJ, Taylor DJ, et al. Abnormalities in skeletal muscle metabolism in cyanotic patients with congenital heart disease: a 31P nuclear magnetic resonance spectroscopy study. *Clin Sci (Lond).* 1993;85:105-109.

137. Bjarke B, Eriksson BO, Saltin B. ATP, CP, and lactate concentrations in muscle tissue during exercise in male patients with tetralogy of Fallot. *Scand J Clin Lab Invest.* 1974;33:255-260.

138. Greene NM, Talner NS. Blood lactate, pyruvate and lactate-pyruvate ratios in congenital heart disease. *N Engl J Med.* 1964;270:1331-1336.

139. Eriksson BO, Bjarke B. Oxygen uptake arterial blood gases and blood lactate concentration during submaximal and maximal exercise in adult subjects with shunt-operated tetralogy of Fallot. *Acta Med Scand.* 1975;197:187-193.

140. Okubo S, Mortola JP. Control of ventilation in adult rats hypoxic in the neonatal period. *Am J Physiol.* 1990;259:R836-841.

141. Blesa MI, Lahiri S, Rashkind WJ, Fishman AP. Normalization of the blunted ventilatory response to acute hypoxia in congenital cyanotic heart disease. *N Engl J Med.* 1977;296:237-241.

142. Edelman NH, Lahiri S, Braudo L, et al. The blunted ventilatory response to hypoxia in cyanotic congenital heart disease. *N Engl J Med.* 1970;282:405-411.

143. Sorensen SC, Severinghaus JW. Respiratory insensitivity to acute hypoxia persisting after correction of tetralogy of Fallot. *J Appl Physiol.* 1968;25:221-223.

144. Habeck JO. The carotid bodies in cyanotic heart disease. *Pathol Res Pract.* 1994;190:650-655.

145. Fishman AP. The enigma of hypoxic pulmonary vasoconstriction. In: Fishman AP, ed. *The Pulmonary Circulation. Normal and Abnormal.* Philadelphia: University of Pennsylvania, 1990.

146. Driscoll DJ, Staats BA, Heise CT, et al. Functional single ventricle: cardiorespiratory response to exercise. *J Am Coll Cardiol.* 1984;4:337-342.

147. Taylor MR. The ventilatory response to hypoxia during exercise in cyanotic congenital heart disease. *Clin Sci.* 1973;45:99-105.

148. Barber G, Danielson GK, Puga FJ, et al. Pulmonary atresia with ventricular septal defect: preoperative and postoperative responses to exercise. *J Am Coll Cardiol.* 1986;7:630-638.

149. Hansen JE, Stelter GP, Vogel JA. Arterial pyruvate, lactate, pH, and PCO2 during work at sea level and high altitude. *J Appl Physiol.* 1967;23:523-530.

150. Burrows FA. Physiologic dead space, venous admixture, and the arterial to end-tidal carbon dioxide difference in infants and children undergoing cardiac surgery. *Anesthesiology.* 1989;70:219-225.

151. Yates AP, Lindahl SG, Hatch DJ. Pulmonary ventilation and gas exchange before and after correction of congenital cardiac malformations. *Br J Anaesth.* 1987;59:170-178.

152. Cottrell JJ. Altitude exposures during aircraft flight. Flying higher. *Chest.* 1988;93:81-84.

153. Harinck E, Hutter PA, Hoorntje TM, et al. Air travel and adults with cyanotic congenital heart disease. *Circulation.* 1996;93:272-276.

CHAPTER 13

Psychiatric and Psychosocial Disorders in Congenital Heart Disease

BARRY H. GUZE ▪ ELISA A. MORENO ▪ JOSEPH K. PERLOFF

Congenital heart disease (CHD) can generate significant stress because of the perceived implications of its presence and because of hospital admissions and readmissions, diagnostic studies, invasive and noninvasive procedures, and recurrent surgery. Emotional responses vary in degree from within the normal range of expectations to overt mental illness, especially when there is a psychiatric predisposition.[1] As more patients with CHD survive into adulthood, increasing numbers confront the prospect of premature mortality and experience difficulties in adjustment with despair because of social, educational, and occupational limitations incurred by postoperative residua and sequelae (see Chapter 20). Responses are further influenced by the severity of the lesion (simple versus complex), the degree of functional disability, and the presence of visible physical abnormalities such as cyanosis, digital clubbing, and surgical scars.[2] However, the frequency and assessment of psychopathology in this patient population is limited by the relatively small number of studies and by diagnostic and severity rating scales that include overlap between symptoms of cardiovascular disease per se and symptoms of disordered mental health.[3]

MECHANISMS OF CENTRAL NERVOUS SYSTEM INJURY IN CONGENITAL HEART DISEASE

Although the intelligence and cognitive abilities of children with CHD may be within the normal range, they often exhibit neurodevelopmental abnormalities and performance significantly below mean values.[4-6] Behavioral problems and deficits in attention, motor control, visual and spatial processing, executive functioning, and higher order thought processes have been documented.[7,8] Risk factors for neurodevelopmental sequelae have been identified in preoperative, intraoperative, and postoperative patients, underscoring the multifactorial etiologies and complex interactions between patient and environment. Postnatal factors such as structural brain lesions, genetic syndromes, deficits in cerebral blood flow, and the type and complexity of the congenital cardiac lesion contribute to long-term adverse neurologic and cognitive outcomes. Reparative versus palliative surgery, intraoperative methods of vital organ support, acid-base regulation, duration of cardiopulmonary bypass, and depth and duration of hypothermia contribute to neurologic vulnerability.[9] Repeated hospitalizations, length of stay in the intensive care unit, and limited physical interaction with the environment are thought to have deleterious effects on neurologic and cognitive development. As the number of children with CHD surviving into adulthood increases, it is crucial to develop strategies that promote neuropsychiatric protection.

PREOPERATIVE AND INTRINSIC FACTORS

Neurologic morbidity in neonates and infants with CHD includes hypotonia, developmental delay, failure to thrive, difficulties with visual and auditory orientation, fine and gross motor delay, abnormal muscle tone, cranial nerve abnormalities, feeding difficulties, irritability and lethargy. Mechanisms responsible for central nervous system injury have been proposed.[5,7,10-13]

Chromosomal Abnormalities and Genetic Polymorphisms: Apoliprotein E

CHD commonly coexists with genetic disorders.[14-18] Wernovsky[8] emphasized high comorbidity with structural central nervous system abnormalities in what he refers to as *congenital brain disease*. Genetic syndromes such as trisomy 13, 18, and 21 (Down syndrome), Williams and DiGeorge syndromes, and the CHARGE and VACTERL associations coexist with congenital cardiac lesions. Microdeletion of chromosome 22 and the 22q11 deletion found in the velo-cardiofacial and DiGeorge syndromes are associated with cardiac lesions involving the ventricular septum, the aortic arch, and conotruncal defects including tetralogy of Fallot and truncus arteriosus.[8,18,19]

An association between genetic polymorphisms and abnormal neurologic development has also been reported. Apoliprotein E (ApoE) is important in cholesterol metabolism and neuronal repair, and the presence of the ApoE e2 allele predicts poorer neurodevelopment in year-old infants who have undergone surgical repair of CHD.[20,21]

Structural Brain Abnormalities: Microcephaly, Open Operculum, and White Matter Injury

Microcephaly

Brain malformations often occur in infants with CHD, and congenital cardiac anomalies are predictors of neurodevelopmental outcome. Wernovsky[22] proposed that brain and heart abnormalities coexist because the central nervous system and cardiovascular system develop approximately in tandem. Neuropathologic reports describe cerebral atrophy, enlarged ventricles, agenesis of the corpus callosum, and hypoplasia of the temporal lobe.[12,23] In one imaging study, one quarter of infants with CHD had structural brain abnormalities such as holoprosencephaly and agenesis of the corpus callosum.[24] Microcephaly was the second most common structural abnormality of the brain,[25] occurring in one fourth to one third of these children.[12,14,26] Microcephaly persisting through infancy has been identified as an independent predictor of developmental delay and of problematic academic performance and is an important marker of brain injury and neurodevelopmental sequelae in patients with CHD.[27] Neonatal autopsies reveal that almost one third of infants with hypoplastic left heart syndrome have central nervous system abnormalities, including microcephaly.[22]

Open Operculum

The operculum (Latin for *little lid*) includes portions of the frontal, parietal, and temporal lobes covering the insula is believed to be related to hand-mouth coordination, taste, and expressive language; and includes Broca's area, which plays an important role in conversation, speech, reading, and writing. An open or underdeveloped operculum has been identified on imaging studies in approximately 25% of neonates with complex congenital cardiac lesions and is considered a marker of functional brain immaturity. Underdevelopment of this area of the brain in children with complex CHD is believed to contribute to feeding difficulties, delays in expressive language, and oral-motor apraxia.[22]

Periventricular Leukomalacia and White Matter Injury

Cerebral white matter injury revealed by neuroimaging is prevalent in infants with CHD and is accompanied by ischemia-related neurologic deficits.[13] Periventricular leukomalacia (PVL) that results from ischemic injury to immature oligodendroglia occurs in infants with CHD[20] and is associated with developmental delay and attention-deficit/hyperactivity disorder (ADHD).[20] Preoperative magnetic resonance imaging (MRI) scans revealed mild ischemic changes in 16% of these patients and infarcts in 8%.[20] Magnetic resonance spectroscopy found elevated brain lactate in 53%. PVL was present in more than 50% of postoperative infants,[13] and more than 50% demonstrated new or worsened PVL.[20] Postoperative MRI scans identified new periventricular leukomalacia in 48%, a new infarct in 19%, and new parenchymal hemorrhage in 33%. Decreased cerebral blood flow has been implicated as the mechanism of white matter injury.[25]

Cerebral Blood Flow

Fetal brain growth depends on adequate oxygen supply[11] and adequate cerebral blood flow, which are functions of many factors, including the type of CHD.[23] Complex malformations, such as the hypoplastic left heart syndrome (HLHS), have especially abnormal flow dynamics that risk cerebral hypoxemia and adverse neurodevelopmental outcomes.[11,23,28] Hypoxemia and hypotension result in white matter injury and global ischemia.[23,25] More specifically, cerebral hypoxia is associated with deficits in visual-spatial function, memory, expressive language, and executive function.[9]

Acyanotic Versus Cyanotic Congenital Heart Disease

Even relatively mild degrees of oxygen desaturation in children with cyanotic CHD are believed to exert adverse effects on neurologic development, cognition, behavior, and academic achievement.[29] Lower IQ scores and defects in motor skills and visual reaction times have been documented in children with cyanotic versus acyanotic lesions, and chronic hypoxia is thought to be the mechanism of injury.[30] However, these studies lacked adequate control for intrinsic neurologic injury, genetic syndromes, or age, and subsequent studies that controlled for these factors yielded conflicting results. Some studies reported that children with cyanotic lesions had significantly lower IQ scores than those with acyanotic lesions and exhibited preoperative differences in cognitive functioning,[31] whereas other studies revealed no significant differences between the two groups. Age at repair of complete transposition of the great arteries was found to be inversely related to IQ scores, and delayed surgical repair correlated with worse cognitive functioning.[32] However, in other types of cyanotic CHD, a relationship between delayed surgical intervention and IQ scores was not identified.[33,34] There was no significant relationship between IQ and age at which a Fontan procedure was done, and intellectual development was within normal range.[35] Yet approximately one fifth of these children had below-average Visual Motor Integration scores. Despite this conflicting evidence, it is generally believed that prolonged hypoxia has deleterious effects on neurologic development and cognitive functioning, regardless of the type of congenital heart lesion.

INTRAOPERATIVE RISK FACTORS

Management of pH

When infants were randomized to alpha-stat or pH-stat management of blood gases during deep hypothermia with circulatory arrest (DHCA), there was no consistent relationship between either management strategy or short-term neurodevelopmental outcome.[36] Patients with complete transposition of the great arteries (TGA) and tetralogy of Fallot who were randomized to pH-stat management revealed higher scores on tests of psychomotor and mental development, and the same effect was found in patients with ventricular septal defect randomized to alpha-stat management. Interestingly, scores on the Bayley Scales of Infant Development were significantly higher in patients with TGA versus other congenital lesions. Thus, a relationship between pH management and neurodevelopmental outcomes in CHD infants undergoing surgical repair is equivocal.

Hematocrit

One randomized trial in infants suggested that hematocrit levels have a protective effect on the brain during cardiopulmonary bypass.[37] Neonates whose hematocrit

levels were maintained at approximately 30% during surgery had higher scores on tests of developmental outcome at age 1 year compared with neonates whose hematocrits were maintained at approximately 20%.[37]

Type of Vital Organ Support: Deep Hypothermic Circulatory Arrest Versus Low-Flow Cardiopulmonary Bypass

Cardiopulmonary bypass (CPB) and DHCA are commonly used during intraoperative repair of congenital heart lesions in infants. Both methods result in transient disruption of cerebral vascular reactivity to oxygen and in blood pressure changes that may contribute to hypoxemia and hypotension, and both methods have been associated with neurodevelopmental abnormalities.[38] DHCA has been implicated in ischemic reperfusion injury, and duration of circulatory arrest has been identified as an independent risk factor for adverse neurologic sequelae. Differences in verbal, quantitative, and general cognitive IQ scores between control subjects and infants and young children undergoing profound hypothermia and circulatory arrest correlate with the duration of arrest.[39] Deep hypothermic circulatory arrest for longer than 45 minutes was followed by increased risk of postoperative seizures, elevated creatinine kinase, electroencephalographic abnormalities, cerebral palsy, and full-scale IQ less than 85.[5] Although the IQ scores of children who underwent intracardiac repair of congenital heart defects were within the normal range, DHCA for longer than 39 minutes was associated with visual-motor and fine motor skill deficits, diminished full-scale IQ, and deficits in higher-order nonverbal processing.[10,19] Cardiopulmonary bypass is also associated with microemboli[12] and with an inflammatory cascade caused by contact of blood with prosthetic surfaces, resulting in white matter injury.[38]

Cardiopulmonary bypass precipitates a systemic inflammatory response associated with the release of the pro-inflammatory cytokines interleukin-1, -6, and -8 and tumor necrosis factor-alpha[40,41] and is also associated with platelet activation, resulting in an increase in the surface density of glycoprotein Ib, the formation of platelet-leukocyte aggregates, and the expression of P-selectin on the platelet surface.[42-45] Platelet degranulation and platelet-leukocyte adhesion may contribute to the complications of CPB through the release of peripheral inflammatory cytokines[45,46] that can enter the central nervous system and produce vasoactive changes and inflammation, which have the potential to modulate cognitive processes.[47-49] In adults undergoing cardiac surgery on CPB, there is evidence of a significant association between "transcerebral platelet activation and neurocognitive decline."[45] Children with CHD who undergo CPB are at particular risk of the inflammatory complications of CPB because their relatively small intravascular volumes and the high flow rates of the circuit may increase the degree of cellular injury.[46]

Since the 1960s, extensive investigations have employed platelets as a peripheral model of central nervous system neuronal function to investigate the neurobiology of psychiatric disorders.[50] Biologic markers in these tiny formed elements can, in theory, be used to subcategorize psychiatric disorders into more neurobiologically homogeneous subgroups. Platelets possess receptors, and messenger systems that make them an attractive model of monoaminergic neurons that possess serotonin$_2$ receptors that are similar to brain 5-HT$_{2A}$ receptors and serotonin transporter and vesicular monoamine transporters that are identical to those of the brain.[50] These characteristics of platelets and the advancement of the monoamine hypothesis of mood disorders, the hypothesis of noradrenergic dysregulation in anxiety disorders, the dopamine hypothesis in schizophrenia, and neuronal mechanisms of action of psychotropic medications have spurred promising research using platelets as a tool.[50]

Platelets may play yet another role. In cyanotic CHD, whole megakaryocytes circulating in the systemic venous bed are delivered into the systemic arterial circulation through right-to-left shunts and randomly lodge in systemic capillaries where their cytoplasmic platelet-derived growth factor and transforming growth factor ß are released (see Chapter 12). Theoretically, shunted systemic venous megakaryocytes might lodge in the brain and release these active cytokines and mitogens, producing localized inflammatory responses and neuronal injury.

Young patients who may be neurologically compromised before cardiac surgery may experience further neurologic injury as a result of cardiopulmonary bypass. The Boston Circulatory Arrest Trial was concerned with the neurodevelopmental status of children randomized to DHCA or cardiopulmonary bypass during the arterial switch operation for complete transposition of the great arteries. In both categories, subjects of various ages experienced an increased risk of neurodevelopmental disability. Deficits tended to be most striking in the areas of visual-spatial skills and motor function, with the circulatory arrest group at significantly higher risk. In the immediate postoperative period, children in the DHCA group experienced more seizures and more clinical neurologic abnormalities. At 1 year of age, motor development scores were lower, and at 2.5 years, deficits in expressive language and fine and gross motor function were more frequent.[9] At 4 years, the full-scale IQ of both cohorts was approximately one half standard deviation below the mean, and in both groups, performance was below the mean, especially in the domains of visual-motor and visual-spatial skills. Compared with a healthy population, these children displayed more deficits in expressive language, visual-motor, and visual-spatial skills. At 8 years of age, deficits in visual-spatial processing and language persisted, in addition to deficits in memory,

hypothesis generation, attention, and executive functioning. When performing tasks that required structuring, pacing, and monitoring behavior, the children became "lost in the details" and had difficulty determining how the various elements of the task fit into a synthetic whole. Many had difficulty with reading comprehension and in applying basic mathematical concepts. Children assigned to total circulatory arrest performed worse in tasks of manual dexterity, penmanship, speech production, visual motor tracking, and verbal fluency. The cardiopulmonary bypass cohort exhibited more impulsive behavior patterns and scored worse on measures of vigilance.[8,9] It is worth noting that test results at age 1 year correlated only modestly with results at 8 years. Accordingly, testing at 1 year may leave undetected poor neurodevelopmental outcomes later in life.[51]

EFFECTS OF SURGICAL INTERVENTION IN INFANTS AND CHILDREN WITH CONGENITAL HEART DISEASE

Although patients with CHD may have preoperative neurologic deficits, their mean intellectual function is reportedly within normal range. Postoperatively, however, significant deficits are confined to children with cyanotic CHD. Regardless of the severity of CHD, children who undergo surgical intervention are at risk for adverse neurodevelopmental and cognitive sequelae.[27] Cerebral palsy, mental retardation, and hypoxic-ischemic abnormalities on MRI are common in children after open heart surgery. Abnormal scans were found in 74% of these patients and were more likely in those who were operated on during early infancy and who underwent hypothermic circulatory arrest for longer than 45 minutes.[52] Patients who underwent surgical repair of acyanotic lesions had impaired intellectual development, particularly complex integration, and were rated by parents as prone to aggressive, impulsive, and hyperactive behavior.[53]

Neuropsychological testing of children after surgical versus transcatheter device closure of a secundum atrial septal defect revealed normal-range IQ and achievement scores in both groups. However, surgical repair group was associated with a 9.5-point deficit in Full-Scale IQ and a 9.7-point deficit in performance IQ.[53] After repair of cyanotic lesions, children experienced a drop in IQ scores and impaired cognitive function. Although mean IQ scores were within the normal range for children with repaired cyanotic lesions, the scores were lower than expected.[30]

Children with cyanotic CHD have lower postoperative IQ scores and a higher incidence of learning disabilities than those with acyanotic malformations or normal children. Children with severe malformations perform worse on verbal IQ and performance IQ and score lower in reading, spelling, and arithmetic.[54] A significant difference was found in full-scale IQ scores and academic performance in children with transposition of the great arteries or tetralogy of Fallot surgically repaired between ages 2 and 5, compared with a control group of children with heart murmurs that required no treatment. The arterial switch operation for transposition of the great arteries was associated with deficits in motor function and visual-spatial skills,[9] and 3 to 5 years after neonatal arterial switch operations, neurologic impairment was more common than in normal peers. In older children who had undergone neonatal TGA repair, IQ scores did not differ from the normal population, but there were significant impairments in motor function, learning, language, and academic achievement.[30,55]

Children who have undergone repair of total anomalous pulmonary venous connection have deficits in fine motor function and visual-motor integration, as well as impairment across other domains, including intelligence, academic achievement, and attention.[55,56] Full-scale IQ was significantly lower in those who experienced hypothermic circulatory arrest for longer than 40 minutes.[19] After the Fontan procedure, children have IQ scores within normal range, but their scores are still significantly lower than the mean for the general population.[10] Patients with hypoplastic left heart syndrome are especially destined for poor neurodevelopmental outcomes, which may in part be related to the peculiar complexity of the malformation and the need for surgical procedures before Fontan repair.[5,10,11,27]

IMMEDIATE POSTOPERATIVE CONCERNS

The brain is vulnerable in the early postoperative period.[30] Seizures, cranial nerve abnormalities, hypotonia and hypertonia, motor asymmetry, and feeding difficulties have been reported immediately following surgery for CHD.[12,30] Infants who experienced postoperative seizures had worse outcomes at 1 year.[57] Extracorporeal membrane oxygenation has been cited as a cerebral hypoxic-ischemic risk that prefigures subsequent neurodevelopmental impairment. Fifty percent of patients so exposed had IQ scores one or more standard deviations below the mean.[30]

Hospitalization per se exerts an adverse effect both emotionally and cognitively in children between the ages of 6 months and 4 years.[30] Early postoperative reregulation from hypothermic body temperature is believed to have an adverse effect on neurologic development.[58] Neurohormonal changes have also been cited, and lower levels of thyroid hormone secondary to transient hypothyroidism in children who have undergone CHD surgery are associated with longer periods of mechanical ventilation and longer ICU stays. These changes are in turn significantly related to poorer neurodevelopmental outcomes. The Boston Circulatory Arrest Study cited

earlier reported that longer ICU stays correlated with lower full-scale, verbal, and performance IQ scores, as well as lower mathematics achievement scores. Long postoperative hospitalization is associated with worse cognitive function, even when adjusted for perioperative events, perfusion time, and sociodemographic variables. Specifically, each additional day in hospital resulted in a 0.9-point reduction in full-scale IQ score.[38] Multiple hospitalizations, length of hospitalization, and repetition of procedures requiring general anesthesia are significantly related to subsequent neurodevelopmental abnormalities.[5] Frequent prolonged hospitalizations and exposure to the various personnel involved in care result in "inconsistency of the physical environment," which can compromise development.[4]

SURGICAL INTERVENTION AND COGNITIVE IMPAIRMENT

Impaired brain function following cardiac surgery was first recognized in patients after valvuloplasty for rheumatic mitral valve disease.[59] The three major categories of central nervous system complications of cardiac surgery (see Chapter 14) include stroke, acute encephalopathy, and chronic cognitive decline.[60] The neurologic manifestations of acute stroke reflect the specific sites of brain injury. Acute encephalopathy includes delirium, confusion, inattention, and drowsiness in addition to stupor, coma, and seizures. Chronic cognitive decline consists of amnesia, aphasia, inattention, and apraxia and is often associated with symptoms of depression such as disturbed sleep, apathy, sadness, and anhedonia. Cognitive decline is the most important complication confronting cardiac surgical patients and affects a significant minority. The prevalence of cognitive decline after coronary artery bypass ranges from 8% to 53% at discharge to 36% at 6 weeks, 24% at 6 months, and 42% at 5 years.[61,62] From its inception, extracorporeal circulation was implicated in brain damage.[63-65] Because cerebral emboli were proposed as the major mechanism of neurological damage, inline filtration systems were installed.[66,67] Extracardiac surgery (coronary artery bypass) was subsequently implicated as a cause of neurologic complications.[68] The risk of cerebral dysfunction was believed to be lower with off-pump coronary artery bypass grafting than with conventional bypass grafting. However, in elderly, high-risk patients, no significant difference in the incidence of cognitive dysfunction was evident between the two groups 3 months after surgery, raising questions about the mechanisms of neurologic injury.

Investigations of central nervous system injury in patients without overt stroke have employed intraoperative transcranial Doppler and diffusion-weighted MRI that disclose cerebral emboli in terminal arterial territories.[69,70] These microemboli are the main source of brain injury and the major source of cognitive impairment.[60] The low incidence of macroembolic stroke (<3%) underscores the success of inline filtration systems. However, the risk of cognitive damage is not eliminated because inline filtration systems are not effective in arresting microemboli that are responsible for the immediate consequences characterized by inattention, confusion, agitation, and delirium and the later consequences characterized by depression and dementia.[60] Microemboli, by reducing the reserve of functioning cerebral neurons, result in changes in regional brain function. However, in patients with significant preexisting cognitive impairment, cerebrovascular disease, advanced age, and systemic hypertension, neuronal loss may be sufficient to cause overt clinical dementia.[60]

Large strokes occur in less than 3% of cases and produce major deficits such as hemiplegia, but in about 10% of cases, the large quantity of embolic material results in acute encephalopathy.

DEVELOPMENT ACROSS THE LIFE SPAN

Approximately 85% of children with CHD now live to adulthood, and this number will increase (see Chapters 4 and 5). Nevertheless, CHD must be regarded as a chronic illness not only because of the obligatory residua and sequelae of operation but also because this growing population has unique concerns, is at higher risk for emotional disturbances, and, with few exceptions, requires specialized long-term care.[71]

Patients not only confront direct consequences of their illness, such as physical limitations, recurrent hospitalizations, operations, and reoperations, but they also confront the emotional consequences of chronic illness. During childhood, the primary concerns are related to parental and sibling attachments, functioning at school, and physically keeping up with peers. During adolescence, the primary concerns are body image, sexuality, and struggle with separation from parents. Adult concerns include education, employment, insurability, marriage, and pregnancy. An overarching issue throughout these stages is the obligatory need for continuity of care and identification of obstacles to achieving it.

Infancy

The birth of a child with CHD may not be the anticipated experience of happiness and hopefulness but instead an experience of parental distress and feelings of loss, circumstances beyond one's control, and fearfulness about the future.[72,73] Parents may react with anger, sadness, guilt, feelings of worthlessness, helplessness, hopelessness, and decreased self-esteem,[74,75] experiences that have a negative impact on the parent-child relationship, especially the maternal-infant bond.[73,76,77] Mothers of infants

with CHD are less likely to smile at their offspring, make eye contact with or touch their babies, or sing to them during feeding, and infants of these mothers are less responsive to parental cues.[78] Insecure attachments during infancy have been correlated with subsequent inability to form secure attachments throughout developmental stages of life.[79]

Childhood

School-age children with complex congenital cardiac malformations that require surgical intervention as neonates or infants have significantly higher rates of learning disabilities and academic difficulties.[22,80,81] Deficits in motor function and visual-spatial processing are common, as are disorders of speech and executive function[9] and behavioral abnormalities including disinhibition, inattention, and hyperactivity, which are criteria of ADHD.[20,29] Learning disabilities result in academic failure, poor classroom performance, and problems with social skills, self-esteem, behavioral disinhibition, and delinquency.[28,56] These children are likely to require special school services as they grow older.[9,56]

Repeated hospitalizations and surgical procedures in early life result in depression and withdrawal and in feelings of rejection and of being punished by parents.[82,83] Children who experience painful invasive procedures, prolonged ICU stays, multiple hospitalizations, and cardiac surgeries often perceive the doctor as perpetrator of their trauma.[84,85] Psychiatric symptoms in children after cardiac surgery are prevalent and include a posttraumatic response characterized by anxiety, fearful withdrawal, and restlessness. Some patients are combative when confronted with ICU procedures, whereas others are passively cooperative.[84,86]

Children with complex CHD are often too ill to attend school regularly, resulting in home tutoring or being held back, with subsequent feelings of social isolation and awkwardness. Young boys with cyanotic heart disease, because they are unable to participate in sports, are teased, excluded from activities, and called names; they feel different, inferior, and rejected.[87]

Adolescence

Adolescence is characterized by physical and emotional growth. Adolescents struggle with issues of identity, body image, self-esteem, sexuality, separation from parents, formation of peer relationships, and the establishment of value systems.[88–92] Patients with CHD confront these developmental tasks with the obstacles of repeated hospitalizations and surgical procedures, interrupted education, and parental overprotection.

Overt stigmata of illness, including physical limitations, cyanosis, short stature, and surgical scars, have a negative impact on peer relationships and socialization.[93,94] In an attempt to be like their peers, adolescents with CHD may engage in risk-taking behavior.

A major task of adolescence is separation and individuation from parents, processes complicated by insecure attachments earlier in life.[88,95,96] Adolescents attend cardiology clinics accompanied by their parents (see Chapter 3) and, more often than not, assume a passive role while the parent relates to the health care provider.[71,97] Adolescents must be encouraged to be active participants.

Parental Stress and Emotional Health

High levels of stress experienced by parents of children with CHD affect the parent-child relationship and the psychological health of the patient.[75,96,98-102] Parents, especially mothers, experience fear, difficulties in coping, pessimism, exhaustion, isolation, decreased socialization,[103] and a sense of helplessness.[75,102,104] The disproportionate burden of maternal caregiving accounts for a higher rate of psychiatric symptoms in mothers compared with fathers of children with CHD.[75]

Maternal Mental Health

Maternal mental health is a strong predictor of the child's emotional health and psychosocial development.[82,105-110] A child's awareness of maternal anxiety has been found to affect the child's perception of illness more than the severity of the cardiac lesion. Parental reports of posttraumatic stress disorder (PTSD) have been correlated with their perception of the intensity of their child's treatment, the greater the perceived treatment intensity, the greater and more adverse the parental response.[111] Young women with CHD have their activities curtailed because of parental fear of adverse consequences and because fear of death resulting from constant parental vigilance makes them feel that they might "die at any moment."[107,109,112,113] Heightened concern and overprotection can lead to a dependent lifestyle in which the child is not stimulated and exploratory behavior is curtailed.[95,114,115]

Comprehension of Illness and Risk-Taking Behavior

Adolescents have difficulty understanding the nature of their CHD, especially if it is complex,[116] yet understanding is essential to psychological health, medical compliance, and avoidance of risk-taking behavior. In one study, less than a quarter of the patients could state their diagnosis, and one third had a poor or incorrect understanding of their illness.[117] Patients must be made aware of symptoms of deterioration of cardiac function; cautioned regarding the harmful effects of tobacco and alcohol; and must know infective endocarditis risk factors and prophylaxis, medication side effects, exercise

limitations, and risks of heritability.[118-120] Nearly 30% of cardiac surgical patients expressed concern about transmission of CHD to their offspring, 50% could not name a single risk factor for infective endocarditis, and nearly 20% had never been to a dentist.[121,122] Sexually active young women with CHD are rarely referred to gynecologists until their second or third decade or until they become pregnant.[123]

These many barriers to the comprehension of illness have been attributed to a number of factors. First, parents themselves may have an inadequate understanding of their child's illness. One study reported that nearly two thirds of parents overestimated their child's physical ability,[124] resulting in an impact on the child's perception of his or her physical limitations, a perception that may not coincide with cardiologists' recommendations. Nonacceptance of physical limitations and denial of illness severity are common.[76] One third of patients believed their condition was less severe than defined by their cardiologist and engaged in higher levels of physical activity than medically recommended. Approximately 80% of patients for whom light physical activity was advised believed that they could participate in physically intense exercise.[125] Second, IQ and developmental delays can limit an adolescent's ability to comprehend the nature of illness and the imperative for healthy behaviors.[117] Third, even when adolescents comprehend the nature of their congenital cardiac disease and of the need for appropriate behavior, risk taking often results from peer pressure and the desire to conform or from frank rebellion against the restrictions demanded by their heart disease. Adherence to medications is difficult for adolescents with long-term illnesses.[91,116,126] Chronically ill adolescents seldom report ever having sexual intercourse, and age of first sexual relations was significantly older than in the general population. Alcohol and tobacco use are prevalent.[127,128] More than half of young adults with complex CHD engage in binge drinking.[129] Adolescents with chronic illness who are isolated due to school absences or whose physical activities are restricted use cigarette smoking as a way to "reconnect" and gain peer approval.[130] Tattooing and piercing are common among chronically ill adolescents, incurring the risk of infective endocarditis.[131]

Self-Image

Self-image, or self-concept, defined as "the totality of an individual's description and valuation of himself or herself," is complex and multifaceted.[87] High self-esteem is associated with positive relationships, academic and occupational success, and psychological health, whereas low self-esteem is associated with risk taking and poor mental health, including depression and suicide attempts.[87,116,132]

Body image refers specifically to one's concept of physical appearance. Patients with physical handicaps have lower self-esteem, a disintegrated view of self, feelings of inferiority, negative self-evaluation, and a sense of "feeling different" from their peers.[87,91,92,133] Children with CHD have a constricted body image, seeing themselves as weak and ill. Although the cardiac defect may be hidden from view, its effects on physical appearance, including small stature, scoliosis, cyanosis, clubbing, sternotomy, or thoracotomy scars, have a profound effect on self-image. Chronic illnesses that limit physical activity affect self-perception, especially in males.[90,134]

Adolescents with CHD avoid physical exposure and intimacy and hesitate to divulge their illness for fear of rejection,[135] especially female adolescents, who feel stigmatized and are particularly self-conscious about surgical scars. They strive to hide physical faults, which are constant reminders of their illness and which have a negative impact on body image and self-esteem during a sensitive developmental period when intimate relationships begin.[83,94] Females who are unable to conceive or bear children experience feelings of self-hatred and a sense of inadequacy.[112]

Sexual maturation is a major developmental milestone of adolescence and is related to the formation of self-image.[92,126] For adolescents with CHD, sexuality is an especially important issue, but parents often see their child as "asexual,"[123] and discussions about sexuality and sexual reproduction are either postponed or avoided by parents, as well as physicians.[133] As a result, adolescents have fears and misinformation about sexual activity, conception, and heritability of their disease. Males in particular report fear of dying during sexual arousal and intercourse, and females fear a perceived inability to conceive and bear children. Both sexes fear transmitting CHD to their offspring.[112,122,123] Female nurse practitioners and physician assistants play useful, practical roles in dealing with female adolescents (see Chapter 3) who need counseling about contraception, family planning, and heritability.[97] Patients engaged in substance abuse and other risk-taking behaviors may require counseling and enrollment in rehabilitation programs.

Psychological functioning in adolescents and adults with CHD is reportedly comparable to healthy peers,[71] but high levels of depression and anxiety have been reported in 30% to 40% of this patient population.[82,93,94,109,116,134,136–140] Depression and anxiety rather than the complexity of the heart disease have the strongest effect on social relationships.[137] Female sex is a specific predictor for psychopathology in adults with CHD.[110] Adolescent females have higher rates of depression than their male counterparts, which in part may reflect the higher incidence of depression in females in the general population.[88] Concern over body image may affect sexual relationships, and more than 40% of females report that their CHD influenced their decision not to have children.[83]

Transition to Adult Care

Adults with CHD should be managed in adult settings whether outpatient or inpatient. Pediatric cardiology clinics are not designed for adults and instead reinforce a sense of dependency that must be overcome if adult maturity is to be achieved. Information should be provided on how to contact the Adult Congenital Heart Association (ACHA) to be informed regarding transfer to an adult facility and the obligatory need for long-term care (see Chapter 2). A formal process involving both patients and parents should be in place before adolescence to anticipate the transition to adult care.[141] Patients and parents should be made aware that the referring pediatric cardiologist will be kept informed. Transfer is facilitated when a visit to the adult clinic is arranged to provide an opportunity to meet the cardiologist who will assume responsibility for continuing care. It is important to inform the patient and parent that the new cardiologist is specially trained in adult CHD and also has knowledge of adult medicine that is required to provide the best overall long-term care. Transition is usually at age 18 years, but mature 16-year-olds and immature 19-year-olds should be judged individually. The transfer should be carried out during a period of medical stability.

The transition from pediatric to adult care takes on special meaning for patients who are emotionally attached to their pediatric cardiologists who have officiated from birth and seen them through many diagnostic procedures and more than one operation. Support groups for patients and parents are helpful, and access to the ACHA Web site can be invaluable (see Chapters 2 and 3).

Adulthood

As patients undergo the transition into adulthood, the central issues become education, employment, insurability, functional status, pregnancy, and childbirth (see Chapters 2 and 3).[95,97,134,136,142–145] Disability and functional status are important concerns[83,106,109,146–148] because patients correctly consider physical health as an important determinant of the quality of life.[149]

Patients with complex lesions are confronted with an uncertain future, shortened life expectancy, and exposure to the traumatic experience of further hospitalizations and operations.[82,91,94,97,136,144,150] Low self-esteem and uncertainty about the future are correlated with a higher incidence of suicide.[151]

Employability and Insurability

Gainful employment is an important determinant of quality of life. Employment is looked on as more than just a means of earning a living and is understandably regarded as an intrinsic value, a means of socialization, and a source of motivation to live.[95,143,152,153] However, adults with congenital heart malformations are more likely to be unemployed regardless of disease severity.[152,153] Patients with mild lesions reported a 50% increase in job application rejection rates, whereas those with complex lesions reported a 400% increase.[71,97,154] Physical disability has an impact on workload and work time, and interrupted education or lower levels of educational achievement result in lower levels of employment and decreased opportunities.[114] Employers are understandably concerned about productivity and reliability.[97] Preexisting disease epitomized by CHD makes health insurance difficult to obtain, and employers are reluctant to assume responsibility for health insurance.[97,122,150] Patients who are insured are reluctant to change jobs because of the risk of losing their coverage, and others are obliged to pay higher premiums.[155] Even patients with minor lesions that carry no functional disability may not be cleared in preemployment and insurance physical examinations.[71] Patients with complex lesions are often refused insurance unless they are on disability, which can discourage them from seeking work.[71] They may also delay follow-up medical visits and discontinue expensive medications they cannot afford.[97]

CLINICAL PSYCHIATRIC ISSUES

Genetic Abnormalities

Genetic abnormalities result in both CHD and psychiatric morbidity. Williams syndrome, Down syndrome, CHARGE (Hall-Hittner syndrome), VACTERL and velo-cardio-facial (VCFS or DiGeorge) syndromes, and trisomy 13, 18, and 21 typically coexist with congenital cardiac disease.[156] A heightened risk of psychiatric disorders such as schizophrenia is thought to be due to coexisting structural abnormalities of the brain (see Chapter 14).[157,158]

The VCFS is an example of a genetic disorder associated with CHD and psychopathology. Schizotypal traits and problems with attention, concentration, and anxiety are common, but the most prevalent psychiatric concern is ADHD, which affects 35% to 55% of patients.[159-161] There is also an increased prevalence of ADHD in first-degree relatives, suggesting that ADHD in VCFS has a genetic basis independent of the VCFS-related abnormalities.[162]

The CHARGE syndrome (Coloboma, Heart disease, Atresia of the choanae, Renal abnormality, Growth, mental retardation, genital anomalies, and Ear malformations and hearing loss) is a heterogeneous disorder. Extensive bilateral coloboma results in poor vision, microcephaly, brain malformations, and poor intellectual outcome.[163] Patients with CHARGE syndrome are hyperactive, socially disinterested, withdrawn, and exhibit impairments in language and social skills believed to be related to the genetic syndrome rather than a direct result of the cardiac malformation.[164]

Mental retardation is common in individuals with genetically confirmed 22q11 deletion (CATCH 22—Cardiac anomaly, Anomalous face, Thymus hypoplasia/aplasia, Cleft palate, and Hypocalcaemia). One study reported that 50% of these patients have IQs <70,[165] and many have ADHD and/or autism spectrum problems with characteristic behavioral profiles of low mental energy and deficits in sustained attention and social interaction.

Psychiatric Disorders

There are four domains predictive of behavioral disorders in children with CHD: child health, child temperament, parent-child relationships, and family environment, the last of which is the most powerful predictor.[166-168] Low economic status and large families increase the risk of anxiety and depression. CHD can disrupt developmental achievements in school or work and give rise to concerns about premature mortality.[141]

Social and emotional maladjustment in CHD increase after cardiac surgery,[169] but significant improvement in self-perception can follow successful repairs.

Children with CHD and physical handicaps have lower IQ scores,[170] feelings of inferiority and anxiety, and consider themselves weak, frightened, and ill.[87] Adults struggle to be normal despite physical limitations.[114]

Depression and Anxiety

CHD is a risk factor for cognitive and behavioral disorders,[171] as well as psychiatric illness. Depression and anxiety are the most common psychiatric disorders in these patients.[93,138,172] Depression is associated with a poor functional state, lower levels of education, unemployment, and older age and is more likely in patients who have undergone multiple cardiac operations with deep hypothermic circulatory arrest.[136,173] Depression affects quality of life and is linked to awareness of increased risk of cardiac and all-cause mortality.[174-177] Depression is common in children and adolescents undergoing heart and heart-lung transplantation (see Chapter 17).[178,179]

In patients with chronic cyanotic CHD, the incidence of self-rated depression was 34%.[138] When adults with CHD who were devoid of overt symptoms of depression or anxiety and who were considered well adjusted were examined with a semistructured psychiatric interview,[142] more than one third met the criteria for a psychiatric diagnosis, most commonly depression or anxiety, and more than one quarter had scores consistent with significant severity.

Posttraumatic Stress Disorder

PTSD consists of a cluster of symptoms following exposure to a traumatic event that involves "actual or threatened death or serious injury, or a threat to the physical integrity of self or others" and that results in "intense fear, helplessness, or horror."[180] There is a state of hyperarousal, a reliving of the event, and avoidance of situations or stimuli associated with the event. Prolonged exposure to a traumatic event increases the likelihood of a posttraumatic response. PTSD symptoms after cardiac surgery are closely associated with the length of ICU stay, during which children are surrounded by critically ill patients, separated from their parents, and subjected to painful and invasive procedures. Longer duration of symptoms in children with chronic PTSD is associated with decreased cerebral volume and lower IQ,[181] and childhood traumatic experiences increase the risk of subsequent substance abuse and suicide attempts in adolescence and adulthood. Symptoms of PTSD in medically ill children include disorganized behavior, poor concentration, sleep disturbances, nightmares, distressing thoughts, and agitation.[84] Trait anxiety—an intrinsic proneness to anxiety—is an independent predictor of PTSD symptoms in medically ill children. Intensity of treatment appears to be associated with PTSD in children, but it is the child's perception of treatment rather than the treatment per se that matters.[111,183] Events such as driving to the hospital or smells associated with treatment act as triggers of physiologic and emotional reactions. Patients who avoid associations that trigger awareness of their illness become medication noncompliant.

Trauma-focused cognitive-behavioral therapy is currently the most effective treatment in children and adolescents with PTSD.[184] There is a lack of randomized, double-blind controlled trials studying the safety and efficacy of pharmacologic agents in otherwise healthy children and adolescents suffering from PTSD. Despite the lack of data, there is a tendency to use medications in conjunction with psychodynamic and cognitive therapies.[84,185]

Onychophagia

Chronic nail biting constitutes a significant risk in patients with CHD because staphylococcal paronychial infection and bacteremia are responsible for infective endocarditis (see Chapter 8). The incidence of nail biting peaks at 45% in adolescence and then declines to a low of 10% by age 60.[186] Treatment has focused largely on behavioral techniques, including competing responses and self-monitoring and aversion therapy such as applying ill-tasting substances to the nails.[139,187,188] As early as the 1970s, a 13-component multifaceted treatment package was developed. The habit reversal program is believed to be the most useful behavioral treatment for nail biting.[188]

Because onychophagia is believed to be part of a spectrum of obsessive-compulsive disorders and because of the efficacy of selective serotonin reuptake inhibitors (SSRIs) for these disorders, pharmacologic

treatment has been considered.[189] Nail biting and hair pulling (trichotillomania) may be similar disorders, both of which might respond to SSRIs,[188] but therapeutic results are inconclusive.[191-193] Behavioral treatment seems to be the better therapeutic option, with an SSRI used as an adjunct.

PHARMACOLOGIC TREATMENT

Selective Serotonin Reuptake Inhibitors

The SSRIs include citalopram, escitalopram, fluoxetine, paroxetine, sertraline, and fluvoxamine. These medications as a class are first-line treatment for depression in otherwise healthy individuals and are used in cardiac patients because of their favorable side-effect profile, minimal drug-drug interactions, low risk of toxicity from overdose, and minimal cardiac risk. However, certain SSRIs carry greater risks. Fluoxetine can lead to higher plasma levels of benzodiazepines in patients being treated concomitantly for anxiety disorders. Fluvoxamine causes significant inhibition of CYP2C19, which can cause elevated plasma levels of propranolol and can inhibit CYP3A4, which elevates levels of calcium channel blockers.[194] Sertraline dilatates coronary arteries, protects endothelium, and is safe and effective in post–myocardial infarction patients.[195] Of the SSRIs, citalopram and escitalopram have only modest degrees of cytochrome p450 inhibition and relatively benign interaction and side-effect profiles, and thus they should be considered first-line agents for the treatment of depression, anxiety, and PTSD.

Tetracyclic Antidepressants

Mirtazapine is a selective alpha-2 adrenergic antagonist that enhances noradrenergic and serotonergic neurotransmission, has little cytochrome P450 inhibition, and blocks 5-HT3.[194] The medication is useful in treating anxiety, depression, insomnia, and anorexia.[196]

Atypical Antidepressants

Venlafaxine is associated with elevation of supine diastolic blood pressure. Clearance is significantly decreased in patients with renal or liver dysfunction. Bupropion, a significant inhibitor of CYP2D6, is contraindicated in patients with electroencephalographic abnormalities.

In patients with liver or renal dysfunction, elevated plasma levels of bupropion increase the risk of seizures.[197]

Duloxetine has a dual action, blocking both serotonin and norepinephrine transporters, and is useful in depressed patients with pain, particularly neuropathic pain. The medication reportedly causes increased heart rate.[194]

Tricyclic Antidepressants

The tricyclic antidepressants (TCAs), which include imipramine, desipramine, amitriptyline, clomipramine, and nortriptyline, have been used in the treatment of depression and PTSD. In general, TCAs should be reserved for depression unresponsive to first-line agents.[196] Their effects on the nondenervated cardiovascular system are well documented and include conduction delay and inhibition of sodium, calcium, and potassium channels. They have the same electrophysiologic profile and risks as type 1A antiarrhythmic drugs, namely, prolongation of the PR and QT intervals and the QRS duration. The physiologic effects on denervated hearts are unknown.[196] Nortriptyline, which has less hepatic metabolism compared with other TCAs, is the only TCA in which therapeutic serum levels have been established and may be preferable to other tricyclic agents.[194]

Monoamine Oxidase Inhibitors

Monoamine oxidase inhibitors (MAOIs), represented by phenelzine and tranylcypromine, require dietary restrictions and have significant side effects that include hypotension, interactions with anesthetic agents and pressors,[196] and hypertensive crisis if tyramine-containing foods are consumed.[194]

CARDIAC TRANSPLANTATION IN CHILDREN AND ADOLESCENTS

Approximately 2% to 3% of patients with CHD undergo cardiac transplantation (see Chapter 17) that epitomizes an event "outside the range of usual human experience" and is responsible for PTSD.[198] Although pediatric and adolescent heart transplant patients can exhibit good postoperative adaptation, they often experience difficulties with school-reintegration, behavioral disturbances, anxiety, and depression.[105,106] A longitudinal study found that more than 25% had posttransplant emotional problems.[106,178,179] The psychiatric morbidity that occurs shortly after transplantation is associated with poor medication compliance, infections, and acute and chronic rejection.[199,200]

The mortality rate for patients on a heart transplant waiting list approaches 30%[201] (see Chapter 17). The wait for a donor organ is an extremely stressful period that can bring patients "to the brink of despair."[198] There is often a feeling of guilt because another must die for a heart to become available.[198] Reports are conflicting regarding the effects of transplantation wait-time on neurodevelopmental outcome.[202,203]

Most pediatric transplant patients experience at least one episode of acute cellular rejection, usually in the first 2 months after transplantation. Repeated endomyocardial biopsies are traumatic,[204] and the complex regimen of immunosuppressants that must be strictly adhered to for the rest of a patient's life can be oppressive.[205]

Neurocognitive Development

Long-term neurocognitive development in children with hypoplastic left heart syndrome who underwent cardiac transplantation as infants is below normal on intelligence and developmental tests. One third of subjects in one study had impaired intellectual functioning with scores over two standard deviations below the mean. Children had demonstrable deficits in mathematic ability, expressive and receptive language, and visual and motor performance.[202] Those who underwent cardiac transplantation and had behavior scores statistically within normal range still had behavioral problems, especially with attention, sometimes relatively severe.

Depression

Depression is common in pediatric cardiac transplant patients. Depression before transplantation is a predictor of depression in the posttransplant period. Nineteen percent of cardiac transplant candidates 18 years or older experienced one or more depressive episodes before transplantation, and 13% to 14% experienced one or more depressive episodes in the first 12 to 18 months posttransplantation. The rate of a major depressive episode rose to 26% by the third posttransplant year.[199]

The meticulous daily treatment with immunosuppressants and the rigorous unremitting schedule of medical follow-ups correlates with depressive symptomatology.[206] In addition to serving as constant reminders of mortality, the medications have undesirable side effects. Corticosteroids alter physical appearance; impair growth; cause weight gain, moon facies, hirsutism, striae, and acne; and in themselves can result in depression, agitation, and psychosis.[201] Although failure to take daily medications is life threatening, nonadherence is common and has been reported in one third of pediatric and adolescent patients.[207-209]

Posttraumatic Stress Syndrome

This psychiatric disorder reportedly afflicts 10% to 17% of cardiac transplantation patients.[204] Occurrence is especially prevalent in the first postoperative year, with a cumulative incidence of 17% over the first 3 posttransplantation years. PTSD in the first postoperative year was a predictor of long-term morbidity and mortality.[200] Patients often reexperience the traumatic event(s) through flashbacks and nightmares; in an attempt to avoid reexperience triggered by association, medical appointments are missed and immunosuppressant medications are neglected, despite the known risks of doing so. There is increased risk of PTSD in patients with a history of psychiatric illness and low family cohesiveness. Cardiac transplant patients who experienced PTSD in their first post-transplant year were 13 times more likely to die by the third posttransplant year.[198]

Impact of Transplantation on the Family

Parents are prone to anxiety and feelings of helplessness while waiting for the donor organ, and the postoperative threats of infection and organ rejection are causes of intense parental anxiety with fear that their child will die. The rates of PTSD in parents was equivalent to the rates in the transplant recipient.[198] Parental mental health correlates with psychological and physical morbidity and patient mortality.[73,208,209] In a very real sense, the family becomes the patient.[209]

Cardiac Transplantation Psychopharmacology

In the first year after cardiac transplantation, depression rates decline, but by the third year the rate increases to approximately 25%,[196] and within 10 years, 33% of patients have depressive symptoms that can present atypically as irritability, headache, gastrointestinal disturbance, and cognitive decline. There is only one current review of the efficacy and safety of pharmacotherapy for depression in heart transplant recipients. In general, the pharmacologic treatment of depression, anxiety, and PTSD is similar in transplantation and nontransplantation patients (see earlier discussion).[196] The SSRIs are again the agents of choice, especially citalopram and escitalopram, which have limited CYP450 interactions. However, certain SSRIs have significant cytochrome P450 inhibition that warn against use in heart transplant recipients. Cyclosporine has a narrow therapeutic index and is metabolized by CYP450. Fluoxetine is thought to affect plasma levels of cyclosporine, cause significant CYP2D6 and CYP3A4 inhibition, and prevent conversion of codeine to its active metabolite, potentially preventing pain relief.[194] For these reasons, this SSRI is not recommended. The tetracyclic antidepressant mirtazapine has shown promise in the treatment of depression and anxiety disorders in cardiac transplant patients.[196]

The atypical antidepressants are not considered first-line agents in this population because of their cardiovascular risk profile, and MAOIs should be avoided in the treatment of depression in cardiac transplant patients.[196]

Tricyclic antidepressants reduce the seizure threshold; this is a relative contraindication in the transplant population, which is already at risk for seizures triggered by encephalopathy and calcineurin inhibitors. If these agents are used in transplant patients with hepatic dysfunction, lower doses are required because the TCAs are hepatically metabolized. In general, however, TCAs should be reserved for depression unresponsive to first-line agents.[196]

St. John's Wort

Twenty percent to 30% of surgical and transplant patients are believed to use homeopathic substances.[196] St. John's Wort, which is not regulated by the Food and Drug Administration, carries potential risks of contamination with toxic substances such as pesticides and heavy metals and has a significant drug-drug interaction profile.[196] An interaction between cyclosporine and St. John's Wort leads to decreased plasma levels of cyclosporine, with the risk of acute rejection. There are also significant drug-drug interactions with St. John's Wort and anticoagulants, resulting in decreased plasma levels of warfarin and interactions with sirolimus and tacrolimus, resulting in decreased plasma levels and the risk of transplant rejection. St. John's Wort also interacts with antidepressants, including the SSRIs, which increases the risk of the serotonin syndrome with hypertension, hyperthermia, myoclonus, and mental status changes.[196]

SUMMARY

Psychiatric disorders are common in adults with CHD. Structural brain abnormalities, chromosomal disorders, and open heart surgery with cardiopulmonary bypass and deep hypothermia contribute to neurologic sequelae that affect developmental and cognitive outcomes. Parental stress, especially maternal anxiety, affects the parent-child relationship and the child's mental health from birth. Children with CHD exhibit learning and behavioral disorders, and repeated hospitalizations have an impact on their socialization. The developmental challenges of adolescence can be difficult for these patients, particularly separation from parents, assuming responsibility for their health, discovering their sexuality, and avoiding risk-taking behavior. As adults, these patients have difficulty with employment and health insurance and often report poor quality of life. Depression, anxiety, and a posttraumatic response have been reported in patients with CHD, especially those who have undergone cardiac transplantation. Clinicians should be aware of and screen for these disorders in this special patient population and their family members. Early detection and treatment are associated with reduced morbidity and mortality.

References

1. Foster E, Graham TP. Task force 2: Special health care needs of adults with congenital heart disease. *JACC.* 2001;37:116–1198.
2. Connelly MS, Webb GD, Somerville J, et al. Canadian Consensus Conference on Adult Congenital Heart Disease 1996. *Can J Cardiol.* 1998;14:395–452.
3. Casey FA, Sykes DH, et al. Behavioral adjustment of children with surgically palliated complex congenital heart disease. *J Pediatr Psychol.* 1996;21:335–352.

4. Wray J, Sensky T. Controlled study of preschool development after surgery for congenital heart disease. *Arch Dis Child.* 1999;80: 511–516.

5. Limperopoulos C, Majnemer A, Shevell MI, et al. Predictors of developmental disabilities after open heart surgery in young children with congenital heart defects. *J Pediatr.* 2002;141:51–58.

6. Wernovsky G. Outcomes regarding the central nervous system in children with complex congenital cardiac malformations. *Cardiol Young.* 2005;15(1 Suppl):132–133.

7. Forbess JM, Visconti KJ, Hancock-Friesen C, et al. Neurodevelopmental outcome after congenital heart surgery: results from an institutional registry. *Circulation.* 2002;106(1 Suppl):I95–I102.

8. Wernovsky G, Shillingford AJ, Gaynor JW. Central nervous system outcomes in children with complex congenital heart disease. *Curr Opin Cardiol.* 2005;20:94–99.

9. Bellinger DC, Wypij D, duDuplessis AJ, et al. Neurodevelopmental status at eight years in children with dextro-transposition of the great arteries: the Boston Circulatory Arrest Trial. *J Thorac Cardiovasc Surg.* 2003;126:1385–1396.

10. Forbess JM, Visconti KJ, Bellinger DC, Jonas RA. Neurodevelopmental outcomes in children after the Fontan operation. *Circulation.* 2001;104(1 Suppl):I127–I132.

11. Kaltman JR, Di H, Tian Z, Rychik J. Impact of congenital heart disease on cerebrovascular blood flow dynamics in the fetus. *Ultrasound Obstet Gynecol.* 2005;25:32–36.

12. Limperopoulos C, Majnemer A, Shevell MI, et al. Neurodevelopmental status of newborns and infants with congenital heart defects before and after open heart surgery. *J Pediatr.* 2000;137:638–645.

13. Mahle WT, Tavani F, Zimmerman RA, et al. An MRI study of neurological injury before and after congenital heart surgery. *Circulation.* 2002;106(1 Suppl):I109–I114.

14. Glauser TA, Rorke LB, Weinberg PM, Clancy RR. Congenital brain anomalies associated with the hypoplastic left heart syndrome. *Pediatrics.* 1990;85:984–990.

15. Jones M. Anomalies of the brain and congenital heart disease: a study of 52 necropsy cases. *Pediatr Pathol.* 1991;11:721–736.

16. Kramer HH, Majewski F, Trampisch HJ, et al. Malformation patterns in children with congenital heart disease. *Am J Dis Child.* 1987;141: 789–795.

17. van Houten JP, Rothman A, Bejar R. High incidence of cranial ultrasound abnormalities in full-term infants with congenital heart disease. *Am J Perinatol.* 1996;13:47–53.

18. Fenton KN, Freeman K, Glogowski K, et al. The significance of baseline cerebral oxygen saturation in children undergoing congenital heart surgery. *Am J Surg.* 2005;190:260–263.

19. Forbess JM, Visconti KJ, Bellinger DC, et al. Neurodevelopmental outcomes after biventricular repair of congenital heart defects. *J Thorac Cardiovasc Surg.* 2002;123:631–639.

20. Galli KK, Zimmerman RA, Jarvik GP, et al. Periventricular leukomalacia is common after neonatal cardiac surgery. *J Thorac Cardiovasc Surg.* 2004;127:692–704.

21. Gaynor JW, Gerdes M, Zackai EH, et al. Apolipoprotein E genotype and neurodevelopmental sequelae of infant cardiac surgery. *J Thorac Cardiovasc Surg.* 2003;126:1736–1745.

22. Wernovsky G. Current insights regarding neurological and developmental abnormalities in children and young adults with complex congenital cardiac disease. *Cardiol Young.* 2006;16 Suppl 1:92–104.

23. Donofrio MT, Bremer YA, Schieken RM, et al. Autoregulation of cerebral blood flow in fetuses with congenital heart disease: the brain sparing effect. *Pediatr Cardiol.* 2003;24:436–443.

24. Miller G, Eggli KD, Contant C, et al. Postoperative neurologic complications after open heart surgery on young infants. *Arch Pediatr Adolesc Med.* 1995;149:764–768.

25. Licht DJ, Wang J, Silvestre DW, et al. Preoperative cerebral blood flow is diminished in neonates with severe congenital heart defects. *J Thorac Cardiovasc Surg.* 2004;128:841–849.

26. Clancy RR, McGaurn SA, Goin JE, et al. Allopurinol neurocardiac protection trial in infants undergoing heart surgery using deep hypothermic circulatory arrest. *Pediatrics.* 2001;108:61–70.

27. Majnemer A, Limperopoulos C, Shevell M, et al. Long-term neuromotor outcome at school entry of infants with congenital heart defects requiring open-heart surgery. *J Pediatr.* 2006;148:72–77.

28. Mahle WT, Clancy RR, Moss EM, et al. Neurodevelopmental outcome and lifestyle assessment in school-aged and adolescent children with hypoplastic left heart syndrome. *Pediatrics.* 2000;105:1082–1089.

29. Bass JL, Corwin M, Gozal D, et al. The effect of chronic or intermittent hypoxia on cognition in childhood: a review of the evidence. *Pediatrics.* 2004;114:805–816.

30. Wray J. Intellectual development of infants, children and adolescents with congenital heart disease. *Dev Sci.* 2006;9:368–378.

31. DeMaso DR, Beardslee WR, Silbert AR, Fyler DC. Psychological functioning in children with cyanotic heart defects. *J Dev Behav Pediatr.* 1990;11:289–294.

32. Newburger JW, Silbert AR, Buckley LP, Fyler DC. Cognitive function and age at repair of transposition of the great arteries in children. *N Engl J Med.* 1984;310:1495–1499.

33. Oates RK, Simpson JM, Cartmill TB, Turnbull JA. Intellectual function and age of repair in cyanotic congenital heart disease. *Arch Dis Child.* 1995;72:298–301.

34. Wray J, Sensky T. Congenital heart disease and cardiac surgery in childhood: effects on cognitive function and academic ability. *Heart.* 2001;85:687–691.

35. Uzark K, Lincoln A, Lamberti JJ, et al. Neurodevelopmental outcomes in children with Fontan repair of functional single ventricle. *Pediatrics.* 1998;101:630–633.

36. du Plessis AJ, Jonas RA, Wypij D, et al. Perioperative effects of alpha-stat versus pH-stat strategies for deep hypothermic cardiopulmonary bypass in infants. *J Thorac Cardiovasc Surg.* 1997;114: 991–1000.

37. Jonas RA, Wypij D, Roth SJ, et al. The influence of hemodilution on outcome after hypothermic cardiopulmonary bypass: results of a randomized trial in infants. *J Thorac Cardiovasc Surg.* 2003;126:1765–1774.

38. Newburger JW, Wypij D, Bellinger DC, et al. Length of stay after infant heart surgery is related to cognitive outcome at age 8 years. *J Pediatr.* 2003;143:67–73.

39. Wells FC, Coghill S, Caplan HL, Lincoln C. Duration of circulatory arrest does influence the psychological development of children after cardiac operation in early life. *J Thorac Cardiovasc Surg.* 1983;86:823–831.

40. Halter J, Steinberg J, Fink G, et al. Evidence of systemic cytokine release in patients undergoing cardiopulmonary bypass. *J Extra Corpor Technol.* 2005;37:272–277.

41. Kalman J, Juhasz A, Bogats G, et al. Elevated levels of inflammatory biomarkers in the cerebrospinal fluid after coronary artery bypass surgery are predictors of cognitive decline. *Neurochem Int.* 2006;48:177–180.

42. Defraigne JO, Pincemail J, Dekoster G, et al. SMA circuits reduce platelet consumption and platelet factor release during cardiac surgery. *Ann Thorac Surg.* 2000;70:2075–2081.

43. Guay J, Ruest P, Lortie L. Cardiopulmonary bypass induces significant platelet activation in children undergoing open-heart surgery. *Eur J Anaesthesiol.* 2004;21:953–956.

44. Ichinose F, Uezono S, Muto R, et al. Platelet hyporeactivity in young infants during cardiopulmonary bypass. *Anesth Analg.* 1999;88: 258–262.

45. Mathew JP, Rinder HM, Smith BR, et al. Transcerebral platelet activation after aortic cross-clamp release is linked to neurocognitive decline. *Ann Thorac Surg.* 2006;81:1644–1649.

46. Rinder CS, Gaal D, Student LA, Smith BR. Platelet-leukocyte activation and modulation of adhesion receptors in pediatric patients with congenital heart disease undergoing cardiopulmonary bypass. *J Thorac Cardiovasc Surg.* 1994;107:280–288.

47. Ramlawi B, Rudolph JL, Mieno S, et al. C-reactive protein and inflammatory response associated to neurocognitive decline following cardiac surgery. *Surgery.* 2006;140:221–226.

48. Ramlawi B, Rudolph JL, Mieno S, et al. Serologic markers of brain injury and cognitive function after cardiopulmonary bypass. *Ann Surg.* 2006;244:593–601.

49. Zhu CB, Blakely RD, Hewlett WA. The proinflammatory cytokines interleukin-1beta and tumor necrosis factor-alpha activate serotonin transporters. *Neuropsychopharmacology.* 2006;31:2121–2131.

50. Gurguis G. Psychiatric disorders. In: Michelson A, ed. *Platelets.* 2nd ed. New York: Elsevier; 2007:791.

51. McGrath E, Wypij D, Rappaport LA, et al. Prediction of IQ and achievement at age 8 years from neurodevelopmental status at age 1 year in children with D-transposition of the great arteries. *Pediatrics.* 2004;114:e572–576.

52. Miller G, Mamourian AC, Tesman JR, et al. Long-term MRI changes in brain after pediatric open heart surgery. *J Child Neurol.* 1994;9:390–397.

53. Visconti KJ, Bichell DP, Jonas RA, et al. Developmental outcome after surgical versus interventional closure of secundum atrial septal defect in children. *Circulation.* 1999;100(19 Suppl):II145–II150.

54. Griffin KJ, Elkin TD, Smith CJ. Academic outcomes in children with congenital heart disease. *Clin Pediatric.* 2003;42:401–409.

55. Hovels-Gurich HH, Seghaye MC, et al. Cognitive and motor development in preschool and school-aged children after neonatal arterial switch operation. *J Thorac Cardiovasc Surg.* 1997;114:578–585.

56. Kirshbom PM, Flynn TB, Clancy RR, et al. Late neurodevelopmental outcome after repair of total anomalous pulmonary venous connection. *J Thorac Cardiovasc Surg.* 2005;129:1091–1097.

57. Bellinger DC, Wypij D, Kuban KC, et al. Developmental and neurological status of children at 4 years of age after heart surgery with hypothermic circulatory arrest or low-flow cardiopulmonary bypass. *Circulation.* 1999;100:526–532.

58. Cottrell SM, Morris KP, Davies P, et al. Early postoperative body temperature and developmental outcome after open heart surgery in infants. *Ann Thorac Surg.* 2004;77:66–71.

59. Fox HM, Rizzo ND, Gifford S. Psychological observations of patients undergoing mitral surgery; a study of stress. *Am Heart J.* 1954;48:645–670.

60. Samuels MA. Can cognition survive heart surgery? *Circulation.* 2006;113:2784–2786.

61. Jensen BO, Hughes P, Rasmussen LS, et al. Cognitive outcomes in elderly high-risk patients after off-pump versus conventional coronary artery bypass grafting: a randomized trial. *Circulation.* 2006;113:2790–2795.

62. Newman MF, Kirchner JL, Phillips-Bute B, et al. Longitudinal assessment of neurocognitive function after coronary-artery bypass surgery. *N Engl J Med.* 2001;344:395–402.

63. Aberg T. Effect of open heart surgery on intellectual function. *Scand J Thorac Cardiovasc Surg.* 1974;1–63.

64. Gilman S. Cerebral disorders after open-heart operations. *N Engl J Med.* 1965;272:489–498.

65. Javid H, Tufo HM, Najafi H, et al. Neurological abnormalities following open-heart surgery. *J Thorac Cardiovasc Surg.* 1969;58:502–509.

66. Aberg T, Kihlgren M. Cerebral protection during open-heart surgery. *Thorax.* 1977;32:525–533.

67. Sotaniemi KA. Brain damage and neurological outcome after open-heart surgery. *J Neurol Neurosurg Psychiatry.* 1980;43:127–135.

68. Shaw PJ, Bates D, Cartlidge NE, et al. Early neurological complications of coronary artery bypass surgery. *Br Med J.* 1985;291:1384–1387.

69. Pugsley W. The use of Doppler ultrasound in the assessment of microemboli during cardiac surgery. *Perfusion.* 1989;4:115–122.

70. Wityk RJ, Goldsborough MA, Hillis A, et al. Diffusion- and perfusion-weighted brain magnetic resonance imaging in patients with neurologic complications after cardiac surgery. *Arch Neurol.* 2001;58:571–576.

71. Kovacs AH, Sears SF, Saidi AS. Biopsychosocial experiences of adults with congenital heart disease: review of the literature. *Am Heart J.* 2005;150:193–201.

72. Garson A Jr, Benson RS, Ivler L, Patton C. Parental reactions to children with congenital heart disease. *Child Psychiatry Human Dev.* 1978;9:86–94.

73. Uzark K, Jones K. Parenting stress and children with heart disease. *J Pediatr Health Care.* 2003;17:163–168.

74. Goldbeck L, Melches J. Quality of life in families of children with congenital heart disease. *Qual Life Res.* 2005;14:1915–1924.

75. Lawoko S, Soares JJ. Distress and hopelessness among parents of children with congenital heart disease, parents of children with other diseases, and parents of healthy children. *J Psychosom Res.* 2002;52:193–208.

76. Daliento L, Mapelli D, Volpe B. Measurement of cognitive outcome and quality of life in congenital heart disease. *Heart.* 2006;92:569–574.

77. Maunder RG, Hunter JJ. Attachment and psychosomatic medicine: developmental contributions to stress and disease. *Psychosom Med.* 2001;63:556–567.

78. Lobo ML. Parent-infant interaction during feeding when the infant has congenital heart disease. *J Pediatr Nurs.* 1992;7:97–105.

79. Goldberg S, Simmons RJ, Newman J, et al. Congenital heart disease, parental stress, and infant-mother relationships. *J Pediatr.* 1991;119:661–666.

80. Miller G, Vogel H. Structural evidence of injury or malformation in the brains of children with congenital heart disease. *Sem Pediatr Neurol.* 1999;6:20–26.

81. Wernovsky G, Wypij D, Jonas RA, et al. Postoperative course and hemodynamic profile after the arterial switch operation in neonates and infants. A comparison of low-flow cardiopulmonary bypass and circulatory arrest. *Circulation.* 1995;92:2226–2235.

82. Garson A Jr, Williams RB Jr, Reckless J. Long-term follow-up of patients with tetralogy of Fallot: physical health and psychopathology. *J Pediatr.* 1974;85:429–433.

83. van Rijen EH, Utens EM, Roos-Hesselink JW, et al. Medical predictors for psychopathology in adults with operated congenital heart disease. *Eur Heart J.* 2004;25:1605–1613.

84. Connolly D, McClowry S, Hayman L, et al. Posttraumatic stress disorder in children after cardiac surgery. *J Pediatric.* 2004;144:480–484.

85. Stuber ML, Shemesh E. Post-traumatic stress response to life-threatening illnesses in children and their parents. *Child Adolesc Psychiatr Clin N Am.* 2006;15:597–609.

86. Danilowicz DA, Gabriel HP. Postoperative reactions in children: "normal" and abnormal responses after cardiac surgery. *Am J Psychiatry.* 1971;128:185–188.

87. Wray J, Sensky T. How does the intervention of cardiac surgery affect the self-perception of children with congenital heart disease? *Child Care Health Dev.* 1998;24:57–72.

88. Cyranowski JM, Frank E, Young E, Shear MK. Adolescent onset of the gender difference in lifetime rates of major depression: a theoretical model. *Arch Gen Psychiatry.* 2000;57:21–27.

89. Kools S, Tong EM, Hughes R, et al. Hospital experiences of young adults with congenital heart disease: divergence in expectations and dissonance in care. *Am J Crit Care.* 2002;11:115–125.

90. Salzer-Muhar U, Herle M, Floquet P, et al. Self-concept in male and female adolescents with congenital heart disease. *Clin Pediatric.* 2002;41:17–24.

91. Tong EM, Sparacino PS, Messias DK, et al. Growing up with congenital heart disease: the dilemmas of adolescents and young adults. *Cardiol Young.* 1998;8:303–309.

92. Uzark K, VonBargen-Mazza P, Messiter E. Health education needs of adolescents with congenital heart disease. *J Pediatr Health Care.* 1989;3:137–143.

93. Green A. Outcomes of congenital heart disease: a review. *Pediatr Nurs.* 2004;30:280–284.

94. Horner T, Liberthson R, Jellinek MS. Psychosocial profile of adults with complex congenital heart disease. *Mayo Clin Proc.* 2000;75: 31–36.

95. Kokkonen J, Paavilainen T. Social adaptation of young adults with congenital heart disease. *Int J Cardiol.* 1992;36:23–29.

96. Sparacino PS, Tong EM, Messias DK, et al. The dilemmas of parents of adolescents and young adults with congenital heart disease. *Heart Lung.* 1997;26:187–195.

97. Rhodes LA, Gustafson RA, Phillips JP, et al. The adult with congenital heart disease. *W V Med J.* 2006;102:310–313.

98. Goldbeck L, Melches J. The impact of the severity of disease and social disadvantage on quality of life in families with congenital cardiac disease. *Cardiol Young.* 2006;16:67–75.

99. Lawoko S, Soares JJ. Quality of life among parents of children with congenital heart disease, parents of children with other diseases and parents of healthy children. *Qual Life Res.* 2003;12: 655–666.

100. Lawoko S, Soares JJ. Psychosocial morbidity among parents of children with congenital heart disease: a prospective longitudinal study. *Heart Lung.* 2006;35:301–314.

101. Van Horn M, DeMaso DR, Gonzalez-Heydrich J, Erickson JD. Illness-related concerns of mothers of children with congenital heart disease. *J Am Acad Child Adolesc Psychiatry.* 2001;40:847–854.

102. Wray J, Sensky T. Psychological functioning in parents of children undergoing elective cardiac surgery. *Cardiol Young.* 2004;14: 131–139.

103. Brown MD, Wernovsky G, Mussatto KA, Berger S. Long-term and developmental outcomes of children with complex congenital heart disease. *Clin Perinatol.* 2005;32:1043–1057.

104. Davis CC, Brown RT, Bakeman R, Campbell R. Psychological adaptation and adjustment of mothers of children with congenital heart disease: stress, coping, and family functioning. *J Pediatr Psychol.* 1998;23:219–228.

105. DeMaso DR, Campis LK, Wypij D, et al. The impact of maternal perceptions and medical severity on the adjustment of children with congenital heart disease. *J Pediatr Psychol.* 1991;16:137–149.

106. DeMaso DR, Douglas Kelley S, Bastardi H, et al. The longitudinal impact of psychological functioning, medical severity, and family functioning in pediatric heart transplantation. *J Heart Lung Transplant.* 2004;23:473–480.

107. Gupta S, Mitchell I, Giuffre RM, Crawford S. Covert fears and anxiety in asthma and congenital heart disease. *Child Care Health Dev.* 2001;27:335–348.

108. Kamphuis M, Ottenkamp J, Vliegen HW, et al. Health related quality of life and health status in adult survivors with previously operated complex congenital heart disease. *Heart.* 2002;87:356–362.

109. Linde LM, Rasof B, Dunn OJ, Rabb E. Attitudinal factors in congenital heart disease. *Pediatrics.* 1966;38:92–101.

110. van Rijen EH, Utens EM, Roos-Hesselink JW, et al. Longitudinal development of psychopathology in an adult congenital heart disease cohort. *Int J Cardiol.* 2005;99:315–323.

111. Stuber ML. Psychiatric sequelae in seriously ill children and their families. *Psychiatric Clin North Am.* 1996;19:481–493.

112. Gantt LT. Growing up heartsick: the experiences of young women with congenital heart disease. *Health Care Women Int.* 1992;13: 241–248.

113. van Rijen EH, Utens EM, Roos-Hesselink JW, et al. Styles of coping and social support in a cohort of adults with congenital heart disease. *Cardiol Young.* 2004;14:122–130.

114. Claessens P, Moons P, de Casterle BD, et al. What does it mean to live with a congenital heart disease? A qualitative study on the lived experiences of adult patients. *Eur J Cardiovasc Nurs.* 2005;4:3–10.

115. Wray J, Radley-Smith R. Developmental and behavioral status of infants and young children awaiting heart or heart-lung transplantation. *Pediatrics.* 2004;113:488–495.

116. Masi G, Brovedani P. Adolescents with congenital heart disease: psychopathological implications. *Adolescence.* 1999;34:185–191.

117. Veldtman GR, Matley SL, Kendall L, et al. Illness understanding in children and adolescents with heart disease. *Heart.* 2000;84: 395–397.

118. Cheuk DK, Wong SM, Choi YP, et al. Parents' understanding of their child's congenital heart disease. *Heart.* 2004;90:435–439.

119. Moons P, De Volder E, Budts W, et al. What do adult patients with congenital heart disease know about their disease, treatment, and prevention of complications? A call for structured patient education. *Heart.* 2001;86:74–80.

120. Cetta F, Bell TJ, Podlecki DD, Ros SP. Parental knowledge of bacterial endocarditis prophylaxis. *Pediatr Cardiol.* 1993;14:220–222.

121. Cetta F, Warnes CA. Adults with congenital heart disease: patient knowledge of endocarditis prophylaxis. *Mayo Clin Proc.* 1995;70: 50–54.

122. Immer FF, Althaus SM, Berdat PA, et al. Quality of life and specific problems after cardiac surgery in adolescents and adults with congenital heart diseases. *Eur J Cardiovasc Prev Rehabil.* 2005;12: 138–143.

123. Canobbio MM. Health care issues facing adolescents with congenital heart disease. *J Pediatr Nurs.* 2001;16:363–370.

124. Hager A, Hess J. Comparison of health related quality of life with cardiopulmonary exercise testing in adolescents and adults with congenital heart disease. *Heart.* 2005;91:517–520.

125. Falk B, Bar-Mor G, Zigel L, et al. Daily physical activity and perception of condition severity among male and female adolescents with congenital heart malformation. *J Pediatr Nurs.* 2006;21:244–249.

126. Rew L. Sexual health promotion in adolescents with chronic health conditions. *Fam Community Health.* 2006;29(1 Suppl):61S–69S.

127. Britto MT, Garrett JM, Dugliss MA, et al. Risky behavior in teens with cystic fibrosis or sickle cell disease: a multicenter study. *Pediatrics.* 1998;101:250–256.

128. Cox CL, McLaughlin RA, Rai SN, et al. Adolescent survivors: a secondary analysis of a clinical trial targeting behavior change. *Pediatr Blood Cancer.* 2005;45:144–154.

129. Reid GJ, Irvine MJ, McCrindle BW, et al. Prevalence and correlates of successful transfer from pediatric to adult health care among a cohort of young adults with complex congenital heart defects. *Pediatrics.* 2004;113(3 Part1):197–205.

130. Tyc VL, Throckmorton-Belzer L. Smoking rates and the state of smoking interventions for children and adolescents with chronic illness. *Pediatrics.* 2006;118:471–487.

131. Cetta F, Graham LC, Lichtenberg RC, Warnes CA. Piercing and tattooing in patients with congenital heart disease: patient and physician perspectives. *J Adolesc Health.* 1999;24:160–162.

132. Biro FM, Striegel-Moore RH, Franko DL, et al. Self-esteem in adolescent females. *J Adolesc Health.* 2006;39:501–507.

133. Lyon ME, Kuehl K, McCarter R. Transition to adulthood in congenital heart disease: missed adolescent milestones. *J Adolesc Health.* 2006;39:121–124.

134. Rietveld S, Mulder BJ, van Beest I, et al. Negative thoughts in adults with congenital heart disease. *Int J Cardiol.* 2002;86:19–26.

135. Lawrence JW, Fauerbach JA, Heinberg L, Doctor M. Visible vs hidden scars and their relation to body esteem. *J Burn Care Rehabil.* 2004;25:25–32.

136. Brandhagen DJ, Feldt RH, Williams DE. Long-term psychologic implications of congenital heart disease: a 25-year follow-up. *Mayo Clin Proc.* 1991;66:474–479.

137. Kendall L, Lewin RJ, Parsons JM, et al. Factors associated with self-perceived state of health in adolescents with congenital cardiac disease attending paediatric cardiologic clinics. *Cardiol Young.* 2001;11:431–438.

138. Popelova J, Slavik Z, Skovranek J. Are cyanosed adults with congenital cardiac malformations depressed? *Cardiol Young.* 2001; 11:379–384.

139. Saliba Z, Butera G, Bonnet D, et al. Quality of life and perceived health status in surviving adults with univentricular heart. *Heart.* 2001;86:69–73.

140. Utens EM, Verhulst FC, Meijboom FJ, et al. Behavioural and emotional problems in children and adolescents with congenital heart disease. *Psychol Med.* 1993;23:415–424.

141. Foster E, Graham TP Jr, Driscoll DJ, et al. Task Force 2: special health care needs of adults with congenital heart disease. *J Am Coll Cardiol.* 2001;37:1176–1183.

142. Bromberg JI, Beasley PJ, D'Angelo EJ, et al. Depression and anxiety in adults with congenital heart disease: a pilot study. *Heart Lung.* 2003;32:105–110.

143. Gersony WM, Hayes CJ, Driscoll DJ, et al. Second natural history study of congenital heart defects. Quality of life of patients with aortic stenosis, pulmonary stenosis, or ventricular septal defect. *Circulation.* 1993;87:I52–I65.

144. Simko LC, McGinnis KA. Quality of life experienced by adults with congenital heart disease. *AACN Clin Issues.* 2003;14:42–53.

145. van Rijen EH, Utens EM, Roos-Hesselink JW, et al. Current subjective state of health, and longitudinal psychological well-being over a period of 10 years, in a cohort of adults with congenital cardiac disease. *Cardiol Young.* 2005;15:168–175.

146. Lane DA, Lip GY, Millane TA. Quality of life in adults with congenital heart disease. *Heart.* 2002;88:71–75.

147. Simko LC, McGinnis KA. What is the perceived quality of life of adults with congenital heart disease and does it differ by anomaly? *J Cardiovasc Nurs.* 2005;20:206–214.

148. Ternestedt BM, Wall K, Oddsson H, et al. Quality of life 20 and 30 years after surgery in patients operated on for tetralogy of Fallot and for atrial septal defect. *Pediatr Cardiol.* 2001;22:128–132.

149. Moons P, Van Deyk K, Marquet K, et al. Individual quality of life in adults with congenital heart disease: a paradigm shift. *Eur Hear J.* 2005;26:298–307.

150. Moons P, Van Deyk K, De Geest S, et al. Is the severity of congenital heart disease associated with the quality of life and perceived health of adult patients? *Heart.* 2005;91:1193–1198.

151. Nollert G, Fischlein T, Bouterwek S, et al. Long-term survival in patients with repair of tetralogy of Fallot: 36-year follow-up of 490 survivors of the first year after surgical repair. *J Am Coll Cardiol.* 1997;30:1374–1383.

152. Crossland DS, Jackson SP, Lyall R, et al. Employment and advice regarding careers for adults with congenital heart disease. *Cardiol Young.* 2005;15:391–395.

153. Kamphuis M, Vogels T, Ottenkamp J, et al. Employment in adults with congenital heart disease. *Arch Pediatr Adolesc Med.* 2002;156:1143–1148.

154. van Rijen EH, Utens EM, Roos-Hesselink JW, et al. Psychosocial functioning of the adult with congenital heart disease: a 20–33 years follow-up. *Eur Heart J.* 2003;24:673–683.

155. Crossland DS, Jackson SP, Lyall R, Hamilton JR, Hasan A, Burn J, O'Sullivan JJ. Life insurance and mortgage application in adults with congenital heart disease. *Eur J Cardiothorac Surg.* 2004;25:931–934.

156. Gibson D, Groeneweg G, Jerry P, Harris A. Age and pattern of intellectual decline among Down syndrome and other mentally retarded adults. *Int J Rehabil Res.* 1988;11:47–55.

157. van Amelsvoort T, Henry J, Morris R, et al. Cognitive deficits associated with schizophrenia in velo-cardio-facial syndrome. *Schizophr Res.* 2004;70:223–232.

158. Barnea-Goraly N, Menon V, Krasnow B, et al. Investigation of white matter structure in velocardiofacial syndrome: a diffusion tensor imaging study. *Am J Psychiatry.* 2003;160:1863–1869.

159. Arnold PD, Siegel-Bartelt J, Cytrynbaum C, et al. Velo-cardio-facial syndrome: implications of microdeletion 22q11 for schizophrenia and mood disorders. *Am J Med Genet.* 2001;105:354–362.

160. Gothelf D, Presburger G, Levy D, et al. Genetic, developmental, and physical factors associated with attention deficit hyperactivity disorder in patients with velocardiofacial syndrome. *Am J Med Genet B Neuropsychiatr Genet.* 2004;126:116–121.

161. Prinzie P, Swillen A, Vogels A, et al. Personality profiles of youngsters with velo-cardio-facial syndrome. *Genet Couns.* 2002;13:265–280.

162. De Smedt B, Swillen A, Ghesquiere P, et al. Pre-academic and early academic achievement in children with velocardiofacial syndrome (del22q11.2) of borderline or normal intelligence. *Genet Couns.* 2003;14:15–29.

163. Raqbi F, Le Bihan C, Morisseau-Durand MP, et al. Early prognostic factors for intellectual outcome in CHARGE syndrome. *Dev Med Child Neurol.* 2003;45:483–488.

164. Graham JM Jr, Rosner B, Dykens E, Visootsak J. Behavioral features of CHARGE syndrome (Hall-Hittner syndrome) comparison with Down syndrome, Prader-Willi syndrome, and Williams syndrome. *Am J Med Genet.* 2005;133:240–247.

165. Niklasson L, Rasmussen P, Oskarsdottir S, Gillberg C. Chromosome 22q11 deletion syndrome (CATCH 22): neuropsychiatric and neuropsychological aspects. *Dev Med Child Neurol.* 2002;44:44–50.

166. Goldberg S, Janus M, Washington J, et al. Prediction of preschool behavioral problems in healthy and pediatric samples. *J Dev Behav Pediatr.* 1997;18:304–313.

167. Gupta S, Giuffre RM, Crawford S, Waters J. Covert fears, anxiety and depression in congenital heart disease. *Cardiol Young.* 1998;8:491–499.

168. Yildiz S, Savaser S, Tatlioglu GS. Evaluation of internal behaviors of children with congenital heart disease. *J Pediatr Nurs.* 2001;16:449–452.

169. Kong SG, Tay JS, Yip WC, Chay SO. Emotional and social effects of congenital heart disease in Singapore. *Aust Paediatr J.* 1986;22:101–106.

170. Kramer HH, Awiszus D, Sterzel U, et al. Development of personality and intelligence in children with congenital heart disease. *J Child Psychol Psychiatry.* 1989;30:299–308.

171. Huang JF, Wang HC, Chen H. [The influential factors of formation and development of personality in children with congenital heart disease]. *Chinese J Nurs.* 1996;31:128–130.

172. Cox D, Lewis G, Stuart G, Murphy K. A cross-sectional study of the prevalence of psychopathology in adults with congenital heart disease. *J Psychosom Res.* 2002;52:65–68.

173. Utens EM, Verhulst FC, Duivenvoorden HJ, et al. Prediction of behavioural and emotional problems in children and adolescents with operated congenital heart disease. *Eur Heart J.* 1998;19:801–807.

174. Denollet J, Brutsaert DL. Personality, disease severity, and the risk of long-term cardiac events in patients with a decreased ejection fraction after myocardial infarction. *Circulation.* 1998;97:167–173.

175. Frasure-Smith N, Lesperance F, Talajic M. The impact of negative emotions on prognosis following myocardial infarction: is it more than depression? *Health Psychol.* 1995;14:388–398.

176. Kawachi I, Colditz GA, Ascherio A, et al. Prospective study of phobic anxiety and risk of coronary heart disease in men. *Circulation.* 1994;89:1992–1997.

177. Moser DK, Dracup K. Is anxiety early after myocardial infarction associated with subsequent ischemic and arrhythmic events? *Psychosom Med.* 1996;58:395–401.

178. Wray J, Radley-Smith R. Depression in pediatric patients before and 1 year after heart or heart-lung transplantation. *J Heart Lung Transplant.* 2004;23:1103–1110.

179. Wray J, Radley-Smith R. Longitudinal assessment of psychological functioning in children after heart or heart-lung transplantation. *J Heart Lung Transplant.* 2006;25:345–352.

180. *Diagnostic and Statistical Manual of Mental Disorders.* 4th ed. Washington, DC: American Psychiatric Association; 2000.

181. Cohen JA. Treating acute posttraumatic reactions in children and adolescents. *Biol Psychiatry.* 2003;53:827–833.

182. Hobbie WL, Stuber M, Meeske K, et al. Symptoms of posttraumatic stress in young adult survivors of childhood cancer. *J Clin Oncol.* 2000;18:4060–4066.

183. Stuber ML, Kazak AE, Meeske K, et al. Predictors of posttraumatic stress symptoms in childhood cancer survivors. *Pediatrics.* 1997; 100:958–964.

184. Personal communication with Dr. Margaret Stuber, UCLA School of Medicine, November 2006.

185. Seedat S, Stein DJ, Ziervogel C, et al. Comparison of response to a selective serotonin reuptake inhibitor in children, adolescents, and adults with posttraumatic stress disorder. *J Child Adolesc Psychopharmacol.* 2002;12:37–46.

186. Odenrick L, Brattstrom V. Nailbiting: frequency and association with root resorption during orthodontic treatment. *Br J Orthod.* 1985;12:78–81.

187. Azrin NH, Nunn RG. Habit-reversal: a method of eliminating nervous habits and tics. *Behav Res Ther.* 1973;11:619–628.

188. Peterson AL, Campise RL, Azrin NH. Behavioral and pharmacological treatments for tic and habit disorders: a review. *J Dev Behav Pediatr.* 1994;15:430–441.

189. Leonard HL, Lenane MC, Swedo SE, et al. A double-blind comparison of clomipramine and desipramine treatment of severe onychophagia (nail biting). *Arch Gen Psychiatry.* 1991;48:821–827.

190. Alexander RC. Fluoxetine treatment of trichotillomania. *J Clin Psychiatry.* 1991;52:88.

191. Christenson GA, Mackenzie TB, Mitchell JE, Callies AL. A placebo-controlled, double-blind crossover study of fluoxetine in trichotillomania. *Am J Psychiatry.* 1991;148:1566–1571.

192. Streichenwein SM, Thornby JI. A long-term, double-blind, placebo-controlled crossover trial of the efficacy of fluoxetine for trichotillomania. *Am J Psychiatry.* 1995;152:1192–1196.

193. Swedo SE, Leonard HL, Rapoport JL, et al. A double-blind comparison of clomipramine and desipramine in the treatment of trichotillomania (hair pulling). *N Engl J Med.* 1989;321:497–501.

194. Lawrence A, Hang R, Reist C. *Handbook of Psychiatric Drugs.* Laguna Beach, CA: Current Clinical Strategies 2004.

195. Glassman AH, O'Connor CM, Califf RM, et al. Sertraline treatment of major depression in patients with acute MI or unstable angina. *JAMA.* 2002;288:701–709.

196. Fusar-Poli P, Picchioni M, Martinelli V, et al. Anti-depressive therapies after heart transplantation. *J Heart Lung Transplant.* 2006;25: 785–793.

197. Lewis BR, Aoun SL, Bernstein GA, Crow SJ. Pharmacokinetic interactions between cyclosporine and bupropion or methylphenidate. *J Child Adolesc Psychopharmacol.* 2001;11:193–198.

198. Stukas AA Jr, Dew MA, Switzer GE, et al. PTSD in heart transplant recipients and their primary family caregivers. *Psychosomatics.* 1999;40:212–221.

199. Dew MA, Kormos RL, DiMartini AF, et al. Prevalence and risk of depression and anxiety-related disorders during the first three years after heart transplantation. *Psychosomatics.* 2001;42:300–313.

200. Dew MA, Kormos RL, Roth LH, et al. Early post-transplant medical compliance and mental health predict physical morbidity and mortality one to three years after heart transplantation. *J Heart Lung Transplant.* 1999;18:549–562.

201. Qvist E, Jalanko H, Holmberg C. Psychosocial adaptation after solid organ transplantation in children. *Pediatr Clin North Am.* 2003;50:1505–1519.

202. Baum M, Freier MC, Freeman K, et al. Neuropsychological outcome of infant heart transplant recipients. *J Pediatr.* 2004;145:365–372.

203. Ikle L, Hale K, Fashaw L, Boucek M, Rosenberg AA. Developmental outcome of patients with hypoplastic left heart syndrome treated with heart transplantation. *J Pediatr.* 2003;142:20–25.

204. Kollner V, Schade I, Maulhardt T, et al. Posttraumatic stress disorder and quality of life after heart or lung transplantation. *Transplant Proc.* 2002;34:2192–2193.

205. Russo LM, Webber SA. Pediatric heart transplantation: immunosuppression and its complications. *Curr Opin Cardiol.* 2004;19: 104–109.

206. Wray J, Long T, Radley-Smith R, Yacoub M. Returning to school after heart or heart-lung transplantation: how well do children adjust? *Transplantation.* 2001;72:100–106.

207. Serrano-Ikkos E, Lask B, Whitehead B, Eisler I. Incomplete adherence after pediatric heart and heart-lung transplantation. *J Heart Lung Transplant.* 1998;17:1177–1183.

208. Dew MA, Myaskovsky L, DiMartini AF, et al. Onset, timing and risk for depression and anxiety in family caregivers to heart transplant recipients. *Psychol Med.* 2004;34:1065–1082.

209. Young GS, Mintzer LL, Seacord D, et al. Symptoms of posttraumatic stress disorder in parents of transplant recipients: incidence, severity, and related factors. *Pediatrics.* 2003;111:e725–e731.

CHAPTER 14

Neurologic Disorders

JOSEPH K. PERLOFF ▪ JEFFREY L. SAVER

Neurologic disorders in adults with congenital heart disease (CHD) are classified as infectious, ischemic, hemorrhagic, hypoxic, seizure related, congenital neurologic, and related to sequelae of cardiac surgery (Table 14–1). Neurodevelopmental disabilities are the most common untoward sequelae of complex CHD. Psychosocial disorders, including mental retardation, disorders of intellectual development and cognition, and disorders of higher cortical function after open heart surgery are discussed in Chapter 13.

INFECTIOUS DISORDERS

Brain Abscess

In 1814, Farre proposed a causal relationship between brain abscess and CHD,[1] and in 1880, Ballet confirmed the association.[2] During the first half of the 20th century, the antemortem diagnosis of brain abscess was rarely established but was included in an extensive 1951 necropsy review of cerebral lesions associated with CHD.[3] Postmortem incidence has been estimated at 2% of patients with cyanotic malformations.[4] An abscess should be suspected when a cyanotic patient experiences protracted headache, focal neurologic signs, seizures, and fever.[5,6] The diagnosis of a fresh brain abscess, which may occur initially in adulthood, is readily made by computed tomography, which identifies the lesion itself and the distinctive ring enhancement (Figs. 14–1, A and 14–2, A). Seizures caused by a fresh abscess often persist after healing or may recur years later because of focal scarring (see Fig. 14–2, B).

Brain abscess may be due to a septic cerebral embolus[7]; (Fig. 14–3) contiguous extension of infection from otitis media, mastoiditis, sinusitis, or a facial or dental infection;

or direct mechanical introduction of infectious organisms by a surgical procedure or trauma.[4,7,8] Less clear is the pathogenesis of a "hematogenous" brain abscess.[4,6,7,9] Two preconditions appear necessary: (1) bacteremia that includes the cerebral circulation and (2) a focal zone of cerebral vulnerability (injury).[4,7,9] Cyanotic CHD lends itself to both of these pathogenetic preconditions. A right-to-left shunt permits bloodborne bacteria normally filtered by the pulmonary circulation to enter the systemic, and therefore cerebral circulation. A focus of vulnerability might result from a silent sterile paradoxical cerebral embolus or from encephalomalacia.[4,9] In the presence of a vulnerable focus that is receptive to infection, the chance occurrence of cerebral bacteremia may culminate in the formation of a brain abscess. If diagnosed in the early phase of cerebritis, treatment with antibiotic therapy alone can be adequate.[10] Most frequently, however, treatment requires aspiration employing computed tomographic or magnetic resonance–directed stereotactic control. Culture and sensitivity tests of the aspirate set the stage for specific antibiotic therapy. Delay in surgical drainage and organism identification can increase morbidity and mortality (see Fig. 14–3). Resection of the abscess is rarely required.

Septic Cerebral Aneurysm

The term *mycotic* is commonly used to refer to septic cerebral aneurysms, but with few exceptions, the term is a misnomer. Mycotic, as defined in *Dorland's Illustrated Medical Dictionary*, means "pertaining to a mycosis; caused by fungi." The appropriate term is *septic aneurysm* or, more specifically, *bacterial aneurysm.*

These aneurysms usually result from an embolus originating at a systemic site of infective endocarditis.[11,12] A patient with infective endocarditis and focal neurologic signs or meningitis should undergo cerebral

Table 14-1 Neurologic Disorders in Adults with Congenital Heart Disease

Infectious

Brain abscess
Septic cerebral aneurysm

Ischemic

Cerebral emboli (paradoxical, systemic)
Cerebral thrombosis (venous, arterial)
Subclavian steal (post–Blalock-Taussig shunt, congenital)
Cerebral arterial vasospasm
Intracranial fibromuscular dysplasia

Hemorrhagic

Intracerebral hemorrhage
Subarachnoid hemorrhage

Hypoxic

Syncope
Spells associated with tetralogy of Fallot

Seizure disorders

Congenital neurologic disorders

Neurologic sequelae of cardiac surgery

angiography.[12] If an infective septic aneurysm is identified (Fig. 14–4, A and B), tailored multimodal therapy is applied. Patients with unruptured aneurysms may be treated initially with antibiotics alone, and serially monitored. Patients with ruptured aneurysms that do not have a hematoma-producing mass effect that requires evacuation and that do not involve vital regions can be treated with endovascular occlusion of a parent artery or coil occlusion of the aneurysm itself. Neurosurgical intervention is undertaken for patients with hematomas needing decompression or aneurysms in vessels supplying vital brain regions. With this approach, good outcomes can often be obtained[13] (see Fig. 14–4, C).

ISCHEMIC DISORDERS

Cerebral Emboli

Cerebral emboli can be bland (which is usually the case) or septic (which is exceptional as noted earlier) and originate in the systemic arterial circulation[14] or from peripheral or pelvic veins as paradoxical emboli.[15,16] A common source of bland cerebral emboli that originates in the systemic arterial circulation in adults with CHD is a left-sided prosthetic valve (see Chapter 16). A relatively common source of emboli is the left atrial appendage in patients with atrial fibrillation (Fig. 14–5). Balloon atrial septostomy in neonates with complete transposition of the great arteries is accompanied by focal brain injury consistent with embolism.[17] A less common but important and potentially correctable source of systemic emboli is an atrial septal aneurysm, a congenital malformation characterized by a local mobile outpouching in the region of the fossa ovalis[16,18-21] (Fig. 14–6). Atrial septal aneurysms were initially identified by angiography and have been found in 1% of necropsies.[20] With the advent of two-dimensional echocardiography and transesophageal echocardiography, atrial septal aneurysms have been detected in up to 4% of unselected patients undergoing cardiac ultrasound investigation and up to

FIGURE 14-1 **(A)** Fresh brain abscess with typical ring enhancement *(arrows)* in a 28-year-old cyanotic woman with tetralogy of Fallot and pulmonary atresia.

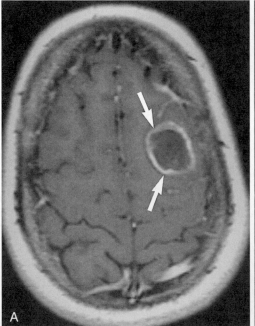

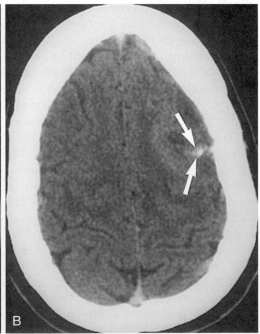

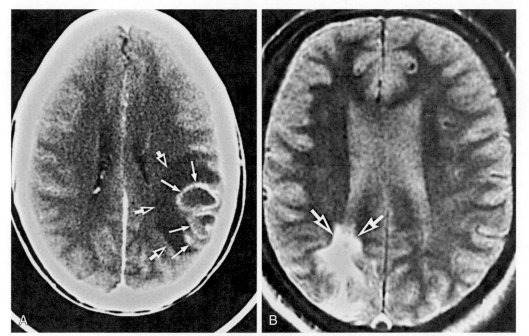

FIGURE 14-2 **(A)** Fresh brain abscess that announced itself as a seizure in a 39-year-old cyanotic woman with double-outlet right ventricle, ventricular septal defect, and pulmonary stenosis. The computed tomographic scan shows the typical ring enhancement *(small inner arrows)* surrounded by edema *(large outer arrows)*. **(B)** Computed tomographic scan from a 29-year-old man with surgically repaired double-outlet left ventricle, ventricular septal defect, and pulmonary stenosis. A brain abscess in childhood presented in the healed state *(arrows)* as a seizure disorder.

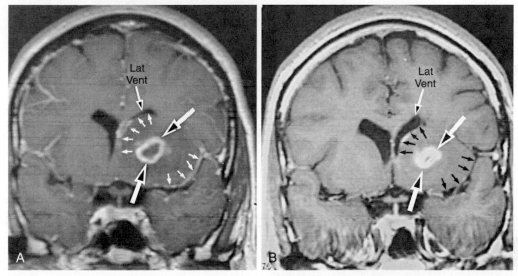

FIGURE 14-3 **(A)** Magnetic resonance image from a 23-year-old man with culture of positive meningitis caused by a brain abscess that encroached on the lateral ventricle (Lat Vent). The outer small arrows identify the extent of edema surrounding the fresh abscess, which exhibits typical ring enhancement *(larger inner arrows)*. **(B)** Antibiotic therapy resulted in a decrease in the central core of the aneurysm *(large inner arrows)*, a decrease in surrounding edema *(outer small black arrows)*, and less encroachment on the lateral ventricle. The congenital cardiac malformation was discrete subaortic stenosis with mild to moderate aortic regurgitation. The brain abscess was believed to have resulted from a septic cerebral embolus (vegetation).

15% of patients with a stroke.[21] Atrial septal aneurysms have been classified according to their intrusion into the left or right atrium and according to their motion during the respiratory cycle.[20] Best seen with transesophageal echocardiography (see Fig. 14–6), the aneurysm may either bulge persistently into the right or left atrium or may exhibit striking oscillations from right atrium to left atrium during respiration.[20,21] The association between atrial septal aneurysms and systemic emboli—including

cerebral emboli—was identified in 1985[22] and has been amply confirmed.[18-21,23] The emboli are believed to originate from fibrin tags or thrombotic material attached to the left atrial surface of the aneurysm.[18,20] Although suspicion of an atrial septal aneurysm as the source of a cerebral embolus is higher in young patients, these aneurysms have been incriminated in patients in their seventh and eighth decades.[18] Because aneurysms of the atrial septum reside in the region of the fossa ovalis, they often

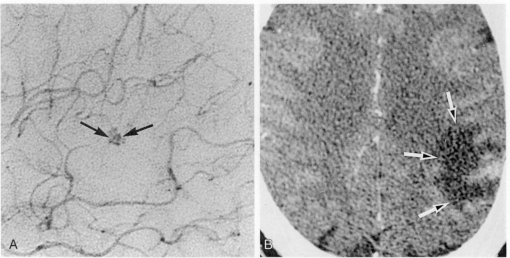

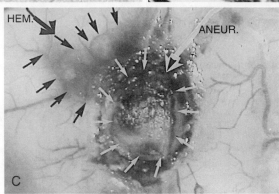

FIGURE 14–4 **(A)** Cerebral arteriogram from a 27-year-old man who had undergone intracardiac repair of congenitally corrected transposition of the great arteries, ventricular septal defect, and pulmonary stenosis. He presented with *Streptococcus viridans* infective endocarditis and a septic-cerebral aneurysm *(arrows)*. **(B)** Arrows identify hemorrhage surrounding the perforating aneurysm. **(C)** Surgical view of the septic aneurysm (ANEUR., *inner arrows*) with surrounding hemorrhage (HEM., *black arrows*) of impending rupture.

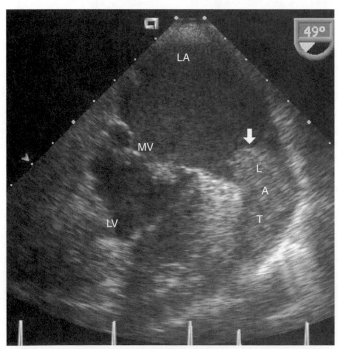

FIGURE 14–5 Transesophageal echocardiogram (TEE) showing a left atrial thrombus (LAT) in the appendage. LV, left ventricle; MV, mitral valve.

coexist with a patent foramen ovale, which sets the stage for a coexisting paradoxical embolus (discussed later).[16,18,20,21] Alternate bulging of an atrial septal aneurysm into the left or right atrium (see Fig. 14–6) is believed to coincide with transient reversal of the interatrial pressure gradient during each respiratory cycle.

Uncommonly, a cerebral embolus originates solely from fibrin/thrombus deposits on the left atrial side of an atrial septal aneurysm (no patent foramen ovale). A relationship is believed to exist between the oscillatory movements of an atrial septal aneurysm and the risk of dislodging a systemic embolus. Anticoagulants or antiplatelet agents are employed as the initial treatment when an atrial septal aneurysm is incriminated as the sole source of a cerebral embolus.[18,20,24] Should anticoagulants and antiplatelet agents fail, especially if recurrence takes the form of an embolic stroke rather than a transient ischemic attack, excision of the offending atrial septal aneurysm is curative.[18]

Uncommon if not rare sources of cerebral emboli originating in the systemic arterial circulation of patients with congenital cardiac disease include an unruptured aneurysm of a sinus of Valsalva[25] and, even less commonly, spontaneous calcific embolization from a bicuspid aortic valve.[26]

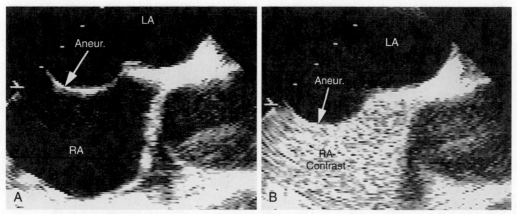

FIGURE 14–6   Transesophageal echocardiographic images from a 29-year-old man with an asymptomatic, mobile atrial septal aneurysm that was an incidental finding. **(A)** The aneurysm (Aneur.), which was devoid of detectable thrombotic material, is shown bowing into the right atrium (RA). LA, left atrium. **(B)** Echo-contrast medium (agitated saline) outlines the aneurysm and shows no right-to-left shunt, indicating that the foramen ovale was not demonstrably patent.

Paradoxical Embolization

Somewhat more unique to CHD are paradoxical emboli described by Connheim[27] in 1887. *Paradoxic* refers to an embolus that originates in the *systemic venous* circulation and enters the *systemic arterial* circulation by way of a right-to-left shunt (Fig. 14-7). The most common pathophysiologic substrate is cyanotic CHD because systemic venous blood continuously flows into the systemic

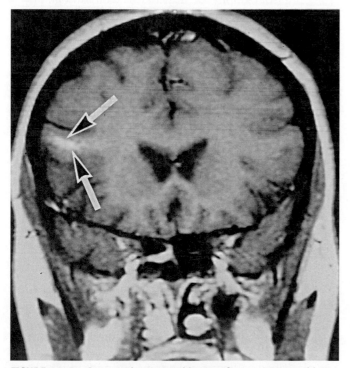

FIGURE 14-7   Computed tomographic scan from a 39-year-old cyanotic woman with an ostium secundum atrial septal defect and supra-systemic pulmonary vascular resistance. Arrows identify a cerebral infarct caused by a paradoxical embolus.

arterial circulation via the shunt.[15] The embolus usually originates in veins of the lower extremities, less commonly in pelvic veins. The increased incidence of lower-extremity varicose veins in patients with cyanotic CHD combines the risk of a systemic venous source with the risk of an obligatory right-to-left shunt. Varicose veins should be carefully sought by inspecting the legs and medial aspect of the thighs with the patient standing upright. Patients with varices should avoid sitting with knees flexed and legs dependent, should avoid crossing their legs when sitting, and should avoid passive standing. Support hose are useful provided that they fit properly and are high enough to avoid creating a proximal tourniquet.

In the absence of cyanosis, the morphologic and physiologic substrate for a paradoxical embolus is a communication in the midportion of the atrial septum—an ostium secundum atrial septal defect[28] or a patent foramen ovale[29-34] (Fig. 14-8)—because inferior vena caval blood tends to stream in that direction. In the fetus, approximately one third of systemic venous return received by the right atrium normally crosses the foramen ovale and enters the left atrium and left ventricle for distribution in the systemic circulation, including cerebral. The fetal eustachian valve is designed to channel blood from the inferior vena cava across the foramen ovale. Postnatal persistence of a well-formed fetal eustachian valve continues to direct inferior vena caval blood toward the midportion of the atrial septum, and if an interatrial communication exists, flow continues into the left atrium and systemic circulation, increasing the likelihood of a paradoxical embolus.[31] The prevalence of a patent foramen ovale among the cryptogenic stroke population is about 40% to 50%,[35] whereas a general population necropsy study of 965 normal hearts disclosed a 27.3% overall incidence of patent foramen ovale, with a progressive decline from 34.3% during the first 3 decades of life to 25.4% during the fourth through the eighth decades, to 20.2% during the ninth and tenth

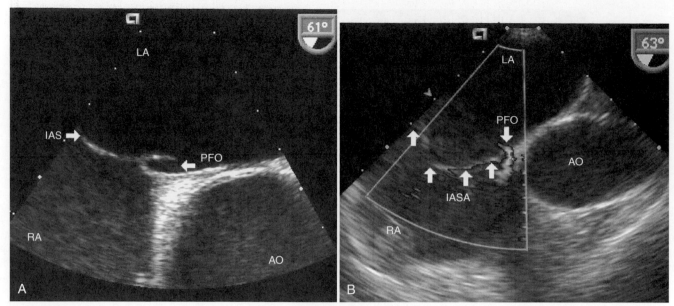

FIGURE 14-8 **(A)** Transesophageal echocardiogram showing a patent foramen ovale (PFO) guarded by its valve. IAS, interatrial septum; LA, left atrium; RA, right atrium. **(B)** Color image showing an interatrial septal aneurysm (IASA) and right-to left flow across a PFO. AO, aorta.

decades.[36] A patent foramen ovale tends to increase in size with age from a mean of 3.4 mm in the first decade to 5.8 mm in the tenth decade.[36]

Delivery of a paradoxical embolus through a patent foramen ovale is more likely to occur in response to physiologic mechanisms that transiently increase the volume and pressure differences between the right and left atria. The straining phase of the Valsalva maneuver is accompanied by a transient rise in right atrial pressure, which reverses the interatrial gradient and induces a right-to-left shunt.[31] More frequently, the right-to-left shunt coincides with release of the Valsalva maneuver because a sudden increase of systemic venous return into the right atrium reverses the interatrial pressure relationships or reinforces the gradient created during the straining phase. Lifting or pushing heavy objects, straining at defecation, and vigorous repetitive cough duplicate the physiologic conditions of the Valsalva maneuver, reversing the normal interatrial pressure gradient and causing transient right-to-left shunting.[37] Rarely, the platypnea-orthodeoxia syndrome, which is defined as an orthostatic right-to-left shunt across an atrial septal defect or patent foramen ovale, is a potential substrate for a paradoxical embolus.[38]

These provoking physiologic mechanisms are important for two reasons. First, when a cerebrovascular ischemic event caused by a right-to-left shunt through a foramen ovale is suspected, the history should include specific questions that define the circumstances immediately preceding the event so that the patient can be instructed on how to avoid the provoking circumstances. Second, the Valsalva maneuver with contrast echocardiography is routinely used for diagnostic purposes[31-33,39] (see Fig. 14–6). When a satisfactory Valsalva maneuver cannot be accomplished in a sedated patient undergoing transesophageal echocardiography, application of positive end-inspiratory pressure serves

the purpose.[31] Transcranial contrast Doppler ultrasonography employs the Valsalva maneuver but with the Doppler probe placed against the side of the cranium just above the zygomatic arch, that is, over the middle cerebral artery.[39]

When a lower extremity source of a paradoxical embolus is sought in patients with a patent foramen ovale and a Valsalva-induced right-to-left shunt, the diagnostic yield from ultrasonography or impedance plethysmography is low. However, these techniques are sensitive only to very large, deep lower extremity thrombi. Contrast venography demonstrates many more lower extremity venous lesions, but is not usually pursued because it causes patient discomfort.[40] Other patients harbor pelvic venous thrombi that can be demonstrated with MR or CT pelvic venography.[41] It has been proposed that fibrin-platelet thrombi are present in the systemic venous circulation and are removed by the efficient lytic system in the lungs. Because the cerebral circulation does not have a significant lytic system, the small emboli that cross an interatrial communication and lodge in the cerebral circulation are not lysed, resulting in an ischemic stroke or transient ischemic attack.

The frequency of recurrent ischemic stroke associated with a patent foramen ovale appears low, only about 0.6% per year on aspirin therapy[23]; hence optimal treatment designed to prevent recurrence is unclear. A coexisting atrial septal aneurysm increases the risk of recurrent stroke six-fold.[16,23] Additional likely, but less well-established, potentiators of risk include large size of the patent foramen ovale, greater physiologic right to left shunt, and a coexisting hypercoagulable state.[16] Because the physical maneuvers described earlier provoke transient right-to-left shunting through an interatrial communication, it seems intuitive that patients at risk should minimize or refrain from straining at defecation, lifting or pushing heavy objects, or vigorous repetitive cough. In light of the possibility that the offending thromboembolus might originate from lower extremity veins, patients should avoid sitting for prolonged periods with knees flexed and legs dependent, should not cross their legs when sitting, and should avoid passive standing as noted earlier.

Treatment options include antiplatelet agents, chronic anticoagulation, and surgical or endovascular device closure of the patent foramen ovale. In unselected older stroke patients with patent foramen ovale, aspirin and warfarin are equally efficacious, but warfarin may be more effective in patients with infarcts that are likely to have been due to paradoxical embolism (otherwise cryptogenic, superficial embolic cerebral territory, absence of hypertension).[24] If recurrent strokes occur on antithrombotic therapy, then surgical closure or catheter device closure of the interatrial communication (see Chapter 18) are rational options.[16,42,43]

Epidemiologic studies have established that patent foramen ovale is not a major risk factor for first stroke in the general population, although a modest association has not been excluded.[44-46] More than 30 million Americans have a patent foramen ovale, but only 1 in 1000 are destined to experience a cerebrovascular event of "unknown cause".[44] A coexisting atrial septal aneurysm substantially increases the risk.[46] Currently, active treatment of patent foramen ovale for stroke prevention should only be considered in patients who have had a first transient ischemic attack or ischemic stroke.

Delivery of whole megakaryocytes from systemic venous to systemic arterial circulation in cyanotic CHD is a special form of "paradoxical embolus." Whole mature megakaryocytes normally migrate from bone marrow sinusoids and enter the systemic venous circulation.[47] These largest of formed elements enter the pulmonary circulation and lodge in the capillary bed where their cytoplasm is fragmented into platelets. In cyanotic CHD, systemic venous megakaryocytes are delivered into the systemic arterial circulation via the right-to-left shunt and randomly lodged in systemic capillary beds where they release their cytoplasmic platelet-derived growth factor and transforming growth factor ß.[48] When these cytokines and mitogens are released in the digits, they cause clubbing of the fingers and toes; when they are released in the periosteum, they cause hypertrophic osteoarthropathy; and when they are released in glomeruli, they cause a nonvascular glomerular abnormality.[49] What might be the result if shunted systemic venous megakaryocytes lodge in cerebral capillaries and release their locally active cytokines and mitogens in the brain?

Cerebral Thrombosis

Distinctions are made between cerebral *venous* and cerebral *arterial* thromboses. In cyanotic patients younger than 4 years of age, intracranial venous thrombosis of the superior sagittal or lateral (transverse) sinus, the great vein of Galen, and the meningeal veins (Fig. 14–9) is virtually always accompanied by iron-deficient microspherocytosis.[50-52] It is therefore important to recognize and preemptively treat the

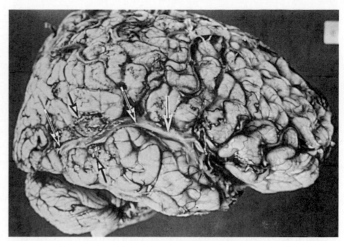

FIGURE 14–9 Necropsy photograph of the brain of a cyanotic, erythrocytotic, iron-deficient infant who died after a transverse (lateral) cerebral venous sinus thrombosis *(black-on-white arrows)*. White-on-black arrows identify a cerebral infarct. *(Courtesy of Dr. Samuel Kaplan, UCLA Division of Pediatric Cardiology.)*

iron deficiency. Dehydration increases the risk of intracranial venous thrombosis, and thus febrile illnesses, especially when accompanied by the dehydrating effects of vomiting and diarrhea, should be treated promptly.

Until relatively recently, a direct relationship was assumed to exist between stroke and the viscous properties of the erythrocytosis of cyanotic CHD. Phlebotomy was routinely employed to reduce the assumed risk of cerebral arterial thrombosis—a risk that has not withstood scrutiny.[53] In a long-term study of more than 100 cyanotic adults, no patient—irrespective of hematocrit level, iron stores, or the presence, degree, or recurrence of cerebral hyperviscosity symptoms—progressed to a completed stroke due to cerebral arterial thrombosis (see Chapter 12).[53] These conclusions have withstood the test of time.

Nonatherosclerotic Arteriopathies

Subclavian Steal

The subclavian steal was originally defined as a causal relationship between stenosis of a subclavian artery proximal to the origin of the vertebral artery and reversal of blood flow in the ipsilateral vertebral artery, thus diverting blood from the basilar system.[54] It subsequently became evident that a classic Blalock-Taussig subclavian-to-pulmonary artery shunt occasionally created an anatomic and physiologic substrate for a subclavian steal identical to that caused by acquired proximal atherosclerotic obstruction of a subclavian artery.[55] However, reversal of flow in the vertebral artery is not invariable because cervical and intrathoracic collaterals connect to the subclavian artery.[55] Importantly, the anatomic and physiologic consequences of a symptomatic subclavian steal are not necessarily eliminated when the Blalock-Taussig anastomosis is divided during subsequent intracardiac repair.[55] Subclavian steal has also been reported when repair of coarctation of the aorta results in suture line distortion or thrombosis of the orifice of the left subclavian artery.[56] The steal has not been observed when unoperated coarctation narrows the orifice of the left subclavian artery (see Chapter 4).

A symptomatic *congenital subclavian steal* (Fig. 14–10) refers to congenital isolation of the left subclavian artery with vertebrobasilar insufficiency[57] causing dizziness, vertigo, headache, visual disturbances, tinnitus, ataxia, and occasionally syncope often exacerbated by exercising the involved upper extremity.[58] Importantly, the symptoms are not always related to vertebrobasilar insufficiency but instead may result from a space-occupying intracranial aneurysm that sometimes coexists.[59] When a congenital subclavian steal is asymptomatic, which is usually the case, the vascular malformation can be suspected because of the combination of a right aortic arch with diminished pulse and blood pressure in the ipsilateral upper extremity.[60]

Migraine

Migraine headaches are relatively common among both cyanotic and acyanotic adults with CHD. Rarely, a protracted migraine is accompanied by ischemic or hemorrhagic cerebral infarction[61-63] (Fig. 14–11). Basilar artery migraine, an uncommon disorder of adolescents, can be associated with symptoms of brainstem ischemia. The mechanism responsible for ischemic "migrainous" strokes is poorly understood. In some cases, vasospasm plays a key role.[61,62] Arterial spasm is a well-known and feared side effect of ergotamine, which is used for treating acute migrainous attacks.[64] Atrial arrhythmias have been attributed to autonomic discharge provoked by migraine headache, and recurrences predispose to cerebral thromboembolism originating in the left atrial appendage (see Fig. 14–5). Individuals experiencing migraine with aura have an increased incidence of patent foramen ovale.[23,65] Passage of microemboli or vasoactive substances through the interatrial septum to the cerebrum may incite migrainous events, and passage of macroemboli in the same patients may cause cerebral infarcts.[66]

Additional Arteriopathies

Fibromuscular dysplasia can cause atypical coarctation of the aorta, dysgenesis of cervicocerebral arteries, and cerebral infarction.[67,68]

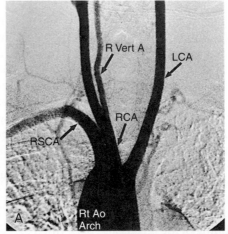

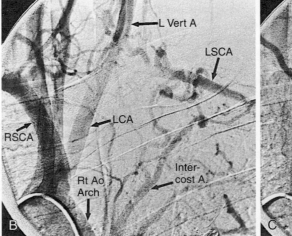

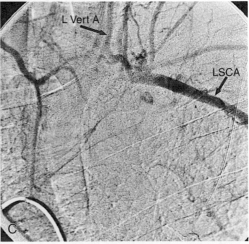

FIGURE 14–10 Arteriograms from a 21-year-old man with a symptomatic congenital subclavian steal. **(A)** Early phase showing a right aortic arch (Rt Ao Arch) from which arose a right subclavian artery (RSCA), a right carotid artery (RCA), a right vertebral artery (R Vert A), and a left carotid artery (LCA). The left subclavian artery is conspicuous by its absence. **(B)** Subsequent phase showing the left subclavian artery (LSCA) filling from the left vertebral artery (L Vert A). Intercost. A, intercostal artery. **(C)** Still later phase showing further filling of the left subclavian artery from the left vertebral artery.

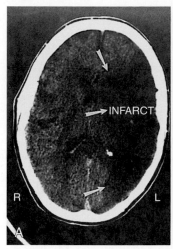
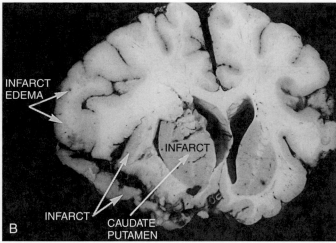

FIGURE 14–11 **(A)** Brain scan without contrast medium enhancement of a cyanotic 44-year-old woman with a nonrestrictive ventricular septal defect and pulmonary vascular disease. Intractable migraine headache culminated in a large left middle cerebral artery infarct involving the left frontal, parietal, and temporal lobes *(arrows)*. **(B)** Section of brain showing extensive infarction *(arrows)*.

Moyamoya syndrome is a progressive, multifocal stenosing arteriopathy of the intracranial vessels that can produce cerebral infarction and hemorrhage. Moyamoya pattern changes have been reported in association with a variety of congenital cardiac defects, including coarctation of the aorta, ventricular septal defect, and tetralogy of Fallot.[69] Moyamoya is also a well-described complication of Down syndrome.[70]

HEMORRHAGIC DISORDERS

Intracranial hemorrhage can be intracerebral or extracerebral (subarachnoid). Two congenital malformations—patent ductus arteriosus and coarctation of the aorta—are associated with intracranial hemorrhage. In the neonate, major fluctuations of blood flow velocity (opening and closing of the ductus) and increased pulse pressure associated with a large patent ductus may rupture capillaries of the germinal matrix and cause intraventricular hemorrhage. Surviving infants experience significant central nervous system residua.

In coarctation of the aorta, intracerebral or subarachnoid hemorrhage is caused by rupture of a congenital aneurysm of the circle of Willis (Fig. 14–12) or, much less commonly, by rupture of an aneurysm in other cerebral arteries.[71-73] The majority of coarctation patients who die from cerebral hemorrhage do so in their second or third decade. Hypertension is not a necessary precondition because cerebral hemorrhage occurs in normotensive patients long after successful coarctation repair.[73] Direct coiling or clipping of an intracranial aneurysm is the most definitive treatment.[74,75] In endovascular coiling, the aneurysm sac is packed with coils, reducing flow and inducing thrombosis. In neurosurgical clipping, a metal clip of proper strength, shape, and size is placed across the neck of the aneurysm. Both approaches obliterate blood flow into the aneurysm while preserving the parent artery.

An additional neurologic disorder that occasionally accompanies aortic coarctation is related to collateral arteries within the spinal canal.[7,76] These dilatated arteries may compress the spinal cord, causing paraparesis or quadraparesis,[77] or may rupture, resulting in the clinical picture of subarachnoid hemorrhage.[78]

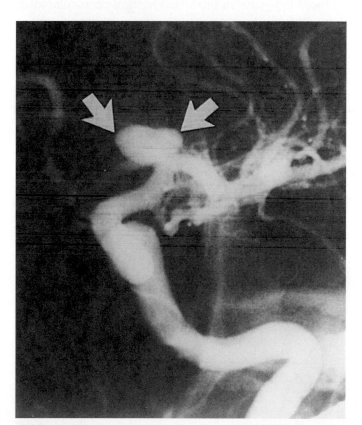

FIGURE 14–12 An 11-mm aneurysm of the circle of Willis *(arrows)* in a 28-year-old cyanotic woman with tetralogy of Fallot and pulmonary atresia. The aneurysm was first suspected when a computed tomographic scan was performed because of a clinical diagnosis of brain abscess. The aneurysm was confirmed on the cerebral arteriogram shown here. The neck of the aneurysm was surgically obliterated with a clip after treatment of the brain abscess (see Fig. 14–1).

A septic cerebral aneurysm can rupture with catastrophic consequences[12] (see previous discussion). Early identification (see Figs.14–4, *A* and *B*) sets the stage for prompt neurosurgical excision (see Fig. 14–4, *C*).

Inappropriate use of antithrombotic agents in adults with cyanotic CHD is a preventable cause of intracranial hemorrhage (Fig. 14–13; see earlier discussion and Chapter 12). Because the risk of cerebral arterial thrombosis in cyanotic CHD is negligible if not absent,[53] anticoagulants and antiplatelet agents provide no tangible benefit while increasing the risk of bleeding by reinforcing the intrinsic hemostatic defects (see Chapter 12).

SYNCOPE

Syncope in *congenital aortic stenosis* is principally due to an exaggerated, prolonged exercise-induced fall in systemic vascular resistance, the effects of which are aggravated by reflex bradycardia mediated by left ventricular baroreceptors.[79] Ventricular tachyarrhythmias seldom initiate syncope in aortic stenosis but are probably the chief cause of death in older patients *after* a faint because syncope-induced hypotension provokes electrical ventricular instability in adults with coexisting coronary atherosclerosis.

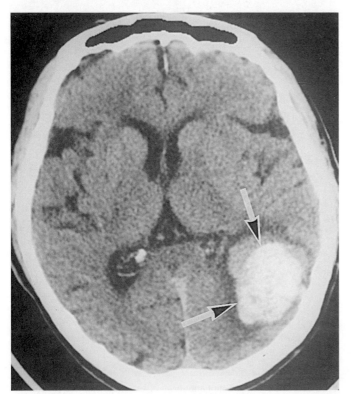

FIGURE 14–13 Computed tomographic scan of a left posterior temporal lobe hemorrhage *(arrows)* in a 36-year-old cyanotic woman with a nonrestrictive ventricular septal defect and suprasystemic pulmonary vascular resistance. The hemorrhage followed warfarin anticoagulation given because of a perceived risk of cerebral arterial thrombotic stroke.

Three electrophysiologic disturbances cause syncope in patients with CHD. Accessory pathways (Wolff-Parkinson-White bypass tracts) permit rapid ventricular responses to atrial flutter or fibrillation, provoking weakness, lightheadedness, or syncope. The most common setting is Ebstein's anomaly of a right-sided tricuspid valve[73] (see Chapter 20). In congenitally corrected transposition of the great arteries with Ebstein's anomaly of the *left* atrioventricular valve, syncope is more likely to be caused by high-degree heart block,[57] analogous to syncope in patients with isolated congenital complete heart block[73] (see Chapters 4 and 20). After intracardiac repair of congenital cardiac malformations, syncope may be due to monomorphic ventricular tachycardia originating in the incised right ventricle[80] or to surgically induced complete heart block (see Chapter 22).

HYPOXIC DISORDERS

In infants with tetralogy of Fallot, hypoxic spells are alarming episodes that typically begin with a progressive increase in the rate and depth of respiration and culminate in worsening cyanosis, limpness, syncope, convulsions, and occasionally cerebrovascular accidents and death.[7,81,82] Electroencephalographic changes during a spell are similar to those recorded in acute hypoxic episodes.[83] After a prolonged hypoxic spell, a cerebral venous sinus thrombosis may become manifest, or cerebral venous thromboses can be small and occult.[84] Surviving infants sometimes experience neurologic deficits and seizures.

SEIZURE DISORDERS

Seizures sometimes follow syncope, and persistent loss of consciousness sometimes follows seizures. As primary cerebral disorders, seizures are likely to occur in the presence of focal organic lesions of the brain but may be sequelae of hypoxic episodes with tetralogy of Fallot (discussed earlier). Seizures occur in the immediate postoperative period in as many as one fifth of neonates, depending on the method used for detection.[85] Seizures detected by continuous electroencephalographic monitoring are significantly more prevalent than clinically overt seizures.[85] In patients with cyanotic CHD, convulsive seizures are features of both fresh and healed brain abscesses (see Fig. 14–2). Seizures may announce a fresh brain abscess and may persist or reappear years later as a result of focal scarring[5] (see Fig. 14–2, *B*) Transient seizure activity sometimes occurs in infants and young children after open heart surgery[86] and is occasionally followed by permanent neurologic injury, including motor disorders and recurrence of seizures.[87]

CONGENITAL NEUROLOGIC DISORDERS

In light of the fact that the central nervous system and the cardiovascular system form nearly simultaneously in early gestation, it is not surprising that there is an increased incidence of structural abnormalities of the brain in children with structural abnormalities of the heart.[85] The more complex cardiac malformations have a proportionately higher incidence of congenital microcephaly, and one third of infants with hypoplastic left heart syndrome have congenital central nervous system disorder.[85] The brain of a full-term neonate with CHD resembles the brain of a preterm neonate.[85] Congenital neurologic disorders that coexist with CHD include chromosomal[7] or genetic abnormalities such as the CHARGE association,[88] Dandy-Walker syndrome,[89] Kallmann's syndrome,[90] and de Lange's syndrome.[91] Cerebral dysgenesis has been reported at necropsy in 10% to 29% of children with CHD, with incidence varying by cardiac lesion.[92] Cerebral lesions range from microdysgenesis to gross abnormalities such as agenesis of the corpus callosum, incomplete operculization, and microcephaly.[92] Among 40 patients with hypoplastic left heart, 29% had major or minor abnormalities of the central nervous system, and 10% had holoprosencephaly or agenesis of the corpus callosum.[93] In a necropsy study of 52 patients with a variety of congenital cardiac diseases, 68% had abnormalities of the lobes, gyri, and fissures.[94]

NEUROLOGIC SEQUELAE OF CARDIAC SURGERY

Neurologic sequelae were common during the early years of extracorporeal circulation, but technical refinements have substantially reduced the incidence.[7,95,96]

Nevertheless, current postoperative neuroimaging has identified a disturbing frequency of hypoxic-ischemic encephalopathy, periventricular leukomalacia, cerebral atrophy, and subdural hematoma,[87,97,98] and a small but not insignificant number of postoperative patients experience alterations of consciousness, local neurologic deficits, choreoathetoid syndromes, and seizures.[82,99,100] Horner's syndrome—usually but not necessarily transient—occasionally follows a Blalock-Taussig shunt or a subclavian flap aortoplasty for coarctation of the aorta.[101] Vocal cord palsy, not to be confused with hoarseness induced by intraoperative endotracheal intubation, is usually self-limiting and usually resolves in a matter of weeks.[7] Inability to wean from the respirator after open heart surgery arouses suspicion of phrenic nerve palsy with diaphragmatic paralysis.[102]

Spinal cord injury is a particular concern during repair of coarctation of the aorta.[103] Inadequate collateral circulation in the presence of aortic cross-clamping is held responsible for ischemic injury. Somatosensory-evoked potentials are now monitored routinely during repair of coarctation, especially when the adequacy of collateral circulation is questionable[104] (Fig. 14–14).

PERIPHERAL MODEL OF CENTRAL NERVOUS SYSTEM NEURONAL FUNCTION

There are substantial similarities between platelets and central nervous system neurons.[105] Accordingly, platelets have been employed as a peripheral model of central nervous system neuronal function to investigate the neurobiology of psychiatric disorders (see Chapter 13).

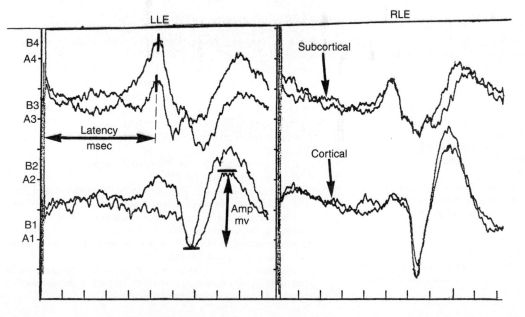

FIGURE 14–14 Somatosensory evoked potentials during repair of coarctation of the aorta in a 39-year-old man. The potentials were evoked (triggered) by stimulation of the tibialis posterior of the left lower extremity (LLE) and right lower extremity (RLE) at 34°C. Latency (msec) and amplitude (Amp mv) recorded by subcortical and cortical electrodes are normal in these tracings.

References

1. Farre JR. *Malformations of the heart.* London; 1814.
2. Ballet G. Des abscës du cerveau consecutifs ä certaines malformation cardiaques. *Arch Gen Med.* 1880;5:659.
3. Berthrong M, Sabiston DC. Cerebral lesions in congenital heart disease. *J Neuropathol Exp Neurol.* 1951;10:98–99.
4. Fischbein CA, Rosenthal A, Fischer EG, et al. Risk factors of brain abscess in patients with congenital heart disease. *Am J Cardiol.* 1974;34:97–102.
5. Kurlan R, Griggs RC. Cyanotic congenital heart disease with suspected stroke. Should all patients receive antibiotics? *Arch Neurol.* 1983;40:209–212.
6. Perloff JK, Marelli A. Neurological and psychosocial disorders in adults with congenital heart disease. *Heart Dis Stroke.* 1992;1:218–224.
7. Park SC, Neches WH. The neurologic complications of congenital heart disease. *Neurol Clin.* 1993;11:441–462.
8. Goodkin HP, Harper MB, Pomeroy SL. Intracerebral abscess in children: historical trends at Children's Hospital Boston. *Pediatrics.* 2004;113:765–770.
9. Shahler RM, Deuchar DC. Hematogenous brain abscess in cyanotic congenital heart disease. Report of three cases, with complete transposition of the great vessels. *Am J Med.* 1972;52:349–355.
10. Saez-Llorens X. Brain abscess in children. *Semin Pediatr Infect Dis.* 2003;14:108–114.
11. Yamada M, Miyasaka Y, Takagi H, Yada K. Cerebral bacterial aneurysm and indications for cerebral angiography in infective endocarditis. *Neurol Med Chir (Tokyo).* 1994;34:697–699.
12. Patel RL, Richards P, Chambers DJ, Venn G. Infective endocarditis complicated by ruptured cerebral mycotic aneurysm. *J R Soc Med.* 1991;84:746–747.
13. Chun JY, Smith W, Halbach VV, et al. Current multimodality management of infectious intracranial aneurysms. *Neurosurgery.* 2001;48:1203–1213.
14. Cerebral Embolization Task Force: cardiogenic brain embolism. *Arch Neurol.* 1986;43:71.
15. Corrin B. Paradoxical embolism. *Br Heart J.* 1964;26:549–553.
16. Kim D, Saver JL. Patent foramen ovale and stroke: what we do and don't know. *Reviews in Neurological Diseases.* 2005;2(1):1–7.
17. McQuillen PS, Hamrick SE, Perez MJ, et al. Balloon atrial septostomy is associated with preoperative stroke in neonates with transposition of the great arteries. *Circulation.* 2006;113:280–285.
18. Mugge A, Daniel WG, Angermann C, et al. Atrial septal aneurysm in adult patients. A multicenter study using transthoracic and transesophageal echocardiography. *Circulation.* 1995;91:2785–2792.
19. Belkin RN, Kisslo J. Atrial septal aneurysm: recognition and clinical relevance. *Am Heart J.* 1990;120:948–957.
20. Pearson AC, Nagelhout D, Castello R, et al. Atrial septal aneurysm and stroke: a transesophageal echocardiographic study. *J Am Coll Cardiol.* 1991;18:1223–1229.
21. Cabanes L, Mas JL, Cohen A, et al. Atrial septal aneurysm and patent foramen ovale as risk factors for cryptogenic stroke in patients less than 55 years of age. A study using transesophageal echocardiography. *Stroke.* 1993;24:1865–1873.
22. Gallet B, Malergue MC, Adams C, et al. Atrial septal aneurysm—a potential cause of systemic embolism. An echocardiographic study. *Br Heart J.* Mar 1985;53:292–297.
23. Mas JL, Arquizan C, Lamy C, et al. Patent Foramen Ovale and Atrial Septal Aneurysm Study Group. Recurrent cerebrovascular events associated with patent foramen ovale, atrial septal aneurysm, or both. *N Engl J Med.* 2001;345(24):1740–1746.
24. Homma S, Sacco RL, Di Tullio MR, et al. PFO in Cryptogenic Stroke Study (PICSS) Investigators. Effect of medical treatment in stroke patients with patent foramen ovale: patent foramen ovale in Cryptogenic Stroke Study. *Circulation.* 2002;105:2625–2631.

25. Shahrabani RM, Jairaj PS. Unruptured aneurysm of the sinus of Valsalva: a potential source of cerebrovascular embolism. *Br Heart J.* 1993;69:266–267.
26. O'Donoghue ME, Dangond F, Burger AJ, et al. Spontaneous calcific embolization to the supraclinoid internal carotid artery from a regurgitant bicuspid aortic valve. *Neurology.* 1993;43:2715–2717.
27. Connheim J. Thrombose and embolie. *Vorlesung uber Allgemeine Pathologie.* Vol 1. Berlin: Hirschwald; 1877;144–145.
28. Harvey JR, Teague SM, Anderson JL, et al. Clinically silent atrial septal defects with evidence for cerebral embolization. *Ann Intern Med.* 1986;105:695–697.
29. Biller J, Johnson MR, Adams HP Jr, et al. Further observations on cerebral or retinal ischemia in patients with right-left intracardiac shunts. *Arch Neurol.* 1987;44:740–743.
30. de Belder MA, Tourikis L, Leech G, Camm AJ. Risk of patent foramen ovale for thromboembolic events in all age groups. *Am J Cardiol.* 1992;69:1316–1320.
31. Movsowitz C, Podolsky LA, Meyerowitz CB, et al. Patent foramen ovale: a nonfunctional embryological remnant or a potential cause of significant pathology? *J Am Soc Echocardiogr.* 1992;5:259–270.
32. Wilmshurst PT, de Belder MA. Patent foramen ovale in adult life. *Br Heart J.* Mar 1994;71:209–212.
33. Di Tullio M, Sacco RL, Gopal A, et al. Patent foramen ovale as a risk factor for cryptogenic stroke. *Ann Intern Med.* 1992;117:461–465.
34. Van Camp G, Schulze D, Cosyns B, Vandenbossche JL. Relation between patent foramen ovale and unexplained stroke. *Am J Cardiol.* 1993;71:596–598.
35. Tobis MJ, Azarbal B. Does patent foramen ovale promote cryptogenic stroke and migraine headache? *Tex Heart Inst J.* 2005;32:362–365.
36. Hagen PT, Scholz DG, Edwards WD. Incidence and size of patent foramen ovale during the first 10 decades of life: an autopsy study of 965 normal hearts. *Mayo Clin Proc.* 1984;59:17–20.
37. Langholz D, Louie EK, Konstadt SN, et al. Transesophageal echocardiographic demonstration of distinct mechanisms for right to left shunting across a patent foramen ovale in the absence of pulmonary hypertension. *J Am Coll Cardiol.* 1991;18:1112–1117.
38. Seward JB, Hayes DL, Smith HC, et al. Platypnea-orthodeoxia: clinical profile, diagnostic workup, management, and report of seven cases. *Mayo Clin Proc.* 1984;59:221–231.
39. Karnik R, Stollberger C, Valentin A, et al. Detection of patent foramen ovale by transcranial contrast Doppler ultrasound. *Am J Cardiol.* 1992;69:560–562.
40. Stollberger C, Slany J, Schuster I, et al. The prevalence of deep venous thrombosis in patients with suspected paradoxical embolism. *Ann Intern Med.* 1993;119(6):461–465.
41. Cramer SC, Rordorf G, Maki JH, et al. Increased pelvic vein thrombi in cryptogenic stroke: results of the Paradoxical Emboli from Large Veins in Ischemic Stroke (PELVIS) study. *Stroke.* 2004;35(1):46–50.
42. Bartz PJ, Cetta F, Cabalka AK, et al. Paradoxical emboli in children and young adults: role of atrial septal defect and patent foramen ovale device closure. *Mayo Clin Proc.* 2006;81:615–618.
43. Windecker S, Wahl A, Chatterjee T, et al. Percutaneous closure of patent foramen ovale in patients with paradoxical embolism: long-term risk of recurrent thromboembolic events. *Circulation.* 2000;101:893–898.
44. Lock JE. Patent foramen ovale is indicted, but the case hasn't gone to trial. *Circulation.* 2000;101:838.
45. Petty GW, Khandheria BK, Meissner I, et al. Population-based study of the relationship between patent foramen ovale and cerebrovascular ischemic events. *Mayo Clin Proc.* 2006;81:602–608.
46. Meissner I, Khandheria BK, Heit JA, et al. Patent foramen ovale: innocent or guilty? Evidence from a prospective population-based study. *J Am Coll Cardiol.* 2006;47:440–445.
47. Italiano JE, Hartwig JH. Megakaryocyte development and platelet formation. In: Michelson AD. *Platelets.* 2nd ed. London: Elsevier; 2007;23–44.

48. Lill MC, Perloff JK, Child JS. Pathogenesis of thrombocytopenia in cyanotic congenital heart disease. *Am J Cardiol.* 2006;98: 254–258.

49. Perloff JK, Latta H, Barsotti P. Pathogenesis of the glomerular abnormality in cyanotic congenital heart disease. *Am J Cardiol.* 2000;86:1198–1204.

50. Cottrill CM, Kaplan S. Cerebral vascular accidents in cyanotic congenital heart disease. *Am J Dis Child.* 1973;125:484–487.

51. Phornphutkul C, Rosenthal A, Nadas AS, Berenberg W. Cerebrovascular accidents in infants and children with cyanotic congenital heart disease. *Am J Cardiol.* 1973;32:329–334.

52. Amitai Y, Blieden L, Shemtov A, Neufeld H. Cerebrovascular accidents in infants and children with congenital cyanotic heart disease. *Isr J Med Sci.* 1984;20:1143–1145.

53. Perloff JK, Marelli AJ, Miner PD. Risk of stroke in adults with cyanotic congenital heart disease. *Circulation.* 1993;87:1954–1959.

54. Reivich M, Holling HE, Roberts B, Toole JF. Reversal of blood flow through the vertebral artery and its effect on cerebral circulation. *N Engl J Med.* 1961;265:878–885.

55. Kurlan R, Krall RL, Deweese JA. Vertebrobasilar ischemia after total repair of tetralogy of Fallot: significance of subclavian steal created by Blalock-Taussig anastomosis. Vertebrobasilar ischemia after correction of tetralogy of Fallot. *Stroke.* 1984;15:359–362.

56. Saalouke MG, Perry LW, Breckbill DL, et al. Cerebrovascular abnormalities in postoperative coarctation of aorta. Four cases demonstrating left subclavian steal on aortography. *Am J Cardiol.* 1978; 42:97–101.

57. Massumi RA. The congenital variety of the "subclavian steal" syndrome. *Circulation.* 1963;28:1149–1152.

58. Luetmer PH, Miller GM. Right aortic arch with isolation of the left subclavian artery: case report and review of the literature. *Mayo Clin Proc.* 1990;65:407–413.

59. Savastano S, Feltrin GP, Chiesura-Corona M, Miotta D. Cerebral ischemia due to congenital malformations of brachiocephalic arteries—case reports. *Angiology.* 1992;43:76–83.

60. Kajinami K, Mori K, Masuda S, et al. Asymptomatic congenital subclavian steal in a young male patient with right aortic arch. *Chest.* 1990;97:481.

61. Bogousslavsky J, Regli F, Van Melle G, et al. Migraine stroke. *Neurology.* 1988;38:223–227.

62. Rothrock JF, Walicke P, Swenson MR, et al. Migrainous stroke. *Arch Neurol.* 1988;45:63–67.

63. Henrich JB, Sandercock PA, Warlow CP, Jones LN. Stroke and migraine in the Oxfordshire Community Stroke Project. *J Neurol.* 1986;233:257–262.

64. Lindboe CF, Dahl T, Rostad B. Fatal stroke in migraine: a case report with autopsy findings. *Cephalalgia.* 1989;9:277–280.

65. Schwerzmann M, Nedeltchev K, Lagger F, et al. Prevalence and size of directly detected patent foramen ovale in migraine with aura. *Neurology.* 2005;65(9):1415–1418.

66. Azarbal B, Tobis J, Suh W, et al. Association of interatrial shunts and migraine headaches: impact of transcatheter closure. *J Am Coll Cardiol.* 2005;45(4):489–492.

67. Janzen J, Vuong PN, Rothenberger-Janzen K. Takayasu's arteritis and fibromuscular dysplasia as causes of acquired atypical coarctation of the aorta: retrospective analysis of seven cases. *Heart Vessels.* 1999;14(6):277–282.

68. Malloy DS, Sangalang VE, Fraser GM. Cerebral infarction secondary to unsuspected intracranial fibromuscular dysplasia following bypass of aortic coarctation. *Stroke.* 1984;15:908–911.

69. Lutterman J, Scott M, Nass R, Geva T. Moyamoya syndrome associated with congenital heart disease. *Pediatrics.* 1998;101(1 Pt 1):57–60.

70. Jea A, Smith ER, Robertson R, Scott RM. Moyamoya syndrome associated with Down syndrome: outcome after surgical revascularization. *Pediatrics.* 2005;116(5):e694–e701.

71. Connolly HM, Huston J 3rd, Brown RD Jr, et al. Intracranial aneurysms in patients with coarctation of the aorta: a prospective magnetic resonance angiographic study of 100 patients. *Mayo Clin Proc.* 2003;78(12):1491–1499.

72. Hodes HL, Steinfeld L, Blumenthal S. Congenital cerebral aneurysms and coarctation of the aorta. *Arch Peds.* 1959;76:28–43.

73. Perloff JK. *Clinical Recognition of Congenital Heart Disease.* Philadelphia: W.B. Saunders; 1994.

74. Meyer FB, Morita A, Puumala MR, Nichols DA. Medical and surgical management of intracranial aneurysms. *Mayo Clin Proc.* 1995;70: 153–172.

75. Molyneux AJ, Kerr RS, Yu LM, et al. International Subarachnoid Aneurysm Trial (ISAT) Collaborative Group. International subarachnoid aneurysm trial (ISAT) of neurosurgical clipping versus endovascular coiling in 2143 patients with ruptured intracranial aneurysms: a randomised comparison of effects on survival, dependency, seizures, rebleeding, subgroups, and aneurysm occlusion. *Lancet.* 2005;366(9488):809–817.

76. Chadduck WM, Cathey SL, Gearhart AT, et al. Paraplegia caused by coarctation of the aorta and hydrocephalus. *Childs Nerv Syst.* 1986;2:162–164.

77. Peters P, Brennan JW, Hughes CF, et al. Late quadriplegia after adult coarctation repair. *Ann Thorac Surg.* 2003;75(1):268–270.

78. Banna MM, Rose PG, Pearce GW. Coarctation of the aorta as a cause of spinal subarachnoid hemorrhage. Case report. *J Neurosurg.* 1973; 39:761–763.

79. Mark AL, Kioschos JM, Abboud FM, et al. Abnormal vascular responses to exercise in patients with aortic stenosis. *J Clin Invest.* 1973;52:1138–1146.

80. Perloff JK, Middlekauff H, Child J, et al. Usefulness of post-ventriculotomy signal averaged electrocardiograms in congenital heart disease. *Am J Cardiol.* 2006;98:1646–1651.

81. Morgan BC, Guntheroth WG, Bloom RS, Fyler DC. A clinical profile of paroxysmal hyperpnea in cyanotic congenital heart disease. *Circulation.* 1965;31:66–69.

82. Shinebourne EA, Anderson RH, Bowyer JJ. Variations in clinical presentation of Fallot's tetralogy in infancy. Angiographic and pathogenetic implications. *Br Heart J.* 1975;37:946–955.

83. Daniels SR, Bates SR, Kaplan S. EEG monitoring during paroxysmal hyperpnea of tetralogy of Fallot: an epileptic or hypoxic phenomenon? *J Child Neurol.* 1987;2:98–100.

84. Rowe RD, Vlad P, Keith JD. Experiences with 180 cases of tetralogy of Fallot in infants and children. *Can Med Assoc J.* 1955;73: 23–30.

85. Wernovsky G. Current insights regarding neurological and developmental abnormalities in children and young adults with complex congenital cardiac disease. *Cardiol Young.* 2006;16 Suppl 1:92–104.

86. Bellinger DC, Wypij D, Kuban KC, et al. Developmental and neurological status of children at 4 years of age after heart surgery with hypothermic circulatory arrest or low-flow cardiopulmonary bypass. *Circulation.* 1999;100:526–532.

87. Ferry PC. Neurologic sequelae of open-heart surgery in children. An "irritating question." *Am J Dis Child.* 1990;144:369–373.

88. Kaplan LC. Choanal atresia and its associated anomalies. Further support for the CHARGE Association. *Int J Pediatr Otorhinolaryngol.* 1985;8:237–242.

89. Sautreaux JL, Giroud M, Dauvergne M, et al. Dandy-Walker malformation associated with occipital meningocele and cardiac anomalies: a rare complex embryologic defect. *J Child Neurol.* 1986;1:64–66.

90. Moorman JR, Crain B, Osborne D. Kallman's syndrome with associated cardiovascular and intracranial anomalies. *Am J Med.* 1984;77: 369–372.

91. Rao PS, Sissman NJ. Congenital heart disease in the de Lange syndrome. *J Pediatr.* 1971;79:674–677.

92. Newburger JW, Bellinger DC. Brain injury in congenital heart disease. *Circulation.* 2006;113:183–185.

93. Glauser TA, Rorke LB, Weinberg PM, Clancy RR. Congenital brain anomalies associated with the hypoplastic left heart syndrome. *Pediatrics.* 1990;85:984–990.

94. Jones M. Anomalies of the brain and congenital heart disease: a study of 52 necropsy cases. *Pediatr Pathol.* 1991;11:721–736.

95. Bozoky B, Bara D, Kertesz E. Autopsy study of cerebral complications of congenital heart disease and cardiac surgery. *J Neurol.* 1984;231:153–161.

96. Bellinger DC, Wypij D, Kuban KCK, et al. Developmental and neurological status of children at 4 years of age after heart surgery with hypothermic circulatory arrest or low-flow cardiopulmonary bypass. *Circulation.* 1999;100:526–532.

97. Galli KK, Zimmerman RA, Jarvik GP, et al. Periventricular leukomalacia is common after neonatal cardiac surgery. *J Thorac Cardiovasc Surg.* 2004;127(3):692–704.

98. Tavani F, Zimmerman RA, Clancy RR, et al. Incidental intracranial hemorrhage after uncomplicated birth: MRI before and after neonatal heart surgery. *Neuroradiology.* 2003;45(4):253–258.

99. Trittenwein G, Nardi A, Pansi H, et al. Verein zur Durchfuhrung wissenschaftlicher Forschung auf dem Gebeit der Neonatologie und Padiatrischen Intensivmedizin. Early postoperative prediction of cerebral damage after pediatric cardiac surgery. *Ann Thorac Surg.* 2003;76(2):576–580.

100. Ferry PC. Neurologic sequelae of cardiac surgery in children. *Am J Dis Child.* 1987;141:309–312.

101. Baudet E, al-Qudah A. Late results of the subclavian flap repair of coarctation in infancy. *J Cardiovasc Surg (Torino).* 1989;30:445–449.

102. Hamilton JR, Tocewicz K, Elliott MJ, et al. Paralysed diaphragm after cardiac surgery in children: value of plication. *Eur J Cardiothorac Surg.* 1990;4:487–490.

103. Serfontein SJ, Kron IL. Complications of coarctation repair. *Semin Thorac Cardiovasc Surg Pediatr Card Surg Annu.* 2002;5:206–211.

104. Pollock JC, Jamieson MP, McWilliam R. Somatosensory evoked potentials in the detection of spinal cord ischemia in aortic coarctation repair. *Ann Thorac Surg.* 1986;41:251–254.

105. Gurguis GN. Psychiatric disorders. In: Michelson AD. *Platelets.* 2nd ed. London: Elsevier, 2007;791–821.

SURGICAL CONSIDERATIONS

Cardiac Surgery in Adults with Congenital Heart Disease: Operation and Reoperation

DANIEL MARELLI ▪ MARK D. PLUNKETT ▪ JOSEPH K. PERLOFF ▪ HILLEL LAKS

The three general categories of adults with congenital heart disease (CHD) include those who have not undergone cardiac surgery, those who have undergone palliative cardiac surgery, and those who have undergone physiologic or anatomic repair. In the United States today, about 20,000 open operations are performed annually for CHD. Repair in neonates and infants sets the stage for adult survival, but the early operation may be followed by reoperation in adulthood[1-20] (see Chapter 5). This chapter is devoted to cardiac surgery in an evolving patient population—the adult with CHD.

Unoperated adults are, with few exceptions, from developing countries (see Chapter 4). Patients who have undergone only an early palliative operation are relatively uncommon and include those with systemic-to-pulmonary arterial shunts, cavopulmonary shunts, and pulmonary artery bands. Most commonly, adults with CHD have undergone physiologic or anatomic repairs in infancy or childhood.

SYSTEMIC-TO-PULMONARY ARTERIAL SHUNTS

Relatively rare are patients surviving to adulthood with a classic Blalock-Taussig (BT) shunt as the only source of pulmonary blood flow. In contrast to the original subclavian-to-pulmonary arterial connections, shunts now employ polytetrafluoroethylene (GORE-TEX®) grafts that do not grow and are designed to serve as a bridge to subsequent intracardiac repair for tetralogy of Fallot and physiologically analogous malformations or a Fontan repair for univentricular hearts.

Before initiating cardiopulmonary bypass (CPB), BT shunts must be ligated or snared, and modified (GORE-TEX®) shunts must be divided to avoid pulmonary arterial distortion by relatively rigid synthetic material. Distorted pulmonary arteries are reconstructed, usually with a pericardial patch.

POTTS OR WATERSTON SHUNTS

These direct aortic-to-pulmonary arterial shunts are no longer used, but older patients in whom Potts or Waterston shunts were placed in infancy or childhood occasionally present for reparative surgery in adulthood. The Potts shunt connects the descending aorta to the proximal left pulmonary artery, whereas the Waterston shunt connects the ascending aorta to the right pulmonary artery. Pulmonary blood flow is usually excessive but is occasionally curtailed by the development of pulmonary vascular disease, which renders the patient inoperable. Takedown requires cardiopulmonary bypass and patch closure from within. Before initiating bypass, runoff is controlled by bilaterally snaring the pulmonary arteries distal to the shunt.

GLENN SHUNT

Typically constructed early in life in patients with a functionally single ventricle, the superior vena cava was originally connected to a divided right pulmonary artery. To be effective, the central venous pressure must be less than 18 to 20 mm Hg and the transpulmonary gradient less than 10 to 12 mm Hg. Because the superior vena cava provides about 30% of an infant's venous return, the Glenn shunt is effective yet avoids left-sided volume overload associated with systemic arterial shunts. Survival to adulthood is common, but classic Glenn shunts are often followed years later by right lower lobe pulmonary arteriovenous fistulae that can be occluded with coil devices (see Chapter 18). The incidence of these fistulae has been reduced by attaching the superior vena cava to an undivided right pulmonary artery—the bilateral Glenn shunt—that often serves as the first stage of a Fontan repair.

PULMONARY ARTERIAL BANDING

The purpose of this procedure is to curtail excessive pulmonary blood flow in patients with a ventricular septal defect (VSD), a complete common atrioventricular (AV) canal, and/or a univentricular heart without pulmonary stenosis. Banding of the pulmonary trunk distorts the origins of the right or left branches in up to 25% of patients, and, rarely, a proximal band distorts the pulmonary valve. Reconstruction of a banded pulmonary artery or a major branch is achieved with pericardium or polytetrafluoroethylene (GORE-TEX®). Rarely, a pulmonary arterial false aneurysm develops because the band cuts through the pulmonary trunk. Rupture is exceptional, but repair is warranted because the false aneurysm can enlarge considerably. Reoperation is usually prompted by the need to address residua and sequelae (see Chapters 20 and 21). Redo procedures are usually complex and incur increased risk.

GENERAL MANAGEMENT

The remainder of this chapter is devoted to lesions that are most common in unoperated or postoperative adults with CHD. Proper care of patients after operation requires knowledge of the preoperative CHD; the type and effects of surgical or catheter intervention; and the presence, type, and degree of postoperative or postinterventional residua and sequelae. Cure in the literal sense is rarely achieved. The wide range of residua and sequelae are coupled with cardiac and noncardiac diseases that are acquired decade by decade and must be considered in preoperative planning. Cardiac surgeons trained to deal with CHD usually adapt to addressing acquired coronary artery disease and acquired valvular disease, but cardiac surgeons trained only in acquired heart disease of adults seldom adapt to dealing with CHD, especially complex CHD.

Reoperation

Median sternotomy can be hazardous during reoperation. Massive hemorrhage can occur when thin-walled vascular structures are adherent to the posterior sternum. Computed tomography (CT) scans provide retrosternal images that anticipate potential complications and assist in planning (see Chapter 7). If the aorta, right atrium, or a conduit is adherent to the sternum, the femoral artery and vein can be exposed before sternotomy, and cardiopulmonary bypass initiated with thin-walled cannulae for femoral artery and vein. Aortic regurgitation may require decompression of the left ventricle, accomplished by cannulating the apex through a small submammary incision. In cyanotic patients, excessive bleeding can be expected because of large vessels throughout the mediastinum, increased tissue vascularity, and inherent hemostatic defects (see Chapter 12). Antifibrinolytic agents are used in high-risk patients.

Myocardial Protection

Myocardial protection is crucial to the outcome of complex procedures. A left ventricular vent and hypothermia to 24°C may be employed and antegrade or retrograde cardioplegia (or both) administered at 10- to 20-minute intervals to avoid washout. A pursestring suture is placed around the coronary sinus to secure the retrograde catheter and improve flow distribution.

Postoperative Care

Postoperative adults with CHD may present more complex problems than adults with acquired heart disease. Right atrial, pulmonary arterial, and left atrial pressure-monitoring lines are employed. Transesophageal echocardiography is used to assess left and right ventricular function to evaluate left- and right-sided valve function and to identify residual shunts. Pulmonary vascular resistance can be lowered with inhaled nitric oxide or milrinone. Ventilator control may be used to reduce PCO_2 to about 35 mm Hg to further control pulmonary artery pressure.

Associated Procedures

Patients older than 40 years of age, especially men, may require coronary bypass grafts. Diseased aortic, mitral, or tricuspid valves may require repair or replacement, and a Maze procedure can be used to address atrial tachyarrhythmias. Implantation of epicardial pacemaker leads with a generator may be nececessary.[21-33] Transvenous leads are not used in the systemic circulation because of the risk of thromboembolism.

SPECIFIC CONGENITAL MALFORMATIONS

Aortic Valve Disease

Aortic valve repair is usually feasible when aortic regurgitation is due to cusp prolapse associated with VSD or tetralogy of Fallot. Stenotic mobile noncalcified congenital bicuspid aortic valves may be amenable to balloon dilatation (see Chapter 18). In older adults, calcified stenotic bicuspid aortic valves account for approximately one half of cases that require surgery for isolated calcific aortic stenosis. With few exceptions, relief of obstruction requires replacement. In the Ross operation, the patient's own normal pulmonary valve (autograft) is excised and inserted in the aortic position, and the excised pulmonary valve is replaced by a homograft (allograft) or xenograft, which is treated with anticalcification agents (see Chapter 16).

Ostium Secundum Atrial Septal Defect

This type of interatrial communication (Fig. 15–1) accounts for up to 40% of acyanotic shunt lesions in unoperated patients older than age 40 years (see Chapter 4). Ostium primum and sinus venosus defects are occasionally represented. The malformation may go unrecognized for decades because symptoms are absent and physical signs are subtle. Age-related mitral valve abnormalities sufficient to cause significant regurgitation occur in approximately 15% of adults with an ostium secundum atrial septal defect (ASD).[34] Older patients deteriorate chiefly on three counts. First, because an age-related decrease in left ventricular distensibility augments the left-to-right shunt. Second, because atrial fibrillation, atrial flutter, and, less commonly, reentrant atrial tachycardia increase in frequency after the fourth decade, augment the left-to-right shunt, and precipitate right ventricular failure. Third, because symptomatic adults older than 40 years of age often have mild to moderate elevations of pulmonary arterial pressure, so the aging volume overloaded right ventricle is beset by both pressure and volume overload. Pulmonary vascular disease with reversed shunt occurs in less than 10% of patients with an ostium secundum ASD and is believed to represent the coincidence of idiopathic pulmonary hypertension rather than the sequel of the ASD shunt.

There is general agreement on the benefits of closure between the early 20s and the early 40s (discussed later). Although there is no consensus regarding the benefits of closure in middle-aged and elderly patients, current evidence supports the conclusion that closure improves longevity and reduces functional limitations.[34-40] However, the risk of atrial fibrillation and flutter and the attendant risk of thromboembolic events may not be reduced.[41]

Operation is performed using cardiopulmonary bypass and moderate hypothermia. For cosmetic purposes in young women, a submammary skin incision with median sternotomy is preferred. Alternatively, a small right anterolateral thoracotomy (Fig. 15–2) or a midline incision in the lower half of the sternum can be employed. There is growing use of thoracoscopic closure as a reliable alternative to percutaneous management for closure of these defects.[42]

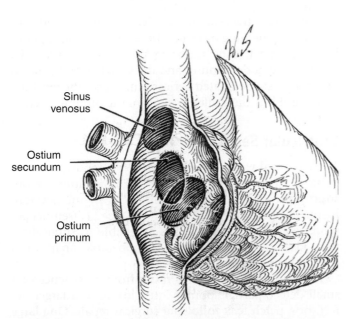

FIGURE 15–1 Diagram showing locations of the most common types of atrial septal defects.

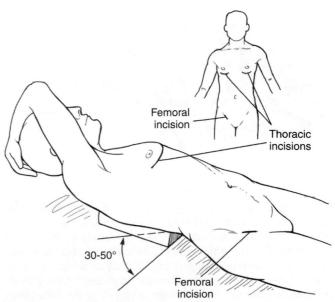

FIGURE 15–2 Patient position for minimally invasive right thoracotomy approach for repair of an atrial septal defect. A 5- to 7-cm incision is made in the submammary crease. An additional incision is made in the groin crease for femoral artery cannulation.

Closure is either primary or with a pericardial patch that baffles right-sided pulmonary veins into the left atrium. Redundant right atrial wall is excised and a regurgitant tricuspid valve is repaired with an annuloplasty if annular dilatation is greater than 34 to 38 mm. A Maze procedure is performed in patients with chronic atrial flutter/fibrillation.[43, 44] Current interest focuses on intravascular devices to close smaller ASDs[45-49] (see Chapter 18).

There is uniform agreement that closure of an isolated nonrestrictive ostium secundum ASD with a large left-to-right shunt during or before the early 20s is followed by long-term survival not significantly different from an age- and sex-matched control population. Repair between 25 and 41 years of age is followed by long-term survival that is good but shorter than normal, and closure after age 41 years is associated with a substantial increase in late mortality and morbidity.[50-54]

Ostium Primum Defect Atrial Septal Defects

Survival in ostium primum defects is analogous to survival in ostium secundum ASDs of equivalent size and shunt volume. The suture line is placed on the tricuspid aspect of the defect outside the conduction tissue, which remains beneath the patch (Fig. 15-3). Atrioventricular valve regurgitation, usually left-sided, is repaired with excellent long-term results.[55-59]

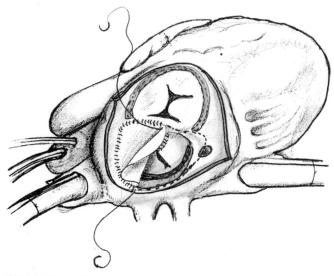

FIGURE 15-3 Diagram showing closure of primum atrial septal defect, mitral valve repair, and tricuspid annuloplasty. The cleft in the anterior mitral leaflet is closed with interrupted sutures. Mitral annuloplasty can be used or the commissures can be plicated. Autologous pericardium is employed to close the atrial septal defect. The suture line is placed on the tricuspid valve side, continued inferiorly on the atrial wall outside the conduction tissue (shown by the dotted line), and then under the lip of the coronary sinus and back to the edge of the ASD. The conduction tissue remains under the patch, and the coronary sinus drains into the right atrium. A tricuspid annuloplasty is sometimes performed.

Reoperation for Atrioventricular Septal Defects

About 10% to 30% of these patients develop postoperative left AV valve malfunction, the commonest cause of which is a residual or recurrent cleft in the anterior leaflet.[60,61] Annuloplasty or commissuroplasty involves isolated stitches along the annulus or a band along the posterior aspect of the annulus.[62-65] The dysplastic superior and inferior bridging leaflets are detached radially along the anterior annulus and augmented with glutaraldehyde-treated autologous pericardium, improving leaflet coaptation. Experience with creating a double orifice valve is limited.[66,67]

Valve Replacement

The annulus projects toward the left ventricle outflow tract because the inlet septum is shortened and the outlet septum is lengthened. A crescent-shaped patch is used to lengthen mitral to aortic continuity along the circumference of the annulus, permitting placement of a low-profile mechanical valve positioned away from the left ventricle outflow with projection into the left atrium.[68] Leaflet remnants are used to anchor the valve along the other segments of the annulus.

Left ventricular outflow tract (LVOT) obstruction caused by tunnel-like narrowing is relatively uncommon[69,70] but may require a Konno procedure for adequate enlargement. LVOT obstruction can also be caused by a subaortic membrane, by abnormal position of a papillary muscle,[69,70] by attachment of left superior leaflet chordae to the outlet septum, or by accessory valve tissue that can be excised. Obstructing chordae require division and reattachment, repair, or valve replacement.

The outflow tract can be effectively shortened and widened by augmenting or lifting the left side of the superior bridging leaflet, thus restoring the angle between the plane of the outlet septum and the septal crest.[71] A patch of glutaraldehyde-treated pericardium closes the resulting defect and lifts the leaflet away from the outflow tract.

Ventricular Septal Defects

Adult survival with a nonrestrictive VSD requires curtailment of excessive pulmonary blood flow either by obstruction to right ventricular outflow or by the development of pulmonary vascular disease (Eisenmenger syndrome). The obstruction is amenable to surgical repair. Eisenmenger syndrome is inoperable apart from lung transplantation.

Restrictive VSDs in adults result from persistence of a small defect, partial spontaneous closure of a larger defect, or a patch leak following surgical repair. One large study reported an 87% 25-year survival but a significant risk of high-degree heart block and sudden death.[72] A study of 1448 patients with VSDs disclosed a 22% incidence of associated defects with development of aortic regurgitation and infundibular pulmonary stenosis.[73] By age 30 years, 89% of patients had aortic regurgitation.

The right cusp of the aortic valve tends to prolapse into a subarterial VSD because of proximity of the aortic annulus, reducing the effective defect size and limiting the shunt but at the price of aortic regurgitation.[74] The prolapsing aortic leaflet requires suspension (Fig. 15–4), and the sinotubular junction may require reduction to a size appropriate to the annulus.

An AV septal type of VSD is located in the inlet septum beneath the septal and posterior tricuspid leaflets. Closure of the defect is usually accompanied by repair of a cleft anterior mitral leaflet and may require reduction of a dilatated annulus.

Double-chambered right ventricle is characterized by a high-pressure proximal chamber and a low-pressure distal chamber that are the result of obstructive fibromuscular proliferation within the right ventricle caused by the jet of a restrictive VSD as it strikes myocardium. The VSD tends to close spontaneously as the fibromuscular tissue proliferates around and over the defect. When spontaneous closure fails to occur, the defect is repaired at the time of surgery for resection of the obstructing tissue within the right ventricle.

The merit of closing a small VSD is questionable; medical surveillance is current policy. Infective endocarditis associated with a small VSD is considered a reason for repair (see Chapter 8). Transcatheter closure is currently investigational.[75,76] When the Qp:Qs is greater than 1.5:1 and the pulmonary vascular resistance is less than 3 to 4 units/m², surgical closure is recommended and can be performed safely. VSD with double-chambered right ventricle is an indication for operation. In adults with VSD and Eisenmenger syndrome, heart-lung transplantation or lung transplantation with closure of the defect is an option (see Chapter 17).

VSD repairs are performed on cardiopulmonary bypass with moderate systemic hypothermia. An appropriately sized patch is created and sewn in place using either interrupted, pledgeted horizontal mattress sutures or a continuous running suture. The patch is cut slightly larger than the defect so that the sutures can be placed away from the edge of the defect and away from the conduction system. Most adults with a perimembranous, inlet, or muscular VSD undergo repair through the tricuspid valve annulus. If the edges of the defect are difficult to visualize because of attachments of the septal leaflet to the edge of the defect, the leaflet can be incised at its base adjacent to the annulus, exposing the VSD beneath. Subarterial VSDs can be approached through the pulmonary valve or the right ventricular outflow tract. Exposure through the pulmonary valve is particularly helpful in placing sutures through the annulus without damaging the valve. The patch material for closure is synthetic such as GORE-TEX or Dacron, or glutaraldehyde-treated autologous pericardium, which we prefer. GORE-TEX® is associated with less hemolysis than pericardial patches but tends to be less well incorporated so that small patch leaks do not readily close.

When preoperative pulmonary artery pressure is moderately elevated, an adjustable ASD can be created (see Fig. 15–15). Alternatively, a fenestrated VSD patch allows transient right-to-left shunting and maintenance of cardiac output. Fenestrated patches can subsequently be closed in the interventional catheterization laboratory.

Among 52 patients between 16 and 67 years of age with VSDs repaired at UCLA, there was no mortality. These repairs were often combined with repairs of the aortic and tricuspid valves and with pulmonary valve replacement. The incidence of postoperative complete heart block was approximately 1% except when the VSD was associated with congenitally corrected transposition of the great arteries (see Chapter 22).

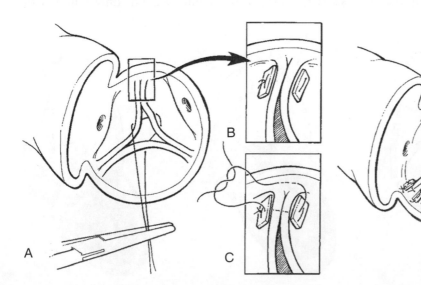

FIGURE 15–4 Technique of aortic valve repair using pericardial pledgeted sutures to resuspend redundant leaflets. Additional apposition can be achieved by adding sutures below the commissures.

Patent Ductus Arteriosus

Closure of an isolated patent ductus arteriosus (PDA) by interventional catheterization is the procedure of choice depending on the size, length, and shape of the ductus[77-81] (see Chapter 18). A technique has been devised in which the ductus is excluded with a stent graft placed in the proximal descending aorta.[82-84] A small PDA is of no hemodynamic importance, but closure is recommended because of susceptibility to infective endocarditis (see Chapter 8). An isolated patent PDA presenting with congestive heart failure in the third or fourth decade is a clear indication for closure.[85] A nonrestrictive ductus with pulmonary vascular disease and reversed shunt precludes closure for the same reasons as with an Eisenmenger VSD (discussed earlier). Lung transplantation with ductal closure is an option.

Surgical closure of a PDA is carried out via a small left posterior thoracotomy. Thoracoscopic procedures are not appropriate in adults because of the frequency of calcification and the corresponding risk of rupture during ligation.[86,87] A ductal aneurysm or major ductal calcification are addressed by surgical intervention best accomplished through a median sternotomy with cardiopulmonary bypass and deep hypothermia.[88,89] The ductus is exposed through an incision in the pulmonary artery and, using low flow, is closed on the pulmonary arterial side with horizontal pledgeted mattress sutures. Alternatively, the pulmonary arterial insertion is patched with glutaraldehyde-treated pericardium or a GORE-TEX® patch. During cooling, the branch pulmonary arteries are snared to prevent steal from the descending aorta.

Coarctation of the Aorta

The majority of coarctation patients who survive infancy can be expected to reach adulthood, but appreciable attrition begins by 20 years of age, and more than three quarters of unoperated patients die by age 50 years. Rupture of

the aorta or dissecting aneurysm is a dramatic complication of aortic coarctation, with a peak incidence in the third and fourth decades. The paracoarctation aorta harbors inherent medial abnormalities qualitatively similar to the Marfan syndrome. The abnormalities pose a special risk during pregnancy (see Chapter 9).

Long-term complications include paracoarctation aneurysm with rupture, dissecting aneurysm of the ascending aortic above a coexisting bicuspid aortic valve,[31] aneurysmal dilatation with rupture of intercostals arteries, premature coronary artery disease, infective endocarditis, and rupture of an intracranial aneurysm (see Chapter 4).

Repair is indicated when the transcoarctation gradient at rest is 30 mm Hg or more[90] and when obstruction recurs after repair or balloon aortoplasty. If the resting gradient is less than 30 mm Hg and the obstruction severe, an exercise test will provoke a larger gradient, and magnetic resonance imaging (MRI) will confirm the severity (see later and see Chapter 7). The majority of infants with unrepaired arch hypoplasia at their initial operation require reoperation as adults. Residual coarctation following childhood repair is due to failure of growth of the anastomosis or technical factors such as a short subclavian flap aortoplasty. Reoperation is common in patients initially treated with a patch because the prosthetic material is necessarily sutured into paracoarctation aorta, which is inherently abnormal.

In patients with coarctation, the left ventricular outflow tract and thoracic aorta must be anatomically defined in their entirety. Previously repaired patients may have additional obstruction because of stenotic bicuspid aortic valve or because a hypoplastic aortic arch failed to grow. Echocardiography focuses on the aortic valve and the ascending aorta (see Chapter 6). Magnetic resonance angiography with three-dimensional computerized reconstruction assesses the transverse arch, isthmus, and descending aorta (see Chapter 7).

The preferred technique of coarctation repair in younger patients is resection with extended end-to-end anastomosis (Fig. 15–5), a procedure that not only removes the

FIGURE 15–5 The first two images illustrate resection of aortic coarctation with end-to-end anastomoses. The third image illustrates excision of the coarctation, reconstruction of the posterior wall with end-to-end anastomosis, and a glutaraldehyde-treated autologous pericardial patch to enlarge the isthmus and the site of repair.

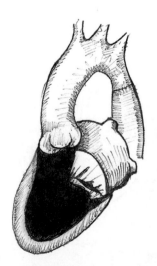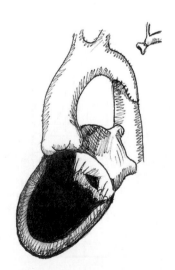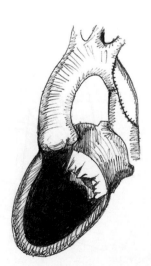

obstruction but also removes the abnormal paracoarctation aorta. Patch augmentation is sometimes appropriate when previous resection has removed the abnormal paracoarctation segments or when collaterals are particularly large and difficult to mobilize.[91-94] Tube-graft interposition is used to relieve long segments of obstruction. Precautions are taken to reduce the risk of spinal cord ischemia. Arterial lines are placed in the upper and lower extremities for blood pressure monitoring during aortic clamping. Distal pressure should be maintained above 50 mm Hg throughout the procedure. Somatosensory evoked potentials are monitored intraoperatively to determine whether extracorporeal circulation should be used to reduce the risk of spinal cord ischemia during aortic cross-clamping (see Chapter 20). Cerebrospinal fluid (CSF) pressure is monitored by catheter, and fluid is allowed to drain if pressure exceeds 10 cm H_2O. The CSF pressure is monitored postoperatively for 48–72 hours.

For patients undergoing operation for recurrent coarctation, mobilization of the aorta for end-to-end anastomosis may be difficult and can cause excessive blood loss. An ascending-to-descending aortic bypass graft can be constructed in these patients. Operation has been performed through either a right thoracotomy or through a median sternotomy and a posterior pericardial approach.[95,96] A 16- to 20-mm graft is used; repair can be performed through the right chest without bypass. Both techniques avoid complications associated with reoperation through a left thoracotomy, including injury to the recurrent laryngeal nerve, the intercostal arteries, and the lung. Bypass permits addressing arch hypoplasia and avoids the need for clamping a potentially thin or calcified aorta. Hypertension is treated aggressively in an intensive care unit. Abdominal pain and distension occur in 5% of patients postoperatively. Management is usually conservative.

A median sternotomy with cannulation of both the ascending aorta and the femoral artery is employed in older patients who require coronary revascularization or repair or replacement of the aortic valve. A Dacron graft can be placed through the diaphragm between the ascending aorta and the proximal abdominal aorta. Alternatively, a clamshell-type incision provides simultaneous access to the mediastinum and the descending thoracic aorta.

Catheter-based techniques are now used for both the primary intervention and for recurrences[97-99] (see Chapter 18). Mild residual gradients are common after angioplasty and stenting,[92] which may not adequately address the abnormal paracoarctation aorta. Surgery achieves long-term elimination of the gradient in most of patients.[100] A residual gradient over 10 mm Hg is associated with an increased risk of adverse cardiovascular events.[100] Because angioplasty alone is followed by a high rate of hypertension and the need for reintervention, stenting is now routinely employed.[100-102] In younger patients, it remains to be seen whether angioplasty with stenting competes with surgery in the long run.

Pulmonary Valve Stenosis

Isolated pulmonary stenosis is typically represented by fusion (nonseparation) of the commissures of a thin mobile trileaflet valve. In older adults, however, the leaflets thicken and occasionally calcify. Right ventriculography and two-dimensional echocardiography identify pliability and doming of the valve and establish the presence and degree of secondary hypertrophic subpulmonary stenosis. Balloon valvuloplasty is the procedure of choice and is almost always feasible in pliant mobile valves. Secondary hypertrophic subpulmonary stenosis usually regresses. A coexisting interatrial communication (patent foramen ovale or ASD) should be closed. When the leaflets are calcified, thickened, and immobile, replacement of the valve is required. A bioprosthesis is the valve of choice (see Chapter 16).

Tetralogy of Fallot

Occasionally, patients with tetralogy of Fallot (TOF) who underwent palliative procedures in childhood present as adults for intracardiac repair.[103] However, the majority of patients reaching adulthood underwent intracardiac repair rather than childhood palliation.[104-113] Aortopulmonary collaterals are common when the tetralogy is accompanied by pulmonary atresia. An occasional acyanotic or mildly cyanotic unoperated patient survives because a nicely balanced degree of obstruction to right ventricular outflow permits adequate but not excessive pulmonary blood flow. Unoperated cyanotic patients occasionally survive to adulthood because of abundant collaterals (discussed later).

Obstruction to right ventricular outflow is typically subvalvular, valvular, and supravalvular because of the rightward and anterior deviation of the infundibular septum inherent with a malaligned ventricular septal defect. The pulmonary valve is often bicuspid and thickened, and the annulus is small. The pulmonary trunk and proximal branch arteries may be inherently obstructed or kinked secondary to palliative shunts. Systemic-to-pulmonary shunts are usually outgrown at an early age, so additional palliation or a more definitive repair is required. The modified BT shunt or a central shunt is currently used for palliation. Potts (descending aorta-to-left pulmonary artery) and Waterston (ascending aorta-to-right pulmonary artery) shunts are no longer used but are occasionally responsible for adult survival.

Residual VSDs, residual or recurrent obstruction to right ventricular outflow, and a major degree of pulmonary regurgitation are indications for reoperation in adults. Right ventricle-to-pulmonary artery conduits require replacement. Aortic valve regurgitation may require repair or valve replacement. Severe pulmonary regurgitation is an immediate sequel of repair with a transannular patch and is a delayed sequel of a subannular incision (Figs. 15–6 and 15–7). Pulmonary valve replacement not only has a hemodynamic purpose but also has an important electrophysiologic effect because severe regurgitation is a trigger for reentrant monomorphic ventricular tachycardia in patients with sites of postventriculotomy-slowed conduction[114] (see Chapter 22). Right ventricular outflow aneurysms are usually sequelae of an excessively large transannular patch (see Fig. 15–6). A QRS duration ≥180 milliseconds or a progressive increase in QRS duration often coincides with foci of slowed conduction,[115,116] but more specific is the signal averaged electrocardiogram (see Chapter 22). Pacemakers are occasionally required in less than 4% of patients late after TOF repair for sick sinus syndrome or high-degree heart block.[116]

Aorta-pulmonary collaterals should be identified and the coil occluded (see Chapter 18). Knowledge of the coronary anatomy avoids injury during a right ventriculotomy. Adults older than age 40 years and those with risk factors for coronary artery disease should undergo coronary angiography. MRI and CT define the morphology of the right ventricular outflow tract and establish the proximity of the right ventricle-to-pulmonary artery conduit or an outflow aneurysm to the sternum (see Chapter 7).

Systemic-to-pulmonary artery shunts should be controlled as soon as cardiopulmonary bypass is instituted. Takedown of a BT shunt is achieved by dissection, proximal and distal ligation, and division. Takedown of a Waterston shunt is accomplished from within the peri-

cardium, and the right pulmonary artery is reconstructed with a pericardial or GORE-TEX® patch. Takedown of a Potts anastomosis (see Fig. 15–9) usually requires low flow or circulatory arrest.[117]

Although residual VSDs can be approached through the right atrium, revision of the right ventricular scar serves the additional purpose of removing sites of slowed conduction that are substrates for monomorphic ventricular tachycardia (see Chapter 22). The pulmonary valve is replaced with an oversized bioprosthesis seated slightly below the annulus of the right ventricular outflow tract (see Fig. 15–7). A transannular hood of pericardium or GORE-TEX® establishes continuity to the pulmonary artery. Homografts may be used as well (Fig. 15–8). The tricuspid valve is usually repaired with an annuloplasty and rarely requires replacement. Survival patterns after operation and reoperation are the subjects of Chapter 5.

Pulmonary Atresia with Ventricular Septal Defect and Major Aortic-to-Pulmonary Collaterals

True pulmonary arteries are absent or hypoplastic, continuous or discontinuous. Collaterals may be the dominant or only blood supply to the lungs. Adequate but not excessive pulmonary blood flow occasionally permits unoperated adult survival. Dilatation of the ascending aorta is common and is the result of an inherent medial abnormality (see Chapter 12) and often responsible for appreciable regurgitation. Stenoses of proximal or distal pulmonary arteries may be sequelae of previous shunts.

Definitive procedures in adults require takedown of previously placed shunts. Systemic-to-pulmonary artery

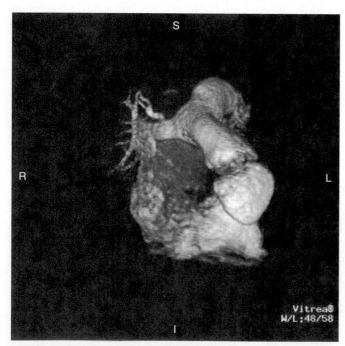

FIGURE 15–6 Three-dimensional image showing aneurysmal dilatation of the right ventricular outflow tract in a patient with repaired tetralogy of Fallot.

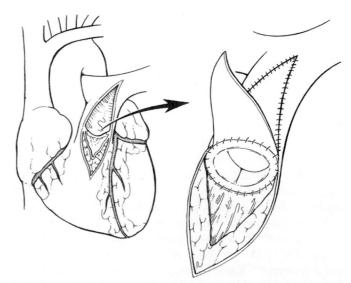

FIGURE 15–7 Pulmonary valve replacement with patch enlargement of the right ventricular outflow tract. The incision extends across the annulus and beyond the bifurcation to the left pulmonary artery.

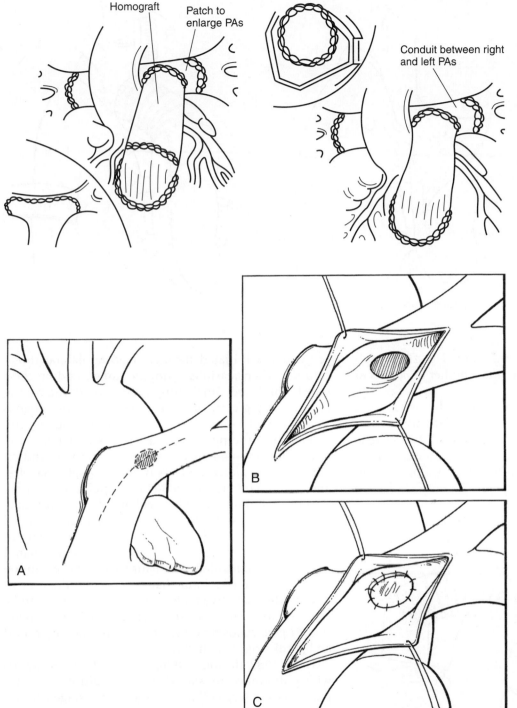

FIGURE 15–8 Repair of tetralogy of Fallot. Ventricular septal defect closure and homograft replacement of the right ventricular outflow tract with hood augmentation of the proximal anastomosis and patch enlargement of the branch pulmonary arteries. A reinforced GORE-TEX® conduit may be placed behind the aorta to reestablish continuity between right and left pulmonary arteries.

FIGURE 15–9 Patch repair of a Potts shunt anastomosis. The main and left pulmonary arteries are incised **(A)** to expose the opening **(B)** in the posterior proximal left pulmonary artery. The defect is closed with a pericardial or prosthetic patch **(C)**.

shunts should be controlled as soon as cardiopulmonary bypass is instituted. Takedown of a Waterston shunt is performed from within the pericardium. The right pulmonary artery is reconstructed with a pericardial or GORE-TEX® patch. Takedown of a Potts anastomosis (Fig. 15–9) usually requires low flow or circulatory arrest.[117] Takedown of a BT shunt is achieved by dissection, proximal and distal ligation, and division at the initiation of cardiopulmonary bypass. Early palliative procedures are designed to create adequate pulmonary blood flow and to encourage growth of the true pulmonary arteries. The goal of surgical management of pulmonary atresia with ventricular septal defect and multiple aortic-to-pulmonary collaterals is to establish continuity between the right ventricle and contiguous pulmonary arteries that permit closure of the ventricular septal defect. To this end, staged unifocalization procedures are employed.[118-123] After unifocalization on one side (Fig. 15–10), the opposite side is

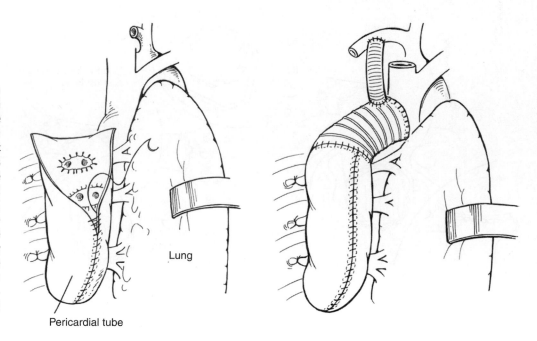

FIGURE 15–10 Unifocalization using a pericardial tube. Through a lateral thoracotomy, a side-to-side anastomosis is created to each major collateral, and an adjacent incision is made in the autologous pericardium placed behind the lung. The pericardium is fashioned into a tube by suturing the edges, and the collaterals are then ligated proximal to the tube. The posterior lying tube is extended by a 16-mm GORE-TEX® graft to the anterior mediastinum. A 6-mm GORE-TEX® shunt is established between the subclavian artery and the 16-mm GORE-TEX® extension.

unifocalized 6 months to 1 year later (Fig. 15–11) followed by the completed repair after another 6 months to 1 year (Fig. 15–12).

Unifocalization procedures join the multifocal sources of pulmonary flow (true pulmonary arteries and aortic-to-pulmonary artery collaterals) into a single source that is ultimately accessed in the anterior mediastinum via median sternotomy. The unifocalization procedure is initiated through a posterolateral thoracotomy. When feasible, a double-lumen endotracheal tube is employed. Single-lung ventilation of the contralateral lung greatly facilitates exposure. Autologous pericardial tube unifocalization of aortopulmonary collaterals and true pulmonary arteries is preferable. Definitive repair entails patch closure of the VSD and establishment of continuity between the right ventricle and pulmonary arteries. Systemic-to-pulmonary artery shunts, including redundant collaterals and surgically created shunts, should previously have been occluded or made readily accessible from the anterior mediastinum for occlusion at the time of biventricular repair. A right ventricular-to-left ventricular systolic pressure ratio of 0.75 or less immediately after termination of cardiopulmonary bypass is acceptable; the ratio can be expected to decrease in the first few days after operation. Higher ratios reflect inadequate pulmonary runoff and predict right ventricular failure.

From 1983 through 2000, 105 children and adults with pulmonary atresia, VSD, and multiple aorta-to-pulmonary artery collaterals underwent staged unifocalization at UCLA. Eight adults underwent uneventful complete repair without mortality or important morbidity. In adults whose blood supply to the lungs is predominantly from collaterals, the multiple-staged approach is preferred. The mortality rate and need for postoperative interventional cardiac catheterization is lower than reports of single-stage repairs. When the blood supply is predominantly from true pulmonary arteries, a one-stage repair is used. As patients age, reoperations are required to replace right ventricular-to-pulmonary artery homografts and degenerated bioprostheses.

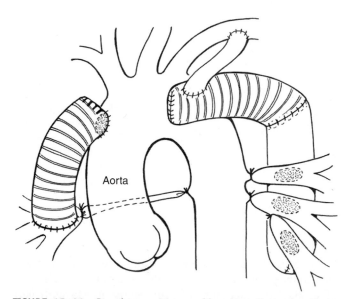

FIGURE 15–11 Based on a 19-year-old male patient who at age 18 years underwent left pericardial tube unifocalization to three collaterals. There was a single collateral to a large pulmonary artery supplying the entire right lung. Right-sided unifocalization was achieved by ligating the collateral and placing a 20-mm GORE-TEX® graft from the right pulmonary artery to the ascending aorta, creating a central restrictive anastomosis.

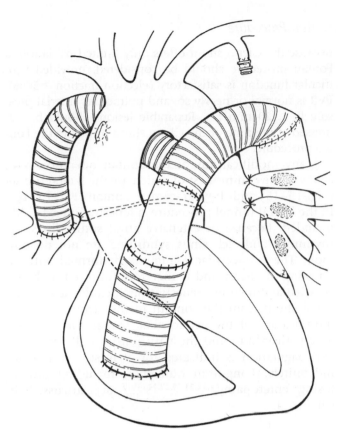

FIGURE 15-12   Complete repair performed after bilateral unifocalizations. The ventricular septal defect was closed. An aortic homograft conduit was placed between the right ventricle and the left unifocalization. The right unifocalization was then connected to the homograft by a 16-mm reinforced GORE-TEX® tube placed behind the aorta.

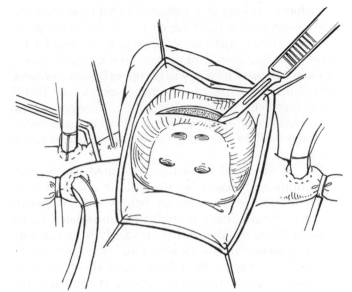

FIGURE 15-13   Takedown of a Mustard baffle. Opening the anatomic right atrium (functional left atrium), discloses the four pulmonary veins surrounded on three sides by the Mustard baffle. The incision enters the atrial chamber that receives systemic venous blood and when completed exposes both caval-atrial junctions and the four pulmonary veins entering a common atrial chamber.

Late Reoperations for Complete Transposition of the Great Arteries

Before introduction of the arterial switch operation in 1982, the Mustard and Senning procedures were the standard surgical interventions for complete transposition. The Mustard procedure uses a pericardial baffle to redirect the systemic and pulmonary venous returns (Fig. 15–13). The Senning procedure uses the atrial septum and wall for the baffle. In both procedures, unoxygenated blood is channeled into the pulmonary circulation, and oxygenated blood is channeled to the systemic circulation. An inherent limitation of atrial switch repairs is the morphologic right ventricle that remains the systemic pump. Long-term survival is dealt with in Chapter 5.

Left ventricular "reconditioning" followed by anatomic correction after atrial switch procedures[124] is conceptually flawed for the following reasons. An immature left ventricle responds to an increase in afterload (reconditioning) by myocyte hyperplasia (replication) coupled with angiogenesis, and thus capillary density remains normal and ventricular function is maintained (see Chapter 23). However, a mature left ventricle responds

to the increased afterload imposed by banding the pulmonary artery by an increase in mass due to an increase in myocyte size (hypertrophy) without angiogenesis, and thus capillary density decreases, and ventricular function is not maintained.

Obstruction of either the systemic or pulmonary veins can almost always be addressed by incision of the site of obstruction and patch augmentation. Repair of the caval part of the baffle enlarges the functional left atrium.[125-139] If the major concern is tricuspid valve regurgitation, the valve can be repaired or replaced.

Single Ventricle—the Univentricular Heart

In the strict anatomic sense, the term *single ventricle* applies to a *univentricular* atrioventricular connection in which both atrioventricular valves are committed to *one ventricular chamber* that qualifies on morphologic grounds as either a right or left ventricle. Functionally analogous but developmentally different is the single ventricle physiology that characterizes tricuspid atresia and mitral atresia. In univentricular hearts as thus defined, unoperated adult survival is uncommon if not rare[31] (see Chapter 4).

Patients with single ventricles are stratified into low-, medium-, and high-risk categories according to pulmonary artery pressure, pulmonary vascular resistance (PVR), ventricular function, and anatomic complexity. In medium- and high-risk patients, connecting the SVC to the superior aspect of the right pulmonary artery (a bidirectional Glenn shunt) can be performed as the first stage of a Fontan procedure or as long-term palliation in anticipation of cardiac transplantation (see Chapter 17). In the Glenn shunt, up to one third of systemic venous return is diverted to the lungs for oxygenation. This proportion is especially true in children who have relatively larger upper bodies compared with adults. In contrast to a systemic-to-pulmonary arterial shunt, the Glenn shunt is tolerated in the presence of impaired ventricular function because blood is channeled to the lungs without increasing the volume delivered to the single ventricle.

The Glenn shunt is usually performed without cardiopulmonary bypass (Fig. 15–14), but repair of additional malformations requires bypass and necessarily increases the risk. Early mortality for an isolated Glenn shunt is 1% to 4% depending on variables such as pulmonary vascular resistance and ventricular function.[140-143] In the long term, the Glenn shunt slowly loses its effectiveness as the lower body grows to adult size and collaterals develop from the superior vena cava to the inferior vena cava.[141-143] These collaterals can be coil embolized by transcatheter intervention (see Chapter 18). Importantly, intrapulmonary AV fistulae develop, resulting in systemic arterial desaturation. Oxygenation can be somewhat improved by constructing an axillary artery-to-vein fistula.[144]

Fontan Procedure

Because the Glenn shunt offers only limited palliation, a Fontan procedure should be considered, provided ventricular function is satisfactory (ejection fraction $\geq 50\%$), PVR is normal or nearly so, and pulmonary arterial pressure is < 20 mm Hg. Reparable lesions should be addressed at the time of the Glenn shunt or before the Fontan procedure.

Many modifications of the Fontan operation have evolved, the commonest of which are the lateral tunnel (Fig. 15–15) and the extracardiac Fontan (Fig. 15–16). In the lateral tunnel procedure, a fenestration is readily included. Because of extensive atrial suture lines, arrhythmias and sick sinus syndrome are not uncommon. The extracardiac Fontan is performed without arresting the heart and is therefore followed by better ventricular function. Fenestration includes a separate small shunt from the conduit to the atrium. A newer modification of the extracardiac Fontan employs Bovine pericardium and the native atrial wall.[9] Warfarin anticoagulation is indicated for at least a year if not indefinitely. Long-term outcomes, including protein losing enteropathy,[7,12,23,25,29,145-150] are discussed in Chapter 5.

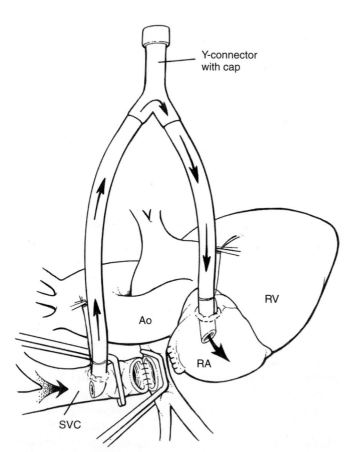

FIGURE 15–14 Creation of a bidirectional Glenn shunt (superior vena cava-to-right pulmonary artery) using an extracorporeal shunt (with systemic heparin) to maintain superior caval flow into the right atrium.

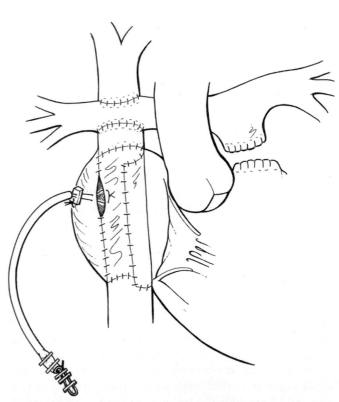

FIGURE 15–15 A lateral tunnel Fontan operation enlarges the right atrium and directs inferior caval flow into the right pulmonary artery using an end-to-side anastomosis to provide bidirectional flow into both pulmonary arteries. A snared pursestring suture adjusts the size of an atrial septal opening used to decompress caval pressures and control the amount of residual right-to-left shunting.

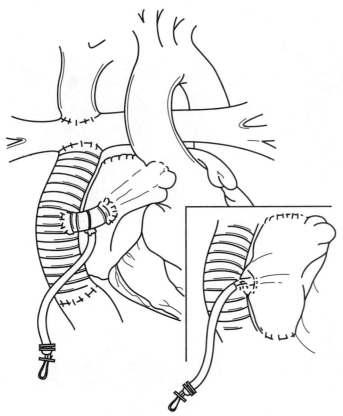

FIGURE 15-16   Extracardiac Fontan with adjustable conduit to atrial connection.

Reoperation is indicated for a failing Fontan circulation, atrial tachyarrhythmias, AV node dysfunction, cyanosis, exercise intolerance, protein-losing enteropathy, and atrioventricular valve regurgitation. Reoperation procedures include Fontan revision, fenestration, pacemaker insertion, a Maze procedure, repair or replacement of an AV valve, and heart transplantation.[152-159] A right atrial-to-pulmonary arterial connection is typically accompanied by massive right atrial enlargement, atrial arrhythmias, and thromboembolism.[145,147,149] Such patients should be considered for conversion into a lateral tunnel or an extracardiac conduit with a right-sided Maze procedure, a reduction of right atrium size, and often a pacemaker.[11,26,27,32,151] If the criteria for Fontan conversion are lacking, cardiac transplantation is an option[152-159] (see Chapter 17).

Ebstein's Anomaly

Right-sided Wolff-Parkinson-White accessory pathways occur in 10% to 18% of these patients[160] and should be mapped and radiofrequency ablated before surgery (see Chapter 22). An accessory pathway with a short antegrade refractory period permits an extremely rapid ventricular response to atrial flutter or fibrillation that can induce ventricular fibrillation.

The atrialized right ventricle is highly arrhythmogenic because it consists of clusters of cardiomyocytes isolated within a fibrous matrix that prevents spiral/scroll reentrant waves from anchoring[161] (see Chapter 22). Excitation provokes polymorphic ventricular tachycardia/fibrillation rather than monomorphic ventricular tachycardia.[161] The arrhythmogenic site must therefore be excluded at operation.[162-166]

Indications for surgical intervention in Ebstein's malformation include New York Heart Association class III or IV, a decline in exercise tolerance, significant or progressive cyanosis, a cardiothoracic ratio greater than 0.65, right ventricular outflow obstruction, a history of paradoxical emboli, and refractory atrial or ventricular tachyarrhythmias. Technical feasibility depends on the presence of a large mobile anterior leaflet that can be identified by echocardiography[165,167-169] (see Chapter 6).

Two techniques of repair have been successfully employed. Danielson[170] reported a repair that includes an annuloplasty and plication of the atrialized right ventricle back to the true annulus (Fig. 15-17). Carpentier[171] then described a technique in which the atrialized right ventricle is plicated perpendicular to the valve annulus toward the cardiac apex, and the displaced leaflets are detached from the right ventricle at their base and reattached to the true annulus (Fig. 15-18). The right atrial appendage is excised together with redundant right atrial wall, and an interatrial communication is closed. When there is a large right-to-left shunt, a snare-controlled adjustable atrial septal defect allows continued right-to-left shunting until the right ventricle recovers. In the presence of severe right ventricular dysfunction and low pulmonary vascular resistance, the right ventricle can be unloaded with a bidirectional Glenn shunt (superior vena cava-to-right pulmonary artery) in addition to the previously described repairs.[172] When operation is not feasible, the valve is replaced with a porcine bioprosthesis (Fig. 15-19). A right atrial Maze procedure may reduce or eliminate atrial arrhythmias. An atrial septal defect or patent foramen ovale is present in more than 50% of patients and is closed at operation.

The Mayo Clinic reported operative experience in more than 500 patients with Ebstein's malformation,[173] with data analyzed for 312 patients undergoing surgical intervention dating from 1972. The tricuspid valve was repaired in 43%, and a bioprosthesis was used in 53%. Of patients who underwent tricuspid repair, 12.6% required reoperation for regurgitation. Patients with porcine bioprostheses experienced a freedom from reoperation of 97% at 5 years and 81% at 15 years.[174] Late deaths occurred in 7.3%. Results using various repair techniques have been reported in smaller series.[175,176] Long-term postoperative outcomes are further dealt with in Chapter 5.

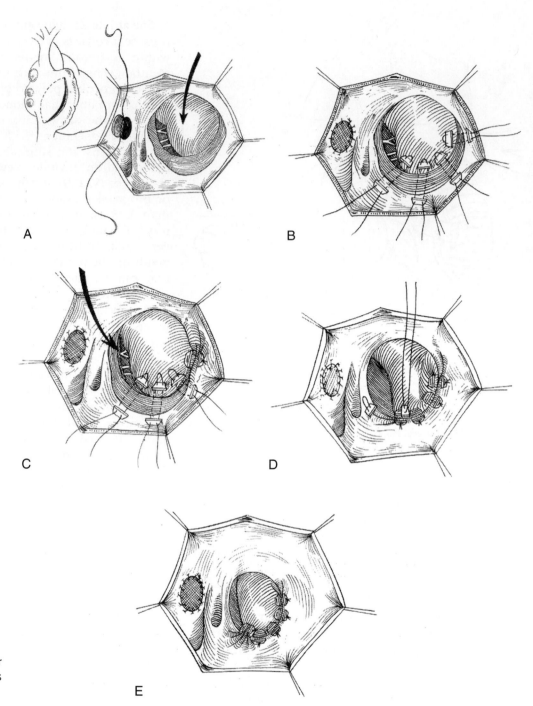

FIGURE 15–17 Danielson repair of the tricuspid valve in Ebstein's anomaly.

Sinus of Valsalva Aneurysms

Closure of a ruptured aortic sinus aneurysm can be accomplished with a primary patch technique from the aortic side. Repair then focuses on an incompetent aortic valve, which may coexist.

Congenital Coronary Artery Fistula

Because surgical mortality in this malformation is less than 1% to 2%, even asymptomatic patients should undergo operation. Preoperative selective coronary ar-

teriography establishes the extent of myocardium served by the feeder vessel of the fistula. The physiologic consequences of occlusion of the distal runoff by proximal fistula ligation are assessed in light of potentially jeopardized myocardium. If the fistula is anterior and relatively small, direct ligation with cardiopulmonary bypass (CPB) standby may be adequate. However, if the fistula is lateral or posterior and is large and tortuous, CPB is required to close the fistula and to perform coronary arterial bypass grafting. Cardiac arrest and myocardial protection are achieved by cardioplegic solution administered antegrade through the aorta while

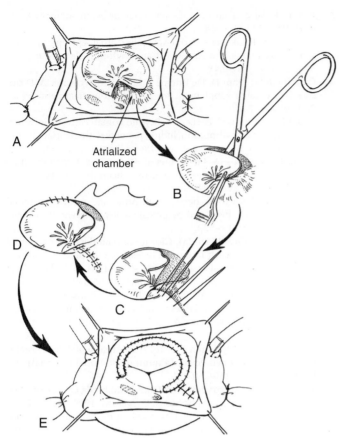

FIGURE 15-18   Carpentier repair of the tricuspid valve in Ebstein's anomaly.

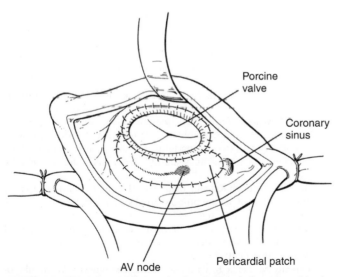

FIGURE 15-19   Injury to the conduction system during tricuspid valve replacement can be avoided by suturing a triangular patch of pericardium over the atrioventricular node and the triangle of Koch.

the fistulous coronary artery is occluded by finger pressure. Combined antegrade-retrograde cardioplegia offers additional protection, particularly to areas of hypoperfused but viable myocardium in the distribution of the fistula.

An aneurysm of the coronary artery feeding the fistula is partially resected and closed when the fistula is oversewn, a procedure that lessens the chance of stasis and clot formation. To obviate myocardial damage, narrowing the lumen just distal to the fistula must be avoided, an objective that can be achieved by keeping the arteriotomy site limited to the proximal dilatated portion of the fistula and by coronary artery bypass grafting to the distal artery or arteries. If the arteriovenous fistula drains into the right atrium (25% of cases) or into the pulmonary artery (15%), closure is achieved by oversewing the distal orifice. When the fistula drains into the right ventricle (40%) or coronary sinus (7%), closure is best accomplished from the proximal aspect. If the fistula is a side branch of a major coronary artery and drains into the left ventricle (approximately 3%), coronary artery bypass grafting should be anticipated. Antiplatelet agents are administered for several months postoperatively if a coronary artery is either opened or bypassed. Surgical risk is low, and symptomatic improvement can be expected even in patients with congestive heart failure.

References

1. Berdat PA, Immer F, Pfammatter JP, Carrel T. Reoperations in adults with congenital heart disease: analysis of early outcome. *Inter J Cardiol.* 2004;93:239–245.
2. Brickner ME, Hillis LD, Lange RA. Congenital heart disease in adults. First of two parts. *N Engl J Med.* 2000;342:256–263.
3. Brili SV, Barberis VI, Karamitros IA, et al. Mild cyanosis due to co-existence of congenitally corrected transposition of the great arteries and Gerbode-type defect. *Cardiology.* 2006;105:41–42.
4. Chessa M, Cullen S, Deanfield J, et al. The care of adult patients with congenital heart defects: a new challenge. *Ital Heart J.* 2004;5:178–182.
5. Deanfield J, Thaulow E, Warnes C, et al. Management of grown up congenital heart disease. *Eur Heart J.* 2003;24:1035–1084.
6. Durack DT. Prevention of infective endocarditis. *N Engl J Med.* 1995;332:38–44.
7. Freed MD. Infective endocarditis in the adult with congenital heart disease. *Cardiol Clin.* 1993;11:589–602.
8. Mavroudis C, Deal BJ, Backer CL. Surgery for arrhythmias in children. *Inter J Cardiol.* 2004;97(1 Suppl):39–51.
9. Moodie DS. Diagnosis and management of congenital heart disease in the adult. *Cardiol Rev.* 2001;9:276–281.
10. Pekdemir H, Gokhan Cin V, Necdet Akkus M, Doven O. Cyanotic tetralogy of Fallot with its infective endocarditis complication on the tricuspid and pulmonary. *Circ J.* 2004;68:178–180.
11. Perloff JK. *Congenital Heart Disease in Adults.* Philadelphia: W.B. Saunders; 1996.
12. Perloff JK, Marelli AJ, Miner PD. Risk of stroke in adults with cyanotic congenital heart disease. *Circulation.* 1993;87:1954–1959.
13. Rogozinska-Zawislak A, Kozak J. Congenital pulmonary arteriovenous fistula coexisting with atrial septal defect. A case report. *Kardio Pol.* 2004;60:63–65.
14. Siegel MJ, Bhalla S, Gutierrez FR, Billadello JB. MDCT of postoperative anatomy and complications in adults with cyanotic heart disease. *AJR.* 2005;184:241–247.
15. Simko LC, McGinnis KA. What is the perceived quality of life of adults with congenital heart disease and does it differ by anomaly? *J Cardiovasc Nurs.* 2005;20:206–214.

16. Suda K, Matsumura M, Matsumoto M. Shunt obstruction after an air travel in an adult patient with cyanotic congenital heart disease. *Cardiology.* 2005;103:142.

17. Therrien J, Webb G. Clinical update on adults with congenital heart disease. *Lancet.* 2003;362:1305–1313.

18. Ullrich NJ, Urion DK. Transient global amnesia in a young adult with cyanotic heart disease. *Pediatr Neurol.* 2003;29:334–336.

19. Walker F, Mullen MJ, Woods SJ, Webb GD. Acute effects of 40% oxygen supplementation in adults with cyanotic congenital heart disease. *Heart.* 2004;90:1073–1074.

20. Webb CL, Jenkins KJ, Karpawich PP, et al. Collaborative care for adults with congenital heart disease. *Circulation.* 2002;105:2318–2323.

21. Chintala K, Forbes TJ, Karpawich PP. Effectiveness of transvenous pacemaker leads placed through intravascular stents in patients with congenital heart disease. *Am J Cardiol.* 2005;95:424–427

22. Cohen MI, Rhodes LA, Spray TL, Gaynor JW. Efficacy of prophylactic epicardial pacing leads in children and young adults. *Ann Thorac Surg.* 2004;78:197–202.

23. Cohen MI, Vetter VL, Wernovsky G, et al. Epicardial pacemaker implantation and follow-up in patients with a single ventricle after the Fontan operation. *J Thorac Cardiovasc Surg.* 2001;121:804–811.

24. Epstein MR, Walsh EP, Saul JP, et al. Long-term performance of bipolar epicardial atrial pacing using an active fixation bipolar endocardial lead. *Pacing Clin Electrophysiol.* May 1998;21:1098–1104.

25. Kucharczuk JC, Cohen MI, Rhodes LA, et al. Epicardial atrial pacemaker lead placement after multiple cardiac operations. *Ann Thorac Surg.* 2001;71:2057–2058.

26. Milgalter E, Laks H. Use of a pericardial patch to bridge the conduction tissue during tricuspid valve replacement. *Ann Thorac Surg.* 1991;52:1337–1339.

27. Overgaard CB, Harrison DA, Siu SC, et al. Outcome of previous tricuspid valve operation and arrhythmias in adult patients with congenital heart disease. *Ann Thorac Surg.* 1999;68:2158–2163.

28. Ramesh V, Gaynor JW, Shah MJ, et al. Comparison of left and right atrial epicardial pacing in patients with congenital heart disease. *Ann Thorac Surg.* 1999;68:2314–2319.

29. Rao V, Van Arsdell GS, David TE, et al. Aortic valve repair for adult congenital heart disease: a 22-year experience. *Circulation.* 2000;102: III40–III43.

30. Roberts AD, Sett S, Leblanc J, Sanatani S. An alternate technique to pacing in complex congenital heart disease: assessment of the left thoracotomy approach. *Can J Cardiol.* 2006;22:481–484.

31. Sabet HY, Edwards WD, Tazelaar HD, Daly RC. Congenitally bicuspid aortic valves: a surgical pathology study of 542 cases (1991 through 1996) and a literature review of 2,715 additional cases. *Mayo Clin Proc.* 1999;74:14–26.

32. Van Nooten GJ, Caes F, Taeymans Y, et al. Tricuspid valve replacement: postoperative and long-term results. *J Thorac Cardiovasc Surg.* 1995;110:672–679.

33. Walker F, Siu SC, Woods S, et al. Long-term outcomes of cardiac pacing in adults with congenital heart disease. *J Am Coll Cardiol.* 2004;43:1894–1901.

34. Donti A, Bonvicini M, Placci A, et al. Surgical treatment of secundum atrial septal defect in patients older than 50 years. *Ital Heart J.* 2001;2:428–432.

35. Gatzoulis MA, Redington AN, Somerville J, Shore DF. Should atrial septal defects in adults be closed? *Ann Thorac Surg.* 1996;61: 657–659.

36. Jemielity M, Dyszkiewicz W, Paluszkiewicz L, et al. Do patients over 40 years of age benefit from surgical closure of atrial septal defects? *Heart.* 2001;85:300–303.

37. Landzberg MJ. Closure of atrial septal defects in adult patients: justification of the "tipping point." *J Interven Cardiol.* 2001;14:267–269.

38. Moodie DS, Sterba R. Long-term outcomes excellent for atrial septal defect repair in adults. *Cleve Clin J Med.* 2000;67:591–597.

39. Oakley CM. Closure of atrial septal defect in adult life. *Cardiologia.* 1996;41:31–34.

40. Perloff JK. Surgical closure of atrial septal defect in adults. *N Engl J Med.* 1995;333:513–514.

41. Ad N, Birk E, Barak J, et al. A one-way valved atrial septal patch: a new surgical technique and its clinical application. *J Thorac Cardiovasc Surg.* 1996;111:841–848.

42. Casselman FP, Dom H, De Bruyne B, et al. Thoracoscopic ASD closure is a reliable supplement for percutaneous treatment. *Heart.* 2005;91:791–794.

43. Deal BJ, Mavroudis C, Backer CL. Beyond Fontan conversion: Surgical therapy of arrhythmias including patients with associated complex congenital heart disease. *Ann Thorac Surg.* 2003;76:542–553.

44. Stulak JM, Dearani JA, Puga FJ, et al. Right-sided Maze procedure for atrial tachyarrhythmias in congenital heart disease. *Ann Thorac Surg.* 2006;81:1780–1784.

45. Hein R, Buscheck F, Fischer E, et al. Atrial and ventricular septal defects can safely be closed by percutaneous intervention. *J Interv Cardiol.* 2005;18:515–522.

46. Holzer R, Cao QL, Hijazi ZM. Closure of a moderately large atrial septal defect with a self-fabricated fenestrated Amplatzer septal occluder in an 85-year-old patient with reduced diastolic elasticity of the left ventricle. *Catheter Cardiovasc Interv.* 2005;64:513–518.

47. Khositseth A, Cabalka AK, Sweeney JP, et al. Transcatheter Amplatzer device closure of atrial septal defect and patent foramen ovale in patients with presumed paradoxical embolism. *Mayo Clin Proc.* 2004;79:35–41.

48. Lloyd TR, Rao PS, Beekman RH 3rd, et al. Atrial septal defect occlusion with the buttoned device (a multi-institutional U.S. trial). *Am J Cardiol.* 1994;73:286–291.

49. Rome JJ, Keane JF, Perry SB, et al. Double-umbrella closure of atrial defects. Initial clinical applications. *Circulation.* 1990;82:751–758.

50. Attenhofer Jost CH, Connolly HM, Danielson GK, et al. Sinus venosus atrial septal defect: long-term postoperative outcome for 115 patients. *Circulation.* 2005;112:1953–1958.

51. Horvath KA, Burke RP, Collins JJ Jr, Cohn LH. Surgical treatment of adult atrial septal defect: early and long-term results. *J Am Coll Cardiol.* 1992;20:1156–1159.

52. Kirklin JW, Barratt-Boyes BG. Atrial septal defect and partial anomalous pulmonary venous connection In: Kirklin JW, Barratt-Boyes BG, ed. *Cardiac Surgery.* New York: Churchill-Livingstone; 1993:620.

53. Kirklin JW, Barratt-Boyes BG. Atrioventricular canal defect. In: Kirklin JW, Barratt-Boyes BG, ed. *Cardiac Surgery.* New York: Churchill-Livingstone; 1993:718.

54. Murphy JG, Gersh BJ, McGoon MD, et al. Long-term outcome after surgical repair of isolated atrial septal defect. Follow-up at 27 to 32 years. *N Engl J Med.* 1990;323:1645–1650.

55. Bergin ML, Warnes CA, Tajik AJ, Danielson GK. Partial atrioventricular canal defect: long-term follow-up after initial repair in patients > or = 40 years old. *J Am Coll Cardiol.* 1995;25: 1189–1194.

56. Burke RP, Horvath K, Landzberg M, et al. Long-term follow-up after surgical repair of ostium primum atrial septal defects in adults. *J Am Coll Cardiol.* 1996;27:696–699.

57. El-Najdawi EK, Driscoll DJ, Puga FJ, et al. Operation for partial atrioventricular septal defect: a forty-year review. *J Thorac Cardiovasc Surg.* 2000;119:880–889.

58. Jemielity M, Perek B, Paluszkiewicz L, Dyszkiewicz W. Results of surgical repair of ostium primum atrial septal defect in adult patients. *J Heart Valve Dis.* 2001;10:525–529.

59. Murashita T, Kubota T, Oba J, et al. Left atrioventricular valve regurgitation after repair of incomplete atrioventricular septal defect. *Ann Thorac Surg.* 2004;77:2157–2162.

60. Michielon G, Stellin G, Rizzoli G, et al. Left atrioventricular valve incompetence after repair of common atrioventricular canal defects. *Ann Thorac Surg.* 1995;60:S604–609.

61. Tlaskal T, Hucin B, Marek J, et al. Individualized repair of the left atrioventricular valve in spectrum of atrioventricular septal defect. *J Cardiovasc Surg.* 1997;38:233–239.

62. Alexi-Meskishvili V, Hetzer R, Dahnert I, et al. Results of left atrioventricular valve reconstruction after previous correction of atrioventricular septal defects. *Eur J Cardiothorac Surg.* 1997;12:460–465.

63. Capouya ER, Laks H, Drinkwater DC Jr, et al. Management of the left atrioventricular valve in the repair of complete atrioventricular septal defects. *J Thorac Cardiovasc Surg.* 1992;104:196–201.

64. Ten Harkel AD, Cromme-Dijkhuis AH, Heinerman BC, et al. Development of left atrioventricular valve regurgitation after correction of atrioventricular septal defect. *Ann Thorac Surg.* 2005;79:607–612.

65. Poirier NC, Williams WG, Van Arsdell GS, et al. A novel repair for patients with atrioventricular septal defect requiring reoperation for left atrioventricular valve regurgitation. *Eur J Cardiothorac Surg.* 2000;18:54–61.

66. Lai YQ, Luo Y, Zhang C, Zhang ZG. Utilization of double-orifice valve plasty in correction of atrioventricular septal defect. *Ann Thorac Surg.* 2006;81:1450–1454.

67. Mace L, Dervanian P, Houyel L, et al. Surgically created double-orifice left atrioventricular valve: a valve-sparing repair in selected atrioventricular septal defects. *J Thorac Cardiovasc Surg.* 2001;121:352–364.

68. McGrath LB, Kirklin JW, Soto B, Bargeron LM Jr. Secondary left atrioventricular valve replacement in atrioventricular septal (AV canal) defect: a method to avoid left ventricular outflow tract obstruction. *J Thorac Cardiovasc Surg.* 1985;89:632–635.

69. Gurbuz AT, Novick WM, Pierce CA, Watson DC. Left ventricular outflow tract obstruction after partial atrioventricular septal defect repair. *Ann Thorac Surg.* 1999;68:1723–1726.

70. Mora BN, Daebritz SH, del Nido PJ Atrioventricular canal defects. In: Selke FW del Nido PJ, Swanson SJ, ed. *Sabiston and Spencer Surgery of the Chest,* Vol II. 7th ed. Philadelphia: Elsevier Saunders; 2005:1963.

71. Van Arsdell GS, Williams WG, Boutin C, et al. Subaortic stenosis in the spectrum of atrioventricular septal defects. Solutions may be complex and palliative. *J Thorac Cardiovasc Surg.* 1995;110:1534–1541.

72. Kidd L, Driscoll DJ, Gersony WM, et al. Second natural history study of congenital heart defects. Results of treatment of patients with ventricular septal defects. *Circulation.* 1993;87:I38–I51.

73. Glen S, Burns J, Bloomfield P. Prevalence and development of additional cardiac abnormalities in 1448 patients with congenital ventricular septal defects. *Heart.* 2004;90:1321–1325.

74. Rhodes LA, Keane JF, Keane JP, et al. Long follow-up (to 43 years) of ventricular septal defect with audible aortic regurgitation. *Am J Cardiol.* 1990;66:340–345.

75. Lock JE, Cockerham JT, Keane JF, et al. Transcatheter umbrella closure of congenital heart defects. *Circulation.* 1987;75:593–599.

76. O'Laughlin MP, Mullins CE. Transcatheter occlusion of ventricular septal defect. *Cath Cardiovasc Diag.* 1989;17:175–179.

77. Arora R, Singh S, Dalra GS. Patent ductus arteriosus: catheter closure in the adult patient. *J Interv Cardiol.* 2001;14:255–259.

78. Bridges ND, Perry SB, Parness I, et al. Transcatheter closure of a large patent ductus arteriosus with the clamshell septal umbrella. *J Am Coll Cardiol.* 1991;18:1297–1302.

79. Chessa M, Carrozza M, Butera G, et al. The impact of interventional cardiology for the management of adults with congenital heart defects. *Cath Cardiovasc Interv.* 2006;67:258–264.

80. Hosking MC, Benson LN, Musewe N, et al. Transcatheter occlusion of the persistently patent ductus arteriosus. Forty-month follow-up and prevalence of residual shunting. *Circulation.* 1991;84:2313–2317.

81. Latson LA. Residual shunts after transcatheter closure of patent ductus arteriosus. A major concern or benign "techno-malady"? *Circulation.* 1991;84:2591–2593.

82. Hazama S, Sakamoto I, Yamachika S, et al. Endovascular surgery using an original occluder for patent ductus arteriosus in an adult patient. *Jpn J Thorac Cardiovasc Surg.* 2005;53:58–61.

83. Ozmen J, Granger EK, Robinson D, et al. Operation for adult patent ductus arteriosus using an aortic stent-graft technique. *Heart Lung Circ.* 2005;14:54–57.

84. Roques F, Hennequin JL, Sanchez B, et al. Aortic stent-graft for patent ductus arteriosus in adults: the aortic exclusion technique. *Ann Thorac Surg.* 2001;71:1708–1709.

85. Campbell M. Natural history of persistent ductus arteriosus. *Br Heart J.* 1968;30:4–13.

86. Ho AC, Tan PP, Yang MW, et al. The use of multiplane transesophageal echocardiography to evaluate residual patent ductus arteriosus during video-assisted thoracoscopy in adults. *Surg Endosc.* 1999;13:975–979.

87. Schrader R, Kadel C, Cieslinski G, et al. Non-thoracotomy closure of persistent ductus arteriosus beyond age 60 years. *Am J Cardiol.* 1993;72:1319–1321.

88. Toda R, Moriyama Y, Yamashita M, et al. Operation for adult patent ductus arteriosus using cardiopulmonary bypass. *Ann Thorac Surg.* 2000;70:1935–1937.

89. Tokuda Y, Matsumoto M, Sugita T. Optimal treatment for adult patent ductus arteriosus. *Ann Thorac Surg.* 2001;72:2186.

90. Marx GR. "Repaired" aortic coarctation in adults: not a "simple" congenital heart defect. *J Am Coll Cardiol.* 2000;35:1003–1006.

91. Aris A, Subirana MT, Ferres P, Torner-Soler M. Repair of aortic coarctation in patients more than 50 years of age. *Ann Thorac Surg.* 1999;67:1376–1379.

92. Bauer M, Alexi-Meskishvili VV, Bauer U, et al. Benefits of surgical repair of coarctation of the aorta in patients older than 50 years. *Ann Thorac Surg.* 2001;72:2060–2064.

93. Bouchart F, Dubar A, Tabley A, et al. Coarctation of the aorta in adults: surgical results and long-term follow-up. *Ann Thorac Surg.* 2000;70:1483–1488.

94. Kirklin JW, Barratt-Boyes BG. Coarctation of the aorta and interrupted aortic arch. In: Kirklin JW, Barratt-Boyes BG, ed. *Cardiac Surgery.* New York: Churchill-Livingstone; 1993:1263.

95. Almeida de Oliveira S, Lisboa LA, Dallan LA, et al. Extraanatomic aortic bypass for repair of aortic arch coarctation via sternotomy: midterm clinical and magnetic resonance imaging results. *Ann Thorac Surg.* 2003;76:1962–1966.

96. Arakelyan V, Spiridonov A, Bockeria L. Ascending-to-descending aortic bypass via right thoracotomy for complex (re-) coarctation and hypoplastic aortic arch. *Eur J Cardiothorac Surg.* 2005;27:815–820.

97. Hellenbrand WE, Allen HD, Golinko RJ, et al. Balloon angioplasty for aortic recoarctation: results of Valvuloplasty and Angioplasty of Congenital Anomalies Registry. *Am J Cardiol.* 1990;65:793–797.

98. Rosenthal E. Stent implantation for aortic coarctation: the treatment of choice in adults? *J Am Coll Cardiol.* 2001;38:1524–1527.

99. Walhout RJ, Lekkerkerker JC, Ernst SM, et al. Angioplasty for coarctation in different aged patients. *Am Heart J.* 2002;144:180–186.

100. Zabal C, Attie F, Rosas M, et al. The adult patient with native coarctation of the aorta: balloon angioplasty or primary stenting? *Heart.* 2003;89:77–83.

101. Carr JA. The results of catheter-based therapy compared with surgical repair of adult aortic coarctation. *J Am Coll Cardiol.* 2006;47:1101–1107.

102. Harrison DA, McLaughlin PR, Lazzam C, et al. Endovascular stents in the management of coarctation of the aorta in the adolescent and adult: one year follow up. *Heart.* 2001;85:561–566.

103. Stewart S, Alexson C, Manning J, et al. Long-term palliation with the classic Blalock-Taussig shunt. *J Thorac Cardiovasc Surg.* 1988;96:117–121.

104. Dittrich S, Vogel M, Dahnert I, et al. Surgical repair of tetralogy of Fallot in adults today. *Clin Cardiol.* 1999;22:460–464.

105. Jonsson H, Ivert T, Jonasson R, et al. Work capacity and central hemodynamics thirteen to twenty-six years after repair of tetralogy of Fallot. *J Thorac Cardiovasc Surg.* 1995;110:416–426.

106. Nollert G, Fischlein T, Bouterwek S, et al. Long-term results of total repair of tetralogy of Fallot in adulthood: 35 years follow-up in 104 patients corrected at the age of 18 or older. *Thorac Cardiovasc Surg.* 1997;45:178–181.

107. Oechslin EN, Harrison DA, Harris L, et al. Reoperation in adults with repair of tetralogy of Fallot: indications and outcomes. *J Thorac Cardiovasc Surg.* 1999;118:245-251.

108. Pome G, Rossi C, Colucci V, et al. Late reoperations after repair of tetralogy of Fallot. *Eur J Cardiothorac Surg.* 1992;6:31-35.

109. Rammohan M, Airan B, Bhan A, et al. Total correction of tetralogy of Fallot in adults—surgical experience. *Inter J Cardiol.* 1998;63: 121-128.

110. Rosenthal A. Adults with tetralogy of Fallot—repaired, yes; cured, no. *N Engl J Med.* 1993;329:655-656.

111. Therrien J, Siu SC, McLaughlin PR, et al. Pulmonary valve replacement in adults late after repair of tetralogy of Fallot: are we operating too late? *J Am Coll Cardiol.* 2000;36:1670-1675.

112. van der Weijden P, Baur LH, Kool LJ, et al. Embolization as a treatment of life-threatening haemoptysis in an adult with tetralogy of Fallot with pulmonary atresia. *Inter J Cardiac Imag.* 1998;14: 123-126.

113. Pacifico AD. Reoperations after repair of tetralogy of Fallot. In: Stark J, ed. *Reoperations in Cardiac Surgery.* Berlin: Springer-Verlag; 1989;171-185.

114. Harrison DA, Harris L, Siu SC, et al. Sustained ventricular tachycardia in adult patients late after repair of tetralogy of Fallot. *J Am Coll Cardiol.* 1997;30:1368-1373.

115. Cullen S, Celermajer DS, Franklin RC, et al. Prognostic significance of ventricular arrhythmia after repair of tetralogy of Fallot: a 12-year prospective study. *J Am Coll Cardiol.* 1994;23:1151-1155.

116. Garson A Jr, Nihill MR, McNamara DG, Cooley DA. Status of the adult and adolescent after repair of tetralogy of Fallot. *Circulation.* 1979;59:1232-1240.

117. Kirklin JW, Devloo RA. Hypothermic perfusion and circulatory arrest for surgical correction of tetralogy of Fallot with previously constructed Potts' anastomosis. *Dis Chest.* 1961;39:87-91.

118. Duncan BW, Mee RB, Prieto LR, et al. Staged repair of tetralogy of Fallot with pulmonary atresia and major aortopulmonary collateral arteries. *J Thorac Cardiovasc Surg.* 2003;126:694-702.

119. Ko Y, Nakamura Y, Nomura K, Yamashiro F. Bidirectional cavopulmonary shunt using the azygos vein. *Jpn J Thorac Cardiovasc Surg.* 2005;53:213-216.

120. Marelli AJ, Perloff JK, Child JS, Laks H. Pulmonary atresia with ventricular septal defect in adults. *Circulation.* 1994;89: 243-251.

121. Permut LC, Laks H. Surgical management of pulmonary atresia with ventricular septal defect and multiple aortopulmonary collaterals. In: Karp RB, Laks H, Wechsler AS, ed. *Advances in Cardiac Surgery.* St. Louis: Mosby Year Book; 1999:75.

122. Reichenspurner H, Netz H, Uberfuhr P, et al. Heart-lung transplantation in a patient with pulmonary atresia and ventricular septal defect. *Ann Thorac Surg.* 1994;57:210-212.

123. Trivedi KR, Karamlou T, Yoo SJ, et al. Outcomes in 45 children with ductal origin of the distal pulmonary artery. *Ann Thorac Surg.* 2006;81:950-957.

124. Poirier NC, Yu JH, Brizard CP, Mee RB. Long-term results of left ventricular reconditioning and anatomic correction for systemic right ventricular dysfunction after atrial switch procedures. *J Thorac Cardiovasc Surg.* 2004;127:975-981.

125. Cetta F, Bonilla JJ, Lichtenberg RC, et al. Anatomic correction of dextrotransposition of the great arteries in a 36-year-old patient. *Mayo Clin Proc.* 1997;72:245-247.

126. Chang AC, Wernovsky G, Wessel DL, et al. Surgical management of late right ventricular failure after Mustard or Senning repair. *Circulation.* 1992;86:II140-149.

127. Cochrane AD, Karl TR, Mee RB. Staged conversion to arterial switch for late failure of the systemic right ventricle. *Ann Thorac Surg.* 1993;56:854-861.

128. Connelly MS, Liu PP, Williams WG, et al. Congenitally corrected transposition of the great arteries in the adult: functional status and complications. *J Am Coll Cardiol.* 1996;27:1238-1243.

129. Fredriksen PM, Chen A, Veldtman G, et al. Exercise capacity in adult patients with congenitally corrected transposition of the great arteries. *Heart.* 2001;85:191-195.

130. Hechter SJ, Webb G, Fredriksen PM, et al. Cardiopulmonary exercise performance in adult survivors of the Mustard procedure. *Cardiol Young.* 2001;11:407-414.

131. Kirklin JW, Blackstone EH, Tchervenkov CI, Castaneda AR. Clinical outcomes after the arterial switch operation for transposition. Patient, support, procedural, and institutional risk factors. Congenital Heart Surgeons Society. *Circulation.* 1992;86:1501-1515.

132. Padalino MA, Stellin G, Brawn WJ, et al. Arterial switch operation after left ventricular retraining in the adult. *Ann Thorac Surg.* 2000;70:1753-1757.

133. Peterson RJ, Franch RH, Fajman WA, Jones RH. Comparison of cardiac function in surgically corrected and congenitally corrected transposition of the great arteries. *J Thorac Cardiovasc Surg.* 1988;96:227-236.

134. Presbitero P, Somerville J, Rabajoli F, et al. Corrected transposition of the great arteries without associated defects in adult patients: clinical profile and follow up. *Br Heart J.* 1995;74:57-59.

135. Quaegebeur JM, Rohmer J, Brom AG. Revival of the Senning operation in the treatment of transposition of the great arteries. Preliminary report on recent experience. *Thorax.* 1977;32:517-524.

136. Serraf A, Roux D, Lacour-Gayet F, et al. Reoperation after the arterial switch operation for transposition of the great arteries. *J Thorac Cardiovasc Surg.* 1995;110:892-899.

137. Stark J. Reoperations after Mustard and Senning operations. In: Stark J, Pacifico AD, ed. *Reoperations in Cardiac Surgery.* Berlin: Springer-Verlag; 1989:187.

138. Turina M, Siebenmann R, Nussbaumer P, Senning A. Long-term outlook after atrial correction of transposition of great arteries. *J Thorac Cardiovasc Surg.* 1988;95:828-835.

139. Webb GD, McLaughlin PR, Gow RM, et al. Transposition complexes. *Cardiol Clin.* 1993;11:651-664.

140. Bruckheimer E, Bulbul ZR, Hellenbrand WE, et al. Takedown of Glenn shunts in adults with congenital heart disease with polytetrafluoroethylene grafts: technique and long-term follow-up. *J Thorac Cardiovasc Surg.* 1997;113:607-608.

141. Elizari A, Somerville J. Experience with the Glenn anastomosis in the adult with cyanotic congenital heart disease. *Cardiol Young.* 1999;9:257-265.

142. Jonas RA. Indications and timing for the bidirectional Glenn shunt versus the fenestrated Fontan circulation. *J Thorac Cardiovasc Surg.* 1994;108:522-524.

143. Kopf GS, Laks H, Stansel HC, et al. Thirty-year follow-up of superior vena cava-pulmonary artery (Glenn) shunts. *J Thorac Cardiovasc Surg.* 1990;100:662-670.

144. Glenn WW, Fenn JE. Axillary arteriovenous fistula. A means of supplementing blood flow through a cava-pulmonary artery shunt. *Circulation.* 1972;46:1013-1017.

145. Driscoll DJ, Offord KP, Feldt RH, et al. Five- to fifteen-year follow-up after Fontan operation. *Circulation.* 1992;85:469-496.

146. Gentles TL, Gauvreau K, Mayer JE Jr, et al. Functional outcome after the Fontan operation: factors influencing late morbidity. *J Thorac Cardiovasc Surg.* 1997;114:392-403.

147. Harrison DA, Liu P, Walters JE, et al. Cardiopulmonary function in adult patients late after Fontan repair. *J Am Coll Cardiol.* 1995;26: 1016-1021.

148. Koutlas TC, Harrison JK, Bashore TM, et al. Late conduit occlusion after modified Fontan procedure with classic Glenn shunt. *Ann Thorac Surg.* 1996;62:258-261.

149. Podzolkov VP, Zaets SB, Chiaureli MR, et al. Comparative assessment of Fontan operation in modifications of atriopulmonary and total cavopulmonary anastomoses. *Eur J Cardiothorac Surg.* 1997;11:458-465.

150. Stamm C, Friehs I, Mayer JE Jr, et al. Long-term results of the lateral tunnel Fontan operation. *J Thorac Cardiovasc Surg.* 2001;121:28-41.

151. Deal BJ, Mavroudis C, Backer CL, et al. Comparison of anatomic isthmus block with the modified right atrial maze procedure for late atrial tachycardia in Fontan patients. *Circulation.* 2002;106: 575-579.

152. Dore A, Somerville J. Right atrioventricular extracardiac conduit as a Fontan modification: late results. *Ann Thorac Surg.* 2000;69: 181-185.

153. Fredriksen PM, Therrien J, Veldtman G, et al. Lung function and aerobic capacity in adult patients following modified Fontan procedure. *Heart.* 2001;85:295-299.

154. Gates RN, Laks H, Drinkwater DC Jr, et al. The Fontan procedure in adults. *Ann Thorac Surg.* 1997;63:1085-1090.

155. Gelatt M, Hamilton RM, McCrindle BW, et al. Risk factors for atrial tachyarrhythmias after the Fontan operation. *J Am Coll Cardiol.* 1994;24:1735-1741.

156. Giannico S, Corno A, Marino B, et al. Total extracardiac right heart bypass. *Circulation.* 1992;86:II110-II117.

157. Kirklin JW, Barratt-Boyes BG. Tricuspid atresia and the Fontan operation In: Kirklin JW, Barratt-Boyes BG, ed. *Cardiac Surgery.* New York: Churchill-Livingstone; 1993:1055.

158. Laks H, Pearl JM, Haas GS, et al. Partial Fontan: advantages of an adjustable interatrial communication. *Ann Thorac Surg.* 1991;52: 1084-1094.

159. Veldtman GR, Nishimoto A, Siu S, et al. The Fontan procedure in adults. *Heart.* 2001;86:330-335.

160. Pressley JC, Wharton JM, Tang AS, et al. Effect of Ebstein's anomaly on short- and long-term outcome of surgically treated patients with Wolff-Parkinson-White syndrome. *Circulation.* 1992;86:1147-1155.

161. Tede NH, Shivkumar K, Perloff JK, et al. Signal-averaged electrocardiogram in Ebstein's anomaly. *Am J Cardiol.* 2004;93:432-436.

162. Attie F, Rosas M, Rijlaarsdam M, et al. The adult patient with Ebstein anomaly. Outcome in 72 unoperated patients. *Medicine.* 2000;79:27-36.

163. Frescura C, Angelini A, Daliento L, Thiene G. Morphological aspects of Ebstein's anomaly in adults. *Thorac Cardiovasc Surg.* 2000;48:203-208.

164. Gentles TL, Calder AL, Clarkson PM, Neutze JM. Predictors of long-term survival with Ebstein's anomaly of the tricuspid valve. *Am J Cardiol.* 1992;69:377-381.

165. Oechslin E, Buchholz S, Jenni R. Ebstein's anomaly in adults: Doppler-echocardiographic evaluation. *Thorac Cardiovascr Surg.* 2000;48:209-213.

166. Saxena A, Fong LV, Tristam M, et al. Late noninvasive evaluation of cardiac performance in mildly symptomatic older patients with Ebstein's anomaly of tricuspid valve: role of radionuclide imaging. *J Am Coll Cardiol.* 1991;17:182-186.

167. Celermajer DS, Bull C, Till JA, et al. Ebstein's anomaly: presentation and outcome from fetus to adult. *J Am Coll Cardiol.* 1994;23:170-176.

168. Hebe J. Ebstein's anomaly in adults. Arrhythmias: diagnosis and therapeutic approach. *Thorac Cardiovasc Surg.* 2000;48:214-219.

169. Kirklin JW, Barratt-Boyes BG. Ebstein's malformation. In: Kirklin JW, Barratt-Boyes BG, ed. *Cardiac Surgery.* New York: Churchill-Livingstone; 1993:1105.

170. Mair DD, Seward JB, Driscoll DJ, Danielson GK. Surgical repair of Ebstein's anomaly: selection of patients and early and late operative results. *Circulation.* 1985;72:II70-76.

171. Carpentier A, Chauvaud S, Mace L, et al. A new reconstructive operation for Ebstein's anomaly of the tricuspid valve. *J Thorac Cardiovasc Surg.* 1988;96:92-101.

172. Reddy VM, McElhinney DB, Silverman NH, et al. Partial biventricular repair for complex congenital heart defects: an intermediate option for complicated anatomy or functionally borderline right complex heart. *J Thorac Cardiovasc Surg.* 1998;116:21-27.

173. Attenhofer Jost CH, Connolly HM, Edwards WD, et al. Ebstein's anomaly—review of a multifaceted congenital cardiac condition. *Swiss Med Wkly.* 2005;135:269-281.

174. Kiziltan HT, Theodoro DA, Warnes CA, et al. Late results of bioprosthetic tricuspid valve replacement in Ebstein's anomaly. *Ann Thorac Surg.* 1998;66:1539-1545.

175. Chauvaud S, Berrebi A, d'Attellis N, et al. Ebstein's anomaly: repair based on functional analysis. *Eur J Cardiothorac Surg.* 2003;23: 525-531.

176. Chen JM, Mosca RS, Altmann K, et al. Early and medium-term results for repair of Ebstein anomaly. *J Thorac Cardiovasc Surg.* 2004;127:990-998.

Prosthetic Materials: Selection, Use, and Long-Term Effects

MARK D. PLUNKETT ▪ JOSEPH K. PERLOFF

Prosthetic materials used in cardiovascular surgery include patches, valves, rings, and conduits. Selection of the most appropriate prosthetic materials for repair of a congenital cardiac defect requires a surgical judgment based on an understanding of the currently available options, qualified in part by patient age and candidacy for anticoagulation. The devices, valves, or materials must achieve an immediately successful technical result while taking into account expected durability, need for anticoagulation, and long-term postoperative effects on morbidity and mortality.

ENDOGENOUS AUTOGRAFT BIOPROSTHETIC MATERIALS

The term *autograft* or *autologous graft* refers to tissue derived from the individual receiving the graft. These materials include the patient's own pericardium, arteries, veins, and valves. *Pericardium*, which is by far the most commonly selected endogenous material for use as an intracardiac patch or baffle, can also be fashioned into a tube that is incorporated into unifocalization procedures (see Chapter 15). *Endogenous arteries*—most commonly the left subclavian—are used to create systemic-to-pulmonary arterial shunts or to reconstruct or augment other arteries such as the transverse or descending aorta in patients with aortic arch anomalies and coarctation. An *endogenous valve* removed from its normal position can be used to replace a diseased valve, most commonly for replacement of a malformed aortic valve with the patient's own (endogenous) pulmonary valve (Ross procedure)[1] (discussed later). A prime asset of an endogenous prosthesis is the likelihood that it has the strength, compliance, and handling characteristics similar to those of the structure that it replaces or repairs. Endogenous bioprostheses have or form an endothelial lining that is seldom associated with thrombus or obstruction and that seldom requires anticoagulation. The materials should readily conform to the natural morphology of surfaces to which they are attached and should be sufficiently compliant to adjust to the phasic changes that accompany filling and emptying of the heart and great arteries. Because endogenous bioprostheses are derived from the host, they are nonantigenic and therefore do not incite an immunologic response. The presence of living endothelial cells and fibroblasts permits an endogenous prosthesis to maintain its substance and configuration, to resist infection, and possibly to grow with the patient.

The shortcomings of endogenous tissues are their limited availability, the effects on the host of removal from their normal locations, and the additional procedure required to harvest them. The amount of removed pericardium is likely to suffice for initial repair of a defect, but if reoperation is required, the remaining pericardium may be insufficient. Harvest of native pericardium risks damage to the phrenic nerves, which may result in temporary or permanent diaphragmatic paralysis. The risk of using arterial structures such as a subclavian or common carotid artery is age dependent, with a relatively low risk of ischemia in neonates and a relatively high risk in older patients. An endogenous valve removed from its normal position requires replacement with an exogenous biologic or synthetic prosthesis, a procedure that adds significantly to the technical difficulty and risk of operation and has a potentially significant impact on long-term outcome.

In congenital heart surgery, pericardium used for reconstruction is subject to exposure to pulmonary arterial or systemic arterial pressure. Accordingly, pericardium that is employed to patch a ventricular septal defect is treated with 0.6% glutaraldehyde for 10 minutes to increase collagen cross-linkage and to prevent aneurysmal dilatation. Pericardium used for a transannular right ventricular outflow tract patch is best treated similarly for at least 5 minutes to minimize the risk of long-term aneurysmal dilatation, particularly in the presence of pulmonary regurgitation or elevated pulmonary arterial pressure. In contrast, pericardium used to close an atrial septal defect or to reconstruct an atrial wall or vein is not treated.

EXOGENOUS BIOPROSTHETIC MATERIALS

Homograft or *allograft* refers to exogenous tissue derived from an individual of the same species but of disparate genotype. *Xenograft* or *heterograft* refers to exogenous tissue derived from an organism of a different species. Exogenous bioprosthetic materials are secured from human cadavers (homografts) or animal sources (xenografts). *Homografts* are cryopreserved and stored in liquid nitrogen for preservation within 24 hours of donor death. The valves are incubated in nutrient medium together with antibiotics, then frozen at a controlled rate to 40°C and stored in the vapor phase (180°C) of a liquid nitrogen tank.[2,3] Tissue trimmings are used for microbiologic control cultures. Actual tissue viability remains uncertain. Currently used homografts consist of aortic and pulmonary valves excised in continuity with their annulus and great artery. The hemodynamic characteristics of homograft valves are optimal because their "natural" attachments permit insertion without reduction of valve orifice size and annular area. Calcification of the walls of aortic and pulmonary homografts occurs within a few years but exerts little or no ill effect on valve function. Homograft valve function can be excellent for 10 to 15 years following insertion in adults, after which there is a 10% to 20% probability of progressive failure. Current data for aortic valve replacement in adults indicate 80% to 90% freedom from significant structural deterioration at 15 years, with low (0.6%–2%) operative mortality.[4,5] Homograft failure occurs in 3 to 5 years in neonates and in 5 to 10 years in older children, depending on the size of the valve, whether the valve is a pulmonary or aortic allograft, and whether the valve replaced is pulmonary or aortic.[6]

The pulmonary valve autograft is a variation in the use of homografts.[7,8] In the Ross procedure, the patient's own pulmonary valve replaces the aortic valve, and a homograft is used in the low-pressure pulmonary position.

Mortality for the Ross procedure in most experienced centers is 2% to 4%, but the learning curve for "double" valve replacement is not well documented. The experience of Ross and colleagues is the largest. Eighty-five percent of survivors were free of reoperation for up to 24 years, and the autograft was free from leaflet degeneration.[7-9] Reoperations were occasioned by infective endocarditis, the substrate for which was valvular regurgitation that resulted from technical faults at the time of the original insertion. Follow-up disclosed no need for reoperation in 85% of cases. In the series by Elkins and colleagues,[9] which is the largest in North America, freedom from reoperation for autograft insufficiency was 83% at 9 years.

Xenografts—exogenous bioprosthetic materials from animal sources—are usually prepared and preserved by fixing the tissue with glutaraldehyde.[10,11] More recently, pressure fixation has improved the preservation process. These fixation techniques serve to prevent tissue breakdown, preserve structural integrity, and reduce antigenicity. Unfortunately, fixation eliminates cellular viability and alters the uniformity with which hemodynamic stress is distributed within the allograft tissue. Because of the fixation process, glutaraldehyde-treated bovine pericardium is thicker and stiffer than fresh native pericardium. Recently introduced CardioFix bovine pericardium (Sulzer Carbomedics, Austin, TX) is fixed by a dye-mediated photooxidation process that avoids the use of aldehydes. The resulting product may prove better for handling characteristics, distribution of hemodynamic forces, durability, and freedom from calcification.

The most important xenograft cardiac bioprostheses are porcine and bovine pericardial valves that are composite biologic and synthetic devices. The leaflets are fixed as described earlier and hand sewn to a synthetic, cloth-covered stent.[11] Bioprosthetic valves have the advantages of a wide range of sizes, ready availability, and a sewing ring that is part of the stent structure. However, the stent and sewing ring decrease the effective valve orifice. This shortcoming is most significant with smaller valves, but the deficit has been successfully addressed by using a thinner sewing ring and supra-annular positioning.[12] The leaflets perform similarly to the natural mechanism and have a low incidence of thromboembolic complications (1% to 3% per patient year) even without anticoagulation. The Carpentier-Edwards Perimount bovine pericardial valve (Edwards Lifesciences, Irvine, CA) has favorable hemodynamics because the pericardium is completely mounted within the stent. Whether this feature will translate into superior clinical results remains to be determined.

Long-term function and durability of current bioprosthetic valves is comparable to homograft valves in adults.[13-15] Bioprosthetic tissue valve durability is significantly coupled to patient age at the time of insertion. Fixation of the xenograft alters the natural characteristics of the valve tissue, rendering it prone to fibrocalcific degradation, fusion, and disruption (Fig. 16–1). In preadolescents, the rate of calcification and failure of a bioprosthetic valve in the systemic circulation is approximately

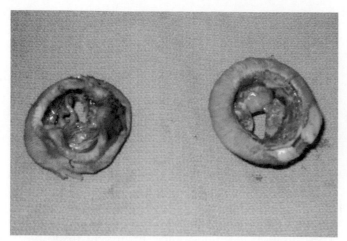

FIGURE 16-1 Calcified Hancock II porcine xenograft valves.

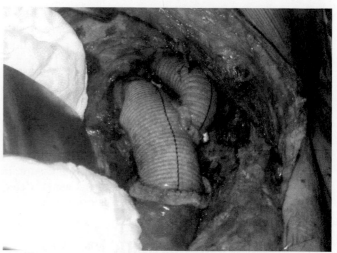

FIGURE 16-2 Dacron graft reconstruction of the distal aorta and left subclavian artery in a 50-year-old woman with aortic aneurysm and recurrent coarctation of the aorta. Flexibility of the graft allows bending which reduces the tendency for kinking at sites of angulation.

10% per year. Degeneration may begin as early as 2 years after implantation and usually occurs by 5 years. In patients aged 35 years or older, the bioprosthetic valve failure rate is between 10% and 20% 10 years after insertion. Bioprosthetic valves possess still greater durability in patients older than 70 years, with a 12-year failure rate of 10%. A bioprosthetic valve tends to have greater longevity in the low-pressure right side of the heart than in the high-pressure left side of the heart and is usually the valve of choice for tricuspid replacement in all ages.[16,17]

The Contegra bovine jugular vein graft (Medtronic, Minneapolis, MN) has recently been approved for use as a right ventricle-to-pulmonary artery graft. The graft incorporates a competent trileaflet valve with associated sinuses, functions well as a valved conduit, and is available in ring-stented and stentless forms in 12-mm to 22-mm sizes. Durability is believed to be comparable to homografts, but long-term results and durability are unknown. There have been reports of aneurysmal dilatation, thrombus formation, and distal stenosis.[18-20]

SYNTHETIC MATERIALS

Dacron fabric (knitted, woven, or double velour) is available as a flat sheet or as a tube graft. Corrugation of the fabric increases its flexibility, allowing natural bending of the graft and a reduced tendency for kinking at areas of angulation (Fig. 16-2). The degree of porosity of the Dacron fabric is an important consideration. More tightly woven fabrics are accompanied by less bleeding through interstices but are somewhat difficult to sew and tend to limit the depth of fibrous ingrowth and the firmness with which the neointimal layer is attached. Conversely, the loosely woven and knitted Dacron fabrics are associated with a significant increase in bleeding through the interstices, especially in cyanotic patients with hemostatic defects, but allow deeper fibrous ingrowth and better anchoring of the neointimal layers. These grafts must be preclotted

with whole blood before use, or the grafts can be autoclaved after bathing with 5% albumen to reduce the porosity. Knitted Dacron grafts rendered impermeable by collagen impregnation (Meadox Medical Inc., Oakland, NJ) are available and have largely eliminated the need for preclotting, albumen impregnation, and autoclaving. Neointimal formation is important in the long-term function of the Dacron prosthesis. Formation of a neointima that is stable and firmly attached to the fabric significantly reduces late complications. Conversely, a neointima characterized by poor fibrous ingrowth and poor attachment to the fabric predisposes to subintimal dissection and excessive thickening that may result in obstruction (Fig. 16-3). The potential for obstruction is increased when turbulence is created by angulation of the conduit or by the presence of a prosthetic valve (Fig. 16-4).

Polytetrafluoroethylene (GORE-TEX®, W. L. Gore and Associates, Flagstaff, AZ) fabric is also available as a flat sheet or tube graft. GORE-TEX® tends to be much less permeable than Dacron and therefore less prone to bleeding through interstices. However, GORE-TEX® fabric may be permeable to plasma, and, on rare occasions, considerable fluid extravasation occurs through the graft. The neointimal layer in GORE-TEX® grafts is usually much thinner than in Dacron grafts (Fig. 16-5) and is therefore less prone to obstruction, although fibrinous material may accumulate at suture lines and at sites of kinking.[21] GORE-TEX® is relatively stiff, has a tendency to kink at sites of acute angulation, and does not adapt well to changes that occur with phasic filling and emptying of the heart. When used as a tube graft in the arterial circulation, GORE-TEX® dampens the propagation of the pulse wave to the downstream artery. A modification called "stretch" GORE-TEX® allows bending of the graft without kinking. Ringed GORE-TEX®

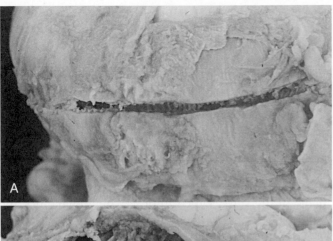

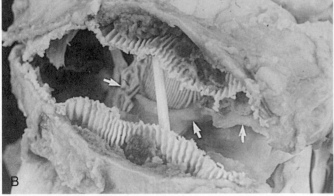

FIGURE 16–3 Specimens from a 42-year-old man with tricuspid atresia and a right atrial-to-pulmonary arterial Dacron Fontan conduit placed at age 20 years. The patient presented moribund after having been lost to follow-up. **(A)** External view of the obstructed conduit at necropsy. **(B)** Opened conduit showing extensive obstructive neointima *(arrows)* and separation of the wall by fresh thrombus.

grafts are tube grafts with riblike rings of rigid polyurethane that prevent kinking or compression of the graft and that maintain a circular form throughout their course. This feature is especially useful for reconstructions prone to compression or distortion from surrounding structures, such as reconstruction of a right pulmonary artery behind the aorta or a right ventricle-to-pulmonary artery conduit that lies behind the sternum.

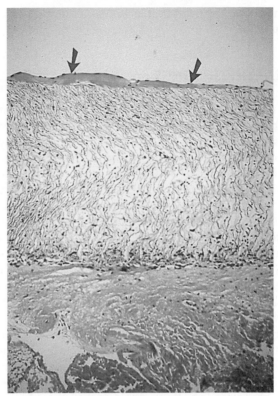

FIGURE 16–5 Hematoxylin and eosin stain of a modified GORE-TEX® Blalock-Taussig shunt 4 years after implantation. The lumen is coated with a thin neointima *(arrows)* (magnification ×25).

Long-term results with GORE-TEX® appear to be more promising than with Dacron.[21–24] The availability of ringed GORE-TEX® and stretch GORE-TEX® has made the materials ideal for extracardiac baffles, as well as for skirt extension of homografts inserted into right ventricular outflow tracts. GORE-TEX® can therefore be used for ventricular septal defect closure and for aortic reconstruction. Placement of a GORE-TEX® pericardial membrane substitute is particularly useful in patients in whom reoperation is anticipated.[25] The GORE-TEX® membrane creates a "safety" layer and a plane of dissection between the

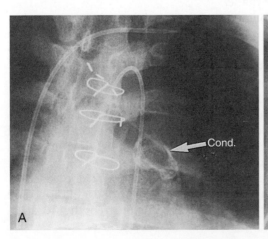

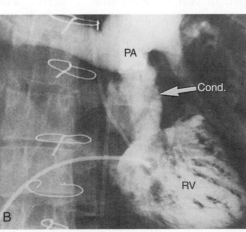

FIGURE 16–4 **(A)** Chest radiograph from a 28-year-old man with double-outlet left ventricle and a calcified obstructed right ventricular-to-pulmonary arterial valved conduit *(arrow Cond)*. **(B)** Right ventriculogram (RV) with opacification of the calcified obstructed conduit. The patient underwent successful reoperation. PA, main pulmonary artery.

sternum and the heart that facilitates a safe sternotomy at reoperation.

PROSTHETIC RINGS

The use of prosthetic rings has increased significantly as improved techniques of mitral and tricuspid valve repairs supplant valve replacement. This is particularly true in adults with congenital malformations such as cleft mitral valve leaflets and Ebstein's anomaly. Successful repair of these valves usually requires both leaflet reconstruction and implantation of an annuloplasty ring. Although annuloplasty techniques using a glutaraldehyde-treated strip of native pericardium are beneficial in some patients, current prosthetic rings provide increased structural integrity for complex valve repairs and achieve long-term durability. These rings are categorized as flexible, semi-rigid, and rigid, and a variety of each type is available. The rings are made of a fabric material (Dacron) that may or may not include a rigid or semi-rigid inner band. Thromboembolism and endocarditis (see Chapter 8) rarely occur following mitral and tricuspid valve repairs with annuloplasty rings. Freedom from thromboembolic events using annuloplasty rings for mitral valve repairs ranges from 87% to 96% at 10 years.[26]

MECHANICAL VALVES

The ideal prosthetic valve should be easy to implant, readily available, nonthrombogenic, resistant to infection, hemodynamically efficient, and resistant to deterioration with lifetime durability. No prosthetic valve fits this description. Despite impressive engineering modifications, thromboembolic complications of mechanical valves have not been resolved. Without anticoagulants, significant thromboembolic events occur at a rate of 15% to 20% per patient year. Warfarin (Coumadin) has reduced this rate to 2.5 events per patient year for the aortic position, and 3.5 events per patient year for the mitral position.[27] However, there is a 2% to 2.5% event per patient year risk of bleeding complications.[28]

All mechanical valves have built-in regurgitation jets that effectively "wash" the hinges of the prosthesis. Intracardiac stasis prevents desirable "washout" within the mechanical valve mechanism and may lead to thrombosis, which is a surgical emergency. Efficacy of thrombolytic agents in occasional patients with valve thromboses has been documented, but restoration of acceptable hemodynamics is yet to be achieved. The *bileaflet* disk valve has an advantage over the formerly used single tilting disk valves because immobilization of one disk or leaflet does not render the entire valve mechanism dysfunctional.[29-32] Opening of the other disk might permit

survival until surgical replacement or thrombolysis is achieved. The On-X valve (Medical Carbon Research Institute, Austin, TX) represents a recent advance in mechanical valve technology. The valve is made from pure Pyrolite carbon that is devoid of the silicon fragment inclusions in other mechanical tilting disk valves, theoretically making the metal structure smoother and the valve less thrombogenic. A flared inlet prevents surrounding tissue from interfering with the valve leaflet mechanism and reduces the likelihood of long-term stenosis secondary to pannus formation and ingrowth. The leaflets achieve a 90-degree opening to the horizontal plane of the valve, which improves hemodynamics and reduces the transvalvular gradient. A multicenter clinical trial is currently under way to assess thromboembolic rates with this valve in the aortic position when left ventricular function is preserved and when the patient is receiving reduced warfarin therapy and aspirin-only therapy.

All prosthetic valves carry a risk of early and late bacterial infection (see Chapter 8). Before the neointimal layer develops on an implanted prosthetic valve-sewing ring, there is a risk of bacterial contamination with infection that is difficult if not impossible to eliminate[33] (see Chapter 8). Late risk of prosthetic valve infection is between 0.5% and 2% per patient year. Antibiotic therapy is seldom successful. Treatment usually requires removal of the prosthesis and replacement with a homograft, a procedure that carries a high mortality rate.

GUIDELINES FOR CHOOSING PROSTHETIC MATERIALS

The choice of prosthetic materials is based on patient age, patient size, the type of congenital malformation, the type of repair, whether subsequent repairs are anticipated, the availability of various synthetic and biologic materials and devices, the risk of infection, and potential complications of anticoagulation. Choices must be individualized, but some general recommendations can be made.

Endogenous autograft materials and exogenous homograft bioprostheses are used with greater frequency in repairs of congenital heart defects, especially if there is a high risk of bacteremia, thromboembolism, or anticipated complications of anticoagulants. The choice of materials is also determined by an attempt to minimize or avoid reoperation. Xenograft bioprosthetic materials are selected when endogenous or homograft materials are unavailable or technically difficult to use. Synthetic cardiac prostheses are chosen when biologic materials are not available; when the risks of bacteremia, thromboembolism, and anticoagulation are judged to be low; and when tensile strength and durability are high priorities.

Mechanical Prosthetic Valves

The Starr-Edwards ball valve prosthesis (Edwards Lifesciences) was introduced in 1966. The current model has a cage made of titanium and a silastic ball. Although the valve is effective and durable, indications for its use are limited because the hemodynamic and thromboembolic profiles compete poorly with newer mechanical valves.[34] However, the Starr-Edwards valve is still implanted in many parts of the world. Tilting disk mechanical valves are either monoleaflet[29-32] (Medtronic-Hall, Medtronic) or bileaflet (St. Jude Medical, Minneapolis, MN; Sulzer CarboMedics; On-X, Medical Carbon Research Institute). Bileaflet valves have low profiles and low mean gradients even in small sizes. All of these valves are made of Pyrolite carbon, which is smooth, relatively nonthrombogenic, and durable. These disk valves are hemodynamically superior to ball-and-cage valves because the effective orifice is only slightly smaller than the annulus.

For the St. Jude prosthesis at 5 years, absence of valve-related events is 84%, absence of valve-related deaths is 94%, and freedom from reoperation is 96%.[29] At 10 years, absence of valve-related events is 75% to 81%, and freedom from valve-related deaths is 84% to 91%. Common to these reports is the paucity of structural valve failure. Similar results have been reported with the CarboMedics bileaflet valve.[32,35]

Stentless Porcine Bioprosthetic Valves

Stentless porcine valves (Toronto SPV, St. Jude Medical; Freestyle, Medtronic; Prima Plus, Edwards) are currently available for use in the aortic and pulmonary positions.[36] Compared with conventional stented porcine valves, these valves have the advantages of an almost complete biologic surface, greater flexibility for compliance, and lower transvalvular gradients. They are, however, more difficult to implant and to explant at reoperation than are stented valves. Early results in older patients are excellent thus far, although there is a small risk of aortic regurgitation. There is more favorable ventricular remodeling after implantation compared with stented bioprosthetic valves.[37] A Dacron cuff on the proximal end facilitates implantation by functioning as a sewing ring but increases the risk of infection when these valves are used in cases of infective endocarditis. Long-term durability is unknown, but data up to 8 years suggests durability that is comparable to stented bioprosthetic valves.[38,39]

Porcine and Bovine Pericardial Bioprosthetic Valves

The Carpentier-Edwards stented bovine pericardial valves have hemodynamic properties that approach those of mechanical low-profile bileaflet valves.[12] Earlier data showed that at 10 years, freedom from reoperation was 95% for patients older than age 65 years of age, and 88% for patients younger than age 65 years. Absence of structural deterioration at 10 years was 91%. More recent data from 12 years of follow-up disclosed a greater than 90% freedom from structural valve dysfunction and a greater than 90% freedom from reoperation.[14] The second-generation Hancock II porcine valve (Medtronic) has similar durability and freedom from structural deterioration.[15] The third-generation Mosaic porcine valve (Medtronic) is treated with zero-pressure glutaraldehyde fixation to maintain leaflet flexibility and alpha-amino oleic acid to achieve antimineralization. Early durability results are promising, but longer follow-up is required to establish the effectiveness of this preparation technique. Other porcine valves are currently available (Magna, St. Jude Medical) with slight variations in structure and preservation techniques designed to improve durability. For all tissue bioprosthetic valves, the rate of structural deterioration is lower in older patients.

GUIDELINES FOR ANTICOAGULATION

The risk of thrombosis and thromboembolic complications always exists when prosthetic materials are used. Guidelines can be generated to assist with treatment strategies, but management must be individualized to meet immediate and long-term needs.

Patches and Conduits

Small pericardial, Dacron, or GORE-TEX® patches do not as a rule require anticoagulants. For short GORE-TEX® shunts, aspirin (325 mg daily) is routine. For baffles or tunnels or for long tortuous GORE-TEX® shunts, warfarin anticoagulation is recommended with an International Normalized Ratio (INR) of 2.5. For smaller prosthetic baffles such as a lateral tunnel Fontan, aspirin alone usually suffices, but additional thrombotic risk factors (Table 16–1) warrant warfarin anticoagulation. Because older patients with Fontan procedures are at increased risk of thromboembolic events, long-term warfarin anticoagulation should be considered.

Bioprosthetic Valves

As a rule, patients with homografts are anticoagulated with aspirin only. Patients with bioprostheses such as porcine and bovine valves are usually treated for 3 months with warfarin followed by lifelong daily aspirin, a regimen that permits formation on the sewing ring of a neo-endothelial lining that resists thrombosis. Alternatively, some surgeons prefer to avoid the risks of warfarin in elderly patients and recommend aspirin from the time of implant. High-flow aortic bioprosthetic valves are much less likely to incur thrombotic complications than

Table 16-1 Risk Factors for Thrombotic Complications with Fontan Physiology

Atrial enlargement and thickening with or without arrhythmias

Elevated transpulmonary gradient that decreases flow within the tunnel

Poor ventricular function irrespective of atrioventricular valve regurgitation

Complex baffling because of unusual venous return

are bioprosthetic valves in the mitral position. Risk is reduced in either position when left ventricular systolic and diastolic functions are preserved. Similar principles apply to bioprostheses in the right side of the heart.

Mechanical Valves

All mechanical valves currently available in the United States require anticoagulation with warfarin. Outcomes of the clinical trial with the On-X valve are under way to determine whether that prosthesis can be managed safely with less anticoagulation. For mechanical bileaflet valves, thrombotic risk is weighed against the hemorrhagic risk of anticoagulation. In the presence of sinus rhythm, the INR should be about 2.5 for a mechanical prosthesis in the aortic position and increased to 3.0 to 3.5 for the mitral position. INR values of 3.5 or more are reserved for patients with atrial fibrillation, multiple mechanical valves, and for mechanical valves in the right side of the heart.

Annuloplasty Ring

For all types of annuloplasty rings in the mitral and tricuspid valve positions, aspirin alone is usually employed, although some surgeons prefer an initial 3 months of warfarin. In the presence of atrial fibrillation or depressed ventricular function, warfarin is indicated.

References

1. Ross DN. Replacement of aortic and mitral valves with a pulmonary autograft. *Lancet.* 1967;2:956–961.
2. Matsuki O, Robles A, Gibbs S, et al. Long-term performance of 555 aortic homografts in the aortic position. *Ann Thorac Surg.* 1988;46: 187–191.
3. Gall K, Smith S, Willmette C, et al. Allograft heart valve sterilization: a six-year in-depth analysis of a twenty-five-year experience with low-dose antibiotics. *J Thorac Cardiovasc Surg.* 1995;110:680–687.
4. Palka P, Harrocks S, Lange A. Primary aortic valve replacement with cryopreserved aortic allograft. *Circulation.* 2002;105:61–66.
5. Vesely I, Gonzalez-Lavin L, Graf D, Boughner D. Mechanical testing of cryopreserved aortic allografts: comparison with xenografts and fresh tissue. *J Thorac Cardiovasc Surg.* 1990;99:119.
6. Forbess JM, Shah AS, St. Louis JD, et al. Cryopreserved homografts in the pulmonary position: determinants of durability. *Ann Thorac Surg.* 2001;71:54–59.
7. Kouchoukos NT, Davila-Roman VG, Spray TL, et al. Replacement of the aortic root with a pulmonary autograft in children and young adults with aortic-valve disease. *N Engl J Med.* 1994;330:1–6.
8. Ross D, Jackson M, Davies J. Pulmonary autograft aortic valve replacement: long-term results. *J Card Surg.* 1991;6(4 Suppl):529–533.
9. Elkins RC. The Ross operation: a 12-year experience. *Ann Thorac Surg.* 1999;68:S14–S18.
10. Starr A, Grunkemeier GL. Expected lifetime of porcine valve. *Ann Thorac Surg.* 1989;48:317–318.
11. Grunkemeier GL, Jamieson WR, Miller DC, Starr A. Actuarial versus actual risk of porcine structural valve deterioration. *J Thorac Cardiovasc Surg.* 1994;108:709–718.
12. Cosgrove DM, Lytle BW, Taylor PC, et al. The Carpentier-Edwards pericardial aortic valve: ten-year results. *J Thorac Cardiovasc Surg.* 1995;110:651–662.
13. Cohn LH, Collins JJ, DiShea VJ, et al. Fifteen-year experience with 1678 Hancock porcine bioprosthetic heart valve replacements. *Ann Surg.* 1989;210:435–443.
14. Dellgren G, David TE, Raanani E, et al. Late hemodynamic and clinical outcomes of aortic valve replacement with the Carpentier-Edwards Perimount pericardial bioprosthesis. *J Thorac Cardiovasc Surg.* 2001;124:146.
15. David TE, Ivanov J, Armstrong S, et al. Late results of heart valve replacement with the Hancock II bioprosthesis. *J Thorac Cardiovasc Surg.* 2001;121:268–278.
16. Van Nooten GJ, Caes F, Taeymans Y, et al. Tricuspid valve replacement: postoperative and long-term results. *J Thorac Cardiovasc Surg.* 1995;110:672–679.
17. Scully HE, Armstrong CS. Tricuspid valve replacement: fifteen years of experience with mechanical prostheses and bioprostheses. *J Thorac Cardiovasc Surg.* 1995;109:1035–1041.
18. Breymann T, Thies WR, Boethig D, et al. Bovine valved venous xenografts for RVOT reconstruction: Results after 71 implantations. *Eur J Cardiothorac Surg.* 2002;21:703–710.
19. Boudjemline Y, Bonnet D, Agnoletti G, et al. Aneurysm of the right ventricular outflow following bovine valved venous conduit insertion. *Eur J Cardiothorac Surg.* 2003;23:122–124.
20. Tiete AR, Sachweh JS, Roemer U, et al. Right ventricular outflow tract reconstruction with the Contegra bovine jugular vein conduit: a word of caution. *Ann Thorac Surg.* 2004;77:2151–2156.
21. Molina JE, Edwards JE, Bianco RW, et al. Composite and plain tubular synthetic graft conduits in right ventricle-pulmonary artery position: fate in growing lambs. *J Thorac Cardiovasc Surg.* 1995;110: 427–435.
22. Bando K, Danielson GK, Schaff HV, et al. Outcome of pulmonary and aortic homografts for right ventricular outflow tract reconstruction. *J Thorac Cardiovasc Surg.* 1995;109:509–517; discussion 517–518.
23. Cerfolio RJ, Danielson GK, Warnes CA, et al. Results of an autologous tissue reconstruction for replacement of obstructed extracardiac conduits. *J Thorac Cardiovasc Surg.* 1995;110:1359–1368.
24. Molina JE. Preliminary experience with Gore-Tex grafting for right ventricle-pulmonary artery conduits. *Texas Heart Institute J.* 1986;13: 137–142.
25. Minale C, Hollweg G, Nikol S, et al. Closure of the pericardium using expanded polytetrafluoroethylene Gore-Tex surgical membrane: clinical experience. *Thorac Cardiovasc Surg.* 1987;35:312–315.
26. Braunberger E, Deloche A, Berrebi A, et al: Very long-term results (more than 20 years) of valve repair with Carpentier's techniques in non-rheumatic mitral valve insufficiency. *Circulation.* 2001;104 (1 Suppl):I8–I11.
27. Akins CW. Results with mechanical cardiac valvular prostheses. *Ann Thorac Surg.* 1995;60;1836–1844.
28. Edmunds LH. Thrombotic and bleeding complications of prosthetic heart valves. *Ann Thorac Surg.* 1987;44:430–445.
29. Khan S, Chaux A, Matloff J, et al. The St. Jude medical valve: experience with 1000 cases. *J Thorac Cardiovasc Surg.* 1994;108: 1010–1020.

30. Horstkotte D, Schulte HD, Bircks W, Strauer BE. Lower intensity anticoagulation therapy results in lower complication rates with the St. Jude Medical prosthesis. *J Thorac Cardiovasc Surg.* 1994;107:1136.

31. Barner HB, Labovitz AJ, Fiore AC. Prosthetic valves for the small aortic root. *J Card Surg.* 1994;9(Suppl):154–157.

32. De Luca L, Vitale N, Giannolo B, et al. Mid-term follow-up after heart valve replacement with CarboMedics bileaflet prostheses. *J Thorac Cardiovasc Surg.* 1993;106:1158–1165.

33. Agnihotri AK, McGiffin DC, Galbraith AJ, O'Brien MF. The prevalence of infective endocarditis after aortic valve replacement. *J Thorac Cardiovasc Surg.* 1995;110:1708–1724.

34. Miller DC, Oyer PE, Mitchell RS, et al. Performance characteristics of the Starr-Edwards model 1260 aortic valve prosthesis beyond ten years. *J Thorac Cardiovasc Surg.* 1984;88:193–207.

35. Lim KH, Caputo M, Ascione R, et al. Prospective randomized comparison of CarboMedics and St. Jude Medical bileaflet mechanical heart valve prostheses: an interim report. *J Thorac Cardiovasc Surg.* 2002;123:21–32.

36. David TE, Feindel CM, Bos J, et al. Aortic valve replacement with a stentless porcine aortic valve. *J Thorac Cardiovasc Surg.* 1994;108:1030–1036.

37. Jin XY, Zhang A, Gibson DG, et al. Changes in left ventricular function and hypertrophy following aortic valve replacement using aortic homograft, stentless, or stented valves. *Ann Thorac Surg.* 1996;62:683–690.

38. Kon ND, Riley RD, Adair SM, et al. Eight-year results of aortic root replacement with the freestyle stentless porcine aortic root bioprosthesis. *Ann Thorac Surg.* 2002;73:1817–1821.

39. Chard RB, Kang N, Andrews DR, et al. Use of the Medtronic Freestyle valve as a right ventricular to pulmonary artery conduit. *Ann Thorac Surg.* 2001;71:361–364.

CHAPTER 17

Cardiac Transplantation in Patients with Congenital Heart Disease

JON A. KOBASHIGAWA ▪ DANIEL MARELLI

The historical events catalogued in Chapter 1 heralded one of the most successful rehabilitation programs that medicine has witnessed. Formidable technical resources permitted remarkably accurate anatomic and physiologic cardiac diagnoses and astonishing feats of reparative surgery. Survival patterns dramatically improved. In the 1950s, only 30% of babies with congenital heart disease (CHD) survived beyond infancy,[1-3] but currently, 75% to 85% survive into adolescence and adulthood.[4-6] It has been estimated, however, that 10% to 20% of this heterogeneous patient population will require cardiac transplantation,[1-8] and those with pulmonary vascular disease will require heart-lung transplantation. CHD patients confront heart transplantation with concerns related to multiple previous operations and to immunologic predispositions that are consequences of frequent exposures to blood products. The transplantation procedure may be technically difficult because of postoperative adhesions, aortopulmonary collaterals, and inherently complex congenital anatomy such as cardiac malpositions, abnormal venous connections, and great arterial positions. The transplant surgeon must adapt the complex recipient anatomy to the normal donor anatomy. Native atrial flaps can be preserved to redirect anomalous systemic venous connections, and morphologic deficiencies or postoperative distortions in recipient anatomy can be compensated by extensive harvesting of donor tissue. This chapter focuses on the indications and special considerations for patients—especially adults—with CHD undergoing heart transplant surgery and the outcomes after transplantation.

INDICATIONS FOR HEART TRANSPLANTATION IN PATIENTS WITH CONGENITAL HEART DISEASE

A prime indication for transplantation is end-stage heart failure with no other surgical or medical therapeutic options provided there is no concurrent illness that would otherwise limit long-term survival. Optimal timing for transplantation can be problematic in a patient with CHD. The decision is usually based on a predicted life expectancy of 2 years or less without transplant, despite lack of secure evidence-based data to support this choice. Rather than predictions of survival, the key determining factors for consideration of transplantation may be a deteriorating quality of life and the need for repeated hospital admissions and complex medical regimens.

CHD anatomy must be taken into consideration before transplant, but no anatomic variation necessarily precludes transplantation. At experienced centers, surgical adjustments can be made for every anomaly. The assessment of pulmonary vascular resistance (by cardiac catheterization) is particularly important because pulmonary hypertension can lead to right heart failure in the transplanted donor heart. In general, pulmonary vascular resistance equal to or less than 5 Wood units or a transpulmonary gradient of less than 15 mm Hg is considered acceptable for heart transplantation, although transplantation centers vary slightly. If higher values are detected, their reversibility should be tested in response to prostacyclin or inhaled nitric oxide. In patients with CHD, assessment of pulmonary vascular resistance may be difficult because of variations in regional pulmonary blood flow and anomalies within the pulmonary vascular bed. In these patients, pulmonary vascular resistance can only be estimated.

The general health of the patient must be carefully assessed. In patients with heart failure, other vital organs may be affected, including the kidney, liver, and lungs. After optimization of cardiac hemodynamics, relative contraindications for heart transplant include creatinine clearance less than 40 ml/min, total bilirubin greater than 3 mg/dl, and pulmonary function less than 50% of predicted. Also important are the psychosocial support and preparation of the patient and the family for life after transplantation.

CHD patients are likely to have undergone one or more previous cardiac operations, entailing homografts and multiple blood transfusions, which can lead to the development of lymphocytotoxic immunoglobulin G antibodies in their circulations. Panel-reactive antibody screening is therefore essential. If these values are higher than 10%, prospective cross-matching should be performed. Finding an immunologically suitable donor organ (no reactivity in the donor-specific cross-match) may be a challenge.

SPECIAL CONSIDERATIONS FOR PATIENTS WITH CONGENITAL HEART DISEASE

Transplantation for Abnormal Situs

Cardiac malpositions may coexist with complex CHD. Right isomerism and left isomerism (the heterotaxies) are prime examples. The complex anatomy poses a number of technical challenges for the transplant surgeon, although almost all anatomic arrangements can be transplanted provided the pulmonary arteries are adequately developed, the pulmonary resistance is low, and pulmonary venous obstruction is absent. Because almost all the cardiac mass is removed at transplantation, the precise intracardiac anatomy is of little relevance. The anatomic arrangements of the great arteries are seldom major concerns, but transplantation can be facilitated by procuring long lengths of donor great arteries. The most challenging problems relate to abnormal venous anatomy. Hepatic veins may enter the lower atrial mass individually (e.g., in some cases of heterotaxy), and it may be necessary to leave the veins attached to a generous button of inferior atrial tissue. In the heterotaxies, the superior caval veins are bilateral. The left superior caval vein may drain into the heart via the coronary sinus (Fig. 17–1). In left isomerism, the inferior vena cava may be interrupted (absence of the suprarenal segment), with the infrarenal segment continuing as the azygous or hemiazygous to join a superior caval vein. It is then critical for the anastomosis of the

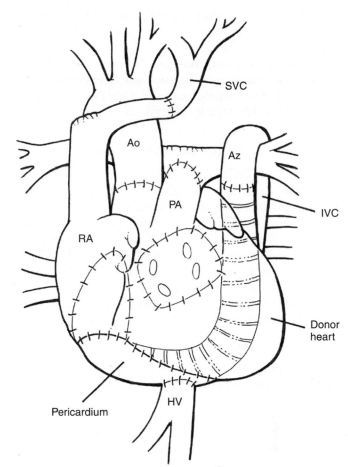

FIGURE 17–1 Heart transplantation after total cavopulmonary connection in a patient with bilateral superior vena cavae. The innominate vein from the donor is used to reconstruct the left superior vena cava. Alternatively (not shown), if the left superior vena cava is too short, a synthetic graft can be used to route left superior vena caval blood along the coronary sinus of the donor heart into the recipient native inferior vena cava.

recipient left cava to the donor right superior caval vein to be widely patent to avoid lower-body venous obstruction. Various surgical techniques have been described to deal with these abnormalities of venous return, all of which are facilitated by procurement of long segments of donor cava and procurement of the donor innominate vein.

Pulmonary venous drainage may also pose technical challenges. In left isomerism, pulmonary venous drainage is generally ipsilateral and can be dealt with by leaving a generous cuff of recipient atrial tissue that incorporates all the pulmonary veins. In right isomerism, pulmonary venous connections are often complex and may be mixed. Obstruction results in increased pulmonary vascular resistance with increased risk of acute failure of the donor right heart. These patients are candidates for transplantation only when there has been prior relief of obstructed pulmonary venous return with no evidence of restenosis. Extracardiac malformations are also matters of concern and must be meticulously identified before embarking on transplantation. In left isomerism, pulmonary arteriovenous malformations cause severe cyanosis, especially after prior bidirectional Glenn shunt, and gastrointestinal abnormalities include biliary and esophageal atresia and congenitally short pancreas. Diffuse arteriovenous malformations contraindicate isolated heart transplantation.[9-13]

Transplantation for the Failed Fontan

Since the early 1970s, the Fontan procedure has provided successful palliation for children with single ventricle physiology. However, a significant number of these patients, particularly those with single morphologic right ventricles, develop late ventricular failure, atrioventricular valve regurgitation, atrial arrhythmias, pleural and pericardial effusions, and protein-losing enteropathy. Many will require heart transplantation, but it is not established whether this group of patients represents a unique transplantation risk.[14-18] There are relatively few adult Fontan patients who have undergone heart transplantation. Much of the failed Fontan experience is derived from the pediatric literature. A large retrospective multi-institutional review consisted of 97 Fontan patients aged younger than 18 years listed at 17 pediatric heart transplant centers from 1993 through 2001.[7] These Fontan data were compared with two additional groups: 747 patients without congenital heart disease (NO-CHD) who were listed for heart transplant during the same time period and 243 patients with CHD who were older than 1 year and who had undergone previous open heart surgery. Mean age for the Fontan patients was 9.7 years (range: 0.5–17.9 years); 25% were younger than 4 years; 53% were UNOS (United Network for Organ Sharing) status one (critically ill); 18% required ventilator support. Pretransplant survival was 78% at 6 months and 74% at 12 months, which was similar to the CHD and NO-CHD groups who were also awaiting cardiac transplantation.

Of the 97 Fontan patients in the multi-institutional study, 70 underwent transplantation. The mean interval from Fontan to transplant was 5.7 years (range: 0.02–15.6 years). Survival was 76% at 1 year, 70% at 3 years, and 68% at 5 years (Fig. 17–2). Survival at 1 year posttransplantation was 8% less than in CHD patients, although the difference was not statistically significant. Survival at 1 year was 14% lower than in NO-CHD patients ($p < .0005$), but after the first posttransplantation year, survival curves of the Fontan and NO-CHD patients were similar, suggesting that the highest risk is in the early posttransplantation period. Causes of death in the Fontan patients included infection (30%), graft failure (17%), rejection (13%), sudden death (13%), and cardiac allograft vasculopathy (9%).

Protein-losing enteropathy was present in 34 patients (37%) at the time of listing for transplantation; the presence of this condition did not influence outcome after listing. Of those patients with protein-losing enteropathy, 73% were transplanted, and 21% died while awaiting transplant compared with 73% and 12%, respectively, in patients without evidence of protein-losing enteropathy. Importantly, the presence of protein-losing enteropathy did not influence survival after transplant. Of the 25 patients with this condition who underwent transplantation, 19 survived more than 30 days posttransplantation, and the enteropathy resolved in all of these patients. Six protein-losing enteropathy patients died less than 30 days after transplantation, too early to determine whether their enteropathy would have eventually resolved.

Heart transplantation is an effective therapy for pediatric patients with a failed Fontan. In a large multicenter study, there was a slight increase in early mortality after

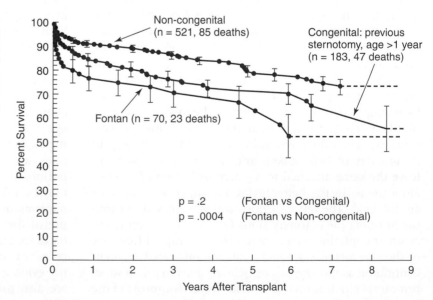

FIGURE 17–2 Comparison of actuarial survival between patients listed for transplantation after a failed Fontan versus those without CHD and those with CHD and previous sternotomy who were older than 1 year of age at the time of listing. There were no differences in survival after listing between groups. *(With permission from Bernstein D, Naftel D, Chin C, et al.: Pediatric heart transplant study. Circulation. 2006;114:273–280.)*

transplant compared with other CHD patients, but the 1-year survival rate of 76% is much better than the high mortality rates reported previously in several small, single-center studies. Complications reported for failed Fontan patients in the peritransplantation period include bleeding due to splanchnic venous congestion and liver dysfunction, microvascular sludging and thromboemboli in the pulmonary vasculature, and false transpulmonary gradients due to arteriovenous malformations, which may predispose to right ventricular failure.[19] Protein-losing enteropathy, one of the major reasons for referral of Fontan patients for transplant, can be expected to resolve in patients who survive beyond the first month after transplant.[7,20-21] It is believed that much of these data can be extrapolated to adults with a failing Fontan.

Transplantation in Patients with Abnormal Pulmonary Anatomy

CHD per se is a risk factor for worse outcome in the first posttransplantation year, with the highest mortality in the early period.[22] Abnormalities of the pulmonary arteries, either native or acquired, are common among patients undergoing transplant for CHD, are regarded as specific risk factors for poor outcome,[2] and include pulmonary artery branch stenosis or hypoplasia, discontinuity of the pulmonary arteries, absence of the right or left pulmonary artery, unilateral pulmonary hypertension, significant aortopulmonary collaterals, a surgically created aortopulmonary shunt, and surgically created structural abnormalities of the pulmonary arteries following a Glenn shunt or Fontan procedure. Careful evaluation of pulmonary artery architecture and flow before transplantation is therefore essential to successful management.

The feasibility of heart transplantation in patients with abnormalities of the pulmonary artery architecture is based on evaluation of the structure, perfusion, and function of the pulmonary vascular bed. Imaging modalities include angiography, magnetic resonance imaging, and ventilation-perfusion radioisotope scanning. Hemodynamic evaluation is employed to assess pulmonary artery pressure and resistance in all lung segments. Pulmonary function testing is often necessary in patients who have had multiple cardiac procedures or prolonged ventilatory support.

Successful heart transplantation has been reported in patients who effectively have a single lung due to absence of the right or left pulmonary artery or unilateral pulmonary vascular disease. Adequacy of the unilateral "good" lung must be established by identifying normal pulmonary artery architecture, normal perfusion to all lung segments, and normal pulmonary function.[23]

Surgical feasibility in patients with structural abnormalities of the pulmonary arteries must be anticipated. Significant pulmonary artery branch stenosis may require stent placement before transplantation to avoid donor right heart failure. Harvesting of additional donor tissue, such as branch pulmonary arteries or systemic veins, may be necessary to permit reconstruction of normal venous and arterial connections, especially in patients who have undergone a Glenn or Fontan procedure. A Waterston or Potts shunt may require temporary occlusion at the time of transplantation to allow the institution of cardiopulmonary bypass.

Recognition of posttransplantation residual abnormalities of pulmonary artery architecture decreases the incidence of heart failure and improves outcomes. If right heart failure occurs and residual stenoses are suspected, early catheterization should be performed with the potential for reoperation. A residual left-to-right shunt through aortopulmonary collaterals can cause high-output heart failure following transplantation. Early intervention to reduce the magnitude of left-to-right shunting by coil occlusion of collateral flow[24] depends on recognition of excessive pulmonary venous return during the transplant procedure and detection of signs of donor heart ventricular volume overload. Aortopulmonary collaterals tend to bleed and cause undesirable perioperative blood loss.

Outcome after Heart Transplantation in Patients with Congenital Heart Disease

Data from the International Society for Heart and Lung Transplantation (ISHLT) reveal that only 2% of adult heart transplants in the previous 2 decades had been for CHD[25] with an 11-year survival of 50%, which is similar to survival in the pediatric population and in adults with acquired heart disease (Fig. 17-3). Although adult CHD is a significant risk factor for posttransplantation 1-year mortality (relative risk = 2.32), there is a subsequent plateau in overall death rate. Long-term survival is then similar to other transplant patients,[1] and the ISHLT Registry data show that CHD is not a risk factor for 10-year mortality. Several small series concluded that the failing Fontan patient has a higher early mortality, thus increasing overall early mortality in the CHD category.[2,4,26,27]

Morbidities for patients specifically transplanted for CHD are not available in the registries but are believed to be similar to morbidities in the majority of other transplant patients. All of these morbidities may be caused or exacerbated by immunosuppression medications. Acute donor heart rejection occurs in approximately one third of patients in the first year after transplantation. By 8 years, more than 97% of recipients have hypertension, more than 14% have significant renal insufficiency (creatinine > 2.5 mg/dl in 10%, long-term dialysis in 4%, and renal transplant in 1%), more than 90% have hyperlipidemia, more than 35% have diabetes, and more than 40% have angiographic evidence of cardiac allograft vasculopathy (an accelerated form of coronary artery disease).[25]

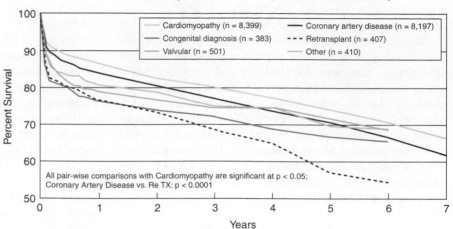

ADULT HEART TRANSPLANTATION
Kaplan-Meier Survival by Diagnosis   (Transplants: 1/1998–6/2004)

FIGURE 17–3 Kaplan-Meier survival curves stratified by recipient diagnosis. In the first year, the type of congenital heart disease is a significant risk factor for mortality. However, after the first year, survival is similar to all other diagnoses except for re-transplants, which have the worst outcome. *(With permission from Taylor DO, Edwards LB, Boucek MM, et al.: Registry of the International Society for Heart and Lung Transplantation: 23rd Official Adult Heart Transplantation Report—2006.* J Heart Lung Transplant. *2006;25:869–879.)*

OPTIMAL IMMUNOSUPPRESSION AFTER HEART TRANSPLANTATION

In the early 1980s, the introduction of cyclosporine, the first oral immunosuppressive agent relatively specific for inhibition of T lymphocytes, resulted in dramatic improvements in survival of all transplanted organs. In the last decade, there has been a major increase in the number of new immunosuppressive agents. A comprehensive review of all aspects of immunosuppressive therapy in heart transplantation has been the subject of several reviews.[28–32]

The increasing number of oral agents used for maintenance therapy has resulted in a large number of drug combinations and potentials for drug interactions (Fig. 17–4).

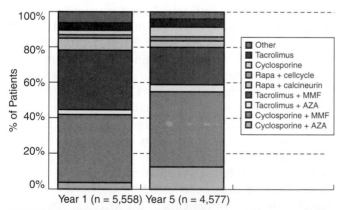

FIGURE 17–4 Combinations of maintenance immunosuppressive agents at 1 and 5 years posttransplantation follow-up from January 2003 to June 2005. Different patients are analyzed in Year 1 and Year 5. In the Year 1 cohort, 76.5% of patients were on prednisone. In the Year 5 cohort, 61% of patients were on prednisone. AZA, azathioprine; MMF, mycophenolate mofetil; Rapa, rapamycin. *(With permission from Taylor DO, Edwards LB, Boucek MM, et al.: Registry of the International Society for Heart and Lung Transplantation: 23rd Official Adult Heart Transplantation Report—2006.* J Heart Lung Transplant. *2006;25:869–879.)*

All immunosuppressive regimens are currently based on the use of calcineurin inhibitors—either cyclosporine or tacrolimus. Cyclosporine was the most commonly used agent prior to 2003, but half of heart transplant recipients are currently receiving tacrolimus,[25] which is generally considered to be associated with a better acute rejection profile, absence of hirsutism, absence of gingival hyperplasia, and a lower incidence of hyperlipidemia.[33,34]

A recent three-arm randomized trial of tacrolimus versus cyclosporine, together with corticosteroids and either sirolimus or mycophenolate mofetil as adjunctive therapy in heart transplantation disclosed lower acute rejection rates in the tacrolimus-treated patients.[35] There is no definitive evidence, however, that either tacrolimus or cyclosporine is associated with less cardiac allograft vasculopathy, less graft loss, or improved survival. Also unsettled are the relative frequencies of posttransplantation diabetes and lymphoproliferative disorders associated with cyclosporine and tacrolimus.

Most transplant centers use a second or third agent as adjunctive therapy, thus allowing enhanced immunosuppressive efficacy while reducing organ toxicities associated with high doses of single agents. Most patients receive some type of antimetabolite/antiproliferative agent. Azathioprine was the most commonly employed adjunctive therapy throughout the 1980s and 1990s, but since 2000, its use has fallen dramatically in favor of mycophenolate mofetil.[25] A phase III study in adults after cardiac transplantation showed a survival benefit for mycophenolate mofetil compared with azathioprine.[36] The newest group of agents used as adjunctive therapies in heart transplantation are the "proliferation signal" or "target of rapamycin" (TOR) inhibitors, which include sirolimus and everolimus.[37,38] The main adverse effects are hyperlipidemia, bone marrow suppression, oral ulcers, and poor wound healing. These agents, when used alone, do not exhibit significant nephrotoxicity, but exacerbation of the calcineurin-inhibitor nephrotoxicity may occur if concomitant dose reduction of the primary immunosuppressant is not initiated.[38]

Pneumonitis and life-threatening pulmonary toxicity have been reported with sirolimus after solid organ transplantation. The most interesting aspect of the use of TOR inhibitors is their potential to prevent posttransplantation cardiac allograft vasculopathy, a serious complication best assessed by coronary artery intravascular ultrasound (IVUS). In separate randomized clinical trials, IVUS demonstrated that coronary arterial intimal proliferation was less pronounced in patients taking mycophenolate mofetil,[39] sirolimus,[37] and everolimus[38] compared with azathioprine.

The weaning or complete avoidance of corticosteroids is one of the most debated topics in adult solid organ transplantation. The benefits of avoiding steroids as part of maintenance immunosuppressive regimens are self-evident. According to the ISHLT registry, 76% of patients were receiving corticosteroids at 1 year and 61% at 5 years after transplantation.[25] The most common maintenance immunosuppression regimens are shown in Figure 17–4.

CONCLUSION

Since the 1970s, heart transplantation has evolved to become a standard treatment for adults with end-stage CHD. Significant advances have been made in performing heart transplantation in patients with complex congenital anatomy and in providing immunosuppression after transplant. Future outcomes depend on improved clinical therapies and on earlier detection and referral for transplantation of CHD patients at high risk.

References

1. Hosseinpour AR, Cullen S, Tsang VT. Transplantation for adults with congenital heart disease. *Eur J Cardiothorac Surg.* 2006;30:508–514.
2. Chen JM, Davies RR, Mital SR, et al. Trends and outcomes in transplantation for complex congenital heart disease: 1984 to 2004. *Ann Thorac Surg.* 2004;78:1352–1361.
3. Dipchand A, Cecere R, Delgado D, et al. Canadian Consensus on cardiac transplantation in pediatric and adult congenital heart disease patients 2004: executive summary. *Can J Cardiol.* 2005;21:1145–1147.
4. Pigula FA, Gandhi SK, Ristich J, et al. Cardiopulmonary transplantation for congenital heart disease in the adult. *J Heart Lung Transplant.* 2001;20:297–303.
5. Mitchell MB, Campbell DN, Boucek MM. Heart transplantation for the failing Fontan circulation. *Semin Thorac Cardiovasc Surg Pediatr Card Surg Annu.* 2004;7:56–64.
6. Perloff JK. Congenital heart disease in adults. A new cardiovascular subspecialty. *Circulation.* 1991;84:1881–1890.
7. Bernstein D, Naftel D, Chin C, et al; Pediatric Heart Transplant Study. Outcome of listing for cardiac transplantation for failed Fontan: a multi-institutional study. *Circulation.* 2006;114:273–280.
8. Chaudhari M, Sturman J, O'Sullivan J, et al. Rescue cardiac transplantation for early failure of the Fontan-type circulation in children. *J Thorac Cardiovasc Surg.* 2005;129:416–422.
9. Schmid C, Tjan TD, Scheld HH. Techniques of pediatric heart transplantation. *Thorac Cardiovasc Surg.* 2005;53(2 Suppl):S141–S145.
10. Vouhe PR, Tamisier D, Le Bidois J, et al. Pediatric cardiac transplantation for congenital heart defects: surgical considerations and results. *Ann Thorac Surg.* 1993;56:1239–1247.
11. Chartrand C. Pediatric cardiac transplantation despite atrial and venous return anomalies. *Ann Thorac Surg.* 1991;52:716–721.
12. Chartrand C, Guerin R, Kangah M, Stanley P. Pediatric heart transplantation: surgical considerations for congenital heart diseases. *J Heart Transplant.* 1990;9:608–616.
13. Menkis AH, McKenzie FN, Novick RJ, et al. Special considerations for heart transplantation in congenital heart disease. The Paediatric Heart Transplant Group. *J Heart Transplant.* 1990;9:602–607.
14. Petko M, Myung RJ, Wernovsky G, et al. Surgical reinterventions following the Fontan procedure. *Eur J Cardiothorac Surg.* 2003;24:255–259.
15. Freedom RM, Hamilton R, Yoo SJ, et al. The Fontan procedure: analysis of cohorts and late complications. *Cardiol Young.* 2000. 10:307–333.
16. Gamba A, Merlo M, Fiocchi R, et al. Heart transplantation in patients with previous Fontan operations. *J Thorac Cardiovasc Surg.* 2004;127:555–562.
17. Michielon G, Parisi F, Di Carlo D, et al. Orthotopic heart transplantation for failing single ventricle physiology. *Eur J Cardiothorac Surg.* 2003;24:502–505.
18. Carey JA, Hamilton JR, Hilton CJ, et al. Orthotopic cardiac transplantation for the failing Fontan circulation. *Eur J Cardiothorac Surg.* 1998;14:7–13.
19. Michielon G, Parisi F, Squitieri C, et al. Orthotopic heart transplantation for congenital heart disease: an alternative for high-risk Fontan candidates? *Circulation.* 2003;108 Suppl 1:II140–9.
20. Brancaccio G, Carotti A, D'Argenio P, et al. Protein-losing enteropathy after Fontan surgery: resolution after cardiac transplantation. *J Heart Lung Transplant.* 2003;22:484–486.
21. Holmgren D, Berggren H, Wahlander H, et al. Reversal of protein-losing enteropathy in a child with Fontan circulation is correlated with central venous pressure after heart transplantation. *Pediatr Transplant.* 2001;5:35–37.
22. Boucek MM, Waltz DA, Edwards LB, et al; International Society for Heart and Lung Transplantation. Registry of the International Society for Heart and Lung Transplantation: ninth official pediatric heart transplantation report—2006. *J Heart Lung Transplant.* 2006;25:893–903.
23. Lamour JM, Hsu DT, Quaegebeur JM, et al. Heart transplantation to a physiologic single lung in patients with congenital heart disease. *J Heart Lung Transplant.* 2004;23:948–953.
24. Krishnan US, Lamour JM, Hsu DT, et al. Management of aortopulmonary collaterals in children following cardiac transplantation for complex congenital heart disease. *J Heart Lung Transplant.* 2004;23:564–569.
25. Taylor DO, Edwards LB, Boucek MM, et al; International Society for Heart and Lung Transplantation. Registry of the International Society for Heart and Lung Transplantation: Twenty-third Official Adult Heart Transplantation Report—2006. *J Heart Lung Transplant.* 2006;25:869–879.
26. Lamour JM, Addonizio LJ, Galantowicz ME, et al. Outcome after orthotopic cardiac transplantation in adults with congenital heart disease. *Circulation.* 1999;100(19 Suppl):II 200–II205.
27. Hasan A, Au J, Hamilton JR, et al. Orthotopic heart transplantation for congenital heart disease. Technical considerations. *Eur J Cardiothorac Surg.* 1993;7:65–70.
28. Kobashigawa JA, Patel JK. Immunosuppression for heart transplantation: where are we now? *Nat Clin Pract Cardiovasc Med.* 2006;3:203–212.
29. Lindenfeld J, Miller GG, Shakar SF, et al. Drug therapy in the heart transplant recipient: part I: cardiac rejection and immunosuppressive drugs. *Circulation.* 2004 14;110:3734–3740.
30. Lindenfeld J, Miller GG, Shakar SF, et al. Drug therapy in the heart transplant recipient: part II: immunosuppressive drugs. *Circulation.* 2004;110:3858–3865.

31. Lindenfeld J, Page RL 2nd, Zolty R, et al. Drug therapy in the heart transplant recipient: part III: common medical problems. *Circulation.* 2005;111:113–117.
32. Page RL 2nd, Miller GG, Lindenfeld J. Drug therapy in the heart transplant recipient: part IV: drug-drug interactions. *Circulation.* 2005;111:230–239.
33. Webber SA. Fifteen years of pediatric heart transplantation at the University of Pittsburgh: lessons learned and future prospects. *Pediatr Transplant.* 1997;1:8–21.
34. Law YM, Yim R, Agatisa P, et al. Lipid profiles in pediatric thoracic transplant recipients are determined by their immunosuppressive regimens. *J Heart Lung Transplant.* 2006;25:276–282.
35. Kobashigawa J, Miller LW, Russell SD, et al; Study Investigators. Tacrolimus with mycophenolate mofetil (MMF) or sirolimus vs. cyclosporine with MMF in cardiac transplant patients: 1-year report. *Am J Transplant.* 2006;6:1377–1386.
36. Kobashigawa J, Miller L, Renlund D, et al. A randomized active-controlled trial of mycophenolate mofetil in heart transplant recipients. Mycophenolate Mofetil Investigators. *Transplantation.* 1998;66:507–515.
37. Keogh A, Richardson M, Ruygrok P, et al. Sirolimus in de novo heart transplant recipients reduces acute rejection and prevents coronary artery disease at 2 years: a randomized clinical trial. *Circulation.* 2004;110:2694–2700.
38. Eisen HJ, Tuzcu EM, Dorent R, et al.; RAD B253 Study Group. Everolimus for the prevention of allograft rejection and vasculopathy in cardiac-transplant recipients. *N Engl J Med.* 2003;349:847–858.
39. Kobashigawa JA, Tobis JM, Mentzer RM, et al. Mycophenolate mofetil reduces intimal thickness by intravascular ultrasound after heart transplant: reanalysis of the multicenter trial. *Am J Transplant.* 2006;5:993–997.

CHAPTER 18

Transcatheter Interventions in Adult Congenital Heart Disease

JAMIL ABOULHOSN ▪ DANIEL LEVI ▪ JOHN W. MOORE

Balloon atrial septostomy, described by Rashkind and Miller[1] in 1966, introduced transcatheter intervention in congenital heart disease (CHD). Shortly thereafter, Portsmann and Wanke[2] performed transcatheter closure of a patent ductus arteriosus, and in 1976, King and Mills[3] published the first report of transcatheter device closure of an atrial septal defect (ASD). Subsequent improvements in device design, catheterization technology, and procedural techniques have brought interventional cardiology to the forefront as a therapeutic method that can delay or obviate surgery in CHD. Because noninvasive cardiovascular imaging and the resolution of computerized tomography (CT) and magnetic resonance imaging (MRI; see Chapter 7) are adequate for anatomic definition in most adults with CHD, diagnostic catheterization is chiefly reserved for hemodynamic assessment. An exception is tetralogy of Fallot with pulmonary atresia (TOF/PA) in which diagnostic catheterization is likely to be superior to MRI/CT scan in delineating the anatomy of aortopulmonary collaterals. Balloon occlusion of collaterals with contrast injection into the true pulmonary arteries delineates overlapping collateral and pulmonary arterial circulations. In patients with single ventricle, diagnostic catheterization, before and after cavopulmonary shunts remain the standard for determining pulmonary arterial pressure, flow, and resistance.

Interventional catheterization can be corrective, reparative, or palliative, an alternative to surgery, or employed to complement and enhance surgical results. It is now the treatment of choice for secundum ASD, coarctation of the aorta, patent ductus arteriosus, and pulmonary valve stenosis. New procedures and devices are continually evolving. Devices are being evaluated for closure of ventricular septal defects (VSD) and for percutaneous valve replacement. This chapter deals with a variety of currently available procedures, with the indications for their use in adults with CHD and with the short- and mid-term outcomes.

INTERVENTIONS FOR SEMILUNAR VALVE AND VENTRICULAR OUTFLOW OBSTRUCTION

Right Ventricular Outflow

Obstruction to right ventricular outflow can be subinfundibular, infundibular, valvular, or supravalvular. Typical mobile pulmonary valve stenosis is most amenable to balloon dilatation. Conduit stenosis and stenoses of main and branch pulmonary arteries can also be addressed through transcatheter techniques. Infundibular obstruction has been effectively relieved in younger patients with stenting, but subpulmonic stenosis is a surgical problem.

Pulmonary Valve Stenosis

Balloon valvuloplasty, a technique first described in 1956 by Rubio and Limon-Lason,[4] is the treatment of choice for isolated mobile dome-shaped pulmonary valve stenosis. The currently employed percutaneous static balloon valvuloplasty technique was reported by Kan et al.[5] in 1982. The procedure has proved safe and efficacious, making balloon valvuloplasty the treatment

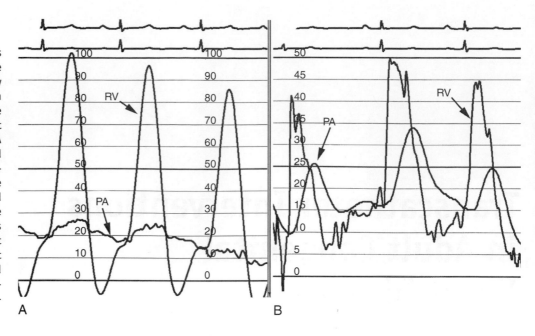

FIGURE 18-1 **(A)** Simultaneous pressures in the right ventricle (RV) and main pulmonary artery (PA) in a 48-year-old female with isolated mobile pulmonary valve stenosis. The maximum gradient approaches 75 mm Hg, and the PA pressure tracing shows the delayed and diminished systolic augmentation of severe pulmonary valve stenosis. **(B)** Simultaneous RV and PA recordings following double balloon valvuloplasty. There is significant reduction in gradient (< 30 mm Hg), reduction in right ventricular systolic pressure, and augmentation of PA systolic pressure indicating successful pulmonary valvuloplasty.

of choice for mobile pulmonary valve stenosis when the Doppler-estimated peak instantaneous gradient is 50 mm Hg or higher.[6-9] Excellent outcomes and low complication rates were reported in more than 800 pulmonary valvuloplasties recorded in the Valvuloplasty and Angioplasty Registry.[8,9] Peak gradients less than 25 mm Hg do not require intervention because these mild gradients do not increase with age, and survival is not curtailed.[7] Nearly 15% of stenotic pulmonary valves are dysplastic and can be distinguished from mobile doming valves by the absence of a pulmonary ejection sound and by echocardiography or MRI. Successful valvuloplasty for severe mobile pulmonary valve stenosis is usually accompanied by gradual regression of secondary hypertrophic subpulmonary stenosis.[10] Dysplastic or heavily calcified pulmonary valves do not lend themselves to valvuloplasty.[8] Isolated infundibular or subinfundibular obstruction to right ventricular outflow is seldom if ever amenable to balloon angioplasty.

The technique of pulmonary valvuloplasty has changed little since early reports, but low-profile catheters have decreased the likelihood of vascular injury at entry sites. Before proceeding with angiography or intervention, simultaneous pressures should be measured in the right ventricle and pulmonary artery (Fig. 18-1). Right ventricular angiography is performed to evaluate outflow tract anatomy, pulmonary valve location, mobility, and annulus size, and supravalvar pulmonary artery anatomy. Measurement of the diameter of the pulmonary valve annulus is an important step before proceeding with balloon selection. The desired balloon to annulus ratio is 1.2 to 1.4.[11] Balloon/annulus ratios that exceed 1.5 risk rupturing the annulus and inducing hemorrhage into right ventricular myocardium.[12] If the annulus is too large for dilatation with a single balloon, two balloons

can be employed. In most instances, the double balloon technique is preferable for pulmonary valvuloplasty in adults (Fig. 18-2). When using two balloons of the same size, each balloon should have a diameter equal to 0.79 of the diameter of the pulmonary annulus, or the combined diameters of the two balloons should be approximately 1.22 times the optimal diameter of a single balloon.[13] Two balloons have the advantage of less trauma at the venous access site, success with larger-diameter pulmonary valves, and potential decompression of the right ventricle during angioplasty through gaps between the balloons.

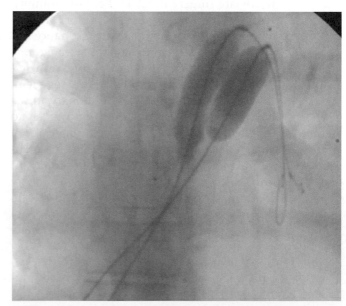

FIGURE 18-2 Cinefluoroscopic image (anteroposterior projection) of double balloon pulmonary valvuloplasty in the patient whose hemodynamics are shown in Figure 18-1.

Immediate and intermediate results have been favorable.[8,9,14] In a study of 25 adolescents and adults, success was achieved in 80% with an immediate decrease in peak gradient from a mean of 94 to 34 mm Hg.[14] Over the subsequent 3 years, the peak gradient decreased further by a mean of 19 mm Hg chiefly because of regression of infundibular hypertrophy (discussed earlier). Twenty-three percent of 533 patients who underwent balloon pulmonary valvuloplasty had a suboptimal outcome over an 8-year follow-up as judged by either a residual peak systolic gradient 36 mm Hg or higher or the need for further transcatheter or surgical intervention.[9] Predictors of suboptimal outcomes included an elevated immediate postprocedure gradient (odds ratio: 1.32 per 10 mm Hg increase) and a lower ratio of balloon-to-annulus diameter. Restenosis is rare. Pulmonary regurgitation is common and is hemodynamically well-tolerated.[15] Compared with surgical valvotomy, transcatheter balloon valvotomy is accompanied by lower morbidity and mortality. Residual systolic gradients are higher, but regurgitation is less.

PULMONARY ARTERY STENOSIS

Stenosis of the pulmonary artery and its branches occurs in William's, Noonan's, and the Alagille syndromes and in patients exposed *in utero* to first-trimester maternal rubella infection. Pulmonary artery and branch stenoses are often associated with other congenital malformations, such as tetralogy of Fallot, or are sequelae of surgical shunts.

Percutaneous static balloon angioplasty technique for treatment of peripheral pulmonary artery stenosis was first described in 1983.[16] The indications for transcatheter intervention include elevation of right ventricular systolic pressure or underperfusion of a lung segment.[17] An adequate result depends on the use of sufficiently large high-pressure balloons that tear the vascular intima and media, leaving a slim safety margin.[18] Elastic recoil of the involved segment is common with balloon angioplasty alone.[19] With the use of stents, the success rate increases from 70% with angioplasty alone to 90% (Fig. 18–3).[18,19] Cutting balloons are often used in addition to conventional static balloons and are more effective in relieving peripheral stenoses that cannot be stented.[20] Sizing the cutting balloons to 200% the minimal luminal diameter results in far greater efficacy at lower inflation pressures than static balloons.[21] Larger-diameter cutting balloons are now commercially available.

In general, the first and second arcade branches of the pulmonary arteries can be effectively treated with stents. It is sometimes necessary to place separate stents simultaneously in adjacent branch pulmonary arteries to prevent obliteration of one branch during stenting of a neighboring artery. Multiple distal stenoses require multiple balloon dilatations. Thorough and aggressive dilatation of these stenoses occasionally drops the right ventricular systolic pressure, but care must be taken to avoid rupture. Diffuse peripheral pulmonary stenosis is not a surgical lesion and at best is problematic for interventional catheterization.

A thorough preintervention right heart catheterization is performed, with particular attention to right ventricular systolic pressure and the pressure gradient across a given stenosis. Magnetic resonance angiography with phase contrast imaging quantifies the relative distribution of blood flow to each lung and is used to identify functionally significant stenosis[22] (see Chapter 7). Although MR and CT angiographic images are sometimes useful to identify the location of a lesion, angiography is the ultimate guide for determining its length, minimal luminal diameter, reference vessel diameter, and lesion distance from branch points.

After transcatheter biplane cineangiography has identified a stenosis and the required measurements are made, a stiff guidewire is advanced past the stenotic area in the largest of the distal branches. Angioplasty without stent placement can be performed in discrete distal lesions, but stenting is preferable for most proximal pulmonary artery segments. High-pressure balloons (Atlas, Bard, Tewksbury, MA; Conquest, Bard, Tewksbury, MA; Mullins, NuMED, Hopkinton, NY) are occasionally required. Third and fourth arcade branch lesions are sometimes better treated with cutting balloons that tear the vessel intima at lower pressure inflations. These segments are often redilatated with larger static balloons that expand the tear introduced by the cutting balloon.

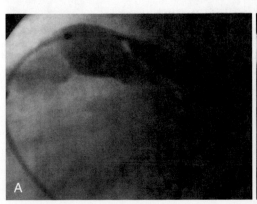
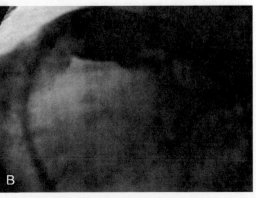

FIGURE 18–3   (A) Cineangiogram (lateral projection) in severe, focal proximal left pulmonary artery stenosis due to surgical scar. **(B)** Cineangiogram following transcatheter stent placement showing a major increase in luminal size.

To prevent elastic recoil of the vessel, stents are favored in branch and medium-sized pulmonary arteries, usually in the first and second arcades of the pulmonary tree.

Stents are mounted on static balloons that are advanced through long sheaths and positioned across a stenotic segment. The balloon diameter generally approximates the reference vessel diameter on either side of the stenosis. Stent deployment across branch points within the pulmonary arterial tree may result in decreased flow to the "jailed" segment and should be avoided.

In a multicenter retrospective analysis of 338 patients who underwent implantation of 664 pulmonary Palmaz stents, the mean systolic pressure gradient decreased from 41 to 8.7 mm Hg immediately following the procedure.[23] Over a mean follow-up period of 5.6 years, the gradient increased to 20 mm Hg. Major complications occurred in less than 1% of patients and included stent migration, hemoptysis, pulmonary edema, and death. Technical means designed to limit complications include conservative serial dilatations, avoidance of overdilatation, and simultaneous placement of right and left pulmonary artery stents in patients with systemic levels of pulmonary blood pressure.

CONDUIT AND PROSTHETIC VALVE STENOSIS

Homografts and bioprosthetic conduits are used extensively to establish communication between the right ventricle and pulmonary artery in a variety of congenital heart defects. Conduits become obstructed because of external compression, calcification, kinking, or exuberant intimal peel (see Chapter 20). The majority of conduits require intervention within a decade after placement, with shorter intervals for smaller conduits.[24,25] Balloon dilatation has met with modest success.[26,27] High-pressure balloons occasionally provide some relief to the obstruction, whereas balloon diameters greater than the original diameter of the conduit risk rupture. Catastrophic hemorrhage is usually controlled by scar tissue surrounding the conduit.

In an effort to improve results and prolong conduit life, balloon-expandable stents have been implanted, with immediate improvement in both angiographic appearance and hemodynamics (Fig. 18–4).[28-30] In a series of 221 patients undergoing transcatheter conduit stent deployment between 1990 and 2004, there was no

FIGURE 18–4 **(A)** Contrast injection into the right ventricle (RV) of a patient with repaired tetralogy of Fallot and severe distal conduit stenosis. The right ventricular systolic pressure was suprasystemic. **(B)** A Palmaz-Genesis 2910 B stent is uncovered within the stenotic conduit. **(C)** Balloon dilatation of the stent to a diameter of 12 mm. **(D)** Angiogram in the RV showing resolution of the conduit stenosis. The RV systolic pressure decreased to half systemic.

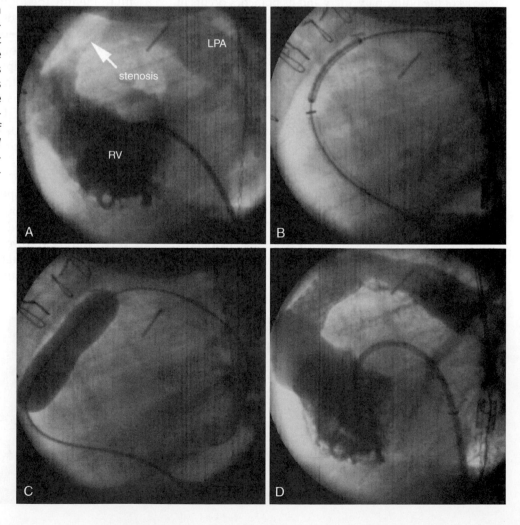

periprocedural mortality and, apart from five malpositioned stents, no procedural complications.[29] During a mean follow-up of 4 years, 83 patients required stent redilatation, and 41 patients required placement of additional stents. Stent fractures occurred in 43% of patients because of compression and retrosternal location. Stent fractures did not cause adverse hemodynamic consequences and did not lead to earlier conduit reoperation. Stent implantation postponed conduit surgery by a mean of 2.7 years. Predictors of shortened freedom from reoperation include a Palmaz-Genesis stent, a homograft conduit, a conduit 10 mm or less, a diagnosis of tetralogy of Fallot, a higher prestent right ventricular systolic pressure, and stent malposition. When coronary arteries are in close proximity to the conduit, selective angiography is often performed with a balloon inflated across a conduit stenosis to ensure freedom from coronary compression by a conduit stent. Stenting in the area of a homograft conduit valve can cause free pulmonary regurgitation.

LEFT VENTRICULAR OUTFLOW AND AORTIC VALVE OBSTRUCTION

Aortic Valve Stenosis

Transcatheter valvuloplasty is the treatment of choice for isolated pulmonary valve stenosis but is palliative for congenital bicuspid aortic valve stenosis. A series of 23 patients was published in 1984.[31] The bicuspid valve necessarily remains bicuspid, albeit functionally improved. Despite acceptable immediate outcomes, recurrent stenosis and progressive regurgitation are common, eventually culminating in surgical intervention.[17]

Balloon valvuloplasty is indicated in patients with mobile congenital bicuspid aortic valve stenosis and a peak left ventricular-to-aortic gradient 50 mm Hg or higher, angina, syncope, effort dyspnea, or ischemic ST/T wave changes on an ambulatory or exercise electrocardiogram.[32]

Asymptomatic patients with peak-to-peak catheter gradients 60 mm Hg or higher are also considered, as are asymptomatic patients with lower gradients who wish to participate in competitive sports or to become pregnant.[32] Balloon valvuloplasty is a useful palliative procedure before or sometimes during pregnancy to defer surgical valve repair or replacement until after delivery (see Chapter 9).[33] Transcatheter valvuloplasty should not be performed in patients in whom aortic regurgitation is more than mild. Patients with calcified or dysplastic aortic valves, annular hypoplasia, or subaortic stenosis are seldom if ever candidates for balloon valvuloplasty.

The most commonly employed procedure in adolescents and adults is retrograde placement of a stiff guidewire across the aortic valve via the femoral artery. The aortic annular diameter is measured by angiography and echocardiography. The recommended initial balloon to annulus ratio is 0.8 to 1.0. Balloons that exceed 120% of aortic annular diameter risk damaging the left ventricle outflow tract and causing significant aortic regurgitation.[34,35] Two retrograde balloons are often employed in larger adults with a recommended combined diameter of 1.35 times the diameter calculated for a single balloon.[13] Double balloons have the advantage of smaller arterial sheaths, thus reducing the risk of arterial injury. There is no difference in complication rate using a single balloon or two balloons.[35] Long balloons (4–5 cm) counter the rocking motion of the balloon during inflation. The balloons are rapidly inflated and deflated to avoid prolonged obstruction to flow. Rapid pacing of the right ventricle during valvuloplasty decreases cardiac output and minimizes undesirable motion of the balloons against the aortic valve during inflation (Fig. 18–5).[36] The waist in the balloon(s) disappears as the leaflets are opened. Aortic valvuloplasty balloons usually have rated burst pressures from 4 to 6 atmospheres. Rupture can cause air

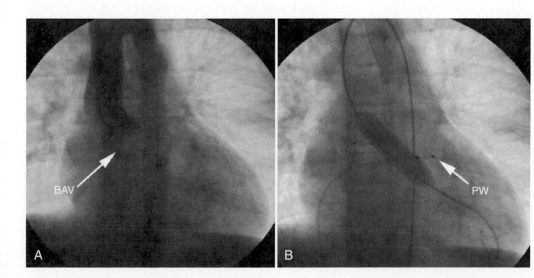

FIGURE 18–5 (A) Anteroposterior cineangiogram in the ascending aorta of a young adult with bicuspid aortic valve stenosis (BAV) and characteristic doming of the mobile bicuspid valve. **(B)** Single balloon valvuloplasty performed retrograde with simultaneous rapid pacing of the right ventricle using a transvenous pacing wire (PW).

embolization and stroke. The pressure gradient across the aortic valve is measured after each dilatation. Additional valvuloplasties are not performed if the gradient is less than 20 to 30 mm Hg or if there is more than mild aortic regurgitation. Transthoracic, intracardiac, and transesophageal echocardiography serve to monitor the degree of aortic regurgitation.[37]

Immediate and short-term results of balloon aortic valvuloplasty in patients with mobile noncalcified bicuspid valves are excellent, with significant decrease in the transvalvular gradient and resolution of symptoms.[34,38] In a multicenter registry of 606 adults who underwent aortic valvuloplasty, the peak transvalvular gradient decreased by 60% immediately following the procedure.[34] The long-term outlook is understandably less favorable, with 50% of patients requiring further intervention during 8 years of follow-up.[38] Even if balloon valvuloplasty eliminates the gradient and induces little or no regurgitation, the bicuspid valve remains bicuspid (see earlier and see Chapter 20).

Coarctation of the Aorta

Both native and recurrent coarctation of the aorta in adults are usually characterized by a discrete narrowing just distal to the left subclavian artery in the region of the ligamentum arteriosum. Less common diffuse forms involve the arch or isthmus. "Significant" coarctation is generally defined as a peak-to-peak catheter gradient 20 mm Hg or higher. However, unimpressive gradients occur when major collaterals exist with anatomically severe coarctation.

Resting and exercise continuous wave Doppler velocities across the site of coarctation are assessed by transthoracic echocardiography (see Chapter 6). MRI and CT angiography with three-dimensional reconstruction demonstrate the degree and extent of coarctation and collateral formation and are widely used for noninvasive imaging before intervention.

Transcatheter balloon angioplasty of aortic coarctation was first performed in 1982[39] and has been applied to discrete native coarctation and to recurrent narrowing with considerable immediate success and a low rate of procedural complications.[40-42] Balloon angioplasty significantly increased the diameter in both native and recurrent coarctation.[42] Procedural success is generally defined as a reduction in peak-to-peak gradient to less than 20 mm Hg. Patients with native coarctation derive greater benefit from angioplasty, as evidenced by increased segment diameter and fewer suboptimal outcomes. Periprocedural death is less than 1%. A higher preprocedural gradient is a risk factor for suboptimal outcomes.

Transcatheter balloon angioplasty of coarctation is performed retrograde from the femoral artery. Pressure gradients across all parts of the aortic arch are carefully sought with an end-hole catheter. Biplane mechanical contrast angiography in the anteroposterior and steep left anterior oblique projections demonstrates the coarctation and arch anatomy. Measurements of the coarctation site and the paracoarctation aorta, the diameters of the transverse and descending aorta at the level of the diaphragm, and the distance from the coarcation site to the takeoff of the left subclavian are guides to balloon and stent selection.

A stiff guidewire is positioned across the site of coarctation in the ascending aorta or right subclavian artery. The balloon employed for dilatation of native or recurrent coarctation should have a diameter equal (± 1-2 mm) to the diameter of the descending aorta at the level of the diaphragm (15-18 mm in most adults). Double balloons can be employed with a combined diameter of 1.21 times that of a single balloon. The catheter(s) are centered at the site of coarctation, and the balloon(s) are inflated with dilute contrast until the waist on the balloon disappears or the maximum safe inflation pressure is reached. The balloon is inflated and deflated quickly, a precaution that is less important in adults with extensive collaterals. Care must be taken to avoid advancing the catheter across the dilatation site without the aid of a previously placed guidewire. A postangioplasty aortogram determines whether or not an intimal tear has been induced. Because the paracoarctation aorta harbors inherent medial abnormalities (see Chapter 20), balloon dilatation further damages these already abnormal segments, risking aneurysm formation.

Stent implantation, first reported in 1995[43] (Fig. 18-6), is performed in a fashion similar to angioplasty, with a few notable exceptions. Heparin is administered to maintain an activated clotting time greater than 220 seconds throughout the procedure. A long sheath is positioned across the coarctation site. The stent is crimped onto a balloon catheter and carefully positioned across the site of stenosis. Careful stent length selection and positioning are imperative so that the abnormal paracoarctation aorta is included, while avoiding placement across the ostium of the left subclavian artery (LSCA). In the presence of hypoplasia of the distal transverse aortic arch, and when the coarctation is immediately distal to the LSCA, it is necessary to cross the LSCA while placing the stent. Open cell stents (MEGA LD, eV3, Plymouth, MN) are always used in these cases and are generally preferred in larger adults. Closed cell stents (Palmaz Genesis, Johnson & Johnson, Warren, NJ; Cordis, Johnson & Johnson, Warren, NJ) are used for adults in whom coarcation is clearly distal to the LSCA and in whom the aorta is less than 17 to 18 mm. The balloon diameter is sized to be equivalent to the diameter of the aorta just proximal to the LSCA or to the diameter of the descending aorta at the level of the diaphragm. The sheath is retracted, and the balloon and stent are exposed after confirming the position of the stent relative to the location of the coarctation and the brachiocephalic arteries.

The balloon is expanded using dilute contrast material, thus deploying the stent. Further dilatation can be

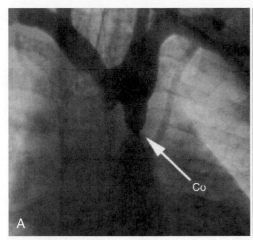
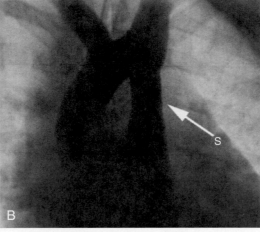

FIGURE 18–6   (A) Anteroposterior cineangiogram of the aortic arch showing a discrete segment of coarctation (Co) distal to the left subclavian artery. There is characteristic dilation of the distal paracoarctation aorta. **(B)** Angiogram following stent implantation that includes the abnormal paracoarctation aorta. There is complete obliteration of the stenotic segment.

achieved with a second larger balloon if additional remodeling of the stent is necessary. Following the procedure, aspirin (usually 325 mg daily) is begun and continued for 6 months to prevent thrombus formation while the stent endothelializes.

Although the immediate results of angioplasty are favorable, the intermediate and long-term results are less impressive. Intermediate results disclose a 3-year freedom from reintervention ranging from 73% to 88%, with a low rate of aneurysm formation.[44,45] Long-term results disclose that 50% of subjects following balloon angioplasty of native coarctation require repeat intervention over a mean follow-up of 10.6 years compared with 12.5% of surgical patients over a similar follow-up period.[46] Repeat interventions were for recurrent stenosis or aneurysm formation. As emphasized earlier, the paracoarctation segments of the aorta harbor medial abnormalities that increase the risk of aneurysm and pseudoaneurysm formation following angioplasty.[47] Aneurysms were detected by MR angiography in 7 of 20 patients (35%) following balloon angioplasty. Four aneurysms were detected within a year of the procedure, and the rest occurred up to 8 years later. No deaths were attributable to aneurysm rupture or thrombosis, and only two of seven patients underwent elective surgical intervention because of aneurysm formation. However, pregnancy increases the risk of rupture (see Chapter 9).

Balloon dilatation with stenting has yielded excellent immediate and intermediate results without significant risk of aneurysm formation. Accordingly, the procedure has become the treatment of choice in adults. In a single-center retrospective analysis of 32 patients who underwent transcatheter stenting for coarctation (9 native and 23 recurrent), the gradient was virtually eliminated in the majority immediately following the procedure.[48] However, gradients increased from a mean of 1.8 to 13 mm Hg during 1.5 years of follow-up chiefly because of neointimal proliferation. Chessa et al.[48] reported intermediate outcomes of stenting in 71 consecutive patients (52 native,

19 recurrent) with a mean age of 22 years. Immediate results were excellent, but over a median follow-up of 3 years, the mean residual Doppler gradient increased from 4 to 13 mm Hg. Four patients required stent dilation at a mean of 21 months after the initial procedure. One death occurred. A multicenter analysis of acute outcomes in 588 stenting procedures disclosed a 98.6% procedural success rate.[49] Complications were encountered in 11.7%, with two procedural deaths. Complications included aneurysm formation, intimal tears, dissection, access site injury, stent migration, balloon rupture, and arterial embolization. The risk of dissection significantly increased in patients older than age 20 years. Long-term outcome of transcatheter stent implantation will not be available for several years, but results thus far appear to be better than angioplasty alone and compare favorably with surgery. With improvement in balloon and stent design, procedural complications are expected to decline.

Central Vein and Venous Baffle Obstruction

Stenoses of large central veins are usually sequelae of surgical procedures or trauma associated with catheterization or indwelling central lines. Venous baffle obstructions are the most frequent cause of reoperation following Mustard/Senning procedures.[50] Balloon angioplasty results in transient improvement at best, with high restenosis rates.[51-53] With intravascular stents (Figs. 18–7 and 18–8), the success rate is high, and the rate of restenosis is low.[51,53,54]

EMBOLIZATION

Transcatheter embolization therapy for cardiovascular collaterals was first performed in 1975 and has become an important therapeutic tool.[55] Embolization of aortopulmonary collaterals in cyanotic patients is performed to palliate complex defects as a part of a collaborative

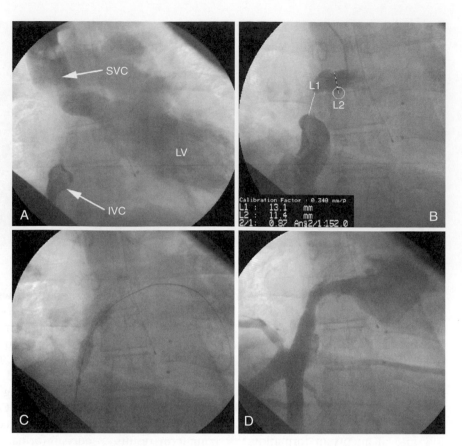

FIGURE 18–7 Thirty-four-year-old patient with D-transposition of the great arteries status post–Mustard atrial switch operation in infancy. There is complete obstruction of the inferior vena caval (IVC) portion of the systemic venous baffle. **(A)** Simultaneous contrast injections into both vena cavae showing an obstructed IVC baffle and a widely patent SVC baffle with contrast filling of the subpulmonary left ventricle (LV). **(B)** Calibrated measurements of the length of the obstruction and the diameter of the distal baffle. **(C)** Successful wiring of the obstruction with subsequent advancement and expansion of a balloon mounted stent. **(D)** Contrast injection into the IVC following placement of two stents (Palmaz-Genesis 2910B and 1910B). There was mild residual stenosis but no pressure gradient.

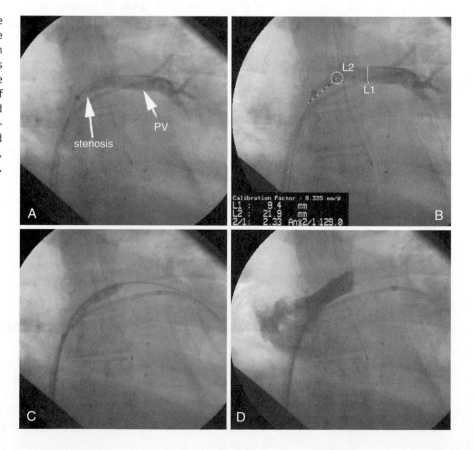

FIGURE 18–8 **(A)** Pulmonary venous (PV) baffle stenosis in a patient with D-transposition of the great arteries status post–Mustard atrial switch operation. A "transseptal" needle puncture was made between the inferior vena cava baffle and the pulmonary venous (PV) baffle, with advancement of a long sheath into the PV baffle. **(B)** Calibrated measurement of the length of stenosis and the diameter of the upstream baffle. **(C)** Balloon-mounted Palmaz-Genesis 2910 B stent (12 mm diameter, 29 mm length) expanded in the area of stenosis. **(D)** Angiogram showing a widely patent PV baffle.

effort with cardiac surgeons[56] and is used as the sole definitive therapy for coronary artery fistulae.

Pulmonary Atresia with Aortopulmonary Collaterals

Tetralogy of Fallot with pulmonary atresia and aortopulmonary collaterals was classified by Collet and Edwards as type IV truncus arteriosus but was reclassified by Van Praagh and Van Praagh[57] as an extreme form of the tetralogy. The spectrum ranges from well-formed confluent pulmonary arteries with small aortopulmonary collaterals to absent central pulmonary arteries with large and extensive collaterals. Three types of systemic collateral arteries have been described[58]: (1) direct aortopulmonary collaterals originate from the descending aorta, join true pulmonary arteries beyond the areas of stenosis, and often develop obstruction secondary to intimal hyperplasia; (2) indirect collaterals emerge from upper arterial branches such as the subclavian, internal mammary, and thyrocervical arteries; and (3) bronchial collaterals emerge from the descending aorta at the hilus and develop extensive intrapulmonary anastomotic networks.

Management requires accurate definition of the collateral anatomy, the degree of overlap with the true pulmonary arterial circulation, and the hemodynamic consequences of collateral elimination.[59] Unifocalization is designed to integrate large aortopulmonary collaterals into the true pulmonary circulation (see Chapter 15). Coil embolization of collaterals is reserved for collaterals distributed to areas of lung with a dual blood supply.[59] Coil embolization of all aortopulmonary collaterals is recommended when the surgical objective is a direct connection between the right ventricle and confluent pulmonary arteries with VSD closure. When a lung lobe has a dual blood supply, embolization of the arteriopulmonary collateral promotes growth of the true pulmonary artery, reduces the risk of hemoptysis, and decreases the volume load to the left ventricle.

Aortopulmonary Collateral in Single Ventricle Physiology

Aortopulmonary collaterals with single ventricle physiology represent enlargement of normal, precapillary anastomoses of bronchial and other systemic arteries or flow through vascular pleural adhesions.[60] Stimuli for development of these collateral arteries include surgical scarring, pulmonary venous occlusion, pulmonary artery branch stenosis, and pulmonary thromboembolism.[61-63] Aortopulmonary collaterals are detected in 36% of patients after a bidirectional Glenn or Fontan procedure, particularly in those with a previous Blalock-Taussig shunt.[64] The majority of these collaterals arise from internal mammary arteries or the thyrocervical trunk (34% and 22%, respectively). Aortopulmonary collaterals can be problematic in patients undergoing Glenn or Fontan procedures because of the volume load to the systemic ventricle and because they are sites of intraoperative and perioperative bleeding.

Currently available embolization agents include four major categories: mechanical devices for occlusion of medium to large vessels, particulates to occlude terminal arterioles, and liquid agents and sclerosing agents to occlude capillary vascular bed collaterals.

The Gianturco stainless steel coil, initially developed in 1975, is the embolization agent most widely used by interventional cardiologists.[65,66] The design of the coil has remained relatively unchanged since its introduction and early modifications.[67,68] A small steel wire is wound tightly into a primary coil, with Dacron strands embedded along the length of the wire to increase thrombogenicity. The coil is packaged in a cylindrical introducer and assumes a compact helical shape as it is extruded from the delivery catheter. The current Gianturco coil is available in a variety of wire sizes, diameters (3-20 mm), and lengths (2-15 mm). The vessel to be embolized is selectively intubated with an end-hole nontapered catheter. Selective angiography is performed to determine the diameter of the vessel. In general, coils are selected with a diameter 20% to 30% larger than the vessel to be occluded. The coils are advanced through the end-hole catheter using the soft end of a guidewire. The catheter lumen and pusher wire should be approximately the same size as the primary coil diameter. Placement of small coils distally with gradual catheter withdrawal while laying down larger coils proximally results in immediate and long-term vessel occlusion. The entire length of the collateral vessels is filled with coils to prevent recanalization.

A wide range of embolization coils are available, including platinum microcoils with or without embedded fibers. These coils are similar in design to the stainless steel coils but are smaller in primary coil diameter, more malleable, more radio-opaque, and can be delivered through a microcatheter system (3-Fr Tracker-18, Target Therapeutics, Boston Scientific, Boston, MA; and Renegade stents, Boston Scientific, Boston, MA), enabling super-selective embolization of distal or tortuous vessels.[69,70] Precise coil position and controlled release are possible with detachable systems.

The Gianturco-Grifka vascular occlusion device introduced in 1995 is a detachable sack that can be filled with coils.[71] The device is used to embolize various vascular connections from pulmonary arteriovenous malformations to patent ductus arteriosus.[72-74] Detachable balloons have been available since 1974[75,76] but have largely been replaced by the Amplatzer plug device designed specifically for use through relatively low profile sheathes (5-6 Fr) and coronary guide catheters. The plugs are made entirely from a Nitinol wire meshwork and are especially useful in occluding large venous and arterial vessels. Because the Amplatzer vascular plug lacks a polyester membrane, high-flow shunts are better closed with the Amplatzer septal occluder or DuctOcclud devices.

Surgical Systemic-to-Pulmonary Arterial Shunts

In patients undergoing cavopulmonary connections (Glenn or Fontan operation), ligation of existing systemic-to-pulmonary arterial shunts may require extensive dissection that adds to the length and complexity of surgery. When an alternative source of blood flow is present, it is advantageous to perform transcatheter occlusion of the systemic-to-pulmonary artery shunt before proceeding with reparative surgery.[77,78] Smaller shunts can be occluded with coils, whereas larger shunts often require occlusion with an Amplatzer plug or DuctOcclud.

Pulmonary Arteriovenous Fistulae

Pulmonary arteriovenous malformations (PAVM) occur in patients with hepatic dysfunction, with hereditary hemorrhagic telangiectasia (Rendu-Osler-Weber syndrome), and when a lung is deprived of "hepatic" pulmonary blood flow.[79-81] PAVMs result in a right-to-left shunt at the precapillary level and in progressive cyanosis. Although the causative agent has not been identified, current data suggest that absence of a "hepatic factor" is the stimulus for development of PAVM in lung segments perfused solely by superior vena caval flow as in a unidirectional Glenn or Fontan.[82,83] Inclusion of hepatic return to an affected lung segment leads to regression of PAVM.[84-86] Surgical creation of a brachial arteriovenous shunt is highly successful in the treatment of PAVM but carries a certain morbidity and mortality, thus providing impetus for the development of minimally invasive percutaneous techniques for the treatment of PAVM. Transcatheter embolization or balloon occlusion decreases the shunt volume in a minority of patients with macroscopic PAVM,[87] but persistent absence of "hepatic factor" to the affected lung leads to fistula reformation. Transcatheter pulmonary artery reconnection by placement of a stent in patients with a unidirectional Fontan can be performed safely, and it significantly improves cyanosis (see Fig. 18–19).[86]

Coronary Artery Fistula

Congenital coronary artery fistulae most often arise from the left coronary artery and drain into the pulmonary artery or right ventricle and, less commonly, into the right atrium or left ventricle.[88-93] The first successful transcatheter closure was performed in 1983.[94] Closure of coronary artery fistulae has subsequently used various embolization or occlusion devices. In 33 patients treated with Gianturco coils, Gianturco-Grafka detachable devices, or double umbrella occluders, complete occlusion was immediately established in 19 patients, 11 of whom had small or minimal residual flow, and two of whom required recatheterization.[95] Procedural complications include transient arrhythmias, coronary spasm, fistula dissection, and coil embolization to the pulmonary artery. It is important to identify all branches of the coronary system so that the fistula can be occluded without sacrificing any of the intrinsic coronary circulation. In some cases, a wire rail is formed through the fistula, and the Amplatzer DuctOcclud device is placed retrograde into the fistula[88] (Fig. 18–9).

OCCLUSION DEVICES

Patent Ductus Arteriosus

Patent ductus arteriosus (PDA) occurs in a wide variety of sizes and shapes but is usually conical. The aortic ampulla is typically larger than the pulmonary artery ampulla. Variations in PDA configuration have been described according to the angiographic classification of Krichenko and colleagues to help guide transcatheter closure procedures.[89] PDA closure is indicated for hemodynamic benefit in patients with significant left-to-right shunts and for elimination of the risk of infective endocarditis when the ductus is restrictive[90-92,96] (see Chapter 8). Closure in the Eisenmenger syndrome is contraindicated.[95,97,98] Transcatheter closure is especially useful in older adults with a calcified moderately restrictive ductus that carries a relatively high surgical risk. Indications for closure of a "silent ductus" detected incidentally by echocardiography remains unresolved. Closure of PDAs are accomplished via interventional catheterization with minimal morbidity and a high rate of success.[99]

Transcatheter occlusion of PDA was initially described by Porstmann et al.[2] in 1967 using an Ivalon plug. The device was fashioned according to the shape and size of the ductus as defined by angiography. Currently available devices include the previously mentioned Gianturco coils (see embolization devices), which continue to be used for closure of a restrictive PDA.[100] Successful coil occlusion depends on sufficient space within the ductus to accommodate enough coil mass to occlude flow without obstructing the aorta or pulmonary artery. A conical duct with a narrow pulmonary end that can be occluded with one or two coils increases the likelihood of long-term success and decreases the likelihood of coil migration.

Coil and device selections are based on the ductal length, diameter of aortic ampulla, and minimum diameter dimensions determined by aortic angiography performed in the right anterior oblique and straight lateral projections (Fig. 18–10). Ideally, coil diameter is at least three times the minimum ductal diameter but must accommodate the aortic ampulla.[101] Coils are positioned by a pushing wire extruded so that there is about three quarters of a loop in the main pulmonary artery with the

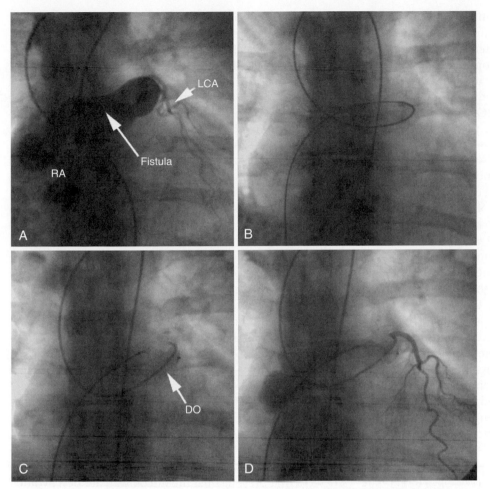

FIGURE 18–9 Left coronary arterial to right atrial fistula. **(A)** Selective left coronary arteriogram identifies an aneurysmal fistula emerging from the left coronary artery (LCA) and draining into the right atrium (RA). The calculated pulmonary-to-systemic flow ratio was 2:1. **(B)** A long wire advanced through the fistula and snared in the inferior vena cava, forming a "wire rail." A long sheath was advanced over the wire rail into the fistula from the right atrium. **(C)** An Amplatzer DuctOcclud (DO) device was advanced through the sheath and deployed within the fistula. **(D)** Left coronary angiography with the device in place showing increased opacification of the left anterior descending coronary artery and decreased contrast flow into the fistula.

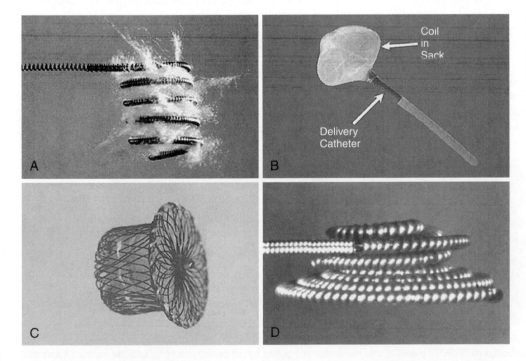

FIGURE 18–10 Devices used for occlusion of patent ductus arteriosus: **(A)** Gianturco coils, **(B)** Gianturco-Grifka vascular occlusion device, **(C)** Amplatzer duct occluder, **(D)** Nit-Occlud coils.

remainder of the coil in the aortic ampulla. Techniques for stabilization of the coil to prevent migration or embolization include use of a balloon catheter, snare, or bioptome to support the coil during delivery or the use of a catheter with a small end hole that results in stabilizing tension between the catheter and coil during delivery.[102-104] Detachable coils, including the NitOcclud coil from pfm Medical (Oceanside, CA), promise to replace the traditional Gianturco coils (see Fig. 18-10). Complete coil closure is achieved in more than 95% of patients.[105] Complications are rare[105] but include stenosis of the left pulmonary artery, stenosis of the proximal descending aorta, hemolysis, and coil migration or embolization.[104]

The Gianturco-Grifka vascular occlusion device consists of a nylon sack filled with wire and is available in various sizes ranging from 3 to 9 mm in diameter (see Fig. 18-10). The device is best suited for an elongated or tubular PDA and is sized to distend the ductus slightly. Device safety and efficacy profiles are excellent,[98] but the AGA DuctOcclud device is now most commonly used for large PDAs.

The Amplatzer duct occluder (AGA Medical, Golden Valley, MN) is now approved by the Food and Drug Administration (FDA) for PDA closure. The device features a Nitinol and mesh plug with a retention skirt at the aortic end (Figs. 18-10 and 18-11) and is delivered through the right femoral vein through a long venous sheath that extends across the ductus. The retention skirt is advanced into the descending aorta and pulled into the ampulla, while the body of the plug is delivered within the body of the PDA by retracting the sheath (see Fig. 18-11). The pivotal study that resulted in FDA approval included 484 patients from 25 centers in the United States and disclosed excellent efficacy and acceptable safety.[106] The Amplatzer ductal occluder was implanted successfully in 99% of patients with immediate angiographic evidence of complete occlusion in 76%. This number increased to 98% in 1 year with excellent long-term results.[107] Four serious complications included two left pulmonary artery obstructions and one death. The device is most suitable for a moderate or large PDA. Occasionally, a nonrestrictive PDA is not amenable to closure even with the largest

Amplatzer duct occluder and may require an Amplatzer septal occluder designed for closure of atrial or ventricular septal defects (discussed later).[108,109]

The NitOcclud device (pfm Medical) is a coil-type mechanism with a controlled delivery system that is the successor to the hourglass-shaped nitinol coil (see Fig. 18-10). The NitOcclud design includes a cone-in-cone constrained configuration that limits migration, graduated loop stiffness, and a disposable delivery system. The device performs best in small to moderate-sized PDAs. Implantation is performed through a long venous sheath advanced into the descending aorta via the PDA. The distal cone is configured in the aorta, the device is then pulled into the ductus, and additional coil loops are delivered into the aortic ampulla with the last loop pulled across the narrowest portion of the ductus. The device consists of a more controlled release system than the Gianturco coils and can be delivered in a flexible 5-Fr catheter. Other devices under investigation or in recent use include the Amplatzer angled PDA occluder, the folding plug buttoned device, and the patch device.

PDA associated with aneurysm must be considered carefully because device placement may apply pressure on the aneurysm, risking dissection or rupture. A covered stent can be used to exclude the aneurysm followed by PDA closure using one of the previously described devices.[110] Patients with abnormalities of the aortic media, as in Marfan syndrome, should also be approached cautiously. Calcified PDA in older adults may be fragile, so devices that press against the ductal wall are best avoided in favor of coil occlusion. When PDA is associated with coarctation, it is best to occlude the ductus first followed by balloon dilatation and stenting of the coarctation.[111] Alternatively, a covered stent has been employed to stent the aorta and close the PDA.[112]

Atrial Septal Defects

Surgical closure an ostium secundum ASD had been standard treatment since the inception of cardiopulmonary bypass. Transcatheter closure was first reported by King and

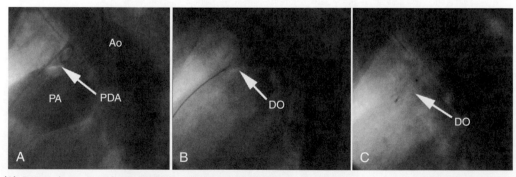

FIGURE 18-11 **(A)** Patent ductus arteriosus (PDA) in a 67-year-old female. Contrast injection through a pigtail catheter placed across the PDA (lateral projection). **(B)** Amplatzer DuctOcclud (DO) device placed within the ductus and pulled by the delivery catheter into the narrow PA ampulla. Aortic angiography shows no significant shunting into the PA. **(C)** The device is detached and is in suitable position.

Mills in 1976, and numerous devices and techniques were subsequently developed.[3] Transcatheter device closure has now supplanted surgery as the standard treatment for most secundum ASDs. Transthoracic and transesophageal echocardiography provide the information necessary for successful percutaneous closure—namely, accurate defect size, adequacy of rims, and presence or absence of associated cardiac anomalies, especially partial anomalous pulmonary venous connections.[105,113,114,115] Echocardiography can image even very thin atrial septal membrane tissue that may not provide a satisfactory rim for device stabilization. Rim adequacy best includes only septal rims with ≥ 2.5 mm thickness.[115] Intracardiac echocardiography (ICE) has also been employed as a method for selection of septal occluder size and for guidance during transcatheter closure.[116,117] Computed tomographic and electron beam angiography with three-dimensional surface reconstruction provides excellent two- and three-dimensional imaging of ASD anatomy.[118]

Advancements in device design and catheterization technology have led to the availability of a variety of transcatheter occlusion devices.[119,120] Closure of small defects (< 1 cm) in asymptomatic patients 25 years of age or older is controversial because there is no demonstrable difference in clinical outcomes between medically and surgically treated patients older than 20 years.[121] However, there is a relatively uniform consensus that ASDs in older patients with Qp:Qs ratio greater than 1.5:1 and low pulmonary vascular resistance should be closed to decrease morbidity and increase longevity. A nonrestrictive ASD with pulmonary vascular disease and reversed shunt is believed to represent a coincidence of ASD and idiopathic pulmonary hypertension. Longevity benefits from the presence of an interatrial communication, which should not be closed. Whether pulmonary vasodilatator therapy will reduce pulmonary vascular resistance sufficiently to permit defect closure is controversial and currently doubtful. Devices that partially close an interatrial communication have been developed for patients with pulmonary vascular disease, but efficacy is unproved.[122-124]

The efficacy of transcatheter device closure compares favorably with surgical closure and is associated with shorter hospital stays and fewer postprocedural complications.[125] The procedure is generally performed under fluoroscopic and transesophageal echocardiographic guidance, although transthoracic echocardiography may suffice in thin young adults.[126] After hemodynamic assessment and confirmation of atrial septal anatomy and pulmonary venous connections, the ASD size is determined with either a static balloon pull-through technique or a compliant sizing balloon inflated across the ASD (Figs. 18–12 and 18–13). The device is then deployed across the defect using a long introducer sheath advanced from the femoral vein (Figs. 18–12 through 18–14). Before final deployment, careful echocardiographic imaging is performed to ensure that the device

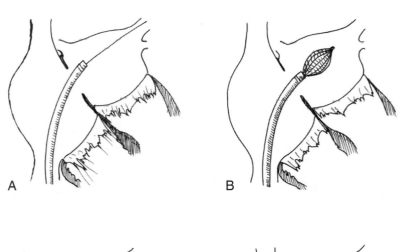

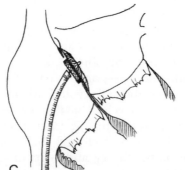

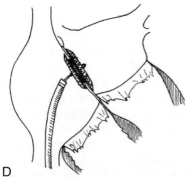

FIGURE 18–12   Artist's rendering of the main steps for transcatheter atrial septal defect (ASD) closure using the Amplatzer Septal Occluder after balloon sizing. **(A)** A long sheath is advanced across the ASD over a guidewire placed in the left superior pulmonary vein. **(B)** The guidewire has been removed and the left atrial disc deployed in the left atrium. **(C)** The delivery sheath and left atrial disc are gently pulled back until resistance is met at the interatrial septum. **(D)** The sheath is pulled back further, and the right atrial disc is deployed, sandwiching the septum and occluding the ASD.

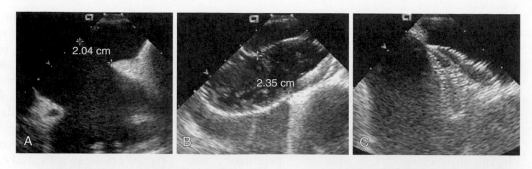

FIGURE 18-13 Transesophageal echocardiographic guidance of ASD occlusion. **(A)** Unstretched ASD diameter showing sufficient anterosuperior rim. **(B)** Balloon sizing. **(C)** Amplatzer Septal Occluder after successful deployment.

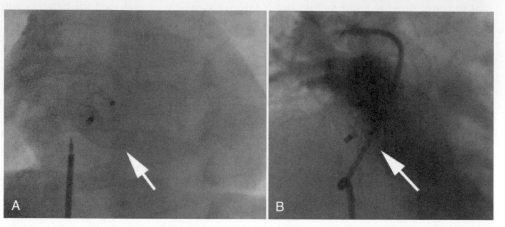

FIGURE 18-14 **(A)** Anteroposterior fluoroscopic appearance of an Amplatzer Septal Occluder (*white arrow*) immediately following release from delivery cable. **(B)** Levophase of mechanical contrast injection into the pulmonary artery following device occlusion of ASD (*white arrow*) showing absence of visible shunt.

does not obstruct pulmonary venous flow, venae caval flow, or coronary sinus drainage or interfere with atrioventricular valve function.

Results vary with each device, but complete closure is usually achieved in 60% to 90% of patients within hours of deployment and in 80% to 100% over a 1-year follow-up.[127] The Amplatzer septal occluder (AGA Medical) is currently the most widely used ASD closure device. Long-term outcome of closure using the Amplatzer septal occluder is excellent as evidenced by minimal complications and no deaths in 151 patients followed for 6.5 years.[128]

Short-term complications are rare, but all devices share the risks of embolization, thrombus formation, aortic root perforation, pericardial effusion, and arrhythmias. Amplatzer septal occluders ranging from 4 to 38 mm have been approved by the FDA, and a 40-mm device has been successfully used, but with increased risk of device embolization.[129] Mid- and long-term complications include endocarditis, thromboembolism, and strut fracture. Thrombus formation is more likely on the CardioSEAL (NMT Medical, Boston, MA), STARFlex (NMT Medical, Boston, MA), PFO-Star (CARDIA, Inc., Burnsville, MN), and ASDOS (Sulzer, Osypka, Germany) than on the Amplatzer septal occluder (AGA, MN).[130,131] The HELEX (Gore) device has a rate of thrombus formation comparable to the AGA ASO device and theoretically causes less erosions because of soft edges. Because the HELEX device is not self-centering, it has advantages in closing fenestrated defects.

Sporadic cases of late erosion of the anterior superior aspect of the Amplatzer septal occluder with perforation into the adjacent ascending aorta prompted AGA Medical to convene a panel of experts to analyze available data in patients with device perforation compared with patients in the U.S. Multicenter Pivotal Study. Patients with perforations were more likely to have a deficient anterior-superior rim and larger device-to-unstretched defect diameter. The panel recommended conservative balloon sizing to achieve flow cessation and to avoid device oversizing in patients with a deficient anterosuperior rim. Pericardial effusion following device placement is more likely to accompany this complication. Atrioventricular block was reported in 10 of 162 patients receiving the Amplatzer septal occluder, six of whom had second- or third-degree heart block that resolved within 6 months.

Following transcatheter closure, prothrombin fragment levels increase, peaking at 7 days and gradually decreasing to normal over 90 days without a detectable effect on platelet activation.[132] These findings call into question the practice of prophylactic antiplatelet therapy. In animal studies and in examination of explanted devices in patients, there is complete endothelialization within weeks to months of implantation. However, a persistent low-grade inflammatory response persists for years.[133,134] Concerns over thrombogenicity and inflammation have spurred efforts to develop bioabsorbable transcatheter closure devices. The BioSTAR Evaluation Study (BEST) is a prospective Phase I clinical trial designed to examine the feasibility, efficacy, and safety of a bioabsorbable device for ASD closure.[135]

Patent Foramen Ovale

A general population necropsy study of 965 normal hearts disclosed a 27.3% overall incidence of patent foramen ovale (PFO).[136-139] A relationship between PFO and stroke was first proposed by Cohnheim in 1877.[136,140] The rationale and efficacy of PFO closure for prevention of cryptogenic stroke[141-144] are discussed in Chapter 14. A potential role of PFO in the pathogenesis of migraine headaches is also discussed in Chapter 14.

Initial percutaneous PFO closure employed the Clamshell device in 36 patients in whom complete closure was achieved in 78%.[145] Transcatheter closure has subsequently employed a variety of devices and has proved to be a safe and efficacious alternative to surgery.[145-148] Newer devices (CardioSEAL and Amplatzer PFO Occluder) specifically designed for PFO closure have improved sealing performance.[149-151] Atrial arrhythmias following device implantation occur in 20% of patients and are usually self-limited. Patients older than 65 years are more likely (7.6%) to develop paroxysmal atrial fibrillation in the 4 weeks following device closure.[151-154]

Ventricular Septal Defect

VSD closure devices must take into account the nonuniform thickness of the ventricular septum, the variable locations of VSDs, the high left ventricular systolic pressure, and the close proximity of the aortic valve and conduction tissue to the membranous septum. Devices also must not predispose to migration, hemolysis, or arrhythmias.[17]

Transcatheter VSD closure was first reported in 1988 in a series of children using an umbrella device.[155] The CardioSEAL device (NMT Medical) used to close ASDs can also be used to close VSDs and is the only device approved in the United States for muscular VSDs. The device is a self-expanding modified Clamshell double umbrella that is advanced through a long venous sheath into the left ventricle. One of the umbrellas is exposed and pulled back against the ventricular septum before exposing the second umbrella. The StarFLEX (NMT Medical) is a newer generation of the same device designed to self-center so that smaller devices can be used to close restrictive VSDs. The triple-jointed legs prevent fracture, maintain a low-profile, and adapt to variations in septal configuration. Efficacy has been demonstrated in perimembranous and muscular VSDs,[156,157] and a 13-year experience has been reported in transcatheter closure of congenital and postoperative muscular VSDs.[158] The three devices used were the Clamshell septal occluder from 1989 to 1995, the CardioSEAL, and StarFLEX septal occluders from 1996 to 2003. Procedural success was high, but adverse events occurred in 90% of patients, including device arm fracture, device embolization, and impingement on valve tissue. All-cause mortality was 8.2%, although only one death was directly attributed to the procedure.

The Amplatzer muscular VSD occluder (AGA Medical) is similar to the Amplatzer ASD occlusion device. A Dacron polyester patch is placed inside two Nitinol disks connected by a waist. The difference lies in the length and diameter of the connecting waist—the muscular VSD device necessarily has a larger connecting waist relative to disc size. The Amplatzer muscular VSD occluder has proved safe and efficacious for closure of congenital and post–myocardial infarction muscular VSDs.[159-162] A U.S. registry of Amplatzer muscular VSD closures including 75 patients who underwent 83 procedures disclosed procedural success in 86.7%.[161] There were two procedure-related deaths, two device embolizations, and one cardiac perforation. A 47% immediate complete closure rate increased to 92% after 12 months. The device is widely used, but concerns regarding safety have held up FDA approval in the United States.

For closure of membranous and perimembranous VSDs, AGA Medical has designed a self-expanding double-disc Nitinol device with a thick waist and an off-center left ventricular disc to limit encroachment on aortic valve leaflets. One hundred patients who underwent perimembranous VSD closure from 2002 to 2004 experienced 93% procedural success and no procedural deaths.[163] Complications occurred in 29% over a median of 182 days, including rhythm or conduction disturbances in 13 patients, two of whom required permanent pacemaker implantation. Trivial to mild aortic and tricuspid regurgitation occurred in 9% of patients. Complete defect closure was achieved immediately in 58% of patients and increased to 83.6% within 6 months.

Membranous VSDs associated with aneurysm formation pose special concerns.[164] The left ventricular margin of the VSD is larger than the right ventricular margin, resembling the aortic margin and ampulla of a PDA, whereas the right ventricular margin and septal aneurysm resemble the narrowing of a PDA at its pulmonary arterial end. This geometric configuration makes closure of VSD with septal aneurysm possible with the Amplatzer duct occluder (Fig. 18–15).[165]

TRANSCATHETER VALVE PROCEDURES

Transcatheter Mitral Valve Repair

Two techniques are under investigation: the edge-to-edge technique and the prosthetic ring annuloplasty (Fig. 18–16). The edge-to-edge technique resembles the Alfieri surgical procedure, which consists of placing stitches between the anterior and posterior mitral valve leaflets to create a double orifice mitral valve.[166] In 2003, a novel transcatheter technique was reported in animals for percutaneous repair of regurgitant mitral valves demonstrating

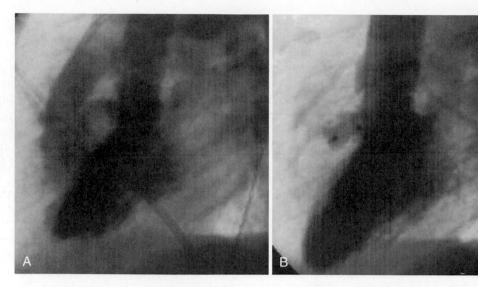

FIGURE 18–15 **(A)** Lateral projection of a left ventricular angiogram showing left-to-right shunting across a perimembranous ventricular septal defect with a septal aneurysm. **(B)** The left ventricular angiogram after release of the Amplatzer duct occluder showing the device in good position and absence of visible shunt. The septal aneurysm persists.

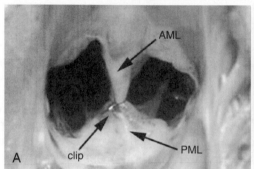
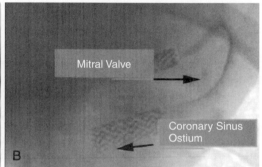

FIGURE 18–16 Techniques under investigation for transcatheter mitral valve repair. **(A)** Photograph of the mitral apparatus viewed from the left atrium illustrating the edge-to-edge method by which a clip is placed between the anterior (AML) and posterior (PML) mitral leaflets. **(B)** Anteroposterior cranial fluoroscopic image of a prosthetic ring annuloplasty device placed in the coronary sinus.

the feasibility of an Alfieri-like mitral repair by advancing a catheter from a peripheral vein across the interatrial septum followed by delivery of a polyester-covered clip device (Evalve, Evalve, Inc., Menlo Park, CA) to the mitral valve leaflets.[167] Using transesophageal echocardiographic guidance, the opened clip is positioned centrally and perpendicular to mitral leaflet coaptation and withdrawn until the leaflets are grasped. The clip is then closed, and the anterior and posterior leaflets are approximated. If relief of regurgitation is not achieved, the clip can be opened and repositioned. The human feasibility study, EVEREST I (Endovascular Valve Edge-to-Edge Repair Study), included 27 patients with severe noncongenital mitral regurgitation.[168] There were no major procedural complications, and the degree of mitral regurgitation improved significantly in 67% of patients. A randomized trial comparing percutaneous and surgical techniques, EVEREST II, is ongoing. Another design for achieving approximation of the mitral leaflets involves transcatheter sutures (Edwards Lifesciences, Irvine, CA). The MILANO II trial to evaluate this transcatheter system is under way. Edge-to-edge techniques thus far are restricted to mitral valves with localized prolapse of the medial portions of either the anterior or posterior leaflet and do not address annular dilation. There are

no data on the efficacy of these techniques for other mitral valve abnormalities.

Transcatheter Mitral Annuloplasty

Prosthetic or pericardial ring annuloplasty is widely used for surgical repair of annular dilatation that accompanies chronic severe mitral regurgitation. The coronary sinus (CS) is 1 to 2 cm posterior to the atrioventricular groove, so a partial annuloplasty can be achieved by placing a stiff device within the sinus. The anatomy of the CS lends itself to device deployment localized to the posterior half of the annulus, leaving the posteromedial commissure and the anterior portion of the annulus unsupported. Imaging with CT or MRI is important to determine coronary sinus anatomy before transcatheter annuloplasty. Most devices are inserted into the coronary sinus through the jugular vein to decrease the anteroposterior annular dimension, thus improving leaflet coaptation. In 2003, a feasibility study was reported in an animal model.[169] The first human study included five patients with chronic mitral regurgitation and anular dilatation.[170] The multicenter EVOLUTION (Clinical Evaluation of the Edwards Lifesciences Percutaneous Mitral Annuloplasty for the Treatment of Mitral Regurgitation) trial is a registry of transcatheter annuloplasty in patients with ischemic mitral regurgitation and coronary sinus anatomy amenable for device implantation.

The technique has not been tested in congenital mitral regurgitation.

Transcatheter Aortic Valve Replacement

The first percutaneous aortic valve replacement in a human was performed in 2002 using a device composed of equine pericardium mounted on a balloon-expandable stent (Fig. 18–17).[171] A recent follow-up reported 36 patients with severe calcific aortic stenosis who had been declined for surgery.[172,173] The percutaneous stented valve was successfully implanted in 27 patients, usually through a venous approach with transseptal catheter advancement. The technique has the advantage of reducing arterial vascular complications but can be technically difficult. Immediate results are encouraging with a decrease in mean gradient from 37 to 9 mm Hg and improved ventricular function and functional class. However, there were six deaths (22%) at 30 days.

A retrograde method using a steerable catheter achieved successful implantation in 47 patients with a dramatic reduction in transvalvular gradient and improvement in ventricular function and functional class.[174] A procedural death was due to obstruction of the ostium of the left coronary artery by an excrescence from a native valve leaflet. There were four other deaths at 30 days. A multicenter European registry is under way to assess further the safety and efficacy of transcatheter aortic valve placement, and a multicenter study for FDA approval is anticipated in the United States.

A self-expanding aortic valve prosthesis intended for retrograde delivery across the aortic valve has been developed by CoreValve (Paris, France). The device was successfully implanted in 17 of 25 patients with immediate hemodynamic improvement and sustained valve performance at 30 days.[175] There was no valve migration, thrombosis, myocardial ischemia, or stroke.

Transcatheter Pulmonary Valve Replacement

A percutaneous stent-based expandable pulmonary valve was designed using a glutaraldehyde-treated bovine jugular venous valve sewn into a balloon expandable stent.[176] *In vitro* and animal studies disclosed that this valve can be compacted into a catheter and deployed without untoward consequences. The device has been experimentally implanted in humans with favorable short-term outcomes, low complications rates, and no deaths.[177]

Under general anesthesia, access is achieved through the femoral or right internal jugular vein. Standard right heart catheterization with systemic arterial pressure monitoring is performed for hemodynamic assessment. Biplane angiography is used to determine the anatomy of the right ventricular outflow tract and branch pulmonary arteries, to select the appropriate site of deployment, and to aid in the choice of the delivery system. After positioning of a stiff guidewire in the pulmonary artery, the valved stent is mounted on a delivery system consisting of a balloon catheter front loaded into a long sheath. The system is then connected to the guidewire and advanced into the pulmonary artery through the obstructed or regurgitant conduit. The stent is uncovered and deployed by balloon inflation (Fig. 18–18). The procedure is currently performed by only a small number of experienced interventionalists, but transcatheter replacement of pulmonary valves is destined to increase in the next few years because of the excellent preliminary human results, the substantial increase in number of available valves, and the increase in trained interventionalists and the number of clinical trials. In 59 consecutive cases, only two stent dislodgments and one homograft dissection were reported.[177] During follow-up, device-related problems occurred in 14 patients, including stent fracture in seven, valve stenosis in three, endocarditis in one, and stent embolization in one. Freedom from valve failure or explantation was 69.8% at 36 months.

Various techniques have been reported for placing percutaneous valves in large pulmonary trunks and right

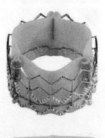
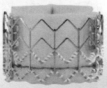

FIGURE 18–17 The Cribier-Edwards percutaneous aortic valve consisting of equine pericardium mounted on a balloon expandable stent.

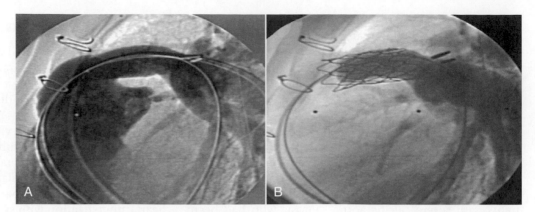

FIGURE 18-18 Transcatheter pulmonary valve replacement. **(A)** Lateral angiogram showing severe regurgitation. **(B)** Regurgitation is absent following transcatheter placement of a stent-mounted bovine valve.

ventricular outflow tracts (> 22 mm). An expandable Nitinol stent was deployed with a central constriction into which the bovine jugular venous valve was directly mounted.[178] An alternative two-step procedure involved a self-expanding Nitinol-covered stent placed in the right ventricular outflow tract followed by placement of the balloon-mounted expandable bovine jugular venous valve. Hybrid techniques have emerged, such as surgical banding of the main pulmonary artery followed by transcatheter placement of the stent-mounted jugular venous valve.[179] Yet to confirm are the feasibility and efficacy of these techniques in patients with aneurysmal right

ventricular outflow tracts after transannular patch repair of tetralogy of Fallot.

TRANSCATHETER APPLICATIONS TO THE SINGLE VENTRICLE

Surgery for hearts with one functional ventricle usually involves three or more complex operations accompanied by significant morbidity and mortality. Transcatheter procedures potentially supplant one or more of the major surgeries in these patients. A combined strategy involving

FIGURE 18-19 Pulmonary artery reconnection in a patient with unidirectional Fontan (F). **(A)** Anteroposterior cineangiography performed simultaneously in the right atrium/Fontan (F) and the superior vena cava/Glenn (G). The right inferior pulmonary artery (RIPA) is connected to the Fontan (F), and the right superior pulmonary artery (RSPA) is connected to the Glenn. Cyanosis was the result of arteriovenous malformations (PAVM) in the right upper lobe (not shown). The right atrium (F) is connected to the left pulmonary artery via a previously stented conduit (St). There is evidence of prior coil embolization of left-sided venous collaterals (C). **(B)** A transseptal needle is advanced from the femoral vein toward a contrast-filled balloon inflated in the RSPA. **(C)** A stent (St-2) is deployed between the right atrium (F) and RSPA. **(D)** Angiography following stent placement discloses a patent connection between the RIPA/F and the RSPA. Six months following this procedure, the peripheral oxygen saturation increased to 94%, implying regression of the PAVM.

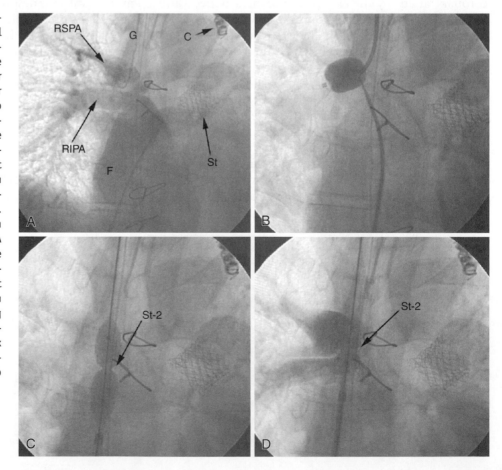

both surgical and transcatheter techniques[180-182] employs a standard Norwood 1 operation for hypoplastic left heart or pulmonary artery banding for double-inlet ventricle followed by a Glenn anastomosis and a hemi-Fontan created by banding the superior vena cava to the right atrial junction and placing a perforated baffle from the inferior vena cava to the roof of the right atrium. Blood flow from the inferior vena cava is preferentially directed through the perforated baffle into the systemic circulation. The construction is amenable to percutaneous completion of the Fontan circulation by stenting the banded right atrium-to-superior vena cava junction and occluding the baffle perforations with coils or closure devices. Alternatively, a total cavopulmonary connection can be achieved by deploying a long covered stent from the inferior vena cava to the right pulmonary artery in the presence of a preexisting Glenn connection.[183] A third alternative involves a special surgical technique for bidirectional Glenn anastomosis in which the proximal aspect of the superior vena cava is sutured to but not connected with the right pulmonary artery; a covered stent subsequently completes the Fontan operation.[184] In the presence of a unidirectional Fontan operation with pulmonary arteriovenous malformations, transcatheter reconnection of the pulmonary arteries is feasible with uncovered stents (Fig. 18-19).[86]

References

1. Rashkind WJ, Miller WW. Creation of an atrial septal defect without thoracotomy. A palliative approach to complete transposition of the great arteries. *JAMA.* 1966;196:991-992.
2. Porstmann W, Wierny L, Warnke H. Closure of persistent ductus arteriosus without thoracotomy. *Ger Med Mon.* 1967;12:259-261.
3. King TD, Thompson SL, Steiner C, Mills NL. Secundum atrial septal defect. Nonoperative closure during cardiac catheterization. *JAMA.* 1976;235:2506-2509.
4. Rubio V, Limon-Lason R. Treatment of pulmonary valvular stenosis and tricuspid stenosis using a modified catheter. Presented before the Second World Conference on Cardiology. Washington, DC, Program 1956.
5. Kan JS, White RI Jr, Mitchell SE, Gardner TJ. Percutaneous balloon valvuloplasty: a new method for treating congenital pulmonary-valve stenosis. *N Engl J Med.* 1982;307:540-542.
6. Allen HD, Beekman RH 3rd, Garson A Jr, et al. Pediatric therapeutic cardiac catheterization: a statement for healthcare professionals from the Council on Cardiovascular Disease in the Young, American Heart Association. *Circulation.* 1998;97:609-625.
7. Hayes CJ, Gersony WM, Driscoll DJ, et al. Second natural history study of congenital heart defects. Results of treatment of patients with pulmonary valvar stenosis. *Circulation.* 1993;87:I28-I37.
8. Stanger P, Cassidy SC, Girod DA, et al. Balloon pulmonary valvuloplasty: results of the Valvuloplasty and Angioplasty of Congenital Anomalies Registry. *Am J Cardiol.* 1990;65:775-783.
9. McCrindle BW. Independent predictors of long-term results after balloon pulmonary valvuloplasty. Valvuloplasty and Angioplasty of Congenital Anomalies (VACA) Registry Investigators. *Circulation.* 1994;89:1751-1759.
10. Fawzy ME, Galal O, Dunn B, et al. Regression of infundibular pulmonary stenosis after successful balloon pulmonary valvuloplasty in adults. *Cathet Cardiovasc Diagn.* 1990;21:77-81.
11. Rao PS. Transcatheter treatment of pulmonary outflow tract obstruction: a review. *Prog Cardiovasc Dis.* 1992;35:119-158.
12. Ring JC, Kulik TJ, Burke BA, Lock JE. Morphologic changes induced by dilation of the pulmonary valve anulus with overlarge balloons in normal newborn lambs. *Am J Cardiol.* 1985;55:210-214.
13. Butto F, Amplatz K, Bass JL. Geometry of the proximal pulmonary trunk during dilation with two balloons. *Am J Cardiol.* 1986;58:380-381.
14. Sharieff S, Shah-e-Zaman K, Faruqui AM. Short- and intermediate-term follow-up results of percutaneous transluminal balloon valvuloplasty in adolescents and young adults with congenital pulmonary valve stenosis. *J Invasive Cardiol.* 2003;15:484-487.
15. Rao PS, Galal O, Patnana M, et al. Results of 3- to 10-year follow-up of balloon dilatation of the pulmonary valve. *Heart.* 1998;80:591-595.
16. Lock JE, Castaneda-Zuniga WR, Fuhrman BP, Bass JL. Balloon dilation angioplasty of hypoplastic and stenotic pulmonary arteries. *Circulation.* 1983;67:962-967.
17. Schneider DJ, Levi DS, Serwacki MJ, et al. Overview of interventional pediatric cardiology in 2004. *Minerva Pediatr.* 2004;56:1-28.
18. Nakanishi T, Tobita K, Sasaki M, et al. Intravascular ultrasound imaging before and after balloon angioplasty for pulmonary artery stenosis. *Catheter Cardiovasc Interv.* 1999;46:68-78.
19. Nakanishi T. Balloon dilatation and stent implantation for vascular stenosis. *Pediatr Int.* 2001;43:548-52.
20. Magee AG, Wax D, Saiki Y, et al. Experimental branch pulmonary artery stenosis angioplasty using a novel cutting balloon. *Can J Cardiol.* 1998;14:1037-1041.
21. Suda K, Matsumura M, Hayashi H, Nishimura K. Comparison of efficacy of medium-sized cutting balloons versus standard balloons for dilation of peripheral pulmonary stenosis. *Am J Cardiol.* 2006;97:1060-3.
22. Roman KS, Kellenberger CJ, Farooq S, et al. Comparative imaging of differential pulmonary blood flow in patients with congenital heart disease: magnetic resonance imaging versus lung perfusion scintigraphy. *Pediatr Radiol.* 2005;35:295-301.
23. McMahon CJ, El Said HG, Vincent JA, et al. Refinements in the implantation of pulmonary arterial stents: impact on morbidity and mortality of the procedure over the last two decades. *Cardiol Young.* 2002;12:445-452.
24. Mohammadi S, Belli E, Martinovic I, et al. Surgery for right ventricle to pulmonary artery conduit obstruction: risk factors for further reoperation. *Eur J Cardiothorac Surg.* 2005;28:217-222.
25. Dearani JA, Danielson GK, Puga FJ, et al. Late follow-up of 1095 patients undergoing operation for complex congenital heart disease utilizing pulmonary ventricle to pulmonary artery conduits. *Ann Thorac Surg.* 2003;75:399-410; discussion 410-411.
26. Zeevi B, Keane JF, Perry SB, Lock JE. Balloon dilation of postoperative right ventricular outflow obstructions. *J Am Coll Cardiol.* 1989;14:401-408; discussion 409-412.
27. Sohn S, Kashani IA, Rothman A. Partial and transient relief of conduit obstruction by low-pressure balloon dilation in patients with congenital heart disease. *Cathet Cardiovasc Diagn.* 1995;34:35-40.
28. Powell AJ, Lock JE, Keane JF, Perry SB. Prolongation of RV-PA conduit life span by percutaneous stent implantation. Intermediate-term results. *Circulation.* 1995;92:3282-3288.
29. Peng LF, McElhinney DB, Nugent AW, et al. Endovascular stenting of obstructed right ventricle-to-pulmonary artery conduits: a 15-year experience. *Circulation.* 2006;113:2598-2605.
30. Aggarwal S, Garekar S, Forbes TJ, Turner DR. Is stent placement effective for palliation of right ventricle to pulmonary artery conduit stenosis? *J Am Coll Cardiol.* 2007;49:480-484.
31. Lababidi Z, Wu JR, Walls JT. Percutaneous balloon aortic valvuloplasty: results in 23 patients. *Am J Cardiol.* 1984;53:194-197.
32. Bonow RO, Carabello BA, Kanu C, et al. ACC/AHA 2006 guidelines for the management of patients with valvular heart disease: a report of the American College of Cardiology/American Heart Association

Task Force on Practice Guidelines (writing committee to revise the 1998 Guidelines for the Management of Patients with Valvular Heart Disease): developed in collaboration with the Society of Cardiovascular Anesthesiologists: endorsed by the Society for Cardiovascular Angiography and Interventions and the Society of Thoracic Surgeons. *Circulation*. 2006;114:e84–e231.

33. Myerson SG, Mitchell AR, Ormerod OJ, Banning AP. What is the role of balloon dilatation for severe aortic stenosis during pregnancy? *J Heart Valve Dis*. 2005;14:147–150.

34. McCrindle BW. Independent predictors of immediate results of percutaneous balloon aortic valvotomy in children. Valvuloplasty and Angioplasty of Congenital Anomalies (VACA) Registry Investigators. *Am J Cardiol*. 1996;77:286–293.

35. Bashore TM, Davidson CJ. Follow-up recatheterization after balloon aortic valvuloplasty. Mansfield Scientific Aortic Valvuloplasty Registry Investigators. *J Am Coll Cardiol*. 1991;17:1188–1195.

36. David F, Sanchez A, Yanez L, et al. Cardiac pacing in balloon aortic valvuloplasty. *Int J Cardiol*. 2007;327–330.

37. Teragaki M, Takeuchi K, Toda I, et al. Potential applications of intracardiac echocardiography in the assessment of the aortic valve from the right ventricular outflow tract. *J Am Soc Echocardiogr*. 1999;12:225–230.

38. Moore P, Egito E, Mowrey H, et al. Midterm results of balloon dilation of congenital aortic stenosis: predictors of success. *J Am Coll Cardiol*. 1996;27:1257–1263.

39. Singer MI, Rowen M, Dorsey TJ. Transluminal aortic balloon angioplasty for coarctation of the aorta in the newborn. *Am Heart J*. 1982;103:131–132.

40. Lock JE, Bass JL, Amplatz K, et al. Balloon dilation angioplasty of aortic coarctations in infants and children. *Circulation*. 1983;68:109–116.

41. Kan JS, White RI Jr, Mitchell SE, et al. Treatment of restenosis of coarctation by percutaneous transluminal angioplasty. *Circulation*. 1983;68:1087–1094.

42. McCrindle BW, Jones TK, Morrow WR, et al. Acute results of balloon angioplasty of native coarctation versus recurrent aortic obstruction are equivalent. Valvuloplasty and Angioplasty of Congenital Anomalies (VACA) Registry Investigators. *J Am Coll Cardiol*. 1996;28:1810–1817.

43. Suarez de Lezo J, Pan M, Romero M, et al. Balloon-expandable stent repair of severe coarctation of aorta. *Am Heart J*. 1995;129:1002–1008.

44. Fletcher SE, Nihill MR, Grifka RG, et al. Balloon angioplasty of native coarctation of the aorta: midterm follow-up and prognostic factors. *J Am Coll Cardiol*. 1995;25:730–734.

45. Ovaert C, McCrindle BW, Nykanen D, et al. Balloon angioplasty of native coarctation: clinical outcomes and predictors of success. *J Am Coll Cardiol*. 2000;35:988–996.

46. Cowley CG, Orsmond GS, Feola P, et al. Long-term, randomized comparison of balloon angioplasty and surgery for native coarctation of the aorta in childhood. *Circulation*. 2005;111:3453–3456.

47. Isner JM, Donaldson RF, Fulton D, et al. Cystic medial necrosis in coarctation of the aorta: a potential factor contributing to adverse consequences observed after percutaneous balloon angioplasty of coarctation sites. *Circulation*. 1987;75:689–95.

48. Johnston TA, Grifka RG, Jones TK. Endovascular stents for treatment of coarctation of the aorta: acute results and follow-up experience. *Catheter Cardiovasc Interv*. 2004;62:499–505.

49. Sandhu SK, Forbes T, Amin Z, et al. Procedural results and acute complications in stenting native and recurrent coarctation of the aorta: a multi-institutional study. American Heart Association Scientific Sessions, oral abstract presentation—2449. 2006;114:II–504.

50. Lange R, Horer J, Kostolny M, et al. Presence of a ventricular septal defect and the Mustard operation are risk factors for late mortality after the atrial switch operation: thirty years of follow-up in 417 patients at a single center. *Circulation*. 2006;114:1905–1913.

51. Chatelain P, Meier B, Friedli B. Stenting of superior vena cava and inferior vena cava for symptomatic narrowing after repeated atrial surgery for D-transposition of the great vessels. *Br Heart J*. 1991;66:466–468.

52. Wisselink W, Money SR, Becker MO, et al. Comparison of operative reconstruction and percutaneous balloon dilatation for central venous obstruction. *Am J Surg*. 1993;166:200–204; discussion 204–205.

53. Ward CJ, Mullins CE, Nihill MR, et al. Use of intravascular stents in systemic venous and systemic venous baffle obstructions. Short-term follow-up results. *Circulation*. 1995;91:2948–2954.

54. Redington AN, Weil J, Somerville J. Self expanding stents in congenital heart disease. *Br Heart J*. 1994;72:378–383.

55. Gianturco C, Anderson JH, Wallace S. Mechanical devices for arterial occlusion. *Am J Roentgenol Radium Ther Nucl Med*. 1975;124:428–435.

56. Sim JY, Alejos JC, Moore JW. Techniques and applications of transcatheter embolization procedures in pediatric cardiology. *J Interv Cardiol*. 2003;16:425–448.

57. Thiene G, Frescura C, Gallucci V. Truncus arteriosus type IV. *Circulation*. 1978;58:758–759.

58. Rabinovitch M, Herrera-deLeon V, Castaneda AR, Reid L. Growth and development of the pulmonary vascular bed in patients with tetralogy of Fallot with or without pulmonary atresia. *Circulation*. 1981;64:1234–1249.

59. Permut LC, Laks H. Surgical management of pulmonary atresia with ventricular septal defect and multiple aortopulmonary collaterals. *Adv Card Surg*. 1994;5:75–95.

60. Turner-Warwick M. Precapillary systemic-pulmonary anastomoses. *Thorax*. 1963;18:225–237.

61. Tadavarthy SM, Klugman J, Castaneda-Zuniga WR, et al. Systemic-to-pulmonary collaterals in pathological states: a review. *Radiology*. 1982;144:55–59.

62. Heimburg P. Bronchial collateral circulation in experimental stenosis of the pulmonary artery. *Thorax*. 1964;19:306–310.

63. Smith GT, Hayland JW, Piemme T, Wells RE Jr. Human systemic-pulmonary arterial collateral circulation after pulmonary thromboembolism. *JAMA*. 1964;188:452–458.

64. Triedman JK, Bridges ND, Mayer JE Jr, Lock JE. Prevalence and risk factors for aortopulmonary collateral vessels after Fontan and bidirectional Glenn procedures. *J Am Coll Cardiol*. 1993;22:207–215.

65. Wallace S, Gianturco C, Anderson JH, et al. Therapeutic vascular occlusion utilizing steel coil technique: clinical applications. *Am J Roentgenol*. 1976;127:381–387.

66. Moore JW, Ing FF, Drummond D, et al. Transcatheter closure of surgical shunts in patients with congenital heart disease. *Am J Cardiol*. 2000;85:636–640.

67. Chuang VP, Wallace S, Gianturco C. A new improved coil for tapered-tip catheter for arterial occlusion. *Radiology*. 1980;135:507–509.

68. Anderson JH, Wallace S, Gianturco C, Gerson LP. "Mini" Gianturco stainless steel coils for transcatheter vascular occlusion. *Radiology*. 1979;132:301–303.

69. Morse SS, Clark RA, Puffenbarger A. Platinum microcoils for therapeutic embolization: nonneuroradiologic applications. *Am J Roentgenol*. 1990;155:401–403.

70. Kaufman SL, Martin LG, Zuckerman AM, et al. Peripheral transcatheter embolization with platinum microcoils. *Radiology*. 1992;184:369–372.

71. Grifka RG, Mullins CE, Gianturco C, et al. New Gianturco-Grifka vascular occlusion device. Initial studies in a canine model. *Circulation*. 1995;91:1840–1846.

72. Ing FF, Mullins CE, Wolfe SB, Grifka RG. Relief of factitious coarctation following occlusion of large patent ductus arteriosus with Gianturco-Grifka vascular occluder. *Cathet Cardiovasc Diagn*. 1998;45:409–412.

73. Befeler B, Justiniano A, Zahn E. Transcatheter closure of a patent ductus arteriosus in an elderly patient with the Gianturco-Grifka vascular occlusion device. *Clin Cardiol.* 2000;23:790-791.

74. Ebeid MR, Braden DS, Gaymes CH, Joransen JA. Closure of a large pulmonary arteriovenous malformation using multiple Gianturco-Grifka vascular occlusion devices. *Catheter Cardiovasc Interv.* 2000;49:426-429.

75. White RI Jr, Lynch-Nyhan A, Terry P, et al. Pulmonary arteriovenous malformations: techniques and long-term outcome of embolotherapy. *Radiology.* 1988;169:663-669.

76. Reidy JF, Anjos RT, Qureshi SA, et al. Transcatheter embolization in the treatment of coronary artery fistulas. *J Am Coll Cardiol.* 1991;18:187-192.

77. Perry SB, Radtke W, Fellows KE, et al. Coil embolization to occlude aortopulmonary collateral vessels and shunts in patients with congenital heart disease. *J Am Coll Cardiol.* 1989;13:100-108.

78. Sharma S, Kothari SS, Krishnakumar R, et al. Systemic-to-pulmonary artery collateral vessels and surgical shunts in patients with cyanotic congenital heart disease: perioperative treatment by transcatheter embolization. *Am J Roentgenol.* 1995;164:1505-1510.

79. Krowka MJ, Cortese DA. Pulmonary aspects of liver disease and liver transplantation. *Clin Chest Med.* 1989;10:593-616.

80. Vase P, Holm M, Arendrup H. Pulmonary arteriovenous fistulas in hereditary hemorrhagic telangiectasia. *Acta Med Scand.* 1985;218:105-109.

81. Chang RK, Alejos JC, Atkinson D, et al. Bubble contrast echocardiography in detecting pulmonary arteriovenous shunting in children with univentricular heart after cavopulmonary anastomosis. *J Am Coll Cardiol.* 1999;33:2052-2058.

82. Srivastava D, Preminger T, Lock JE, et al. Hepatic venous blood and the development of pulmonary arteriovenous malformations in congenital heart disease. *Circulation.* 1995;92:1217-1222.

83. Cloutier A, Ash JM, Smallhorn JF, et al. Abnormal distribution of pulmonary blood flow after the Glenn shunt or Fontan procedure: risk of development of arteriovenous fistulae. *Circulation.* 1985;72:471-479.

84. Uemura H, Yagihara T, Hattori R, et al. Redirection of hepatic venous drainage after total cavopulmonary shunt in left isomerism. *Ann Thorac Surg.* 1999;68:1731-1735.

85. Lee J, Menkis AH, Rosenberg HC. Reversal of pulmonary arteriovenous malformation after diversion of anomalous hepatic drainage. *Ann Thorac Surg.* 1998;65:848-849.

86. Aboulhosn J, Danon S, Levi DS, et al. Regression of pulmonary arteriovenous malformations after transcatheter reconnection of the pulmonary arteries in patients with unidirectional Fontan. *Congenital Heart Disease.* 2007;2:179-184.

87. Gomes AS, Benson L, George B, Laks H. Management of pulmonary arteriovenous fistulas after superior vena cava-right pulmonary artery (Glenn) anastomosis. *J Thorac Cardiovasc Surg.* 1984;87:636-639.

88. Behera SK, Danon S, Levi DS, Moore JW. Transcatheter closure of coronary artery fistulae using the Amplatzer duct occluder. *Catheter Cardiovasc Interv.* 2006;68:242-248.

89. Krichenko A, Benson LN, Burrows P, et al. Angiographic classification of the isolated, persistently patent ductus arteriosus and implications for percutaneous catheter occlusion. *Am J Cardiol.* 1989;63:877-880.

90. Fisher RG, Moodie DS, Sterba R, Gill CC. Patent ductus arteriosus in adults—long-term follow-up: nonsurgical versus surgical treatment. *J Am Coll Cardiol.* 1986;8:280-284.

91. Balzer DT, Spray TL, McMullin D, et al. Endarteritis associated with a clinically silent patent ductus arteriosus. *Am Heart J.* 1993;125:1192-1193.

92. Parthenakis FI, Kanakaraki MK, Vardas PE. Images in cardiology: silent patent ductus arteriosus endarteritis. *Heart.* 2000;84:619.

93. Pas D, Missault L, Hollanders G, et al. Persistent ductus arteriosus in the adult: clinical features and experience with percutaneous closure. *Acta Cardiol.* 2002;57:275-278.

94. Reidy JF, Sowton E, Ross DN. Transcatheter occlusion of coronary to bronchial anastomosis by detachable balloon combined with coronary angioplasty at same procedure. *Br Heart J.* 1983;49:284-287.

95. Armsby LR, Keane JF, Sherwood MC, et al. Management of coronary artery fistulae. Patient selection and results of transcatheter closure. *J Am Coll Cardiol.* 2002;39:1026-1032.

96. Ing FF, Sommer RJ. The snare-assisted technique for transcatheter coil occlusion of moderate to large patent ductus arteriosus: immediate and intermediate results. *J Am Coll Cardiol.* 1999;33:1710-1718.

97. Roy A, Juneja R, Saxena A. Use of Amplatzer duct occluder to close severely hypertensive ducts: utility of transient balloon occlusion. *Indian Heart J.* 2005;57:332-336.

98. Schneider DJ, Moore JW. Patent ductus arteriosus. *Circulation.* 2006;114:1873-1882.

99. Moore JW, Khan M. Gianturco coil occlusion of patent ductus arteriosus. *Curr Interv Cardiol Rep.* 2001;3:80-85.

100. Moore JW, Levi DS, Moore SD, et al. Interventional treatment of patent ductus arteriosus in 2004. *Catheter Cardiovasc Interv.* 2005;64:91-101.

101. Berdjis F, Moore JW. Balloon occlusion delivery technique for closure of patent ductus arteriosus. *Am Heart J.* 1997;133:601-604.

102. Grifka RG. Transcatheter PDA closure using the Gianturco-Grifka vascular occlusion device. *Curr Interv Cardiol Rep.* 2001;3:174-182.

103. Kuhn MA, Latson LA. Transcatheter embolization coil closure of patent ductus arteriosus—modified delivery for enhanced control during coil positioning. *Cathet Cardiovasc Diagn.* 1995;36:288-290.

104. Galal MO. Advantages and disadvantages of coils for transcatheter closure of patent ductus arteriosus. *J Interv Cardiol.* 2003;16:157-163.

105. Magni G, Hijazi ZM, Pandian NG, et al. Two- and three-dimensional transesophageal echocardiography in patient selection and assessment of atrial septal defect closure by the new DAS-Angel Wings device: initial clinical experience. *Circulation.* 1997;96:1722-1728.

106. Pass RH, Hijazi Z, Hsu DT, et al. Multicenter USA Amplatzer patent ductus arteriosus occlusion device trial: initial and one-year results. *J Am Coll Cardiol.* 2004;44:513-519.

107. Masura J, Tittel P, Gavora P, Podnar T. Long-term outcome of transcatheter patent ductus arteriosus closure using Amplatzer duct occluders. *Am Heart J.* 2006;151:755.e7-755.e10.

108. Eicken A, Balling G, Gildein HP, et al. Transcatheter closure of a non-restrictive patent ductus arteriosus with an Amplatzer muscular ventricular septal defect occluder. *Int J Cardiol.* 2007;117:e40-e42.

109. Spies C, Ujivari F, Schrader R. Transcatheter closure of a 22 mm patent ductus arteriosus with an Amplatzer atrial septal occluder. *Catheter Cardiovasc Interv.* 2005;64:352-355.

110. Roques F, Hennequin JL, Sanchez B, et al. Aortic stent-graft for patent ductus arteriosus in adults: the aortic exclusion technique. *Ann Thorac Surg.* 2001;71:1708-1709.

111. Hakim F, Hawelleh AA, Goussous Y, Hijazi ZM. Simultaneous stent implantation for coarctation of the aorta and closure of patent ductus arteriosus using the Amplatzer duct occluder. *Catheter Cardiovasc Interv.* 1999;47:36-38.

112. Sadiq M, Malick NH, Qureshi SA. Simultaneous treatment of native coarctation of the aorta combined with patent ductus arteriosus using a covered stent. *Catheter Cardiovasc Interv.* 2003;59:387-390.

113. Varma C, Benson LN, Silversides C, et al. Outcomes and alternative techniques for device closure of the large secundum atrial septal defect. *Catheter Cardiovasc Interv.* 2004;61:131-139.

114. Cooke JC, Gelman JS, Harper RW. Echocardiologists' role in the deployment of the Amplatzer atrial septal occluder device in adults. *J Am Soc Echocardiogr.* 2001;14:588-594.

115. Carcagni A, Presbitero P. Transcatheter closure of secundum atrial septal defects with the Amplatzer occluder in adult patients. *Ital Heart J.* 2002;3:182-187.

116. Butera G, Chessa M, Bossone E, et al. Transcatheter closure of atrial septal defect under combined transesophageal and intracardiac echocardiography. *Echocardiography.* 2003;20:389–390.

117. Zanchetta M, Rigatelli G, Pedon L, et al. Transcatheter atrial septal defect closure assisted by intracardiac echocardiography: 3-year follow-up. *J Interv Cardiol.* 2004;17:95–98.

118. Aboulhosn J, French WJ, Buljubasic N, et al. Electron beam angiography for the evaluation of percutaneous atrial septal defect closure. *Catheter Cardiovasc Interv.* 2005;65:565–568.

119. Banerjee A, Bengur AR, Li JS, et al. Echocardiographic characteristics of successful deployment of the Das AngelWings atrial septal defect closure device: initial multicenter experience in the United States. *Am J Cardiol.* 1999;83:1236–1241.

120. Walsh KP, Tofeig M, Kitchiner DJ, et al. Comparison of the Sideris and Amplatzer septal occlusion devices. *Am J Cardiol.* 1999;83: 933–936.

121. Shah D, Azhar M, Oakley CM, et al. Natural history of secundum atrial septal defect in adults after medical or surgical treatment: a historical prospective study. *Br Heart J.* 1994;71:224–227; discussion 228.

122. O'Loughlin AJ, Keogh A, Muller DW. Insertion of a fenestrated Amplatzer atrial septostomy device for severe pulmonary hypertension. *Heart Lung Circ.* 2006;15:275–277.

123. Holzer R, Cao QL, Hijazi ZM. Closure of a moderately large atrial septal defect with a self-fabricated fenestrated Amplatzer septal occluder in an 85-year-old patient with reduced diastolic elasticity of the left ventricle. *Catheter Cardiovasc Interv.* 2005;64:513–518; discussion 519–521.

124. Fraisse A, Chetaille P, Amin Z, et al. Use of Amplatzer fenestrated atrial septal defect device in a child with familial pulmonary hypertension. *Pediatr Cardiol.* 2006;27:759–762.

125. Du ZD, Koenig P, Cao QL, et al. Comparison of transcatheter closure of secundum atrial septal defect using the Amplatzer septal occluder associated with deficient versus sufficient rims. *Am J Cardiol.* 2002;90:865–869.

126. Kardon RE, Sokoloski MC, Levi DS, Perry JS, 2nd, Schneider DJ, Allada V, Moore JW. Transthoracic echocardiographic guidance of transcatheter atrial septal defect closure. *Am J Cardiol.* 2004;94: 256–260.

127. Rao PS. Comparative summary of atrial septal defect occlusion devices. Philadelphia: Lippincott, Williams & Wilkins, 2003:91–101.

128. Masura J, Gavora P, Podnar T. Long-term outcome of transcatheter secundum-type atrial septal defect closure using Amplatzer septal occluders. *J Am Coll Cardiol.* 2005;45:505–507.

129. Lopez K, Dalvi BV, Balzer D, et al. Transcatheter closure of large secundum atrial septal defects using the 40 mm Amplatzer septal occluder: results of an international registry. *Catheter Cardiovasc Interv.* 2005;66:580–584.

130. Anzai H, Child J, Natterson B, et al. Incidence of thrombus formation on the CardioSEAL and the Amplatzer interatrial closure devices. *Am J Cardiol.* 2004;93:426–431.

131. Krumsdorf U, Ostermayer S, Billinger K, et al. Incidence and clinical course of thrombus formation on atrial septal defect and patient foramen ovale closure devices in 1,000 consecutive patients. *J Am Coll Cardiol.* 2004;43:302–309.

132. Rodes-Cabau J, Palacios A, Palacio C, et al. Assessment of the markers of platelet and coagulation activation following transcatheter closure of atrial septal defects. *Int J Cardiol.* 2005;98: 107–112.

133. Sigler M, Jux C, Ewert P. Histopathological workup of an Amplatzer atrial septal defect occluder after surgical removal. *Pediatr Cardiol.* 2006;27:775–776.

134. Sigler M, Jux C. Biocompatibility of septal defect closure devices. *Heart.* 2007;93:444–449.

135. Mullen MJ, Hildick-Smith D, De Giovanni JV, et al. BioSTAR Evaluation Study (BEST): a prospective, multicenter, Phase I clinical trial to evaluate the feasibility, efficacy, and safety of the BioSTAR bioabsorbable septal repair implant for the closure of atrial-level shunts. *Circulation.* 2006;114:1962–1967.

136. Lechat P, Mas JL, Lascault G, et al. Prevalence of patent foramen ovale in patients with stroke. *N Engl J Med.* 1988;318:1148–1152.

137. Steiner MM, Di Tullio MR, Rundek T, et al. Patent foramen ovale size and embolic brain imaging findings among patients with ischemic stroke. *Stroke.* 1998;29:944–948.

138. Overell JR, Bone I, Lees KR. Interatrial septal abnormalities and stroke: a meta-analysis of case-control studies. *Neurology.* 2000;55: 1172–1179.

139. Cujec B, Mainra R, Johnson DH. Prevention of recurrent cerebral ischemic events in patients with patent foramen ovale and cryptogenic strokes or transient ischemic attacks. *Can J Cardiol.* 1999;15: 57–64.

140. Wu LA, Malouf JF, Dearani JA, et al. Patent foramen ovale in cryptogenic stroke: current understanding and management options. *Arch Intern Med.* 2004;164:950–956.

141. Hanna JP, Sun JP, Furlan AJ, et al. Patent foramen ovale and brain infarct. Echocardiographic predictors, recurrence, and prevention. *Stroke.* 1994;25:782–786.

142. Mas JL, Zuber M. Recurrent cerebrovascular events in patients with patent foramen ovale, atrial septal aneurysm, or both and cryptogenic stroke or transient ischemic attack. French Study Group on Patent Foramen Ovale and Atrial Septal Aneurysm. *Am Heart J.* 1995;130:1083–1088.

143. Homma S, Di Tullio MR, Sacco RL, et al. Surgical closure of patent foramen ovale in cryptogenic stroke patients. *Stroke.* 1997;28: 2376–2381.

144. Dearani JA, Ugurlu BS, Danielson GK, et al. Surgical patent foramen ovale closure for prevention of paradoxical embolism-related cerebrovascular ischemic events. *Circulation.* 1999;100:II171–II175.

145. Bridges ND, Hellenbrand W, Latson L, et al. Transcatheter closure of patent foramen ovale after presumed paradoxical embolism. *Circulation.* 1992;86:1902–1908.

146. Hara H, Virmani R, Ladich E, et al. Patent foramen ovale: current pathology, pathophysiology, and clinical status. *J Am Coll Cardiol.* 2005;46:1768–1776.

147. Ende DJ, Chopra PS, Rao PS. Transcatheter closure of atrial septal defect or patent foramen ovale with the buttoned device for prevention of recurrence of paradoxic embolism. *Am J Cardiol.* 1996;78:233–236.

148. Du ZD, Cao QL, Joseph A, et al. Transcatheter closure of patent foramen ovale in patients with paradoxical embolism: intermediate-term risk of recurrent neurological events. *Catheter Cardiovasc Interv.* 2002;55:189–194.

149. Chatterjee T, Petzsch M, Ince H, et al. Interventional closure with Amplatzer PFO occluder of patent foramen ovale in patients with paradoxical cerebral embolism. *J Interv Cardiol.* 2005;18: 173–179.

150. Thanopoulos BV, Dardas PD, Karanasios E, Mezilis N. Transcatheter closure versus medical therapy of patent foramen ovale and cryptogenic stroke. *Catheter Cardiovasc Interv.* 2006;68:741–746.

151. Kiblawi FM, Sommer RJ, Levchuck SG. Transcatheter closure of patent foramen ovale in older adults. *Catheter Cardiovasc Interv.* 2006;68:136–142; discussion 143–144.

152. Azarbal B, Tobis J, Suh W, et al. Association of interatrial shunts and migraine headaches: impact of transcatheter closure. *J Am Coll Cardiol.* 2005;45:489–492.

153. Tobis MJ, Azarbal B. Does patent foramen ovale promote cryptogenic stroke and migraine headache? *Tex Heart Inst J.* 2005;32: 362–365.

154. Reisman M, Christofferson RD, Jesurum J, et al. Migraine headache relief after transcatheter closure of patent foramen ovale. *J Am Coll Cardiol.* 2005;45:493–495.

155. Bridges ND, Perry SB, Keane JF, et al. Preoperative transcatheter closure of congenital muscular ventricular septal defects. *N Engl J Med.* 1991;324:1312–1317.

156. Pienvichit P, Piemonte TC. Percutaneous closure of postmyocardial infarction ventricular septal defect with the CardioSEAL septal occluder implant. *Catheter Cardiovasc Interv.* 2001;54:490–494.

157. Lock JE, Block PC, McKay RG, et al. Transcatheter closure of ventricular septal defects. *Circulation.* 1988;78:361–368.

158. Knauth AL, Lock JE, Perry SB, et al. Transcatheter device closure of congenital and postoperative residual ventricular septal defects. *Circulation.* 2004;110:501–507.

159. Chessa M, Carminati M, Cao QL, et al. Transcatheter closure of congenital and acquired muscular ventricular septal defects using the Amplatzer device. *J Invasive Cardiol.* 2002;14:322–327.

160. Thanopoulos BD, Karanassios E, Tsaousis G, et al. Catheter closure of congenital/acquired muscular VSDs and perimembranous VSDs using the Amplatzer devices. *J Interv Cardiol.* 2003;16:399–407.

161. Holzer R, Balzer D, Cao QL, et al. Device closure of muscular ventricular septal defects using the Amplatzer muscular ventricular septal defect occluder: immediate and mid-term results of a U.S. registry. *J Am Coll Cardiol.* 2004;43:1257–1263.

162. Holzer R, Balzer D, Amin Z, et al. Transcatheter closure of postinfarction ventricular septal defects using the new Amplatzer muscular VSD occluder: results of a U.S. Registry. *Catheter Cardiovasc Interv.* 2004;61:196–201.

163. Holzer R, de Giovanni J, Walsh KP, et al. Transcatheter closure of perimembranous ventricular septal defects using the Amplatzer membranous VSD occluder: immediate and midterm results of an international registry. *Catheter Cardiovasc Interv.* 2006;68: 620–628.

164. Pedra CA, Pedra SR, Esteves CA, et al. Percutaneous closure of perimembranous ventricular septal defects with the Amplatzer device: technical and morphological considerations. *Catheter Cardiovasc Interv.* 2004;61:403–410.

165. Tan CA, Levi DS, Moore JW. Percutaneous closure of perimembranous ventricular septal defect associated with a ventricular septal aneurysm using the Amplatzer ductal occluder. *Catheter Cardiovasc Interv.* 2005;66:427–431.

166. Kherani AR, Cheema FH, Casher J, et al. Edge-to-edge mitral valve repair: the Columbia Presbyterian experience. *Ann Thorac Surg.* 2004;78:73–76.

167. St Goar FG, Fann JI, Komtebedde J, et al. Endovascular edge-to-edge mitral valve repair: short-term results in a porcine model. *Circulation.* 2003;108:1990–1993.

168. Feldman T, Wasserman HS, Herrmann HC, et al. Percutaneous mitral valve repair using the edge-to-edge technique: six-month results of the EVEREST Phase I Clinical Trial. *J Am Coll Cardiol.* 2005;46:2134–2140.

169. Kaye DM, Byrne M, Alferness C, Power J. Feasibility and short-term efficacy of percutaneous mitral annular reduction for the therapy of heart failure-induced mitral regurgitation. *Circulation.* 2003;108: 1795–1797.

170. Webb JG, Harnek J, Munt BI, et al. Percutaneous transvenous mitral annuloplasty: initial human experience with device implantation in the coronary sinus. *Circulation.* 2006;113:851–855.

171. Cribier A, Eltchaninoff H, Bash A, et al. Percutaneous transcatheter implantation of an aortic valve prosthesis for calcific aortic stenosis: first human case description. *Circulation.* 2002;106:3006–3008.

172. Cribier A, Eltchaninoff H, Tron C, et al. Percutaneous implantation of aortic valve prosthesis in patients with calcific aortic stenosis: technical advances, clinical results and future strategies. *J Interv Cardiol.* 2006;19:S87–S96.

173. Cribier A, Eltchaninoff H, Tron C, et al. Treatment of calcific aortic stenosis with the percutaneous heart valve: mid-term follow-up from the initial feasibility studies: the French experience. *J Am Coll Cardiol.* 2006;47:1214–1223.

174. Webb JG, Chandavimol M, Thompson CR, et al. Percutaneous aortic valve implantation retrograde from the femoral artery. *Circulation.* 2006;113:842–850.

175. Grube E, Laborde JC, Gerckens U, et al. Percutaneous implantation of the CoreValve self-expanding valve prosthesis in high-risk patients with aortic valve disease: the Siegburg first-in-man study. *Circulation.* 2006;114:1616–1624.

176. Bonhoeffer P, Boudjemline Y, Saliba Z, et al. Transcatheter implantation of a bovine valve in pulmonary position: a lamb study. *Circulation.* 2000;102:813–816.

177. Khambadkone S, Coats L, Taylor A, et al. Percutaneous pulmonary valve implantation in humans: results in 59 consecutive patients. *Circulation.* 2005;112:1189–1197.

178. Boudjemline Y, Agnoletti G, Bonnet D, et al. Percutaneous pulmonary valve replacement in a large right ventricular outflow tract: an experimental study. *J Am Coll Cardiol.* 2004;43:1082–1087.

179. Boudjemline Y, Schievano S, Bonnet C, et al. Off-pump replacement of the pulmonary valve in large right ventricular outflow tracts: a hybrid approach. *J Thorac Cardiovasc Surg.* 2005;129:831–837.

180. Konertz W, Schneider M, Herwig V, et al. Modified hemi-Fontan operation and subsequent nonsurgical Fontan completion. *J Thorac Cardiovasc Surg.* 1995;110:865–867.

181. Hausdorf G, Schneider M, Konertz W. Surgical preconditioning and completion of total cavopulmonary connection by interventional cardiac catheterisation: a new concept. *Heart.* 1996;75:403–409.

182. Klima U, Peters T, Peuster M, et al. A novel technique for establishing total cavopulmonary connection: from surgical preconditioning to interventional completion. *J Thorac Cardiovasc Surg.* 2000; 120:1007–1009.

183. Crystal MA, Yoo SJ, Mikailian H, Benson LN. Images in cardiovascular medicine. Catheter-based completion of the Fontan circuit: a nonsurgical approach. *Circulation.* 2006;114:e5–e6.

184. Galantowicz M, Cheatham JP. Fontan completion without surgery. *Semin Thorac Cardiovasc Surg Pediatr Card Surg Annu.* 2004;7:48–55.

CHAPTER 19

Noncardiac Surgery

JOSEPH K. PERLOFF ▪ MICHAEL SOPHER

When adults with congenital heart disease (CHD) undergo noncardiac surgery, perioperative safety can be increased, often appreciably, if inherent risks are anticipated. The first section of this chapter deals with general considerations, including collaboration with anesthesiologist and surgeon; the types of noncardiac operations that are most prevalent in this adult population; coexisting acquired cardiovascular disease; coexisting medical disorders; medications; hemostatic abnormalities in cyanotic patients; the risk of infective endocarditis; and whether the noncardiac surgery is elective or urgent, major or minor. The second section of the chapter is a discussion of management of unoperated adults with CHD, and the third section focuses on management of patients who have undergone reparative or palliative cardiac surgery.

GENERAL CONSIDERATIONS

It is important to select an anesthesiologist with experience in the specific problems associated with CHD, especially in the adult. The noncardiac surgeon need not have special knowledge of the congenital cardiac malformation, but the attending cardiologist and anesthesiologist who have this knowledge should brief the surgeon regarding the relative risks of operation, including risks of perioperative bleeding, ventricular dysfunction, cyanosis, pulmonary hypertension, arrhythmias, and infective endocarditis. It is the anesthesiologist who is largely, if not wholly, responsible for the physiologic integrity of the patient during noncardiac surgery and who plays a central postoperative role, especially in pain management.[1] When anesthesia is undertaken by a noncardiac anesthesiologist, a broad understanding of the anatomy and physiology of the relevant congenital cardiac malformation should be provided by the attending cardiologist.

The types of noncardiac operations performed in adults with CHD, in order of prevalence, are oral surgery; abdominal surgery (especially gall bladder); neurosurgery (e.g., cerebral abscess or cerebral aneurysm); plastic surgery; genitourinary surgery in males; tubal ligation, abortion, and hysterectomy in females; inguinal herniorrhaphy; vascular surgery for varicose veins; hemorrhoidectomy; and orthopedic surgery (especially for kyphoscoliosis). Nonsurgical procedures, such as radiofrequency ablation and placement of pacemakers and defibrillators, are becoming increasingly frequent in these patients.

Central to risk stratification and perioperative planning are the type of CHD, coexisting acquired cardiovascular disorders or medical disorders either intrinsic to or independent of the congenital cardiac malformation, and whether the noncardiac operation is urgent or elective, major or minor. Age-related acquired disorders of the heart and circulation include ischemic heart disease, systemic hypertension, disturbances in cardiac rhythm and conduction, ventricular failure, carotid artery disease, peripheral vascular disease, and varicosities.[2-6] Major risk factors associated with perioperative morbidity include cyanosis, pulmonary hypertension, and ventricular failure and its catabolic consequences.[7]

Commonly encountered medical disorders include renal and pulmonary diseases and diabetes mellitus. Medications for heart disease and for associated medical disorders must be reviewed in detail, and administration and dosage must be adjusted in anticipation of operation. Planning is especially important in patients with symptomatic coronary artery disease, systemic hypertension, rhythm and conduction disturbances, ventricular failure, and diabetes.

When noncardiac surgery is elective, decisions must be made regarding pre-operative diagnostic tests, such as echocardiography, stress tests, coronary angiography, and pulmonary function. Invasive intraoperative monitoring should be considered on the basis of the type of CHD and the type of surgery, particularly when there is the risk of blood loss or major fluid shifts.[8] Intraoperative transesophageal echocardiography is selectively employed, especially for monitoring ventricular function.

Cyanotic patients may initially experience acute gouty arthritis after operation, or quiescent gout may recur postoperatively (see Chapter 12). Increased tissue vascularity and inherent hemostatic defects including thrombocytopenia and loss of the largest von Willebrand multimers are prevalent. Perioperative bleeding should therefore be anticipated and management carefully planned (see Chapter 12). Anticoagulants are the most problematic medications. It is essential to have protocols for the management of anticoagulants, including presurgical conversion from warfarin to heparin and reinitiation of warfarin postoperatively.

Infective endocarditis prophylaxis is based on the cardiac substrate and whether the type of noncardiac surgery is likely to be accompanied by bacteremia (see Chapter 8). Application of these general principles depends in large part on whether noncardiac surgery is elective or urgent. Emergency surgery with its attendant risks should be avoided if at all possible.

UNOPERATED ACYANOTIC CONGENITAL HEART DISEASE

Situs Inversus with Dextrocardia

This cardiac malposition is characterized by mirror-image locations of thoracic and abdominal viscera.[9] The heart resides in the right hemithorax, the stomach is beneath the right hemidiaphragm, the liver and gallbladder are beneath the left hemidiaphragm, and the vermiform appendix is in the left lower quadrant of the abdomen. Because the malposition usually occurs with hearts that are otherwise structurally and functionally normal, it may go unrecognized until noncardiac surgery brings the patient to medical attention. The risk of noncardiac surgery lies in misconstruing the location of the mirror-image abdominal viscera. The pain of biliary colic is in the left upper quadrant of the abdomen (Fig. 19–1), and the pain of acute appendicitis is in the left lower quadrant.

Congenital Complete Heart Block

In this disorder of conduction, there is no arithmetic relationship between atrial and ventricular activation[9,10] (see Chapter 22). The scalar electrocardiogram is all that is necessary to make a secure diagnosis of complete heart block, which is likely to be congenital if the slow ventricular rate is known to have been present from infancy. The QRS duration is usually normal because the

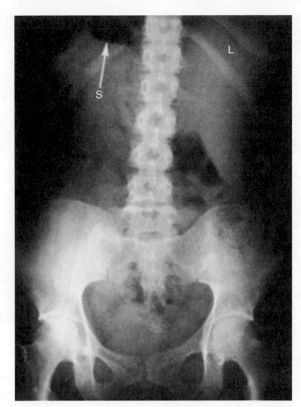

FIGURE 19–1   Abdominal radiograph from a 28-year-old woman with biliary colic that was in the left upper quadrant because of situs inversus. The liver (L) (and therefore the gallbladder) was on the left, and the stomach (S) was on the right. The mirror-image heart was otherwise normal. The patient underwent uneventful cholecystectomy.

subsidiary pacemaker is located above the bifurcation of the bundle of His.[10] Patients usually require a pacemaker before the sixth decade (Fig. 19–2).[9,11,12] Circulatory integrity in isolated congenital complete heart block is determined by the ventricular rate, by ventricular function (which is usually normal), and by the limited hemodynamic adjustments to stress. A substantial majority of young patients are asymptomatic, but the heart and circulation may not necessarily respond appropriately to sudden increases in demand that might accompany noncardiac surgery.[9] In patients with relatively slow heart rates or with subnormal responses to exercise, circulatory adequacy is less likely, and serious complications are more likely to occur (Chapter 11). This is especially so in the presence of wide QRS complexes (pacemaker below the bifurcation of the bundle of His) and a history of syncope or near-syncope.[11] In these high-risk patients, a temporary right ventricular pacemaker should be inserted before noncardiac surgery. Patients who are judged to be at relatively low risk should have electrocardiographic monitoring during and immediately after operation. Intraoperative vagotonic stimuli during ophthalmic or gastrointestinal surgery should be minimized and treated promptly with intravenous atropine or glycopyrrolate, which usually suffices.

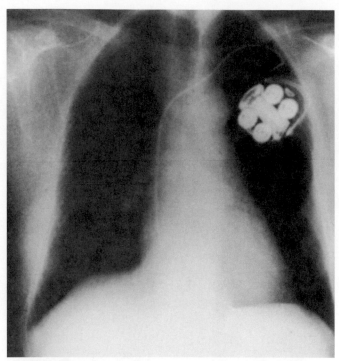

FIGURE 19–2 Chest radiograph from a 60-year-old man with congenital complete heart block and an otherwise normal heart. A pacemaker was implanted at age 51 years.

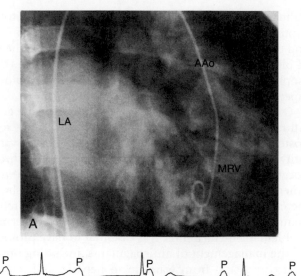

FIGURE 19–3 **(A)** Contrast medium injected into a morphologic right ventricle (MRV) that gave rise to the ascending aorta (AAo) in a 41-year-old man with congenitally corrected transposition of the great arteries. The left atrium (LA) filled because of incompetence of the left atrioventricular valve. Systolic function of the subaortic ventricle was depressed. **(B)** Rhythm strip from the same patient showing complete heart block with a slow ventricular response despite a narrow QRS complex.

Congenitally Corrected Transposition of the Great Arteries

Ventriculo–great arterial malalignment (transposition) is accompanied by atrioventricular malalignment, the double discordance physiologically correcting the discordance intrinsic to each malalignment. This malformation poses four potential risks in patients undergoing noncardiac surgery: (1) disturbances in atrioventricular conduction and atrial rhythm, (2) depressed function of the subaortic morphologic right ventricle, (3) systemic (tricuspid) atrioventricular valve regurgitation, and (4) infective endocarditis because of coexisting pulmonary stenosis, ventricular septal defect, or regurgitation of the left atrioventricular valve.[10] Figure 19–3 refers to a patient who had combined risks of depressed ventricular function, left atrioventricular valve incompetence, and complete heart block.

High-degree heart block in congenitally corrected transposition of the great arteries is a corollary to isolated congenital complete heart block (discussed earlier).[13,14] Conduction defects can reside in the atrioventricular node, the penetrating bundle, or the bundle branches and are potential risks even when coexisting congenital cardiac malformations are absent. Complete atrioventricular block accrues at a rate of about 2% per year.[10,14] When all ages are considered, more than 75% of patients ultimately exhibit atrioventricular block ranging from PR interval prolongation to complete

heart block.[10] Conduction intervals on the surface electrocardiogram coincide with electrophysiologic conduction intervals.[10] It is prudent to monitor the electrocardiogram during and immediately after noncardiac surgery even if the PR interval is normal or only moderately prolonged. In patients with 2:1 atrioventricular block or a history of intermittent changes from PR interval prolongation to 2:1 heart block, a temporary transvenous pacing wire should be in place during and immediately after operation.[13] When the subsidiary pacemaker is proximal to the bifurcation of the His bundle (normal sequence of ventricular activation; see Fig. 19–3), patients should be managed as those with isolated congenital complete heart block (see earlier discussion). Congenitally corrected transposition of the great arteries may be complicated by supraventricular tachycardia, atrial fibrillation, or atrial flutter. These tachyarrhythmias occasionally occur with accelerated conduction through left accessory pathways.[15] Limited functional reserve of a subaortic systemic morphologic right ventricle is a potential risk during noncardiac surgery even if ventricular inversion is otherwise uncomplicated (see Chapters 4 and 11). Left atrioventricular valve regurgitation (see Fig. 19–3) is a substrate for infective endocarditis, imposes volume overload on the functionally limited subaortic right ventricle, and increases the likelihood of disturbances in atrial rhythm, especially atrial fibrillation.

Bicuspid Aortic Stenosis

If the bicuspid aortic valve is functionally normal or only moderately stenotic, the main risk of noncardiac surgery is infective endocarditis (see Chapter 8). If there is severe stenosis of a thin mobile bicuspid valve, the hemodynamic risk of noncardiac surgery can be substantially reduced by balloon dilatation (see Chapter 18). More problematic is severe calcific bicuspid aortic stenosis, which accounts for approximately half of surgically important cases of aortic stenosis in adults.[16] The risks of noncardiac surgery are determined by the degree of obstruction, the functional state of the afterloaded left ventricle, and the presence and degree of acquired coronary artery disease.[2-6] Surgical risks and clinical management are similar to those in adults with acquired calcific aortic stenosis of trileaflet aortic valves.[17] Balloon angioplasty is usually inadequate. Coronary angiography helps to determine whether angina pectoris is due to coexisting coronary artery disease or to the increased oxygen demands of an hypertrophied left ventricle. Preoperative coronary angioplasty reduces the risk of noncardiac surgery. The margin of perioperative safety may be improved by employing a pulmonary artery catheter, by intraoperative transesophageal echocardiography, and by using an arterial line for blood pressure monitoring supervised by the anesthesiologist. A sudden fall in systemic vascular resistance may not be offset by an increase in stroke volume because of fixed obstruction to left ventricular outflow, and rapid infusion of intravenous fluids to counter the fall in blood pressure may cause pulmonary edema.[17] Pharmacologic support of systemic resistance is safer and more efficacious. Sudden intraoperative left ventricular failure requires swift completion of the noncardiac surgical procedure.

Because the stenotic bicuspid aortic valve is susceptible to infective endocarditis, patients undergoing noncardiac surgery that might result in bacteremia should receive appropriate antibiotic prophylaxis (see Chapter 8).

Bicuspid Aortic Regurgitation

The major risks of noncardiac surgery in patients with congenital bicuspid aortic regurgitation are infective endocarditis (Chapter 8) and the functional status of the volume-loaded left ventricle. If left ventricular function is normal, noncardiac surgery should be well tolerated. Coronary artery disease is rarely a problem because patients are likely to be young adults with normal or even large extramural coronary arteries. Moderate intraoperative hypotension is not a hazard because it decreases regurgitant flow and reduces left ventricular volume overload.

Infective endocarditis, to which the incompetent bicuspid aortic valve is susceptible, can suddenly and catastrophically augment the degree of regurgitation, imposing an additional volume load on a functionally adequate left ventricle or, still worse, on a depressed left ventricle.[18] Meticulous prophylaxis is therefore obligatory (see Chapter 8).

If left ventricular function is depressed, elective noncardiac surgery raises the prospect of preemptive aortic valve repair or replacement (Chapter 16). Risk reduction for emergency noncardiac surgery in patients with severe bicuspid aortic regurgitation and a dilated, depressed left ventricle can be achieved by hemodynamic monitoring with a pulmonary artery catheter, intraoperative transesophageal echocardiography, an arterial line, and postoperative pharmacologic afterload reduction.

Coarctation of the Aorta

Five perioperative considerations confront patients with coarctation of the aorta who require noncardiac surgery: (1) the presence and functional status of a coexisting bicuspid aortic valve (discussed earlier), (2) systemic blood pressure and left ventricular function, (3) the presence of premature coronary artery disease, (4) the risk of infective endocarditis, and (5) the risk of dissection of the ascending aorta. Of particular concern is the occasional older patient in whom coarctation is accompanied by depressed left ventricular function, a significantly stenotic or incompetent bicuspid aortic valve, and atherosclerotic coronary artery disease. In an attempt to reduce the risk and depending on the urgency of noncardiac surgery, priority is assigned to aortic valve replacement, coronary artery angioplasty, and repair of the coarctation. Even if coarctation repair is achieved, pharmacologic management of systemic hypertension and depressed left ventricular function must still be addressed. An arterial line and a pulmonary artery catheter should be inserted for monitoring during and immediately after noncardiac surgery, and intraoperative transesophageal echocardiography should be considered. There is a small but significant risk of infective endocarditis at the coarctation site, but the principle risk is on a coexisting bicuspid aortic valve (see Chapter 8).[10]

Pulmonary Valve Stenosis

Mild pulmonary valve stenosis incurs no risk during noncardiac surgery, and moderate stenosis incurs little more than the risk of infective endocarditis (see Chapter 8). If noncardiac surgery is elective and pulmonary stenosis is severe, especially if right ventricular function is depressed, operative risk is materially reduced by balloon valvuloplasty (see Chapter 18). When urgent noncardiac surgery precludes balloon valvuloplasty, hemodynamic monitoring of the right ventricle can be achieved by inserting a central venous catheter into the right atrium and by intraoperative transesophageal echocardiography for assessing right ventricular function. Systemic arterial blood pressure should be monitored in the operating room and postoperatively because severe pulmonary stenosis limits or precludes appropriate responses of the systemic circulation to major hemodynamic fluctuations.

Ebstein's Anomaly of the Tricuspid Valve

Three risks are incurred by noncardiac surgery in patients with acyanotic Ebstein's anomaly: (1) atrial tachyarrhythmias (fibrillation or flutter) with or without accessory pathways (see Chapter 22), (2) paradoxical embolization through an interatrial communication, and (3) the functionally inadequate right ventricle. The major perioperative hazard is atrial fibrillation or flutter with accelerated conduction through accessory pathways. A history of rapid heart action or delta waves on the scalar electrocardiogram requires perioperative electrocardiographic monitoring. The anesthesiologist must be prepared for pharmacologic intervention or intraoperative cardioversion. The risk of postoperative paradoxical embolization from leg veins is minimized by the use of support hose and early ambulation. There is no documented susceptibility of the malformed incompetent tricuspid valve for infective endocarditis in the absence of a pacemaker.

Ostium Secundum Atrial Septal Defect

In young adults, an isolated, uncomplicated ostium secundum atrial septal defect incurs comparatively little risk during noncardiac surgery, with two caveats. First is the response to hemorrhage that provokes a rise in systemic resistance and a fall in venous return, a combination that augments the left-to-right interatrial shunt, sometimes appreciably. A second risk is paradoxical embolization from leg veins because thrombi that enter the inferior vena cava tend to stream across the atrial septal defect into the systemic circulation.[10] Postoperative leg care and early ambulation minimize venous stasis.

In older patients with an ostium secundum atrial septal defect, noncardiac surgery incurs significant risks. The effect of the large left-to-right shunt on pulmonary compliance and on the work of breathing increases anesthetic risk.[1] Advancing age is accompanied by decreased left ventricular distensibility, which augments the left-to-right interatrial shunt.[10,19] Beginning in the fourth decade, there is an increase in the incidence of atrial arrhythmias, especially atrial fibrillation, and, less commonly, atrial flutter or supraventricular tachycardia.[10] Noncardiac surgery may serve as an arrhythmogenic trigger, so electrocardiographic monitoring is desirable even in patients without a history of disturbances in atrial rhythm.

The majority of symptomatic adults aged 40 years or older with ostium secundum atrial septal defect have mild to moderate pulmonary hypertension that exists with a persistent, large left-to-right shunt, and thus the aging right ventricle is doubly beset by both pressure and volume overload.[10] However, a pulmonary artery catheter for hemodynamic monitoring is more likely to find its way across the atrial septal defect than into the right ventricle or pulmonary artery or if thrombi or air bubbles were to develop, could result in paradoxical embolism and stroke. Monitoring of the overloaded right ventricle is best accomplished with intraoperative transesophageal echocardiography.

UNOPERATED CYANOTIC CONGENITAL HEART DISEASE

Anesthetic Risk

Because the ventilatory response to hypoxemia is blunted in cyanotic patients,[20] systemic hypoxemia can be seriously aggravated by the superimposition of alveolar hypoxia associated with general anesthesia. Basal state hyperventilation in cyanotic patients prevents a rise in PCO_2 (Chapter 12), but hyperventilation is suppressed by general anesthesia. An experienced anesthesiologist is aware of these risks, which can be obviated by controlled ventilation.

Acute Cholecystitis

Adults with cyanotic CHD have an increased incidence of acute cholecystitis caused by calcium bilirubinate gallstones (Figs. 19–4, *A*, and 19–5, *A*).[21] Bilirubin is formed from the breakdown of heme, a process that is excessive because of the increase in red cell mass (Chapter 12). Unconjugated bilirubin is virtually insoluble in water at physiologic pH, so when the unconjugated form appears in bile, it tends to solidify and form calcium bilirubinate gallstones[21] (see Fig. 19–5, *A*). Acute cholecystitis is important not only because of its prevalence in cyanotic adults but also because noncardiac surgery is seldom elective and because the acutely inflamed gallbladder (see Fig. 19–5, *B*) is a source of gram-negative bacteremia that incurs the risk of infective endocarditis (see Chapter 8). Importantly, biliary colic and acute cholecystitis may become clinically manifest years after the elimination of cyanosis by cardiac surgery.[21]

Acute Gouty Arthritis

The stress of noncardiac surgery may induce a first attack of gout or may induce a recurrence. The incidence of acute gouty arthritis in cyanotic adults is similar to that in other forms of secondary hyperuricemia, but management differs (see Chapter 12).[22] It is important to control the pain of the acute attack without provoking the undesirable dehydrating gastrointestinal side effects of oral colchicine. Fluid loss results in hemoconcentration, which is undesirable in cyanotic patients with erythrocytosis. Intravenous colchicine avoids the nausea and diarrhea that frequently accompany oral colchicine in full therapeutic dose.[21] Intravenous colchicine (1–2 mg slowly

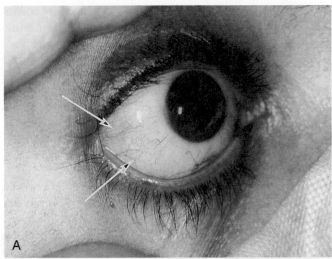

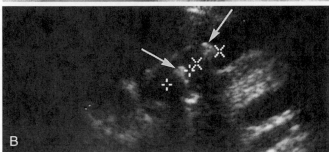

FIGURE 19–4 **(A)** A 32-year-old woman with complex cyanotic congenital heart disease and acute cholecystitis presented with scleral icterus superimposed upon cyanosis. Note the increased vascularity of the sclera. **(B)** Ultrasonogram of the gallbladder in a 32-year-old cyanotic woman with single ventricle, pulmonary vascular disease, and recurrent biliary colic. Arrows indicate calcium bilirubinate gallstones.

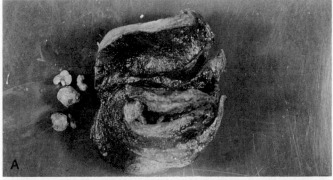

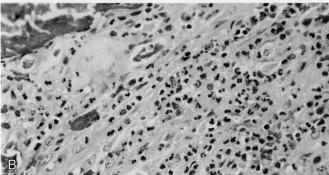

FIGURE 19–5 **(A)** Surgical specimen of a thick-walled gallbladder and calcium bilirubinate gallstones from a 45-year-old cyanotic man with a nonrestrictive ventricular septal defect, Eisenmenger syndrome, and acute cholecystitis. **(B)** Histologic section of the thick-walled gallbladder shows the inflammatory reaction of acute cholecystitis that incurred the risk of gram-negative bacteremia.

over 5 minutes) is followed by 1-mg oral doses at 6- and 12-hour intervals, with the total dose not exceeding 4 mg in 24 hours. Corticosteroids are efficacious in acute gouty arthritis and are legitimate alternatives to colchicine in selected patients.[21]

Perioperative Management of Hemostasis

Abnormal hemostasis and its perioperative management in cyanotic patients are dealt with in detail in Chapter 12. The bleeding tendency is due to a combination of intrinsic hemostatic defects acting in concert with the risk inherent in increased tissue vascularity.[21,23,24] If the hematocrit level is greater than 65% in an iron-replete state, and if the timing (urgency) of noncardiac surgery permits, a 250 to 500 ml isovolumetric phlebotomy should be performed, followed in 24 hours by an additional withdrawal designed to reduce the hematocrit to just below 65%.[21] This policy achieves an appropriate balance between desirable hemostatic effects of preoperative phlebotomy and the undesirable effects of iron depletion. Phlebotomized units should be reserved for potential autologous transfusion.

The accuracy of clinical laboratory determinations of coagulation parameters is compromised in cyanotic patients. Prothrombin time, International Normalized Ratio (INR), and thromboplastin time laboratory results are likely to be spurious and therefore misleading. Tubes for determining these coagulation parameters contain a fixed amount of citrate as an anticoagulant based on normal hematocrit levels, but that fixed amount of citrate is excessive for erythrocytotic blood, which contains less plasma. Tubes with the correct amount of citrate can be prepared if clinical laboratory technicians are informed of the patient's hematocrit. The correction should be made when hematocrit levels exceed 55%.

Excessive intraoperative or postoperative blood loss is analogous to excessive phlebotomy (see Chapter 12).[21] The management of perioperative bleeding (assuming that the noncardiac surgery is otherwise uncomplicated) employs fresh frozen plasma, cryoprecipitate, and platelet transfusion (see Chapter 12).

Intravenous Access

Peripheral intravenous lines, infusions, and intravenous drugs in cyanotic patients risk introducing air or particles into peripheral veins with delivery into the systemic circulation by the right-to-left shunt. Accordingly, air and particle filters should be routine, with the filter device inserted into the distal end of the intravenous line (Fig. 19–6) to minimize trapped air or particles in the long proximal segment of the line. If these filters are not available, great care should be taken to remove all air bubbles from these lines.

Elevated Pulmonary Vascular Resistance

Noncardiac surgery in cyanotic patients with elevated pulmonary vascular resistance incurs the risks inherent in cyanosis and the more formidable risks of pulmonary vascular disease. Fixed pulmonary vascular resistance precludes rapid adaptive responses to labile intraoperative or postoperative hemodynamic fluctuations. A sudden major fall in systemic resistance may precipitate intense cyanosis and even death. A sudden rise in systemic resistance may abruptly and dangerously depress systemic, and therefore cerebral, blood flow. The simplest and most useful way for the anesthesiologist to monitor systemic vascular resistance is with an arterial line and a fingertip pulse oximeter that reflects moment-to-moment variations in systemic resistance because oxygen saturation tends to fall as systemic resistance falls and vice versa. In patients with Eisenmenger physiology, inserting a pulmonary artery catheter incurs risk without benefit.[24] Percutaneous entry incurs the risk of bleeding (discussed earlier), and intracardiac monitoring provides little or no useful information that is not more safely and readily secured by the pulse oximeter.

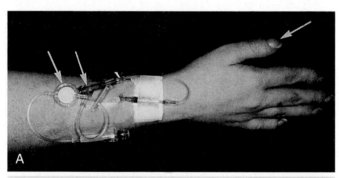

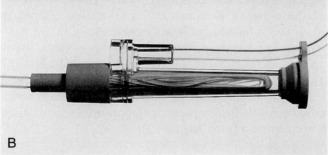

FIGURE 19–6 **(A)** Air/particle filter system *(oblique paired arrows)* inserted into an intravenous line of a cyanotic adult. Note clubbing of the thumb *(single arrow on right)* and digits. The filter system was placed in the distal end of the intravenous line to minimize air or particles trapped in the long proximal segment of the line. **(B)** Close-up of a second type of air/particle filter.

Postural hypotension often occurs during early convalescence from noncardiac surgery with general anesthesia. The postural drop in systemic resistance suddenly augments the right-to-left shunt. Convalescent cyanotic patients with pulmonary vascular disease should change positions slowly (lying to sitting, sitting to standing, standing to walking) until postoperative postural hypotension has abated.

Oxygen Inhalation

It seems intuitive that oxygen inhalation is desirable in cyanotic patients during and immediately after noncardiac surgery. Administration of high levels of inspired oxygen may raise arterial oxygen saturation in the presence of a right-to-left shunt by increasing the partial pressure of alveolar oxygen, but there is little evidence that routine perioperative use of inhaled oxygen is beneficial.[21] Unhumidified oxygen causes drying of the nasal mucous membranes and predisposes to epistaxis in cyanotic patients with intrinsic hemostatic defects and increased mucous membrane vascularity (see earlier and Chapter 12).

Tetralogy of Fallot

Unoperated tetralogy of Fallot is no longer a common cause of cyanotic CHD in adults.[10] Should that eventually arise, intraoperative and postoperative monitoring of systemic vascular resistance are readily achieved with a systemic arterial line and a pulse oximeter. A slower heart rate and increased preload are important in maintaining adequate flow through a dynamic right ventricular outflow tract. Susceptibility to infective endocarditis requires antibiotic prophylaxis if the noncardiac surgical procedure incurs the risk of bacteremia (see Chapter 8). Early postoperative postural hypotension is managed as just described.

SURGICALLY REPAIRED CONGENITAL HEART DISEASE

This category comprises an increasing percentage of congenital cardiac patients who require noncardiac operations. With few exceptions, repair leaves behind residua and sequelae that vary from innocuous to serious (see Chapter 20). Certain concerns are unique to patients who have undergone reparative surgery for complex cyanotic CHD, whereas other concerns derive from acquired cardiovascular disease and from noncardiac medical illnesses.

Aortic Valve

Direct surgical repair or balloon valvuloplasty for isolated congenital bicuspid aortic stenosis at best creates a functionally normal bicuspid valve that retains the risk of infective endocarditis (Chapter 8). Surgical techniques for creating a trileaflet aortic valve are evolving, but repair may leave residual stenosis or incompetence. Noncardiac surgery may incur the risk of dissection of an ascending aorta that is significantly dilatated because of the inherent medial abnormality associated with a bicuspid aortic valve.[25] Aortic regurgitation as a residuum following repair of tetralogy of Fallot, perimembranous ventricular septal defect, or discrete subaortic stenosis is usually a concern because of susceptibility to infective endocarditis rather than because of the volume load imposed on the left ventricle.

Pulmonary Valve

Mild residual obstruction or mild low-pressure pulmonary regurgitation imposes no hemodynamic burden and does not require antibiotic prophylaxis for infective endocarditis (Chapter 8). However, prophylaxis is prudent after repair of complex right ventricular outflow obstruction (e.g., tetralogy of Fallot) because of potential residual obstruction and regurgitation.

Atrioventricular Valves

A cleft but competent mitral valve is a functionally unimportant residuum after repair of an atrioventricular septal defect. Although the risk of infective endocarditis during noncardiac surgery is low, prophylaxis is advisable because the valve is structurally abnormal. A similar case can be made for ideal reconstruction of the tricuspid valve in right-sided Ebstein's anomaly or for an inherently competent left-sided Ebstein valve in congenitally corrected transposition of the great arteries.

Prosthetic Valves

Prosthetic mechanical valves in the left side of the heart, whether in the inflow or outflow position (Chapter 16), significantly complicate the management of noncardiac surgery. The most compelling concern is anticoagulation. Perioperative management of anticoagulants depends chiefly on the type and location of the prosthesis and on the atrial rhythm.[26] Currently employed low-profile mechanical valves (Chapter 16) carry a lower risk of thromboembolic complications than older generations of mechanical valves. Mechanical mitral prostheses are at higher risk of thromboembolism than are mechanical aortic prostheses, especially if the mitral prosthesis is associated with atrial fibrillation.

If noncardiac surgery is elective, and if the prosthesis carries a relatively high thromboembolic risk, warfarin should be replaced with either subcutaneous enoxaparin or other low-molecular-weight heparins, or with an in-hospital continuous intravenous infusion of heparin at a rate that achieves an activated partial thromboplastin time of 1.5 to 2 times control. The infusion is continued until the prothrombin time or INR approaches normal. Intravenous heparin is discontinued 4 to 6 hours before the elective operation, restarted within 48 hours postoperatively, and replaced by warfarin as soon as safety permits. For a lower-risk prosthetic valve in the aortic location (Chapter 16), warfarin is discontinued 2 to 3 days before noncardiac surgery and is resumed 2 to 3 days postoperatively.

More problematic is emergency noncardiac surgery in a patient receiving warfarin for a mechanical prosthesis. Rapid reversal of the warfarin-induced hemostatic defect or defects requires infusion of fresh frozen plasma and vitamin K. However, if vitamin K is used preoperatively, response to the readministration of warfarin postoperatively may be seriously blunted.

Ventricular Function

Ventricular function is a major concern in the management of surgically repaired patients with CHD undergoing noncardiac surgery. The functional adequacy of the subaortic ventricle is, as a rule, more important than the function of the subpulmonary ventricle. Cases in point are the functional adequacy of a subaortic morphologic right ventricle in congenitally corrected transposition of the great arteries (see Fig. 19–3), the subaortic right ventricle after an atrial switch repair for complete transposition of the great arteries, and the systemic ventricle after a Fontan repair. There is concern regarding the long-term patency of reimplanted coronary arteries after the arterial switch operation for complete transposition of the great arteries, and impaired myocardial blood flow has been reported in response to vasodilatation with adenosine in asymptomatic children 10 years or more after surgery.[27] In another study, 74% of asymptomatic children 9 years after the arterial switch operation had wall motion abnormalities unmasked by dobutamine stress echocardiography.[28] Intraoperative transesophageal echocardiography is usually the best means of monitoring systolic ventricular function. Inotropic support and afterload reduction may be necessary. Undesirable perioperative fluid overload must be balanced against the need for adequate preload.

Electrophysiologic Sequelae and Residua

Among the most prevalent and important concerns in the management of postoperative congenital cardiac patients undergoing noncardiac surgery are electrophysiologic sequelae and residua (Chapter 22). Electrophysiologic sequelae after intraatrial repair vary from atrial flutter or fibrillation after closure of an ostium secundum atrial septal defect to complex disturbances in rhythm and conduction after atrial switch repairs for complete transposition of the great arteries (Chapters 20 and 22).

Intraventricular surgery can be followed by electrophysiologic sequelae that originate from the ventriculotomy per se and from the intracardiac repair (Chapter 20). With current surgical techniques for repair of tetralogy of Fallot, bifascicular block and complete heart block are uncommon but are often present in patients who were operated on decades earlier and now require noncardiac surgery. If operation is elective, preoperative insertion of a dual-chamber pacemaker reduces perioperative risk. When noncardiac surgery is urgent, a temporary transvenous pacemaker wire should be placed. A more frequent electrophysiologic concern is electrical instability of the incised right ventricle that may harbor a slowed conduction reentrant substrate capable of sustained monomorphic ventricular tachycardia.[29] Less well known but no less important are atrial arrhythmias in adults who have undergone repair of tetralogy of Fallot (Chapters 20 and 22). Supraventricular tachycardia, atrial fibrillation, or atrial flutter occurred in 34% of these patients, and sinus node dysfunction occurred in 36%.[30] Antiarrhythmic therapy should be reviewed before noncardiac surgery, the rhythm should be continuously monitored perioperatively, acute perioperative arrhythmias should be promptly treated, and antiarrhythmic medications should be restarted as soon as possible after operation.

Pulmonary Hypertension and Pulmonary Vascular Disease

Even minor noncardiac surgery in patients with pulmonary vascular disease is potentially hazardous. Accordingly, elective surgery, with certain exceptions, is to be avoided. In a report of 144 pulmonary hypertensive patients undergoing noncardiac surgical procedures, 42% had short-term morbidity including respiratory failure (28%), cardiac arrhythmias (12%), and congestive heart failure (11%), and 10 (7%) experienced perioperative death.[31] Multivariate predictors of morbidity and mortality included right axis deviation, right ventricular hypertrophy, right ventricular systolic pressure $\geq$ 0.66 of systemic, intraoperative use of dopamine or epinephrine, New York Heart Association class $\geq$ II, anesthesia longer than 3 hours, and nonsurgical procedures that are inherently higher risk.[31] Elevated, if not fixed, pulmonary vascular resistance limits or precludes intraoperative or postoperative circulatory adjustments to hemodynamic fluctuations, such as the formidable risk of hypotension. Systemic blood pressure should be monitored with an arterial line, and moment-to-moment fluctuations in the degree of right-to-left shunting can be monitored with a pulse oximeter. Insertion of a pulmonary catheter is in itself a risk that must be carefully weighed in the balance and inserted with extreme caution, if at all. Intraoperative transesophageal echocardiography is a safer and useful means of monitoring right ventricular function (Chapter 6).

Current treatment modalities for pulmonary vascular disease include prostacyclin analogues, the endothelin receptor antagonist bosentan, inhaled iloprost, intravenous epoprostenol, and inhaled nitric oxide. In managing patients with pulmonary hypertension perioperatively, it is useful to have available inhaled nitric oxide delivery modalities. Because most patients with primary pulmonary hypertension are young women, the most frequent noncardiac surgical procedure is tubal ligation or abortion, which are recommended because of the formidable hazards of pregnancy (see Chapter 9).

Acquired Cardiovascular Diseases and Noncardiac Medical Illnesses

These diseases and illnesses can be major concerns when postoperative adults with CHD require noncardiac surgery. The patients not only have surgically modified congenital cardiac malformations but also age-related acquired cardiovascular or noncardiovascular diseases, especially coronary artery disease, systemic hypertension, renal disease, pulmonary disease, diabetes mellitus, or gastrointestinal disorders.

References

1. Baum VC, Perloff JK. Anesthetic implications of adults with congenital heart disease. *Anesth Analg.* 1993;76:1342–1358.
2. Detsky AS, Abrams HB, Forbath N, et al. Cardiac assessment for patients undergoing noncardiac surgery. A multifactorial clinical risk index. *Arch Int Med.* 1986;146:2131–2134.
3. Eagle KA, Berger PB, Calkins H, et al. ACC/AHA guideline update for perioperative cardiovascular evaluation for noncardiac surgery—executive summary: a report of the American College of Cardiology/American Heart Association Task Force on Practice Guidelines (Committee to Update the 1996 Guidelines on Perioperative Cardiovascular Evaluation for Noncardiac Surgery). *J Am Coll Card.* 2002;39:542–553.
4. Eagle KA, Brundage BH, Chaitman BR, et al. Guidelines for perioperative cardiovascular evaluation for noncardiac surgery: an abridged version of the report of the American College of Cardiology/American Heart Association Task Force on Practice Guidelines. *Mayo Clin Proc.* 1997;72:524–531.
5. Freeman WK, Gibbons RJ, Shub C. Preoperative assessment of cardiac patients undergoing noncardiac surgical procedures. *Mayo Clin Proc.* 1989;64:1105–1117.
6. Lee TH, Marcantonio ER, Mangione CM, et al. Derivation and prospective validation of a simple index for prediction of cardiac risk of major noncardiac surgery. *Circulation.* 1999;100:1043–1049.
7. Warner MA, Lunn RJ, O'Leary PW, Schroeder DR. Outcomes of noncardiac surgical procedures in children and adults with congenital heart disease. Mayo Perioperative Outcomes Group. *Mayo Clin Proc.* 1998;73:728–734.
8. Foster E, Graham TP Jr, Driscoll DJ, et al. Task Force 2: special health care needs of adults with congenital heart disease. *J Am Coll Card.* 2001;37:1176–1183.
9. Esscher E. Review article. Congenital complete heart block. *Acta Paediatr Scand.* 1981;70:131–136.
10. Perloff JK. *The Clinical Recognition of Congenital Heart Disease.* 5th ed. Philadelphia: W.B. Saunders, 2003.

11. Pinsky WW, Gillette PC, Garson A Jr, McNamara DG. Diagnosis, management, and long-term results of patients with congenital complete atrioventricular block. *Pediatrics.* 1982;69:728–733.

12. Reid JM, Coleman EN, Doig W. Complete congenital heart block. Report of 35 cases. *Br Heart J.* 1982;48:236–239.

13. Gillette PC, Busch U, Mullins CE, McNamara DG. Electrophysiologic studies in patients with ventricular inversion and "corrected transposition." *Circulation.* 1979;60:939–945.

14. Huhta JC, Maloney JD, Ritter DG, et al. Complete atrioventricular block in patients with atrioventricular discordance. *Circulation.* 1983;67:1374–1377.

15. Bharati S, Rosen K, Steinfield L, Miller RA, Lev M. The anatomic substrate for preexcitation in corrected transposition. *Circulation.* 1980;62:831–842.

16. Subramanian R, Olson LJ, Edwards WD. Surgical pathology of pure aortic stenosis: a study of 374 cases. *Mayo Clin Proc.* 1984;59:683–690.

17. O'Keefe JH Jr, Shub C, Rettke SR. Risk of noncardiac surgical procedures in patients with aortic stenosis. *Mayo Clin Proc.* 1989;64:400–405.

18. Morganroth J, Perloff JK, Zeldis SM, Dunkman WB. Acute severe aortic regurgitation. Pathophysiology, clinical recognition, and management. *Ann Intern Med.* 1977;87:223–232.

19. Tikoff G, Kuida H. Pathophysiology of heart failure in congenital heart disease. *Mod Concepts Cardiovas Dis.* 1972;41:1–6.

20. Edelman NH, Lahiri S, Braudo L, et al. The blunted ventilatory response to hypoxia in cyanotic congenital heart disease. *N Engl J Med.* 1970;282:405–411.

21. Perloff JK. Systemic complications of cyanosis in adults with congenital heart disease. Hematologic derangements, renal function, and urate metabolism. *Cardiol Clin.* 1993;11:689–699.

22. Ross EA, Perloff JK, Danovitch GM, et al. Renal function and urate metabolism in late survivors with cyanotic congenital heart disease. *Circulation.* 1986;73:396–400.

23. Colon-Otero G, Gilchrist GS, Holcomb GR, et al. Preoperative evaluation of hemostasis in patients with congenital heart disease. *Mayo Clin Proc.* 1987;62:379–385.

24. Devitt JH, Noble WH, Byrick RJ. A Swan-Ganz catheter related complication in a patient with Eisenmenger's syndrome. *Anesthesiology.* 1982;57:335–337.

25. Larson EW, Edwards WD. Risk factors for aortic dissection: a necropsy study of 161 cases. *Am J Cardiol.* 1984;53:849–855.

26. Tinker JH, Noback CR, Vlietstra RE, Frye RL. Management of patients with heart disease for noncardiac surgery. *JAMA.* 1981;246:1348–1350.

27. Hauser M, Bengel FM, Kuhn A, et al. Myocardial blood flow and flow reserve after coronary reimplantation in patients after arterial switch and Ross operation. *Circulation.* 2001;103:1875–1880.

28. Hui L, Chau AK, Leung MP, et al. Assessment of left ventricular function long term after arterial switch operation for transposition of the great arteries by dobutamine stress echocardiography. *Heart.* 2005;91:68–72.

29. Perloff JK, Middlekauf HR, Child JS, et al. Usefulness of postventriculotomy signal averaged electrocardiograms in congenital heart disease. *Am J Cardiol.* 2006;98:1646–1651

30. Perloff JK, Natterson PD. Atrial arrhythmias in adults after repair of tetralogy of Fallot. *Circulation.* 1995;91:2118–2119.

31. Ramakrishna G, Sprung J, Ravi BS, et al. Impact of pulmonary hypertension on the outcomes of noncardiac surgery: predictors of perioperative morbidity and mortality. *J Am Coll Cardiol.* 2005;45:1691–1699.

RESIDUA
AND SEQUELAE
AFTER SURGERY
OR INTERVENTIONAL
CATHETERIZATION

CHAPTER 20

Residua and Sequelae: A Perspective

JOSEPH K. PERLOFF

The residua and sequelae after surgery for congenital heart disease (CHD) have long been matters of interest.[1] *A residuum* (pl. *residua*) is defined as "that which remains, a residue, what is left over" (*Oxford English Dictionary*).[1] *Residua* are therefore extrinsic to—that is, apart from—the design of the surgical procedure and take the form of cardiac, vascular, and noncardiovascular disorders intentionally left behind at the time of reparative cardiac surgery (Table 20-1). With few exceptions, these residua are obligatory and do not result from an operation having fallen short of its objective, at least in a technical sense.[2] A *sequel* (pl. *sequelae*) is defined as "what follows or arises out of an earlier event."[1] *Sequelae* are therefore intrinsic to the operative design and are represented by alterations or disorders intentionally incurred—occasionally or invariably—at the time of cardiac surgery. Sequelae are obligatory consequences of operation and are not necessarily acceptable or desirable (Table 20-2). *Complications* are unintentional, nonobligatory aftermaths of reparative surgery that range from inconsequential to fatal (Fig. 20-1). Complications are not dealt with here, although sequelae and complications imperceptibly merge.

Surgery is *curative* when no postoperative residua, sequelae, or complications are incurred,[3] implying that normal cardiovascular structure and function are achieved and maintained. Further medical or surgical management (treatment) for CHD is no longer necessary. However, curative cardiac surgery does not preclude noncardiac residua (see Table 20-1), some of which have major impacts on morbidity and longevity.

RESIDUA

Electrophysiologic residua are inherent components of certain congenital cardiac malformations, are often present in preoperative 12-lead scalar electrocardiograms, and persist—sometimes harmlessly, sometimes not so harmlessly—after reparative surgery (see Chapter 22). The four major electrophysiologic residua include (1) axis deviation, especially left; (2) conduction defects, especially atrioventricular; (3) disorders of impulse formation, especially involving the sinus node; and (4) disturbances in atrial and ventricular rhythm.

Left-axis deviation is an electrocardiographic feature of atrioventricular septal defect, double-outlet right ventricle with subaortic ventricular septal defect, tricuspid atresia with pulmonary stenosis and normally related great arteries, univentricular hearts of the left ventricular type without inversion of the outlet chamber, congenitally corrected transposition of the great arteries with normal subpulmonary ventricular pressure, and bypass tracts with Ebstein's anomaly of the tricuspid valve.[4] When cardiac surgery does not alter the electrophysiologic mechanism responsible for left-axis deviation, the axis deviation and its substrate persist as postoperative residua. However, when accessory pathways express themselves as left-axis deviation, the substrate can be intentionally eliminated by catheter ablation or surgical revision.

Right-axis deviation that accompanies right ventricular hypertrophy is not the result of a congenital electrophysiologic substrate. When surgery or interventional catheterization is followed by regression of hypertrophy, as

Table 20-1   Residua after Reparative Surgery for Congenital Heart Disease
Electrophysiologic
Valvular
Ventricular
Vascular
Noncardiovascular

Table 20-2   Sequelae after Reparative Surgery for Congenital Heart Disease
Electrophysiologic
Valvular
Prosthetic materials
Myocardial and endocardial
Vascular
Neurologic

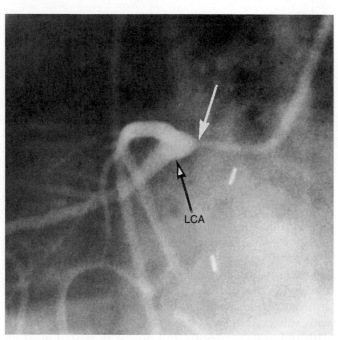

FIGURE 20-1   Selective coronary arteriogram from a 17-year-old female patient with left ostial obstruction *(white arrow)* caused by a coronary artery cannula employed at intracardiac repair of tetralogy of Fallot. The ostial obstruction represents a complication, not a sequel of operation. LCA, left coronary artery.

after repair of pulmonary valve stenosis, right-axis deviation decreases but seldom disappears altogether.

Conduction defects, overt or potential, may persist as residua after reparative cardiac surgery. A case in point is congenitally corrected transposition of the great arteries in which conduction defects range from PR interval prolongation, to second-degree atrioventricular block (typically 2:1), to complete heart block.[5] Less common and less important is the mild to moderate PR interval prolonga-

tion that persists after closure of an ostium secundum atrial septal defect.[6] Still less common but potentially grave is first-degree atrioventricular block that sometimes accompanies *familial* ostium secundum atrial septal defect and persists postoperatively.[6]

Residual abnormalities of *impulse formation* generally reside in the sinus node. In an ostium secundum atrial septal defect, for example, sinus node dysfunction has been identified as early as the first years of life[7] and persists as a postoperative residuum. In a sinus venosus atrial septal defect of the superior vena caval type, the defect occupies the site of the normal sinoatrial node, which is therefore absent. The ectopic atrial rhythm is reflected in a leftward shift of the P wave axis.[5]

Preoperative *atrial tachyarrhythmias* in ostium secundum atrial septal defect or Ebstein's anomaly of the tricuspid valve may persist as postoperative residua and are represented by atrial fibrillation or flutter and supraventricular tachycardia. Atrial fibrillation also results from preoperative atrial enlargement caused by large left-to-right shunts or atrioventricular valve regurgitation.

Valvular Residua

Structural and functional abnormalities of cardiac valves that persist as residua after surgery or interventional catheterization fall into three general categories (see Chapter 21): (1) congenitally malformed but functionally normal valves that persist unchanged as postoperative residua, (2) intrinsically normal cardiac valves that are rendered incompetent by physiologic stress inherent in the congenital malformation that prompted surgical repair, and (3) congenitally malformed stenotic or incompetent cardiac valves that do not lend themselves to repair and therefore harbor the postoperative residua of incomplete repair. Aortic valve abnormalities that persist as physiologically unimportant postoperative residua include a functionally normal bicuspid aortic valve with coarctation of the aorta (Fig. 20-2) and mild aortic regurgitation that persists after repair of tetralogy of Fallot, perimembranous ventricular septal defect, or truncus arteriosus.

An intrinsically normal cardiac valve rendered incompetent by the physiologic stress of the congenital malformation that prompted surgical repair is represented by tricuspid regurgitation in response to pulmonary hypertension or obstruction to right ventricular outflow. These anatomically normal tricuspid valves lend themselves to functional repair during cardiac surgery, leaving behind morphologic residua of the reparative technique.

Congenitally malformed cardiac valves that do not lend themselves to anatomic repair are represented by the mitral valve abnormality of atrioventricular septal defect. Surgery can render the valve competent but leaves behind an obligatory postoperative anatomic residuum. Another case in point is balloon dilatation or direct repair of congenital bicuspid aortic stenosis. Assuming complete relief

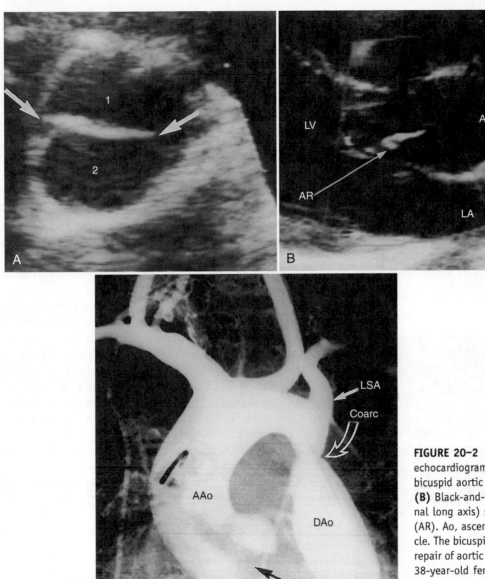

FIGURE 20–2   (A) Diastolic frame of a two-dimensional echocardiogram (short axis) showing a functionally normal bicuspid aortic valve *(arrows)* with its two leaflets (1, 2). **(B)** Black-and-white copy of a color flow image (parasternal long axis) showing mild bicuspid aortic regurgitation (AR). Ao, ascending aorta; LA, left atrium; LV, left ventricle. The bicuspid aortic valve persisted as a residuum after repair of aortic coarctation. **(C)** Thoracic aortogram from a 38-year-old female patient with coarctation of the aorta (Coarc) and a moderately incompetent bicuspid aortic valve that persisted as a residuum after the coarctation was repaired. AAo, ascending aorta; DAo, descending aorta; LSA, left subclavian artery.

of obstruction with little or no incompetence, the valve remains bicuspid albeit functionally normal and represents an important residuum (see Chapter 21).

After cardiac surgery, *ventricular residua* can be permanent, such as inherently abnormal chamber morphology, or can change with the passage of time, such as alterations in chamber mass (see Table 20–1 and Chapter 23). Permanent postoperative ventricular morphologic residua occur in hearts with either one or two ventricles. The chamber morphology inherent in a univentricular heart necessarily persists as a postoperative residuum in which functional expression differs according to whether the morphology of the single chamber is left or right ventricular,[8] differences that are reflected in survival patterns after a Fontan repair (see Chapter 5).

A postoperative ventricular morphologic residuum of fundamental importance is the persistence of an anatomic right ventricle in the systemic location after an atrial switch operation for complete transposition of the great arteries or after operation for congenitally corrected transposition of the great arteries. The systemic circulation is served by a morphologic subaortic right ventricle that is not designed to serve the systemic circulation (see Chapter 5).

An increase in ventricular mass and its regression after operation or catheter intervention are fundamental properties of ventricular myocardium (see Chapter 23). An increase in mass in excess of the normal growth process is determined by the type of inciting stimulus (hemodynamic or hypoxic), cardiomyocyte immaturity or maturity at the time the inciting stimulus is imposed, the duration of the stimulus, and the type of myocardial cell involved in the increased mass. Neonatal cardiac myocytes temporarily retain their intrauterine capacity to replicate—*hyperplasia*—which is the cellular response to hemodynamic overload or hypoxia imposed on an immature heart. Within a few months after birth, myocytes begin to lose their capacity to replicate. Hypoxia then exerts a deleterious effect, and pressure or volume overload provokes an increase in ventricular mass due to myocyte enlargement—*hypertrophy*—without capillary angiogenesis leading to an undesirable *decrease* in capillary density. A variation on this theme occasionally occurs many years after an atrial switch operation for complete transposition of the great arteries, when hypertrophic subpulmonary stenosis provokes an increase in left ventricular mass due to myocyte hypertrophy (Fig. 20–3).

An important objective of reparative surgery is elimination of the stimulus that provoked the increase in ventricular mass, whether the increase was caused by myocyte hyperplasia or hypertrophy. The precise cellular basis for postoperative regression of increased ventricular mass is not entirely clear. When an increase in mass is caused by hypertrophy, regression implies a decrease in size of normal numbers of enlarged (hypertrophied) cardiac myocytes. When an increase in mass is caused by hyperplasia, regression of mass implies a decrease in size of greater numbers of normal-sized (replicated) cardiomyocytes (see Chapter 23). These different patterns of regression have important functional implications (discussed later). The response of *fibroblast hyperplasia* to operative elimination of the overload or hypoxic stimulus is unknown, but there is evidence that connective tissue cells do not regress as do cardiac myocytes.[9]

Maintenance or restoration of normal ventricular function is an important objective of cardiac surgery. After a Fontan repair for tricuspid atresia, left ventricular function is better than after a Fontan repair for single ventricle of left ventricular morphology, which in turn is better than the function of a single ventricle of right ventricular morphology.[8] In hearts equipped with two ventricles, the ejection fraction of a morphologic right ventricle is inherently lower than the ejection fraction of a morphologic left ventricle, whether the right ventricle is subpulmonary (noninverted) or subaortic (inverted). Accordingly, a postoperative residuum of considerable importance is the relative functional inadequacy of a subaortic morphologic right ventricle after an atrial switch operation for complete transposition of the great arteries, or the functional inadequacy of a subaortic morphologic right ventricle after surgery for congenitally corrected transposition of the great arteries.

Interestingly and importantly, preoperative left ventricular systolic function that *exceeds* normal may persist as a presumably innocent and perhaps desirable postoperative ventricular functional residuum.[9] Witness the *supranormal* left ventricular systolic function that accompanies congenital aortic stenosis when the increased afterload is imposed during the stage of myocyte immaturity. The increase in ventricular mass is due chiefly to an increase in the number of cardiomyocytes—hyperplasia—which is accompanied by a proportionate growth in the microvascular bed—capillary angiogenesis. Increased numbers of normal myocytes accompanied by normal capillary density are responsible for supranormal ejection performance (see Chapter 23).[9] After interventional catheterization or surgical relief of aortic stenosis, left ventricular mass decreases, capillary density increases, and supranormal left ventricular ejection fraction persists as a potentially desirable postoperative left ventricular functional residuum.

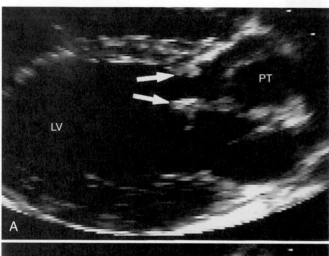

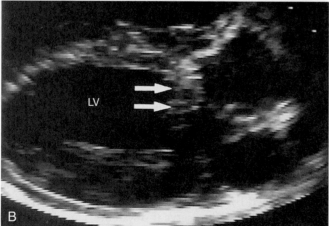

FIGURE 20–3 Two-dimensional echocardiographic images (parasternal long axis) from a 20-year-old female patient with complete transposition of the great arteries and a Mustard repair at age 4 months. Hypertrophic left ventricular (LV) outflow obstruction (paired arrows) was progressive, culminating in the severe obstruction shown in diastole (above) and in systole (below) during which the outflow tract virtually sealed. PT, pulmonary trunk.

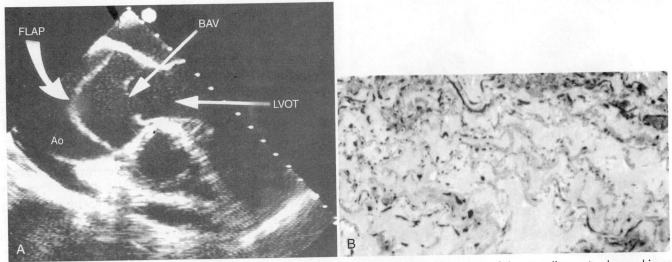

FIGURE 20–4   (A) Transesophageal echocardiogram from a 21-year-old male with dissecting aneurysm of the ascending aorta above a bicuspid aortic valve. **(B)** Fragmentation of medial elastic fibers in the aortic root of a patient with bicuspid aortic stenosis.

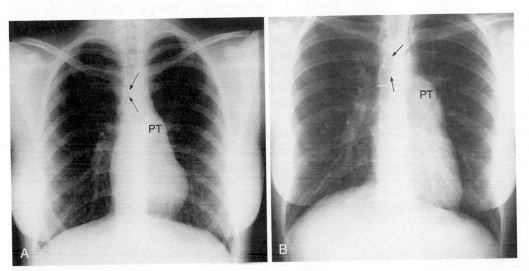

FIGURE 20–5   (A) X-ray of a 16-year-old female patient who underwent surgical closure of an ostium secundum atrial septal defect at age 5 years. The x-ray is normal except for mild dilatation of the pulmonary trunk (PT) and the metal sutures *(arrows)*. **(B)** Marked residual dilatation of the pulmonary trunk (PT) in a 24-year-old female patient who underwent surgical closure of an ostium secundum atrial septal defect at age 6 years. The x-ray is otherwise normal except for metal sutures *(arrows)*.

Vascular Residua

There are two principal categories of vascular residua after repair of congenital cardiac malformations: (1) anatomic residua that involve the aorta, pulmonary trunk, cerebral arteries, and coronary arteries and (2) elevated resistance or pressure in the systemic or pulmonary vascular beds.

A relationship exists between inherent medial abnormalities of the ascending aorta (Fig. 20–4) and a congenitally bicuspid aortic valve.[10,11] The proximal and distal paracoarctation aorta harbor similar medial abnormalities.[12] Both sites are susceptible to rupture or dissection,[10–13] a predisposition that remains as an important postoperative residuum.

An analogous but benign residuum is persistent dilatation of the pulmonary trunk after closure of an atrial septal defect (Fig. 20–5). Dilatation of the pulmonary trunk as a residuum after relief of typical mobile pulmonary valve stenosis occasionally merges imperceptibly with aneurysmal dilatation (Fig. 20–6) attributed to an inherent abnormality of the media of the pulmonary trunk.[14,15]

Aneurysm of the circle of Willis is an important cerebral vascular residuum after repair of coarctation of the aorta.[5] Predisposition to rupture persists after operation and may announce itself in normotensive patients long after ideal coarctation repair.[13] Coronary artery anomalies occur in tetralogy of Fallot in 2% to 10% of patients.[5] Barring accidental injury at operation, these anomalous coronaries persist as functionally unimportant postoperative vascular residua. Similarly, the dilatated, tortuous coronary arteries in adults with cyanotic CHD (see Chapter 12) persist as presumably benign vascular residua after surgical relief of cyanosis[5] (Fig. 20–7). Not so benign is the coronary artery intimal proliferation,

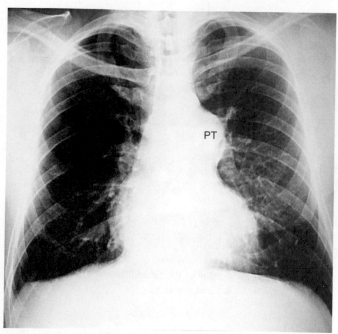

FIGURE 20-6 Striking residual dilatation of the pulmonary trunk (PT) 23 years after surgical pulmonary valvotomy for isolated mobile pulmonary valve stenosis.

medial thickening, and premature atherosclerosis that persists after repair in older patients with coarctation of the aorta or supravalvular aortic stenosis (Fig. 20–8). Persistent systemic hypertension, usually systolic, is an important vascular residuum after repair of coarctation of the aorta. The older the patient at the time of repair, the more likely is long-term elevation of blood pressure.[16] Even if the postoperative basal blood pressure is normal, the systolic pressure may rise disproportionately during exercise, implying a residual decrease in compliance of the proximal aortic and systemic arterial walls[16] (see Chapter 11). Systemic hypertension occasionally persists as a postoperative residuum after repair of supravalvular aortic stenosis in Williams syndrome.[17]

The preoperative status of the resistance vessels of the pulmonary vascular bed is a major determinant of residual postoperative pulmonary vascular disease. There are three principal age-related characteristics of a normally evolving pulmonary vascular bed: (1) remodeling of neonatal medial muscular thickness, (2) distal extension of medial muscle, and (3) replication (proliferation) of peripheral acinar units with an increase in the number of intraacinar arteries that is proportionate to the increase in acinar units.[4] Early operation sets the stage for normal evolution (maturation) of the pulmonary vascular bed and lessens the likelihood of residual postoperative pulmonary vascular disease. Technical refinements and relative safety of surgical repair within the first year of life have created an air of optimism regarding the prevalence of pulmonary vascular disease as a postoperative residuum. An exception is Down syndrome, which has an independent proclivity for pulmonary vascular disease because of an inadequate increase in intraacinar arteries.[18]

Noncardiovascular residua are represented by developmental abnormalities, abnormalities of the central nervous

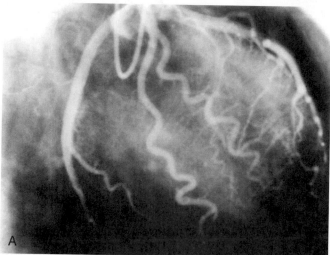

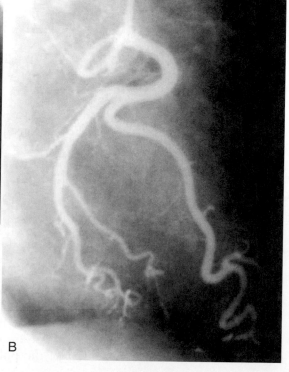

FIGURE 20-7 Dilatated and tortuous left **(A)** and right **(B)** coronary arteries in a 32-year-old female patient with a nonrestrictive ventricular septal defect and Eisenmenger syndrome.

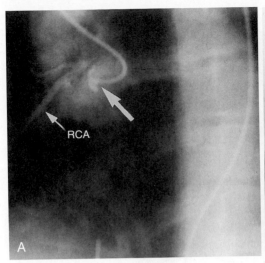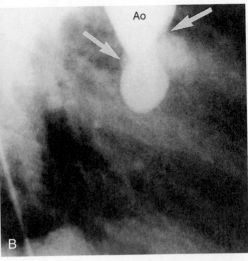

FIGURE 20–8 **(A)** Right coronary artery (RCA) ostial occlusion *(large unmarked arrow)* that resulted from a thickened ridge of aortic intimal proliferation in a patient with supravalvular aortic stenosis (as shown in **(B)** *(paired arrows)*. The ostial obstruction was bypassed during repair of the supravalvular stenosis, leaving the bypassed right coronary as a postoperative vascular residuum. Ao, aorta.

system and of the special senses, and medical and dental disorders. These residua vary from minor alterations in thoracic configuration (pectus excavatum, scoliosis, kyphosis) to major central nervous system residua that exert profound effects on the quality of life long after cardiac surgery[15,19-21] (see Chapter 14).

Hypoplastic left heart syndrome and complete transposition of the great arteries are accompanied by decreases in intrauterine cerebral blood flow and organic brain disease[21] (see Chapter 14). Mental retardation is inherent in Down syndrome, and premature Alzheimer's disease tends to be additive when survival extends into the fourth decade[22] (see Chapter 13). Physical retardation (dwarfism) is a feature of Turner syndrome and the Ellis-van Creveld syndrome and persists as a postoperative residuum, although patients with XO Turner syndrome sometimes respond to hormone replacement with development of secondary sex characteristics and normal phenotype (Fig. 20–9) but persistence of small stature. Somatic abnormalities such as facial dysmorphism (Fig. 20–10), cleft lip, cleft palate, and the musculoskeletal limb abnormalities accompanying the Holt-Oram syndrome (Fig. 20–11) persist as obligatory undesirable postoperative residua.[23]

Focal neurologic deficits and seizure disorders are important noncardiovascular postoperative residua (see Table 20–1). Spinal cord injuries incurred during repair of aortic coarctation are avoidable complications rather than residua[24] (see Chapter 14). Paradoxical emboli in patients with cyanotic CHD (Fig. 20–12, *A* and *B*) may target the brain (Fig. 20–12, *C*) and result in permanent neurologic residua after repair of the malformation that set the stage for the embolus. A healed brain abscess (Fig. 20–13) serves as the residual focus of a late postoperative seizure disorder (see Chapter 14).

Abnormalities of special senses (visual, auditory) persist as postoperative residua (see Table 20–1). Cataracts and deafness are intrinsic to the rubella syndrome and

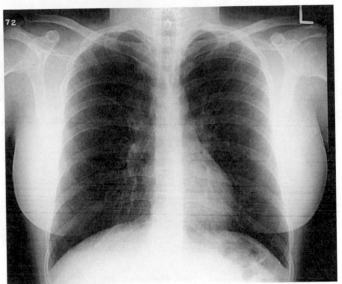

FIGURE 20–9 X-ray of a 28-year-old woman with XO Turner syndrome. She experienced an ideal response to hormone replacement with normal breast development, development of secondary sex characteristics, and normal phenotype except for small stature. There was no cardiovascular disease.

persist as major residua after division of a coexisting patent ductus arteriosus.[5] However, residua related to special senses are occasionally salutary, as in Williams syndrome, in which visual and conceptual deficits are counterbalanced by hyperacusis and exceptional auditory and musical skills, including perfect pitch.[25] Dental abnormalities as postoperative residua include premature eruption of malformed maxillary incisors in the Ellis-van Creveld syndrome and the malformed teeth and abnormal bite (malocclusion) of Williams syndrome[5] (Fig. 20–14).

Medical disorders may or may not be related to the congenital cardiac malformation for which an operation was performed and may or may not be cardiovascular. Diabetes, acquired coronary artery disease, and essential

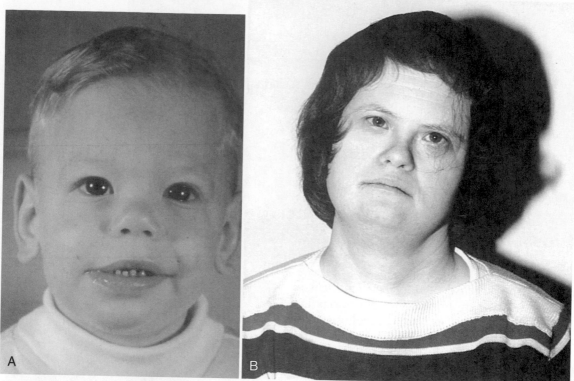

FIGURE 20–10 Facial dysmorphism characteristic of Williams syndrome **(A)** and Down syndrome **(B)**. These dysmorphic facies persist as obligatory postoperative residua.

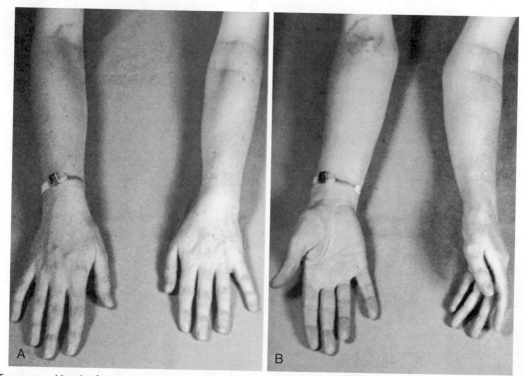

FIGURE 20–11 Forearms and hands of a 34-year-old female patient with the Holt-Oram syndrome and an ostium secundum atrial septal defect. **(A)** The left thumb is moderately hypoplastic; the left arm is shorter than the right. **(B)** Supination of the left hand is limited by radial hypoplasia. The "crooked" appearance of the hypoplastic thumb becomes apparent. The limb abnormality persisted postoperatively as an obligatory noncardiovascular residuum.

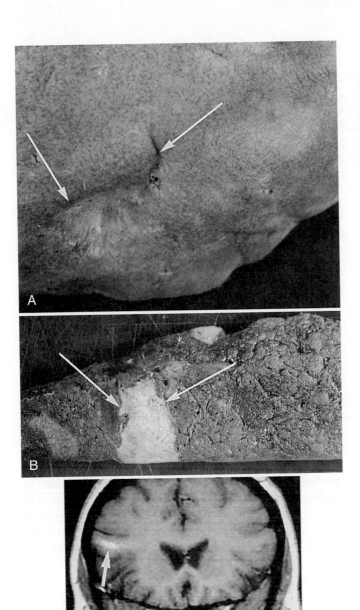

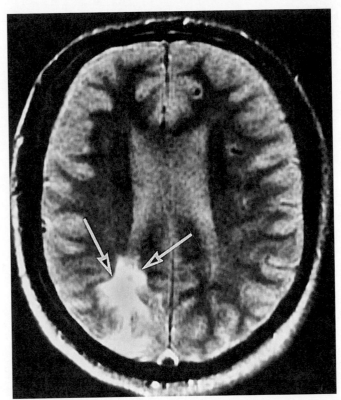

FIGURE 20-13   Computed tomographic scan from a 26-year-old male patient with tetralogy of Fallot. A healed brain abscess *(paired arrows)* caused a childhood seizure disorder that persisted as a residuum after subsequent intracardiac repair.

FIGURE 20-12   **(A)** Renal infarct *(paired arrows)* from a paradoxical embolus, an incidental residuum discovered at necropsy in a 47-year-old male patient who had undergone a Fontan repair for univentricular heart. **(B)** Splenic infarct *(paired arrows)* from a paradoxical embolus, an incidental residuum discovered at necropsy in a 42-year-old cyanotic woman with Eisenmenger syndrome. **(C)** Healed cerebral infarct *(arrow)* from a paradoxical embolus, a neurologic residuum in a 39-year-old cyanotic woman with Eisenmenger syndrome.

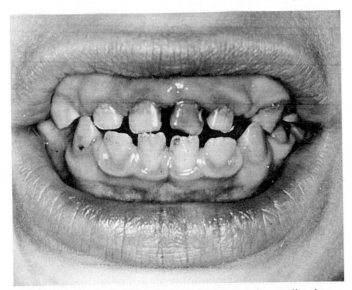

FIGURE 20-14   Williams syndrome, typical dental abnormality characterized by small, malformed, widely spaced teeth with malocclusion.

hypertension are age-related disorders that persist as postoperative residua. The association between autoimmune hypothyroidism and Down syndrome is widely accepted[26] and may express itself as a postoperative residuum. Cyanotic adults have a predisposition to calcium bilirubinate gallstones that may announce themselves as acute cholecystitis years after successful cardiac operation (Fig. 20-15; see Chapter 19). Conversely, preoperative hyperuricemia and gouty arthritis do not persist after surgical relief of cyanosis[27] (see Chapter 12).

SEQUELAE

Electrophysiologic sequelae after atriotomy are due less to the atrial incision than to the intraatrial repair for which the atriotomy provides access (see Chapter 15). Closure of an ostium secundum atrial septal defect in older adults may be

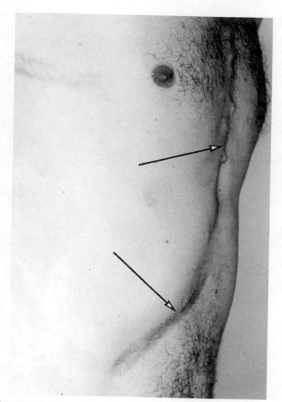

FIGURE 20–15   Thoracic and abdominal scars in a 34-year-old male who underwent intracardiac repair of cyanotic congenital heart disease via a midline sternotomy (*upper arrow*). Three years later, a cholecystectomy (right upper quadrant scar, *lower arrow*) was done for biliary colic caused by residual calcium bilirubinate gallstones.

preceded or followed (or both) by atrial tachyarrhythmias that represent residua rather than sequelae. However, atrial tachyarrhythmias that appear late postoperatively are probably sequelae of preexisting chronic volume overload of the right atrium. Sinus node injury during closure of an atrial septal defect, especially a superior vena caval sinus venosus defect, is less a sequel than a complication. Mustard or Senning operations for complete transposition of the great arteries are replete with postoperative sequelae of impulse formation and rhythm that represent subtle mergers of sequelae and complications (see Chapter 15). A right atrial incision provides access for intraventricular repair of tetralogy of Fallot or perimembranous ventricular septal defect (see Chapter 15). Operative injury to the proximal right bundle branch alone or in combination with injury to the left anterior fascicle is a complication rather than a sequel.

An authentic sequel after right ventriculotomy is prolongation of right ventricular activation manifested in the 12-lead scalar electrocardiogram as "right bundle branch block," although the conduction defect usually reflects prolonged *intraventricular* conduction rather than interruption of the proximal right bundle branch[28] (see Chapter 22). However, when the surface electrocardiogram exhibits the combination of right bundle branch block *and* left anterior fascicular block, the

conduction defect is likely to be bifascicular because of the proximity of the right bundle branch and the left anterior fascicle. Bifascicular block sets the stage for complete heart block, a potentially hazardous postoperative electrophysiologic sequel if not complication (see Chapter 22). A second important electrophysiologic sequel of ventriculotomy is a slowed conduction substrate for reentrant monomorphic ventricular tachycardia (see Chapter 22).[29]

Cardiac Valves

Sequelae involving cardiac valves result from surgery or interventional catheterization on left ventricular or right ventricular *outflow* or *inflow* tracts (see Table 20–2 and see Chapter 21).

Outflow Repair

Mild aortic regurgitation is a common sequel of balloon dilatation or direct repair of congenital bicuspid aortic stenosis—a small price to pay for relief of obstruction. Similarly, balloon dilatation or surgical repair of mobile congenital pulmonary valve stenosis may be followed by mild pulmonary regurgitation, a physiologically minor and altogether acceptable sequel. Conversely, surgical repair of complex obstruction to right ventricular outflow represented by tetralogy of Fallot tends to be followed by significant degrees of pulmonary regurgitation, which when severe, serve as a trigger for monomorphic ventricular tachycardia (see Chapter 22) and have a negative impact on the functional state of the incised right ventricle.

Inflow Repair

Sequelae of inflow valve repairs are more prevalent and functionally more significant than sequelae of outflow repairs, because the mitral and tricuspid mechanisms are much more complex than the aortic and pulmonary valve mechanisms. Even if reconstruction of the malformed mitral valve associated with an atrioventricular septal defect eliminates regurgitation altogether, the left ventricular inflow remains guarded by a morphologically abnormal mitral apparatus for which subsequent competence is influenced by changes in left ventricular geometry that accompany advancing age. The reconstructed tricuspid apparatus of Ebstein's anomaly creates a functionally adequate but structurally abnormal valve mechanism that is an obligatory sequel of repair (see Chapter 15).

Prosthetic Materials

Biologic and nonbiologic materials employed as components of surgical procedures for CHD represent a special category of sequelae (see Table 20–2). Patches, prosthetic valves, and conduits are the subjects of Chapter 16.

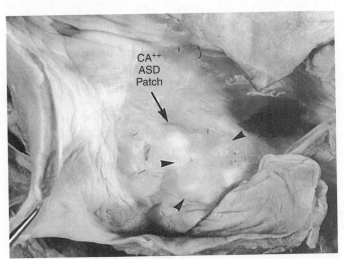

FIGURE 20–16 Three black arrowheads bracket a calcified atrial septal defect patch (Ca^{++} ASD Patch) in a 47-year-old male with tricuspid atresia and a Fontan repair at age 32.

Patches

An endogenous pericardial patch for closure of an ostium secundum atrial septal defect is, as a rule, devoid of sequelae, although the patch occasionally calcifies (Fig. 20–16). Glutaraldehyde-treated pericardium and polytetrafluoroethylene (GORE-TEX®) fabric are employed for closure of ventricular septal defects to avoid a patch aneurysm that might otherwise occur because of the large pressure difference between left and right ventricles (Fig. 20–17; see Chapter 16). These relatively

strong yet compliant materials conform to the ventricular septum while exerting the least stress on fragile myocardial sutures. A neointimal layer covers the patch within a few months. Aneurysm formation is an uncommon if not rare sequel.

Prosthetic valves are themselves obligatory sequelae of valve replacement. Inherent faults in the prostheses vary in frequency and significance according to the physical and hemodynamic characteristics of the device (endogenous, homografts, xenografts, or mechanical), the site of insertion, and patient age at the time of insertion (see Chapter 16). An endogenous valve is represented by the Ross procedure in which the patient's normal pulmonary valve replaces an abnormal aortic valve. When an endogenous pulmonary valve is placed in the aortic position, the inherent cuspal inequality of the pulmonary valve is offset by superior tensile strength of the leaflets (see Chapter 21). Degeneration and calcification of xenograft bioprosthetic valves (Fig. 20–18) are major sequelae significantly coupled with younger patient age at the time of insertion (see Chapter 16).

Thromboembolism, infective endocarditis, and anticoagulant-induced bleeding, the incidence of which can be minimized but not eliminated, are complications rather than sequelae of mechanical prosthetic valves.

Conduits are either nonvalved (generally synthetic) or valved (exogenous bioprostheses). Homograft valve leaflets in conduits are less prone to degeneration than xenograft leaflets (see Chapter 16). An especially undesirable sequel is formation within the conduit of excessively thickened neointima (peel) (Fig. 20–19).

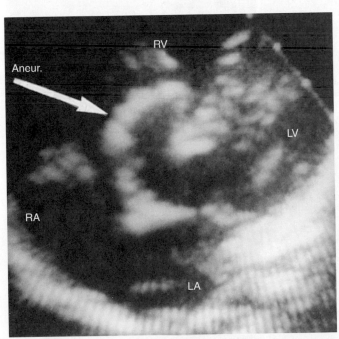

FIGURE 20–17 Septal aneurysm *(arrow)* following repair of a perimembranous ventricular septal defect. LA, left atria; LV, left ventricle, RA, right atria; RV, right ventricle.

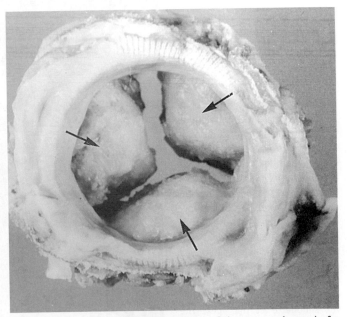

FIGURE 20–18 Fibrocalcific degeneration of three cusps *(arrows)* of a pericardial aortic valve bioprosthetic xenograft removed from a 19-year-old male 4 years after insertion.

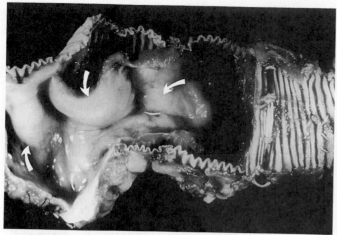

FIGURE 20–19 Excised external valved conduit from a 19-year-old male with congenitally corrected transposition of the great arteries, ventricular septal defect, and pulmonary stenosis. Excessive neointimal proliferation *(curved arrows)* caused conduit obstruction.

Myocardial and Endocardial Sequelae

A sequel of open heart surgery decades ago was depressed ventricular function because of inadequate myocardial protection. With current methods of protection, that sequel has become a thing of the past.

Myocardial sequelae generally originate at the site of a ventriculotomy incision. Morphologic and mechanical sequelae at these sites are usually negligible, although repair of the right ventricular outflow tract can be followed by aneurysm formation, which is more properly considered a complication (Figs. 20–20 and 20–21). An aneurysm at the site of right ventricular outflow reconstruction can adversely affect ventricular function, but the incisional scar can harbor the slowed conduction substrate for reentrant monomorphic ventricular tachycardia (see Chapter 22).[29]

Endocardial sequelae after intraventricular repair have been called surgical fibroelastosis.[30] The cause and functional significance of this uncommon, if not rare, endo-

FIGURE 20–20 Right ventricular angiocardiograms after intracardiac repair of tetralogy of Fallot. **(A)** Incisional aneurysm of the right ventricular outflow tract (RVOT) in diastole *(arrows)*. PT, pulmonary trunk. **(B)** The dyskinetic incisional aneurysm expanded during systole *(arrows)*.

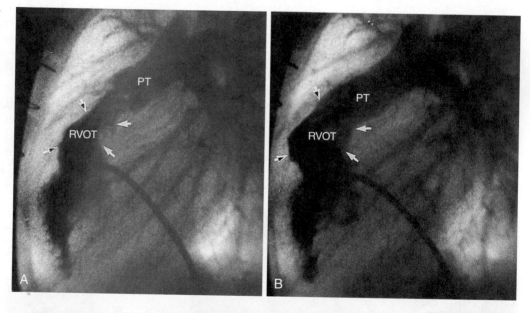

FIGURE 20–21 **(A)** X-ray in an 18-year-old male with tetralogy of Fallot. The cardiac configuration is typically boot shaped because a small underfilled left ventricle is located above a right ventricle (RV) that occupies the apex. The pulmonary trunk is not border forming. RA, right atrium. **(B)** After intracardiac repair, there is a right ventricular incisional aneurysm *(paired arrows)*. Postoperative pulmonary regurgitation enlarged the right ventricle (RV), which forms a convex silhouette at the apex. The right atrium (RA) is enlarged.

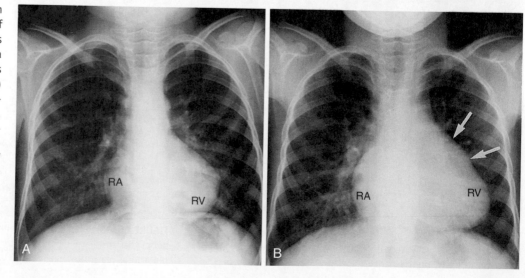

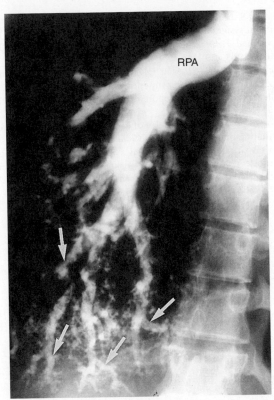

FIGURE 20–22   Pulmonary arteriogram showing right lower lobe arteriovenous fistulae *(arrows)* seven years after a classic Glenn operation in a 20-year-old female with tricuspid atresia and pulmonary stenosis. RPA, right pulmonary artery.

cardial lesion, which is not necessarily confined to the chamber in which the intracardiac repair was performed, have not been established.

Vascular Sequelae

Two vascular sequelae occur years after a classic Glenn shunt (superior vena cava to divided right pulmonary artery): (1) right lower lobe pulmonary arteriovenous fistulae[31] (Fig. 20–22) and (2) collateral veins to the inferior vena cava.

Neurologic Sequelae

The incidence of postoperative neurologic sequelae has declined as cardiac surgical techniques have improved (see Chapter 15).[32] However, cardiopulmonary bypass, circulatory arrest, and hypothermia in neonates and infants are responsible for neurologic and psychiatric sequelae[21] (see Chapters 13 and 14). The central nervous system and the cardiovascular system form nearly simultaneously in early gestation. Accordingly, in children with congenital malformations of the heart, there is an increased incidence of congenital malformations of the brain[33] (see Chapter 14).

References

1. Engle MA, Perloff JK, ed. *Congenital Heart Disease after Surgery.* New York: Yorke Medical Books; 1983.
2. Preminger TJ, Sanders SP, van der Velde ME, et al. "Intramural" residual interventricular defects after repair of conotruncal malformations. *Circulation.* 1994;89:236–242.
3. Stark J. Do we really correct congenital heart defects? *J Thorac Cardiovasc Surg.* 1989;97:1–9.
4. Perloff JK, Roberts NK, Cabeen WR Jr. Left axis deviation: a reassessment. *Circulation.* 1979;60:12–21.
5. Perloff JK. *The Clinical Recognition of Congenital Heart Disease.* 5th ed. Philadelphia: W.B. Saunders; 2003.
6. Pease WE, Nordenberg A, Ladda RL. Familial atrial septal defect with prolonged atrioventricular conduction. *Circulation.* 1976;53:759–762.
7. Karpawich PP, Antillon JR, Cappola PR, Agarwal KC. Pre- and postoperative electrophysiologic assessment of children with secundum atrial septal defect. *Am J Cardiol.* 1985;55:519–521.
8. Sano T, Ogawa M, Yabuuchi H, et al. Quantitative cineangiographic analysis of ventricular volume and mass in patients with single ventricle: relation to ventricular morphologies. *Circulation.* 1988;77:62–69.
9. Assey ME, Wisenbaugh T, Spann JF Jr, Gillette PC, Carabello BA. Unexpected persistence into adulthood of low wall stress in patients with congenital aortic stenosis: is there a fundamental difference in the hypertrophic response to a pressure overload present from birth? *Circulation.* 1987;75:973–979.
10. Holmes KW, Lehmann CU, Dalal D, et al. Progressive dilation of the ascending aorta in children with isolated bicuspid aortic valve. *Am J Cardiol.* 2007;99:978–983.
11. Hahn RT, Roman MJ, Mogtader AH, Devereux RB. Association of aortic dilation with regurgitant, stenotic and functionally normal bicuspid aortic valves. *J Am Coll Cardiol.* 1992;19:283–288.
12. Isner JM, Donaldson RF, Fulton D, et al. Cystic medial necrosis in coarctation of the aorta: a potential factor contributing to adverse consequences observed after percutaneous balloon angioplasty of coarctation sites. *Circulation.* 1987;75:689–695.
13. Simon AB, Zloto AE. Coarctation of the aorta. Longitudinal assessment of operated patients. *Circulation.* 1974;50:456–464.
14. Jaffin BW, Gundel WD, Capeless MA, et al. Aneurysm of the pulmonary artery as a cause of severe chest pain. *Arch Intern Med.* 1983;143:1484–1485.
15. Niwa K, Perloff JK, Bhuta SM, et al. Structural abnormalities of great arterial walls in congenital heart disease: light and electron microscopic analyses. *Circulation.* 2001;103:393–400.
16. Sehested J, Baandrup U, Mikkelsen E. Different reactivity and structure of the prestenotic and poststenotic aorta in human coarctation. Implications for baroreceptor function. *Circulation.* 1982;65:1060–1065.
17. Ino T, Nishimoto K, Iwahara M, et al. Progressive vascular lesions in Williams-Beuren syndrome. *Pediatr Cardiol.* 1988;9:55–58.
18. Chi TPL, Krovetz J. The pulmonary vascular bed in children with Down syndrome. *J Pediatr.* 1975;86:533–538.
19. Farley FA, Phillips WA, Herzenberg JE, et al. Natural history of scoliosis in congenital heart disease. *J Pediatr Orthop.* 1991;11:42–47.
20. Greenwood RD, Rosenthal A, Parisi L, et al. Extracardiac abnormalities in infants with congenital heart disease. *Pediatrics.* 1975;55:485–492.
21. Wernovsky G. Current insights regarding neurological and developmental abnormalities in children and young adults with complex congenital cardiac disease. *Cardiol Young.* 2006;16(1 Suppl):92–104.
22. Scinto LF, Daffner KR, Dressler D, et al. A potential noninvasive neurobiological test for Alzheimer's disease. *Science.* 1994;266:1051–1054.
23. Lin AE, Perloff JK. Upper limb malformations associated with congenital heart disease. *Am J Cardiol.* 1985;55:1576–1583.

24. Pollock JC, Jamieson MP, McWilliam R. Somatosensory evoked potentials in the detection of spinal cord ischemia in aortic coarctation repair. *Ann Thorac Surg.* 1986;41:251–254.

25. Sacks O. Musical ability. *Science.* 1995;268:621–622.

26. Friedman DL, Kastner T, Pond WS, O'Brien DR. Thyroid dysfunction in individuals with Down syndrome. *Arch Intern Med.* 1989;149: 1990–1993.

27. Ross EA, Perloff JK, Danovitch GM, et al. Renal function and urate metabolism in late survivors with cyanotic congenital heart disease. *Circulation.* 1986;73:396–400.

28. Horowitz LN, Alexander JA, Edmunds LH Jr. Postoperative right bundle branch block: identification of three levels of block. *Circulation.* 1980;62:319–328.

29. Perloff JK, Middlekauf HR, Child JS, et al. Usefulness of post-ventriculotomy signal averaged electrocardiograms in congenital heart disease. *Am J Cardiol.* 2006;98:1646–1651.

30. Bharati S, Lea M. Sequelae of atriotomy on the endocardium, conduction system and coronary arteries. In: Engle MA, Perloff JK, ed. *Congenital Heart Disease after Surgery.* New York: Yorke Medical Books; 1983:229–246.

31. McFaul RC, Tajik AJ, Mair DD, et al. Development of pulmonary arteriovenous shunt after superior vena cava-right pulmonary artery (Glenn) anastomosis. Report of four cases. *Circulation.* 1977;55: 212–216.

32. Ferry PC. Neurologic sequelae of open-heart surgery in children. An "irritating question." *Am J Dis Child.* 1990;144:369–373.

33. Hovels-Gurich HH, Seghaye MC, Schnitker R, et al. Long-term neurodevelopmental outcomes in school-aged children after neonatal arterial switch operation. *J Thorac Cardiovasc Surg.* 2002;124: 448–458.

Residua and Sequelae Involving Cardiac Valves

JOSEPH K. PERLOFF ▪ MARK D. PLUNKETT

The general topic of residua and sequelae is the subject of Chapter 20. This chapter focuses on residua and sequelae involving cardiac valves. Prosthetic valves and materials are discussed in Chapter 16.

RESIDUA

Aortic Valve

Congenitally abnormal aortic valves are unicuspid, bicuspid, tricuspid, or quadricuspid. *Bicuspid aortic valves* can be functionally normal, stenotic, or incompetent.[1,2] Bicuspid aortic stenosis can present in infancy, or a functionally normal bicuspid aortic valve can await late adulthood to manifest itself as fibrocalcific stenosis (Fig. 21–1). Bicuspid aortic regurgitation tends to be progressive, typically reaching functional significance in adults. The bicuspid aortic valve is also important for two additional reasons, namely, a lifetime susceptibility to infective endocarditis (see Chapter 8) and because of the coexisting abnormality inherent in the ascending aortic media that predisposes to dilatation and aneurysm formation.[3,4]

The structural valvular abnormality in early life is characterized by two thin, pliant, mobile leaflets without commissural separation (see Fig. 21–1). Although surgical repair or balloon dilatation (see Chapter 18) can reduce if not eliminate the gradient while inducing little or no regurgitation, the inherent bicuspid condition is an obligatory residuum. Alternatively, a surgical attempt can be made to convert the bicuspid valve into a trileaflet mechanism using native pericardial leaflet extensions.[5] The short-term results are promising, but long-term durability is uncertain. In the UCLA experience with 128 aortic valve repairs that used pericardial leaflet extension, the mean interval between original repair and reoperation for congenital (including bicuspid aortic valve) and acquired aortic valve disease was less than 4 years in both groups, with the early reoperation rate significantly higher in the congenital group.[6] Even if surgical or interventional catheterization transforms a stenotic bicuspid aortic valve into a functionally normal bicuspid valve, the susceptibility to infective endocarditis, the potential development of fibrocalcific stenosis, and the inherent fibrillin-1 abnormality of the ascending aorta media[3,7] persist as postoperative residua. A coexisting bicuspid aortic valve after repair of aortic coarctation is an important postoperative residuum[1] (Fig. 21–2). The morphology of a bicuspid aortic valve has prognostic relevance. Fusion of the right and left coronary cusps is associated with coarctation of the aorta, whereas fusion of the right and noncoronary cusps is associated with a propensity for cuspal pathology.[8,9]

Supravalvar aortic stenosis occurs at the level of the sinotubular junction or proximal ascending aorta and may present either as a component of Williams syndrome, as an isolated sporadic disorder, or as an autosomal dominant familial form. Any of these varieties can be clinically manifest in infancy or in later life, but most patients present in their first or second decade with progressive obstruction and left ventricular hypertrophy. The coronary ostia originate proximal to obstruction, are subjected to suprasystemic systolic pressure, fill predominantly during systole, and may be displaced or distorted by the stenotic ring. The ostial changes are progressive and, combined with left ventricular hypertrophy, incur an increased risk of sudden death. Surgical treatment consists of patch enlargement of

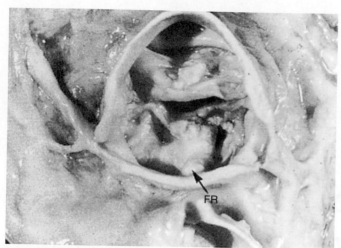

FIGURE 21-1 Functionally normal bicuspid aortic valve (left). Calcific bicuspid aortic stenosis (right). *(From Tatsuna et al.: Circulation 1973;48:1028. With permission of the American Heart Association.)*

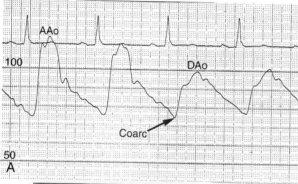

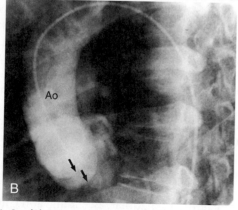

FIGURE 21-2 **(A)** Pressure pulses from a 24-year-old man who at age 7 years underwent resection with end-to-end anastomosis of coarctation of the aorta. Mild residual obstruction is reflected in the peak systolic pressure difference as the catheter was advanced from ascending aorta (AAo) into descending aorta (DAo). Coarc, coarctation. **(B)** Contrast injection into ascending aorta (Ao) discloses a bicuspid aortic valve *(arrows)* with dilatation of the ascending aorta.

one or more aortic sinuses with augmentation of the sinotubular ring. Postoperative residua include myocardial ischemia that results from coronary ostial displacement or progressive ostial fibrosis, and aneurysm formation when repair includes resection of the sinotubular ridge.[10]

Incompetence of a trileaflet aortic valve occurs as a residuum after intracardiac repair of tetralogy of Fallot, an aortic/left ventricular tunnel, a ventricular septal defect (VSD; Figs. 21-3 and 21-4), and discrete subaortic stenosis (Fig. 21-5). Aortic regurgitation with the tetralogy tends to be mild and occurs later in life than does aortic regurgitation with an isolated VSD because the powerful jet generated by a left-to-right shunt (see Fig. 21-4) is not present with the tetralogy in which the left ventricle ejects directly into the biventricular aorta.[11] Patient age influences the incidence of residual postoperative aortic regurgitation.[12] Inherent abnormalities of the aortic valve cusps reportedly develop in 77% of adults when the tetralogy of Fallot is associated with pulmonary atresia,[12] and the regurgitation tends to be progressive.[13] Much less common is late development of aortic valve calcification (Fig. 21-6).

The incidence of aortic regurgitation with VSDs (see Fig. 21-3) depends chiefly on the relative prevalence of perimembranous versus doubly committed subarterial defects.[14-17] Perimembranous defects are much more common in Caucasians and are associated with a relatively low incidence of aortic regurgitation, whereas subarterial defects are much more common in Asians and are associated with a relatively high incidence.[14,16] In either case, the regurgitation is acquired[16] and is a potentially important postoperative residuum.

When the VSD is doubly committed and subarterial, a structurally normal aortic valve lacks adequate annular support, so the right and left coronary cusps become displaced into the right ventricular outflow tract, rendering the valve incompetent. Hemodynamic factors are also believed to play an important role in the development of aortic regurgitation,[11] as illustrated in Figure 21-4. The corollary to these observations is that patient age significantly affects the incidence of residual postoperative aortic regurgitation. If the defect is closed while the aortic valve is competent, the valve remains competent. New-onset aortic regurgitation is considered an indication for surgical closure even of a restrictive VSD. Closures of VSDs in infants and young children have appreciably decreased aortic regurgitation as a functionally significant postoperative residuum (see Chapter 15).

The valve mechanism in *truncus arteriosus* is usually quadricuspid (Fig. 21-7, A) and believed to represent a morphogenetic combination of aortic and pulmonary valves.[18] In addition to abnormalities of size and number, truncal cusps are usually focally or diffusely thickened and poorly supported.[19,20] Even a trileaflet truncal valve (50%-60% of cases) differs from a normal trileaflet aortic valve.[1,20] Not surprisingly, truncal valves tend to function abnormally and are usually incompetent (Fig. 21-7, B)[20] and much less commonly stenotic.[21] Because truncal valves are inherently abnormal, early repair of the basic malformation does not influence the function of the malformed valve, which remains an important postoperative residuum.[22]

Discrete (fixed) subaortic stenosis is accompanied by aortic regurgitation in 30% to 55% of patients aged 18 years

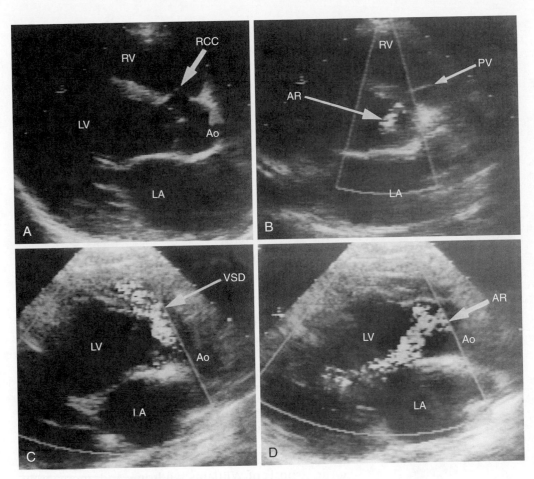

FIGURE 21-3 **(A)** Two-dimensional echocardiogram (parasternal long axis) showing herniation of the right coronary cusp (RCC) into the outflow tract of the right ventricle (RV) in a patient with aortic regurgitation and a restrictive perimembranous ventricular septal defect. Ao, aorta; LA, left atrium; LV, left ventricle. **(B)** Black-and-white rendition of a color flow image shows mild aortic regurgitation (AR). PV, pulmonary valve. **(C)** Black-and-white rendition of a color flow image (parasternal long axis) from another patient with a restrictive perimembranous ventricular septal defect (VSD) and aortic regurgitation (AR) as shown in **D.**

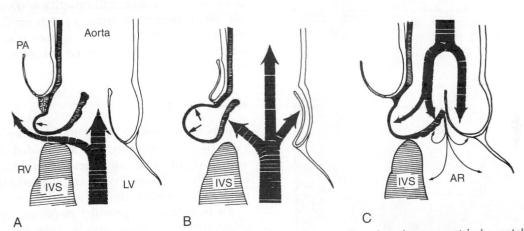

FIGURE 21-4   Proposed pathogenetic mechanism of aortic regurgitation in the presence of a perimembranous ventricular septal defect. **(A)** During early systole, an anatomically unsupported aortic valve and sinus are drawn into the right ventricular (RV) outflow tract by high-velocity shunt flow through the ventricular septal defect. Small arrow points to the herniated aortic cusp. IVS, interventricular septum; LV, left ventricle; PA, pulmonary artery. **(B)** Ejection from the left ventricle distends the unsupported sinus, creating a larger bulge *(paired arrows).* **(C)** The free margin of the elongated, herniated cusp does not properly appose the other two cusps during diastole, rendering the valve mechanism incompetent.

or younger and in up to two thirds of older patients[16,17] (see Fig. 21-5). Aortic cusp abnormalities result from either proximity to or direct extension of the subaortic membrane or fibromuscular collar or from injury and scarring caused by a high-velocity eccentric jet that strikes the ventricular surface of the cusps.[23] In either event, the degree of aortic regurgitation is progressive and is a substrate for infective endocarditis (see Chapter 8). Selection of patients for surgical resection of discrete subaortic stenosis depends in part on the degree of obstruction but also on the desire to preempt the progression of aortic regurgitation. As with subarterial VSDs, new-onset aortic regurgitation is an indication for surgical resection (see Chapter 15).

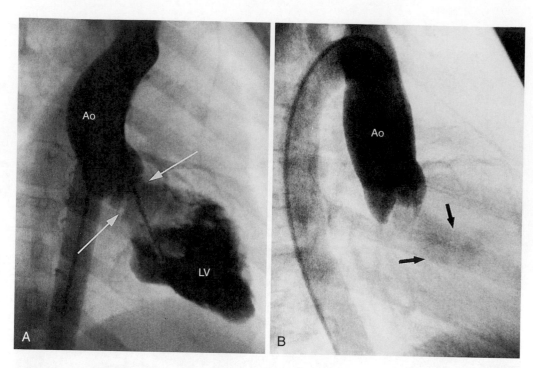

FIGURE 21-5 **(A)** Left ventriculogram (LV) showing discrete subaortic stenosis *(paired arrows)*. **(B)** The thoracic aortogram discloses mild aortic regurgitation *(paired arrows)*. Ao, ascending aorta.

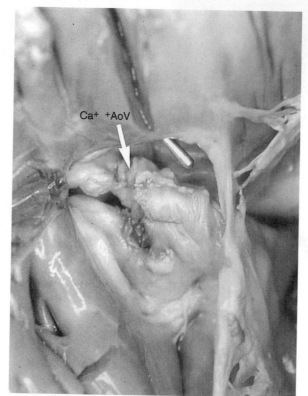

FIGURE 21-6 Necropsy specimen of aortic valve calcification ($Ca^{++}AoV$) in a 32-year-old man with tetralogy of Fallot.

Aortic/left ventricular tunnel is a rare congenital malformation characterized by a vascular channel that originates immediately above the right sinus of Valsalva, tunnels through the ventricular septum, and enters the left ventricle just inferior to the right and noncoronary cusps.[24,25] Incompetence due to injury to aortic leaflets augments regurgitant flow through the tunnel. Residual postoperative aortic regurgitation is the rule.[26]

Stenosis of the pulmonary artery and its branches (supravalvular) occurs in combination with the supravalvular aortic stenosis of Williams syndrome and, more rarely, as an isolated lesion. Balloon dilatation is of little benefit; repair usually requires a patch similar to the technique for supravalvular aortic stenosis. Postoperative residua include persistent or recurrent supravalvular obstruction.

Mitral Valve

Postoperative residua involving a morphologic mitral valve (not synonymous with a left-sided atrioventricular valve) fall into two categories: (1) residua involving an inherently malformed valve and (2) residua involving an inherently normal mitral valve.

An *inherently (congenitally) malformed mitral valve* is a component of an *atrioventricular septal defect* (ASD).[1] What has been called a *cleft* in the anterior leaflet is in fact an abortive commissure between the anterior and posterior bridging leaflets, a deformity identified by its orientation toward the ventricular septum in contrast to a true isolated cleft, which is oriented toward the left ventricular outflow tract[27] (see Chapter 6). In complete common atrioventricular canal, the atrioventricular orifice is guarded by a five-leaflet valve mechanism.[1] Not surprisingly, the more severe the regurgitation, the more likely there will be residual regurgitation after repair. Irrespective of the success of the surgical intervention, postoperative morphologic abnormalities are obligatory residua. Regurgitation sometimes

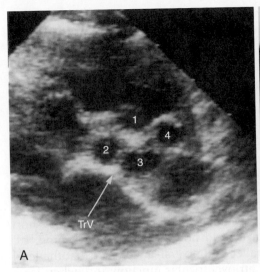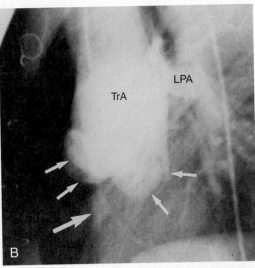

FIGURE 21-7 **(A)** Two-dimensional echocardiogram (short axis) showing the four leaflets (1, 2, 3, 4) of a quadricuspid truncal valve (Tr.V). **(B)** Lateral angiogram with contrast medium injected into a truncus arteriosus (TrA) outlines the four cusps *(four small arrows)* of a quadricuspid valve that is mildly incompetent *(large arrow)*. LPA, left pulmonary artery that originated from the truncus. Metal sutures (upper left) are in the sternum.

develops or worsens years after successful repair, in part because of changes in left ventricular geometry caused by ischemic heart disease or systemic hypertension. Residual postoperative regurgitation is less likely after surgical repair of a true isolated mitral cleft.[27]

The incidence of congenital abnormalities of the mitral apparatus associated with *coarctation of the aorta* is estimated at 26% to 58%.[28-30] The abnormalities vary from clinically occult to grossly overt and are expressed as stenosis or incompetence. Echocardiographic assessment immediately to 14 years after coarctation repair disclosed residual mitral valve abnormalities in approximately 50% of patients,[29] but clinically significant regurgitation was infrequent.[31] A stenotic mitral orifice may be one component of Shone's complex, a constellation of left heart obstructive lesions including coarctation and subaortic stenosis.

Incompetence of an inherently normal mitral valve is a common accompaniment of *anomalous origin of the left coronary artery from the pulmonary trunk* because of ischemic dysfunction of papillary muscles and adjacent myocardium[1] (Fig. 21-8). Regurgitation develops from within a few months of age to young adulthood and may require reconstruction if not replacement[32] (see Chapter 15).

Ostium secundum atrial defect is associated with an age-related incidence of structural abnormalities of mitral valve leaflets,[33-36] principally the medial half of the anterior leaflet, which develops a surface layer of fibrosis.[36] Chordae tendineae are thickened and occasionally fused. Mitral valve lesions with secundum ASDs have been attributed to abnormal cusp movement associated with left ventricular cavity deformity (abnormal position and motion of the ventricular septum in response to right ventricular volume overload).[34,37] The incidence of residual postoperative regurgitation varies with patient age.[37]

When an ASD is associated with acquired (rheumatic) mitral stenosis—Lutembacher's syndrome[1]—closure of the interatrial communication and repair of the stenotic

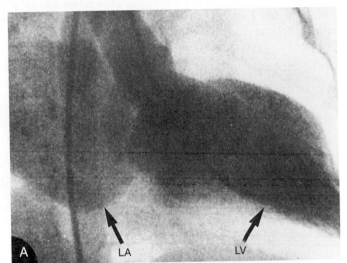

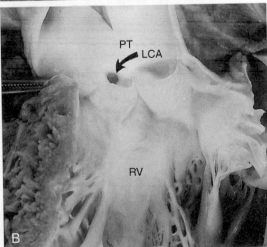

FIGURE 21-8 **(A)** Left ventriculogram (LV) showing mitral regurgitation and a moderately dilatated left atrium (LA) in an 11-year-old boy with anomalous origin of the left coronary artery from the pulmonary trunk. **(B)** Necropsy specimen from a 5-year-old boy with anomalous origin of the left coronary artery (LCA) from the pulmonary trunk (PT). RV, right ventricle.

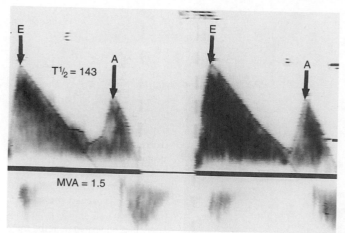

FIGURE 21-9 Postoperative mitral valve inflow Doppler recording in a 47-year-old man with Lutembacher's syndrome. An ostium secundum atrial septal defect had been surgically closed. The stenotic rheumatic mitral valve was reconstructed, leaving a residual morphologic abnormality of the mitral valve and mild residual mitral stenosis. A, late diastolic peak velocity due to atrial contraction; E, early diastolic peak velocity; MVA, mitral valve area; $T^{1}/_{2}$, pressure half-time.

mitral valve leave the rheumatic mitral valve as a postoperative residuum (Fig. 21-9) even if reconstruction is functionally ideal.

Tricuspid Valve

Residua involving a *tricuspid valve* (not synonymous with a right-sided atrioventricular valve) are related to an inherently malformed mechanism or to an inherently normal tricuspid valve rendered incompetent by hemodynamic stress and annular dilatation.

In *Ebstein's anomaly of the tricuspid valve*, the basal attachments of the septal and posterior leaflets are apically displaced, and leaflet movement is impaired by short chordae tendineae and nodular fibrotic thickening.[38-41] The anterior leaflet is almost always attached at the level of the normal atrioventricular junction and, when large and mobile, lends itself to surgical reconstruction into a relatively competent tricuspid mechanism guarded by a single cusp[40,41] (see Chapter 15). Residual incompetence is common, but even assuming ideal reconstruction with little or no regurgitation (Fig. 21-10), morphologic residua necessarily remain.

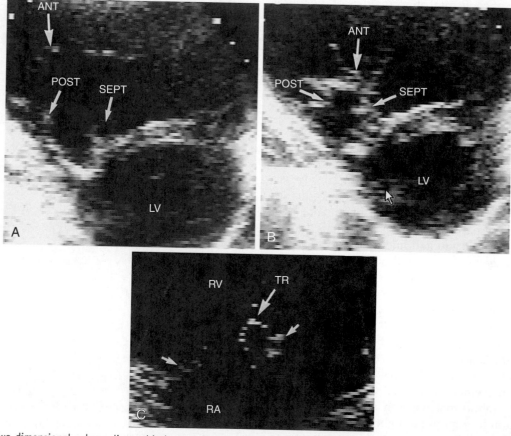

FIGURE 21-10 Two-dimensional echocardiographic images from a 34-year-old man after reconstruction of Ebstein's anomaly of the tricuspid valve. **(A)** Diastolic frame shows the open position of the large anterior (ANT) tricuspid leaflet. The posterior (POST) and septal (SEPT) leaflets are relatively immobile. **(B)** Systolic frame showing closure of the functionally unicuspid right atrioventricular valve. **(C)** Black-and-white photograph of color flow image showing trivial residual tricuspid regurgitation (TR). RA, right atrium; RV, right ventricle. Two small, unmarked arrows identify the posterior and septal tricuspid leaflets.

Structural abnormalities of the inverted tricuspid valve occur in 50% to 90% of necropsy cases of *congenitally corrected transposition of the great arteries.*[42,43] Although characterized as *Ebstein-like*, these abnormalities differ substantially from Ebstein's anomaly of a noninverted tricuspid valve. The small malformed anterior leaflet of an inverted tricuspid valve usually consists of multiple cusps or a tensor apparatus comprising multiple or compound papillary muscles and anomalous chordal attachments.[42,43] Accordingly, surgical reconstruction is seldom feasible. Instead, an incompetent valve must be replaced (see Chapter 15), leaving the prosthesis as an obligatory residuum.

In an atrioventricular septal defect (discussed earlier), whether with a common atrioventricular orifice or separate right and left atrioventricular orifices, surgical repair leaves the right-sided component guarded by an inherently abnormal morphologic residuum even if competence is achieved.

Congenital tricuspid stenosis is characterized by a small but well-formed tricuspid valve that joins an underdeveloped inlet portion of the right ventricle and is believed to represent a less severe form of tricuspid atresia in which a transilluminated dimple separates the right atrium from the right ventricle.[1,44] Surgical repair of a congenitally stenotic tricuspid valve usually leaves some degree of residual obstruction, even if repair is accomplished with comparatively little regurgitation (Fig. 21–11).

An inherently normal tricuspid valve may be rendered incompetent by high systolic pressure imposed on a right ventricle by the congenital malformation for which intracardiac repair is primarily intended. Because the incompetent valve is inherently structurally normal, repair is generally feasible during operation that focuses on the basic congenital cardiac defect. Successful tricuspid reconstruction coupled with decline if not normalization of right ventricular systolic pressure decreases the incidence and degree of residual postoperative regurgitation.

SEQUELAE

Aortic Valve

Stenosis of the aortic valve is more often than not the major or only site of congenital obstruction to left ventricular outflow and is most frequently caused by a bicuspid aortic valve[2] (discussed earlier). Surgical repair of a thin, mobile stenotic bicuspid valve permits precise separation of the commissures under direct vision, achieving the maximum aortic valve area with the minimum risk of inducing regurgitation (see Chapter 15). Percutaneous balloon valvuloplasty ideally achieves the same result (see Chapter 18). The best outcome that can be achieved from either surgical repair or balloon dilatation is a bicuspid valve that functions normally, but has a mechanism that confronts the same fate as an inherently functionally normal bicuspid aortic valve, namely, fibrocalcific thickening or progressive regurgitation (discussed earlier).

The most common immediate sequel of a therapeutic intervention on a stenotic bicuspid aortic valve is regurgitation, the prevalence and degree of which is greater if the obstruction is addressed by balloon valvuloplasty rather than by direct repair.[45] Meticulous monitoring of balloon dilatation with transesophageal echocardiography improves the margin of safety, minimizing the risk of significant balloon-induced regurgitation (see Chapter 18). Echocardiographic or angiographic distinction between a bicuspid and a unicommissural unicuspid aortic valve can be difficult if not impossible[46] (see Chapter 6). If surgical repair or balloon dilatation is attempted on a stenotic unicommissural unicuspid aortic valve mistaken for a bicuspid aortic valve, serious regurgitation is a common immediate sequel.[45-47] The presence of aortic stenosis from birth does not distinguish a unicommissural valve from a bicuspid aortic valve, and fibrocalcific obstruction of a unicommissural aortic valve may follow the same time course as a bicuspid aortic valve.[47,48]

Congenital aortic valve regurgitation, whether caused by a bicuspid, unicommissural unicuspid, or quadricuspid valve mechanism,[44,48,49] can be repaired by a valve-sparing operation that employs glutaraldehyde-treated autologous pericardium[50] (see Chapter 15). A pulmonary autograft, a homograft, or a prosthetic valve is an obligatory sequel of replacement (see Chapter 16).

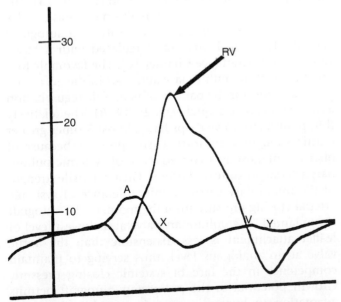

FIGURE 21–11   Right ventricular (RV) and right atrial pressure pulses from a 47-year-old woman with congenital tricuspid stenosis. The presystolic gradient reflects augmented right atrial contraction and an increase in A wave. The Y descent is gentle because of tricuspid obstruction. Mild tricuspid regurgitation was a sequel of intracardiac repair.

Pulmonary Valve

Typical *pulmonary valve stenosis* is characterized as a thin, pliant, mobile, conical or dome-shaped structure with a narrow outlet at its apex. Three rudimentary raphes extend from a central orifice to the pulmonary sinuses. Surgical separation of the commissures by incision of the raphes was the technique of choice[51] until the advent of balloon valvuloplasty, which now competes with repair under direct vision[52] (see Chapter 18). Complete or virtually complete relief of obstruction can be achieved with either technique, while inducing no more than mild to moderate pulmonary regurgitation, a sequel that does not adversely affect long-term outcome.[52] Secondary hypertrophic subpulmonary stenosis generally regresses after successful surgery or balloon dilatation of the stenotic valve.[53,54]

A much less common variety of pulmonary stenosis is a dysplastic valve characterized by thick immobile cusps without commissural fusion, often accompanied by a small annulus.[55,56] Partial or total valvectomy alone or in combination with a transannular patch reduces the obstruction, but the inevitable sequel is significant pulmonary regurgitation. Balloon valvuloplasty is of little or no value in dysplastic pulmonary stenosis because obstruction is caused by thickened cusps rather than commissural fusion (see Chapter 18).

Complex Obstruction to Right Ventricular Outflow

In tetralogy of Fallot, stenosis of the pulmonary valve (often bicuspid) is one component of complex obstruction to right ventricular outflow that consists of rightward and anterior deviation (malalignment) of the infundibular septum, which is the primary cause of obstruction, hypertrophy of septoparietal trabeculations, and hypertrophy of the trabecula septomarginalis.[1] Postoperative pulmonary regurgitation is a common sequel of intracardiac repair and is invariable when repair employs a transannular patch, followed by immediate and severe regurgitation (see Chapters 15 and 16). Importantly, an infundibular incision per se tends to be followed by progressive pulmonary regurgitation because the infundibulum supports the pulmonary valve during diastole. Mild to moderate postoperative pulmonary regurgitation is generally well tolerated,[57] but severe regurgitation (Fig. 21–12) results in progressive dilatation and depressed right ventricular function. Severe pulmonary regurgitation also serves as a trigger for monomorphic ventricular tachycardia in the presence of a susceptible slowed conduction reentrant substrate[58] (see Chapter 22).

The Jatene[59] and Norwood[60] operations, performed respectively for complete transposition of the great arteries and hypoplastic left heart syndrome, relocate the

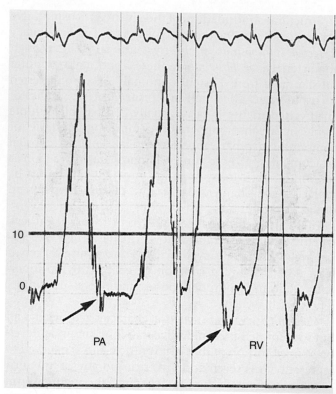

FIGURE 21–12 Pulmonary arterial (PA) and right ventricular (RV) pressure pulses after transannular patch repair of tetralogy of Fallot. The pulmonary arterial pressure pulse falls to a diastolic pressure of zero *(arrow)*. The right ventricular pressure pulse exhibits a prominent early diastolic dip *(arrow)*. These pressure pulse configurations are typical of severe pulmonary regurgitation.

pulmonary valve to the aortic position (Fig. 21–13). The Ross procedure replaces the malformed aortic valve with the patient's own pulmonary valve (an autograft) (Fig. 21–14), which in turn is replaced with a tissue valve or homograft (see Chapter 16). The favorable biomechanics of the pulmonary autograft in the aortic position account for the paucity of neoaortic regurgitation as a postoperative sequel (Fig. 21–14, *B*). The relatively thin pulmonary valve cusps have almost 3 times greater tensile strength than aortic cusps, possibly because of fiber orientation as a consequence of systemic pulmonary arterial pressure in the fetus. Greater tensile strength of the pulmonary cusps permits tolerance of systemic arterial closing pressure from the moment the autograft is implanted. The pulmonary valve at its lowest level of leaflet attachment is less distensible than the aortic valve at an analogous level, thus serving to maintain competence in the face of systemic closing pressure. Growth potential of the pulmonary autograft permits adaptation to hydraulic conditions within the aortic root. Early and late development of pulmonary autograft regurgitation in the aortic position is almost invariably associated with annular dilatation and loss of central leaflet coaptation.

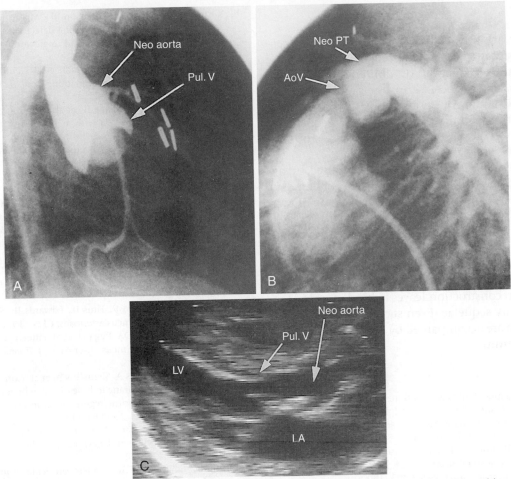

FIGURE 21–13 **(A)** Thoracic aortogram from a 5-week-old neonate after a Jatene arterial switch repair for complete transposition of the great arteries. The left ventricular outflow tract is guarded by the pulmonary valve autograft (Pul.V). The transplanted coronary arteries arise from the neoaorta. **(B)** Contrast injection into the right ventricle (RV) shows the outflow tract giving rise to the transplanted neopulmonary trunk (NeoPT) beneath which resides the aortic valve (AoV). **(C)** Two-dimensional echocardiogram (parasternal long-axis) showing the neoaorta above the pulmonary valve. LA, left atrium; LV, left ventricle.

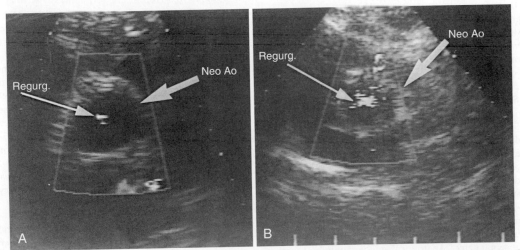

FIGURE 21–14 **(A)** Black-and-white rendition of a color flow image (short axis) from a 32-year-old woman who underwent a Ross procedure for bicuspid aortic regurgitation. The transplanted pulmonary valve autograft is now the neoaortic valve (NeoAo) that exhibits trivial regurgitation (Regurg). **(B)** Black-and-white rendition of a color flow image (short axis) from a 17-year-old girl who underwent a Ross procedure following balloon dilatation of a stenotic bicuspid aortic valve that resulted in acute severe aortic regurgitation. The pulmonary valve autograft is now the neoaortic valve, which is moderately regurgitant (Regurg).

Mitral Valve

Surgical repair achieves only limited success when *congenital mitral stenosis* is characterized by short chordae tendineae, fibrous reduction or obliteration of interchordal spaces, and a decrease in interpapillary muscle distance[1] (see Chapter 5). Residual obstruction is likely, and postoperative mitral regurgitation is a frequent sequel. Balloon valvuloplasty is even less successful than surgical repair[61-63] (see Chapter 18).

Isolated *congenital mitral regurgitation* is caused by defects in leaflet tissue (isolated clefts), absent or redundant chordae tendineae, and abnormal size or location of papillary muscles.[64] Mitral regurgitation caused by an isolated congenital cleft lends itself to surgical repair, a procedure generally devoid of postoperative sequelae.[64-66] With that exception, congenital mitral regurgitation typically involves more than one component of the mitral apparatus, so surgical reconstruction leaves behind morphologic faults as necessary sequelae. Even successful complex mitral valve repairs are accompanied by the persistent risk of infective endocarditis.

References

1. Perloff JK. Congenital aortic regurgitation. *The Clinical Recognition of Congenital Heart Disease.* 5th ed. Philadelphia: W.B. Saunders; 2003.
2. Roberts WC. The congenitally bicuspid aortic valve. A study of 85 autopsy cases. *Am J Cardiol.* 1970;26:72–83.
3. Niwa K, Perloff JK, Bhuta SM, et al. Structural abnormalities of great arterial walls in congenital heart disease: light and electron microscopic analyses. *Circulation.* 2001;103:393–400.
4. Beroukhim RS, Roosevelt G, Yetman AT. Comparison of the pattern of aortic dilation in children with the Marfan's syndrome versus children with a bicuspid aortic valve. *Am J Cardiol.* 2006;98:1094–1095.
5. Prêtre R, Kadner A, Dave H, et al. Tricuspidisation of the aortic valve with creation of a crown-like annulus is able to restore a normal valve function in bicuspid aortic valves. *Eur J Cardiothorac Surg.* 2006;29:1001–1006.
6. De La Zerda D, Cohen O, Fishbein M, et al. Aortic valve-sparing repair with autologous pericardial leaflet extension has a greater early re-operation rate in congenital versus acquired valve disease. *Eur J Cadiothoracic Surg.* 2007;31:256–260.
7. Fedak PW, Verma S, David TE, et al. Clinical and pathophysiological implications of a bicuspid aortic valve. *Circulation.* 2002;106:900–904.
8. Folger GM Jr, Stein PD. Bicuspid aortic valve morphology when associated with coarctation of the aorta. *Cathet Cardiovasc Diagn.* 1984;10:17–25.
9. Ciotti GR, Vlahos AP, Silverman NH. Morphology and function of the bicuspid aortic valve with and without coarctation of the aorta in the young. *Am J Cardiol.* 2006;98:1096–1102.
10. Myers JL, Waldhausen JA, Cyran SE, et al. Results of surgical repair of congenital supravalvular aortic stenosis. *J Thorac Cardiovasc Surg.* 1993;105:281–287.
11. Tatsuno K, Konno S, Ando M, Sakakibara S. Pathogenetic mechanisms of prolapsing aortic valve and aortic regurgitation associated with ventricular septal defect. Anatomical, angiographic, and surgical considerations. *Circulation.* 1973;48:1028–1037.
12. Marelli AJ, Perloff JK, Child JS, Laks H. Pulmonary atresia with ventricular septal defect in adults. *Circulation.* 1994;89:243–251.
13. Capelli H, Ross D, Somerville J. Aortic regurgitation in tetrad of Fallot and pulmonary atresia. *Am J Cardiol.* 1982;49:1979–1983.
14. Griffin ML, Sullivan ID, Anderson RH, Macartney FJ. Doubly committed subarterial ventricular septal defect: new morphological criteria with echocardiographic and angiocardiographic correlation. *Br Heart J.* 1988;59:474–479.
15. Hisatomi K, Kosuga K, Isomura T, et al. Ventricular septal defect associated with aortic regurgitation. *Ann Thorac Surg.* 1987;43:363–367.
16. Rhodes LA, Keane JF, Keane JP, et al. Long follow-up (to 43 years) of ventricular septal defect with audible aortic regurgitation. *Am J Cardiol.* 1990;66:340–345.
17. Schmidt KG, Cassidy SC, Silverman NH, Stanger P. Doubly committed subarterial ventricular septal defects: echocardiographic features and surgical implications. *J Am Coll Cardiol.* 1988;12:1538–1546.
18. Van Mierop LH, Patterson DF, Schnarr WR. Pathogenesis of persistent truncus arteriosus in light of observations made in a dog embryo with the anomaly. *Am J Cardiol.* 1978;41:755–762.
19. Butto F, Lucas RV Jr, Edwards JE. Persistent truncus arteriosus: pathologic anatomy in 54 cases. *Pediatr Cardiol.* 1986;7:95–101.
20. Fuglestad SJ, Puga FJ, Danielson GK, Edwards WD. Surgical pathology of the truncal valve: a study of 12 cases. *Am J Cardiovasc Pathol.* 1988;2:39–47.
21. Ledbetter MK, Tandon R, Titus JL, Edwards JE. Stenotic semilunar valve in persistent truncus arteriosus. *Chest.* 1976;69:182–187.
22. Di Donato RM, Fyfe DA, Puga FJ, et al. Fifteen-year experience with surgical repair of truncus arteriosus. *J Thorac Cardiovasc Surg.* 1985;89:414–422.
23. Motro M, Schneeweiss A, Shem-Tov A, et al. Correlation of distance from subaortic membrane to base of the right aortic valve cusp and the development of aortic regurgitation in mild discrete subaortic stenosis. *Am J Cardiol.* 1989;64:395–396.
24. Hovaguimian H, Cobanoglu A, Starr A. Aortico-left ventricular tunnel: a clinical review and new surgical classification. *Ann Thorac Surg.* 1988;45:106–112.
25. Tuna IC, Edwards JE. Aortico-left ventricular tunnel and aortic insufficiency. *Ann Thorac Surg.* 1988;45:5–6.
26. Serino W, Andrade JL, Ross D, et al. Aorto-left ventricular communication after closure. Late postoperative problems. *Br Heart J.* 1983;49:501–506.
27. Smallhorn JF, de Leval M, Stark J, et al. Isolated anterior mitral cleft. Two dimensional echocardiographic assessment and differentiation from "clefts" associated with atrioventricular septal defect. *Br Heart J.* 1982;48:109–116.
28. Bruno E, Juaneda E, Moreyra E, Alday LE. The mitral middiastolic rumble in isolated coarctation of the aorta: cross-sectional and Doppler echocardiographic study. *J Cardiovasc Tech.* 1990;9:143.
29. Celano V, Pieroni DR, Morera JA, et al. Two-dimensional echocardiographic examination of mitral valve abnormalities associated with coarctation of the aorta. *Circulation.* 1984;69:924–932.
30. Rosenquist GC. Congenital mitral valve disease associated with coarctation of the aorta: a spectrum that includes parachute deformity of the mitral valve. *Circulation.* 1974;49:985–993.
31. Freed MD, Keane JF, Van Praagh R, et al. Coarctation of the aorta with congenital mitral regurgitation. *Circulation.* 1974;49:1175–1184.
32. Laborde F, Marchand M, Leca F, et al. Surgical treatment of anomalous origin of the left coronary artery in infancy and childhood. Early and late results in 20 consecutive cases. *J Thorac Cardiovasc Surg.* 1981;82:423–428.
33. Boucher CA, Liberthson RR, Buckley MJ. Secundum atrial septal defect and significant mitral regurgitation: incidence, management and morphologic basis. *Chest.* 1979;75:697–702.
34. Davies MJ. Mitral valve in secundum atrial septal defects. *Br Heart J.* 1981;46:126–128.
35. Liberthson RR, Boucher CA, Fallon JT, Buckley MJ. Severe mitral regurgitation: a common occurrence in the aging patient with secundum atrial septal defect. *Clin Cardiol.* 1981;4:229–232.

36. Nagata S, Nimura Y, Sakakibara H, et al. Mitral valve lesion associated with secundum atrial septal defect. Analysis by real time two dimensional echocardiography. *Br Heart J.* 1983;49:51–58.

37. Schreiber TL, Feigenbaum H, Weyman AE. Effect of atrial septal defect repair on left ventricular geometry and degree of mitral valve prolapse. *Circulation.* 1980;61:888–896.

38. Anderson KR, Zuberbuhler JR, Anderson RH, et al. Morphologic spectrum of Ebstein's anomaly of the heart: a review. *Mayo Clin Proc.* 1979;54:174–180.

39. Leung MP, Baker EJ, Anderson RH, Zuberbuhler JR. Cineangiographic spectrum of Ebstein's malformation: its relevance to clinical presentation and outcome. *J Am Coll Cardiol.* 1988;11:154–161.

40. Marino JP, Mihaileanu S, el Asmar B, et al. Echocardiography and color-flow mapping evaluation of a new reconstructive surgical technique for Ebstein's anomaly. *Circulation.* 1989;80:I197–I202.

41. Attenhofer Jost CH, Connolly HM, Dearani JA, et al. Ebstein's anomaly. *Circulation.* 2007;115:277–285.

42. Gerlis LM, Wilson N, Dickinson DF. Abnormalities of the mitral valve in congenitally corrected transposition (discordant atrioventricular and ventriculoarterial connections). *Br Heart J.* 1986;55:475–479.

43. Losekoot TG, Anderson RH, Becker AE, et al. *Congenitally Corrected Transposition.* London: Churchill Livingstone; 1983.

44. Roberts WC, Morrow AG, McIntosh CL, et al. Congenitally bicuspid aortic valve causing severe, pure aortic regurgitation without superimposed infective endocarditis. Analysis of 13 patients requiring aortic valve replacement. *Am J Cardiol.* 1981;47:206–209.

45. Sholler GF, Keane JF, Perry SB, et al. Balloon dilation of congenital aortic valve stenosis. Results and influence of technical and morphological features on outcome. *Circulation.* 1988;78:351–360.

46. Simon AL, Reis RL. The angiographic features of bicuspid and unicommissural aortic stenosis. *Am J Cardiol.* 1971;28:353–358.

47. Falcone MW, Roberts WC, Morrow AG, Perloff JK. Congenital aortic stenosis resulting from a unicommissural valve. Clinical and anatomic features in twenty-one adult patients. *Circulation.* 1971;44:272–280.

48. Olson LJ, Subramanian R, Edwards WD. Surgical pathology of pure aortic insufficiency: a study of 225 cases. *Mayo Clin Proc.* 1984;59:835–841.

49. Matsumoto M, Miki S, Kusuhara K, et al. Quadricuspid aortic valve associated with severe aortic regurgitation. *Jpn Circ J.* 1985;49:190–191.

50. Odim J, Laks H, Allada V, et al. Results of aortic valve-sparing and restoration with autologous pericardial leaflet extensions in congenital heart disease. *Ann Thorac Surg.* 2005;80:647–653.

51. Kopecky SL, Gersh BJ, McGoon MD, et al. Long-term outcome of patients undergoing surgical repair of isolated pulmonary valve stenosis. Follow-up at 20–30 years. *Circulation.* 1988;78:1150–1156.

52. Rao PS, Fawzy ME, Solymar L, Mardini MK. Long-term results of balloon pulmonary valvuloplasty of valvar pulmonic stenosis. *Am Heart J.* 1988;115:1291–1296.

53. Fontes VF, Esteves CA, Sousa JE, et al. Regression of infundibular hypertrophy after pulmonary valvuloplasty for pulmonic stenosis. *Am J Cardiol.* 1988;62:977–979.

54. Robertson M, Benson LN, Smallhorn JS, et al. The morphology of the right ventricular outflow tract after percutaneous pulmonary valvotomy: long term follow up. *Br Heart J.* 1987;58:239–244.

55. Schneeweiss A, Blieden LC, Shem-Tov A, et al. Diagnostic angiocardiographic criteria in dysplastic stenotic pulmonic valve. *Am Heart J.* 1983;106:761–762.

56. Watkins L Jr, Donahoo JS, Harrington D, et al. Surgical management of congenital pulmonary valve dysplasia. *Ann Thorac Surg.* 1977;24:498–507.

57. Ilbawi MN, Idriss FS, DeLeon SY, et al. Factors that exaggerate the deleterious effects of pulmonary insufficiency on the right ventricle after tetralogy repair. Surgical implications. *J Thorac Cardiovasc Surg.* 1987;93:36–44.

58. Perloff JK, Middlekauf HR, Child JS, et al. Usefulness of post-ventriculotomy signal averaged electrocardiograms in congenital heart disease. *Am J Cardiol.* 2006;98:1646–1651.

59. Jatene AD, Fontes VF, Paulista PP, et al. Anatomic correction of transposition of the great vessels. *J Thorac Cardiovasc Surg.* 1976;72:364–370.

60. Norwood WI, Lang P, Casteneda AR, Campbell DN. Experience with operations for hypoplastic left heart syndrome. *J Thorac Cardiovasc Surg.* 1981;82:511–519.

61. Alday LE, Juaneda E. Percutaneous balloon dilatation in congenital mitral stenosis. *Br Heart J.* 1987;57:479–482.

62. Grifka RG, Nihill MP, Mullins CE. Percutaneous transseptal double balloon valvuloplasty for congenital mitral stenosis. *Am J Cardiol.* 1990;66:522.

63. Spevak PJ, Bass JL, Ben-Shachar G, et al. Balloon angioplasty for congenital mitral stenosis. *Am J Cardiol.* 1990;66:472–476.

64. Carpentier A, Branchini B, Cour JC, et al. Congenital malformations of the mitral valve in children. Pathology and surgical treatment. *J Thorac Cardiovasc Surg.* 1976;72:854–866.

65. Okita Y, Miki S, Kusuhara K, et al. Early and late results of reconstructive operation for congenital mitral regurgitation in pediatric age group. *J Thorac Cardiovasc Surg.* 1988;96:294–298.

66. Stellin G, Bortolotti U, Mazzucco A, et al. Repair of congenitally malformed mitral valve in children. *J Thorac Cardiovasc Surg.* 1988;95:480–485.

CHAPTER 22

Electrophysiologic Abnormalities: Unoperated Occurrence and Postoperative Residua and Sequelae

KALYANAM SHIVKUMAR ▪ JOSEPH K. PERLOFF

Electrophysiologic abnormalities in congenital heart disease (CHD) fall into three general categories: (1) disturbances in rhythm and conduction that are inherent components of certain unoperated malformations and that persist as obligatory residua after reparative surgery; (2) electrophysiologic abnormalities that develop as consequences of the hemodynamic or hypoxic effects imposed on the heart by the basic unoperated malformation and that may or may not persist as postoperative residua; and (3) electrophysiologic abnormalities that are postoperative sequelae of reparative surgery. This chapter begins with a historical review of the physiologic bases and pathophysiology of arrhythmias and then focuses on specific malformations.

In the 19th century, cardiac arrhythmias were characterized by clinicians such as Wenckebach,[1] and a series of morphologic discoveries laid the foundation for applying concepts of the electrical system of the heart to clinical settings.[1] In 1839, Jan Evangelista Purkinje discovered the fibers that bear his name, Willem His discovered the bundle of His in 1893, and in 1906, Sunao Tawara, while working in Ludwig Aschoff's laboratory in Marburg, published his epoch-making monograph. The introduction of electrocardiography by Willem Einthoven in 1911 was a key contribution to cardiology as a discipline and to modern medicine as a whole.[2,3] Einthoven's invention still resonates.

Fundamental scientific concepts of electrophysiology have stood the test of time. In a series of remarkable experiments, George Ralph Mines described the "vulnerable period" and developed a theoretical basis for reentry.[4] Walter Garrey proposed the "critical mass hypothesis" of cardiac fibrillation.[5] Walter Gaskell introduced the concept of atrioventricular (AV) block and described the influence of the autonomic system on the heart and circulation.[6] Meticulous clinical observations by investigators such as Sir Thomas Lewis correlated electrocardiograms (ECGs) with clinical syndromes, laying the foundation of a new clinical specialty.[7,8] A relatively recent milestone was the recording of the His bundle potential in animals and subsequently in human beings,[9] paving the way for understanding the mechanisms of commonly encountered arrhythmias.[10] After mechanisms were reasonably well established, therapies were tested and introduced into clinical practice. Accessory AV connections identified by invasive electrophysiologic studies were initially addressed surgically.[11] In the 1980s and 1990s, the introduction of catheter-based direct current and subsequently radiofrequency ablation obviated the need for surgery and dramatically transformed the field, allowing diagnosis and treatment during a single nonsurgical procedure.[12] Cardiac electrophysiology continues to evolve at a lively pace and has changed from providing treatment *after* the clinical expression of arrhythmias to preventive interventions such as using implantable cardioverter using defibrillators (ICDs) before a life-threatening arrhythmia is documented.[13]

PATHOPHYSIOLOGY—MECHANISMS OF CARDIAC ARRHYTHMIAS

Cardiac arrhythmias involve disturbances of impulse formation, impulse propagation, or both and occur in the presence or absence of structural heart disease. An understanding of electrocardiography and arrhythmia mechanisms requires an understanding of cardiac electrical function at a cellular level.

Cellular Electrophysiology

The resting membrane potential of cardiac cells is governed by potassium conductance and, to a lesser extent, by several other ion channels and ion exchange proteins. Figure 22–1 shows an action potential (AP) and the inward and outward membrane currents that are responsible for the changes in membrane potential. The action potential itself is a plot of membrane voltage over time.[14] The resting membrane potential is governed by the Nernst equation and predominantly by potassium conductance at baseline (phase 4). The action potential is "sculpted" by the balance between inward and outward currents. When there is a net inward current, the membrane potential moves in a positive direction (depolarization). The converse is the case when there is a net outward current (repolarization). Phase 0 of the AP is due to rapid influx of Na via the voltage gated Na channels in response to a depolarizing stimulus followed by activation of inward calcium currents (via L-type calcium channels). Phase 2 is created in large part by the activation of the inward calcium currents. Repolarization involves the concerted activation of several potassium currents (phase 3), which is a tightly regulated process that governs electrical excitation in cardiac cells. The major repolarizing currents in ventricular myocytes are I_{Ks} (slow component of the delayed rectifier current), I_{Kr} (rapid component of the delayed rectifier current), and I_{to} (the transient outward current). The molecular basis

of these currents has been established, and alterations have been held responsible for long QT1 (I_{Ks}) and long QT2 (I_{Kr}) syndromes.[14] Drugs that increase the duration of the action potential (sotalol, dofetilide, erythromycin, sertraline, etc.) block K currents. Almost all antiarrhythmic medications alter one or more of these transmembrane currents.

Correlation of Cellular Electrophysiology with the Electrocardiogram

Since the mid–1990s, studies have revealed distinct myocardial cell types with unique cellular and ionic characteristics across the ventricular wall that contribute to electrical heterogeneity in the form of dispersion of repolarization and refractoriness. The ST segment and T wave are expressions of transventricular electrical differences in repolarizing currents. These differences play an important role in the genesis of normal and abnormal waves in the ECG and allow ready extrapolation with the clinical and physiologic relevance of various changes in pathophysiologic milieu and genetic mutations. Differences between these cell types are thought to play a role in the genesis of the J-wave (Osborn) in the ECG of patients during hypothermia.[15] In congenital and drug-induced long QT syndromes, a disproportionate prolongation of the action potential duration (APD) of the Purkinje fibers and M cells of the deep subendocardium/mid-myocardium is held responsible for the development of long QT intervals, abnormal T-wave morphologies, and U waves. The resulting dispersions of repolarization have also been shown to contribute to the polymorphic ventricular arrhythmias in this syndrome.[16]

MECHANISMS OF CARDIAC ARRHYTHMIAS

See Tables 22–1 through 22–4. Arrhythmias can occur in the absence of structural heart disease due purely to functional changes (e.g., congenital and acquired long QT syndromes, electrolyte disturbances) or can occur in the presence of structural heart disease (ventriculotomy scars, infarction scars, chamber dilatation, or hypertrophy). Ventricular dysfunction is both a structural and functional cause of arrhythmias.[17]

Structural Basis of Cardiac Arrhythmias

Cardiac structure and electrical function are intimately related (Fig. 22–2). Ventriculotomy scars, infarction scars, and the stretch of cardiac chambers can create arrhythmogenic substrates. Regions of slowed conduction set the stage for macroreentrant arrhythmias.[18] Congenital diseases that create a substrate for macroreentry include the Wolff-Parkinson-White syndrome and its variants. It has long been known that an accessory AV

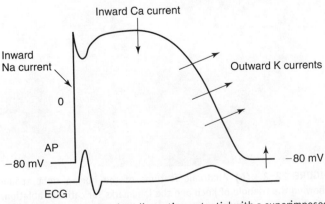

FIGURE 22–1 A stylized cardiac action potential with a superimposed electrocardiogram (ECG). Ca, calcium; K, potassium; Na, sodium.

Table 22-1 Mechanisms of Cardiac Arrhythmias

FUNCTIONAL	STRUCTURAL	COMPLEX MECHANISMS
Genetic	**Genetic**	e.g., Congestive heart failure
1. Long QT syndromes	1. Arrhythmogenic RV dysplasia	
2. Ryanodine receptor mutations	2. Hypertrophic cardiomyopathy	
3. Brugada syndrome	3. Familial Wolff-Parkinson-White syndrome	
Acquired	**Acquired**	
1. Electrolyte disturbances	1. Post–myocardial infarction scar	
2. Drug-induced arrhythmias	2. Postsurgical scar	

Table 22-4 Clinical Clues to Arrhythmia Mechanism

	REENTRY	FOCAL
Onset and termination	Abrupt	"Warm-up"
Effect of overdrive pacing	Termination	Transient suppression ("overdrive suppression") focal arrhythmias, and EAD-driven arrhythmias or worsening (DAD-driven)
Entrainment	Yes	No
Autonomic modulation	+	+++
Therapy	Drugs (+/−) Ablation (+++)	Drugs (+) Ablation (+++)

DAD, delayed after-depolarization; EAD, early after-depolarization.

Table 22-2 Mechanisms of Cardiac Arrhythmias

SUPRAVENTRICULAR ARRHYTHMIAS	VENTRICULAR ARRHYTHMIAS
Reentry	**Reentry**
Atrioventricular nodal reentrant tachycardia	Ventricular tachycardia (postinfarction)
Atrioventricular reentrant tachycardia	Polymorphic VT/torsades (Long QT syndrome)
"Incisional" tachycardias (postsurgical)	Ventricular fibrillation
Atrial fibrillation	
Focal	**Focal**
Atrial ectopic tachycardia	Idiopathic right ventricle and left ventricle ventricular tachycardia
Atrial fibrillation	Idiopathic ventricular fibrillation

Table 22-3 Mechanisms of Cardiac Arrhythmias

SINGLE CELL	MULTICELLULAR/WHOLE ORGAN
Disorders of impulse formation	Disorders of impulse propagation
Focal	Reentry
Triggered activity (DAD and EAD)	Macroreentry (scars)
	Functional reentry
	Reflection
	Phase 2 reentry

DAD, delayed after-depolarization; EAD, early after-depolarization.

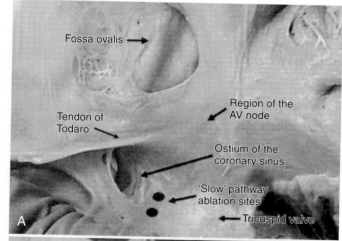

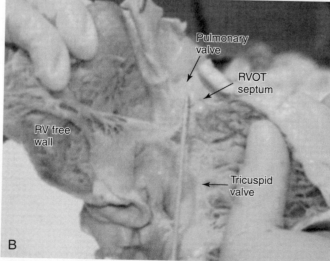

FIGURE 22-2 **(A)** Anatomic features of the human right atrium showing the triangle of Koch and the landmarks for catheter ablation. **(B)** Outflow tract of the right ventricle. All known regular arrhythmias are encountered in adults with congenital heart disease.

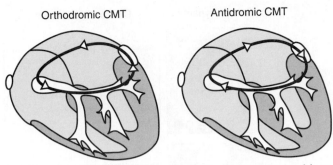

FIGURE 22-3 Mechanistic basis of arrhythmias in patients with accessory pathways.

connection predisposes to cardiac arrhythmias, and accessory pathways have provided a useful clinical model of the functional characteristics of macroreentrant tachycardias. Orthodromic atrioventricular reentrant tachycardia is characterized by a narrow QRS complex with antegrade conduction of impulses down the AV node/His Purkinje system and retrograde activation of the atria through the accessory AV connection (Fig. 22-3). Other arrhythmias in this setting include antidromic tachycardia characterized by antegrade activation of the ventricles through the accessory AV connection and retrograde activation of the atria through the AV node (see Fig. 22-3) and atrial fibrillation with ventricular conduction through an accessory pathway (Fig. 22-4). Before the advent of catheter ablation, treatment of drug-refractory arrhythmias and Wolff-Parkinson-White syndrome required surgical ablation.[19]

In complex disease processes such as heart failure, structural abnormalities can be accompanied by important functional changes such as repolarizing currents that lead to prolongation of the cardiac action potential and abnormal calcium handling.[20,21] Cardiac ultrastructural changes secondary to pathophysiologic processes such as the apoptosis accompanying heart failure can affect the pattern of electrical excitation,[22,23] and apoptosis has been implicated in the genesis of diverse cardiac arrhythmias.[24] Multiple factors can therefore act in concert to cause clinical arrhythmias.

Functional Changes Underlying the Genesis and Perpetuation of Cardiac Arrhythmias

The early 1990s witnessed dramatic advances in our understanding of the molecular biology and genetics of ion channels and the molecular causes of cardiac arrhythmias.[25,26] The genetic basis of certain congenital diseases that cause sudden death, such as the long QT syndrome, has been established,[27] and specific therapies have been designed and tested. Studies at the cellular level and animal experimental studies simulating clinical disease states are now routine.

Cardiac arrhythmias unaccompanied by structural alterations are represented by long QT syndromes characterized by abnormal cardiac repolarization, lengthening the QT interval, and a propensity for lethal arrhythmias.[28] The molecular basis of almost all the long QT syndromes has been determined. Alterations in potassium currents are responsible for LQT1 (I_{Ks}) and LQT2 (I_{Kr}), whereas alteration in a sodium current is responsible for LQT3 (SCN5a).[29,30] Potentially proarrhythmic drugs (sotalol, dofetilide, erythromycin, quinidine, and sertraline) block K currents and increase the duration of the action potential. Functional disorders that predispose to cardiac arrhythmias are powerfully modulated by autonomic influences and by alterations in ionic homeostasis such as changes in extracellular potassium concentration.[31] *Hyper*kalemia is pro-arrhythmic in part because of inactivation of sodium channels that occurs when the resting membrane potential becomes less negative (i.e., depolarized as predicted by the Nernst equation). Inactivation of Na channels predisposes to slowed conduction, a prerequisite for reentry.

After an arrhythmia occurs, a series of electrophysiologic changes ensue, collectively referred to as electrical remodeling, a dynamic phenomenon that reflects rapid physiologic changes in the electrical behavior of atrial and ventricular cells.[32] The atrial effective refractory period shortens even after a brief episode of atrial fibrillation, lending credence to the concept that "atrial fibrillation begets atrial fibrillation."[33] Recordings from excised atrial appendages and from human atrial myocytes of

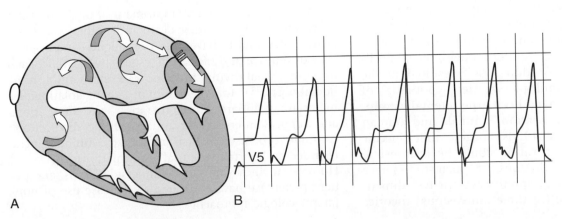

FIGURE 22-4 Mechanistic basis of arrhythmias in patients with accessory pathways. Antegrade conduction of atrial fibrillation.

explanted hearts have been studied in great detail to determine the ionic currents that regulate the atrial action potential.[34-36] These data are being used to strengthen mathematical models of atrial arrhythmias.[37-39]

ARRHYTHMIAS IN THE SETTING OF ACUTE MYOCARDIAL ISCHEMIA

No matter how often observed, a heart that suddenly goes into ventricular fibrillation is an awesome sight. The kind heart, one that has been beating faithfully and uncomplainingly for millions and millions of beats, is suddenly betrayed by the hand that feeds it, its coronary arteries.

Arrhythmias due to acute myocardial ischemia are catastrophic, with the vast majority presenting as out-of-hospital cardiac arrest.[40] Myocardial ischemia is characterized by a dramatic change in cellular electrophysiological behavior and ionic homeostasis. One of the major consequences is the perturbation of ionic fluxes across the cardiac sarcolemmal membrane, resulting in net potassium loss from the intracellular space.[41] As early as 1954, potassium was suspected as an excitant responsible for cardiac arrhythmias.[42] An increase in extracellular K concentration is a hallmark of acute myocardial ischemia and is thought to play an important role in the genesis of lethal arrhythmias following acute coronary events.[43] The accumulation of K in the extracellular space due to lack of washout by vascular flow has profound electrophysiologic effects. Membrane depolarization results in slowed conduction and altered refractoriness, which, in concert with other factors, triggers reentrant ventricular tachycardia and sudden cardiac death. Reentry has been postulated as the mechanistic basis of so-called Harris phase I tachyarrhythmias that occur within 30 minutes of coronary occlusion.[43]

RECENT ADVANCES

Healed ventriculotomy scars are especially prone to harbor substrates for reentry.[18] Mathematical modeling of arrhythmias using computers has had a dramatic impact on understanding and designing research studies. As early as 1964, a computer model of atrial fibrillation introduced by Gordon Moe[44] resulted in the formulation of the "multiple wavelet hypothesis" of atrial fibrillation, which has been experimentally evaluated.[45] Theoretical, simulation, animal, and human studies since the mid–1990s suggest that specific patterns of electrical activation could be responsible for functional reentrant rhythms.[46-49] Such studies have led to the application of spiral wave (in two dimensions) and scroll wave (in three dimensions) theories

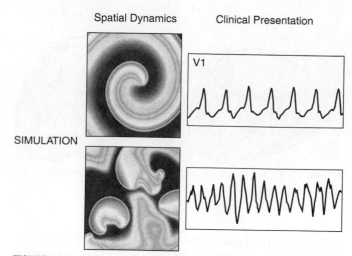

FIGURE 22–5 Simulation of arrhythmias in two dimensions showing a stable spiral wave and its clinical counterpart (monomorphic ventricular tachycardia) and spiral wave breakup and its clinical counterpart (ventricular fibrillation). *(Courtesy UCLA Cardiac Simulation Group.)*

to electrical activation in the heart. Changes in the biologic behavior of these activation patterns have been correlated with changes in clinical expressions of arrhythmias. For example, spiral/scroll wave breakup has been shown to correlate with transition of ventricular tachycardia to ventricular fibrillation (Fig. 22–5).[50,51] An ongoing research effort has been designed to identify specific targets for therapy that prevent lethal arrhythmias such as ventricular fibrillation. Functional patterns of arrhythmias use preexisting heterogeneity in cardiac structure (endocardial structures) to "anchor" waves of reentrant excitation,[52] highlighting the complex interplay between structure and function. One of the exciting developments in computational biology is the simulation of cardiac arrhythmias using mathematical models that may eventually permit formulation of rational pharmacologic and nonpharmacologic therapies.[51]

MANAGEMENT

Arrhythmias range from asymptomatic at one end of the spectrum to sudden cardiac death at the other end. Atrial arrhythmias tend to have dire consequences in the presence of ventricular dysfunction, especially diastolic. Lack of normal atrial rhythm predisposes to stasis and thromboembolism.[53] Before the advent of catheter ablation, the mainstays of antiarrhythmic therapy[54] were medications and surgical intervention; antiarrhythmic medications continue to be used as first-line therapy. Amiodarone is regarded as "mortality neutral" but inferior to ICDs.[55,56] However, inefficacy, proarrhythmia, side effects, and patient preference have conspired to increase use of nonpharmacologic approaches.

Invasive Electrophysiologic Studies

Electrophysiologic studies provide valuable information regarding the sinoatrial (SA) node, the AV node, and the His Purkinje system and provide controlled settings for investigating the mechanisms of supraventricular and ventricular arrhythmias. Simple pacing techniques and drug interventions can help distinguish arrhythmia mechanisms (see Table 22–2). The capability of inducing arrhythmias lends itself to targeting areas of the myocardium that are crucial in the genesis or maintenance of arrhythmias and to deciding the optimal therapeutic approach.

Nonpharmacologic arrhythmia management is "mechanism based." Whether an arrhythmia is "focal" or "reentrant" is a useful distinction in deciding the approach during invasive electrophysiologic studies for treatment. Before ablation, well-established techniques of pacing and drug interventions are employed to determine whether an arrhythmia is reentrant (see Table 22–3). Entrainment mapping helps distinguish the exact location of the pacing catheter in relation to the tachycardia circuit. Similarly, origin of focal arrhythmias can be accurately mapped. Recently, specialized electroanatomic mapping systems have improved the spatial resolution of mapping and have increased the success of catheter-based techniques for arrhythmia therapy.

Catheter Ablation

The energy source used for catheter ablation was initially direct current shocks,[57,58] which are now replaced by a radiofrequency (RF) current that has revolutionized the field of cardiac electrophysiology. An accurate diagnosis and a cure for the targeted arrhythmia can be provided during a single invasive electrophysiologic study.

How Does Radiofrequency Work?

RF is the most widely used energy source for catheter ablation. Application of RF current (approximately 460 KHz) through an electrode causes resistive heating at the electrode-tissue interface, resulting in controlled thermal injury. A typical lesion delivered through a 4-mm catheter tip is about 5 to 6 mm in diameter and 2 to 3 mm deep.[59-61] Irrigating the tips of RF catheters has recently been used to increase lesion size.[62] Other energy sources that are under investigation for catheter ablation include ultrasound, cryoinjury, and microwave.[63]

Specific Arrhythmias

Atrioventricular Nodal Reentrant Tachycardia (AVNRT)

This common cause of paroxysmal supraventricular tachycardia (SVT) can be cured by catheter ablation. The arrhythmia is thought to be due to reentry within a confined region of the AV node complex. Functionally distinct conduction pathways—fast and slow—are held responsible for the arrhythmia, which can present in its "typical" slow-fast AVNRT form with narrow QRS complexes and retrograde P waves that are "hidden" within the QRS complex. An atypical "fast-slow" form is characterized by retrograde P waves that fall well after each QRS complex and are inverted in leads II, III, and aVF.[64,65] Both forms of AVNRT are thought to be reentry within the AV node and can be cured by "slow pathway" ablation. The tissue that participates in the "slow" limb of the circuit is typically near the ostium of the coronary sinus and is ablated by application of RF energy (see Fig. 22–2). Success rates are 98% to 100% in experienced hands, and the risk of creating heart block is less than 1%.[66-68]

Accessory Pathways

Catheter ablation has had a significant impact on management, with success rates of 90% to 100%. Right-sided accessory pathways are approached from the venous side, left-sided accessory pathways require a transaortic or transseptal approach, and posteroseptal accessory pathways are a challenge because of inaccessibility to endocardially placed catheters. Accessory pathways require treatment when they cause symptoms or have electrophysiologic characteristics that indicate a need for treatment.[69]

Atrial Tachycardias and Flutter

Atrial tachycardias can be due to focal or reentrant mechanisms, most of which are successfully managed by catheter ablation.[70] "Typical" or "atypical" forms of atrial flutter are a prototypical reentrant atrial arrhythmia that is now curable by catheter ablation.[71] The typical form is characterized by "saw-tooth waves" in the inferior leads and counterclockwise activation through the isthmus between the tricuspid valve and the inferior vena cava, which is a critical limb of the tachycardia circuit. RF energy ablation of this isthmus cures the tachycardia and is employed as first-line treatment.[72] Other types of reentrant atrial tachycardias that use this isthmus can also be successfully ablated. Macroreentrant right and left atrial tachycardias that reside in healed atrial surgical scars require careful mapping to delineate the circuits and permit successful ablation.[73,74]

Idiopathic Right and Left Ventricular Tachycardias

Monomorphic tachycardias arising from the right ventricular outflow tract can be mapped and effectively ablated.[75] Similarly, left ventricular tachycardias that originate at a focal site within the left ventricle have also been successfully ablated.[18,76,77]

Atrial Fibrillation

Atrial fibrillation is one of the commonest arrhythmias encountered in clinical practice and is a leading arrhythmic cause of hospitalization. Morbidity includes decreased exercise tolerance and thromboembolic risk. Management has previously focused on pharmacologic rhythm or rate control and on prevention of thromboembolism with warfarin. Several carefully conducted clinical trials have defined the roles of these therapeutic options.[53] Antiarrhythmic drugs have limitations, modest efficacy, and proarrhythmic propensities. An exciting new development is the recognition of sleeves of atrial myocardium that extend into the pulmonary veins and harbor arrhythmogenic foci[78,79] that have been successfully ablated with RF.[80] Alternative energy sources such as ultrasound are being tested for electrical ablation in pulmonary veins.[81] Other foci that cause atrial fibrillation amenable to catheter ablation reside at the ligament of Marshall and the junction between the superior vena cava and the right atrium.[82]

Little is known about the cellular behavior of "triggers" of atrial fibrillation. Why atrial fibrillation sometimes persists and sometimes is self-limiting is also poorly understood. Because brief episodes can be followed by electrical remodeling, an argument has been made for ablation of the triggers.[39] Ongoing studies and practice patterns seek to establish criteria for catheter ablation.

Patients with persistent or permanent atrial fibrillation may be candidates for a surgical "maze" procedure (see Chapter 15). Catheter-based techniques are not yet sufficiently reliable for creating the required linear ablative lesions.

Ventricular Tachycardias in the Setting of Structural Heart Disease

Standard management of ventricular tachycardia (VT) in patients with postventriculotomy, postinfarction, cardiomyopathy ventricular scars, or arrhythmogenic right ventricular dysplasia[83] has been antiarrhythmic drugs and ICDs (discussed later). Mapping and catheter ablation have also been attempted using standard electrophysiologic techniques, newer electroanatomic mapping systems, myocardial voltage maps,[84,85] and percutaneous access to pericardial space.[86] Attention has recently focused on the signal averaged ECG (SAECG) as a more sensitive and specific means than QRS duration for detecting slow conduction substrates of reentrant monomorphic ventricular tachycardia (MVT).[18] The technique has been employed in electrophysiologic assessment after right ventriculotomy for intracardiac repair of CHD.[18] A positive SAECG connotes the presence of a slow conduction substrate and the potential for reentrant MVT. A negative SAECG indicates absence of a reentrant substrate (discussed later).[18]

Catheter Ablation of Ventricular Fibrillation

Primary idiopathic ventricular fibrillation in some patients has recently been shown to originate from the distal His Purkinje system. In resuscitated patients, focal delivery of radiofrequency has effectively prevented further episodes of VF.[87,88]

Implanted Devices

The impact of implanted cardiac defibrillator devices, especially the ICD in the management of cardiac arrhythmias has been profound. Clinical trials have convincingly established the superiority of ICDs compared with medical therapy in the prevention of sudden death in patients surviving an out-of-hospital cardiac arrest and in patients with left ventricular dysfunction following myocardial infarction.[89] In addition to secondary prevention, results of the recent MADIT2 study disclosed that ICDs reduce mortality even in asymptomatic patients with left ventricular dysfunction[13] (Table 22–5). "Resynchronization" of the ventricles by simultaneous right and left ventricular pacing in patients with heart failure has provided further therapeutic options.[90]

Table 22–5 Management of Cardiac Arrhythmias
Pharmacologic
1. Drugs that modulate autonomic influences (beta-blockers, digoxin)
2. Antiarrhythmic drugs: class I (sub-classes a, b, c), class II–IV
3. Ancillary therapy to prevent morbidity related to arrhythmia (e.g., warfarin in atrial fibrillation)
Nonpharmacologic
1. Catheter Ablation
Cure: WPW, AVNRT, Atrial flutter, "focal tachycardias," idiopathic RVOT and LV tachycardias
Adjunctive: Macro-reentrant atrial and ventricular tachycardia (e.g., post infarction, post-surgery, arrhythmogenic RV dysplasia)
2. Implanted Devices
a. Established value in SCD prevention
b. Prevent occasional episodes of reentrant arrhythmias by anti-tachycardia pacing
c. Yet to be determined effect on arrhythmias by resynchronization (e.g., biventricular pacing)
3. Cardiac Surgery
a. Maze procedure (effective for management of "permanent" atrial fibrillation
b. Effective for rare cases of incessant monomorphic atrial and ventricular tachycardias

AVNRT, atrioventricular nodal reentrant tachycardia; LV, left ventricle; RVOT, right ventricular outflow tract ventricular tachycardia; SCD, sudden cardiac death; WPW, Wolff-Parkinson-White syndrome.

Cardiac Surgery

Before the introduction of catheter ablation, cardiac surgery was the sole nonpharmacologic method for managing arrhythmias associated with accessory atrioventricular connections.[90] The surgical "Maze" procedure introduced by Cox is now a standard technique for the nonpharmacologic management of certain atrial tachyarrhythmia, especially but not only those associated with CHD.[91] Modifications of the Maze procedure using handheld probes for creating radiofrequency lesions, cryogenics, and microwave have also been employed.

FUTURE

The future management of cardiac arrhythmias will undoubtedly involve combinations and refinements of currently available methods and the development of new methodologies. Recognition of the mechanisms of action of antiarrhythmic drugs has prompted a reclassification to provide a framework for understanding complex drug effects.[92] Molecular targets for critical parameters that affect cardiac arrhythmias promise to result in the development of "designer" antiarrhythmic drugs.[93]

Electrophysiologic abnormalities arise from disorders of impulse generation, impulse conduction, or combinations thereof.[94-97] The mechanisms reviewed here are well supported by animal models, and persuasive evidence for these mechanisms is rapidly accumulating for humans, primarily by means of intracardiac recordings and mapping techniques.

Reentry can occur in any cardiac tissue but is most commonly associated with the atrioventricular node or with ventricular or atrial scars (discussed earlier). Slow conduction that facilitates reentry in areas of myocardial scar are due to anisotropic conduction or to damaged or partially depolarized myocytes that have slow response action potentials.[98-100] In CHD, atriotomy and ventriculotomy scars create the substrate for a reentry circuit (see earlier and later discussions).

Programmed electrical stimulation provides controlled stimuli that initiate reentrant arrhythmias. However, initiation of an arrhythmia does not necessarily indicate that the arrhythmogenic substrate is reentrant, because programmed stimulation can theoretically initiate arrhythmias due to triggered automaticity. Arrhythmias arising from anatomically fixed regions include atrioventricular nodal reentrant tachycardia, circus movement tachycardia involving accessory pathway conduction, atrial flutter, and monomorphic ventricular tachycardia (discussed earlier).[19,101-105] Mechanical disruption of critical portions of the reentrant circuit serves to eliminate the arrhythmogenic substrate (discussed earlier).

Myocardial hypertrophy in animal models is accompanied by higher excitability thresholds, depressed membrane potential, prolonged action potential,[106,107] and depressed rates of rise of action potential upstroke, all of which serve to slow conduction velocity.[108,109] Pressure overload hypertrophy can be accompanied by focal areas of myocardial fibrosis, slow conduction, and heterogeneous refractoriness that facilitate reentry.[107,110-112] Chamber mass may regress when the hemodynamic consequences of the congenital cardiac malformation are eliminated by surgery, but preexisting areas of fibrosis persist (see Chapters 20 and 23). In TOF, the presence and degree of right ventricular fibrosis increase with age and may in part explain why atrial and ventricular arrhythmias that occur late after repair are more common in patients who are older at the time of surgery.[113-118] Similarly, patients with atrial septal defects who experience preoperative atrial fibrillation or atrial flutter may continue to do so after surgical repair.[119]

Conduction Defects

Conduction defects originate in the sinus node (SA block), in the AV node, in the bundle of His, in the bundle branches, or in the Purkinje system. The clinically important conduction defects that cause bradyarrhythmias are SA block, AV nodal block, or infranodal block. Other congenital conduction defects are innocently expressed in the surface ECG as left-axis deviation or right bundle branch block. Congenital complete heart block can either be isolated or an inherent component of certain malformations such as left isomerism or congenitally corrected transposition of the great arteries (see later).

Isolated congenital complete heart block is diagnosed if the conduction defect is known to have existed from infancy or *in utero*.[120] The P wave axis is normal because atrial depolarization originates in a normal sinus node. The QRS configuration exhibits a normal pattern of ventricular excitation (narrow complexes) when the pacemaker is above the bifurcation of the bundle of His, which is usually the case.[121] Permanent anatomic interruption of conduction is not always present, as indicated by occasional changes from complete to incomplete heart block or even to sinus rhythm.[121] Intracardiac electrophysiologic assessment identifies the level of block, which in itself is not a predictor of malignant bradyarrhythmias.[120] However, a relatively slow resting heart rate, bundle branch block QRS morphology, ventricular arrhythmias on ambulatory ECGs or in response to exercise stress, and suboptimal ventricular rate response to exercise are risk factors for syncope or sudden death and therefore warrant consideration for implantation of a permanent pacemaker.[120,122] However, only prolongation of the corrected QT interval predicts an unfavorable outcome.[123] Because of the difficulty in identifying high-risk patients and because the first syncopal episode may be fatal, prophylactic permanent pacemaker implantation has been recommended for all adults with congenital complete heart block.[123]

Conduction defects are common sequelae of intracardiac repair of CHD and may be evident immediately after operation or may emerge years later. Incisions or sutures can disrupt the sinus node, the specialized interatrial conduction tissue, the AV node, infranodal specialized conduction tissue, and the His-Purkinje system.[124] Incisions may isolate areas of myocardium, creating anatomic substrates for reentry, or may heal with fibrosis that subsequently progresses and provides arrhythmic foci.[125,126] Foreign-body reactions around suture sites may set the stage for arrhythmias.[127,128] Subendocardial fibrosis after cardiopulmonary bypass has been attributed to disruption of myocardial lymphatics.[124]

In brief, arrhythmias and conduction disturbances after surgical repair of congenital cardiac malformations can represent electrophysiologic residua inherent in the basic malformation or can be sequelae of an operation (see Chapter 20). The postoperative presence of or susceptibility to arrhythmias and conduction defects depends on the preoperative electrophysiologic substrates and the type and timing of reparative surgery.

MALFORMATIONS INVOLVING INTRAATRIAL SURGERY

Ostium Secundum Atrial Septal Defect

A normal preoperative P wave axis is directed downward and to the left, indicating depolarization from a right sinus node.[129] Sinus arrhythmia depends on separation of the systemic and pulmonary venous returns. Accordingly, sinus arrhythmia is absent or minimal in children with an atrial septal defect and does not occur in adults.[129] When the interatrial communication is closed, sinus arrhythmia becomes manifest. Ventricular activation is characterized by a slightly prolonged, rightward, superior, and anterior terminal force derived from the outflow tract of the volume overloaded right ventricle.[130] Terminal force prolongation may progress to a wide QRS complex.[120,130] The term *crochetage* (French for "notch"), the work of a crochet needle, has been applied to the notching typically seen near the apex of the R waves in the inferior limb leads of the scalar ECG of patients with ostium secundum or sinus venous atrial septal defects (Fig. 22–6).[131] The electrophysiologic mechanism of the notch is unknown, but it correlates with the presence of a left-to-right interatrial shunt. The combination of the crochetage notch with incomplete right bundle branch block considerably increases the specificity of the ECG in the diagnosis of an ostium secundum or sinus venous atrial septal defect.[131] Minor abnormalities of sinus node function can be elicited by electrophysiologic testing in 41% to 83% of patients, but symptomatic bradyarrhythmias are uncommon.[131-136] Mild PR interval prolongation has an incidence of 20% to 30% and is usually due to prolonged intraatrial conduction time with normal atrioventricular nodal and infranodal conduction,[131,137-141] although

prolongation of AV nodal conduction time occasionally occurs in older patients.[135,142] AV block is rare except in older adults or in patients with familial atrial septal defects.[143-151] Infranodal conduction is normal, as indicated by a normal His-ventricular (HV) interval.[135,137,138,152]

Atrial tachyarrhythmias are uncommon in children with unoperated ostium secundum atrial septal defects,[150,153-158] but the incidence increases with age probably because of the development of focal fibrosis in the dilatated right atrium and because augmentation of the left-to-right shunt in older age increases the dilatation still further.[119,143,156,159-164] Approximately one half of patients who survive to age 60 years experience atrial arrhythmias, the most common of which are fibrillation and flutter.[143,150,153-158,160,164-166]

Electrocardiographic monitoring early after operation often discloses transient atrial tachyarrhythmias and AV junctional rhythms.[154,160] Patients with preoperative atrial arrhythmias frequently manifest recurrences early postoperatively and are likely to experience late recurrences (discussed later).[166,167] Accelerated junctional rhythms are common, are generally well tolerated, and usually resolve without specific therapy.[150,153,155,157,158]

Sinus node dysfunction, generally manifested as sinus bradycardia or sinus pauses, is not uncommon early after operation because the sinus node is vulnerable to damage from cannulation of the superior vena cava. Mild sinus node dysfunction often improves after repair provided there is no significant intraoperative injury to the node.[132,152] Prolonged episodes of sinus bradycardia or sinus arrest occur in approximately 5% of postoperative patients,[150,153,155,157,158,168] the majority of whom have stable junctional escape rhythms. The sinus node usually recovers, but occasionally sinus bradycardia persists and requires a permanent pacemaker.[169,170]

The P wave amplitude decreases postoperatively,[160,171] and PR interval prolongation frequently resolves, presumably because of a reduction in right atrial size.[131,139] Postoperative normalization of intraatrial and AV nodal conduction is reflected in shortening of the atrial-His (AH) interval and in shortening of the AV Wenckebach cycle length.[152] Second- or third-degree AV block is uncommon and usually resolves early postoperatively.[131,139,154,165] Pacemaker implantation is rarely required.[165,169]

Patients can experience atrial tachyarrhythmias long after surgical repair, although the risk of this is highly variable. Preoperative atrial arrhythmias, older age at the time of repair, and postoperative right ventricular dysfunction increase the probability of atrial fibrillation late after operation (see Chapter 20).[165,172] In an analysis of 104 patients who underwent atrial septal defect closure at age 14 years or less, 89% remained in sinus rhythm 9 to 20 years after surgery,[169] 96% who underwent repair at or before age 11 years were free of atrial fibrillation or flutter at long-term follow-up, but 45% who underwent repair at age 41 years or older did not remain in sinus rhythm.[84] Of 18 adults who experienced paroxysmal atrial arrhythmias preoperatively, only three remained in sinus rhythm 3 to 25 years after surgery.[119]

Atrial tachycardia or flutter is often due to macroreentry around the atriotomy incision, around the atrial septal defect patch, or through the inferior vena caval–tricuspid annulus isthmus.[173] When anatomic barriers create isthmuses, catheter ablation can interrupt reentry. Occasionally, sinus bradycardia or, rarely, AV block develops late postoperatively and requires pacemaker implantation.[165,166,170,174] In four patients who died suddenly late after surgery, necropsy identified foreign body reactions with fibrosis at suture sites near the SA node and at the approaches to the AV node, suggesting that late-onset bradyarrhythmias may have been the mechanism of sudden death.[128]

Experience to date suggests that transcatheter closure of secundum atrial septal defects (see Chapter 18) is followed by fewer electrophysiologic sequelae than surgical closure. First-degree AV block, premature atrial contractions, atrial tachyarrhythmias, and junctional arrhythmias may disappear.[175]

Sinus Venosus Atrial Septal Defect

The superior vena caval variety of sinus venosus defect, which is the more common variety, abuts or occupies the site of the SA node,[176] so the P wave axis is often leftward, indicating an ectopic atrial (nonsinus) focus (see Fig. 22–6).[120] If a sinus P wave is present before operation, the proximity of the defect to the SA node predisposes to injury

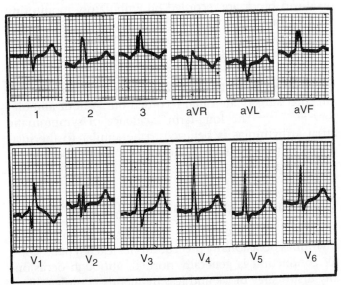

FIGURE 22–6 Electrocardiogram from a 25-year-old woman with a sinus venosus atrial septal defect of the superior vena caval type. Because the defect occupied the site of the normal sinus node, there is an ectopic pacemaker. P waves are inverted in leads 2, 3, and aVF (left superior P wave axis). Intracardiac electrophysiologic study identified the pacemaker in the left atrium. The QRS exhibits the typical pattern of right ventricular volume overload with slight prolongation of terminal forces that are directed to the right, superiorly, and anteriorly (rSr in lead V_1). Note also the "crochetage" or notch near the apex of the R waves in inferior leads 3 and aVF.

during operation and increases the incidence of postoperative sinus or ectopic atrial bradyarrhythmias.[177,178]

Atrioventricular Septal Defect

An ostium primum atrial septal defect is one component of this complex malformation that may occur in isolation or with mitral regurgitation.[121] A nonrestrictive ostium primum defect attenuates the hemodynamic effects of mitral regurgitation on the left side of the heart while augmenting the effects of the left-to-right shunt on the right side of the heart.[121] When mitral regurgitation exists with a restrictive ostium primum atrial septal defect, the dominant hemodynamic effects are those of the regurgitation. When a cleft but competent mitral valve exists with a nonrestrictive ostium primum defect, the dominant hemodynamic effects are analogous to those of an ostium secundum defect of similar size.

The scalar ECG in more than 50% of patients discloses PR interval prolongation owing to a combination of prolonged conduction from sinus node to atrioventricular node (enlarged right atrium) and to disruption of interatrial pathways by the defect with displacement of the AV node posteroinferiorly toward the ostium of the coronary sinus.[121,179-181] Conduction times through the AV node and His bundle are typically normal.[181-183]

The distinctive feature of the scalar ECG is a frontal plane QRS axis that is directed leftward and superiorly with counterclockwise depolarization and a change in terminal force direction that causes notching of S waves in the inferior lead (Fig. 22–7).[121] This pattern results from posteroinferior displacement of the common bundle of His and of the left bundle fascicles and to relative hypoplasia of the anterior fascicle of the left bundle branch.[178,180,183] The inferior portion of the left ventricle is therefore activated earlier than the anterior portion.[184-186]

Atrial tachyarrhythmias in isolated ostium primum atrial septal defects occur with a frequency and age range similar to that in ostium secundum defects of equivalent size and shunt volume.[121] High-degree heart block occasionally occurs in older patients, with an incidence somewhat greater than that of secundum defects.[187,188]

Surgical closure of ostium primum atrial septal defects is followed by electrophysiologic sequelae similar to those after repair of secundum defects of equivalent size. Early postoperative atrial tachyarrhythmias and bradyarrhythmias generally resolve within days.[139,150,189,190] AV block early after operation usually disappears spontaneously, but high-degree block persists in up to 11% of patients.[189-193] Late-onset high-degree block is uncommon.[183,189,191,194,195] The increased incidence of postoperative AV block in ostium primum defects is probably related to proximity of the displaced AV node and bundle of His to the site of surgical repair. Persistent sinus node dysfunction, sometimes accompanied by atrial flutter or fibrillation, is detected on ambulatory ECGs or exercise testing in up to

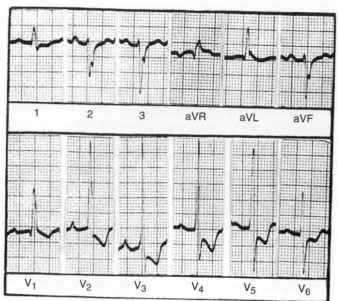

FIGURE 22-7 Electrocardiogram from an acyanotic 24-year-old man with complete common atrioventricular canal and pulmonary vascular disease. The PR interval is 0.20 sec. P waves are peaked (right atrial) in leads V_{2-3}. The QRS complex exhibits left-axis deviation with counterclockwise depolarization. The S waves are notched in leads 2, 3, and aVF, reflecting the change in terminal force direction typical of an atrioventricular septal defect. Right ventricular hypertrophy is indicated by tall right precordial R waves and deep left precordial S waves. The Q wave in lead V_1 indicates right atrial enlargement.

18% of postoperative patients and occasionally requires pacemaker implantation.[189,190]

In *complete common atrioventricular canal*, the incidence of PR interval prolongation is more than 50%[120] (see Fig. 22-7) because of a combination of intraatrial conduction delay (right atrial enlargement), disruption of intraatrial pathways, and displacement of the AV node posteriorly toward the ostium of the coronary sinus.[120,179-181,183] Conduction time through the AV node is occasionally prolonged,[183] but complete heart block is rare.[181,188,196] The distinctive frontal plane QRS pattern of left-axis deviation with counterclockwise depolarization and notching of S waves in the inferior leads is the same as described earlier for ostium primum atrial septal defects.[179,180,184-186] In Down syndrome, the frontal plane QRS axis is distinctively even more leftward, not uncommonly between −90 and −150 degrees.[174]

Early postoperatively, transient atrial tachyarrhythmias and junctional rhythms are relatively common. The incidence of atrial flutter or fibrillation late after repair is approximately 5% with atrial premature beats occurring in up to 10% of patients.[174,197] A major postoperative electrophysiologic complication reflects damage to the AV conduction system.[196,198-201] Transient complete AV block occurs in as many as a third of patients, but the incidence has progressively declined because of better understanding of the anatomy of the conduction system

and improved surgical techniques.[174,199,200] Persistent complete AV block occurs immediately after surgery in 1% to 7% of patients and develops late after operation in approximately 2%.[197-199,201] Prolonged infranodal conduction may be a marker for increased risk of late-onset heart block and can be present even if the PR interval on the scalar ECG is normal.[183] The most common postoperative intraventricular conduction abnormality is right bundle branch block,[174,197,201] but more than 50% of patients have a reduction in QRS duration.[197] Whether postoperative right bundle branch block (central or peripheral) together with preoperative left-axis deviation has the same significance as acquired bifascicular block is unclear. Although late-onset ventricular arrhythmias occur in up to one third of patients,[197] complex ventricular arrhythmias or ventricular tachycardia are generally associated with impaired left ventricular function and are rarely detected on ambulatory monitoring.[197]

Anomalous Pulmonary Venous Connection

Partial anomalous pulmonary venous connection occurs in isolation or with an ostium secundum atrial septal defect[120] but is almost always present when there is a superior vena caval sinus venous atrial septal defect. In *total* anomalous pulmonary venous connection, an atrial septal defect is the only pathway by which pulmonary venous blood can enter the left side of the heart. Atrial arrhythmias and sinus node dysfunction are electrophysiologic sequelae of repair.[178,202-205] Intraoperative and perioperative heart block are recorded on ambulatory monitoring more commonly in younger patients with up to 8% developing perioperative heart block that ultimately requires a permanent pacemaker.[206] Early postoperative atrial fibrillation, atrial flutter, or junctional rhythm occurs in more than 40% of patients.[204] Asymptomatic atrial arrhythmias late after surgery are often recorded on 24-hour ambulatory ECGs.[202] The long-term incidence of symptomatic atrial arrhythmias is believed to be similar to the incidence in patients with nonrestrictive ostium secundum atrial septal defects.

Complete Transposition of the Great Arteries

Sinus node dysfunction and a predisposition to atrial arrhythmias occasionally precede atrial switch repairs.[207-211] AV conduction is generally normal, although occasionally first-degree block and less frequently complete heart block occur.[211-213]

Transient supraventricular arrhythmias commonly coincide with balloon atrial septotomy, but whether the procedure predisposes to an increased incidence of subsequent atrial arrhythmias is unclear.[207,214] Also unclear is the effect of a Blalock-Hanlon atrial septectomy on subsequent atrial arrhythmias.[214-217] The following remarks focus on the electrophysiologic sequelae of intraatrial baffle operations (Mustard and Senning). The arterial switch operation is subsequently discussed.[218,219]

Mustard Operation

The Mustard repair involves excision of the atrial septum and insertion of a pericardial or Dacron baffle that directs systemic and coronary venous return across the mitral valve into the left ventricle and pulmonary artery and directs pulmonary venous return across the tricuspid valve into the right ventricle and aorta (see Chapter 15).[220] Electrophysiologic sequelae of this extensive reconstruction come as no surprise and include atrial arrhythmias, damage to the sinus node either directly or by transection or compression of the sinus node artery, and damage to the AV node.[221-224] Atrial arrhythmias are sequelae of sinus node dysfunction and surgical disruption of atrial tissue, which result in areas of delayed atrial activation and dispersion of refractoriness.[221,223,225-227] Disruption of atrial conduction can be so extensive that portions of the atria become electrically isolated, allowing the simultaneous presence of independent atrial rhythms in the pulmonary venous and systemic venous atria.[125] Canine models of the Mustard operation have demonstrated multiple regional substrates for the development of atrial fibrillation and flutter.[228] The Senning modification of the atrial switch procedure does not reduce the type or incidence of atrial arrhythmias.[213,222,227,229-232]

The postoperative P wave amplitude may decrease dramatically after an atrial switch because of a reduction in size of the systemic venous atrium, with little change in P axis.[228,233] In 30% to 75% of patients, atrial tachyarrhythmias and bradyarrhythmias, most frequently accelerated junctional rhythms (Fig. 22–8), junctional escape rhythms, ectopic atrial rhythms, and sinus node dysfunction manifested by sinus bradycardia or sinus pauses, occur early postoperatively.[208,211,213,231,232,234-238] The majority of these arrhythmias are tolerated satisfactorily and resolve within a few weeks. Early postoperative first-degree AV block occurs in 5% to 13% of patients and often resolves within a few weeks.[212,222,233] Second- or third-degree heart block becomes manifest in 3% to 16% of patients, is more frequent after closure of a coexisting ventricular septal defect, and often resolves within days.[208,211,213,231,232,234-238] Implantation of a permanent pacemaker is rarely necessary.[239,240]

By the time of hospital discharge, sinus rhythm is present in 80% to 95% of patients, many of whom nevertheless continue to experience episodic junctional and atrial ectopic rhythms and sinus node dysfunction.[212-214,217,222,232,236,241,242] Intracardiac electrophysiologic testing discloses impaired sinus node function in 37% to 100% of patients, but abnormal sinus node recovery times and SA conduction times lack sensitivity and specificity in predicting clinical sinus node dysfunction.[212,222,223,226,243-245] Some degree of chronotropic inadequacy in response to exercise is almost invariably present.[246] With the passage of time, progressive sinus node dysfunction develops in the majority of patients.[208,217,235,238,247-249] In a multicenter study involving 372 patients, 76% were in sinus rhythm during the first postoperative year, but the incidence decreased to 57% 8 years later.[235] The majority of electrophysiologic disorders were sinus bradycardia, junctional escape rhythms, and AV block.

During the first 10 postoperative years, 2% to 10% of patients experience atrial tachyarrhythmias (Fig. 22–9), chiefly atrial flutter/tachycardia, atrial fibrillation, and junctional tachycardia.[226,250,251] Dysfunction of the

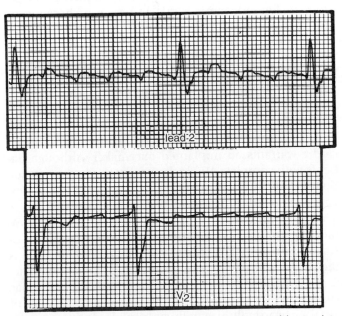

FIGURE 22–9 Rhythm strips from a 25-year-old man with complete transposition of the great arteries and a Mustard repair in infancy. In addition to late-onset atrial flutter with a slow ventricular response (impaired atrioventricular conduction) shown here, there was sinus node dysfunction.

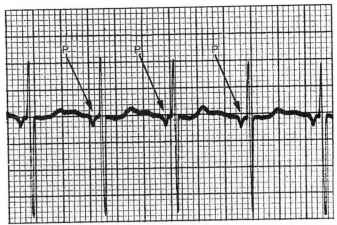

FIGURE 22–8 Rhythm strip demonstrating a junctional ectopic rhythm early after a Mustard repair for complete transposition of the great arteries.

sinus node and right ventricle are risk factors for the development of late atrial arrhythmias.[226,247] The coexistence of sinus bradycardia or high-degree AV block with paroxysmal atrial arrhythmias is not uncommon.[217,247,250,252,253] It is important to stress that atrial tachyarrhythmias are poorly tolerated because of the appreciably reduced size of the atrial compartments, and require prompt attention (discussed later).

Intracardiac mapping has disclosed that atrial tachycardia or flutter after a Mustard operation is often due to macroreentry around a surgical incision site. Zones critical to the development and maintenance of intraatrial reentry occur between the atrial baffle and the coronary sinus and between the atriotomy incision and the tricuspid annulus.[173]

During long-term follow-up, 2% to 8% of patients die suddenly.[211,217,229,231,233,235,244,245,254,255] An anatomic cause of sudden death is seldom established, suggesting that a fatal arrhythmia is the mechanism.[211,221,244,256] Sudden death is more likely in patients whose prevailing rhythm is atrial flutter/tachycardia.[235,247] In a multicenter study of young patients who had undergone a Mustard repair, there was a 10% risk of sudden death when an episode of atrial flutter was documented.[216] In a single-center study of 249 consecutive patients who underwent a Mustard procedure (mean follow-up, 11.7 years), the risk of late death—73% of which were sudden—increased 4.7-fold after occurrence of atrial flutter and 2.6-fold after the onset of right ventricular failure.[247] The majority of sudden deaths were in patients with documented junctional rhythms or AV block.[211,231,244,255] It is unclear whether atrial tachyarrhythmias predispose to sudden death because of hemodynamic sequelae per se or because the arrhythmia itself identifies patients with the poorest hemodynamic substrates. A relationship between sudden death and bradyarrhythmias has not been identified. Sudden death occasionally occurs in patients with satisfactorily functioning pacemakers.[216,235]

These observations argue for aggressive suppression of atrial tachyarrhythmias and careful evaluation of sinus node function and AV conduction. Symptomatic bradycardia warrants an implanted pacemaker. Although patients with complete AV block often have adequate escape rhythms and are asymptomatic,[235] they are at risk of syncope and sudden death, so pacemaker implantation is generally warranted. The risk is of particular concern if AV block is due to infranodal damage incurred during closure of a coexisting ventricular septal defect. Unknown is the prognostic significance of impaired sinus node function or impaired AV conduction identified by intracardiac electrophysiologic study, but the frequent coexistence of atrial tachyarrhythmias with sinus node dysfunction demands particularly close attention.[222,223,226,243,245]

For permanent pacing, transvenous leads can be placed in the left atrial appendage and onto the left ventricular endocardium, with access by means of the atrial baffle

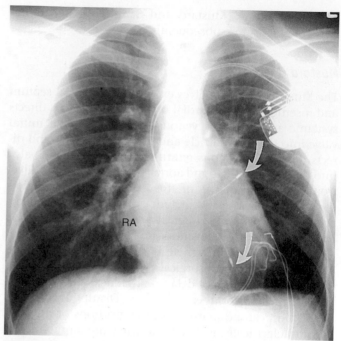

FIGURE 22–10 Chest radiograph from a 28-year-old man with complete transposition of the great arteries. Atrial flutter with high-degree atrioventricular block developed 23 years after a Mustard repair. The rhythm was converted to sinus, and a dual-chamber transvenous pacemaker was implanted with leads in the left atrial appendage (*upper arrow*) and the left ventricular endocardium (*lower arrow*). The right atrium (RA) is enlarged.

(Fig. 22–10).[240,257,258] Although atrial tachycardia is occasionally well tolerated, conversion to sinus rhythm is still warranted. Atrial tachycardia, even with controlled ventricular rates (see Fig. 22–9), limits exercise capacity.[259] Intracardiac mapping for identification and ablation of critical conduction zones within the atria (most commonly around surgical incisions) are employed for definitive treatment of the arrhythmia, potentially avoiding the need for antiarrhythmic drugs, which may be ineffective, cause unacceptable side effects, or exacerbate bradyarrhythmias.[173,260]

Senning Repair

The Senning operation is functionally similar to but technically different from the Mustard.[261] The sinus node is displaced inferomedially into the pulmonary venous portion of the reconstructed atrium in contrast to the Mustard operation in which the position of the sinus node is not altered.[234] The P wave amplitude is reduced with little or no change in its frontal plane axis, and the PR interval usually remains normal (discussed earlier). Extensive atrial reconstruction is associated with electrophysiologic sequelae similar to those of the Mustard repair.[208,262-269] Medial and caudad placement of the sinus node in the Senning operation may account for a reportedly lower incidence of sinus node dysfunction.[234,270] Atrial tachyarrhythmias arising from reentrant loops around surgical incisions are similar to those after the Mustard procedure.[173,260] Of 220 patients surviving the Senning repair, permanent pacemaker implantation was required in 7% at 10 years and in 10.5% 15 years after surgery.[271] Late sudden death occurred in 4% to 6%.[208,267,270]

Arterial Switch

The *arterial switch* operation involves transecting and reattaching the pulmonary arterial and aortic trunks to the concordant ventricles with implantation of the coronary arteries into the neoaorta (see Chapter 15).[272] The risk of injury to atrial tissue and to the sinus and AV nodes is determined by repair of coexisting atrial or ventricular septal defects. Early postoperative atrial premature beats occur in up to 60% of patients and may be related to prior atrial septostomy or septectomy.[207,209,219,268] Antiarrhythmic therapy or temporary pacing is rarely necessary.[242] Mild prolongation of sinus node recovery time was found in 3% to 30% of patients who underwent electrophysiologic investigation.[268,273] AV conduction is usually unimpaired, but first-degree AV block has been reported.[207,268,273-275] In 364 survivors of arterial switch operations, 24-hour ambulatory monitoring at a mean of 2.1 years after operation disclosed sinus rhythm in 98%, first-degree AV block in 2.0%, second-degree atrioventricular block in 0.7%, and complete heart block that necessitated a permanent pacemaker in 1.7%.[273]

The major long-term concerns after the arterial switch operation relate to myocardial ischemia associated with transfer of the coronary arteries to the neoaorta (see Chapter 5).[276-278] The incidence of late atrial arrhythmias or ischemic ventricular arrhythmias has been low, although major obstruction of the transferred coronary arteries incurs the risk of sudden death.[207,268,278,279]

Single Ventricle

Because the inlet portion of a ventricular septum is absent, the position of AV conducting tissue is altered.[280-283] In a single *left* ventricle with a rudimentary outlet chamber, the posterior AV node is hypoplastic and makes no ventricular connection. An accessory anterior AV node connects with the His bundle, the course of which varies depending on the position of the outlet chamber. If the outlet chamber resides at the right basal aspect of the heart (noninverted position), a relatively long bundle of His runs down the right wall of the left ventricle toward the outlet foramen before giving rise to right and left bundle branches. The PR interval is usually normal despite an elongated, nonbranching, penetrating bundle. The frontal plane QRS axis is directed leftward and either superiorly (left-axis deviation) or inferiorly. When the outlet chamber resides at the left basal aspect of the heart (inverted position), the AV conduction bundle encircles the outflow tract of the left ventricle before giving rise to

the right and left bundle branches near the outlet foramen. AV conduction time is often prolonged and occasionally culminates in complete heart block. Ventricular depolarization is clockwise (Q waves in leads 2, 3, and aVF), and the frontal plane QRS axis is directed inferiorly and to the left or right. In a univentricular heart of the *right* ventricular type, ventricular myocardium extends to the crux, so there is a normally placed posterior atrioventricular node. AV conduction is normal with a normal PR interval. The frontal plane QRS axis is directed to the right.

In a univentricular heart of the *indeterminate* type, the AV node is located anteriorly or anterolaterally. Multiple Purkinje fiber fascicles connect the AV node to the ventricular chamber. Death attributed to arrhythmias, which remains to be proved, has been reported in up to 30% of patients regardless of surgical palliation.[284,285]

Tricuspid Atresia

Sinus rhythm is the rule, but older patients occasionally experience atrial fibrillation.[286] The mechanism responsible for the distinctive left-axis deviation in the common variety of tricuspid atresia with normally related great arteries, a restrictive ventricular septal defect, and a small right ventricle is not clear, but when tricuspid atresia is accompanied by a large ventricular septal defect and a well-formed right ventricle, the QRS axis is normal.[120] The AV node and the AV conducting bundle are normally located despite an abnormal central fibrous skeleton. The left bundle branch originates close to the AV node, and the right bundle branch is elongated.[287]

Fontan Procedure

The Fontan procedure (Fig. 22-11), originally designed for tricuspid atresia and pulmonary stenosis, has undergone a number of modifications and is now applied to a variety of complex cyanotic malformations in which a biventricular repair is not feasible (see Chapter 15).[288-297] Common to all modifications is a circulation in series without a subpulmonary ventricle. A modified Fontan repair is now the procedure of choice for single ventricle or tricuspid atresia (see Chapter 15).

Sinus rhythm is an important precondition because atrial tachyarrhythmias adversely affect left ventricular function, provoking a rise in left atrial pressure that compromises the Fontan circulation. Persistent preoperative atrial arrhythmias are considered relative contraindications to operation (see Chapter 15), but atrial fibrillation or flutter is occasionally controlled after surgery.[225]

Early postoperatively, 20% to 30% of patients experience atrial arrhythmias, most commonly ectopic or junctional tachycardia that usually resolves without specific therapy.[292,296,298,299] Atrial fibrillation or flutter with an

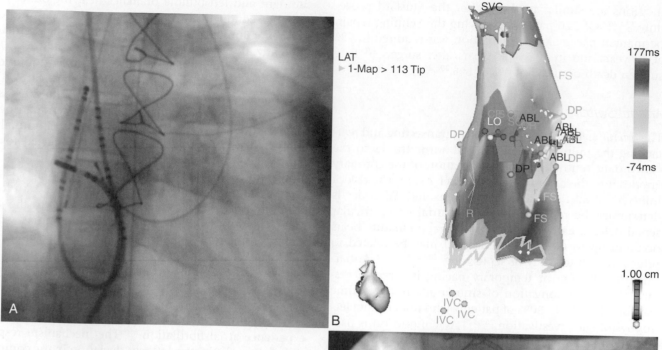

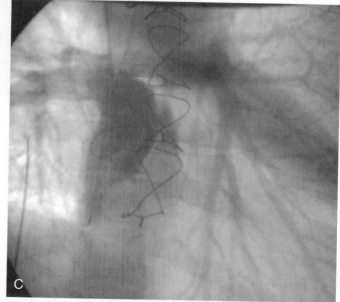

FIGURE 22–11 Electroanatomic map and fluoroscopic images of mac-roreentrant atrial tachycardia following a Fontan repair. **(B)** After a lateral tunnel repair, the patient presented with atrial tachycardia that was electroanatomically mapped and successfully ablated. **(A)** The panel on the left side of the map shows a fluoroscopic image of the site of successful ablation. **(C)** The panel on the right shows an angiogram of the chamber. The map itself depicts the site of early activation as a red signal with the late activated regions encoded in blue. The arrhythmia was successfully ablated at a relatively restricted zone near the site of early activation. Although the arrhythmia was in a "focal" location, the mechanism was probably reentry within a restricted zone.

accelerated ventricular rate risks rapid hemodynamic deterioration and death.[292,296,300] Atrial tachyarrhythmias occur less commonly after total cavopulmonary connections than after atriopulmonary connections (see Chapter 15) because right atrial size does not increase in the former.[298,301] Sustained accelerated junctional rhythms are associated with a mortality of 20% to 100%.[299,300,302,303] Symptomatic sinus bradycardia or complete AV block that necessitates pacemaker implantation occurs early postoperatively in up to 10% of patients.[290,292,295–297,300,302] Supraventricular tachyarrhythmias late after atriopulmonary connections reportedly occur in 20% to 40% of patients, may cause rapid hemodynamic deterioration, and are difficult to treat.[288–290,292,296–298,304,305]

Late onset of atrial arrhythmias after a classic Fontan procedure implies obstruction to right atrial flow. Eighty-six percent of patients so affected had obstruction in the right atrial to pulmonary arterial connection, and 57% had a right atrial thrombus requiring anticoagulation and reoperation (see Chapter 5).[305] Conversion to a cavopulmonary anastomosis provides hemodynamic relief.[306]

More than 50% of patients experience sinus node dysfunction late after a Fontan operation.[292,296,297,307,308] In tricuspid atresia, the artery to the SA node arises from the left coronary artery in 59% of cases and is susceptible to injury from insertion of a Fontan venous conduit into the roof of the right atrium.[309] When symptomatic bradycardias occur, dual-chamber pacing is the treatment of choice. Rate-responsive single-chamber pacing has not provided hemodynamic or functional advantage compared with fixed-rate ventricular pacing.[310] If the need for permanent pacing is anticipated at the time of surgery, atrial and ventricular epicardial leads should be placed.

Late sudden death has been attributed to disturbances in ventricular rhythm, although arrhythmias of ventricular origin are generally not inducible during electrophysiologic study.[294,295,298,307,311,312] The functional adequacy of the systemic ventricle is probably the chief determinant of late postoperative ventricular arrhythmias.[292]

MALFORMATIONS REQUIRING INTRAVENTRICULAR SURGERY

Ventricular Septal Defect

Ventricular tachyarrhythmias occur in 3% to 6% of patients with unoperated ventricular septal defects, including restrictive defects.[313,314] Spontaneous closure of a perimembranous ventricular septal defect with aneurysm formation is sometimes associated with AV conduction abnormalities and occasionally with late-onset complete heart block (Fig. 22–12).

A major electrocardiophysiologic complication of operation is damage to the AV conducting system.[315] The

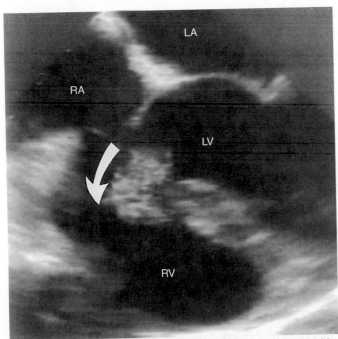

FIGURE 22–12 Two-dimensional echocardiogram (black-and-white photograph of color flow image) from a 22-year-old woman who experienced spontaneous closure of a perimembranous ventricular septal defect with aneurysm formation. Arrow identifies flow into the aneurysm. She subsequently developed complete heart block that required a dual-chamber pacemaker. RA and LA, right and left atria; RV and LV, right and left ventricles.

His bundle penetrates the intact AV node portion of the membranous septum and runs close to the edge of a perimembranous defect, giving rise to the bundle branches.[316,317] Repair through a right ventriculotomy typically results in a right bundle branch block pattern,[318-323] which usually resides in peripheral Purkinje fibers and only occasionally in the proximal or distal right bundle.[320,324,325] Repair through a transatrial incision is accompanied by proximal right bundle branch block in up to one third of patients.[318,320,323,326] Postoperative left anterior fascicular block, usually in conjunction with proximal right bundle branch block (bifascicular block), occurs in 4% to 26% of patients and occasionally develops late after operation.[318,319,322,323,327] Concern has been expressed that proximal conduction system injury, especially bifascicular, predisposes to late-onset complete heart block and sudden death, a risk that is realized in less than 5% of patients.[318,323,328-331] Although the transatrial approach reduces the likelihood of postoperative left anterior fascicular block, the incidence of complete heart block is not necessarily reduced.[326]

Transient complete heart block becomes manifest early postoperatively in 4% to 28% of patients[318,319,329] and persists in 1% to 2%.[189] Those who recover AV conduction are at increased risk for late development of high-degree heart block.[329,332,333] His-ventricular interval prolongation and block below the His bundle during atrial pacing are believed to incur a higher risk of late complete heart block.[329,330] Permanent pacemaker implantation is warranted for persistent complete heart block even if there is a stable escape rhythm, because the risks of syncope and sudden death are as high as 30% during relatively short follow-up.[332,334-336] Postoperative first-degree AV block occurs in 6% of patients and is usually caused by conduction delay above the bundle of His.[327,330,333] Infranodal conduction delay is seldom accompanied by prolongation of the PR interval.

Early postoperatively, transient junctional rhythms, ectopic atrial rhythms, and premature ventricular contractions occur in one third of patients and usually resolve without specific therapy.[318] Significant ventricular arrhythmias late after surgery are uncommon with a higher incidence after ventriculotomy.[321,326,333]

Tetralogy of Fallot

Bradyarrhythmias and Atrioventricular Block

The bundle of His is located inferior and posterior to the malaligned ventricular septal defect and gives rise to a right bundle branch that courses anteriorly along the inferior edge of the defect.[337,338] The branching bundle of His is either separated from the rim of the defect by muscular tissue or is located close to the subendocardium immediately adjacent to the defect.[339-341] Conduction tissue in the latter location is more susceptible to injury during patch closure. Fibers of the posterior division of the left bundle branch leave the bundle of His after a relatively short distance, whereas fibers to the anterior division leave the common bundle after a longer distance and are closer to the ventricular septal defect.

Sinus node dysfunction is uncommon immediately after repair, and late-onset bradyarrhythmias are rare.[115,342-344] However, 36% of patients in one report had sinus node dysfunction identified on late ambulatory electrocardiographic recordings,[117] and 4 of 53 patients at a mean postoperative follow-up of 9.1 years had sinus node dysfunction of sufficient severity to warrant permanent pacemaker implantation.[117]

PR interval prolongation in 8% of postoperative patients was attributed to prolongation of the atrial-His interval or prolongation of both the atrial-His and His-ventricular intervals.[345-347] When PR prolongation resulted from conduction delay above the His bundle (atrial-His interval prolongation), the risk of progression to high-degree AV block appeared to be low.

A right bundle branch block pattern occurred in 59% to 100% of patients after repair[174,343,344,348] and resided in the peripheral right ventricular Purkinje fibers or in the distal or proximal right bundle branch.[324,349,350] There are distinctive regional delays in epicardial right ventricular activation depending on location of the block.[174,324] Epicardial activation mapping before and after repair has linked the right bundle branch block appearance and prolonged right ventricular activation to the ventriculotomy incision and the infundibular resection and not to closure of the ventricular septal defect.[351] Despite the various patterns of right ventricular conduction delay detected by epicardial mapping, the surface ECG does not distinguish the type of delay unless left anterior fascicular block coexists.[174,328,352] Bifascicular block (Fig. 22–13) implies damage to the anterior fascicle of the left bundle branch and to the proximal portion of the right bundle branch. The combination of left anterior hemiblock and right bundle branch block occurs early postoperatively in up to 10% of patients.[174,330,331,348,352-357] Although an early study of bifascicular block disclosed a 21% incidence of subsequent complete heart block (see Fig. 22–13) and a 12.5% risk of sudden death, the current consensus is a 1% to 11% incidence of complete heart block and a 0% to 1% risk of sudden death during follow-up averaging 4 to 8.5 years.[331,344,346,348,353,355,357-359] Late-onset complete heart block develops in less than 1% of patients who have bifascicular block without a history of early transient complete AV block.

Early postoperatively, up to 22% of patients have complete heart block,[327,348,355,357,360-363] but normal AV conduction returns spontaneously in the majority, leaving less than 2% with permanent complete heart block.[348,352,363,364] When high-degree heart block persists, a stable escape rhythm is often present initially. However,

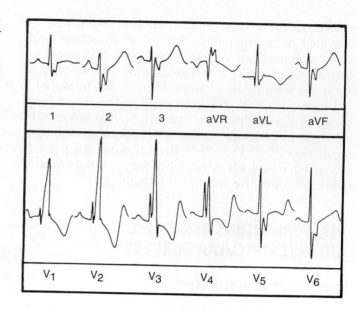

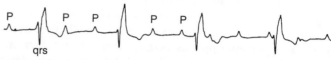

FIGURE 22–13 Twelve-lead electrocardiogram and rhythm strip from a patient with tetralogy of Fallot after intracardiac repair. Bifascicular block *(top panel)* progressed to complete atrioventricular block *(bottom panel).*

without an implantable pacemaker, nearly a third of these patients experience syncope or sudden death within 5 to 10 years.[336,345,348,365] Transient postoperative AV block appears to be a significant risk factor for late AV block.[329,345,348] Approximately one half of patients with early transient complete heart block have bifascicular block after resolution of complete heart block.[348,351] Late-onset AV block that is occasionally manifest a decade or more after repair occurs in only 1% to 2% of patients previously in sinus rhythm, but the block can announce itself with syncope or sudden death.[345,346,348,363,365,366]

Electrophysiologic assessment of infranodal conduction can be useful in identifying patients at particularly high risk of late-onset complete AV block (Fig. 22–14).[345,367] Up to one half of patients with postoperative bifascicular block have His-ventricular interval prolongation and experience a high incidence of perioperative complete heart block.[329] Patients with normal His-ventricular intervals remained free of heart block over a mean follow-up of 6.5 years. Among 59 consecutive patients, only 1 of 9 with His-ventricular interval prolongation developed late complete heart block.[346] Among 51 postoperative children who had electrophysiologic studies at a mean follow-up of 3 years, only one developed complete heart block.[368]

In brief, persistent complete heart block after intracardiac repair of tetralogy of Fallot warrants pacemaker implantation. Transient postoperative complete heart block

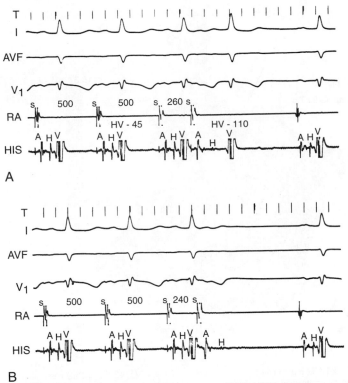

A

B

FIGURE 22–14 Atrial pacing in a patient who experienced syncope after intracardiac repair of tetralogy of Fallot. From the top down of panels A and B are 20-msec time lines (T); surface electrocardiogram leads 1, aVF, and V_1; and intracardiac recordings from the high right atrium (RA) and His bundle position (His). Stimulus artifacts (s) are seen in the RA tracings. In the His bundle tracing the atrial (A), His bundle (H), and ventricular (V) deflections are labeled. In both panels, a paced atrial drive at a cycle length of 500 msec is followed by a single premature stimulus. During the basic drive, the His-ventricular (HV) interval is normal (45 msec). **(A)** A premature stimulus follows the last beat of the basic drive by 260 msec. With the premature stimulus, the atrial-His interval is prolonged, the HV interval is markedly prolonged to 110 msec, and the amplitude of the His deflection is diminished. **(B)** A premature stimulus shown 20 msec earlier. Block occurs within or below the His bundle, as indicated by the His deflection without a subsequent ventricular depolarization. The H1–H2 interval is 310 msec, strongly suggesting impaired infranodal conduction.

incurs a significant risk of late-onset complete heart block. Electrophysiologic evaluation of infranodal conduction can identify highest-risk patients in whom pacemaker implantation is a legitimate option. At least one postoperative exercise stress test and one 24-hour ambulatory ECG are recommended. The risk of high-degree heart block increases slightly when right bundle branch block coexists with left anterior fascicular block.

Tachyarrhythmias

In *unoperated* patients, episodes of supraventricular tachycardia cause an increase in right-to-left shunting that may precipitate hypercyanotic episodes.[369,370] Accessory pathway conduction is rare and coincidental.[348,371] Ventricular

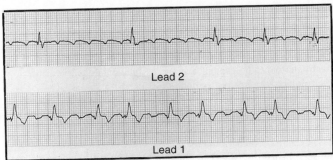

FIGURE 22–15 Rhythm strips from a 68-year-old woman with tetralogy of Fallot who had undergone intracardiac repair at age 33 years. Thirty-five years later, she developed atrial tachycardia/flutter (atrial cycle length of 280 msec) with variable atrioventricular conduction, as shown here.

arrhythmias are infrequent in unoperated patients younger than 8 years, but the incidence increases with age.[358,372] On 24-hour ambulatory recordings, premature ventricular contractions (30 per hour) or repetitive premature ventricular beats have been detected in 20% of patients between the ages of 8 and 15 years and in approximately one half of patients older than age 15.[358,372,373] Syncope and sudden death attributed to ventricular tachycardia have been reported in unoperated patients, albeit rarely.[117,347,358]

Repair through an atriotomy predisposes to late development of atrial arrhythmias. The incidence of atrial tachyarrhythmias, which ranges from less than 2% to as high as 23% after reparative surgery, may cause significant morbidity (Fig. 22–15).[117,347,374]

The incidence of atrial tachyarrhythmias ranges from less than 2% to as high as 23% after reparative surgery and may cause significant morbidity. Among 53 patients late after repair, ambulatory recordings identified 6 cases of supraventricular tachycardia and 12 cases of atrial fibrillation or flutter.[117] It is unclear whether atrial tachyarrhythmias predispose to sudden death because of the hemodynamic sequelae per se or whether the arrhythmia itself identifies patients with the poorest hemodynamic substrates. Up to 5.5% of patients who have had a right ventriculotomy die suddenly or require treatment for nonfatal sustained monomorphic ventricular tachycardia 4 years or more after intracardiac repair.[114,115,344,363,371,375] Although sudden death is occasionally caused by late-onset complete heart block (discussed earlier) and although atrial tachyarrhythmias may cause significant morbidity (discussed earlier), there is a uniform consensus that ventricular tachyarrhythmias—more specifically reentrant monomorphic ventricular tachycardia—are chiefly responsible for postventriculotomy sudden cardiac death.[114,115,376] Programmed electrical stimulation disclose that sustained ventricular tachycardia usually arises either from the area of the right ventriculotomy scar or from the ventricular septal patch, sites prone to developing extensive fibrosis (Fig. 22–16).[114,377-385] Right ventricular fibrosis detected by magnetic resonance imaging might prove be a risk factor

FIGURE 22–16 Electroanatomic map and electrocardiograms from a patient with ventricular tachycardia originating at the edge of the ventricular septal defect patch (VSD) following repair of tetralogy of Fallot (TOF). The ventricular tachycardia was electroanatomically mapped and successfully ablated. The map itself depicts the scarred regions (VSD patch) as areas of low voltage, and the comparatively healthy regions as blue/purple. The arrhythmia, which was successfully ablated at a relatively restricted zone near the inferior margin of the VSD patch, was a classic reentrant tachycardia that showed two discrete exits from the scar, hence the two VT morphologies shown in the electrocardiograms. The red areas are of radiofrequency energy application. The pink and blue tags mark the location of the conduction system fibers.

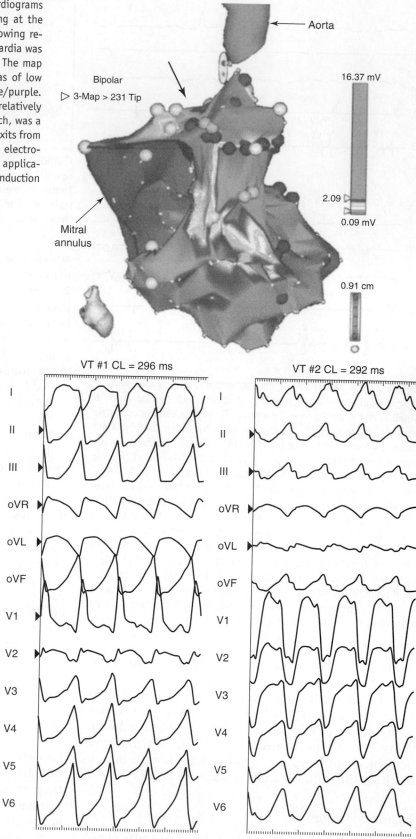

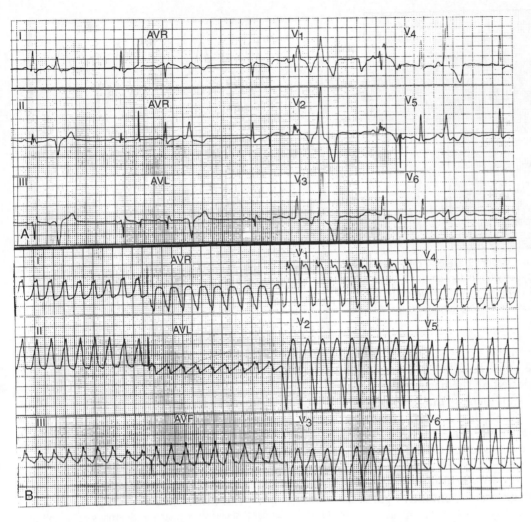

FIGURE 22–17 Electrocardiograms from a 51-year-old man 20 years after intracardiac repair of tetralogy of Fallot. **(A)** Sinus rhythm with ventricular bigeminy. The QRS complex shows right bundle branch block with left-axis deviation (bifascicular block). **(B)** Spontaneous sustained monomorphic ventricular tachycardia in the same patient. The QRS has a left bundle branch block inferior-axis configuration consistent with origin of the tachycardia in the right ventricular outflow tract.

(discussed earlier). An important mission is identification of patients at risk for sudden death due to postoperative monomorphic ventricular tachycardia (Fig. 22–17). Let us examine the following relevant information.

The long-term incidence of ventricular ectopic beats sufficiently frequent to appear on routine 12-lead ECGs is reportedly 19%.[344,371] Thirty percent of patients with ectopic ventricular beats on 12-lead ECGs recorded any time after ventriculotomy repair die suddenly, whereas patients without these ectopic beats do not experience sudden death.[386] Twenty-four-hour ambulatory ECGs disclose frequent or repetitive ventricular ectopic beats in 17% to 44% of patients, especially after complex repairs,[344,347,358,387,388] although these ventricular arrhythmias per se do not necessarily indicate an increased risk of sudden death.[389]

Repairs through the right atrium and pulmonary artery are associated with a lower incidence of ventricular arrhythmias than are repairs through a ventriculotomy despite similar right ventricular/left ventricular systolic pressure ratios.[387] Age at repair is an important arrhythmogenic factor, with only 1% of patients undergoing operation before 18 months of age exhibiting ventricular ectopic

beats on routine 12-lead ECGs compared with 5% to 19% repaired at an older age.[113,115,116,118,344,358,388,390,391] Exercise-induced ventricular arrhythmias occur in up to 38% of patients who do not have ventricular ectopic rhythms on 24-hour ambulatory ECGs (Fig. 22–18).[113,118,376,388,390,392] Programmed electrical stimulation initiates ventricular tachycardia in virtually all patients who experience spontaneous sustained monomorphic ventricular tachycardia. When repair is performed without a ventriculotomy, the incidence of induced sustained monomorphic ventricular tachycardia at electrophysiologic study is significantly reduced.[387] The prognostic significance of inducibility or noninducibility in patients with ambient ventricular ectopic beats remains uncertain.[377,380,391]

Electrophysiologic mechanisms of ventricular tachyarrhythmias include reentry, automaticity, and triggered activity. The commonest tachyarrhythmic cause of postventriculotomy sudden cardiac death—a relatively rare but dreaded sequel of right ventriculotomy—is reentrant monomorphic ventricular tachycardia (MVT).[378,381,384,393] Two major variables set the stage:(1) a susceptible slow conduction myocardial substrate, that is, focal areas of slow conduction that can sustain reentry and (2) a trigger

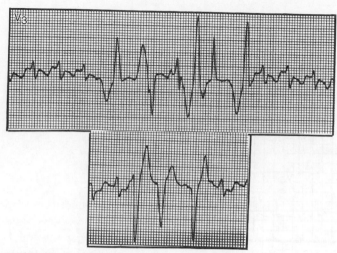

FIGURE 22-18 Rhythm strips during treadmill exercise testing of a 52-year-old man with tetralogy of Fallot who underwent initial intracardiac repair at age 13 years and re-repair at age 51 years. Strips demonstrate exercise-induced nonsustained polymorphic ventricular tachycardia.

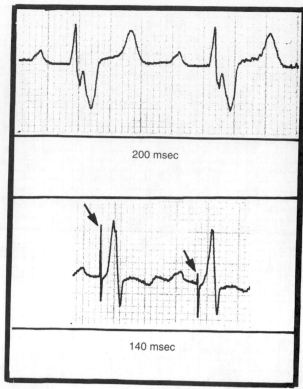

FIGURE 22-19 Rhythm strips from a 26-year-old woman with tetralogy of Fallot and absent pulmonary valve who underwent ventricular septal defect closure and placement of a right ventricular to pulmonary artery valved conduit in childhood. At age 26 years, conduit regurgitation prompted reoperation, during which a pacemaker was implanted for symptomatic bradyarrhythmias. The upper panel shows sinus rhythm with first-degree atrioventricular block and striking QRS prolongation (200 msec). The lower panel shows sinus rhythm with atrial sensing and ventricular pacing. The QRS duration has decreased from 200 to 140 msec.

mechanism that activates the substrate.[375,391] Slow conduction substrates can be suspected on the basis of a scalar QRS duration ≥180 msec or an increase in QRS duration 30 msec over 6 months or less. All else being equal, prolongation of the QRS ≥180 msec (Fig. 22–19) is a significant independent predictor of sudden death.[394]

The signal averaged ECG (SAECG) is a sensitive and specific method for detecting slow conduction[395-397] and is now used for electrophysiologic assessment after right ventriculotomy for intracardiac repair of CHD.[18] A positive SAECG indicates the presence of a slow conduction substrate and the attendant risk of reentrant MVT. A negative SAECG connotes absence of a reentrant substrate. The common site of slow conduction substrates is along the ventriculotomy scar, a site that can be established by mapping. Radiofrequency ablation or revision of the ventriculotomy scar can render a positive SAECG negative, thus eliminating the arrhythmogenic focus. Orthogonal X, Y, Z body surface electrodes are used to detect ventricular late potentials by permitting examination of portions of the ECG otherwise obscured by noise and artifacts. Interpretation of the SAECG is based on criteria derived from three-time domain variables calculated by an automated algorithm and visually inspected: (1) filtered QRS duration in milliseconds, which indicates the degree to which late potentials prolong the QRS; (2) root-mean-square (RMS) voltage in microvolts of the terminal 40 msec of the filtered QRS, which represents the amount of late potential energy; and (3) duration in milliseconds of low amplitude signals (LAS) 40 μV in the terminal filtered QRS. A positive SAECG is defined as a filtered QRS duration 145 msec plus RMS duration of the terminal 40 msec of the filtered QRS <17.5 microvolts (μV) and/or LAS of the terminal filtered QRS

50 msec. These criteria and conclusions reflect the recommendations of the American Heart Association, the American College of Cardiology, the European Society of Cardiology, and independently published sources.[18]

Importantly, a slow conduction substrate remains dormant unless activated by a trigger. Accordingly, a susceptible substrate *and* an effective trigger are necessary for the overt expression of reentrant MVT. A well-recognized trigger is severe postventriculotomy pulmonary regurgitation, but triggers also take the form of impaired autonomic nervous system regulation after intracardiac repair of TOF or increased adrenergic discharge. Fright can provoke a catecholaminergic surge that triggers a susceptible substrate—literally "scared to death."

A positive SAECG in conjunction with severe pulmonary regurgitation warrants pulmonary valve replacement with revision of the ventriculotomy scar. Postoperative normalization of the SAECG signifies that both substrate and trigger have been eliminated together with the risk of MVT. If pulmonary regurgitation is insufficient to warrant valve replacement, the slow conduction substrate(s) can be localized by mapping and eliminated with radiofrequency ablation as stated earlier.

Sudden death and ventricular tachyarrhythmias are infrequent when intracardiac repair is performed before age 5 years or when repair in adults is followed by little or no right ventricular pressure or volume overload and good right ventricular function.[115,344,374] Most patients who die suddenly have right ventricular systolic pressures over 60 mm Hg and poor right ventricular function.[113,115,116,118,151,376,386,388,390,391,398-400] Interestingly, pacing may reduce QRS duration (see Fig. 22–19) but without known effect on risk.

In brief, the most common cause of sudden death after intracardiac repair of TOF is sustained monomorphic ventricular tachycardia, which requires for its genesis both a susceptible substrate (slow conduction capable of sustaining reentry) and a trigger (severe pulmonary regurgitation, catecholamine stimulation, ventricular ectopic beats) that activates the reentrant substrate. Ventricular ectopic rhythms that might trigger a susceptible substrate should be sought with an exercise stress test and 24-hour ambulatory ECGs, especially in postoperative patients with depressed function of a dilatated, overloaded right ventricle. If a signal-averaged ECG detects slow conduction, an intracardiac electrophysiologic study can determine whether that substrate is potentially inducible.[391] If monomorphic ventricular tachycardia is inducible, radiofrequency catheter ablation is an attractive option (see Fig. 22–16) unless the patient has severe pulmonary regurgitation that requires reoperation, during which excision of the ventriculotomy scar serves to remove the slow conduction substrate. If a signal-averaged ECG detects slow conduction, but the potential reentrant substrate is not inducible on electrophysiologic study, it is unlikely that ectopic ventricular beats or catecholamines will initiate monomorphic ventricular tachycardia. The patient should remain under careful surveillance because the noninducible substrate may change. These recommendations are relevant in patients who have had a ventriculotomy for repair of other malformations. Patients who experience spontaneous sustained ventricular tachycardia or syncope or who are resuscitated from ventricular fibrillation require evaluation to determine the most appropriate antiarrhythmic therapy, that is, re-repair with surgical excision, catheter ablation of the tachycardia focus, or an implantable cardioverter/defibrillator.

Congenitally Corrected Transposition of the Great Arteries

Congenitally corrected transposition of the great arteries regardless of coexisting anomalies is associated with an abnormal AV conduction system.[401-405] A posterior AV node is either absent or does not join infranodal conduction tissue.[404] An accessory anterior AV node joins a long nonbranching bundle of conducting tissue that passes anterior to the pulmonary artery through the conus septum and bifurcates into inverted right and left bundle branches. If the anterior AV node fails to join the infranodal conduction tissue, AV block exists from birth.[401,406] When complete heart block is present, the QRS complex pattern is supraventricular as in isolated congenital complete heart block.[120] Accessory AV connections that produce preexcitation and circus movement tachycardia occasionally occur, particularly in association with Ebstein's anomaly of the systemic (tricuspid) AV valve. The bypass tracts are then left sided.[407-409]

The PR interval is prolonged in approximately one half of cases.[120,402] First-degree AV block is caused by prolongation of the atrial-His interval in approximately 50% of patients, by prolongation of the His-ventricular interval in 33%, and by prolonged intraatrial conduction in the remainder.[403,408,410] Second-degree AV block is almost always 2:1. A change from PR interval prolongation to 2:1 block to complete heart block is a pattern of particular diagnostic significance.[406,411] Complete AV block that is present from birth or that developed later occurred in 22% of 107 patients.[406] The risk of complete AV block accrues at about 2% per year regardless of associated abnormalities.[411] A rapid deflection similar to the His bundle deflection is recorded in the majority of patients at electrophysiologic study; the site of block is most commonly above or within the area that generates the His bundle–like electrogram.[408,410,412] These findings are consistent with a narrow QRS and with histologic findings that disclose fibrosis of the common nonbranching bundle.[410,413,414] Complete AV block often coexists with a stable escape rhythm,[406,407] although syncope and sudden death sometimes occur after long periods of stability. Accordingly, pacemaker implantation is a strong consideration.[406,407,412,415,416]

Because of inversion of the ventricles and the bundle branches, septal activation is initially right to left. Septal Q waves are therefore absent in left precordial leads and present in right precordial leads. Left-axis deviation is a feature of the ECG when systolic pressure in the subpulmonary morphologic left ventricle is not elevated.[120,411]

Intracardiac repair of the ventricular septal defect incurs complete heart block in more than one fourth of patients [406,417-419] because the nonpenetrating AV conduction bundle runs along the superior margin of the defect.[402,412,417] Patients who are spared intraoperative heart block are apparently not at risk of developing late postoperative heart block.[406,419]

Discrete Subaortic Stenosis

Proximity of the site of obstruction to the bundle of His and bundle branches places the specialized conduction tissues at risk during surgical repair. Left bundle branch block, left anterior hemiblock, or right bundle branch block are incurred in approximately 20% of patients, and complete heart block in 8%.[420,421]

CONGENITAL DISEASES OF CARDIAC VALVES

Congenital Aortic Valve Stenosis

Supraventricular premature beats in excess of 0.5 per hour occur in approximately 20% of unoperated patients with congenital aortic valve stenosis.[314] Serious ventricular arrhythmias are associated with high left ventricular end-diastolic pressure, peak systolic gradients greater than 50 mm Hg, and aortic regurgitation.[314,422] Following balloon valvuloplasty, premature ventricular beats occur in nearly a third of patients and occur in 17% following direct aortic valve repair.[314] Multiform ectopic ventricular contractions and nonsustained or sustained ventricular tachycardia are respectively recorded on 24-hour ambulatory ECGs in 44% and 64% of cases after balloon valvotomy or aortic valve replacement.[422] Among all operated patients, 12.3% have ventricular tachycardia on late ambulatory electrocardiographic recordings.[422]

Ebstein's Anomaly of the Tricuspid Valve

The electrophysiologic features of Ebstein's anomaly relate to its morphologic substrates (Table 22-6). The right side of the heart consists of three anatomic components: the right atrium proper, the functional right ventricle, and an intervening zone that is anatomically and electrically right ventricle but functionally a right atrium.[120] The atrialized right ventricle generates an intracavitary right ventricular electrogram but an atrial pressure pulse.[423] Mechanical stimulation of this site provokes a right ventricular QRS complex and risks inducing ventricular tachycardia. Nevertheless, spontaneous ventricular tachycardia is uncommon, if not rare.[424]

The surface ECG is often virtually diagnostic of Ebstein's anomaly.[120,411] P waves are characteristically strikingly tall and broad and have been characterized as "Himalayan"

(Fig. 22-20). The duration of the P wave and the long PR interval are caused chiefly by prolonged conduction in the large right atrium. Delayed conduction through the bundle of His and distal bundle branches has been ascribed to lengthened, stretched conduction fibers within the atrialized right ventricle. Despite prolonged His-ventricular intervals and marked PR interval prolongation, complete heart block is rare.[425,426] Should an implantable pacemaker be required, however, the ventricular lead should be applied to the left ventricular epicardium to avoid the risk of inducing ventricular tachycardia by inadvertently stimulating the atrialized right ventricle with a transvenous lead (discussed later).

The QRS complex typically exhibits a right bundle branch block pattern (see Fig. 22-20),[120,423,425] which is largely the result of abnormal activation and prolonged conduction in the atrialized right ventricle, a conclusion in accord with the occasional but distinctive appearance of a bizarre "second" QRS complex attached to the preceding "normal" complex.[120,423,426]

Precordial initial force abnormalities are important features of the ECG of Ebstein's anomaly, apart from preexcitation. Q waves commonly appear in lead V_1 and occasionally extend as far as lead V_4 (see Fig. 22-20).[120,427] This pattern reflects right ventricular intracavitary potentials recorded unusually far to the left because of striking enlargement of the right atrium.[120] The benign significance of Q waves in right precordial leads is important to recognize in adults with Ebstein's anomaly who present with chest pain.[120]

Reentrant supraventricular tachycardia, atrial fibrillation, atrial flutter, and junctional tachycardia occur in 25% to 30% of patients, and preexcitation caused by right-sided accessory AV pathways (i.e., on the same side as the malformed tricuspid valve)[424,426] occurs in 5% to 25% of surface ECGs (Fig. 22-21).[120,423,424,427-429] The high incidence

---

Table 22-6 Major Electrophysiologic Abnormalities in Ebstein's Anomaly

- Intraatrial conduction disturbances: right atrial P wave abnormalities, PR interval prolongation
- Atrioventricular nodal conduction disturbance: PR interval prolongation
- Infranodal conduction disturbances
- Intra- or infra-His delay
- Right bundle branch block
- Bizarre "second" QRS attached to preceding "normal" complex
- Wolff-Parkinson-White syndrome accessory pathways
- Supraventricular tachycardia
- Atrial fibrillation or flutter
- Electromechanical dissociation in atrialized right ventricle
- Irritability of atrialized right ventricle (inducible ventricular tachycardia)
- Q waves in leads V_{1-4}

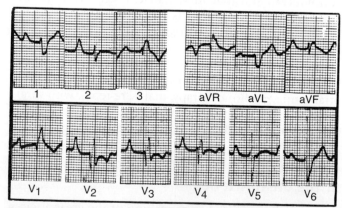

FIGURE 22-20 Electrocardiogram from an 18-year-old man with Ebstein's anomaly of the tricuspid valve. The P waves are strikingly tall and peaked, the PR interval is prolonged, and there is the QRS configuration of complete right bundle branch block. The QR pattern in leads V_{1-4} is due to enlargement of the right atrium. This electrocardiogram is virtually diagnostic of Ebstein's anomaly.

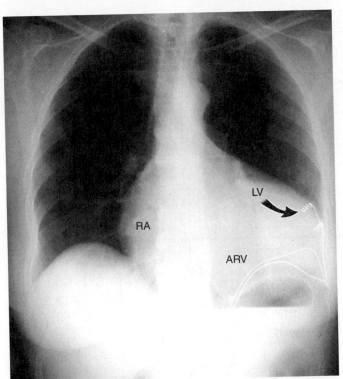

FIGURE 22-21 Chest radiograph from a 63-year-old woman with Ebstein's anomaly of the tricuspid valve and complete heart block. A transvenous pacemaker induced right ventricular tachycardia because of stimulation of the atrialized right ventricle. A left ventricular (LV) epicardial pacemaker lead (*arrow*) was subsequently placed. The cardiac configuration is typical of Ebstein's anomaly. ARV, atrialized right ventricle; RA, right atrium.

of accessory pathways is attributed to failure of the AV annulus to fuse with the hypoplastic central cardiac fibrous skeleton, allowing persistence of fetal accessory AV connections. Accessory pathways are located with equal frequency in the posterior septum and free wall.[426] Approximately one third of patients with preexcitation have more than one bypass tract and usually have QRS patterns that resemble septal accessory pathways.[424] Antegrade conduction through an accessory pathway can be intermittent.[424] Some pathways conduct only in a retrograde (ventriculoatrial) direction and produce orthodromic circus movement tachycardia but no preexcitation in sinus rhythm.

The most common overt manifestation of accessory AV connections in Ebstein's anomaly is orthodromic circus movement reentry tachycardia with the AV node conducting in the antegrade direction and the accessory pathway conducting in the retrograde direction (Fig. 22-22).[424,427,429] Preexcitation caused by antegrade conduction through the accessory pathway may become evident after restoration of sinus rhythm. Conduction through the AV node and His-Purkinje system during tachycardia produces a QRS complex of right ventricular conduction delay inherent in the basic Ebstein ECG. The ventriculoatrial conduction time during tachycardia is longer (150-300 msec) than the

conduction time for patients with right-sided accessory pathways in the absence of Ebstein's anomaly, probably because of slow conduction through the atrialized right ventricle and right atrium near the insertion of the accessory tracts.[426] Antidromic circus movement tachycardia and antegrade conduction through the accessory pathway with retrograde conduction through the AV node is an alternative pattern (Fig. 22-23, *A* and *B*).[424,430] Some patients with preexcitation never experience tachyarrhythmias, whereas others experience recurrent supraventricular tachycardia, atrial fibrillation, or atrial flutter with or without bypass tracts.[424,425,427]

An accessory pathway with a short antegrade refractory period permits an extremely rapid ventricular response to atrial flutter or fibrillation that may precipitate ventricular fibrillation, which is held responsible for the occasional occurrence of syncope and sudden death.[427,429,431] In the presence of rapidly conducting accessory tissue, antiarrhythmic medications that slow conduction and prolong refractoriness in that pathway (type Ia or Ic or amiodarone) should be administered. Drugs that slow conduction through the AV node, including digoxin, adrenergic blockers, and calcium channel antagonists, serve to accelerate the ventricular response to atrial fibrillation through an accessory pathway and are contraindicated unless the antegrade refractory period of the accessory pathway is known to be relatively long.[432-434] Patients with rapidly conducting accessory pathways are candidates for catheter ablation or surgical division of the bypass tracts. When there are accessory pathway–mediated supraventricular tachyarrhythmias in patients with a mild tricuspid malformation, radiofrequency catheter ablation of the bypass tract eliminates the tachycardia substrate without operation (Fig. 22-24). Preoperative invasive electrophysiologic assessment with catheter ablation of accessory pathways is also recommended for patients scheduled to undergo tricuspid valve repair or replacement to avoid the need for intraoperative AV disconnection and to reduce the need for postoperative electrophysiologic evaluation, especially in the presence of a prosthetic tricuspid valve.[435]

Ventricular tachycardia occurs in less than 7% of patients with unoperated Ebstein's anomaly.[428] Macroreentrant ventricular tachycardia involving the bundle branches has been identified, and primary ventricular tachycardia has been mapped to the atrialized right ventricle.[436,437] Ventricular fibrillation can be induced by catheter manipulation in the atrialized right ventricle (see Fig. 22-21) and may occur during induction of general anesthesia.[423-425,429] Reentry is related to spiral (in two-dimensional) and scroll (in three-dimensional) waves of excitation.[50] Reentrant monomorphic ventricular tachycardia depends on a combination of slow conduction, unidirectional block, and a substrate that permits anchoring of spiral/scroll waves. When spiral/scroll waves are not anchored, they meander erratically as polymorphic ventricular tachycardia

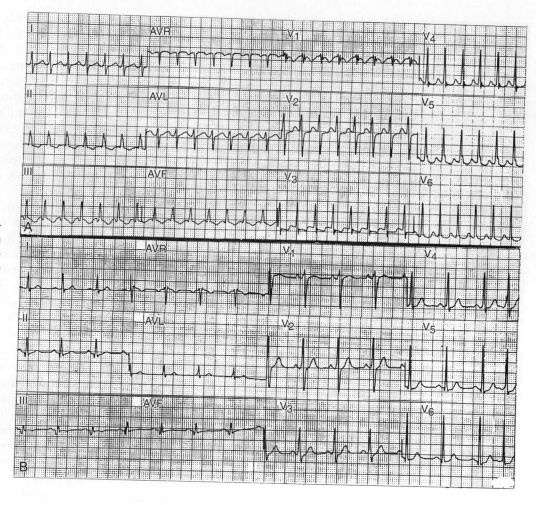

FIGURE   22–22 Electrocardiograms from a 19-year-old man with Ebstein's anomaly and Wolff-Parkinson-White syndrome. **(A)** There is narrow QRS orthodromic circus movement tachycardia. The atrioventricular node is the antegrade limb of the circuit, and the right-sided accessory pathway provides retrograde (ventriculoatrial) conduction. Hence, there is no preexcitation on the surface electrocardiogram. **(B)** Sinus rhythm after termination of the tachycardia. The PR interval is 0.14 sec, and the delta wave forces are appropriate for a right posterior location of the accessory pathway.

or break up into ventricular fibrillation.[50] In Ebstein's anomaly, the atrialized right ventricle consists of clusters of cardiomyocytes that are isolated within a fibrous matrix, thus preventing spiral/scroll reentrant waves from anchoring. (Fig. 22–25, *A* and *B*). Accordingly, excitation of the arrhythmogenic atrialized right ventricle does not result in monomorphic ventricular tachycardia but instead in polymorphic ventricular tachycardia/fibrillation.[50]

Reparative surgery for Ebstein's anomaly involves either reconstruction or replacement of the tricuspid valve, closure of an atrial septal defect or patent foramen ovale, and division of nonablated accessory pathways.[438–443] The atrialized right ventricle must be excluded to eliminate the potential arrhythmogenic site.[50] Early postoperatively, atrial fibrillation and flutter are common.[425,444] Premature ventricular contractions occur in approximately 15% of patients and ventricular fibrillation in 8%.[425,439] Transient heart block develops in 20% of patients who undergo tricuspid reconstruction, but persistent complete heart block seldom follows.[425] As many as 25% of patients undergoing tricuspid valve replacement experience persistent high-grade AV block.[438,444] The occurrence rate of late-onset high-degree heart block is less than 3%.[425]

The incidence of late postoperative supraventricular tachyarrhythmias is related to the preoperative incidence.[425] Of patients with atrial fibrillation or flutter, one third experience recurrences within 2 to 3 years after operation, but successful surgical division or ablation of accessory pathways precludes rapid circus movement tachycardia.[425,441,443] Sinus bradycardia necessitating pacemaker implantation is infrequent.[425] Premature ventricular contractions and ventricular tachycardia are rare (discussed earlier).[441,444] Late postoperative sudden death occurs in up to 7% of patients, with those who experienced preoperative ventricular fibrillation at greatest risk.[425,438,442] Surgical exclusion of the arrhythmogenic atrialized right ventricle reduces or eliminates the risk.

MYOCARDIAL DISEASES

Arrhythmogenic Right Ventricular Dysplasia

Characterized by fibro-fatty replacement of right ventricular myocardium, congenital arrhythmogenic right ventricular dysplasia is a poorly understood disease that is familial in nearly a third of cases (see Chapter 10).[445–447]

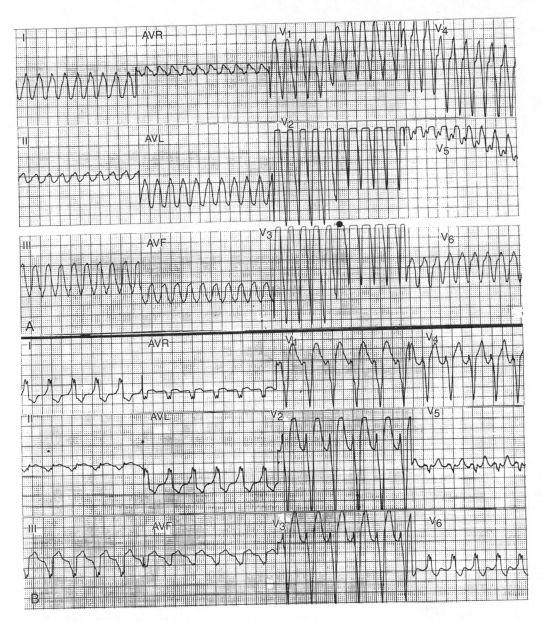

FIGURE 22-23   **(A)** Atrial fibrillation. Ventricular activation through the accessory pathway produces maximal preexcitation. **(B)** Antidromic circus movement tachycardia. The accessory pathway provides the antegrade limb of the circuit, with retrograde conduction (ventriculoatrial) involving the His-Purkinje system and the atrioventricular node.

The diagnosis should be entertained in young patients with frequent ventricular arrhythmias of a left bundle branch block configuration (Fig. 22–26). Magnetic resonance imaging improves diagnostic sensitivity by identifying fatty infiltration, thinning, and wall motion abnormalities (see Fig. 22–26).[448]

The surface ECG generally shows normal sinus node function and normal AV conduction, although sick sinus syndrome and AV conduction abnormalities have been described.[449] QRS prolongation may occur with partial or complete right bundle branch block,[450] and T waves may be inverted in right precordial leads. An "epsilon wave" is occasionally seen in the anterior precordial leads after the termination of the QRS complex.[451] Although approximately 90% of patients have abnormalities on the surface ECG, these abnormalities correlate poorly with the extent of right ventricular dysplasia.[452]

Late potentials on signal-averaged ECGs occur in approximately 75% of patients.[453-455] The combination of time domain and frequency domain analysis has excellent predictive value, with a sensitivity of 100% and a specificity of 94% for the presence of arrhythmogenic right ventricular dysplasia.[453] Supraventricular arrhythmias, although rarely the primary presentation, occur in one fourth of patients.[456]

The primary presenting symptoms range from palpitations to syncope and sudden death. Ventricular tachyarrhythmias, sustained or nonsustained, often triggered by exertion, have a left bundle branch block pattern (see Fig. 22–26).[457] Twelve of 60 patients who died suddenly before age 35 years had morphologic characteristics of right ventricular dysplasia on postmortem examination.[458] Sudden death was the first sign of disease in 5 of the 12 patients.[458]

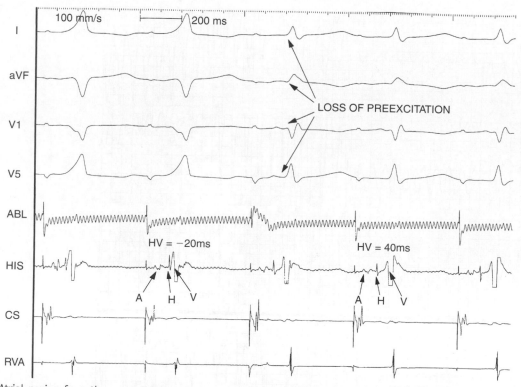

FIGURE 22–24 Atrial pacing from the coronary sinus during radiofrequency catheter ablation of a right paraseptal accessory pathway in a 13-year-old girl with Ebstein's anomaly of the tricuspid valve and Wolff-Parkinson-White syndrome. From top down are surface electrocardiogram leads 1, aVF, V_1, and V_5, together with intracardiac recordings from the ablation catheter (ABL), His bundle position (HIS), coronary sinus (CS), and right ventricular apex (RVA). In the His bundle tracing, the atrial (A), His bundle (H), and ventricular (V) deflections are labeled. During pacing at a cycle length of 500 msec (120 bpm), a delta wave representing ventricular preexcitation (note the negative His-ventricular [HV] interval from the His bundle electrogram (H) to the onset of the QRS complex on the surface leads) is seen on the first two beats. On the third beat, the accessory pathway is successfully ablated with loss of the delta wave and normalization of the HV interval to 40 msec. Retrograde accessory pathway conduction was also ablated, eliminating the substrate for accelerated atrioventricular conduction. Pacing artifact is seen in all leads.

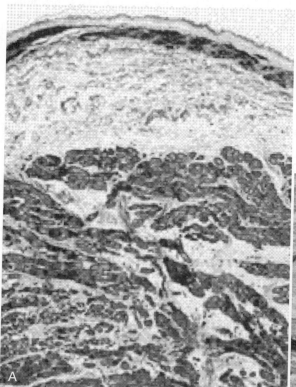

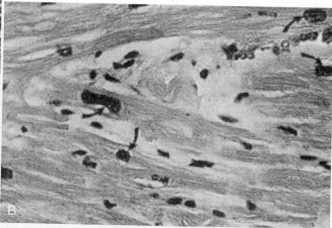

FIGURE 22–25 Ebstein's anomaly. **(A)** In the atrialized right ventricle *(blue area)*, fibrous tissue separates and isolates bundles of cardiomyocytes *(red area)* (trichrome stain). The endocardium *(top)* is thickened and fibrotic. **(B)** In contrast, in the true right atrium, fibrosis is scant, and there is a normal array of cardiomyocytes with enlarged hyperchromic nuclei *(curved arrows)* indicating hypertrophy (hemoxatoxylin eosin stain).

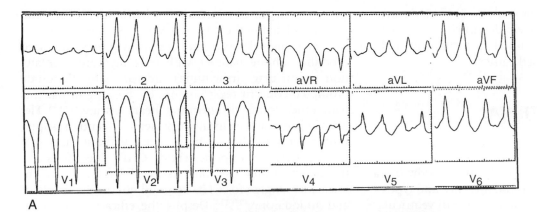

A

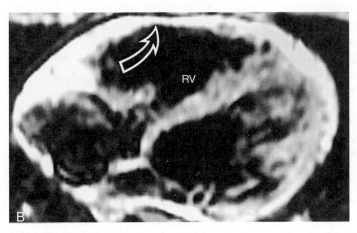

B

FIGURE 22-26   (A) Twelve-lead scalar electrocardiogram from a 27-year-old woman with arrhythmogenic right ventricular dysplasia. The ventricular tachycardia has a left bundle branch block configuration. **(B)** Magnetic resonance image shows a segment of thinned (dysplastic) right ventricle free wall *(arrow)* with fatty infiltration (density) typical of arrhythmogenic right ventricular (RV) dysplasia. The contiguous dense zones represent pericardial fat.

Up to 90% of patients with right ventricular dysplasia and previously documented ventricular arrhythmias have inducible ventricular tachycardia on electrophysiologic study, although induction is much less frequent in the absence of spontaneous ventricular tachycardia.[455,459] Infusion of isoproterenol during testing increases sensitivity.[460]

Therapeutic options for patients with serious ventricular arrhythmias associated with arrhythmogenic right ventricular dysplasia include antiarrhythmic drugs, implantable cardioverter/defibrillator placement, resection of the site of earliest ventricular activation, catheter ablation, and total disconnection of the right ventricular free wall.[461–465] Sotalol, a nonselective adrenergic blocking agent with class III antiarrhythmic properties (prolongation of repolarization), or amiodarone (a class III agent) in combination with adrenergic blockade, may render the ventricular tachycardia noninducible and suppress ventricular arrhythmias seen on ambulatory electrocardiography.[464–466] When antiarrhythmic therapy renders ventricular tachycardia noninducible, the recurrence rate of spontaneous ventricular arrhythmias is low.[465] ICDs are appropriate for high-risk patients and for survivors of sudden death. Intracardiac direct current ablation has largely been replaced by radiofrequency ablation because of the risk of barotraumas, cardiac perforation, and hemopericardium.[463] The widespread distribution of right ventricular dysplasia limits the efficacy of catheter ablation techniques, and right ventricular thinning increases the risk of perforation during catheter manipulation. Regional sur-

gical resection at sites of earliest epicardial ventricular activation is of little or no value because ventricular tachycardia recurs at other sites. Electrical isolation using right ventricular disconnection[461,462,467] is soon followed by left ventricular failure because of interruption of ventricular-ventricular interaction.

Isolated Noncompaction of Left Ventricular Myocardium

This rare disorder is characterized by prominent left ventricular trabeculations with deep intertrabecular recesses and is associated with ventricular tachycardia.[468–470] Electrocardiographic abnormalities include sinus bradycardia, broad or peaked P waves, first-degree AV block, right- or left-axis deviation, and left ventricular conduction delay.[469] Among eight patients with isolated noncompaction of left ventricular myocardium, ventricular arrhythmias occurred in five and were the initial presentation in two.[469] Wolff-Parkinson-White syndrome was present in one patient who presented with ventricular fibrillation and cardiac arrest. An additional patient died of ventricular fibrillation.[469]

Uhl's Anomaly

Uhl's anomaly is characterized by abnormalities of right ventricular free wall ranging from focal thinning to complete absence of myocardium that results in apposition of endocardial and epicardial layers.[120,471,472] This "parchment" right ventricle has been described as "inexcitable."[120] Focal thinning is believed to merge with right ventricular dysplasia (discussed earlier).[471]

THERAPY FOR ARRHYTHMIAS

Antiarrhythmic Drugs

Attention must be directed not only to the arrhythmia under consideration but also to the presence and type of reparative surgery, the presence and degree of ventricular dysfunction, the risk of impairment of sinus node and AV conduction, potential proarrhythmic effects, and negative inotropic properties. Patients must be carefully monitored when receiving negative inotropic agents such as adrenergic and calcium channel blocking agents, sotalol, and type I antiarrhythmic drugs, including disopyramide, flecainide, and propafenone.[466,473-476]

Virtually all antiarrhythmic drugs have the potential for impairing impulse formation in the sinus node, in the AV node, and in ectopic pacemakers, as well as for impeding conduction through the AV node and His-Purkinje system. Because mild impairment of sinus node or AV node function is common after intraatrial surgery, antiarrhythmic drugs may precipitate sinus node arrest or AV block or suppress atrial or AV nodal escape rhythms. Adrenergic blockers, calcium channel blockers, digoxin, amiodarone, flecainide, moricizine, propafenone, and sotalol are particularly potent suppressors of sinus node or AV node impulse generation and conduction.[477-482] Antiarrhythmic therapy should be initiated only after excluding potentially serious bradyarrhythmias. Therapy is started in a monitored setting in which prompt drug withdrawal and institution of supportive measures can be provided if bradyarrhythmias become manifest. Antiarrhythmic therapy to suppress tachyarrhythmias may require implantation of a permanent pacemaker.

Any antiarrhythmic drug may aggravate the rhythm disturbance that it is intended to remedy.[483-486] Drugs that prolong ventricular refractoriness and hence the QT interval (quinidine, procainamide, disopyramide, amiodarone, and sotalol) can precipitate the rapid polymorphic ventricular tachycardia called torsades de pointes.[487] Fortunately, the incidence is no more than 1.5% to 2% per year of therapy with quinidine and sotalol and probably lower with other agents.[466,488] A 25% prolongation of the corrected QT interval generally warrants reduction in dosage or discontinuation of the drug. Amiodarone is an exception to this rule in both adult and pediatric patients because moderate QT interval prolongation is usual and torsades de pointes is rare.[489,490] Serious proarrhythmic responses occur most commonly in the presence of structural heart disease and depressed ventricular function.[425,426] Flecainide, which slows conduction through all cardiac

tissues, may provoke incessant arrhythmias[484-486,491] and is best initiated in the hospital, especially in patients considered at high risk of ventricular arrhythmias. Increased mortality among patients with post–myocardial infarction ventricular arrhythmias treated with flecainide prompted concern regarding use of the drug in patients with other forms of structural heart disease.[492,493] Flecainide is efficacious in the treatment of reentrant supraventricular arrhythmias in patients without structural heart disease, but in postoperative CHD, side effects and the proarrhythmic risk limit its use.[493-495] Atrial arrhythmias after surgery for CHD respond effectively to sotalol and amiodarone.[496-498] Despite the efficacy of amiodarone and the relative infrequency of significant side effects in the young, there is concern because of adverse long-term effects.[499-502]

Nonpharmacologic Therapies

A variety of nonpharmacologic alternatives can be considered when antiarrhythmic drugs are ineffective. Radiofrequency catheter ablation is the treatment of choice for the Wolff-Parkinson-White syndrome associated with congenital heart defects (discussed earlier). In structurally normal hearts, ablation is low risk and highly effective for AV nodal reentrant tachycardia. In patients with CHD and AV nodal reentrant tachycardia, ablation carries an increased risk of inducing complete heart block. Catheter ablation is the best choice for incessant ectopic atrial tachycardia, as well as for atrial arrhythmias originating in regions of scar. Reentrant arrhythmias may arise from surgical scar sites after atriotomy or ventriculotomy and can be eliminated by targeting zones of slow conduction or isthmuses in the reentrant pathway. The signal averaged ECG identifies the presence of slow conduction substrates, and mapping sets the stage for radiofrequency ablation.[18] Intraatrial reentrant tachycardias can arise from multiple circuits. Twenty-six intraatrial reentrant tachycardias were studied in 18 patients late after surgery (nine atrial septal defect repairs, four Fontan procedures, two Mustard procedures, two Senning procedures, and one Rastelli procedure); successful ablation was achieved in 15 patients with 21 tachycardia circuits.[173] In each case, a surgical incision or barrier played a crucial role in creating the reentrant circuit and in providing a border for interruption of the circuit.[173] In 10 patients, including six after Fontan procedures, two after atrial baffle procedures (Senning and Mustard), and two after repair of tetralogy of Fallot, reentrant tachycardia circuits were successfully altered.[260] Supraventricular tachycardias associated with accessory pathway conduction in CHD are treated with catheter-guided intracardiac mapping and radiofrequency ablation (see Fig. 22–24). Thirteen of 15 accessory pathways were successfully ablated in 11 patients, including seven with Ebstein's anomaly.[503] As mentioned earlier, ventricular tachyarrhythmias occurring late after intracardiac repair of congenital malformations can be treated with radio-frequency ablation, but experience is less extensive.[18,504]

Arrhythmias not amenable to catheter ablation can be managed surgically by excision of ectopic atrial foci or excision of foci along a right ventriculotomy scar.[505] Patients with Wolff-Parkinson-White syndrome undergo transection of accessory AV connections with a high success rate.[425,441,443,505] Arrhythmia surgery is especially appropriate when there are additional indications for cardiac surgery, such as reoperation for TOF or repair of Ebstein's anomaly. The Maze procedure involves creation of multiple atrial incisions designed to eliminate the atrial fibrillation/flutter circuits (see Chapter 15) and has been employed for refractory paroxysmal or chronic atrial fibrillation or flutter.[506] The basis for the procedure originates in the 1914 observations of Garrey on the nature of fibrillary contraction of the heart: "Sufficiently narrow bridges of any portion of the musculature of the auricles or ventricles will prevent the extension of the fibrillatory process."[507] Because of high success rates in patients without structural heart disease (98% cure rate, including patients controlled postoperatively on antiar-rhythmic medications),[506] the Maze procedure is being used for refractory atrial arrhythmias in patients requiring surgery for CHD (Fig. 22–27).

An ICD is an option for adult and pediatric patients with recurrent life-threatening ventricular tachycardia or for those who have been resuscitated from ventricular fibrillation.[508] Experience with implantation in young patients and in patients with CHD is increasing as new-generation devices become more compact and offer both bradycardia and antitachycardia pacing in addition to low-energy cardioversion and high-energy defibrillation.[509,510] Implanted antitachycardia pacemakers are also options for atrial flutter, AV nodal reentry tachycardia, or circus movement reentry tachycardia.[511,512] In patients with refractory atrial arrhythmias and rapid ventricular rates, radiofrequency catheter ablation of AV conduction in conjunction with permanent pacemaker implantation can result in symptomatic relief but does not provide effective therapy for the atrial arrhythmia per se.

References

1. Upshaw CB Jr, Silverman ME. The Wenckebach phenomenon: a salute and comment on the centennial of its original description. *Ann Intern Med.* 1999;130:58–63.
2. Hurst JW. Naming of the waves in the ECG, with a brief account of their genesis. *Circulation.* 1998;98:1937–1942.
3. Wellens HJ. Bishop lecture. The electrocardiogram 80 years after Einthoven. *J Am Coll Cardiol.* 1986;7:484–491.
4. DeSilva RA. George Ralph Mines, ventricular fibrillation and the discovery of the vulnerable period. *J Am Coll Cardiol.* 1997;29:1397–1402.
5. Garrey W. Auricular fibrillation. *Physiol Rev.* 1924;4:215–250.
6. Silverman ME, Upshaw CB Jr. Walter Gaskell and the understanding of atrioventricular conduction and block. *J Am Coll Cardiol.* 2002;39:1574–1580.
7. Davies MK, Hollman A. Sir Thomas Lewis (1881–1945). *Heart.* 1996;76:383.
8. Fye WB. Sir Thomas Lewis: pioneer cardiologist and clinical scientist. *Bull History Med.* 1998;72:789–790.
9. Scherlag BJ, Lau SH, Helfant RH, et al. Catheter technique for recording His bundle activity in man. *Circulation.* 1969;39:13–18.
10. Damato AN, Lau SH, Helfant R, et al. A study of heart block in man using His bundle recordings. *Circulation.* 1969;39:297–305.
11. Gallagher JJ. Wolff-Parkinson-White syndrome: surgery to radiofrequency catheter ablation. *Pacing Clin Electrophysiol.* 1997;20:512–533.
12. Calkins H, Sousa J, el-Atassi R, et al. Diagnosis and cure of the Wolff-Parkinson-White syndrome or paroxysmal supraventricular tachycardias during a single electrophysiologic test. *N Engl J Med.* 1991;324:1612–1618.
13. Moss AJ, Zareba W, Hall WJ, et al. Prophylactic implantation of a defibrillator in patients with myocardial infarction and reduced ejection fraction. *N Engl J Med.* 2002;346:877–883.
14. Weiss JN. Ion channels in cardiac muscle. In: Langer GA, ed. *The Mammalian Myocardium.* 2nd ed. San Diego: Academic Press; 1997.
15. Yan GX, Antzelevitch C. Cellular basis for the electrocardiographic J wave. *Circulation.* 1996;93:372–379.
16. Antzelevitch C, Shimizu W, Yan GX, et al. The M cell: its contribution to the ECG and to normal and abnormal electrical function of the heart. *J Cardiovasc Electrophysiol.* 1999;10:1124–1152.
17. Janse MJ. Electrophysiology of arrhythmias. *Arch Mal Coeur Vaiss.* 1999;92:9–16.

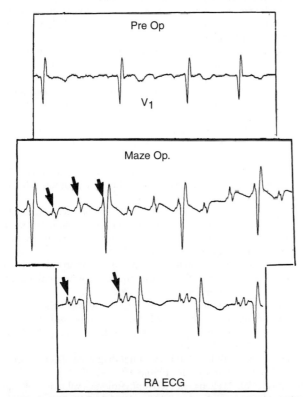

FIGURE 22–27 Rhythm strips from a 45-year-old man with Ebstein's anomaly and chronic atrial fibrillation. He underwent tricuspid valve reconstruction and a modified Maze procedure. The upper strip, recorded preoperatively, shows atrial fibrillation. The middle strip, recorded on the second postoperative day, shows atrial tachycardia (atrial rate 215/min) with 3:1 atrioventricular conduction. The lower strip, recorded on the third postoperative day, shows a fractionated atrial electrogram at 85 beats per minute that may represent sinus rhythm.

18. Perloff JK, Middlekauf HR, Child JS, et al. Usefulness of post-ventriculotomy signal averaged electrocardiograms in congenital heart disease. *Am J Cardiol.* 2006;98:1646–1651.

19. Gallagher JJ, Pritchett EL, Sealy WC, et al. The preexcitation syndromes. *Prog Cardiovasc Dis.* 1978;20:285–327.

20. Tomaselli GF, Marban E. Electrophysiological remodeling in hypertrophy and heart failure. *Cardiovasc Res.* 1999;42:270–283.

21. Tomaselli GF, Rose J. Molecular aspects of arrhythmias associated with cardiomyopathies. *Curr Opin Cardiol.* 2000;15:202–208.

22. Colucci WS. Apoptosis in the heart. *N Engl J Med.* 1996;335:1224–1226.

23. Narula J, Haider N, Virmani R, et al. Apoptosis in myocytes in end-stage heart failure. *N Engl J Med.* 1996;335:1182–1189.

24. Nerheim P, Krishnan SC, Olshansky B, Shivkumar K. Apoptosis in the genesis of cardiac rhythm disorders. *Cardiol Clin.* 2001;19:155–163.

25. Priori SG, Barhanin J, Hauer RN, et al. Genetic and molecular basis of cardiac arrhythmias: impact on clinical management part III. *Circulation.* 1999;99:674–681.

26. Priori SG, Barhanin J, Hauer RN, et al. Genetic and molecular basis of cardiac arrhythmias: impact on clinical management parts I and II. *Circulation.* 1999;99:518–528.

27. Janse MJ, Wilde AA. Molecular mechanisms of arrhythmias. *Rev Port Cardiol.* 1998;17(2 Suppl):II41–II46.

28. Viskin S. Long QT syndromes and torsade de pointes. *Lancet.* 1999;354:1625–1633.

29. Roden DM, Spooner PM. Inherited long QT syndromes: a paradigm for understanding arrhythmogenesis. *J Cardiovasc Electrophysiol.* 10:1664–1683.

30. Towbin JA, Vatta M. Molecular biology and the prolonged QT syndromes. *Am J Med.* 2001;110:385–398.

31. Siscovick DS, Raghunathan TE, Psaty BM, et al. Diuretic therapy for hypertension and the risk of primary cardiac arrest. *N Engl J Med.* 1994;330:1852–1857.

32. Nattel S. Atrial electrophysiological remodeling caused by rapid atrial activation: underlying mechanisms and clinical relevance to atrial fibrillation. *Cardiovasc Res.* 42:298–308.

33. Wijffels MC, Kirchhof CJ, Dorland R, Allessie MA. Atrial fibrillation begets atrial fibrillation. A study in awake chronically instrumented goats. *Circulation.* 1995;92:1954–1968.

34. Bosch RF, Zeng X, Grammer JB, et al. Ionic mechanisms of electrical remodeling in human atrial fibrillation. *Cardiovasc Res.* 1999;44:121–131.

35. Le Grand BL, Hatem S, Deroubaix E, et al. Depressed transient outward and calcium currents in dilated human atria. *Cardiovasc Res.* 1994;28:548–556.

36. Workman AJ, Kane KA, Rankin AC. The contribution of ionic currents to changes in refractoriness of human atrial myocytes associated with chronic atrial fibrillation. *Cardiovasc Res.* 2001;52:226–235.

37. Courtemanche M, Ramirez RJ, Nattel S. Ionic mechanisms underlying human atrial action potential properties: insights from a mathematical model. *Am J Physiol.* 1998;275:H301–321.

38. Harrild D, Henriquez C. A computer model of normal conduction in the human atria. *Circ Res.* 2000;87:E25–36.

39. Shivkumar K, Weiss JN. Atrial fibrillation: from cells to computers. *Cardiovasc Res.* 2001;52:171–173.

40. Zipes DP, Wellens HJ. Sudden cardiac death. *Circulation.* 1998;98:2334–2351.

41. Weiss J, Shine KI. [K+]o accumulation and electrophysiological alterations during early myocardial ischemia. *Am J Physiol.* 1982;243:H318–327.

42. Harris AS, Bisteni A, Russell RA, et al. Excitatory factors in ventricular tachycardia resulting from myocardial ischemia; potassium a major excitant. *Science.* 1954;119:200–203.

43. Janse MJ, Wit AL. Electrophysiological mechanisms of ventricular arrhythmias resulting from myocardial ischemia and infarction. *Physiol Rev.* 1989;69:1049–1169.

44. Moe GK, Rheinboldt WC, Abildskov JA. A computer model of atrial fibrillation. *Am Heart J.* 1964;67:200–220.

45. Allessie MA, Lammers WJEP, Bonke FIM, Hollen J. Experimental evaluation of Moe's multiple wavelet hypothesis of atrial fibrillation. In: Zipes DP, Jalife J, ed. *Cardiac Arrhythmias.* New York: Grune & Stratton; 1985:265–276.

46. Garfinkel A, Chen PS, Walter DO, et al. Quasiperiodicity and chaos in cardiac fibrillation. *J Clin Invest.* 1997;99:305–314.

47. Gray RA, Jalife J, Panfilov AV, et al. Mechanisms of cardiac fibrillation. *Science.* 1995;270:1222–1223; author reply 1224–1225.

48. Jalife J. *Mathematical Approaches to Cardiac Arrhythmias* New York: New York Academy of Science; 1990.

49. Winfree AT. Electrical turbulence in three-dimensional heart muscle. *Science.* 1994;266:1003–1006.

50. Tede NH, Shivkumar K, Perloff JK, et al. Signal-averaged electrocardiogram in Ebstein's anomaly. *Am J Cardiol.* 2004;93:432–436.

51. Weiss JN, Chen PS, Qu Z, et al. Ventricular fibrillation: how do we stop the waves from breaking? *Circ Res.* 2000;87:1103–1107.

52. Wu TJ, Yashima M, Xie F, et al. Role of pectinate muscle bundles in the generation and maintenance of intra-atrial reentry: potential implications for the mechanism of conversion between atrial fibrillation and atrial flutter. *Circ Res.* 1998;83:448–462.

53. Narayan SM, Cain ME, Smith JM. Atrial fibrillation. *Lancet.* 1997;350:943–950.

54. Freemantle N, Cleland J, Young P, et al. beta Blockade after myocardial infarction: systematic review and meta regression analysis. *BMJ.* 1999;318:1730–1737.

55. Naccarelli GV, Wolbrette DL, Patel HM, Luck JC. Amiodarone: clinical trials. *Curr Opin Cardiol.* 2000;15:64–72.

56. Roy D, Talajic M, Dorian P, et al. Amiodarone to prevent recurrence of atrial fibrillation. Canadian Trial of Atrial Fibrillation Investigators. *N Engl J Med.* 2000;342:913–920.

57. Gallagher JJ, Svenson RH, Kasell JH, et al. Catheter technique for closed-chest ablation of the atrioventricular conduction system. *N Engl J Med.* 1982;306:194–200.

58. Scheinman MM, Morady F, Hess DS, Gonzalez R. Catheter-induced ablation of the atrioventricular junction to control refractory supraventricular arrhythmias. *JAMA.* 1982;248:851–855.

59. Haines DE, Watson DD, Verow AF. Electrode radius predicts lesion radius during radiofrequency energy heating. Validation of a proposed thermodynamic model. *Circ Res.* 1990;67:124–129.

60. Simmers TA, Wittkampf FH, Hauer RN, Robles de Medina EO. In vivo ventricular lesion growth in radiofrequency catheter ablation. *Pacing Clin Electrophysiol.* 1994;17:523–531.

61. Simmers TA, Wittkampf FH, de Bakker JMT, Hauer RN. Relation between myocardial temperature-gradient and volume of permanently and transiently effected tissue—implications for radiofrequency ablation. *Circulation.* 1993;88:I399.

62. Jais P, Haissaguerre M, Shah DC, et al. Successful irrigated-tip catheter ablation of atrial flutter resistant to conventional radiofrequency ablation. *Circulation.* 1998;98:835–838.

63. Langberg JJ, Wonnell T, Chin MC, et al. Catheter ablation of the atrioventricular junction using a helical microwave antenna: a novel means of coupling energy to the endocardium. *Pacing Clin Electrophysiol.* 1991;14:2105–2113.

64. Josephson ME, Wellens HJ. Differential diagnosis of supraventricular tachycardia. *Cardiol Clin.* 1990;8:411–442.

65. Josephson ME, Wellens HJ. Electrophysiologic evaluation of supraventricular tachycardia. *Cardiol Clin.* 1997;15:567–586.

66. Jackman WM, Beckman KJ, McClelland JH, et al. Treatment of supraventricular tachycardia due to atrioventricular nodal reentry, by radiofrequency catheter ablation of slow-pathway conduction. *N Engl J Med.* 1992;327:313–318.

67. Jazayeri MR, Hempe SL, Sra JS, et al. Selective transcatheter ablation of the fast and slow pathways using radiofrequency energy in patients with atrioventricular nodal reentrant tachycardia. *Circulation.* 1992;85:1318–1328.

68. Wellens HJ. Catheter ablation of cardiac arrhythmias: usually cure, but complications may occur. *Circulation*. 1999;99:195–197.

69. Wellens HJ, Rodriguez LM, Timmermans C, Smeets JP. The asymptomatic patient with the Wolff-Parkinson-White electrocardiogram. *Pacing Clin Electrophysiol*. 1997;20:2082–2086.

70. Lesh MD, Van Hare GF, Epstein LM, et al. Radiofrequency catheter ablation of atrial arrhythmias. Results and mechanisms. *Circulation*. 1994;89:1074–1089.

71. Wellens HJ. Contemporary management of atrial flutter. *Circulation*. 2002;106:649–652.

72. Natale A, Newby KH, Pisano E, et al. Prospective randomized comparison of antiarrhythmic therapy versus first-line radiofrequency ablation in patients with atrial flutter. *J Am Coll Cardiol*. 2000;35:1898–1904.

73. Nakagawa H, Shah N, Matsudaira K, et al. Characterization of reentrant circuit in macroreentrant right atrial tachycardia after surgical repair of congenital heart disease: isolated channels between scars allow "focal" ablation. *Circulation*. 2001;103:699–709.

74. Markowitz SM, Brodman RF, Stein KM, et al. Lesional tachycardias related to mitral valve surgery. *J Am Coll Cardiol*. 2002;39: 1973–1983.

75. Movsowitz C, Schwartzman D, Callans DJ, et al. Idiopathic right ventricular outflow tract tachycardia: narrowing the anatomic location for successful ablation. *Am Heart J*. 1996;131:930–936.

76. Callans DJ, Menz V, Schwartzman D, et al. Repetitive monomorphic tachycardia from the left ventricular outflow tract: electrocardiographic patterns consistent with a left ventricular site of origin. *J Am Coll Cardiol*. 1997;29:1023–1027.

77. Nakagawa H, Beckman KJ, McClelland JH, et al. Radiofrequency catheter ablation of idiopathic left ventricular tachycardia guided by a Purkinje potential. *Circulation*. 1993;88:2607–2617.

78. Chen PS, Wu TJ, Ikeda T, et al. Focal source hypothesis of atrial fibrillation. *J Electrocardiol*. 1998;31(Suppl):32–34.

79. Haissaguerre M, Jais P, Shah DC, et al. Spontaneous initiation of atrial fibrillation by ectopic beats originating in the pulmonary veins. *N Engl J Med*. 1998;339:659–666.

80. Oral H, Knight BP, Tada H, et al. Pulmonary vein isolation for paroxysmal and persistent atrial fibrillation. *Circulation*. 2002;105: 1077–1081.

81. Natale A, Pisano E, Shewchik J, et al. First human experience with pulmonary vein isolation using a through-the-balloon circumferential ultrasound ablation system for recurrent atrial fibrillation. *Circulation*. 2000;102:1879–1882.

82. Hwang C, Wu TJ, Doshi RN, et al. Vein of Marshall cannulation for the analysis of electrical activity in patients with focal atrial fibrillation. *Circulation*. 2000;101:1503–1505.

83. Marchlinski FE, Callans DJ, Gottlieb CD. Electroanatomic substrate for ventricular tachycardia in the setting of right ventricular cardiomyopathy. *Circulation*. 1998;98:1823.

84. Marchlinski FE, Callans DJ, Gottlieb CD, Zado E. Linear ablation lesions for control of unmappable ventricular tachycardia in patients with ischemic and nonischemic cardiomyopathy. *Circulation*. 2000;101:1288–1296.

85. Soejima K, Stevenson WG. Ventricular tachycardia associated with myocardial infarct scar: a spectrum of therapies for a single patient. *Circulation*. 2002;106:176–179.

86. Sosa E, Scanavacca M, d'Avila A, Oliveira F, Ramires JA. Nonsurgical transthoracic epicardial catheter ablation to treat recurrent ventricular tachycardia occurring late after myocardial infarction. *J Am Coll Cardiol*. May 2000;35:1442–1449.

87. Haissaguerre M, Shah DC, Jais P, et al. Role of Purkinje conducting system in triggering of idiopathic ventricular fibrillation. *Lancet*. 2002;359:677–678.

88. Haissaguerre M, Shoda M, Jais P, et al. Mapping and ablation of idiopathic ventricular fibrillation. *Circulation*. 2002;106:962–967.

89. Glikson M, Friedman PA. The implantable cardioverter defibrillator. *Lancet*. 2001;357:1107–1117.

90. Harken AH, Horowitz LN, Josephson ME. The surgical treatment of ventricular tachycardia. *Ann Thorac Surg*. 1980;30:499–508.

91. Cox JL, Boineau JP, Schuessler RB, et al. Electrophysiologic basis, surgical development, and clinical results of the maze procedure for atrial flutter and atrial fibrillation. *Adv Card Surg*. 1995;6:1–67.

92. The 'Sicilian Gambit'. A new approach to the classification of antiarrhythmic drugs based on their actions on arrhythmogenic mechanisms. The Task Force of the Working Group on Arrhythmias of the European Society of Cardiology. *Eur Heart J*. 1991;12: 1112–1131.

93. Weiss JN, Garfinkel A, Karagueuzian HS, et al. Chaos and the transition to ventricular fibrillation: a new approach to antiarrhythmic drug evaluation. *Circulation*. 1999;99:2819–2826.

94. Hoffman BF, Cranefield PF. *Electrophysiology of the Heart*. New York: McGraw-Hill Book; 1960.

95. Hoffman BF, Rosen MR. Cellular mechanisms for cardiac arrhythmias. *Circ Res*. 1981;49:1–15.

96. Rosen MR. The links between basic and clinical cardiac electrophysiology. *Circulation*. 1988;77:251–263.

97. Zipes DP. Cardiac electrophysiology: promises and contributions. *J Am Coll Cardiol*. 1989;13:1329–1352.

98. de Bakker JM, van Capelle FJ, Janse MJ, et al. Reentry as a cause of ventricular tachycardia in patients with chronic ischemic heart disease: electrophysiologic and anatomic correlation. *Circulation*. 1988;77:589–606.

99. Spear JF, Horowitz LN, Hodess AB, et al. Cellular electrophysiology of human myocardial infarction. 1. Abnormalities of cellular activation. *Circulation*. 1979;59:247–256.

100. Spear JF, Michelson EL, Moore EN. Cellular electrophysiologic characteristics of chronically infarcted myocardium in dogs susceptible to sustained ventricular tachyarrhythmias. *J Am Coll Cardiol*. 1983;1:1099–1110.

101. Akhtar M, Jazayeri MR, Sra J, et al. Atrioventricular nodal reentry. Clinical, electrophysiological, and therapeutic considerations. *Circulation*. 1993;88:282–295.

102. Josephson ME, Almendral JM, Buxton AE, Marchlinski FE. Mechanisms of ventricular tachycardia. *Circulation*. 1987;75LIII41–III47.

103. Klein GJ, Guiraudon GM, Sharma AD, Milstein S. Demonstration of macroreentry and feasibility of operative therapy in the common type of atrial flutter. *Am J Cardiol*. 1986;57:587–591.

104. Waldo AL, MacLean WA, Karp RB, et al. Entrainment and interruption of atrial flutter with atrial pacing: studies in man following open heart surgery. *Circulation*. 1977;56:737–745.

105. Wellens HJ, Duren DR, Lie KI. Observations on mechanisms of ventricular tachycardia in man. *Circulation*. Aug 1976;54: 237–244.

106. Aronson RS, Nordin C. Electrophysiologic properties of hypertrophied myocytes isolated from rats with renal hypertension. *Eur Heart J*. 1984;5(Suppl F):339–345.

107. Cameron JS, Myerburg RJ, Wong SS, et al. Electrophysiologic consequences of chronic experimentally induced left ventricular pressure overload. *J Am Coll Cardiol*. 1983;2:481–487.

108. Gelband H, Bassett AL. Depressed transmembrane potentials during experimentally induced ventricular failure in cats. *Circ Res*. 1973;32:625–634.

109. White CW, Mirro MJ, Lund DD, et al. Alterations in ventricular excitability in conscious dogs during development of chronic heart failure. *Am J Physiol*. 1986;250:H1022–1029.

110. Bing OH, Matsushita S, Fanburg BL, Levine HJ. Mechanical properties of rat cardiac muscle during experimental hypertrophy. *Circ Res*. 1971;28:234–245.

111. Cheitlin MD, Robinowitz M, McAllister H, et al. The distribution of fibrosis in the left ventricle in congenital aortic stenosis and coarctation of the aorta. *Circulation*. 1980;62:823–830.

112. Bishop SP, Melsen LR. Myocardial necrosis, fibrosis, and DNA synthesis in experimental cardiac hypertrophy induced by sudden pressure overload. *Circ Res*. 1976;39:238–245.

113. Burns RJ, Liu PP, Druck MN, et al. Analysis of adults with and without complex ventricular arrhythmias after repair of tetralogy of Fallot. *J Am Coll Cardiol.* 1984;4:226–233.

114. Deanfield JE, Ho SY, Anderson RH, et al. Late sudden death after repair of tetralogy of Fallot: a clinicopathologic study. *Circulation.* 1983;67:626–631.

115. Garson A Jr, Randall DC, Gillette PC, et al. Prevention of sudden death after repair of tetralogy of Fallot: treatment of ventricular arrhythmias. *J Am Coll Cardiol.* 1985;6:221–227.

116. Kobayashi J, Hirose H, Nakano S, et al. Ambulatory electrocardiographic study of the frequency and cause of ventricular arrhythmia after correction of tetralogy of Fallot. *Am J Cardiol.* 1984;54:1310–1313.

117. Roos-Hesselink J, Perlroth MG, McGhie J, Spitaels S. Atrial arrhythmias in adults after repair of tetralogy of Fallot. Correlations with clinical, exercise, and echocardiographic findings. *Circulation.* 1995;91:2214–2219.

118. Wessel HU, Bastanier CK, Paul MH, et al. Prognostic significance of arrhythmia in tetralogy of Fallot after intracardiac repair. *Am J Cardiol.* Nov 1980;46:843–848.

119. Brandenburg RO Jr, Holmes DR Jr, Brandenburg RO, McGoon DC. Clinical follow-up study of paroxysmal supraventricular tachyarrhythmias after operative repair of a secundum type atrial septal defect in adults. *Am J Cardiol.* 1983;51:273–276.

120. Jayaprasad N, Johnson F, Venugopal K. Congenital complete heart block and maternal connective tissue disease. *Int J Cardiol.* 2006;112:153–158.

121. Perloff JK. *The Clinical Recognition of Congenital Heart Disease.* 4th ed. Philadelphia: W.B. Saunders; 1994.

122. Ross BA. Congenital complete atrioventricular block. *Pediatr Clin North Am.* 1990;37:69–78.

123. Michaelsson M, Jonzon A, Riesenfeld T. Isolated congenital complete atrioventricular block in adult life. A prospective study. *Circulation.* 1995;92:442–449.

124. Bharati S, Lev M. The myocardium, the conduction system and general sequelae after surgery for congenital heart disease. In: Engle MA, Perloff JK, ed. *Congenital Heart Disease after Surgery.* New York: Yorke Medical Books; 1983.

125. Stark SI, Rosenfeld LE, Kleinman CS, Batsford WP. Atrial dissociation: an electrophysiologic finding in a patient with transposition of the great arteries. *J Am Coll Cardiol.* 1986;8:236–238.

126. Bharati S, Lev M. Sequelae of atriotomy on the endocardium, conduction system and coronary arteries. In: Engle MA, Perloff JK, ed. *Congenital Heart Disease after Surgery.* New York: Yorke Medical Books; 1983;229–246.

127. Bharati S, Lev M. Conduction system in cases of sudden death in congenital heart disease many years after surgical correction. *Chest.* Dec 1986;90:861–868.

128. Bharati S, Lev M. Conduction system in sudden unexpected death a considerable time after repair of atrial septal defect. *Chest.* Jul 1988;94:142–148.

129. Finley JP, Nugent ST, Hellenbrand W, et al. Sinus arrhythmia in children with atrial septal defect: an analysis of heart rate variability before and after surgical repair. *Br Heart J.* 1989. 61:280–284.

130. Sung RJ, Tamer DM, Agha AS, et al. Etiology of the electrocardiographic pattern of "incomplete right bundle branch block" in atrial septal defect: an electrophysiologic study. *J Pediatr.* 1975;87:1182–1186.

131. Heller J, Hagege AA, Besse B, et al. "Crochetage" (notch) on R wave in inferior limb leads: a new independent electrocardiographic sign of atrial septal defect. *J Am Coll Cardiol.* 1996;27:877–882.

132. Bolens M, Friedli B. Sinus node function and conduction system before and after surgery for secundum atrial septal defect: an electrophysiologic study. *Am J Cardiol.* 1984;53:1415–1420.

133. Cascos AS. Holt-Oram syndrome. *Acta Paediatr Scand.* 1967;56:313–317.

134. Clark EB, Kugler JD. Preoperative secundum atrial septal defect with coexisting sinus node and atrioventricular node dysfunction. *Circulation.* May 1982;65:976–980.

135. Ruschhaupt DG, Khoury L, Thilenius OG, et al. Electrophysiologic abnormalities of children with ostium secundum atrial septal defect. *Am J Cardiol.* 1984;53:1643–1647.

136. Benedini G, Affatato A, Bellandi M, et al. Pre-operative sinus node function in adult patients with atrial septal defect (ostium secundum type). *Eur Heart J.* 1985;6:261–265.

137. Anderson PA, Rogers MC, Canent RV Jr, Spach MS. Atrioventricular conduction in secundum atrial septal defects. *Circulation.* 1973;48:27–31.

138. Bagger JP, Thomsen PE, Bjerregaard P, et al. Intracardiac electrography in patients before and after surgical repair of secundum atrial septal defect. *J Electrocardiol.* 1984;17:347–352.

139. Chen S, Arcilla RA, Moulder PV, Cassels DE. Postoperative conduction disturbances in atrial septal defect. *Am J Cardiol.* 1968;22:636–644.

140. Sherron P, Torres-Arraut E, Tamer D, et al. Site of conduction delay and electrophysiologic significance of first-degree atrioventricular block in children with heart disease. *Am J Cardiol.* 1985;55:1323–1327.

141. Shiku DJ, Stijns M, Lintermans JP, Vliers A. Atrioventricular conduction and right atrial volume in children with and without secundum atrial septal defects. *Br Heart J.* 1981;46:69–73.

142. Sobrino JA, de Lombera F, del Rio A, et al. Atrioventricular nodal dysfunction in patients with atrial septal defect. Abnormalities of conduction and reciprocal rhythms. *Chest.* 1982;81:477–482.

143. John Sutton MG, Tajik AJ, McGoon DC. Atrial septal defect in patients ages 60 years or older: operative results and long-term postoperative follow-up. *Circulation.* 1981;64:402–409.

144. Bizarro RO, Callahan JA, Feldt RH, Kurland LT, et al. Familial atrial septal defect with prolonged atrioventricular conduction. A syndrome showing the autosomal dominant pattern of inheritance. *Circulation.* 1970;41:677–683.

145. Bjornstad PG. Secundum type atrial septal defect with prolonged PR interval and autosomal dominant mode of inheritance. *Br Heart J.* 1974;36(12):1149–1154.

146. Emanuel R, O'Brien K, Somerville J, et al. Association of secundum atrial septal defect with abnormalities of atrioventricular conduction or left axis deviation. Genetic study of 10 families. *Br Heart J.* 1975;37:1085–1092.

147. Lev M, Paul MH, Cassels DE. Complete atrioventricular block associated with atrial septal defect of the fossa ovalis (secundum) type. A histopathologic study of the conduction systems. *Am J Cardiol.* 1967;19:266–274.

148. Maron BJ, Borer JS, Lau SH, et al. Association of secundum atrial septal defect and atrioventricular nodal dysfunction. A genetically transmitted syndrome. *Br Heart J.* 1978;40:1293–1299.

149. Pease WE, Nordenberg A, Ladda RL. Familial atrial septal defect with prolonged atrioventricular conduction. *Circulation.* 1976;53:759–762.

150. Reid JM, Stevenson JC. Cardiac arrhythmias following successful surgical closure of atrial septal defect. *Br Heart J.* 1967;29:742–747.

151. Scanlon PJ, Pryor R, Blount SG Jr. Right bundle-branch block associated with left superior or inferior intraventricular block. Clinical setting, prognosis, and relation to complete heart block. *Circulation.* 1970;42:1123–1133.

152. Kano Y, Abe T, Tanaka M, Takeuchi E. Electrophysiological abnormalities before and after surgery for atrial septal defect. *J Electrocardiol.* 1993;26:225–229.

153. Bink-Boelkens MT, Meuzelaar KJ, Eygelaar A. Arrhythmias after repair of secundum atrial septal defect: the influence of surgical modification. *Am Heart J.* 1988;115:629–633.

154. Bink-Boelkens MT, Velvis H, van der Heide JJ, et al. Dysrhythmias after atrial surgery in children. *Am Heart J.* 1983;106:125–130.

155. Cohn LH, Morrow AG, Braunwald E. Operative treatment of atrial septal defect: clinical and haemodynamic assessments in 175 patients. *Br Heart J.* 1967;29:725–734.

156. Liberthson RR, Boucher CA, Strauss HW, et al. Right ventricular function in adult atrial septal defect. Preoperative and postoperative assessment and clinical implications. *Am J Cardiol.* 1981;47: 56–60.

157. Popper RW, Knott JM, Selzer A, Gerbode F. Arrhythmias after cardiac surgery. I. Uncomplicated atrial septal defect. *Am Heart J.* 1962;64:455–461.

158. Young D. Later results of closure of secundum atrial septal defect in children. *Am J Cardiol.* 1973;31:14–22.

159. Craig RJ, Selzer A. Natural history and prognosis of atrial septal defect. *Circulation.* 1968;37:805–815.

160. Forfang K. Electrocardiographic findings before and after surgery for atrial septal defect of the secundum type in middle-aged patients. *Cardiology.* 1978;63:94–106.

161. Kuzman WJ, Yuskis AS. Atrial septal defects in the older patient simulating acquired valvular heart disease. *Am J Cardiol.* 1965;15: 303–309.

162. Paolillo V, Dawkins KD, Miller GA. Atrial septal defect in patients over the age of 50. *Int J Cardiol.* 1985;9:139–147.

163. Sealy WC, Farmer JC, Young WG Jr, Brown IW Jr. Atrial dysrhythmia and atrial secundum defects. *J Thorac Cardiovasc Surg.* 1969; 57:245–250.

164. Tikoff G, Schmidt AM, Hecht HH. Atrial fibrillation in atrial septal defect. *Arch Intern Med.* 1968;121:402–405.

165. Horvath KA, Burke RP, Collins JJ Jr., Cohn LH. Surgical treatment of adult atrial septal defect: early and long-term results. *J Am Coll Cardiol.* 1992;20:1156–1159.

166. Murphy JG, Gersh BJ, McGoon MD, et al. Long-term outcome after surgical repair of isolated atrial septal defect. Follow-up at 27 to 32 years. *N Engl J Med.* 1990;323:1645–1650.

167. Saksena FB, Aldridge HE. Atrial septal defect in the older patient. A clinical and hemodynamic study in patients operated on after age 35. *Circulation.* 1970;42:1009–1020.

168. Solti F, Szabo Z, Bodor E, Renyi-Vamos F Jr. Changes in the pacemaker function of the sinus node after closure of atrial septal defect. Temporary and stable iatrogenic sick sinus syndrome. *Cor Vasa.* 1979;21:242–248.

169. Meijboom F, Hess J, Szatmari A, et al. Long-term follow-up (9 to 20 years) after surgical closure of atrial septal defect at a young age. *Am J Cardiol.* 1993;72:1431–1434.

170. Ohnishi S, Kasanuki H, Takamizawa K, et al. Long-term management of bradyarrhythmias following open heart surgery: surgical A-V block and sick sinus syndrome after surgery for secundum atrial septal defects treated with permanent cardiac pacing. *Jpn Circ J.* 1986;50:903–917.

171. McNamara DG, Latson LA. Long-term follow up of patients with malformations for which definitive surgical repair has been available for 25 years or more. In: Engle MA, Perloff JK, ed. *Congenital Heart Disease after Surgery.* New York: Yorke Medical Books; 1983;77–99.

172. Cowen ME, Jeffrey RR, Drakeley MJ, et al. The results of surgery for atrial septal defect in patients aged fifty years and over. *Eur Heart J.* 1990;11:29–34.

173. Kalman JM, VanHare GF, Olgin JE, et al. Ablation of "incisional" reentrant atrial tachycardia complicating surgery for congenital heart disease. Use of entrainment to define a critical isthmus of conduction. *Circulation.* 1996;93:502–512.

174. Vetter VL, Horowitz LN. Electrophysiologic residua and sequelae of surgery for congenital heart defects. *Am J Cardiol.* 1982;50: 588–604.

175. Schenck MH, Sterba R, Foreman CK, Latson LA. Improvement in noninvasive electrophysiologic findings in children after transcatheter atrial septal defect closure. *Am J Cardiol.* 1995;76: 695–698.

176. Davia JE, Cheitlin MD, Bedynek JL. Sinus venosus atrial septal defect: analysis of fifty cases. *Am Heart J.* 1973;85:177–185.

177. Kyger ER 3rd, Frazier OH, Cooley DA, et al. Sinus venosus atrial septal defect: early and late results following closure in 109 patients. *Ann Thorac Surg.* 1978;25:44–50.

178. Trusler GA, Kazenelson G, Freedom RM, et al. Late results following repair of partial anomalous pulmonary venous connection with sinus venosus atrial septal defect. *J Thorac Cardiovasc Surg.* 1980;79:776–781.

179. Feldt RH, DuShane JW, Titus JL. The atrioventricular conduction system in persistent common atrioventricular canal defect: correlations with electrocardiogram. *Circulation.* 1970;42:437–444.

180. Lev M. The architecture of the conduction system in congenital heart disease. I. Common atrioventricular orifice. *AMA Arch Pathol.* 1958;65:174–191.

181. Waldo AL, Kaiser GA, Bowman FO Jr, Malm JR. Etiology of prolongation of the P-R interval in patients with an endocardial cushion defect. Further observations on internodal conduction and the polarity of the retrograde P wave. *Circulation.* 1973;48:19–26.

182. Goodman DJ, Harrison DC, Cannom DS. Atrioventricular conduction in patients with incomplete endocardial cushion defect. *Circulation.* 1974;49:631–637.

183. Jacobsen JR, Gillette PC, Corbett BN, et al. Intracardiac electrography in endocardial cushion defects. *Circulation.* 1976;54:599–603.

184. Boineau JP, Moore EN, Patterson DF. Relationship between the ECG, ventricular activation, and the ventricular conduction system in ostium primum ASD. *Circulation.* 1973;48:556–564.

185. Campbell RM, Dick M 2nd, Hees P, Behrendt DM. Epicardial and endocardial activation in patients with endocardial cushion defect. *Am J Cardiol.* 1983;51:277–281.

186. Durrer D, Roos JP, van Dam RT. The genesis of the electrocardiogram of patients with ostium primum defects (ventral atrial septal defects). *Am Heart J.* 1966;71:642–650.

187. Eckberg DL, Ross J Jr, Morgan JR. Acquired right bundle-branch block and left anterior hemiblock in ostium primum atrial septal defect. *Circulation.* 1972;45:658–662.

188. Somerville J. Ostium primum defect: factors causing deterioration in the natural history. *Br Heart J.* 1965;27:413–419.

189. Losay J, Rosenthal A, Castaneda AR, et al. Repair of atrial septal defect primum. Results, course, and prognosis. *J Thorac Cardiovasc Surg.* 1978;75:248–254.

190. Portman MA, Beder SD, Ankeney JL, et al. A 20-year review of ostium primum defect repair in children. *Am Heart J.* 1985;110: 1054–1058.

191. Fryda RJ, Kaplan S, Helmsworth JA. Postoperative complete heart block in children. *Br Heart J.* 1971;33:456–462.

192. Goodman DJ, Harrison DC, Schroeder JS. Ostium primum defect in the adult: postoperative follow-up studies. *Chest.* 1975;67: 185–189.

193. King RM, Puga FJ, Danielson GK, et al. Prognostic factors and surgical treatment of partial atrioventricular canal. *Circulation.* 1986;74:I42–I46.

194. Fasting H, Axelsen F, Sondergaard T. Atrial septal defect, primum type. Results of surgical closure in 46 patients. *Scand J Thorac Cardiovasc Surg.* 1980;14:165–168.

195. Squarcia U, Merideth J, McGoon DC, Weidman WH. Prognosis of transient atrioventricular conduction disturbances complicating open heart surgery for congenital heart defects. *Am J Cardiol.* 1971;28:648–652.

196. Ho SY, Rossi MB, Mehta AV, et al. Heart block and atrioventricular septal defect. *Thorac Cardiovasc Surg.* 1985;33:362–365.

197. Daliento L, Rizzoli G, Marchiori MC, et al. Electrical instability in patients undergoing surgery for atrioventricular septal defect. *Int J Cardiol.* 1991;30:15–21.

198. McGrath LB, Gonzalez-Lavin L. Actuarial survival, freedom from reoperation, and other events after repair of atrioventricular septal defects. *J Thorac Cardiovasc Surg.* 1987;94:582–590.

199. Rastelli GC, Ongley PA, Kirklin JW, McGoon DC. Surgical repair of the complete form of persistent common atrioventricular canal. *J Thorac Cardiovasc Surg.* 1968;55:299–308.

200. Singh AK, Corwin RD, Cooper GN Jr, Karlson KE. Early and late results following repair of partial atrioventricular (AV) canal. *Thorac Cardiovasc Surg.* 1984;32:89–91.

201. Culpepper W, Kolff J, Lin CY, et al. Complete common atrioventricular canal in infancy—surgical repair and postoperative hemodynamics. *Circulation.* 1978;58:550–558.

202. Davis JT, Ehrlich R, Hennessey JR, et al. Long-term follow-up of cardiac rhythm in repaired total anomalous pulmonary venous drainage. *Thorac Cardiovasc Surg.* 1986;34:172–175.

203. DeLeon SY, Freeman JE, Ilbawi MN, et al. Surgical techniques in partial anomalous pulmonary veins to the superior vena cava. *Ann Thorac Surg.* 1993;55:1222–1226.

204. Stewart S, Alexson C, Manning J. Early and late results of repair of partial anomalous pulmonary venous connection to the superior vena cava with a pericardial baffle. *Ann Thorac Surg.* 1986;41:498–501.

205. Yee ES, Turley K, Hsieh WR, Ebert PA. Infant total anomalous pulmonary venous connection: factors influencing timing of presentation and operative outcome. *Circulation.* 1987;76:III83–87.

206. Wilson WR Jr, Ilbawi MN, DeLeon SY, et al. Technical modifications for improved results in total anomalous pulmonary venous drainage. *J Thorac Cardiovasc Surg.* 1992;103:861–870; discussion 870–861.

207. Arensman FW, Bostock J, Radley-Smith R, Yacoub MH. Cardiac rhythm and conduction before and after anatomic correction of transposition of the great arteries. *Am J Cardiol.* 1983;52:836–839.

208. Deanfield J, Camm J, Macartney F, et al. Arrhythmia and late mortality after Mustard and Senning operation for transposition of the great arteries. An eight-year prospective study. *J Thorac Cardiovasc Surg.* 1988;96:569–576.

209. Martin RP, Radley-Smith R, Yacoub MH. Arrhythmias before and after anatomic correction of transposition of the great arteries. *J Am Coll Cardiol.* 1987;10:200–204.

210. Nagashima M, Matsushima M, Ogawa A, et al. Cardiac arrhythmias in healthy children revealed by 24-hour ambulatory ECG monitoring. *Pediatr Cardiol.* 1987;8:103–108.

211. Southall DP, Keeton BR, Leanage R, et al. Cardiac rhythm and conduction before and after Mustard's operation for complete transposition of the great arteries. *Br Heart J.* 1980;43:21–30.

212. Beerman LB, Neches WH, Fricker FJ, et al. Arrhythmias in transposition of the great arteries after the Mustard operation. *Am J Cardiol.* 1983;51:1530–1534.

213. Ullal RR, Anderson RH, Lincoln C. Mustard's operation modified to avoid dysrhythmias and pulmonary and systemic venous obstruction. *J Thorac Cardiovasc Surg.* 1979;78:431–439.

214. Cornell WP, Maxwell RE, Haller JA, Sabiston DC. Results of the Blalock-Hanlon operation in 90 patients with transposition of the great vessels. *J Thorac Cardiovasc Surg.* 1966;52:525–532.

215. Blalock A, Hanlon CR. The surgical treatment of complete transposition of the aorta and the pulmonary artery. *Surg Gynecol Obstet.* 1950;90:1–15.

216. Garson A Jr, Bink-Boelkens M, Hesslein PS, et al. Atrial flutter in the young: a collaborative study of 380 cases. *J Am Coll Cardiol.* 1985;6:871–878.

217. Hayes CJ, Gersony WM. Arrhythmias after the Mustard operation for transposition of the great arteries: a long-term study. *J Am Coll Cardiol.* 1986;7:133–137.

218. Bove EL, Beekman RH, Snider AR, et al. Arterial repair for transposition of the great arteries and large ventricular septal defect in early infancy. *Circulation.* 1988;78:III26–III31.

219. Lange PE, Pulss W, Sievers HH, et al. Cardiac rhythm and conduction after two-stage anatomic correction of simple transposition of the great arteries. *Thorac Cardiovasc Surg.* 1986;34:22–24.

220. Mustard WT. Successful two-stage correction of transposition of the great vessels. *Surgery.* 1964;55:469–472.

221. Edwards WD, Edwards JE. Pathology of the sinus node in d-transposition following the Mustard operation. *J Thorac Cardiovasc Surg.* 1978;75:213–218.

222. El-Said GM, Gillette PC, Cooley DA, et al. Protection of the sinus node in Mustard's operation. *Circulation.* 1976;53:788–791.

223. Gillette PC, Kugler JD, Garson A Jr, et al. Mechanisms of cardiac arrhythmias after the Mustard operation for transposition of the great arteries. *Am J Cardiol.* 1980;45:1225–1230.

224. Sunderland CO, Henken DP, Nichols GM, et al. Postoperative hemodynamic and electrophysiologic evaluation of the interatrial baffle procedure. *Am J Cardiol.* 1975;35:660–666.

225. Isaacson R, Titus JL, Merideth J, et al. Apparent interruption of atrial conduction pathways after surgical repair of transposition of great arteries. *Am J Cardiol.* 1972;30:533–535.

226. Vetter VL, Tanner CS, Horowitz LN. Inducible atrial flutter after the Mustard repair of complete transposition of the great arteries. *Am J Cardiol.* 1988;61:428–435.

227. Wittig JH, Stark J. Intraoperative mapping of atrial activation before, during, and after the Mustard operation. *J Thorac Cardiovasc Surg.* 1977;73:1–13.

228. Cronin CS, Nitta T, Mitsuno M, et al. Characterization and surgical ablation of acute atrial flutter following the Mustard procedure. A canine model. *Circulation.* 1993;88:II461–II471.

229. Clarkson PM, Barratt-Boyles BG, Neutze JM. Late dysrhythmias and disturbances of conduction following Mustard operation for complete transposition of the great arteries. *Circulation.* 1976;53:519–524.

230. Duster MC, Bink-Boelkens MT, Wampler D, et al. Long-term follow-up of dysrhythmias following the Mustard procedure. *Am Heart J.* 1985;109:1323–1326.

231. Lewis AB, Lindesmith GG, Takahashi M, et al. Cardiac rhythm following the Mustard procedure for transposition of the great vessels. *J Thorac Cardiovasc Surg.* 1977;73:919–926.

232. Stewart S, Alexson C, Manning J. Late results of the Mustard procedure in transposition of the great arteries. *Ann Thorac Surg.* 1986;42:419–424.

233. El-Said GM, Rosenberg HS, Mullins CE, et al. Dysrhythmias after Mustard's operation for transposition of the great arteries. *Am J Cardiol.* 1972;30:526.

234. Byrum CJ, Bove EL, Sondheimer HM, et al. Sinus node shift after the Senning procedure compared with the Mustard procedure for transposition of the great arteries. *Am J Cardiol.* 1987;60:346–350.

235. Flinn CJ, Wolff GS, Dick M 2nd, et al. Cardiac rhythm after the Mustard operation for complete transposition of the great arteries. *N Engl J Med.* 1984;310:1635–1638.

236. Furuta N, Luhmer I, Oelert H. Clinical experience with atrial inversion using a Gore-Tex baffle in 52 cases of transposition of the great arteries. *Ann Thorac Surg.* 1985;40:50–56.

237. Ihenacho HN, Patel RG, Singh SP, et al. Transposition of the great arteries. A review of 37 cases after Mustard's operation. *Thorax.* 1973;28:448–452.

238. Janousek J, Paul T, Luhmer I, et al. Atrial baffle procedures for complete transposition of the great arteries: natural course of sinus node dysfunction and risk factors for dysrhythmias and sudden death. *Z Kardiol.* 1994;83:933–938.

239. Aghaji MA, Litwin SB. Results of Mustard's repair for dextro-transposition of the great arteries. *J Cardiovasc Surg (Torino).* 1990;31:7–13.

240. Kratz JM, Gillette PC, Crawford FA, et al. Atrioventricular pacing in congenital heart disease. *Ann Thorac Surg.* 1992;54:485–489.

241. Egloff LP, Freed MD, Dick M, et al. Early and late results with the Mustard operation in infancy. *Ann Thorac Surg.* 1978;26:474–484.

242. Thies WR, Breymann T, Kleikamp G, et al. Early rhythm disorders after arterial switch and intraatrial repair in infants with simple

transposition of the great arteries. *Thorac Cardiovasc Surg.* 1991;39 (2 Suppl):190–193.

243. Haemmerli M, Bolens M, Friedli B. Electrophysiological studies after the Mustard and Senning operations for complete transposition. Do they have prognostic value? *Int J Cardiol.* 1990;27: 167–173.

244. Mair DD, Danielson GK, Wallace RB, McGoon DC. Long-term follow-up of Mustard operation survivors. *Circulation.* 1974; 50(2 Suppl):II46–II53.

245. Saalouke MG, Rios J, Perry LW, et al. Electrophysiologic studies after Mustard's operation for d-transposition of the great vessels. *Am J Cardiol.* 1978;41:1104–1109.

246. Hesslein PS, Gutgesell HP, Gillette PC, McNamara DG. Exercise assessment of sinoatrial node function following the Mustard operation. *Am Heart J.* 1982;103:351–357.

247. Gewillig M, Cullen S, Mertens B, et al. Risk factors for arrhythmia and death after Mustard operation for simple transposition of the great arteries. *Circulation.* 1991;84(5 Suppl):III187–III192.

248. Warnes CA, Somerville J. Transposition of the great arteries: late results in adolescents and adults after the Mustard procedure. *Br Heart J.* 1987;58:148–155.

249. Hramer HH, Rammos S, Krogmann O, et al. Cardiac rhythm after Mustard repair and after atrial switch operation for complete transposition. *Int J Cardiol.* 1992;32:5.

250. Myridakis DJ, Ehlers KH, Engle MA. Late follow-up after venous switch operation (Mustard procedure) for simple and complex transposition of the great arteries. *Am J Cardiol.* 1994;74: 1030–1036.

251. Penkoske PA, Westerman GR, Marx GR, et al. Transposition of the great arteries and ventricular septal defect: results with the Senning operation and closure of the ventricular septal defect in infants. *Ann Thorac Surg.* 1983;36:281–288.

252. Ferrer MI. The sick sinus syndrome. *Circulation.* 1973;47:635–641.

253. Schiller MS, Levin AR, Haft JI, et al. Electrophysiologic studies in sick sinus syndrome following surgery for d-transposition of the great arteries. *J Pediatr.* 1977;91:891–896.

254. Ashraf MH, Cotroneo J, DiMarco D, Subramanian S. Fate of long-term survivors of Mustard procedure (inflow repair) for simple and complex transposition of the great arteries. *Ann Thorac Surg.* 1986;42:385–389.

255. Champsaur GL, Sokol DM, Trusler GA, Mustard WT. Repair of transposition of the great arteries in 123 pediatric patients: early and long-term results. *Circulation.* 1973;47:1032–1041.

256. Bharati S, Molthan ME, Veasy LG, Lev M. Conduction system in two cases of sudden death two years after the Mustard procedure. *J Thorac Cardiovasc Surg.* 1979;77:101–108.

257. Gillette PC, Wampler DG, Shannon C, Ott D. Use of cardiac pacing after the Mustard operation for transposition of the great arteries. *J Am Coll Cardiol.* 1986;7:138–141.

258. Ward DE, Clarke B, Schofield PM, et al. Long term transvenous ventricular pacing in adults with congenital abnormalities of the heart and great arteries. *Br Heart J.* 1983;50:325–329.

259. Wessel HU, Benson DW Jr, Braunlin EA, et al. Exercise response before and after termination of atrial tachycardia after congenital heart disease surgery. *Circulation.* 1989;80:106–111.

260. Triedman JK, Saul JP, Weindling SN, Walsh EP. Radiofrequency ablation of intra-atrial reentrant tachycardia after surgical palliation of congenital heart disease. *Circulation.* 1995;91: 707–714.

261. Senning A. Surgical correction of transposition of the great vessels. *Surgery.* 1959;45:966–980.

262. Byrum CJ, Bove EL, Sondheimer HM, et al. Hemodynamic and electrophysiologic results of the Senning procedure for transposition of the great arteries. *Am J Cardiol.* 1986;58:138–142.

263. George BL, Laks H, Klitzner TS, et al. Results of the Senning procedure in infants with simple and complex transposition of the great arteries. *Am J Cardiol.* 1987;59:426–430.

264. Hays MD, Gillette PC. Atrial automatic ectopic tachycardia successfully treated with encainide in a 4-week-old infant after Senning procedure. *Am Heart J.* 1989;117:489–492.

265. Marquez-Montes J, O'Connor F, Burgos R, et al. Comparative electrophysiological evaluation of atrial activation and sinoatrial node function following Senning and Mustard procedures: an experimental study. *Ann Thorac Surg.* 1983;36:692–699.

266. Rubay J, de Leval M, Bull C. To switch or not to switch? The Senning alternative. *Circulation.* 1988;78:III1–III4.

267. Turina M, Siebenmann R, Nussbaumer P, Senning A. Long-term outlook after atrial correction of transposition of great arteries. *J Thorac Cardiovasc Surg.* 1988;95:828–835.

268. Vetter VL, Tanner CS. Electrophysiologic consequences of the arterial switch repair of d-transposition of the great arteries. *J Am Coll Cardiol.* 1988;12:229–237.

269. Weldon CS, Hartmann AF Jr, Kelly JP. Current management of transposition of the great arteries: immediate septostomy, occasional prostaglandin infusion, and early Senning operations. *Ann Thorac Surg.* 1983;36:10–18.

270. Helbing WA, Hansen B, Ottenkamp J, et al. Long-term results of atrial correction for transposition of the great arteries. Comparison of Mustard and Senning operations. *J Thorac Cardiovasc Surg.* 1994;108:363–372.

271. Turina MI, Siebenmann R, von Segesser L, et al. Late functional deterioration after atrial correction for transposition of the great arteries. *Circulation.* 1989;80:I162–II167.

272. Jatene AD, Fontes VF, Paulista PP, et al. Anatomic correction of transposition of the great vessels. *J Thorac Cardiovasc Surg.* 1976;72: 364–370.

273. Rhodes LA, Wernovsky G, Keane JF, et al. Arrhythmias and intra-cardiac conduction after the arterial switch operation. *J Thorac Cardiovasc Surg.* 1995;109:303–310.

274. Losay J, Planche C, Gerardin B, et al. Midterm surgical results of arterial switch operation for transposition of the great arteries with intact septum. *Circulation.* 1990;82(5 Suppl): IV146–IV150.

275. Villafane J, White S, Elbl F, Rees A, Solinger R. An electrocardiographic midterm follow-up study after anatomic repair of transposition of the great arteries. *Am J Cardiol.* 1990;66:350–354.

276. Goor DA, Shem-Tov A, Neufeld HN. Impeded coronary flow in anatomic correction of transposition of the great arteries: prevention, detection, and management. *J Thorac Cardiovasc Surg.* 1982; 83:747–754.

277. Yacoub MH, Radley-Smith R. Anatomy of the coronary arteries in transposition of the great arteries and methods for their transfer in anatomical correction. *Thorax.* 1978;33:418–424.

278. Mayer JE Jr, Sanders SP, Jonas RA, et al. Coronary artery pattern and outcome of arterial switch operation for transposition of the great arteries. *Circulation.* 1990;82(5 Suppl):IV139–IV145.

279. Menahem S, Ranjit MS, Stewart C, et al. Cardiac conduction abnormalities and rhythm changes after neonatal anatomical correction of transposition of the great arteries. *Br Heart J.* 1992;67: 246–249.

280. Becker AE, Wilkinson JL, Anderson RH. Atrioventricular conduction tissues in univentricular hearts of left ventricular type. *Herz.* 1979;4:166–175.

281. Krongrad E, Malm JR. Intraoperative mapping in patients with univentricular hearts. *Herz.* 1979;4:232–238.

282. Wenink AC. The conducting tissues in primitive ventricle with outlet chamber. Two different possibilities. *J Thorac Cardiovasc Surg.* 1978;75:747–753.

283. Wilkinson JL, Keeton B, Dickinson DF, et al. Morphology and conducting tissue in univentricular hearts of right ventricular type. *Herz.* 1979;4:151–160.

284. Moodie DS, Ritter DG, Tajik AH, et al. Long-term follow-up after palliative operation for univentricular heart. *Am J Cardiol.* 1984;53: 1648–1651.

285. Moodie DS, Ritter DG, Tajik AJ, O'Fallon WM. Long-term follow-up in the unoperated univentricular heart. *Am J Cardiol.* 1984;53: 1124–1128.

286. Dick M, Fyler DC, Nadas AS. Tricuspid atresia: clinical course in 101 patients. *Am J Cardiol.* 1975;36:327–337.

287. Guller B, DuShane JW, Titus JL. The atrioventricular conduction system in two cases of tricuspid atresia. *Circulation.* 1969;40: 217–226.

288. Alboliras ET, Porter CB, Danielson GK, et al. Results of the modified Fontan operation for congenital heart lesions in patients without preoperative sinus rhythm. *J Am Coll Cardiol.* 1985;6: 228–233.

289. Behrendt DM, Rosenthal A. Cardiovascular status after repair by Fontan procedure. *Ann Thorac Surg.* 1980;29:322–330.

290. Case CL, Gillette PC, Zeigler V, Sade RM. Problems with permanent atrial pacing in the Fontan patient. *Pacing Clin Electrophysiol.* 1989;12:92–96.

291. Castaneda AR. From Glenn to Fontan. A continuing evolution. *Circulation.* 1992;86(5 Suppl):II80–II84.

292. Chen SC, Nouri S, Pennington DG. Dysrhythmias after the modified Fontan procedure. *Pediatr Cardiol.* 1988;9:215–219.

293. Fontan F, Baudet E. Surgical repair of tricuspid atresia. *Thorax.* 1971;26:240–248.

294. Humes RA, Porter CJ, Mair DD, et al. Intermediate follow-up and predicted survival after the modified Fontan procedure for tricuspid atresia and double-inlet ventricle. *Circulation.* 1987;76: III67–71.

295. Matsuda H, Kawashima Y, Kishimoto H, et al. Problems in the modified Fontan operation for univentricular heart of the right ventricular type. *Circulation.* 1987;76:III45–52.

296. Weber HS, Hellenbrand WE, Kleinman CS, et al. Predictors of rhythm disturbances and subsequent morbidity after the Fontan operation. *Am J Cardiol.* 1989;64:762–767.

297. Ward KE, Moak JP, Garson A Jr. Appearance and disappearance of arrhythmias after the Fontan operation. *J Am Coll Cardiol.* 1985; 5:427.

298. Gelatt M, Hamilton RM, McCrindle BW, et al. Risk factors for atrial tachyarrhythmias after the Fontan operation. *J Am Coll Cardiol.* 1994;24:1735–1741.

299. Kurer CC, Tanner CS, Norwood WI, Vetter VL. Perioperative arrhythmias after Fontan repair. *Circulation.* 1990;82(5 Suppl): IV190–IV194.

300. Gewillig M, Wyse RK, de Leval MR, Deanfield JE. Early and late arrhythmias after the Fontan operation: predisposing factors and clinical consequences. *Br Heart J.* 1992;67:72–79.

301. Balaji S, Gewillig M, Bull C, et al. Arrhythmias after the Fontan procedure. Comparison of total cavopulmonary connection and atriopulmonary connection. *Circulation.* 1991;84(5 Suppl): III162–III167.

302. Cecchin F, Johnsrude CL, Perry JC, Friedman RA. Effect of age and surgical technique on symptomatic arrhythmias after the Fontan procedure. *Am J Cardiol.* 1995;76:386–391.

303. Peters NS, Somerville J. Arrhythmias after the Fontan procedure. *Br Heart J.* 1992;68:199–204.

304. Cromme-Dijkhuis AH, Hess J, Hahlen K, et al. Specific sequelae after Fontan operation at mid- and long-term follow-up. Arrhythmia, liver dysfunction, and coagulation disorders. *J Thorac Cardiovasc Surg.* 1993;106:1126–1132.

305. Driscoll DJ, Offord KP, Feldt RH, et al. Five- to fifteen-year follow-up after Fontan operation. *Circulation.* 1992;85:469–496.

306. Kao JM, Alejos JC, Grant PW, et al. Conversion of atriopulmonary to cavopulmonary anastomosis in management of late arrhythmias and atrial thrombosis. *Ann Thorac Surg.* 1994;58: 1510–1514.

307. Kurer CC, Tanner CS, Vetter VL. Electrophysiologic findings after Fontan repair of functional single ventricle. *J Am Coll Cardiol.* 1991;17:174–181.

308. Sharratt GP, Johnson AM, Monro JL. Persistence and effects of sinus rhythm after Fontan procedure for tricuspid atresia. *Br Heart J.* 1979;42:74–80.

309. Battistessa SA, Ho SY, Anderson RH, et al. The arterial supply to the right atrium and the sinus node in classic tricuspid atresia. *J Thorac Cardiovasc Surg.* 1988;96:816–822.

310. Karpawich PP, Paridon SM, Pinsky WW. Failure of rate responsive ventricular pacing to improve physiological performance in the univentricular heart. *Pacing Clin Electrophysiol.* 1991;14:2058–2061.

311. Balaji S, Johnson TB, Sade RM, et al. Management of atrial flutter after the Fontan procedure. *J Am Coll Cardiol.* 1994;23: 1209–1215.

312. Mair DD, Rice MJ, Hagler DJ, et al. Outcome of the Fontan procedure in patients with tricuspid atresia. *Circulation.* 1985;72: II88–II92.

313. Kidd L, Driscoll DJ, Gersony WM, et al. Second natural history study of congenital heart defects. Results of treatment of patients with ventricular septal defects. *Circulation.* 1993;87(2 Suppl): I38–I51.

314. Wolfe RR, Driscoll DJ, Gersony WM, et al. Arrhythmias in patients with valvar aortic stenosis, valvar pulmonary stenosis, and ventricular septal defect. Results of 24-hour ECG monitoring. *Circulation.* 1993;87(2 Suppl):I89–I101.

315. Lev M. The architecture of the conduction system in congenital heart disease. III. Ventricular septal defect. *Arch Pathol.* 1960;70: 529–549.

316. Milo S, Ho SY, Wilkinson JL, Anderson RH. Surgical anatomy and atrioventricular conduction tissues of hearts with isolated ventricular septal defects. *J Thorac Cardiovasc Surg.* 1980;79:244–255.

317. Titus JL. Cardiac arrhythmias. 1. Anatomy of the conduction system. *Circulation.* 1973;47:170–177.

318. Hobbins SM, Izukawa T, Radford DJ, et al. Conduction disturbances after surgical correction of ventricular septal defect by the atrial approach. *Br Heart J.* 1979;41:289–293.

319. Kulbertus HE, Coyne JJ, Hallidie-Smith KA. Conduction disturbances before and after surgical closure of ventricular septal defect. *Am Heart J.* 1969;77:123–131.

320. Okoroma EO, Guller B, Maloney JD, Weidman WH. Etiology of right bundle-branch block pattern after surgical closure of ventricular-septal defects. *Am Heart J.* 1975;90:14–18.

321. Otterstad JE, Erikssen J, Froysaker T, Simonsen S. Long term results after operative treatment of isolated ventricular septal defect in adolescents and adults. *Acta Med Scand Suppl.* 1986;708:1–39.

322. van Lier TA, Harinck E, Hitchcock JF, et al. Complete right bundle branch block after surgical closure of perimembranous ventricular septal defect. Relation to type of ventriculotomy. *Eur Heart J.* 1985;6:959–962.

323. Ziady GM, Hallidie-Smith KA, Goodwin JF. Conduction disturbances after surgical closure of ventricular septal defect. *Br Heart J.* 1972;34:1199–1204.

324. Horowitz LN, Alexander JA, Edmunds LH Jr. Postoperative right bundle branch block: identification of three levels of block. *Circulation.* 1980;62:319–328.

325. Krongrad E, Malm JR, Bowman FO Jr, et al. Electrophysiological delineation of the specialized A-V conduction system in patients with congenital heart disease. II. Delineation of the distal His bundle and the right bundle branch. *Circulation.* 1974;49: 1232–1238.

326. Houyel L, Vaksmann G, Fournier A, Davignon A. Ventricular arrhythmias after correction of ventricular septal defects: importance of surgical approach. *J Am Coll Cardiol.* 1990;16:1224–1228.

327. Yabek SM, Jarmakani JM, Roberts NK. Diagnosis of trifascicular damage following tetralogy of Fallot and ventricular septal defect repair. *Circulation.* 1977;55:23–27.

328. Abe T, Komatsu S. Conduction disturbances and operative results after closure of ventricular septal defects by three different surgical approaches. *Jpn Circ J.* 1983;47:328–335.

329. Godman MJ, Roberts NK, Izukawa T. Late postoperative conduction disturbances after repair of ventricular septal defect and tetralogy of Fallot. Analysis by His bundle recordings. *Circulation.* 1974;49:214–221.

330. Pahlajani DB, Miller RA, Serratto M. Patterns of atrioventricular conduction in children. *Am Heart J.* 1975;90:165–171.

331. Wolff GS, Rowland TW, Ellison RC. Surgically induced right bundle-branch block with left anterior hemiblock. An ominous sign in postoperative tetralogy of Fallot. *Circulation.* 1972;46:587–594.

332. Blake RS, Chung EE, Wesley H, Hallidie-Smith KA. Conduction defects, ventricular arrhythmias, and late death after surgical closure of ventricular septal defect. *Br Heart J.* 1982;47:305–315.

333. Moller JH, Patton C, Varco RL, Lillehei CW. Late results (30 to 35 years) after operative closure of isolated ventricular septal defect from 1954 to 1960. *Am J Cardiol.* 1991;68:1491–1497.

334. Driscoll DJ, Gillette PC, Hallman GL, et al. Management of surgical complete atrioventricular block in children. *Am J Cardiol.* 1979;43:1175–1180.

335. Hofschire PJ, Nicoloff DM, Moller JH. Postoperative complete heart block in 64 children treated with and without cardiac pacing. *Am J Cardiol.* 1977;39:559–562.

336. Lauer RM, Ongley PA, Dushane JW, Kirklin JW. Heart block after repair of ventricular septal defect in children. *Circulation.* 1960;22:526–534.

337. Feldt RH, DuShane JW, Titus JL. The anatomy of the atrioventricular conduction system in ventricular septal defect and tetralogy of Fallot: correlations with the electrocardiogram and vectorcardiogram. *Circulation.* 1966;34:774–782.

338. Lev M. The architecture of the conduction system in congenital heart disease. II. Tetralogy of Fallot. *AMA Arch Pathol.* 1959;67:572–587.

339. Dickinson DF, Wilkinson JL, Smith A, et al. Variations in the morphology of the ventricular septal defect and disposition of the atrioventricular conduction tissues in tetralogy of Fallot. *Thorac Cardiovasc Surg.* 1982;30:243–249.

340. Kurosawa H, Imai Y. Surgical anatomy of the atrioventricular conduction bundle in tetralogy of Fallot. New findings relevant to the position of the sutures. *J Thorac Cardiovasc Surg.* 1988;95:586–591.

341. Thiene G, Mazzucco A, Anderson RH, et al. Tetralogy of Fallot after surgery: autopsy review of 14 cases. *Hum Pathol.* 1984;15:1018–1024.

342. Niederhauser H, Simonin P, Friedli B. Sinus node function and conduction system after complete repair of tetralogy of Fallot. *Circulation.* 1975;52:214–220.

343. Tamer D, Wolff GS, Ferrer P, et al. Hemodynamics and intracardiac conduction after operative repair of tetralogy of Fallot. *Am J Cardiol.* 1983;51:552–556.

344. Walsh EP, Rockenmacher S, Keane JF, et al. Late results in patients with tetralogy of Fallot repaired during infancy. *Circulation.* 1988;77:1062–1067.

345. Friedli B, Bolens M, Taktak M. Conduction disturbances after correction of tetralogy of Fallot: are electrophysiologic studies of prognostic value? *J Am Coll Cardiol.* 1988;11:162–165.

346. Hougen TJ, Dick M 2nd, Freed MD, Keane JF. His bundle electrogram after intracardiac repair of tetralogy of Fallot. Analysis of data in 59 patients. *Am J Cardiol.* 1978;41:552–558.

347. Zahka KG, Horneffer PJ, Rowe SA, et al. Long-term valvular function after total repair of tetralogy of Fallot. Relation to ventricular arrhythmias. *Circulation.* 1988;78:III14–III19.

348. Sondheimer HM, Izukawa T, Olley PM, et al. Conduction disturbances after total correction of tetralogy of Fallot. *Am Heart J.* 1976;92:278–282.

349. Gelband H, Waldo AL, Kaiser GA, et al. Etiology of right bundle-branch block in patients undergoing total correction of tetralogy of Fallot. *Circulation.* 1971;44:1022–1033.

350. Goor DA, Lavee J, Smolinsky A, et al. Correction of tetrad of Fallot with reduced incidence of right bundle branch block. *Am J Cardiol.* 1981;48:892–896.

351. Horowitz LN, Simson MB, Spear JF, et al. The mechanism of apparent right bundle branch block after transatrial repair of tetralogy of Fallot. *Circulation.* 1979;59:1241–1252.

352. Yabek SM, Jarmakani JM, Roberts N. Postoperative trifascicular block complicating tetralogy of Fallot repair. *Pediatrics.* 1976;58:236–242.

353. Bolens M, Friedli B. Progressive atrioventricular block after total correction of Fallot's tetralogy, documented by repeat electrophysiological studies. *Cardiology.* 1982;69:185–191.

354. Calder AL, Barratt-Boyes BG, Brandt PW, Neutze JM. Postoperative evaluation of patients with tetralogy of Fallot repaired in infancy. Including criteria for use of outflow patching and radiologic assessment of pulmonary regurgitation. *J Thorac Cardiovasc Surg.* 1979;77:704–720.

355. Chesler E, Beck W, Schrire V. Left anterior hemiblock and right bundle branch block before and after surgical repair of tetralogy of Fallot. *Am Heart J.* 1972;84:45–52.

356. Deanfield JE, McKenna WJ, Hallidie-Smith KA. Detection of late arrhythmia and conduction disturbance after correction of tetralogy of Fallot. *Br Heart J.* 1980;44:248–253.

357. Steeg CN, Krongrad E, Davachi F, et al. Postoperative left anterior hemiblock and right bundle branch block following repair of tetralogy of Fallot. Clinical and etiologic considerations. *Circulation.* 1975;51:1026–1029.

358. Deanfield JE, McKenna WJ, Presbitero P, et al. Ventricular arrhythmia in unrepaired and repaired tetralogy of Fallot. Relation to age, timing of repair, and haemodynamic status. *Br Heart J.* 1984;52:77–81.

359. Downing JW Jr, Kaplan S, Bove KE. Postsurgical left anterior hemiblock and right bundle-branch block. *Br Heart J.* 1972;34:263–270.

360. John S, Bhati BS, Shatpathy P, et al. Total surgical correction of tetralogy of Fallot. Results in 45 consecutive cases. *Thorax.* 1972;27:66–69.

361. John S, Sukumar IP, Cherian G, et al. Intracardiac repair in tetralogy of Fallot. Hemodynamic studies following corrective surgery. *Circulation.* 1974;49:958–961.

362. Trimble AS, Morch JE, Froggatt GM, Metni FN. Total intracardiac repair of the adult cyanotic tetralogy of Fallot: clinical experience and late follow-up. *Can Med Assoc J.* 1970;103:911–914.

363. Zhao HX, Miller DC, Reitz BA, Shumway NE. Surgical repair of tetralogy of Fallot. Long-term follow-up with particular emphasis on late death and reoperation. *J Thorac Cardiovasc Surg.* 1985;89:204–220.

364. Anderson PA, Rogers MC, Canent RV Jr, et al. Reversible complete heart block following cardiac surgery. Analysis of His bundle electrograms. *Circulation.* 1972;46:514–521.

365. Rosenthal A, Behrendt D, Sloan H, et al. Long-term prognosis (15 to 26 years) after repair of tetralogy of Fallot: I. Survival and symptomatic status. *Ann Thorac Surg.* 1984;38:151–156.

366. Karpawich PP, Jackson WL, Cavitt DL, Perry BL. Late-onset unprecedented complete atrioventricular block after tetralogy of Fallot repair: electrophysiologic findings. *Am Heart J.* 1987;114:654–656.

367. Neches WH, Park SC, Mathews RA, et al. Tetralogy of Fallot: postoperative electrophysiologic studies. *Circulation.* 1977;56:713–719.

368. Gillette PC, Yeoman MA, Mullins CE, McNamara DG. Sudden death after repair of tetralogy of Fallot. Electrocardiographic and electrophysiologic abnormalities. *Circulation.* 1977;56:566–571.

369. King SB, Franch RH. Production of increased right-to-left shunting by rapid heart rates in patients with tetralogy of Fallot. *Circulation.* 1971;44:265–271.

370. Young D, Elbl F. Supraventricular tachycardia as cause of cyanotic syncopal attacks in tetralogy of Fallot. *N Engl J Med.* 1971;284:1359–1360.

371. Quattlebaum TG, Varghese J, Neill CA, Donahoo JS. Sudden death among postoperative patients with tetralogy of Fallot: a follow-up study of 243 patients for an average of twelve years. *Circulation.* 1976;54:289–293.

372. Sullivan ID, Presbitero P, Gooch VM, et al. Is ventricular arrhythmia in repaired tetralogy of Fallot an effect of operation or a consequence of the course of the disease? A prospective study. *Br Heart J.* 1987;58:40–44.

373. Presbitero P, Demarie D, Aruta E, et al. Results of total correction of tetralogy of Fallot performed in adults. *Ann Thorac Surg.* 1988;46:297–301.

374. Waien SA, Liu PP, Ross BL, et al. Serial follow-up of adults with repaired tetralogy of Fallot. *J Am Coll Cardiol.* 1992;20:295–300.

375. Chandar JS, Wolff GS, Garson A Jr, et al. Ventricular arrhythmias in postoperative tetralogy of Fallot. *Am J Cardiol.* 1990;65: 655–661.

376. Kavey RE, Blackman MS, Sondheimer HM. Incidence and severity of chronic ventricular dysrhythmias after repair of tetralogy of Fallot. *Am Heart J.* 1982;103:342–350.

377. Deal BJ, Scagliotti D, Miller SM, et al. Electrophysiologic drug testing in symptomatic ventricular arrhythmias after repair of tetralogy of Fallot. *Am J Cardiol.* 1987;59:1380–1385.

378. Downar E, Harris L, Kimber S, et al. Ventricular tachycardia after surgical repair of tetralogy of Fallot: results of intraoperative mapping studies. *J Am Coll Cardiol.* 1992;20:648–655.

379. Dunnigan A, Pritzker MR, Benditt DG, Benson DW Jr. Life threatening ventricular tachycardias in late survivors of surgically corrected tetralogy of Fallot. *Br Heart J.* 1984;52:198–206.

380. Garson A Jr, Porter CB, Gillette PC, McNamara DG. Induction of ventricular tachycardia during electrophysiologic study after repair of tetralogy of Fallot. *J Am Coll Cardiol.* 1983;1:1493–1502.

381. Horowitz LN, Vetter VL, Harken AH, Josephson ME. Electrophysiologic characteristics of sustained ventricular tachycardia occurring after repair of tetralogy of Fallot. *Am J Cardiol.* 1980;46: 446–452.

382. Kugler JD, Pinsky WW, Cheatham JP, et al. Sustained ventricular tachycardia after repair of tetralogy of Fallot: new electrophysiologic findings. *Am J Cardiol.* 1983;51:1137–1143.

383. Mehta AV, Sanchez GR. Sustained ventricular tachycardia after repair of tetralogy of Fallot: new electrophysiologic findings. *Am J Cardiol.* 1984;53:989.

384. Oda H, Aizawa Y, Murata M, et al. A successful electrical ablation of recurrent sustained ventricular tachycardia in a postoperative case of tetralogy of Fallot. *Jpn Heart J.* 1986;27:421–428.

385. Swerdlow CD, Oyer PE, Pitlick PT. Septal origin of sustained ventricular tachycardia in a patient with right ventricular outflow tract obstruction after correction of tetralogy of Fallot. *Pacing Clin Electrophysiol.* 1986;9:584–588.

386. Garson A Jr, Nihill MR, McNamara DG, Cooley DA. Status of the adult and adolescent after repair of tetralogy of Fallot. *Circulation.* 1979;59:1232–1240.

387. Dietl CA, Cazzaniga ME, Dubner SJ, et al. Life-threatening arrhythmias and RV dysfunction after surgical repair of tetralogy of Fallot. Comparison between transventricular and transatrial approaches. *Circulation.* 1994;90:II7–II12.

388. Joffe H, Georgakopoulos D, Celermajer DS, et al. Late ventricular arrhythmia is rare after early repair of tetralogy of Fallot. *J Am Coll Cardiol.* 1994;23:1146–1150.

389. Cullen S, Celermajer DS, Franklin RC, et al. Prognostic significance of ventricular arrhythmia after repair of tetralogy of Fallot: a 12-year prospective study. *J Am Coll Cardiol.* 1994;23:1151–1155.

390. Garson A Jr, Gillette PC, Gutgesell HP, McNamara DG. Stress-induced ventricular arrhythmia after repair of tetralogy of Fallot. *Am J Cardiol.* 1980;46:1006–1012.

391. Manolis AS, Chiladakis JA, Malakos JS, et al. Abnormal signal averaged electrocardiogram in patients with incomplete right bundle branch block. *Clin Cardiol.* 1997;20:17–22.

392. Irving JB, Godman MJ. Exercise testing and ambulatory electrocardiographic monitoring following surgical repair of tetralogy of Fallot. *Eur Heart J.* 1980;1:117–121.

393. Kremers MS, Wells PJ, Black WH, Solodyna MA. Entrainment of ventricular tachycardia in postoperative tetralogy of Fallot. *Pacing Clin Electrophysiol.* 1988;11:1310–1314.

394. Gatzoulis MA, Till JA, Somerville J, Redington AN. Mechano-electrical interaction in tetralogy of Fallot. QRS prolongation relates to right ventricular size and predicts malignant ventricular arrhythmias and sudden death. *Circulation.* 1995;92: 231–237.

395. Giroud D, Zimmermann M, Adamec R, et al. Ventricular late potentials and spontaneous ventricular arrhythmias after surgical repair of tetralogy of Fallot: do they have prognostic value? *Br Heart J.* 1994;72:580–583.

396. Simson MB, Untereker WJ, Spielman SR, et al. Relation between late potentials on the body surface and directly recorded fragmented electrograms in patients with ventricular tachycardia. *Am J Cardiol.* 1983;51:105–112.

397. Vaksmann G, el Kohen M, Lacroix D, et al. Influence of clinical and hemodynamic characteristics on signal-averaged electrocardiogram in postoperative tetralogy of Fallot. *Am J Cardiol.* 1993;71:317–321.

398. Chen D, Moller JH. Comparison of late clinical status between patients with different hemodynamic findings after repair of tetralogy of Fallot. *Am Heart J.* 1987;113:767–772.

399. Dreyer WJ, Paridon SM, Fisher DJ, Garson A Jr. Rapid ventricular pacing in dogs with right ventricular outflow tract obstruction: insights into a mechanism of sudden death in postoperative tetralogy of Fallot. *J Am Coll Cardiol.* 1993;21:1731–1737.

400. Kavey RE, Thomas FD, Byrum CJ, et al. Ventricular arrhythmias and biventricular dysfunction after repair of tetralogy of Fallot. *J Am Coll Cardiol.* 1984;4:126–131.

401. Bharati S, McCue CM, Tingelstad JB, et al. Lack of connection between the atria and the peripheral conduction system in a case of corrected transposition with congenital atrioventricular block. *Am J Cardiol.* 1978;42:147–153.

402. Gillette PC, Reitman MJ, Mullins CE, et al. Electrophysiology of ventricular inversion. *Br Heart J.* 1974;36:971–980.

403. Kupersmith J, Krongrad E, Gersony WM, Bowman FO Jr. Electrophysiologic identification of the specialized conduction system in corrected transposition of the great arteries. *Circulation.* 1974;50: 795–800.

404. Waldo AL, Pacifico AD, Bargeron LM, et al. Electrophysiological delineation of the specialized A-V conduction system in patients with corrected transposition of the great vessels and ventricular septal defect. *Circulation.* 1975;52:435–441.

405. Wilkinson JL, Smith A, Lincoln C, Anderson RH. Conducting tissues in congenitally corrected transposition with situs inversus. *Br Heart J.* 1978;40:41–48.

406. Huhta JC, Maloney JD, Ritter DG, et al. Complete atrioventricular block in patients with atrioventricular discordance. *Circulation.* 1983;67:1374–1377.

407. Bharati S, Rosen K, Steinfield L, et al. The anatomic substrate for preexcitation in corrected transposition. *Circulation.* 1980;62: 831–842.

408. Daliento L, Corrado D, Buja G, et al. Rhythm and conduction disturbances in isolated, congenitally corrected transposition of the great arteries. *Am J Cardiol.* 1986;58:314–318.

409. Nakajima K, Bunko H, Tonami N, et al. Congenitally corrected transposition of the great arteries associated with the pre-excitation syndrome. *Clin Nucl Med.* 1986;11:564–567.

410. Gillette PC, Busch U, Mullins CE, McNamara DG. Electrophysiologic studies in patients with ventricular inversion and "corrected transposition." *Circulation.* 1979;60:939–945.

411. Perloff JK. *The Clinical Recognition of Congenital Heart Disease.* 5th ed. Philadelphia: W.B. Saunders; 2003.

412. Amikam S, Lemer J, Kishon Y, et al. Complete heart block in an adult with corrected transposition of the great arteries treated with permanent pacemaker. *Thorax.* 1979;34:547–549.

413. Foster JR, Damato AN, Kline LE, et al. Congenitally corrected transposition of the great vessels: localization of the site of complete atrioventricular block using His bundle electrograms. *Am J Cardiol.* 1976;38:383–387.

414. Rosen KM, Loeb HS, Gunnar RM, Rahimtoola SH. Mobitz type II block without bundle-branch block. *Circulation.* 1971;44:1111–1119.

415. Berman DA, Adicoff A. Corrected transposition of the great arteries causing complete heart block in an adult. Treatment with an artificial pacemaker. *Am J Cardiol.* 1969;24:125–129.

416. Friedberg DZ, Nadas AS. Clinical profile of patients with congenital corrected transposition of the great arteries. A study of 60 cases. *N Engl J Med.* 1970;282:1053–1059.

417. de Leval MR, Bastos P, Stark J, et al. Surgical technique to reduce the risks of heart block following closure of ventricular septal defect in atrioventricular discordance. *J Thorac Cardiovasc Surg.* 1979;78:515–526.

418. Hwang B, Bowman F, Malm J, Krongrad E. Surgical repair of congenitally corrected transposition of the great arteries: results and follow-up. *Am J Cardiol.* 1982;50:781–785.

419. McGrath LB, Kirklin JW, Blackstone EH, et al. Death and other events after cardiac repair in discordant atrioventricular connection. *J Thorac Cardiovasc Surg.* 1985;90:711–728.

420. Champsaur G, Trusler GA, Mustard WT. Congenital discrete subvalvar aortic stenosis. Surgical experience and long-term follow-up in 20 paediatric patients. *Br Heart J.* 1973;35:443–446.

421. Somerville J, Stone S, Ross D. Fate of patients with fixed subaortic stenosis after surgical removal. *Br Heart J.* 1980;43:629–647.

422. Keane JF, Driscoll DJ, Gersony WM, et al. Second natural history study of congenital heart defects. Results of treatment of patients with aortic valvar stenosis. *Circulation.* 1993;87(2 Suppl): I16–I27.

423. Kastor JA, Goldreyer BN, Josephson ME, et al. Electrophysiologic characteristics of Ebstein's anomaly of the tricuspid valve. *Circulation.* 1975;52:987–995.

424. Smith WM, Gallagher JJ, Kerr CR, et al. The electrophysiologic basis and management of symptomatic recurrent tachycardia in patients with Ebstein's anomaly of the tricuspid valve. *Am J Cardiol.* 1982;49:1223–1234.

425. Oh JK, Holmes DR Jr, Hayes DL, et al. Cardiac arrhythmias in patients with surgical repair of Ebstein's anomaly. *J Am Coll Cardiol.* 1985;6:1351–1357.

426. Price JE, Amsterdam EA, Vera Z, et al. Ebstein's disease associated with complete atrioventricular block. *Chest.* 1978;73:542–544.

427. Kumar AE, Fyler DC, Miettinen OS, Nadas AS. Ebstein's anomaly. Clinical profile and natural history. *Am J Cardiol.* 1971;28:84–95.

428. Celermajer DS, Bull C, Till JA, et al. Ebstein's anomaly: presentation and outcome from fetus to adult. *J Am Coll Cardiol.* 1994;23:170–176.

429. Watson H. Natural history of Ebstein's anomaly of tricuspid valve in childhood and adolescence. An international co-operative study of 505 cases. *Br Heart J.* 1974;36:417–427.

430. Inoue H, Matsuo H, Takayanagi K, et al. Antidromic reciprocating tachycardia via a slow Kent bundle in Ebstein's anomaly. *Am Heart J.* 1983;106:147–149.

431. Rossi L, Thiene G. Mild Ebstein's anomaly associated with supraventricular tachycardia and sudden death: clinicomorphologic features in 3 patients. *Am J Cardiol.* 1984;53:332–334.

432. Klein GJ, Bashore TM, Sellers TD, et al. Ventricular fibrillation in the Wolff-Parkinson-White syndrome. *N Engl J Med.* 1979;301:1080–1085.

433. McGovern B, Garan H, Ruskin JN. Precipitation of cardiac arrest by verapamil in patients with Wolff-Parkinson-White syndrome. *Ann Intern Med.* 1986;104:791–794.

434. Wellens HJ, Durrer D. Effect of digitalis on atrioventricular conduction and circus-movement tachycardias in patients with Wolff-Parkinson-White syndrome. *Circulation.* 1973;47:1229–1233.

435. Kocheril AG, Rosenfeld LE. Radiofrequency ablation of an accessory pathway in a patient with corrected Ebstein's anomaly. *Pacing Clin Electrophysiol.* 1994;17:986–990.

436. Andress JD, Vander Salm TJ, Huang SK. Bidirectional bundle branch reentry tachycardia associated with Ebstein's anomaly: cured by extensive cryoablation of the right bundle branch. *Pacing Clin Electrophysiol.* 1991;14:1639–1647.

437. Lo HM, Lin FY, Jong YS, et al. Ebstein's anomaly with ventricular tachycardia: evidence for the arrhythmogenic role of the atrialized ventricle. *Am Heart J.* 1989;117:959–962.

438. Abe T, Komatsu S. Valve replacement for Ebstein's anomaly of the tricuspid valve. Early and long-term results of eight cases. *Chest.* 1983;84:414–417.

439. Danielson GK, Maloney JD, Devloo RA. Surgical repair of Ebstein's anomaly. *Mayo Clin Proc.* 1979;54:185–192.

440. Iwa T, Teranaka M, Tsuchiya K, et al. Simultaneous surgery for Wolff-Parkinson-White syndrome combined with Ebstein's anomaly. Interruption of multiple accessory conduction pathways. *Thorac Cardiovasc Surg.* 1980;28:42–47.

441. Pressley JC, Wharton JM, Tang AS, et al. Effect of Ebstein's anomaly on short- and long-term outcome of surgically treated patients with Wolff-Parkinson-White syndrome. *Circulation.* 1992;86:1147–1155.

442. Ross D, Somerville J. Surgical correction of Ebstein's anomaly. *Lancet.* 1970;2:280–284.

443. Sealy WC, Gallagher JJ, Pritchett EL, Wallace AG. Surgical treatment of tachyarrhythmias in patients with both an Ebstein anomaly and a Kent bundle. *J Thorac Cardiovasc Surg.* 1978;75:847–853.

444. Raj Behl P, Blesovsky A. Ebstein's anomaly: sixteen years' experience with valve replacement without plication of the right ventricle. *Thorax.* 1984;39:8–13.

445. Basso C, Thiene G, Corrado D, et al. Arrhythmogenic right ventricular cardiomyopathy. Dysplasia, dystrophy, or myocarditis? *Circulation.* 1996;94:983–991.

446. Laurent M, Descaves C, Biron Y, et al. Familial form of arrhythmogenic right ventricular dysplasia. *Am Heart J.* 1987;113:827–829.

447. Nava A, Thiene G, Canciani B, et al. Familial occurrence of right ventricular dysplasia: a study involving nine families. *J Am Coll Cardiol.* 1988;12:1222–1228.

448. Carlson MD, White RD, Trohman RG, et al. Right ventricular outflow tract ventricular tachycardia: detection of previously unrecognized anatomic abnormalities using cine magnetic resonance imaging. *J Am Coll Cardiol.* 1994;24:720–727.

449. Nogami A, Adachi S, Nitta J, et al. Arrhythmogenic right ventricular dysplasia with sick sinus syndrome and atrioventricular conduction disturbance. *Jpn Heart J.* 1990;31:417–423.

450. Fontaine G, Umemura J, Di Donna P, et al. [Duration of QRS complexes in arrhythmogenic right ventricular dysplasia. A new non-invasive diagnostic marker]. *Ann Cardiol Angeiol (Paris).* 1993;42:399–405.

451. Fontaine G, Guiraudon G, Frank R, et al. Stimulation studies and epicardial mapping in ventricular tachycardia: study of mechanisms and selection for surgery. In: Kulbertus HE, ed. *Reentrant Arrhythmias.* Lancaster, England: MTP Publishing; 1977:334.

452. Metzger JT, de Chillou C, Cheriex E, et al. Value of the 12-lead electrocardiogram in arrhythmogenic right ventricular dysplasia, and absence of correlation with echocardiographic findings. *Am J Cardiol.* 1993;72:964–967.

453. Kinoshita O, Fontaine G, Rosas F, et al. Time- and frequency-domain analyses of the signal-averaged ECG in patients with arrhythmogenic right ventricular dysplasia. *Circulation.* 1995;91:715–721.

454. Leclercq JF, Coumel P. Late potentials in arrhythmogenic right ventricular dysplasia. Prevalence, diagnostic and prognostic values. *Eur Heart J.* 1993;14(Suppl E):80–83.

455. Lemery R, Brugada P, Janssen J, et al. Nonischemic sustained ventricular tachycardia: clinical outcome in 12 patients with arrhythmogenic right ventricular dysplasia. *J Am Coll Cardiol.* 1989;14:96–105.

456. Tonet JL, Castro-Miranda R, Iwa T, et al. Frequency of supraventricular tachyarrhythmias in arrhythmogenic right ventricular dysplasia. *Am J Cardiol.* 1991;67:1153.

457. Reiter MJ, Smith WM, Gallagher JJ. Clinical spectrum of ventricular tachycardia with left bundle branch morphology. *Am J Cardiol.* 1983;51:113–121.

458. Thiene G, Nava A, Corrado D, et al. Right ventricular cardiomyopathy and sudden death in young people. *N Engl J Med.* 1988;318:129–133.

459. Di Biase M, Favale S, Massari V, et al. Programmed stimulation in patients with minor forms of right ventricular dysplasia. *Eur Heart J.* 1989;10(Suppl D):49–53.

460. Haissaguerre M, Le Metayer P, D'Ivernois C, et al. Distinctive response of arrhythmogenic right ventricular disease to high dose isoproterenol. *Pacing Clin Electrophysiol.* 1990;13:2119–2126.

461. Guiraudon G, Fontaine G, Frank R, et al. Surgical treatment of ventricular tachycardia guided by ventricular mapping in 23 patients without coronary artery disease. *Ann Thorac Surg.* 1981;32:439–450.

462. Guiraudon GM, Klein GJ, Gulamhusein SS, et al. Total disconnection of the right ventricular free wall: surgical treatment of right ventricular tachycardia associated with right ventricular dysplasia. *Circulation.* 1983;67:463–470.

463. Leclercq JF, Chouty F, Cauchemez B, et al. Results of electrical fulguration in arrhythmogenic right ventricular disease. *Am J Cardiol.* 1988;62:220–224.

464. Leclercq JF, Coumel P. Characteristics, prognosis and treatment of the ventricular arrhythmias of right ventricular dysplasia. *Eur Heart J.* 1989;10(Suppl D):61–67.

465. Wichter T, Borggrefe M, Haverkamp W, et al. Efficacy of antiarrhythmic drugs in patients with arrhythmogenic right ventricular disease. Results in patients with inducible and noninducible ventricular tachycardia. *Circulation.* 1992;86:29–37.

466. Hohnloser SH, Woosley RL. Sotalol. *N Engl J Med.* 1994;331:31–38.

467. Sano S, Ishino K, Kawada M, et al. Total right ventricular exclusion procedure: an operation for isolated congestive right ventricular failure. *J Thorac Cardiovasc Surg.* 2002;123:640–647.

468. Chenard J, Samson M, Beaulieu M. Embryonal sinusoids in the myocardium: report of a Case Successfully Treated Surgically. *Can Med Assoc J.* 1965;92:1356–1359.

469. Chin TK, Perloff JK, Williams RG, et al. Isolated noncompaction of left ventricular myocardium. A study of eight cases. *Circulation.* 1990;82:507–513.

470. Jenni R, Goebel N, Tartini R, et al. Persisting myocardial sinusoids of both ventricles as an isolated anomaly: echocardiographic, angiographic, and pathologic anatomical findings. *Cardiovasc Intervent Radiol.* 1986;9:127–131.

471. Gerlis LM, Schmidt-Ott SC, Ho SY, Anderson RH. Dysplastic conditions of the right ventricular myocardium: Uhl's anomaly vs arrhythmogenic right ventricular dysplasia. *Br Heart J.* 1993;69:142–150.

472. Uhl HS. A previously undescribed congenital malformation of the heart: almost total absence of the myocardium of the right ventricle. *Bull Johns Hopkins Hosp.* 1952;91:197–209.

473. de Paola AA, Horowitz LN, Morganroth J, et al. Influence of left ventricular dysfunction on flecainide therapy. *J Am Coll Cardiol.* 1987;9:163–168.

474. Greene HL, Richardson DW, Hallstrom AP, et al. Congestive heart failure after acute myocardial infarction in patients receiving antiarrhythmic agents for ventricular premature complexes (Cardiac Arrhythmia Pilot Study). *Am J Cardiol.* 1989;63:393–398.

475. Podrid PJ, Schoeneberger A, Lown B. Congestive heart failure caused by oral disopyramide. *N Engl J Med.* 1980;302:614–617.

476. Story JR, Abdulla AM, Frank MJ. Cardiogenic shock and disopyramide phosphate. *JAMA.* 1979;242:654–655.

477. Clyne CA, Estes NA 3rd, et al. *N Engl J Med.* 1992;327:255–260.

478. Goldberg D, Reiffel JA, Davis JC, et al. Electrophysiologic effects of procainamide on sinus function in patients with and without sinus node disease. *Am Heart J.* 1982;103:75–79.

479. Hellestrand KJ, Nathan AW, Bexton RS, Camm AJ. Electrophysiologic effects of flecainide acetate on sinus node function, anomalous atrioventricular connections, and pacemaker thresholds. *Am J Cardiol.* 1984;53:30B–38B.

480. Mason JW. Amiodarone. *N Engl J Med.* 1987;316:455–466.

481. Reiffel JA, Bigger JT Jr, Cramer M. Effects of digoxin on sinus nodal function before and after vagal blockade in patients with sinus nodal dysfunction: a clue to the mechanisms of the action of digitalis on the sinus node. *Am J Cardiol.* 1979;43:983–989.

482. Touboul P. Electrophysiologic properties of sotalol and d-sotalol. A current view. *Eur Heart J.* 1993;14(Suppl H):24–29.

483. Anastasiou-Nana MI, Anderson JL, Stewart JR, et al. Occurrence of exercise-induced and spontaneous wide complex tachycardia during therapy with flecainide for complex ventricular arrhythmias: a probable proarrhythmic effect. *Am Heart J.* 1987;113:1071–1077.

484. Morganroth J, Anderson JL, Gentzkow GD. Classification by type of ventricular arrhythmia predicts frequency of adverse cardiac events from flecainide. *J Am Coll Cardiol.* 1986;8:607–615.

485. Perry JC, McQuinn RL, Smith RT Jr, et al. Flecainide acetate for resistant arrhythmias in the young: efficacy and pharmacokinetics. *J Am Coll Cardiol.* 1989;14:185–191; discussion 192–183.

486. Stanton MS, Prystowsky EN, Fineberg NS, et al. Arrhythmogenic effects of antiarrhythmic drugs: a study of 506 patients treated for ventricular tachycardia or fibrillation. *J Am Coll Cardiol.* 1989;14:209–215; discussion 216–207.

487. Surawicz B. Electrophysiologic substrate of torsade de pointes: dispersion of repolarization or early afterdepolarizations? *J Am Coll Cardiol.* 1989;14:172–184.

488. Roden DM, Woosley RL, Primm RK. Incidence and clinical features of the quinidine-associated long QT syndrome: implications for patient care. *Am Heart J.* 1986;111:1088–1093.

489. Paul T, Guccione P. New antiarrhythmic drugs in pediatric use: amiodarone. *Pediatr Cardiol.* 1994;15:132–138.

490. Torres V, Tepper D, Flowers D, et al. QT prolongation and the antiarrhythmic efficacy of amiodarone. *J Am Coll Cardiol.* 1986;7:142–147.

491. Coromilas J, Saltman AE, Waldecker B, et al. Electrophysiological effects of flecainide on anisotropic conduction and reentry in infarcted canine hearts. *Circulation.* 1995;91:2245–2263.

492. Echt DS, Liebson PR, Mitchell LB, et al. Mortality and morbidity in patients receiving encainide, flecainide, or placebo. The Cardiac Arrhythmia Suppression Trial. *N Engl J Med.* 1991;324:781–788.

493. Perry JC, Garson A Jr. Flecainide acetate for treatment of tachyarrhythmias in children: review of world literature on efficacy, safety, and dosing. *Am Heart J.* 1992;124:1614–1621.

494. Kim SS, Lal R, Ruffy R. Treatment of paroxysmal reentrant supraventricular tachycardia with flecainide acetate. *Am J Cardiol.* 1986;58:80–85.

495. Musto B, Cavallaro C, Musto A, et al. Flecainide single oral dose for management of paroxysmal supraventricular tachycardia in children and young adults. *Am Heart J.* 1992;124:110–115.

496. Maragnes P, Tipple M, Fournier A. Effectiveness of oral sotalol for treatment of pediatric arrhythmias. *Am J Cardiol.* 1992;69:751–754.

497. Pfammatter JP, Paul T, Lehmann C, Kallfelz HC. Efficacy and proarrhythmia of oral sotalol in pediatric patients. *J Am Coll Cardiol.* 1995;26:1002–1007.

498. Pongiglione G, Strasburger JF, Deal BJ, Benson DW Jr. Use of amiodarone for short-term and adjuvant therapy in young patients. *Am J Cardiol.* 1991;68:603–608.

499. Coumel P, Lucet V, Do Ngoc D. The use of amiodarone in children. *Pacing Clin Electrophysiol.* 1983;6:930–939.

500. Garson A Jr, Gillette PC, McVey P, et al. Amiodarone treatment of critical arrhythmias in children and young adults. *J Am Coll Cardiol.* 1984;4:749–755.

501. Guccione P, Paul T, Garson A Jr. Long-term follow-up of amiodarone therapy in the young: continued efficacy, unimpaired growth, moderate side effects. *J Am Coll Cardiol.* 1990;15:1118–1124.

502. Herre JM, Ross BA. Amiodarone in children: borrowing from the future? *J Am Coll Cardiol.* 1990;15:1125–1126.

503. Van Hare GF, Lesh MD, Stanger P. Radiofrequency catheter ablation of supraventricular arrhythmias in patients with congenital heart disease: results and technical considerations. *J Am Coll Cardiol.* 1993;22:883–890.

504. Goldner BG, Cooper R, Blau W, Cohen TJ. Radiofrequency catheter ablation as a primary therapy for treatment of ventricular tachycardia in a patient after repair of tetralogy of Fallot. *Pacing Clin Electrophysiol.* 1994;17:1441–1446.

505. Case CL, Crawford FA, Gillette PC, et al. Management strategies for surgical treatment of dysrhythmias in infants and children. *Am J Cardiol.* 1989;63:1069–1073.

506. Cox JL, Boineau JP, Schuessler RB, et al. Five-year experience with the maze procedure for atrial fibrillation. *Ann Thorac Surg.* 1993;56:814–823; discussion 823–814.

507. Garrey WE. The nature of fibrillary contraction of the heart—its relation to tissue mass and form. *Am J Physiol.* 1914;33:397.

508. Winkle RA, Mead RH, Ruder MA, et al. Long-term outcome with the automatic implantable cardioverter-defibrillator. *J Am Coll Cardiol.* 1989;13:1353–1361.

509. Kral MA, Spotnitz HM, Hordof A, et al. Automatic implantable cardioverter defibrillator implantation for malignant ventricular arrhythmias associated with congenital heart disease. *Am J Cardiol.* 1989;63:118–119.

510. Kron J, Oliver RP, Norsted S, Silka MJ. The automatic implantable cardioverter-defibrillator in young patients. *J Am Coll Cardiol.* 1990;16:896–902.

511. Bertholet M, Demoulin JC, Waleffe A, Kulbertus H. Programmable extrastimulus pacing for long-term management of supraventricular and ventricular tachycardias: clinical experience in 16 patients. *Am Heart J.* 1985;110:582–589.

512. Rhodes LA, Walsh EP, Gamble WJ, et al. Benefits and potential risks of atrial antitachycardia pacing after repair of congenital heart disease. *Pacing Clin Electrophysiol.* 1995;18:1005–1016.

Myocardial Growth and the Development and Regression of Increased Ventricular Mass

JOSEPH K. PERLOFF

Three hundred years ago, William Harvey wrote in *De Motu Cordis* that "the left ventricle requires to be stronger, inasmuch as the blood which it propels has to be driven through the whole body . . . and this, too, is the reason why the left ventricle . . . has parities three times thicker and stronger than those of the right."[1] Implicit in these remarks was an awareness of one of the most fundamental biologic properties of the mammalian heart—its capacity to adapt to functional requirements. Ventricular myocardium achieves adaptation because of its capacity to increase mass in response to hemodynamic, hormonal, and genetic stimuli.[2,3]

The *left ventricle* is the ancient systemic pump of the phylum Chordata that includes mammals, amphibians, reptiles, birds, and fish. In non-air-breathing fish and amphibians, gills in pharyngeal clefts serve as organs of gas exchange between water and blood. The *right ventricle*, by contrast, is a "recent" evolutionary adaptation that appeared beneath the conus arteriosus during the Jurassic Period 206 to 144 million years ago as a crucial cardiovascular adaptation to the air-breathing and land-living of Amniotes whose embryonic development is within a membrane, the amniotic sac. The right and left ventricles develop from the same heart tube during morphogenesis, but they evolve into structures with so many different characteristics that, with some justification, they may be regarded as two different organs—"two hearts that beat as one."[4] These comments not withstanding, the newly described "helical heart" is composed of remarkable encircling muscle bundles that bind the two ventricles together into a highly interdependent functional unit[5] (Fig. 23–1; discussed later).

This chapter is concerned with normal intrauterine cardiac growth, normal extrauterine cardiac growth from birth to cardiomyocyte maturity, an increase in growth (ventricular mass) in excess of normal, and finally regression of increased ventricular mass. Congenital malformations of the heart and circulation are inciting stimuli that provoke an increase cardiac mass beyond its normal intrauterine and extrauterine growth potentials. Reparative surgery serves to reduce, if not eliminate, the inciting stimuli, setting the stage for regression of increased cardiac mass.

Ventricular mass is a term that does not beg the question of its biologic basis. From the cell biologic point of view, *hypertrophy* refers to an increase in size of preexisting cells, whereas *hyperplasia* refers to an increase in the number of cells because of mitotic division.[6] From a gross morphologic point of view, an increase in ventricular mass is referred to as hypertrophy.

"... the superbly beautiful and complex molecular machinery that enables the heart to fulfill its crucial role in the circulatory system can only function within an architectural design that allows the contractile apparatus to perform with mechanical efficiency determined by the appropriate integration of the vectors of force generated by shortening of cardiac sarcomeres."[7]

In *Tractatus de Corde* (1669), Richard Lower described the scroll-like structure of cardiac muscle as a spiral apical vortex.[8] Twenty years later, Giovanni Borelli provided physiologic insight into the spiral vortex by applying principles of mechanical physics to muscle movement, characterizing left ventricular ejection as a wringing mechanical motion.[9,10] More than 300 years elapsed

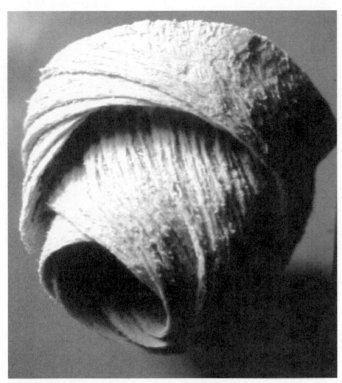

FIGURE 23-1   Biventricular muscle band: a helix with oblique fibers forms the apical loop, and a transverse buttress forms the basal loop. *(From Buckberg, G.D.: Semin Thorac Cardiovasc Surg. 2001;298–319. Used with permission.)*

before the architectural arrangement of ventricular muscle mass—the Gordian knot of cardiac anatomy—was unraveled.[9,10] The beauty of the heart's geometry is its simple bandlike structure characterized by a spiral double helix capable of contraction[10] (Fig. 23-2). Ventricular myocardial mass consists of a muscular band that com-

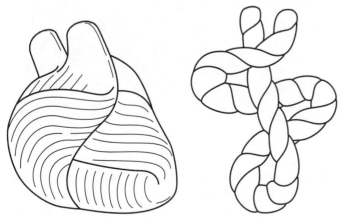

FIGURE 23-2   The heart showing basal and helical loops. The rope model illustrates the three segments of the architectural pattern: (1) the point of origin at the pulmonary artery and termination at the aorta, (2) the circumferential wrap around the basal loop, and (3) the helix that includes the descending and ascending segments of the apical loop. *(From Buckberg, G.D.: Semin Thorac Cardiovasc Surg. 2001;298–319. Used with permission.)*

prises two spirals curling in a helical manner from just below the pulmonary artery to the base of the aorta. Using hand dissection of a boiled heart, Torrent-Guasp unwrapped the organ and uncovered the ventricular myocardial fold[10] (see Figs. 23-1 and 23-2). The anatomic basis of the wringing motion of cardiac contraction was revealed at last (Fig. 23-3).

NORMAL INTRAUTERINE CARDIAC GROWTH

Developmental biology as a discipline was founded by Wilhelm Roux and his colleagues in 1894 and has now come full flower.[11,12] How seemingly homogeneous masses of early embryonic cells are transformed into tissues and organs that form a complex living creature is a process that continues to excite and mystify.[13]

Goethe regarded the human heart as the "most diverse, most changeable, most versatile part of creation." The vertebrate heart is the first organ to form and function[11] and, accordingly, has been of special interest to developmental biologists. There are three stages of intrauterine cardiac development: (1) cytodifferentiation, (2) formation and looping of the straight cardiac tube, and (3) the postlooping stage.[11,14,15] Cytodifferentiation refers to the development of specific cell lines from undifferentiated progenitor cells within the anterior lateral mesoderm.[11,15,16] Before tissues or organs can emerge, cytodifferentiation "informs" cells about who they are and what tissues they are destined to form.[12] The process of gastrulation refers to movements and infoldings of embryonic cells destined to become endoderm in early animal embryos, immediately following the blastoderm stage. Beginning shortly after gastrulation (about human embryonic day 20), progenitor cells are committed to a cardiogenic outcome.[11] However, the molecular factors responsible for that commitment are for the most part unknown.[11,17] Once differentiated, cells have specific destinies that they are bound to fulfill, and thus cardiac morphogenesis can then commence from the first embryonic tissue layers to the completely formed heart. Cytodifferentiation results in myoblastic synthesis of cell-specific contractile proteins (myosin and actin). Thick and thin filaments appear within the cytoplasm of these primitive cells.[18–20] Contractile proteins have been synthesized in cultures of isolated cardiac myocytes before the cells beat. Contractile proteins and myocyte contractility are therefore independent of hemodynamic forces (discussed later).

The primitive straight cardiac tube is derived from precursors that form a bilaterally symmetric cardiogenic "field," which evolves into parallel cardiac primordia that fuse at the midline.[11,21]

The newly formed single straight tubular human heart is composed of a pure population of myocytes and a simple endothelium.[22] Rhythmic contractions begin 18 to 21 days

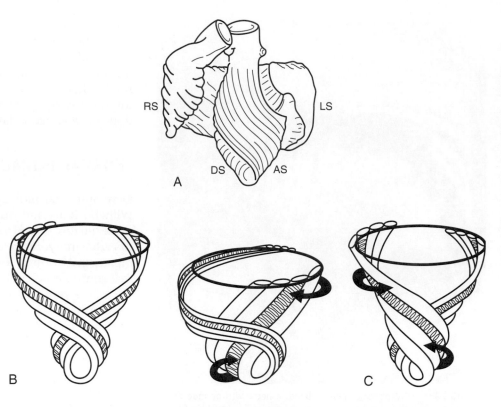

FIGURE 23-3 **(A)** Schematic representation of the ventricular myocardial band with the descending and ascending segments relaxed (no contraction). **(B)** Contraction of the descending segment initiates counterclockwise rotation of the ventricular base *(upper arrow)* and clockwise rotation of the apex *(lower arrow)*, two opposite rotations that are responsible for the agonist twisting of the ventricular mass and descent of the base. **(C)** Contraction of the ascending segment initiates *clockwise rotation of the ventricular base (upper arrow)* and counterclockwise rotation of the apex *(lower arrow)*, opposite rotations that are responsible for the antagonistic untwisting of the ventricular mass and ascent of the base. *(From Buckberg, G.D.: Semin Thorac Cardiovasc Surg. 2001;298–319. Used with permission.)*

after conception. At this stage, the heart serves no circulatory function, but if the beat stops, the fetus dies. The straight tube then undergoes rightward looping, which is the first major morphologic transformation of the developing heart and the first indication in the embryo of left-right asymmetry.[11] Looping to the right occurs in all vertebrate species, but there is little information in animal morphogenesis regarding the cellular or molecular basis for left-right differences.[23]

In the postlooping stage, atrial and ventricular chambers are morphologically identifiable, although cells from these chambers arise from separate lineages that are specified before looping occurs.[11] Atrial and ventricular myocytes express distinct subsets of cardiac muscle genes that confer contractile, electrophysiologic, and pharmacologic properties unique to each chamber.[11] Cardiomyocytes normally comprise 75% of myocardial tissue volume but constitute only 30% to 40% of the cell population, with fibroblasts constituting the majority of nonmyocytes[24-26] (Figs. 23–4 and 23–5). The postlooping stage is accompanied by rapid proliferation of nonmyocytes including fibroblasts that constitute the majority, in addition to endocardial cells, coronary artery endothelial cells, smooth muscle cells from epicardial and intramyocardial coronary arteries and arterioles, lymphatics, macrophages, and mast cells.[24-26] A distinctive feature of the postlooping stage is close coupling between cardiac growth and hemodynamic forces, a relationship that begins in the embryo and continues after birth.[16] Postembryonic cardiac growth is the consequence of both hyperplasia and hypertrophy of myocytes and hyperplasia of nonmyocytes (Table 23–1).

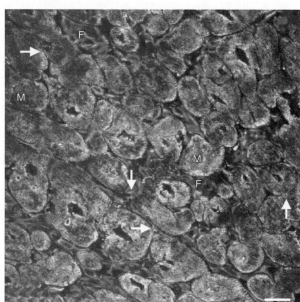

FIGURE 23-4 Structural interrelation of cardiac myocytes and fibroblasts. Spatial arrangements of myocytes (M green antimyomesin label) and fibroblasts (F blue antivimentin label). *(From Kohl, P., Camelliti, P.: Cardiac myocyte-non-myocyte electronic coupling. Heart Rhythm 2007;4:233–235. Used with permission.)*

Neonatal rat myocardium transiently retains its capacity for myocyte hyperplasia[26-28] (cytogenesis, mitosis, and DNA synthesis), and in the newt, terminally differentiated cardiomyocytes retain their ability to enter the cell cycle.[11] In larger mammals, hyperplasia of the cardiomyocyte plays

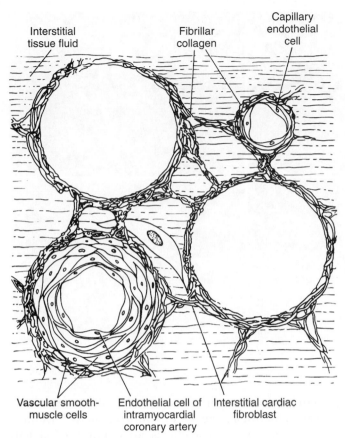

FIGURE 23–5 Schematic illustration of cell composition of the myocardium. Myocytes represent 33% of the cell population but occupy 75% of the volume (structural space). Nonmyocytes include vascular smooth muscle cells, cardiac fibroblasts, endothelial cells, macrophages, and mast cells. *(From Weber, K.T., Brilla, C.J.: Pathological hypertrophy and cardiac interstitium: fibrosis and renin-angiotensin-aldosterone system. Circulation. 1991;83:1849–1865. Used with permission from the American Heart Association.)*

Table 23–1   Cytologic Features of Increased Cardiac Mass

Immature Heart

Muscle cells—hyperplasia and hypertrophy
Non–muscle cells—hyperplasia

Mature Heart

Muscle cells—hypertrophy
Non–muscle cells—hyperplasia

---

a major *intrauterine* role in normal cardiac growth, but toward term the number of mitoses decreases appreciably, and within a finite time after birth, mitoses disappear altogether.[26-28] Accordingly, cardiomyocytes are terminally differentiated and can neither replicate nor regenerate.[2,11] Myocyte enlargement, that is, hypertrophy, results from an increase in contractile protein content per individual myocardial cell and is the principal mechanism of cardiac growth.[2,26]

The heart increases its mass in response to circulatory demands that govern transmission of mechanical information from the sarcolemma to myocyte nuclei.[29] Mechanical stress and cell deformation generate a wide range of signals that originate in membranes and cytoplasm—mechanoreceptors—and modify the rates of RNA and protein synthesis and protein degradation.[29-32] Stress applied to cultured myocytes induces early expression of genes used as markers of myocyte growth.[29,30,32,33] Upregulation of transforming growth factor-β during embryonic heart development and the impact of transforming growth factor-β on cardiac gene expression imply a functional role for this family of regulatory peptides in cardiac organogenesis.[34,35] However, the ultimate phenotype of the cell, organ, or organism is the reflection of the protein products of the genes—the proteomic profile.[36]

NORMAL EXTRAUTERINE CARDIAC GROWTH

The fetal heart is primed to respond to the sudden hemodynamic and respiratory changes at birth. Growth of the heart from early postnatal life to maturity is governed by the gradual increase in circulatory demands of the developing neonate, infant, child, and adolescent. Cardiac dimensions increase with increasing age during the first 20 years of life, correlate with body size, and are larger in males than in females.[37] The relatively low intrauterine oxygen environment and low partial pressure of arterial oxygen in the fetus promote rapid myocyte division and cardiac growth[38] (Fig. 23–6). Conversely, the increase in ambient oxygen and in partial pressure of systemic arterial oxygen accompanying spontaneous respiration are associated with, and in part responsible for, decreasing the rate of cardiomyocyte replication.[38] Although heart muscle cells can cycle only a certain number of times, the long-held conviction that mature myocytes have *entirely* lost their ability to divide must be qualified.[39-42] In the strictest sense, the capability of mature cardiac myocytes to replicate may be suppressed rather than wholly lost.[39,40] As mammals age, increasing numbers of their cardiomyocytes become multinucleated, and large myocytes may contain four times the normal amount of genetic material.[39] The implication is that mature cardiac muscle cells retain a capability, albeit abridged, to synthesize DNA.

A comparison of the extrauterine growth patterns of the right and left ventricles provides insights into the responses of normal cardiac muscle working under different loading conditions.[43,44] "The left ventricle requires to be stronger inasmuch as the blood which it propels has to be driven through the whole body[1]" (discussed earlier). The hemodynamic changes after birth establish a low-resistance low-pressure pulmonary circulation and a relatively high pressure high-resistance systemic circulation. Subsequent differences in growth rates of the right and left ventricles are principally due to different

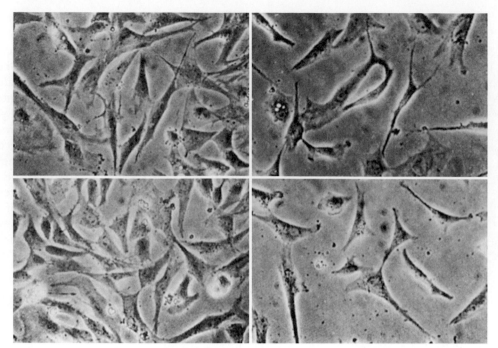

FIGURE 23-6 Cell cultures from 8-day chick embryo ventricles grown for 48 hours in 10% oxygen *(left panels)* and 80% oxygen *(right panels)*. The cells cultured in 10% oxygen are more numerous than cells grown in 80% oxygen. *(From Hollenberg, M.: Effect of oxygen on growth of cultured myocardial cells. Circ Res. 1971;28:148–157. Used with permission from the American Heart Association.)*

workloads, with responses coupled to rapid somatic growth. There is a much slower rate of growth of the right ventricle compared with the left ventricle.[45,46] The major growth is in the left ventricular free wall and the least growth is in the right ventricular free wall, with intermediate growth in the ventricular septum.[47] Although both ventricles continue to increase their mass in the developing child, the left ventricle outgrows the right ventricle culminating in a 20-fold increase in human left ventricular weight from birth to maturity.[26,48]

INCREASE IN VENTRICULAR MASS BEYOND THE PROCESS OF NORMAL GROWTH

Variables that influence an increase in ventricular mass beyond normal intrauterine and extrauterine growth are shown in Table 23–2. Cell types (see Figs. 23–4 and 23–5) and genetic influences were mentioned earlier. Different genes are expressed selectively in different types of

Table 23–2 Variables That Determine Ventricular Mass
Type of inciting stimulus: hemodynamic, nonhemodynamic
Timing of the inciting stimulus relative to myocardial immaturity or maturity
Degree and duration of the stimulus
Cell type: myocyte or nonmyocyte
Genetic regulation of the cell population

hypertrophy and might account for the differences in normal and abnormal increases in ventricular mass.[49] Familial hypertrophic cardiomyopathy is an example of genetic regulation of cardiac mass[50] that may act in concert with inciting stimuli that include a host of growth and mechanical factors.[49] Stressing of mechanoreceptors that reside in cardiomyocyte membranes results in early induction of gene expression.[30,32,51] Clinical stimulation of these mechanoreceptors by hemodynamic overload modifies the expression of cardiac genes, leading to a new phenotype better adapted to the increase in functional demands (discussed later).[51,52]

Catecholamines (norepinephrine), angiotensin II, and aldosterone are nonhemodynamic neurohormonal stimuli that induce an increase in ventricular mass.[29,53] Importantly, hemodynamic and nonhemodynamic neurohormonal stimuli target both myocyte *and* nonmyocyte cellular elements. Induction of hypertrophy does not require contractile activity.[49] When growth factors are tested in culture models, immature rat cardiomyocytes increase in size and protein content when catecholamines are added to the cell culture.[54] A normotensive infusion of norepinephrine in mature animals stimulates hypertrophy of left ventricular myocytes,[54,55] and serum obtained from human subjects during isotonic exercise stimulates hypertrophy of cultured immature rat cardiomyocytes, even though catecholamine levels in the serum are not elevated.[56] Angiotensin II plays a major role in governing fibroblast/collagen turnover in hypertrophied hearts, increasing left ventricular diastolic stiffness.[29,31,53] Insulin-like growth factor I, as well as recombinant human growth hormone, reportedly increase myocardial mass and improve ventricular function in dilatated cardiomyopathy.[57-59] Hypoxia applied during myocardial immaturity of the neonatal period enhances DNA synthesis and myocyte replication.[60] When cultured chick embryo cardiomyocytes are exposed to progressively lower concentrations of oxygen, their rates of cell division increase progressively (see Fig. 23-6).

Now let us examine the timing of the inciting stimulus relative to immaturity or maturity of the myocardium, a concern central to congenital heart disease in which hemodynamic and nonhemodynamic stimuli are commonly imposed on an immature heart. A clinical example of the effect of hypoxemia on the immature heart is represented by anomalous origin of the left coronary artery from the pulmonary trunk in which the hypoperfused but viable region of left ventricular myocardium characteristically and often markedly increases its mass, recognized in the electrocardiogram as hypertrophy (Fig. 23-7). This malformation sheds light on the relationship between hypoxemia and myocardial cell replication in the immature heart, an observation relevant to cultured chick embryo cardiomyocytes exposed to low concentrations of oxygen (see Fig. 23-6). Exposure of the immature rat heart to

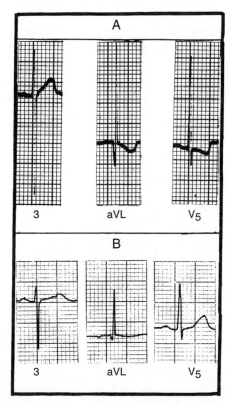

FIGURE 23-7 Leads 3, aVL, and V₅ before and after ligation of an anomalous left coronary artery that arose from the pulmonary trunk. **(A)** Before operation, age 4 months. There is left-axis deviation, with voltage and repolarization criteria of left ventricular hypertrophy in leads aVL and V₅. Lead aVL exhibits a deep but narrow Q wave. **(B)** Five years after operation. Left-axis deviation persists, but left ventricular hypertrophy and the deep Q wave in lead aVL have disappeared.

hypoxia results in hyperplasia (replication) of both cardiac myocytes and fibroblasts (see Figs. 23-4 and 23-5).[60] During early neonatal development, nonmyocytes replicate more vigorously in response to hypoxia than cardiomyocytes, and replication of left ventricular myocytes is greater and persists longer than division of right ventricular myocytes.[47] The difference in responses to hypoxia of nonmyocytes and of immature and mature myocytes underscores the importance of the timing of hypoxia. Excessive replication of fibroblasts in response to hypoxemia in the immature heart and excessive collagen turnover in response to hemodynamic and neurohormonal stimuli in the immature and mature heart may adversely affect diastolic function[24,61,62] (discussed earlier).

The collagen component of extracellular matrix is responsible for the functional integration of ventricular myocardium, permitting interdigitation and transmission of force between contracting myocytes.[63] The increase in stroma reflects collagen hyperplasia rather than connective tissue replacement of injured cardiomyocytes (discussed earlier).

The response of myocardial mass is greater in infants and young children than the response to equivalent stimuli in older children and adults, indicating that the human myocardium manifests an age-dependent change in trophic capacity similar to that observed in animals.[28] Differences in trophic responses are an intrinsic property of myocardium at a given age and occur without neurohormonal mediation.[64] Acute left ventricular afterload in a young child tends to provoke a rapid increase in ventricular mass that plateaus within a week.[65] This response is relevant to the proposed preparation of the left ventricle for a two-stage arterial switch operation for complete transposition of the great arteries (see Chapter 15).

The degree and duration of a given stimulus are reflected in three functionally distinct responses that permit the heart to meet changing demands—namely, acute beat-to-beat regulation (Starling's law), short-term response to physiologic and pharmacologic interventions, and adaptation to chronic hemodynamic overload.[51] Cardiomyocyte growth expresses itself as an increase in myocardial mass and thickness, whereas nonmyocyte growth expresses itself as structural remodeling of the interstitium.[24] Myocyte and nonmyocyte growth are independent of each other, with responses that can be either appropriate (adaptive) or inappropriate (maladaptive) for the degree and duration of a given stimulus.[24,66] A variation on this theme is the response to experimental acute aortic regurgitation in which protein synthesis contributes to the early phase of hypertrophy, but the later phase of chronic volume overload results in progressive hypertrophy due to suppression of protein degradation, culminating in heart failure.[67]

Degree and duration must take into account whether the stimulus is hemodynamic or neurohormonal and whether the principal target is the myocyte or nonmyo-cyte. The response of the myocyte (contractile element) ceases to be compensatory when the loading conditions exceed the growth capacity of terminally differentiated cardiac muscle cells to normalized wall stress or when the contractile performance of hypertrophied myocardium per unit mass is less than that of normal myocardium.[66] These responses are reflected in initial systolic adaptation and subsequent systolic maladaptation (decompensa-tion). When the inciting stimulus results in an adaptive increase in collagen turnover, the response preserves functional and structural integrity of myocardial matrix, whereas an excessive (maladaptive) increase in collagen has a negative impact on ventricular stiffness and dia-stolic function as noted earlier.

ULTRASTRUCTURAL RESPONSES TO OVERLOAD

Let us now examine the ultrastructural responses associ-ated with an increase in ventricular mass, focusing prin-cipally on the relationship between the cardiomyocyte and its microvascular blood supply.[19,20,48,68-70] Myocyte growth (enlargement) is characterized by an increase in cell breadth, length, or both, which are morphometric measures of cell *hypertrophy*.[71] Myocyte *hyperplasia* is char-acterized by an increase in cell number (replication, mi-tosis), a biologic response reserved for the fetal myocyte and the immature postnatal myocyte (see earlier discus-sion). *Angiogenesis* refers to formation of new capillaries, a process designed to keep pace with myocyte replication responsible for the increase in ventricular mass during

normal cardiac growth and in response to hemodynamic overload.[69,70] The landmark study of Roberts and Wearn[72] more than a half century ago demonstrated that (1) capil-laries multiply during postnatal growth, (2) muscle-to-capillary ratio attains a value of approximately 1:1 at maturity, and (3) this ratio persists thereafter. The rela-tively exuberant capillary angiogenesis in infants and young children gradually decreases but is not entirely lost even in adults.[69,70] The biologic significance of the rate of capillary angiogenesis in neonates and infants is propor-tional to myocyte replication (hyperplasia) in the fetus and in the immature postnatal heart, a hypothesis in ac-cord with morphometric analyses of the left ventricular pressure overload hypertrophy of congenital aortic steno-sis in which the relative densities of coronary capillaries and cardiomyocytes remains constant[69] (Fig. 23-8, *A* and *B*). Conversely, in the left ventricular pressure overload hypertrophy of acquired aortic stenosis, there is a de-crease in capillary density reflected in an undesirable in-crease in the cross-sectional myocyte area served by a single capillary[69] (Fig. 23-8, *C* and *D*). Accordingly, coro-nary capillaries proliferate in the immature heart as a part of the process of normal ventricular growth and prolifer-ate as part of accelerated left ventricular growth induced by congenital left ventricular afterload, so that capillary supply remains proportional to myocyte volume.[69]

Enlargement (hypertrophy) of cardiomyocytes is accompanied by changes in ultrastructural (subcellu-lar) components—adenosine triphosphate (ATP) syn-thesis, mitochondria, which are responsible for oxygen consumption, and myofibrils, which contain the con-tractile proteins that utilize ATP. Two factors relevant to the process of increased ventricular mass are the

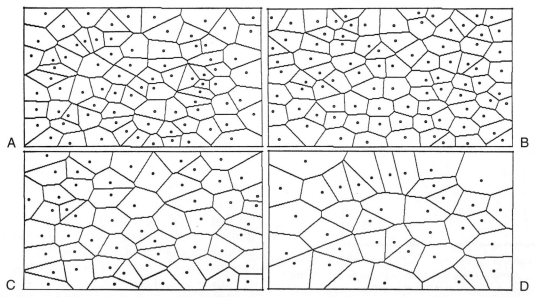

FIGURE 23-8 Computer printouts of results from an image analyzer used to locate positions of all capillaries in tissue cross sections. Each capillary *(central dots)* is surrounded by a polygonal region defined as the domain area. **(A)** Infant control heart. **(B)** Infant with congenital aortic stenosis. **(C)** Adult control heart. **(D)** Adult with acquired aortic stenosis. The corresponding capillary densities in these fields are, respectively, 3040/mm² (A), 3306/mm² in (B), 2052/mm² in (C), 1406/mm² in (D). *(From* Circulation *1992. Used with permission from the American Heart Association.)*

mitochondrial:myofibrillar volume ratios and the expansion of myocardial capillary microvasculature that serves to maintain an adequate supply of oxygen as ventricular mass increases (discussed earlier).

Changes in sarcomeres, mitochondrial:myofibrillar volume ratios, and capillary versus myocyte growth ratios differ in response to pressure or volume overload. When *pressure overload* is the stimulus, an increase in systolic wall stress results in replication of sarcomeres in *parallel* (thickening of myocytes; Fig. 23-9) and hence an increase in wall thickness.[48,73] The mitochondrial:myofibrillar volume ratio decreases, an alteration that potentially impairs energy supply by setting the stage for a disparity between ATP synthesis and utilization.[20,43] When *volume overload* is the inciting stimulus, an increase in end-diastolic wall stress results in replication of sarcomeres in *series* (lengthening of myocytes; see Fig. 23-9), setting the stage for elongation and chamber enlargement (discussed later).[48,73] The mitochondrial:myofibrillar volume ratio remains nearly constant, so that there is little or no disparity between ATP synthesis and utilization.[68]

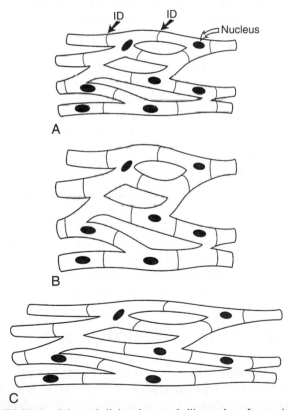

FIGURE 23-9 Schematic light microscopic illustration of normal myocardium. **(A)** Branching fibers (myocardial cells) are demarcated by intercalated disks (ID). **(B)** Replication of sarcomeres in parallel with thickening of myocytes and an increase in wall thickness in response to an increase in systolic wall stress associated with pressure overload. **(C)** Replication of sarcomeres in series with elongation of myocytes and chamber enlargement in response to an increase in end-diastolic wall stress associated with volume overload.

GROSS MORPHOLOGIC AND PHYSIOLOGIC RESPONSES TO OVERLOAD

These two responses to mechanical stress depend on the stage of myocardial maturity or immaturity at the time overload becomes operative; the type of overload (pressure or volume); the rate, degree, and chronicity of overload; and the morphologic ventricle (right versus left) that responds to the overload. Ventricular responses to hemodynamic overload are divided into three stages[74]: (1) the acute response (Starling or Anrep), (2) the chronic response of relatively stable hyperfunction accompanied by normalization of stress per unit of myocardial mass, and (3) the late stage of depressed or decompensated ventricular function. The following remarks deal with the relatively stable adaptive hyperfunction that is achieved when chronic pressure or volume overload is imposed on an immature or mature left or right ventricle, and then with the transition from a desirable adaptive response to an undesirable maladaptive pathologic response.

The "functional morphology" or ventricular modeling of chronic pressure or volume overload reflects the in-parallel or in-series changes in sarcomeres just described[48,73] (see Fig. 23-9). In response to *pressure* overload, replication of sarcomeres in parallel results in an increase in ventricular wall thickness without an increase in chamber volume, an adaptive response appropriate for developing power. In response to *volume* overload, replication of sarcomeres in series results in an increase in chamber volume with a proportional increase in wall thickness,[48,75] an adaptive response appropriate for developing acceleration. Depending on the type of volume overload, the geometry or modeling of the left ventricle varies from ellipsoid (normal shape), as in aortic regurgitation, to spherical, as in mitral regurgitation. The apex of a spherically dilatated left ventricle is globally stretched, so that the apical loop changes from an oblique to a transverse configuration.[5]

The response to exercise in trained athletes sheds light on adaptive and maladaptive increases in ventricular mass.[76-86] Athletes engaged in isometric exercise (weightlifters, shot putters) experience an increase in left ventricular wall thickness with little or no increase in chamber volume, analogous to the response to cardiac lesions that impose pressure overload. Athletes engaged in isotonic exercise (long-distance runners, cyclists, swimmers) experience an increase in left ventricular internal dimensions with a proportional increase in wall thickness, analogous to the response to cardiac lesions that impose volume overload. Swimmers and cyclists engage in both isotonic *and* isometric exercise, so the gross morphologic response of the left ventricle is a combination of ventricular enlargement (volume overload) and increased wall thickness (pressure overload).[48,76,85] In athletes trained in isotonic exercise, the stimulus to volume hypertrophy is believed to balance between the left and right ventricles,[78,87] although in experimental animals, the cellular, subcellular, and microvascular responses of the two chambers differ.[68] When exercise is largely isometric (weightlifters) or triathlon, in which participants compete without stopping in three successive events, usually long-distance swimming, bicycling, and running, the response of the left and right ventricles differs substantially, with the major increase in mass assigned to the left ventricle.[77,87]

Now let us turn to the *physiologic* responses or adaptations to chronic overload, emphasizing the type of loading conditions, the stage of myocardial maturity or immaturity at the time overload is initiated, and the morphologic characteristics of the ventricle confronting the overload stimulus.

In the pressure-overloaded ventricle, replication of sarcomeres in parallel results in a disproportionate increase in wall thickness relative to cavity size (discussed earlier), a response well suited to the physiologic requirements of ejecting a normal stroke volume against a high resistance. In the volume-overloaded ventricle, replication of sarcomeres in series results in an increase in cavity size with a proportional increase in wall thickness, a response well suited to the physiologic requirements of ejecting a large stroke volume against a normal or low resistance (discussed earlier). If the increased afterload is initially imposed on immature left ventricular myocardium, as in congenital aortic stenosis, systolic performance is supranormal and wall stress is low,[88,89] but if equivalent afterload is imposed on mature left ventricular myocardium, systolic performance is normal at best. Importantly, these responses persist into adulthood,[90] reflecting a fundamental difference in the substrate when pressure overload is imposed on an *immature* left ventricle. The difference is believed to reside in the property of immature left ventricular myocytes to respond by hyperplasia *and* hypertrophy and in the property of coronary capillaries to proliferate and maintain a blood supply proportional to myocyte volume (see earlier discussion).[69]

Right ventricular systolic performance is also influenced by the timing of the afterload stimulus. The fetal right ventricle necessarily confronts systemic afterload. When fetal systemic afterload continues after birth, as in tetralogy of Fallot, right ventricular free wall growth keeps pace with that of the left ventricle, and long-term function of the morphologic right ventricle is good. Conversely, when chronic pressure overload is imposed on a *mature* right ventricle that has lost its capacity for myocyte hyperplasia and angiogenesis, ejection performance is not as good, and the right ventricle fails at pressures well below systemic levels.

An additional variable that influences ventricular performance in the presence of an increase in ventricular mass is the coronary circulation, both the microcirculation (see earlier discussion) and the extramural coronary circulation. A morphologic right ventricle is perfused by a concordant morphologic right coronary artery designed to supply a thin-walled, low-resistance pump,[91] a relationship that may incur functional limitations when ejection is against a systemic workload.[92] Failure of a subaortic morphologic right ventricle in isolated congenitally corrected transposition of the great arteries is a case in point (see Chapter 4). When aortic valve replacement is followed by regression of left ventricular mass, the left coronary arterial system decreases in size, whereas the right coronary arterial system remains unchanged.[93] In cyanotic congenital heart disease, flow reserve remains normal despite an appreciable increase in basal coronary blood flow the in dilated extramural coronary arteries.[94] Preservation of normal flow reserve resides in the coronary microcirculation that remodels in hypoxemic erythrocytotic patients with cyanotic CHD, as it does in hypoxemic erythrocytotic residents acclimatized to high altitude.[94] Although microcirculatory remodeling is a key regulator of flow reserve, enhanced vasodilatatory capacity supplements remodeling (see Chapter 12).

The response to ventricular overload is considered adaptive when normalization of stress per unit of myocardial mass is achieved, when cardiac reserve is reestablished, and when further overload is handled normally. However, the heart does not possess an unlimited capacity to adapt its mass to hemodynamic needs.[86] An increase in ventricular mass becomes maladaptive—pathologic—when hypertrophy is no longer compensatory, that is, when overload exceeds the hypertrophic capacity of cardiomyocytes to normalize stress per unit mass, when the contractile performance per unit mass is less than that of normal myocardium,[25,62,66,95] or when myocyte size exceeds capillary supply.[69] Nor can we ignore the potentially maladaptive increase in extracellular matrix, an excess of which exerts a deleterious effect on diastolic ventricular function (discussed earlier).

The response to loading conditions must also take into account the chronically *underloaded* heart.[96] Patients with severe cyanotic tetralogy of Fallot older than 2 years of age have a decrease in left ventricular end-diastolic volume and a decrease in left ventricular ejection fraction related to underfilling of the left side of the heart because of reduced pulmonary arterial blood flow.[96]

REGRESSION OF VENTRICULAR MASS

Pivotal to a discussion of increased ventricular mass is the response when reparative surgery or interventional catheterization eliminates or reduces the inciting mechanical, hypoxic, or neurohumoral stimulus.[24,25,62,63,97–102] A fundamental principle of a therapeutic intervention such as surgery is the alteration of structure to preserve or improve function. Regression of ventricular mass is an active biologic process that does not depend only on removal of the mechanical stimulus.[63,101] Regression is associated with preservation of normal ventricular function when the increased mass was *adaptive*, that is, associated with normal stress per unit of myocardial mass[66] (see Fig. 23-9). When the capacity of myocardium to normalize stress is exceeded, the increase in mass is *maladaptive* (pathologic), and regression is unlikely to be followed by normalization of ventricular function.[24,25,66] If the inciting stimuli were imposed during myocardial immaturity, that is, before terminal differentiation, myocytes respond by an increase in number (mitosis, replication; discussed earlier). Regression of ventricular mass is then characterized by increased numbers of myocytes that are individually reduced in size.[103] The efficiency of the microvascular bed increases because capillary density increases—each capillary supplies a smaller than normal myocyte. At the subcellular level, an important question is whether regression of myocyte hypertrophy after elimination of systolic wall stress (afterload) is associated with a reduction of sarcomeres in parallel and whether regression of hypertrophy after elimination of diastolic wall stress (preload) is associated with a reduction of sarcomeres in series. Evidence of the reversibility of an increase in ventricular mass due to hypertrophy in the gross morphologic sense is reflected in something as simple as the scalar electrocardiogram. After successful relief of severe pulmonary valve stenosis, for example, the electrocardiographic pattern of right ventricular hypertrophy may virtually disappear (see Fig. 23-11).

Anomalous origin of the left coronary artery from the pulmonary trunk is associated with a regional increase in left ventricular mass ascribed to myocyte hyperplasia caused by hypoperfusion (hypoxia) of viable immature myocardium[104] (discussed earlier). When myocardial perfusion is normalized by surgery,[105] scalar electrocardiographic evidence of "left ventricular hypertrophy" decreases, sometimes appreciably (see Fig. 23-7). Assuming that preoperative regional increase in ventricular mass was due to hyperplasia of hypoxemic immature left ventricular myocytes, postoperative regression of ventricular mass should be associated with increased numbers of smaller myocytes (discussed earlier).[103]

When an increase in ventricular mass is accompanied by increased turnover of extracellular matrix, an important concern is the degree to which excess connective tissue is capable of regression, as well as the residual effect of excess connective tissue on long-term ventricular diastolic function. There is evidence that an increase in connective tissue due to fibroblast hyperplasia does not readily regress.[62,98]

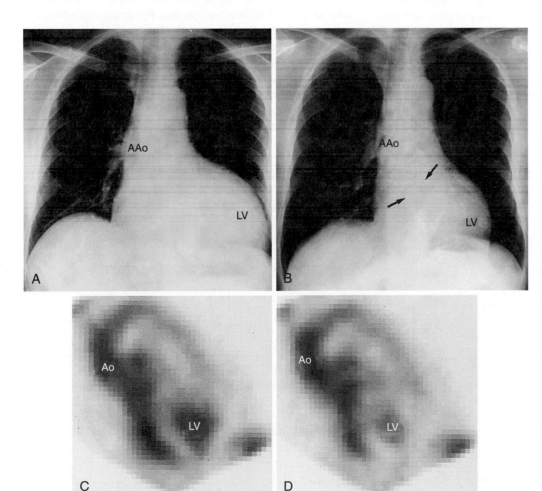

FIGURE 23-10 **(A)** Chest x-ray from a 55-year-old man with severe chronic bicuspid aortic regurgitation. An adaptive response in left ventricular (LV) mass was characterized by a conspicuous increase in internal dimensions with a concordant increase in wall thickness. AAo, ascending aorta. **(B)** Chest x-ray 9 months after aortic valve replacement *(arrows)*. The size and configuration of the left ventricle are virtually normal, indicating regression of ventricular mass. **(C and D)** Radionuclide images showing normal left ventricular internal dimensions and normal ejection fraction of 55%.

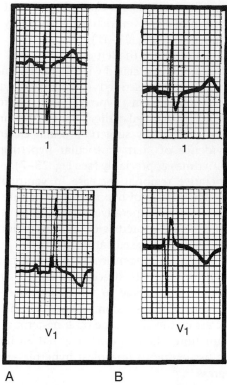

FIGURE 23–11 **(A)** Leads 1 and V_1 from a 2-year-old boy with severe pulmonary valve stenosis, right axis deviation, and right ventricular hypertrophy. **(B)** Seven years after pulmonary valvotomy. Right-axis deviation has resolved, and the prominent R wave in lead V_1 has been replaced with an rSr,', electrocardiographic features of regression of right ventricular hypertrophy.

Observations in humans and in experimental animals leave little doubt that ventricular mass is capable of regression after elimination of inciting stimuli (Figs. 23–7, 23–10, and 23–11). Regression of increased ventricular mass can be as rapid as its rate of development, at least experimentally.[98,106] In humans, however, the time course of regression may be prolonged for years.[99]

Remodeling of a ventricle undergoing regression of mass is related chiefly to the geometric response to the inciting stimulus responsible for the increase in mass. Remodeling of the left ventricle after elimination of the volume overload of aortic regurgitation or isotonic exercise is represented by a greater reduction in internal dimensions than in wall thickness[99] (see Fig. 23–9). Remodeling of the left ventricle after elimination of pressure overload as in aortic stenosis or isometric exercise is characterized by a greater reduction in wall thickness than in internal dimensions.

OBJECTIVES OF OPERATION

A major objective of cardiac surgery or interventional catheterization in congenital heart disease is the reduction or elimination of stimuli responsible for an increase in ventricular mass. There is a prevailing air of optimism when surgery or interventional catheterization is followed by normalization of stress per unit of ventricular mass and normalization of chamber geometry.[102] However, the relationship among ventricular mass, geometry, and function can be capricious. It should not be assumed that regression of ventricular mass ensures normal function or that failure of regression necessarily implies abnormal function. The many variables that bear on regression of ventricular mass are relevant (discussed earlier). Congenital aortic stenosis imposes increased afterload on an immature left ventricle with myocytes capable of replication and coronary capillaries capable of angiogenesis (see Fig. 23–8, A and B). Accordingly, systolic performance is supranormal[89] (Fig. 23–12, A and B). Acquired aortic stenosis that imposes equivalent afterload on mature left ventricular myocytes is associated with normal or subnormal left ventricular systolic function because myocytes increase in size—hypertrophy—without the benefit of angiogenesis, so capillary density decreases.[107,108] In congenital aortic stenosis, reduced wall stress and supranormal left ventricular performance persists postoperatively even into adulthood, because an increase in the number of relatively small myocytes is accompanied by a proportionate increase in number of capillaries, hence capillary density increases, so that the microvasculature is more efficient (discussed earlier).[15] In coarctation of the aorta, left ventricular function may remain supranormal after successful normotensive repair even when regression of left ventricular mass is incomplete,[109] and incomplete regression of ventricular mass in the mature mammalian heart may be accompanied by normal ventricular function. In deconditioned trained greyhounds, left ventricular function may remain normal despite lack of regression of exercise-induced hypertrophy.[110] Nevertheless, there comes a point when hemodynamic overload is no longer innocently borne, and the desirable physiologic adaptation accompanying an increase in ventricular mass is maladaptive—pathologic—a self-evident observation in patients and occasionally in trained athletes.[83] Professional cyclists who continue strenuous training begun in their youth experience slightly depressed left ventricular function after initially normal adaptation.[83]

What is the response of an *underloaded* ventricle when surgery normalizes its loading conditions? The volume-underloaded left ventricle in cyanotic tetralogy of Fallot is an example (discussed earlier). After successful intracardiac repair, left-sided volumes increase, but left ventricular function may not normalize.[96,111]

CONCLUSION

A fundamental property of the mammalian heart is its capacity to adapt to functional requirements by increasing its mass in response to hemodynamic, hormonal,

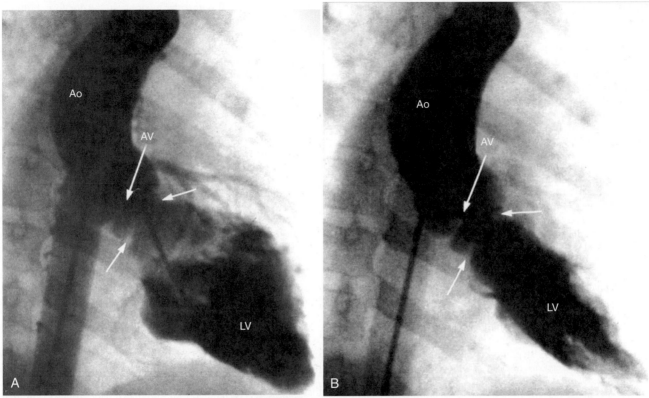

FIGURE 23-12   Left ventricular (LV) angiographic diastolic **(A)** and systolic frames **(B)** from a 19-year-old man with fixed subaortic stenosis *(paired arrows)* and a gradient of 105 mm Hg. The supranormal left ventricular ejection fraction shown here persisted after surgical resection of the subaortic membrane. Ao, ascending aorta; AV, aortic valve.

and genetic stimuli. The heart, which is the first organ to form and to function in vertebrates, continues to fascinate developmental biologists. This chapter was designed to put into perspective normal intrauterine and extrauterine cardiac growth, adaptive and maladaptive increases in cardiac growth (ventricular mass), and regression of ventricular mass.

Congenital heart disease may induce an increase in ventricular mass beyond normal intrauterine and extrauterine growth potentials. Reparative surgery or interventional catheterization reduces, if not eliminates, the inciting stimuli, permitting regression of increased ventricular mass before an adaptive response becomes pathologic.

References

1. Harvey W. *The Circulation of the Blood and Other Writings*, trans. Franklin KJ, with an introduction by Andrew Wear. London: J.M. Dent and Sons; 1963;46–47.
2. van Bilsen M, Chien KR. Growth and hypertrophy of the heart: towards an understanding of cardiac specific and inducible gene expression. *Cardiovasc Res.* 1993;27:1140–1149.
3. Perloff JK. Development and regression of increased ventricular mass. *Am J Cardiol.* 1982;50:605–611.
4. Yacoub MH. Two hearts that beat as one. *Circulation.* 1995;92: 156–157.
5. Buckberg G. Ventricular shape and function in health and disease. *Eur J Cardiothorac Surg.* 2001;29S1:S1.
6. Pardee AB. G1 events and regulation of cell proliferation. *Science.* 1989;246:603–608.
7. Coghlan HC, Coghlan AR, Buckberg GD, et al. The structure and function of the helical heart and its buttress wrapping. III. The electric spiral of the heart: The hypothesis of the anisotropic conducting matrix. *Semin Thorac Cardiovasc Surg.* 2001;13:333–341.
8. Lower R. *Tractatus de Corde.* London: Dawsons of Pall Mall; 1968.
9. Buckberg G. Rethinking the cardiac helix: a structure/function journey. *Eur J Cardiothorac Surg.* 2006;29S1:S1.
10. Torrent-Guasp F, Buckberg GD, Clemente C, et al. The structure and function of the helical heart and its buttress wrapping. I. The normal macroscopic structure of the heart. *Semin Thorac Cardiovasc Surg.* 2001;13:301–319.
11. Olson EN, Srivastava D. Molecular pathways controlling heart development. *Science.* 1996;272:671–676.
12. Barinaga M. Looking to development's future. *Science.* 1994;266: 561–564.
13. Touchette N. Finding clues about how embryo structures form. *Science.* 1994;266:564–565.
14. Reller MD, McDonald RW, Gerlis LM, Thornburg KL. Cardiac embryology: basic review and clinical correlations. *J Am Soc Echocardiogr.* 1991;4:519–532.
15. Srivastava D, Cserjesi P, Olson EN. A subclass of bHLH proteins required for cardiac morphogenesis. *Science.* 1995;270:1995–1999.
16. Icardo JM. Heart anatomy and developmental biology. *Experientia.* 1988;44:910–919.
17. Lyons GE. Vertebrate heart development. *Curr Opin Genet Dev.* 1996;6:454–460.
18. Zak R, Kizu A, Bugaisky L. Cardiac hypertrophy: its characteristics as a growth process. *Am J Cardiol.* 1979;44:941–946.
19. Panidis IP, Kotler MN, Ren JF, et al. Development and regression of left ventricular hypertrophy. *J Am Coll Cardiol.* 1984;3:1309–1320.

20. Anversa P, Ricci R, Olivetti G. Quantitative structural analysis of the myocardium during physiologic growth and induced cardiac hypertrophy: a review. *J Am Coll Cardiol.* 1986;7:1140–1149.

21. DeRuiter MC, Poelmann RE, VanderPlas-de Vries I, et al. The development of the myocardium and endocardium in mouse embryos. Fusion of two heart tubes? *Anat Embryol.* 1992;185:461–473.

22. De La Cruz MV, Gómez CS, Cayré R. The developmental components of the ventricles: their significance in congenital cardiac malformations. *Cardiol Young.* 1991;1:123.

23. Levin M, Johnson RL, Stern CD, et al. A molecular pathway determining left-right asymmetry in chick embryogenesis. *Cell.* 1995;82:803–814.

24. Weber KT, Brilla CG. Pathological hypertrophy and cardiac interstitium. Fibrosis and renin-angiotensin-aldosterone system. *Circulation.* 1991;83:1849–1865.

25. Pfeffer JM. Regression of left ventricular hypertrophy as viewed from the periphery. *Curr Opin Cardiol.* 1994;9:527–533.

26. Zak R. Cell proliferation during cardiac growth. *Am J Cardiol.* 1973;31:211–219.

27. Zak R. Development and proliferative capacity of cardiac muscle cells. *Circ Res.* 1974;35(II Suppl):17–26.

28. Colan SD, Parness IA, Spevak PJ, Sanders SP. Developmental modulation of myocardial mechanics: age- and growth-related alterations in afterload and contractility. *J Am Coll Cardiol.* 1992;19:619–629.

29. Diez J. Current work in the cell biology of left ventricular hypertrophy. *Curr Opin Cardiol.* 1994;9:512–519.

30. Francis GS, Carlyle WC. Hypothetical pathways of cardiac myocyte hypertrophy: response to myocardial injury. *Eur Heart J.* 1993;14(Suppl J):49–56.

31. Miyata S, Haneda T. Hypertrophic growth of cultured neonatal rat heart cells mediated by type 1 angiotensin II receptor. *Am J Physiol.* 1994;266:H2443–H2451.

32. Yamazaki T, Komuro I, Yazaki Y. Molecular mechanism of cardiac cellular hypertrophy by mechanical stress. *J Mol Cell Cardiol.* 1995;27:133–140.

33. Barton PJ, Bhavsar PK, Brand NJ, et al. Gene expression during cardiac development. *Symp Soc Exp Biol.* 1992;46:251–264.

34. MacLellan WR, Brand T, Schneider MD. Transforming growth factor-beta in cardiac ontogeny and adaptation. *Circ Res.* 1993;73:783–791.

35. Sheng Z, Pennica D, Wood WI, Chien KR. Cardiotrophin-1 displays early expression in the murine heart tube and promotes cardiac myocyte survival. *Development.* 1996;122:419–428.

36. Mayr M, Zhang J, Greene AS, et al. Proteomics-based development of biomarkers in cardiovascular disease: mechanistic, clinical, and therapeutic insights. *Mol Cell Proteomics.* 2006;5:1853–1864.

37. Scholz DG, Kitzman DW, Hagen PT, et al. Age-related changes in normal human hearts during the first 10 decades of life. Part I (Growth): a quantitative anatomic study of 200 specimens from subjects from birth to 19 years old. *Mayo Clin Proc.* 1988;63:126–136.

38. Ghani QP, Hollenberg M. Poly(adenosine dephosphate ribose) metabolism and regulation of myocardial cell growth by oxygen. *Biochem J.* 1978;170:387–394.

39. Barnes DM. Joint Soviet-U.S. attack on heart muscle dogma. *Science.* 1988;242:193–195.

40. Claycomb WC, Moses RL. Growth factors and TPA stimulate DNA synthesis and alter the morphology of cultured terminally differentiated adult rat cardiac muscle cells. *Dev Biol.* 1988;127:257–265.

41. Schneider MD, Olson EN. Control of myogenic differentiation by cellular oncogenes. *Mol Neurobiol.* 1988;2:1–39.

42. Varmus HE. The molecular genetics of cellular oncogenes. *Ann Rev Genet.* 1984;18:553–612.

43. Legato MJ. Cellular mechanisms of normal growth in the mammalian heart. I. Qualitative and quantitative features of ventricular architecture in the dog from birth to five months of age. *Circ Res.* 1979;44:250–262.

44. Legato MJ. Cellular mechanisms of normal growth in the mammalian heart. II. A quantitative and qualitative comparison between the right and left ventricular myocytes in the dog from birth to five months of age. *Circ Res.* 1979;44:263–279.

45. De La Cruz MV, Anselmi G, Romero A, Monroy G. A qualitative and quantitative study of the ventricles and great vessels of normal children. *Am Heart J.* 1960;60:675–690.

46. Emery JL, Mithal A. Weights of cardiac ventricles at and after birth. *Br Heart J.* 1961;23:313–316.

47. Anversa P, Olivetti G, Loud AV. Morphometric study of early postnatal development in the left and right ventricular myocardium of the rat. I. Hypertrophy, hyperplasia, and binucleation of myocytes. *Circ Res.* 1980;46:495–502.

48. Grossman W. Cardiac hypertrophy: useful adaptation or pathologic process? *Am J Med.* 1980;69:576–584.

49. Simpson PC. Regulation of hypertrophy and gene transcription in cultured heart muscle cells. In: Chien S, ed. *Molecular Biology of the Cardiovascular System.* Philadelphia: Lea & Febiger; 1990:125.

50. Watkins H, Seidman JG, Seidman CE. Familial hypertrophic cardiomyopathy: a genetic model of cardiac hypertrophy. *Hum Mol Genet.* 1995;4:1721–1727.

51. Schwartz K, Mercadier J, Lompre A, et al. Phenotypic conversions in cardiac hypertrophy. In: Chien S, ed. *Molecular Biology of the Cardiovascular System.* Philadelphia: Lea & Febiger; 1990:103.

52. Schneider MD, Parker TG., Paker SE, et al. Functional role of growth factors and cellular oncogenes in cardiac and skeletal muscle. In: Chien S, ed. *Molecular Biology of the Cardiovascular System.* Philadelphia: Lea & Febiger; 1990:63.

53. Baker KM, Booz GW, Dostal DE. Cardiac actions of angiotensin II: role of an intracardiac renin-angiotensin system. *Ann Rev Physiol.* 1992;54:227–241.

54. Simpson P. Norepinephrine-stimulated hypertrophy of cultured rat myocardial cells is an alpha 1 adrenergic response. *J Clin Invest.* 1983;72:732–738.

55. Laks MM. Norepinephrine—the producer of myocardial cellular hypertrophy and/or necrosis and/or fibrosis. *Am Heart J.* 1977;94:394.

56. Simpson P, McGrath A, Savion S. Myocyte hypertrophy in neonatal rat heart cultures and its regulation by serum and by catecholamines. *Circ Res.* 1982;51:787–801.

57. Fazio S, Sabatini D, Capaldo B, et al. A preliminary study of growth hormone in the treatment of dilated cardiomyopathy. *N Engl J Med.* 1996;334:809–814.

58. Ito H, Hiroe M, Hirata Y, et al. Insulin-like growth factor-I induces hypertrophy with enhanced expression of muscle specific genes in cultured rat cardiomyocytes. *Circulation.* 1993;87:1715–1721.

59. Ohya Y, Abe I, Fujii K, et al. Hyperinsulinemia and left ventricular geometry in a work-site population in Japan. *Hypertension.* 1996;27:729–734.

60. Hollenberg M, Honbo N, Samorodin AJ. Effects of hypoxia on cardiac growth in neonatal rat. *Am J Physiol.* 1976;231:1445–1450.

61. Goldstein S. Replicative senescence: the human fibroblast comes of age. *Science.* 1990;249:1129–1133.

62. Wikman-Coffelt J, Parmley WW, Mason DT. The cardiac hypertrophy process. Analyses of factors determining pathological vs. physiological development. *Circ Res.* 1979;45:697–707.

63. Arita M, Horinaka S, Frohlich ED. Biochemical components and myocardial performance after reversal of left ventricular hypertrophy in spontaneously hypertensive rats. *J Hypertens.* 1993;11:951–959.

64. Cooper Gt, Kent RL, Mann DL. Load induction of cardiac hypertrophy. *J Mol Cell Cardiol.* 1989;21(5 Suppl):11–30.

65. Jonas RA, Giglia TM, Sanders SP, et al. Rapid, two-stage arterial switch for transposition of the great arteries and intact ventricular septum beyond the neonatal period. *Circulation.* 1989;80:I203–I208.

66. Tsutsui H, Ishihara K, Cooper GT. Cytoskeletal role in the contractile dysfunction of hypertrophied myocardium. *Science.* 1993;260:682–687.

67. Magid NM, Borer JS, Young MS, et al. Suppression of protein degradation in progressive cardiac hypertrophy of chronic aortic regurgitation. *Circulation.* 1993;87:1249–1257.

68. Anversa P, Levicky V, Beghi C, et al. Morphometry of exercise-induced right ventricular hypertrophy in the rat. *Circ Res.* 1983;52:57–64.

69. Rakusan K, Flanagan MF, Geva T, et al. Morphometry of human coronary capillaries during normal growth and the effect of age in left ventricular pressure-overload hypertrophy. *Circulation.* 1992; 86:38–46.

70. Tomanek RJ. Age as a modulator of coronary capillary angiogenesis. *Circulation.* 1992;86:320–321.

71. Anversa P, Loud AV, Giacomelli F, Wiener J. Absolute morphometric study of myocardial hypertrophy in experimental hypertension. II. Ultrastructure of myocytes and interstitium. *Lab Invest.* 1978;38: 597–609.

72. Roberts JT, Wearn JT. Quantitative changes in the capillary muscle relationship in human hearts during normal growth and hypertrophy. *Am Heart J.* 1941:617.

73. Grossman W, Jones D, McLaurin LP. Wall stress and patterns of hypertrophy in the human left ventricle. *J Clin Invest.* 1975;56: 56–64.

74. Meerson FZ. The myocardium in hyperfunction, hypertrophy and heart failure. *Circ Res.* 1969;25(Suppl 2):1–163.

75. Lin HL, Katele KV, Grimm AF. Functional morphology of the pressure- and the volume-hypertrophied rat heart. *Circ Res.* 1977;41: 830–836.

76. Bezucha GR, Lenser MC, Hanson PG, Nagle FJ. Comparison of hemodynamic responses to static and dynamic exercise. *J Appl Physiol.* 1982;53:1589–1593.

77. Brown S, Byrd R, Jayasinghe MD, Jones D. Echocardiographic characteristics of competitive and recreational weight lifters. *Cardiovasc Ultrason.* 1983. 2:163.

78. Ehsani AA, Hagberg JM, Hickson RC. Rapid changes in left ventricular dimensions and mass in response to physical conditioning and deconditioning. *Am J Cardiol.* 1978;42:52–56.

79. Fagard R, Van den Broeke C, Amery A. Left ventricular dynamics during exercise in elite marathon runners. *J Am Coll Cardiol.* 1989;14:112–118.

80. Keul J, Dickhuth HH, Simon G, Lehmann M. Effect of static and dynamic exercise on heart volume, contractility, and left ventricular dimensions. *Circ Res.* 1981;48:I162–170.

81. Morganroth J, Maron BJ, Henry WL, Epstein SE. Comparative left ventricular dimensions in trained athletes. *Ann Intern Med.* 1975;82: 521–524.

82. Muntz KH, Gonyea WJ, Mitchell JH. Cardiac hypertrophy in response to an isometric training program in the cat. *Circ Res.* 1981;49:1092–1101.

83. Nishimura T, Yamada Y, Kawai C. Echocardiographic evaluation of long-term effects of exercise on left ventricular hypertrophy and function in professional bicyclists. *Circulation.* 1980;61: 832–840.

84. Roeske WR, O'Rourke RA, Klein A, et al. Noninvasive evaluation of ventricular hypertrophy in professional athletes. *Circulation.* 1976; 53:286–291.

85. Van Decker W, Panidis IP, Boyle K, et al. Left ventricular structure and function in professional basketball players. *Am J Cardiol.* 1989; 64:1072–1074.

86. D'Andrea A, Caso P, Scarafile R, et al. Biventricular myocardial adaptation to different training protocols in competitive master athletes. *Int J Cardiol.* 2007;115:342–349.

87. Douglas PS, O'Toole ML, Hiller WD, Reichek N. Different effects of prolonged exercise on the right and left ventricles. *J Am Coll Cardiol.* 1990;15:64–69.

88. Borow KM, Colan SD, Neumann A. Altered left ventricular mechanics in patients with valvular aortic stenosis and coarctation of the aorta: effects on systolic performance and late outcome. *Circulation.* 1985;72:515–522.

89. Donner R, Carabello BA, Black I, Spann JF. Left ventricular wall stress in compensated aortic stenosis in children. *Am J Cardiol.* 1983;51:946–951.

90. Assey ME, Wisenbaugh T, Spann JF Jr, et al. Unexpected persistence into adulthood of low wall stress in patients with congenital aortic stenosis: is there a fundamental difference in the hypertrophic response to a pressure overload present from birth? *Circulation.* 1987;75:973–979.

91. Murray PA, Vatner SF. Fractional contributions of the right and left coronary arteries to perfusion of normal and hypertrophied right ventricles of conscious dogs. *Circ Res.* 1980;47:190–200.

92. Manohar M, Thurmon JC, Tranquilli WJ, et al. Regional myocardial blood flow and coronary vascular reverse in unanesthetized vascular reserve in unanesthetized young calves with severe concentric right ventricular hypertrophy. *Circ Res.* 1981;48:785–796.

93. Villari B, Hess OM, Meier C, et al. Regression of coronary artery dimensions after successful aortic valve replacement. *Circulation.* 1992;85:972–978.

94. Dedkov EI, Perloff JK, Tomanek RJ, et al. The coronary microcirculation in cyanotic congenital heart disease. *Circulation.* 2006;114: 196–200.

95. Mann DL, Spann JF, Cooper G. Basic mechanisms and models in cardiac hypertrophy. *Mod Concepts Cardiovasc Dis.* 1988;57:7.

96. Jarmakani JM, Graham TP Jr, Canent RV Jr, Jewett PH. Left heart function in children with tetralogy of Fallot before and after palliative or corrective surgery. *Circulation.* 1972;46:478–490.

97. Cooper GT, Satava RM, Harrison CE, Coleman HN 3rd. Normal myocardial function and energetics after reversing pressure-overload hypertrophy. *Am J Physiol.* 1974;226:1158–1165.

98. Cutilletta AF, Dowell RT, Rudnik M, et al. Regression of myocardial hypertrophy. I. Experimental model, changes in heart weight, nucleic acids and collagen. *J Mol Cell Cardiol.* 1975;7:761–780.

99. Monrad ES, Hess OM, Murakami T, et al. Time course of regression of left ventricular hypertrophy after aortic valve replacement. *Circulation.* 1988;77:1345–1355.

100. Sanford CF, Griffin EE, Wildenthal K. Synthesis and degradation of myocardial protein during the development and regression of thyroxine-induced cardiac hypertrophy in rats. *Circ Res.* 1978;43: 688–694.

101. Susic D, Nunez E, Frohlich ED. Reversal of hypertrophy: an active biologic process. *Curr Opin Cardiol.* 1995;10:466–472.

102. Toussaint C, Cribier A, Cazor JL, et al. Hemodynamic and angiographic evaluation of aortic regurgitation 8 and 27 months after aortic valve replacement. *Circulation.* 1981;64:456–463.

103. Bai SL, Campbell SE, Moore JA, et al. Influence of age, growth, and sex on cardiac myocyte size and number in rats. *Anat Rec.* 1990;226:207–212.

104. Perloff JK. Anomalous origin of the left coronary artery from the pulmonary trunk In: Perloff JK, ed. *The Clinical Recognition of Congenital Heart Disease.* 4th ed. Philadelphia: W.B. Saunders; 1994.

105. Finley JP, Howman-Giles R, Gilday DL, et al. Thallium-201 myocardial imaging in anomalous left coronary artery arising from the pulmonary artery. Applications before and after medical and surgical treatment. *Am J Cardiol.* 1978;42:675–680.

106. Marcus ML, Eckberg DL, Braxmeier JL, Abboud FM. Effects of intermittent pressure loading on the development of ventricular hypertrophy in the cat. *Circ Res.* 1977;40:484–488.

107. Gunther S, Grossman W. Determinants of ventricular function in pressure-overload hypertrophy in man. *Circulation.* 1979;59: 679–688.

108. Huber D, Grimm J, Koch R, Krayenbuehl HP. Determinants of ejection performance in aortic stenosis. *Circulation.* 1981;64:126–134.

109. Carpenter MA, Dammann JF, Watson DD, et al. Left ventricular hyperkinesia at rest and during exercise in normotensive patients 2 to 27 years after coarctation repair. *J Am Coll Cardiol.* 1985;6:879–886.

110. Carew TE, Covell JW. Left ventricular function in exercise-induced hypertrophy in dogs. *Am J Cardiol.* 1978;42:82–88.

111. Sandor GG, Patterson MW, Tipple M, et al. Left ventricular systolic and diastolic function after total correction of tetralogy of Fallot. *Am J Cardiol.* 1987;60:1148–1151.

INDEX

Page numbers followed by f indicate figures; t, tables.